Complications in Surgery and Trauma

Complications in Surgery and Trauma

Edited by

Stephen M. Cohn

University of Texas Health Science Center
San Antonio, Texas, U.S.A.

Associate Editors

Erik Barquist

Patricia M. Byers

Enrique Ginzburg

Fahim A. Habib

Mauricio Lynn

Mark McKenney

Nicholas Namias

David Shatz

Danny Sleeman

informa
healthcare

New York   London

Informa Healthcare USA, Inc.
270 Madison Avenue
New York, NY 10016

© 2007 by Informa Healthcare USA, Inc.
Informa Healthcare is an Informa business

No claim to original U.S. Government works
Printed in the United States of America on acid-free paper
10 9 8 7 6 5 4 3 2 1

International Standard Book Number-10: 0-8247-5898-6 (Hardcover)
International Standard Book Number-13: 978-0-8247-5898-1 (Hardcover)

Library of Congress Cataloging-in-Publication Data

Complications in surgery and trauma / edited by Stephen M. Cohn.
    p. ; cm.
  Includes bibliographical references and index.
  ISBN-13: 978-0-8247-5898-1 (hardcover : alk. paper)
  ISBN-10: 0-8247-5898-6 (hardcover : alk. paper)
  1. Surgery--Complications. 2. Wounds and injuries--Complications. I. Cohn, Stephen M.
  [DNLM: 1. Intraoperative Complications--prevention & control. 2. Postoperative Complications--prevention & control. 3. Wounds and Injuries--complications. WO 181 C7373 2006]

RD98.C665 2006
617'.9--dc22

2006044474

Visit the Informa Web site at
www.informa.com

and the Informa Healthcare Web site at
www.informahealthcare.com

This text is dedicated
To my supportive parents, Leland and Iris,
To my wonderful children, Sam and Elizabeth,
To my loving wife, Kelly.

Lechaim (To Life!)

Steve Cohn, 2006

Foreword

Most surgeons would prefer not to talk about surgical complications, much less write about them. If they are written about, unusual complications are frequently published as case reports. For this reason, I know of no single-author books on this topic; multiple-author works on surgical complications are the norm. This book is no exception. The multiple authors of its chapters have been chosen for their specific expertise in a given anatomic or physiologic field.

From the patient's viewpoint, a surgical complication is any unexpected event that occurs after surgical intervention and causes the patient pain or suffering. From the surgeon's viewpoint, many of the occurrences that patients would call complications are seen instead as sequelae. A sequela is an untoward occurrence that is out of the surgeon's control, such as phantom limb pain after amputation, the dumping syndrome after gastric resection, and the onset of diabetes after pancreatic resection. The list is almost endless. Surgeons should warn their patients about potential problems before performing the procedure and should convince the patient that the need for operative intervention outweighs any problems that may result.

A classic example of such a problem is wound infection. Wound infection can be a sequela when the surgeon is forced to operate through an infected site. In fact, one wound classification system is based on the potential that infection may develop. More often, however, wound infections are true complications and can be prevented. Among the many available preventive techniques are nutritional support, prophylactic administration of antibiotics, skin preparation, sterility of the operative environment, and sterile technique. For example, before sterile technique was adopted, compound fractures resulted in amputation and a mortality rate of 50% to 80% because of systemic infection, probably by streptococcus. The patients who survived frequently experienced the development of "laudable pus," which indicated a localized infection, probably due to staphylococcus. War wounds, whether clean contaminated or fully contaminated, were and still are treated with debridement and secondary closure. Appendicitis with rupture is still treated with secondary closure

at many medical centers. Since 1900, long before the development of antibiotics, addressing clean wounds under sterile surgical conditions has been associated with low rates of wound infection.

The example given above, wound infection, cuts across all surgical disciplines and demonstrates the need for a system-oriented approach to minimizing complications. The occurrence and severity of complications are affected by factors related to patient, environment, hospital, nursing, and surgeon. It makes little difference whether one uses the "weakest link" or the "Swiss cheese" model to explain the occurrence of complications due to failure of the system if, during each case, the level of care is optimized and adequate communication between all personnel providing patient care is ensured.

A strong case can be made for the usefulness of the classic surgical mortality and morbidity conference in analyzing the system failures associated with a given complication. The mortality and morbidity discussion addresses approaches that can be used to obviate a surgical complication in the future. The use of a table can be helpful in placing complications related to system failure into such categories as errors in judgment, errors in technique, and delay in diagnosis, treatment, or both because of the disease progress. Such an analysis serves both educational and quantity-of-care goals.

The thrust of this book is to review and classify the complications related to surgery from the standpoints of prevention, recognition, and management so that their impact on the patient's recovery can be minimized. This book analyzes the complications associated with many types of surgical intervention and dissects the optimal manner of preventing each one. It also discusses diagnostic and therapeutic techniques that can be used to minimize the impact of such complications on the welfare of the patient. Therefore, this book should be a standard reference for all surgeons, regardless of specialty.

J. Bradley Aust, M.D., Ph.D.
Department of Surgery, University of Texas Health Science Center at San Antonio, San Antonio, Texas, U.S.A.

Preface

"This was not my patient..."
"I was not present for this case..."
"There is nothing different I would do the next time..."
"Let me have the surgical attending tell you why we did this..."
"I never saw this patient..."
"If you do enough operations you are bound to have this happen"
"It was an act of God..."
"I did a perfect operation...the ungrateful patient died..."

Anonymous Chief Resident

This text was conceived to provide important information regarding the incidence and management of complications encountered in the surgical care of patients. More importantly, the contributing authors have identified methods to prevent or avoid complications. To paraphrase Albert Einstein, "Geniuses learn from other people's mistakes."

This book is dedicated to all the surgeons who have paved the path for surgical success.

Stephen M. Cohn

Contents

Contributors

Håkin Ahlman Gothenberg University, Sahlgrenska Universitetsjukhuset, Goteborg, Sweden

Fotios M. Andreopoulos Departments of Surgery and Biomedical Engineering, University of Miami School of Medicine, Miami, Florida, U.S.A.

Robert W. Bailey Division of Laparoscopic and Bariatric Surgery, Daughtry Family Department of Surgery, Miller School of Medicine, University of Miami, Miami, Florida, U.S.A.

Erik Barquist Ryder Trauma Center, Department of Surgery, University of Miami, Miller School of Medicine, Miami, Florida, U.S.A.

Adam J. Bell Division of Endourology and Laparoscopy, Department of Urology, University of Miami Miller School of Medicine, Miami, Florida, U.S.A.

Edward M. Boyle Division of Cardiothoracic Surgery, University of Washington, Seattle, Washington, U.S.A.

Stephen Brower Department of Surgery, University of Miami Miller School of Medicine, Miami, Florida, U.S.A.

Robert F. Buckman, Jr. Department of Surgery, Temple University School of Medicine, Philadelphia, Pennsylvania, U.S.A.

George W. Burke Division of Transplantation, The DeWitt Daughtry Family Department of Surgery, University of Miami, Miller School of Medicine, Miami, Florida, U.S.A.

Patricia M. Byers Division of Trauma, Burns, and Critical Care, The DeWitt Daughtry Family Department of Surgery, University of Miami, Miller School of Medicine, Miami, Florida, U.S.A.

Denise M. Carneiro-Pla DeWitt Daughtry Family Department of Surgery, Miller School of Medicine, University of Miami, Miami, Florida, U.S.A.

Gaetano Ciancio Division of Transplantation, The DeWitt Daughtry Family Department of Surgery, University of Miami, Miller School of Medicine, Miami, Florida, U.S.A.

Miguel A. Cobas Division of Trauma Anesthesia and Critical Care, Department of Anesthesiology, University of Miami, Miller School of Medicine, Miami, Florida, U.S.A.

Mark Cockburn Department of Surgery, Miller School of Medicine at the University of Miami, Miami, Florida, U.S.A.

Raymond P. Compton Paris Surgical Specialists, Paris, Tennessee, U.S.A.

Victor Cruz Department of Surgery, Stony Brook University Hospital, Stony Brook, New York, U.S.A.

James C. Doherty Division of Trauma Surgery, Advocate Christ Medical Center, Oak Lawn, and Department of Surgery, University of Illinois College of Medicine at Chicago, Chicago, Illinois, U.S.A.

Matthew O. Dolich Division of Trauma and Surgical Critical Care, University of California, Irvine School of Medicine, Irvine, California, U.S.A.

Charles Eaton The Hand Center, Jupiter, Florida, U.S.A.

Akpofure Peter Ekeh Department of Surgery, Wright State University School of Medicine, Dayton, Ohio, U.S.A.

Mohamed Fahim Anesthesia Critical Care, Davis Memorial Hospital, Elkins, West Virginia, U.S.A.

Debra Fertel Division of Pulmonary and Critical Care Medicine, Department of Medicine, University of Miami Miller School of Medicine, Miami, Florida, U.S.A.

Raquel Garcia-Roca University of Miami School of Medicine/Jackson Memorial Hospital, Miami, Florida, U.S.A.

Nicole S. Gibran Department of Surgery, University of Washington, Seattle, Washington, U.S.A.

Enrique Ginzburg   Division of Trauma and Surgical Critical Care, DeWitt Daughtry Family Department of Surgery, University of Miami Miller School of Medicine, Miami, Florida, U.S.A.

Amy J. Goldberg   Department of Surgery, Temple University School of Medicine, Philadelphia, Pennsylvania, U.S.A.

Dean Goldberg   Department of Surgery, Lee Memorial Hospital, Fort Myers, Florida, U.S.A.

Angelo E. Gousse   Department of Urology, Miller School of Medicine at the University of Miami, Miami, Florida, U.S.A.

Barth A. Green   Department of Neurological Surgery & The Miami Project to Cure Paralysis, University of Miami School of Medicine, Miami, Florida, U.S.A.

Fahim A. Habib   Division of Trauma and Surgical Critical Care, DeWitt Daughtry Family Department of Surgery, University of Miami School of Medicine, Miami, Florida, U.S.A.

Allen D. Hamdan   Harvard Medical School and Division of Vascular Surgery, Beth Israel Deaconess Medical Center, Boston, Massachusetts, U.S.A.

Iftikharul Haq   Department of Neurological Surgery & The Miami Project to Cure Paralysis, University of Miami School of Medicine, Miami, Florida, U.S.A.

John J. Hong   Robert Wood Johnson Medical School, University of Medicine and Dentistry of New Jersey, New Brunswick, New Jersey, U.S.A.

Gillian Hotz   Department of Surgery, University of Miami Miller School of Medicine, Miami, Florida, U.S.A.

Kenji Inaba   Department of Surgery, University of Miami Miller School of Medicine, Miami, Florida, U.S.A.

George L. Irvin III   DeWitt Daughtry Family Department of Surgery, Miller School of Medicine, University of Miami, Miami, Florida, U.S.A.

F. Frank Isik   Department of Surgery, University of Washington, Seattle, Washington, U.S.A.

Michael E. Ivy   Hartford Hospital, Hartford, and University of Connecticut School of Medicine, Farmington, Connecticut, U.S.A.

Andrew Jea   Department of Neurological Surgery, University of Miami Miller School of Medicine, Miami, Florida, U.S.A.

Igor Jeroukhimov   Department of Surgery, Assaf Harophe Medical Center, Tel Aviv University, Zerifin, Israel

Dory Jewelewicz   Department of Anesthesiology, University of Miami/Jackson Memorial Hospital, Miami, Florida, U.S.A.

Richard J. Kaplon   Cardiac and Thoracic Surgery Medical Group, Sacramento, California, U.S.A.

Riyad C. Karmy-Jones   Division of Cardiothoracic Surgery, University of Washington, and Thoracic Surgery, Harborview Medical Center, Seattle, Washington, U.S.A.

Rosemary F. Kelly   Cardiovascular and Thoracic Surgery, University of Minnesota, Minneapolis, Minnesota, U.S.A.

Robert R. Kester   Department of Urology, Miller School of Medicine at the University of Miami, Miami, Florida, U.S.A.

Yoram Klein   Division of Trauma and Emergency Surgery, Kaplan Medical Center, Rehovot and Department of Surgery, Hadassah EIN, Kerem Medical Center, Jerusalem, Israel

David S. Lasko   University of Miami School of Medicine/Jackson Memorial Hospital, Miami, Florida, U.S.A.

Raymond J. Leveillee   Division of Endourology and Laparoscopy, Department of Urology, University of Miami Miller School of Medicine, Miami, Florida, U.S.A.

David M. Levi   Department of Surgery, University of Miami, Miami, Florida, U.S.A.

Peter P. Lopez   Division of Trauma and Surgical Critical Care, DeWitt Daughtry Family Department of Surgery, University of Miami Miller School of Medicine, Miami, Florida, U.S.A.

Louis B. Louis IV   Division of Cardiothoracic Surgery, DeWitt Daughtry Family Department of Surgery, University of Miami Miller School of Medicine, Jackson Memorial Hospital, Miami, Florida, U.S.A.

Edward Lubin   Department of Anesthesiology, Yale University School of Medicine, New Haven, Connecticut, U.S.A.

Mauricio Lynn   Division of Trauma and Surgical Critical Care, DeWitt Daughtry Family Department of Surgery, University of Miami, Miller School of Medicine, Miami, Florida, U.S.A.

Jana B. A. MacLeod Division of Trauma and Critical Care, Department of Surgery, Emory University School of Medicine, Atlanta, Georgia, U.S.A.

Sapoora Manshaii St. Louis University School of Medicine, St. Louis, Missouri, U.S.A.

Hussein Mazloum Department of Surgery, McLaren Regional Medical Center and the College of Human Medicine–Michigan State University, Flint, Michigan, U.S.A.

Scott McDonald DeWitt Daughtry Family Department of Surgery, University of Miami School of Medicine, Miami, Florida, U.S.A.

Thomas Mellman Dartmouth Hitchcock Medical Center, Dartmouth Medical School, Lebanon, New Hampshire, U.S.A.

Joshua Miller Division of Transplantation, The DeWitt Daughtry Family Department of Surgery, University of Miami, Miller School of Medicine, Miami, Florida, U.S.A.

Frederick L. Moffat DeWitt Daughtry Family Department of Surgery, University of Miami School of Medicine, Miami, Florida, U.S.A.

John C. Mullen Department of Cardiac Sciences, University of Alberta, Edmonton, Canada

Halperin Nahum Department of Orthopedic Surgery, Tel Aviv University, Sackler Faculty of Medicine, Assaf Harofeh Medical Center, Zeriffin, Israel

Nicholas Namias Miller School of Medicine at the University of Miami, Miami, Florida, U.S.A.

D. Narayan Section of Plastic Surgery, Yale University School of Medicine, New Haven, Connecticut, U.S.A.

Adrian W. Ong Department of Surgery, Allegheny General Hospital, Drexel University College of Medicine, Pittsburgh, Pennsylvania, U.S.A.

Patrick W. Owens Department of Orthopedics and Rehabilitation, University of Miami, Miami, Florida, U.S.A.

Abhijit S. Pathak Department of Surgery, Temple University School of Medicine, Philadelphia, Pennsylvania, U.S.A.

Manuel Penalver Division of Gynecologic Oncology, Department of Obstetrics and Gynecology, Sylvester Comprehensive Cancer Center, University of Miami/ Jackson Memorial Medical Center, Miami, Florida, U.S.A.

James B. Peoples Department of Surgery, Wright State University School of Medicine, Dayton, Ohio, U.S.A.

J. Martin Perez Robert Wood Johnson University Hospital, New Brunswick, New Jersey, U.S.A.

J. A. Persing Section of Plastic Surgery, Yale University School of Medicine, New Haven, Connecticut, U.S.A.

Si M. Pham Division of Cardiothoracic Surgery, DeWitt Daughtry Family Department of Surgery, University of Miami Miller School of Medicine, Jackson Memorial Hospital, Miami, Florida, U.S.A.

Louis R. Pizano DeWitt Daughtry Family Department of Surgery, University of Miami, Miller School of Medicine, Miami, Florida, U.S.A.

Frank B. Pomposelli, Jr. Harvard Medical School and Division of Vascular Surgery, Beth Israel Deaconess Medical Center, Boston, Massachusetts, U.S.A.

Juan Carlos Puyana Surgical/Trauma Intensive Care Unit, University of Pittsburgh Medical Center, Pittsburgh, Pennsylvania, U.S.A.

Xiao-Shi Qi Division of Cardiothoracic Surgery, DeWitt Daughtry Family Department of Surgery, University of Miami Miller School of Medicine, Jackson Memorial Hospital, Miami, Florida, U.S.A.

Josh M. Randall Division of Endourology and Laparoscopy, Department of Urology, University of Miami Miller School of Medicine, Miami, Florida, U.S.A.

Qammar Rashid Department of Surgery, Howard University, Washington, D.C., U.S.A.

Nizam Razack Department of Neurological Surgery, University of Miami Miller School of Medicine, Miami, Florida, U.S.A.

Howard Richter Department of Orthopedics and Rehabilitation, University of Miami, Miller School of Medicine, Miami, Florida, U.S.A.

Michael J. Robbins Department of Anesthesiology, Yale University School of Medicine, New Haven, Connecticut, U.S.A.

Emery M. Salom Division of Gynecologic Oncology, Department of Obstetrics and Gynecology, Sylvester Comprehensive Cancer Center, University of Miami/ Jackson Memorial Medical Center, Miami, Florida, U.S.A.

Yekutiel Sandman   Department of Urology, Jackson Memorial Medical Center, University of Miami Miller School of Medicine, Miami, Florida, U.S.A.

Romualdo J. Segurola, Jr.   Cardiovascular and Thoracic Surgery, University of Minnesota, Minneapolis, Minnesota, U.S.A.

Gennaro Selvaggi   Department of Surgery, University of Miami, Miami, Florida, U.S.A.

Christopher K. Senkowski   Mercer University School of Medicine, Memorial Health University Medical Center, Savannah, Georgia, U.S.A.

Malachi G. Sheahan   Division of Vascular Surgery, Louisiana State University School of Medicine, New Orleans, Louisiana, U.S.A.

J. H. Shin   Section of Plastic Surgery, Yale University School of Medicine, New Haven, Connecticut, U.S.A.

Guatam V. Shrikhande   Department of Surgery, Harvard Medical School and Beth Israel Deaconess Medical Center, Boston, Massachusetts, U.S.A.

Raymond S. Sinatra   Department of Anesthesiology, Yale University School of Medicine, New Haven, Connecticut, U.S.A.

Danny Sleeman   DeWitt Daughtry Family Department of Surgery, Miller School of Medicine, University of Miami, Miami, Florida, U.S.A.

Andreas G. Tzakis   Department of Surgery, University of Miami, Miami, Florida, U.S.A.

Don H. Van Boerum   Section of Trauma Surgery, Department of Surgery, Sutter Roseville Medical Center, Roseville, California, U.S.A.

Albert J. Varon   Division of Trauma Anesthesia and Critical Care, Department of Anesthesiology, University of Miami, Miller School of Medicine, Miami, Florida, U.S.A.

Michael Y. Wang   Department of Neurological Surgery & The Miami Project to Cure Paralysis, University of Miami School of Medicine, Miami, Florida, U.S.A.

Gelfer Yael   Department of Orthopedic Surgery, Tel Aviv University, Sackler Faculty of Medicine, Assaf Harofeh Medical Center, Zeriffin, Israel

Bar Ziv Yaron   Department of Orthopedic Surgery, Tel Aviv University, Sackler Faculty of Medicine, Assaf Harofeh Medical Center, Zeriffin, Israel

Kosashvili Yona   Department of Orthopedic Surgery, Tel Aviv University, Sackler Faculty of Medicine, Assaf Harofeh Medical Center, Zeriffin, Israel

Gregory A. Zych   Department of Orthopedics and Rehabilitation, University of Miami, Miller School of Medicine, Miami, Florida, U.S.A.

The Surgical Mortality and Morbidity Review

INTRODUCTION

We surgeons establish a delightfully rewarding, gratifying, and unique bond with our patients. For our medical colleagues, the stakes are totally different. Without much trepidation, we, the authors, would permit Helen Keller to take our blood pressure or even palpate our edematous ankles. Similarly, if our health maintenance organization (HMO) relegated our primary care to someone with limited intellectual capacity, we would risk a visit or two before complaining.

But when a surgeon suggests that we must go to sleep while he or she clamps our aorta or removes our cancerous tumor, we demand dazzling expertise and total commitment. We may not be able to accurately assess the former (the diplomas on the wall are not sufficient), but we can sense the latter. From our surgeon, we expect knowledge, experience, and technical proficiency; equally important, if things do not go well, we want our surgeon to hurt as much as we do. That is commitment!

WHAT IS HURT?

Physical pain is easy to describe and define. We have all stubbed a toe or bruised an elbow. Calibrating pain is more complex. We have all seen the rancher from Wyoming who brings his traumatically amputated lower limb to the surgeon by bus, and the businessman from New York City who requires morphine for a haircut. Vicarious hurt, on the other hand, may be unique to humans and is more difficult to explain.

In its simplest form, the morbidity and mortality conference examines misadventures; dissects the preoperative, intraoperative, and postoperative events related to them; and derives strategies to prevent their recurrence. The varieties of surgical error are comprehensively explored in this book. Some are "surgeon specific": we may commit an error in the patient's diagnosis, in our surgical technique, or in the perioperative management of the case. Occasionally, these errors are readily apparent: the appendix was normal or the anastomosis leaked. Some problems, however, are "system specific": the Monday morning anesthesiology conference typically runs later than 8:00 A.M. On Mondays, when the rushed anesthesiologists exit their conference, their tardiness prompts an abbreviated preoperative assessment of the patient. The chart clearly states that the patient has diabetes or is being treated with drops for glaucoma, but the anesthesiologist misses this statement. That is a system-specific problem.

To the conscientious surgeon, any problem is always his or her fault. Whenever we, as surgeons, blame the hospital administrator because the ceiling collapsed or blame "patient disease" because our diabetic patient experienced a wound infection, that is a cop-out. We must always strive to eliminate all trouble for our patients. Every mishap is always avoidable and every problem that does occur is our fault. This philosophy greatly simplifies the adjudication of the mortality and morbidity process. This philosophy also defines hurt. If you want to be God, you must accept responsibility. God controls everything. It follows logically that you receive credit for both the good and the bad. If the bad is your fault, it must hurt. Good surgeons hurt—a lot.

WHO IS RESPONSIBLE?

Ultimately, our goal is to make our patients and their families feel better. If we can accomplish this by virtue of our superior comprehension of some subcellular mechanism of disease or by means of some particular therapy, so much the better. We infuse a phosphodiesterase inhibitor to prevent cyclic-adenosine monophosphate degradation and thus to build the contractile strength of cardiomyocytes. We do this because we know that, with age and congestive failure, patients deplete their cardiac beta-adrenergic receptors, and thus we must resort to a different inotropic strategy. That is great! We can tuck our thumbs into our axillae and strut off to the next lucky patient with the full knowledge that this cardiac cripple is incredibly fortunate to have a surgeon with our degree of omniscience.

Conversely, after our patient tiptoes his or her way through the surgical intensive care unit minefield, some well-meaning cardiology fellow or surgical intensive care unit nurse tells the family that Uncle Andy "almost died" and "really has a bag for a heart." The family (and Uncle Andy) is justifiably delighted to be discharged eventually from the surgical intensive care unit (and the hospital). But, in reality, Uncle Andy arrives home on pins and needles, expecting to die at any moment, for he is now obsessed with the knowledge of the horrible condition of his heart. That is a complication! We can have a civil discussion about who is responsible for this travesty of care, but we believe that it is the surgeon. From the moment that a surgical diagnosis is even suggested by the patient, his or her mother-in-law, or the medical consultant, the surgeon must enthusiastically accept responsibility for the patho-physio-psycho-social outcome of his or her surgical endeavors. Transfecting a responsive insulin receptor into an unsuspecting hepatocyte for the purpose of glorifying dysfunctional carbohydrate metabolism is nearly miraculous. Accomplishing this while sacrificing Uncle Andy's comprehension and adding to the confusion of the family is a travesty of surgical or medical skill. Our ultimate surgical goal is to make the family understand that Uncle Andy really does feel better.

ARE DEATH AND DISEASE INEVITABLE?

As conscientious, sensitive, thoughtful, compassionate surgeons, we must not accept the obvious answer to this question of whether death and disease are unavoidable (1). The surgical mortality and morbidity conference is unique in medicine and probably in the civilized world. Short of bank robbery, few events are as independently attributable to their perpetrator as is a surgical procedure. The surgeon meets the patient and family. He or she describes the pathological problem and the proposed surgical solution. If trust and commitment are not immediately emblazoned into this initial interaction, the whole process is fortunate to achieve junior bush league status. If the diagnosis is omniscient, the surgical technique flawless, the perioperative care masterful, and the patient expeditiously returned to the position of a socially responsible contributor to society, but the patient or the family does not comprehend the process, then the surgeon has failed.

Open discussion of this glorious spectrum of therapeutic opportunities is the purpose of a constructively educational surgical mortality and morbidity conference. When we, as surgeons, welcome this amplitude of criticism, we confidently bare our souls in the knowledge that no matter how good we are, we welcome any sacrifice to be even better. And after every patient we are privileged to treat and after every mortality and morbidity conference, we should look ourselves in the mirror, acknowledging that we may not know what profession is second best but that we are incredibly fortunate to be members of the most gratifying, responsible, receptive, critical, rewarding, and fun guild that exists (Polk H, Guandlick S, personal communication, 2002).

Julie Heimbach, M.D.
Mayo Clinic, Rochester, Minnesota, U.S.A.
Jyoti Arya, M.D.
University of Colorado, Denver, Colorado, U.S.A.
Alden H. Harken, M.D.
University of California, San Francisco,
and UCSF-East Bay Surgery Program, Oakland,
California, U.S.A.

REFERENCE

1.   Harken AH. Enough is enough. Arch Surg 1999; 134:1061–1063.

The Surgical Mortality and Morbidity Review: Best Practices and Procedures

The mortality and morbidity conference is an exercise unique to surgeons among all the members of the medical profession. Our colleagues in the medical specialties do not organize such conferences and rarely publicly probe their practices for systematic or individual error. Because surgeons collect data on mortality and morbidity and discuss such events regularly, surgical practice is most frequently analyzed by quality assurance staff. The quality assurance mavens are simply being lazy. They would provide a much greater return, in terms of overall improvement in patient care, if they invested their effort among those, primarily nonsurgeons, who do not engage in regular analysis of potential error.

Sad to say, the mortality and morbidity conference in some institutions I have had the privilege to visit sometimes fails to meet the objective of identifying error so that it may be corrected. Failure most frequently is due to lack of any real discussion in depth about the details of complications and deaths. Cases of senior or powerful attending physicians are not brought up for discussion, or details of errors in such cases are glossed over. No one utters critical remarks; moderators shirk their responsibility to probe. The conference is a sham. Even worse, in some institutions, the mortality and morbidity conference is converted into a presentation of "interesting" cases—an exercise better reserved for Grand Rounds—and investigation of the potential for prevention of deaths and complications does not occur.

If a mortality and morbidity conference is to achieve its desired goal, all cases resulting in any deviation, however minor, from the desired and expected outcome must be identified and be eligible for discussion. There can be no exceptions. Additionally, the conference must be appropriately structured; attendance without exception must be required of all staff, residents, and students assigned to the service or department. The conference must be led by moderators who understand and accept that it is their duty to probe for errors and for the causes of untoward outcomes. The conference should be open to nurses and other members of the hospital staff interested in the presentations and discussions.

To enhance effective discussion and sharing of experience, both the number of cases eligible for review and the size of the audience participating in the discussion should be neither too large nor too small. Between 30 and 50 is about the right number for both parameters. If necessary, because of the great workload of the service or department, multiple mortality and morbidity conferences should be conducted by subunits. The conference should be conducted weekly, be limited to one hour in duration so that the attention of the audience does not wander, start on time, and end on time. The room in which the mortality and morbidity conference is held should be large enough to accommodate the audience comfortably. There should be facilities for displaying X rays—about eight large films simultaneously—and equipment to project occasional pertinent slide or computer illustrations also should be available.

It is not necessary, in my view, to have a pathologist or radiologist in regular attendance. These specialists tend to spend too much time on demonstration of details that are of great interest within their medical niche but do not quickly advance the point of the mortality and morbidity conference: determination of the accuracy and effectiveness of the diagnosis or treatment in the case under discussion.

An agenda listing pertinent statistical and case information should be distributed at the entrance to the meeting room. No information identifiable with a specific patient should be included in the agenda. Material presented at mortality and morbidity conferences is usually protected by quality assurance privileges and regulations. Nonetheless, all copies of the agenda should be collected and destroyed at the end of the conference.

The agenda should include all material for a fixed time period; from eight o'clock Sunday morning to the same time on the following Sunday morning is a convenient interval. The agenda should list the following statistics: numbers of admissions, discharges, open operations, closed (e.g., laparoscopic) procedures, other procedures, complications, and deaths. This statistical information should be followed by a morbidity summary that separately lists each instance of an unexpected or untoward outcome in outline fashion (e.g., wound infection; 64F, colectomy, drained sixth pod). The sketchy information serves simply to remind the audience of the patient involved. The morbidity data are followed by a mortality summary in which each death is individually listed, also in shorthand fashion (e.g., 64F, colectomy; stroke fourth pod; pneumonia; died 10th pod; cause: MOF; no autopsy).

The assignment as moderator should be rotated among several of the most junior members of the staff. These persons are more likely to be up to date in their knowledge base. The moderator chooses from among the cases listed on the agenda those for presentation and discussion, emphasizing cases with unexpected outcomes, teaching value, rarity, etc. The moderator must maintain control of the conference, insisting that presentations be succinct, discussions be pertinent, and no witch-hunting be practiced by the audience. Knowledgeable members of the staff should be called upon for comment, especially if it is likely they will dissent. Residents should be liable to be called upon at any time—a device that helps to keep them awake. The moderator should generate any required minutes or reports soon after the conference has been completed.

Presentations, as requested by the moderator, are made by the resident team involved. All members of the team should stand at the front of the room. Usually a student or intern quickly summarizes the clinical course up to the time of operation or other salient event. These presentations should be rehearsed so that they are short and succinct, no more than a minute or two in length, even for a complicated case. Because all cases are eligible for discussion, all will have to be prepared. Pertinent X rays should be put up during the initial presentation for viewing by the audience; the X rays must be sorted in advance because there is no time within an efficiently conducted mortality and morbidity conference for rummaging through an X-ray file.

The presentation is next taken up and completed, beginning with the operation and continuing through the postoperative course, by the most senior resident involved in the procedure. I advise residents to read *Forgive and Remember* by Bosk (1) and to identify and follow the 15 rules of successful resident behavior identified therein. If they do so, they will acknowledge their errors during their presentation, thus anticipating reaction from the audience and controlling the discussion at the mortality and morbidity conference. If they do not, their experience at mortality and morbidity will sometimes be unnecessarily unpleasant.

I made it a rule that if residents had not disagreed at the time with the attending physician about any decision or other matter, then they carried responsibility for the outcome and had to conduct the presentation and answer questions from the audience. On the other hand, if they had clearly established their position of dissent, all they had to do was say so; the attending physician then had to come forward to complete the presentation and handle the discussion.

After the completed presentation, the moderator may ask the members of the audience whether they have questions that might clarify details of the presentation. Then the moderator initiates discussion of alternatives and possible error. If their presentation has been conducted as it should be, the residents will have left no question unanswered and the conference will simply move on to the next case.

The mortality and morbidity conference should be the best teaching exercise conducted by a surgical service or department. The goal is to have an open, thorough, detailed discussion of untoward outcomes so that all may learn from these events with the aim of improving the excellence of patient care. Properly conducted, the mortality and morbidity conference will, at least sometimes, be an uncomfortable exercise for some participants because no one, save an intellectual masochist, relishes having his or her potential lapses discussed in public. But, if properly conducted in a spirit of open intellectual inquiry, the mortality and morbidity conference will serve to enhance the professional knowledge and conduct of all participants and will help to avoid repetitive error. It is, therefore, "worth the price" of occasional embarrassment.

Robert E. Condon, M.D., M.Sc, FACS
*Department of Surgery, The Medical College
of Wisconsin, Milwaukee, Wisconsin, and
The University of Washington Medical School,
Seattle, Washington, U.S.A.*

REFERENCE

1. Bosk CL. Forgive and Remember: Managing Medical Failure. 2nd ed. Chicago: University of Chicago Press, 2003.

1

Complications of Anesthesia

Miguel A. Cobas and Albert J. Varon

*Division of Trauma Anesthesia and Critical Care, Department of Anesthesiology, University of
Miami, Miller School of Medicine, Miami, Florida, U.S.A.*

The study of complications that follow the administration of
anesthesia is challenging because their occurrence is
infrequent and they are influenced by a number of different
factors attributable to the patient, the surgical procedure, or
the method or agent of anesthesia. Historically, there have been
two common methods of studying complications in anesthesia. The first method is evaluation of cases, preferably
prospectively, albeit many studies have been done retrospectively with a large cohort of cases. However, because the
incidence of major complications in modern anesthesia is very
low, an enormous amount of data set would be required to
provide the study with sufficient power to detect significant
differences. The second method is to study a single complication in an attempt to detect a pattern associated with the
occurrence of that complication.

Many authors have tried to elucidate the real risk of death
for anesthetized patients. In the 1950s, Beecher and Todd's (1)
landmark study of more than 500,000 anesthetics concluded
that anesthesia was a contributory factor in mortality in 1:560
cases, and was the primary cause of death in 1:2680 cases. The
determination that an important contribution to the mortality
rate was residual paralysis by curare was noteworthy.

Since this study by Beecher and Todd, many others
have attempted to determine the mortality rate associated
with anesthesia. Anesthesia was found to be the primary
cause of death in 1 of every 852 cases (2) to 1 in every
14,075 cases (3). A significant number of fatalities occurred
in the patient's hospital room, emphasizing the need for
postoperative monitoring. In fact, in most of the studies
from the 1960s, the main safety recommendation was the
creation of a postanesthesia-care unit. Other anesthesia
complications commonly cited as important causes of
mortality were aspiration, errors in airway management,
hypovolemia, and overdose of anesthetic agents. These
studies also showed that the highest mortality rates
occurred among elderly patients, those with preexisting
diseases, and those who required emergency surgery.

In the 1980s, the landscape of anesthesia started to
change across the world. At that time the work force of
anesthesia in most developed countries consisted of a trained
anesthetist, in most cases a physician. In the United States,
the concept of the anesthesia-care team, in which a physician
supervises a Certified Nurse Anesthetist, was consolidated.
The advent of newer and safer anesthetic drugs and
improvements in patient monitoring, such as the widespread
use of pulse oxymetry, and a few years later, capnography,
lead to a dramatic reduction in mortality rates (3).

Holland studied over one million anesthetics
spanning from 1960 to 1985. According to this study, the
incidence of death attributed to anesthesia decreased from
1:550 in 1960 to 1:10,250 in 1970, and to 1:26,000 in
1984 (4). The shortcomings of this article were its retrospective design and the fact that the authors only reviewed
mortality within the first 24 hours after anesthesia.

Perhaps the most cited study in anesthesia mortality is
the Confidential Enquiry into Perioperative Death
(CEPOD) (5). The authors reported the results of over 500,000
cases in three areas of the United Kingdom over a period of
one year. The report included deaths that occurred within
30 days after the anesthetic was administered, and found that
anesthesia was solely responsible for death in three patients, or
in about one death for every 185,000 cases. It is worth
noting that the criteria for adjudicating a death exclusively to
anesthesia were stricter in the CEPOD study than in other
studies, including those performed by the same authors (6,7).

In 1984, the American Society of Anesthesiologists
(ASA) embarked on a nationwide project to study all the
closed claims related to anesthesia. The goal of the Closed
Claims Project was to discover unappreciated patterns of
anesthesia care that may contribute to patient injury and
subsequent litigation (8). This database represents the
largest resource for the study of adverse outcomes related to
anesthesia care and provides a reliable assessment of
common complications, their consequences, and the
importance that the patient gives to them.

According to this database, death, although extremely
uncommon, remains the most common cause of lawsuits
against anesthesiologists, but its percentual weight has
declined from 56% in the 1970s to 32% in the 1990s.
Emerging as an important liability cause for anesthesiologists is peripheral nerve injury, currently accounting for
16% of all claims.

COMPLICATIONS OF AIRWAY MANAGEMENT
Major Complications

Respiratory events constitute the largest group of claims against anesthesiologists, and they are responsible for the largest proportion of deaths and brain injury settlements. There are three major mechanisms of injury that account for such devastating outcomes: inadequate ventilation, esophageal intubation, and difficult tracheal intubation.

Esophageal intubation is neither uncommon nor disastrous when the patient's airway is difficult to access, but failure to recognize this complication is lethal. It is interesting to note that in 48% of the cases of unrecognized esophageal intubation, breath sounds were auscultated and documented (9). A *sustained* end-tidal CO_2 (ETCO$_2$) is essential to confirming tracheal intubation because brief CO_2 signals can sometimes be detected when the endotracheal tube is placed in the esophagus.

Although the best way to definitely secure the airway is by means of endotracheal intubation, sometimes the rush to intubate makes the clinician forget that with a self-inflating bag and proper technique, it is possible to provide adequate oxygenation and ventilation in most occasions. Even when intubation is the ultimate goal, preoxygenation is extremely valuable. By denitrogenating the lungs and filling the functional residual capacity (FRC) with a high concentration of oxygen, the time the patient can tolerate apnea is greatly prolonged.

It is important to develop a plan for securing the airway in the first attempt and a backup plan if the first option fails. The ASA has developed a comprehensive algorithm for dealing with a potential difficult airway (Fig. 1). In this algorithm, great emphasis is placed on anticipation and preparation.

A suspected difficult airway should ideally be secured with the patient awake and breathing spontaneously because taking away the native respiratory drive with the use of anesthetics and muscle relaxants could prove lethal. The most feared scenario occurs when the trachea cannot be intubated and mask ventilation is not effective. In this "can't intubate, can't ventilate" situation, the practitioner has four options: laryngeal mask airway (LMA), Combitube, transtracheal jet ventilation (TTJV), and cricothyroidotomy.

The LMA and the Combitube are devices that are blindly inserted into the oropharynx and are designed to provide supraglottic oxygenation and ventilation, but do not protect against aspiration. Although their use is limited in the presence of laryngospasm or upper airway obstruction, they are extremely useful in rescue situations, while other options for definitively securing the airway are being contemplated or the patient is allowed to resume spontaneous breathing.

The two other techniques recommended for the above scenario are infraglottic and require more skill and time. TTJV requires the availability of a high-pressure oxygen source and tubing to deliver oxygen into the trachea through a large gauge (i.e., 14 or 15) catheter inserted in the cricoidthyroid membrane.

Cricothyroidotomy is the preferred surgical airway in an emergency situation because the anatomic structures are easier to locate and dissect when compared with the traditional tracheostomy.

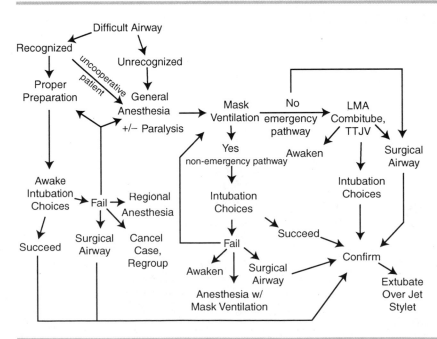

Figure 1 American Society of Anesthesiologists' algorithm for the difficult airway. *Abbreviations*: LMA, laryngeal mask airway; TTJV, transtracheal jet ventilation. *Source*: From American Society of Anesthesiologists on management of the difficult airway.

Airway Trauma

A recent review of airway trauma during anesthesia revealed that claims for this complication rank fourth, after death, brain damage, and nerve damage malpractice claims (10). Interestingly enough, this complication is more likely to occur among female patients than among male patients and among children than adults, and these differences are statistically significant. Difficult intubation played a significant role (38%) in all claims for airway trauma.

When considering airway trauma related to perioperative care, the sites most commonly affected are the larynx, pharynx, esophagus, and trachea. Laryngeal injuries comprise about a third of all airway trauma complications reported in the Closed Claims Project database (8). This type of injury was not associated with difficult intubation. Most of the laryngeal injuries were found in short-term intubations. One-third of all laryngeal injuries resulted in vocal cord paralysis, 16% in granulomas, and 8% in arytenoid dislocation.

Tracheal injuries represented 14% of all the airway complications. Most of these were associated with the creation of a tracheostomy tract in the setting of a lost airway. Forty percent of tracheal injuries involve lacerations that occur during intubation.

A rare but potentially lethal complication of intubation is tracheobronchial disruption. A review of the literature reveals mostly case reports and small series. Risk factors implicated in tracheal rupture include old age, chronic obstructive pulmonary disease, and corticosteroid therapy. Factors related to the intubation may include the use of a stylet, especially if it protrudes at the tip of the endotracheal tube, and forceful entry of the tube into the trachea after a difficult intubation. The disruption usually occurs in the posterior membranous part of the trachea, and physical signs include respiratory distress, stridor, and subcutaneous emphysema. Radiographic confirmation usually reveals a balloon that has been overinflated in an attempt to reduce the air leak, and pneumomediastinum with or without pneumopericardium. Fiberoptic bronchoscopy is the best method to diagnose tracheobronchial disruption. There is considerable controversy regarding the appropriate treatment of this injury. While some authors advocate emergent repair, two recent case reports of conservative treatment in elderly patients suggest that this could be a feasible option (11–13).

Injuries to the esophagus and the oropharynx tend to be more severe because pharyngeal and esophageal tears often result in abscesses or mediastinitis. These entities carry a high mortality rate when there is a delay in the diagnosis. Patients who have had difficult tracheal intubation should be observed carefully for signs of mediastinitis or retropharyngeal abscess.

Aspiration

Aspiration is defined as the passage of stomach contents through the glottic opening, causing varying degrees of lung damage and potential death.

Risk factors for aspiration include emergency surgery, surgery in pregnancy as early as 10 weeks, small bowel obstruction, bleeding ulcers, and autonomic neuropathy delaying gastric emptying.

The classic example of aspiration pneumonitis was described in pregnant patients undergoing general anesthesia for cesarean section. Later studies postulated that an amount of at least 0.4 mL/kg and a pH of less than 2.5 were major determinants of the severity of aspiration pneumonitis.

An ounce of prevention is worth a pound of cure when presented with patients at risk. The most common strategies used for the prevention of aspiration include the administration of drugs designed to increase the pH of the aspirate. H2 blockers are an effective option; however, they must be given at least two hours before surgery for their effect to take place. When premedicating just before surgery, it is more effective to use a nonparticulate antacid such as sodium citrate. Metoclopramide has also been advocated to promote gastric emptying, but is not devoid of side effects. Cricoid pressure has been advocated as the single most effective measure for preventing aspiration during intubation. It is important to remember that the operator applying cricoid pressure should not discontinue the maneuver until verification of appropriate endotracheal intubation and cuff inflation. If a patient is deemed to be at risk of aspiration, it is recommended to delay extubation until the patient is awake and has protective airway reflexes.

If aspiration does occur, treatment is usually supportive. Prompt bronchoscopy is only indicated for retrieval of aspirated particulate matter. Most of the time, the aspiration has no major consequences, and it will manifest itself as a mild hypoxemia, which can be treated with supplemental oxygen. The absence of symptoms in the two first hours after the event usually correlates with a benign course (14). In more severe cases, the patient can present signs of clinical pneumonitis, with wheezing, rales, and rhonchi, but this clinical picture, as well as its X-ray changes, can be delayed up to 12 to 24 hours. In some cases, the syndrome is so severe that it requires mechanical ventilation and positive end-expiratory pressure. Antibiotics are usually not recommended because most of the time the aspirated material is sterile. If there is worsening of the patient status three to five days after the event, bacterial contamination should be suspected, and therapy should be guided by culture data.

Laryngospasm

Laryngospasm is defined as an involuntary contraction of the vocal cords resulting in airway obstruction. It is typically a phenomenon related to airway instrumentation and is described more frequently in the pediatric population. Environmental factors may play an important role in the development of laryngospasm. Lakshmipathy et al. studied

310 healthy children and found a strong association between household smoking and development of laryngospasm under general anesthesia (15). One of the most common causes of laryngospasm is the contact of secretions, blood, or vomitus against the vocal cords, causing reflex closure. Clinical signs of laryngospasm include stridor and an increased respiratory effort with visible tugging at the suprasternal notch.

Laryngospasm is usually short-lived and self-limited, and sometimes there is a valve-like effect of the vocal cords allowing some expiratory flow. The first line of treatment for laryngospasm is positive-pressure ventilation delivered gently by face mask. In children, where short periods of apnea are associated with rapid desaturation, administration of a small dose of succinylcholine (0.25 mg/kg) will relax the vocal cords and allow ventilation. It is worth noting that if pharmacologic paralysis is not feasible, laryngospasm will eventually recede due to hypoxia and hypercarbia.

Minor Complications
Temporomandibular Joint Injuries

Injuries to the temporomandibular joint have a unique set of characteristics. Almost all of these injuries occur in previously healthy young females, and are not associated with prolonged or difficult intubation. The reason for this demographic profile is perhaps the fact that temporomandibular joint disease is more prevalent in young females (16).

Dislocation of the mandible occurs when there is subluxation of the condylar process over the articular eminence of the temporomandibular joint and, characteristically, the patients cannot bring their teeth together. This complication may not be apparent during anesthesia, but will manifest with severe pain and consequent muscle spasm over the temporomandibular joint region.

The treatment for this condition consists of restoring the mandibular condyle back into its socket. Most of the time, this can be accomplished with the patient awake, after administration of a benzodiazepine to improve the muscle spasm. An operator then places the thumbs inside the mouth of the patient, over both the inferior molar surfaces, and then pushes downward and backward to snap the joint back into place. It is obvious that the operator must take great care to avoid damage to his or her thumbs because the patient's teeth may close forcefully.

Dental Injury

Dental damage is the most common type of injury during general anesthesia (17,18), with an incidence ranging from 0.01% to 0.1% (19,20). The upper central incisors are the teeth having the highest risk for dental injury, and damage is much more common if there is a preexistent dental disease. Decidual teeth have shallow roots, which makes them prompt to dislodgment. Therefore, the best strategy to prevent this type of injury is a thorough dental evaluation before surgery. If there is extensive tooth decay, protruding teeth, loose teeth, or prosthesis, the anesthetist should inform the patient that there is a possibility of teeth being dislodged, and some practitioners would advocate the removal of very loose teeth while the patient is awake.

If a tooth becomes dislodged during laryngoscopy, immediate retrieval from the oropharynx is mandated. Sometimes, X-rays of the neck, chest, and abdomen are necessary to locate the piece. If the tooth is located in the lung, a bronchoscopy should be performed promptly. The tooth should be reimplanted immediately when feasible, applying pressure over the piece; this will minimize the risk of root resorption. A dental consult should be requested for as soon as possible.

Sore Throat

The reported incidence of sore throat after anesthesia varies widely, ranging from 6% to 40% (21). This transient minor complaint is not an airway injury, but should be regarded as an important outcome to be avoided for patient satisfaction. A sore throat is one of the most common and least desirable events for patients after anesthesia (22) and appears to be more frequent in women than in men (23).

A study reported that sore throat and coughing on the first postoperative day were significantly less frequent in patients in the low pressure–high volume cuff group. This finding suggests that the pressure exerted to the tracheal mucosa is more important than the total contact area of the cuff. The authors, however, found no differences when comparing voice changes or difficulty in swallowing between the groups (24).

Another factor implicated in the genesis of sore throat after anesthesia is the use of succinylcholine; however, this has not been substantiated (25,26). Inflating the endotracheal tube cuff with lidocaine or lubricating the outer surface of the endotracheal tube with lidocaine gel has been used to prevent sore throat after anesthesia. The utility of these techniques is controversial and, therefore, cannot be advocated as a standard of care (27,28).

COMPLICATIONS OF THE RESPIRATORY SYSTEM
Bronchospasm

Bronchospasm is a reflex constriction of the smooth bronchial muscle leading to increased airway resistance, expiratory flow obstruction, and air entrapment in a fashion similar to that of an acute asthma attack. Perhaps the main difference between a bronchospastic episode under anesthesia and asthma is the presence of inflammation in the latter. Bronchospasm under anesthesia has been recognized as a serious problem;

it is more likely to occur in individuals with asthma or reactive airway disease, smokers, patients with chronic obstructive pulmonary disease, and those with an acute viral respiratory infection; however, it also can occur in healthy individuals.

The underlying mechanism for bronchospasm during anesthesia seems to be related to an increase in bronchomotor tone associated with intubation and laryngoscopy, as demonstrated by Gal and Suratt in healthy volunteers (29). In predisposed individuals, premature manipulation of the airway will result in an exaggerated response.

The preoperative assessment of a patient at risk for bronchospasm should include a detailed history, with emphasis on the severity of symptoms, use of bronchodilators and steroids, and previous intubation. If a patient scheduled for elective surgery is actively wheezing during the preoperative visit, all efforts should be made to optimize the patient's condition; otherwise, surgery should be postponed.

Bronchospasm that develops intraoperatively typically occurs after induction of anesthesia, usually as a result of manipulation of the airway before adequate depth of anesthesia has been established. Minimizing the response to intubation and laryngoscopy is paramount. Several agents have been used with success for this purpose, the most common being β_2 agonists and lidocaine (30). Regarding specific induction agents, it appears that propofol has a slightly more favorable profile than thiopental with respect to airway resistance (31), but this effect seems to be limited to the nongeneric formulation (32). Ketamine is the only induction agent consistently shown to induce bronchodilation, and may be considered as an option when patients need to undergo surgery while actively wheezing. Due to its undesirable side effects, however, this agent cannot be recommended routinely.

The physical signs of bronchospasm that can be recognized during surgery include difficult ventilation ("stiff bag"), wheezing, and elevated peak airway pressures. It is important to remember that wheezing is a nonspecific sign, and can be associated with other conditions, including mechanical obstruction, main stem intubation, pneumothorax, or heart failure.

The treatment includes deepening of anesthesia or sedation, confirmation of the proper position of the endotracheal tube (an endotracheal tube touching the carina is extremely irritating to the airway), continuing positive-pressure ventilation, and aggressive use of β_2 agonists. The use of neuromuscular blocking agents helps decrease chest wall rigidity, but not bronchomotor tone. The amount of β_2 agent that actually reaches the alveoli when given through an endotracheal tube is highly variable because a significant percentage of the dose delivered adheres to the polyvinylchloride of the tube. Therefore treatment must be guided by clinical response, rather than by a fixed number of puffs.

Atelectasis

Arterial oxygenation is impaired during general anesthesia with either spontaneous or controlled ventilation. This impairment in oxygenation is largely due to ventilation–perfusion mismatch and shunt, with the magnitude of the shunt correlating closely with the degree of the atelectasis.

Many factors influence the development of atelectasis during surgery. Induction of general anesthesia is consistently associated with a significant decrease in FRC and the formation of compression atelectasis. These changes occur within minutes of the anesthetic induction. The reduction in FRC correlates well with an increase in the venous admixture and alveoloarterial oxygen gradient. This is a very common cause of decreased arterial oxygen saturation in the recovery room.

Another important factor in the development of intraoperative atelectasis is the type of surgery. Upper abdominal and thoracic procedures predispose the patient to this complication. The mechanical factors inherent to the procedure are compounded by the inability to cough and mobilize secretions. Adequate pain control in the postoperative period is essential to minimize the risk of atelectasis in these patients. Epidural anesthesia is an effective technique for pain control in patients whose respiratory function may be compromised and who require upper abdominal or thoracotomy procedures.

COMPLICATIONS OF THE CARDIOVASCULAR SYSTEM
Perioperative Myocardial Ischemia or Infarction

Coronary artery disease is the most frequent cause of perioperative cardiac morbidity and mortality in noncardiac surgery. Clinicians often need to identify patients at risk for developing cardiac complications. An extensive effort has been done to classify patients according to their risk factors.

A history of prior myocardial infarction is an important predictor of postoperative reinfarction, and its incidence is inversely proportional to the time elapsed since the event. In the 1970s, reinfarction was reported in 30% of patients with recent (less than three months) myocardial infarction (33), but that number decreased to less than 5% in the 1990s (34), presumably due to improved hemodynamic monitoring and a prompt therapy of hemodynamic disturbances. What seemed clear was that the rate of reinfarction did not stabilize until approximately six months after the original myocardial infarction; thus previous recommendations to postpone all elective surgery until that period had passed. Even then, patients with a previous myocardial infarction will have an increased risk of reinfarction when compared to the general population.

In 1996, the American College of Cardiology and the American Heart Association published guidelines for perioperative cardiovascular evaluation for non-cardiac surgery (35). These guidelines provided a framework for considering cardiac risk in a variety of patients and surgical conditions.

The major clinical predictors of increased perioperative cardiovascular risk are unstable coronary syndromes, defined as recent myocardial infarction, unstable or severe angina, decompensated congestive heart failure, significant arrhythmias, and severe valvular disease. Factors considered to be of intermediate significance are mild angina, old myocardial infarction, compensated congestive heart failure, and diabetes. Other factors include advanced age, uncontrolled hypertension, history of stroke, or abnormal nonspecific electrocardiogram findings such as ST segment changes, left ventricular hypertrophy, or left bundle branch block.

When considering the probability of postoperative cardiac ischemic events, it is important to stratify according to the type of surgery. The cardiac risk is high—combined incidence of cardiac death and myocardial infarction more than 5%—in emergent major operation, aortic or peripheral vascular surgery, or any operation with major blood loss. Intermediate surgical risk—cardiac risk less than 5%—is represented by carotid endarterectomy, intraperitoneal and intrathoracic operations, and orthopedic, prostate, and head and neck surgery.

Those patients deemed to be at risk based on either their functional status or the type of surgery should undergo further preoperative evaluation.

From all the interventions attempted to reduce the incidence of postoperative myocardial infarction, the only one that has shown to be effective is the perioperative administration of β blockers (36,37). These agents are extremely useful, yet widely underutilized.

If myocardial infarction does occur, it usually presents in the first 48 to 72 hours postoperatively. Most of these infarctions are subendocardial (non–Q wave); however, the diagnostic criteria are not uniformly defined. Furthermore, therapy with thrombolytic agents or anticoagulation in the setting of recent surgery is often contraindicated. Therefore, the main therapeutic approach in these cases is to maximize oxygen supply and reduce demand. In this setting, β blockers have also proven to be very useful.

Intraoperative Arrhythmias

Intraoperative arrhythmias are very common during anesthesia, occurring in approximately 20% of patients, but only a very small number are considered serious. Not surprisingly, arrhythmias tend to occur more frequently in the elderly, in patients with preexisting heart disease or receiving digitalis, and at times of hemodynamic disturbances such as induction and emergence.

There are important anesthetic interactions that could make the heart more susceptible to arrhythmias. The discussion of specific conduction disturbances is beyond the scope of this chapter; however, it is important to know that various clinical situations can potentiate the arrhythmogenic effects of anesthetics. Although halogenated inhalational agents per se are unlikely to cause a clinically significant arrhythmia, in the presence of hypercarbia, hypoxia, and/or increased catecholamines, there is a higher risk for the development of ventricular ectopy.

The dose of epinephrine required to induce arrhythmias is almost half in the presence of halothane than in the presence of isoflurane, suggesting that halothane reduces the threshold for arrhythmias (38).

Most of the intravenous agents commonly used in anesthetic practice do not produce clinically significant arrhythmias. Perhaps an exception to this is ketamine, which has strong sympathomimetic properties.

Local anesthetics block sodium channels, and thus have antiarrhythmic properties, but at toxic dosages, they become arrhythmogenic. Bupivacaine is especially notorious in this regard, with many reports of induction of ventricular tachycardia, ventricular fibrillation, and cardiac arrest. The proposed mechanism for this cardiac toxicity is that the drug is removed slowly from the sodium channel blocked, causing a delay in repolarization, leading to an increasingly prolonged QT interval and torsade de pointes. Cardiac arrests induced by bupivacaine are considered very difficult to treat, and there is support for using bretylium in this scenario (39).

COMPLICATIONS OF THE RENAL SYSTEM
Renal Toxicity of General Anesthetics

All inhaled anesthetics depress renal function as manifested by a decreased glomerular filtration rate (GFR), a decreased renal blood flow, and electrolyte disturbances. Free fluoride ions produced by the metabolism of these compounds can be directly nephrotoxic. Metoxiflurane, enflurane, and sevoflurane produce free fluoride ions when metabolized. The classic example of fluoride-induced nephrotoxicity was described in 1966 with metoxiflurane. Its toxic effect was manifested by decreased concentrating ability. Later reports confirmed that prolonged exposure to enflurane was also a risk factor for this complication (40). Halothane, isoflurane, and desflurane do not result in the production of fluoride in concentrations large enough to cause any kidney damage (40–42). Methoxiflurane is no longer in use in current human anesthetic practice. Enflurane's use is also very limited due to the widespread acceptance of newer agents.

Sevoflurane is a fluorinated anesthetic used for many years in Japan, which has progressively gained acceptance in the United States. It has a low blood gas partition coefficient, which provides for a rapid onset of action, and it is not an irritant to the airways, making it an attractive choice for inhalation anesthesia. Serum fluoride concentration from the metabolism of this gas sometimes peaks above what is considered a safe threshold; however, because of its rapid elimination, these ions do not, stay around long enough to produce any toxicity (43). Sevoflurane does produce another metabolite, the compound A, after it reacts with carbon dioxide absorbers. Although at low gas flows this metabolite has been shown to be directly nephrotoxic in rats (44), the effect in humans remains unclear (45–48). Currently, the Food and Drug Administration recommends the use of fresh gas flow of at least 2 L/min when using sevoflurane.

Postoperative Renal Dysfunction

The development of acute renal failure results in a significant increase in morbidity and mortality, as well as in health-care costs because renal replacement therapy is expensive and not free of complications. Development of renal failure in the perioperative period is almost always the result of a combination of factors and almost never the result of an anesthetic agent alone.

Whether the cause of renal failure is aortic cross-clamping, cardiopulmonary bypass, radiological contrast agent exposure, or protracted hypotension, the primary mechanism of injury is the ischemia of the outer renal medulla. This area represents a vascular watershed and is the first to manifest injury after a hypoxemic event (49).

One of the challenges facing physicians is to characterize patients at risk for the development of renal failure. These patients include those who undergo procedures requiring cardiopulmonary bypass, with a reported incidence between 1% and 7% (50,51). Vascular surgery patients represent another important risk group for the development of renal failure, where it has traditionally been associated with poor prognosis (52,53). As expected, the incidence of acute renal failure after infrarenal aortic surgery is less than when aortic clamping is above the renal vessels. If the surgery is performed on an emergency basis, the incidence of this complication increases. Emergency operations for ruptured or leaking aneurysms are associated with renal failure in up to 30% of cases (54).

Acute renal failure following trauma is rare. Morris retrospectively reviewed over 70,000 patients admitted to nine trauma centers during a five-year span. These authors found that the incidence of patients who required dialysis was only 0.01%. In the majority of the cases of renal failure presenting after trauma, the signs developed late and were associated with multiple organ failure (55).

Preexistent renal failure has been consistently shown to be an important predictor of postoperative renal failure. Therefore, it is essential to maintain proper renal function throughout the stress of surgery by providing the patient with adequate fluid volume, and using invasive hemodynamic monitoring when necessary. Adequate preoperative hydration of the patient not only ensures an adequate oxygen delivery to the renal tubules, but also diminishes demand by reducing the stimulus for sodium reabsorption. It is appropriate to set euvolemia as a goal while avoiding hypervolemia, in order to optimize oxygen delivery to the outer medulla without increasing the demand.

A theoretical approach to minimize damage to the kidney would be to effectively reduce renal medullary oxygen demand. It is known that inhibitors of the adenosine triphosphatase (ATPase) located in the medullary thick ascending limb, such as furosemide, can dramatically reduce the metabolic demands of this region. In a study of radiocontrast exposure, however, pretreatment with furosemide failed to show a beneficial effect (56). Prophylactic oral administration of *n*-acetylcysteine, along with hydration, has been reported to prevent reduction in the renal function by low-osmolality contrast agents in patients with chronic renal insufficiency (57).

The most controversial agent proposed to offer renal protection is DA at a low dose ("renal dose"). DA has been utilized extensively in doses less than 3 μg/kg/min to provide renal protection by improving renal blood flow. The conventional wisdom has been that at this dose range, only dopaminergic receptors will be stimulated, promoting splanchnic and renal vasodilation, as well as an increase in urine output and sodium excretion. These findings have been corroborated in animals and humans, but do not necessarily translate into an improved clinical outcome. In 1998, a comprehensive review of the literature found no evidence of a renal protective effect of DA in the perioperative period (58). More recently, a multicenter, randomized, double-blind, placebo-controlled study failed to show any benefit in critically ill patients at risk for renal dysfunction (59). A meta-analysis seems to confirm these findings (60). In fact, attempting to "improve" the renal function intraoperatively may actually predispose the kidney to ischemic injury by increasing oxygen requirements, and may result in undesirable cardiovascular side effects, i.e., tachycardia or arrhythmias. The notion of isolated dopaminergic receptor stimulation has been challenged because a study of normal volunteers given weight-based infusions of DA reported an enormous intersubject variability in plasma concentrations (61). Presently, there is insufficient evidence to support the use of DA as a renal protecting agent.

Dopexamine is a pure dopaminergic agonist that has gained some attention because it may improve renal perfusion without the risks of adrenergic stimulation. However, large and well-designed trials are necessary to assess its usefulness.

Fenoldopam is a specific DA 1–receptor agonist. It has been shown to reduce blood pressure in a dose-dependent manner, while preserving renal perfusion and GFR (62). At a low dose, fenoldopam has been reported to improve renal blood flow without changes in systemic blood pressure. However, there is currently insufficient data to support the use of fenoldopam in critically ill patients.

COMPLICATIONS OF THE NEUROLOGIC SYSTEM
Perioperative Stroke

The incidence of perioperative strokes after surgery other than cardiac or neurologic is approximately 0.05% (63). As expected, the incidence is greater in the elderly and in patients with atherosclerosis. The pathophysiology of intraoperative stroke is for the most part thromboembolic. A study of the mechanisms of perioperative cerebral infarction reported that atrial fibrillation was present in 33% of patients (64). On the other hand, the presence of a carotid bruit in an otherwise asymptomatic patient does not seem to be a risk factor (65). A surgical procedure with a higher risk for perioperative stroke is carotid endarterectomy, where the incidence is reported to be about 5%.

It seems reasonable that a general approach to prevent perioperative stroke is to maintain an adequate balance between cerebral oxygen supply and demand. This may be achieved by various interventions including maintaining blood pressure within 20% of baseline values. Because patients with long-standing hypertension have their autoregulatory cerebral perfusion curve shifted toward higher pressures, what could be considered as normotension for most patients might represent hypotension in this population.

If a stroke is suspected, an immediate computed tomography (CT) scan of the brain with contrast should be obtained, along with neurology consultation. Thrombolytic therapy is usually contraindicated in the immediate postoperative period, and instituting anticoagulation must proceed with caution.

Postoperative Cognitive Dysfunction

More than 150 years have passed since the first anesthetic was demonstrated, and the mechanism of action of general anesthetics is still elusive. Although all anesthetic drugs create a temporary dysfunction in the brain, the exact duration of this effect is unknown.

Fine motor coordination is impaired for up to five hours after only a few minutes of exposure to halothane (66), and prolonged exposure to isoflurane may affect behavior up to 48 hours after the event (67). However, these effects are believed to be short-lived and self-limited, especially in a young healthy population.

There is special concern about the possibility of long-lasting cognitive impairment in the elderly.

Although the results in this area of investigation are still controversial, a recent, prospective, randomized trial showed that up to 6% of patients undergoing either general or epidural anesthesia with sedation had some degree of cognitive impairment that was evident even six months after the operation (68).

Another study evaluated 261 patients for five years to determine a long-term cognitive impairment after coronary artery bypass graft surgery using cardiopulmonary bypass. The investigators found cognitive dysfunction in 53% of patients at discharge from the hospital and in 42% at five years, with early cognitive impairment being a strong predictor of long-term impairment. Although there was no control group in this study, the fact that there was such a pronounced cognitive decline immediately after surgery suggests that this type of procedure may hasten cognitive impairment (69).

These results, disturbing as they are, need to be confirmed by other trials evaluating different patient populations, anesthetic regimens, and types of surgery. If that is the case, permanent cognitive impairment will become an important perioperative complication to be considered in the geriatric population.

Perioperative Visual Loss

Perioperative visual loss is rare but one of the most devastating complications that can occur in the immediate postoperative period. This complication has been reported after cardiopulmonary bypass surgery in the prone position, prolonged hypotension, and direct compression of the globe.

The most common diagnosis of this condition is ischemic optic neuropathy (ION), which is a well-known entity affecting patients with risk factors such as hypertension, atherosclerosis, and diabetes.

The ASA established a database for cases of perioperative visual loss. In 23 cases of perioperative visual loss reported up to 1999, ION was present in 20 of them. In all the cases, the anesthetic was longer than five hours, and blood loss was considerable, averaging 2.2 L. Patients were in the prone position in 50% of the cases, and hypotension (systolic blood pressure or mean arterial pressure 40% below baseline) was found in 52% of the cases (70).

The diagnosis of ION should be suspected in any patient with complaints of visual loss immediately after surgery, especially if it is painless. Suspicion of this entity should be followed by early ophthalmologic consultation. Unfortunately, this disorder carries a poor prognosis (70,71). Due to the multifactorial etiology of this complication, there is not a single specific measure to prevent this complication. However, obvious precautions should include intraoperative monitoring of ocular areas, avoiding external compression on the eyes, and aggressive treatment of hypotension.

Awareness

Awareness during anesthesia is defined as the spontaneous recall of intraoperative events. It is a form of explicit memory because patients usually are able to tell exactly what was being said or done during a specific time of the procedure. Awareness has been described as one of the most horrible and traumatic experiences a patient can suffer, especially if they are under the effect of muscle relaxants. Patients have described this experience as the feeling of being buried alive.

The incidence of awareness for noncardiac, nonobstetric surgery has been reported to be 0.2% (72). In cardiac surgery, it can reach up to 1.5%, and has been reported in as high as 11% of emergency trauma cases. In obstetrics, the incidence ranges from 0.4% to 7% (73).

Frequent scenarios for the development of awareness are those in which administration of anesthetics is limited due to hemodynamic instability. Other causes include equipment malfunction or drug errors. A common time for awareness to occur is between induction of general anesthesia and skin incision. This is a period of relative quietness, when there is little stimulation to the patient, and therefore blood pressure tends to drift down. The usual response of anesthesia practitioners in this circumstance is to lower the concentration of anesthetics, increasing the risk of awareness.

It is important to note that the patient can be suffering awareness, and yet nothing seems wrong even when the anesthetic chart is carefully reviewed. Increases in heart rate and blood pressure could represent indirect signs of awareness, but the most reliable indicator of the patient being awake and aware of the surroundings is motion. Therefore, one must carefully consider the use of muscle relaxants, especially when the surgical procedure does not require them.

Patients who experienced awareness will sometimes complain of sleep disturbances, dreams and nightmares, flashbacks, and daytime anxiety. A small percentage of patients will go on to develop post-traumatic stress disorders (74).

According to the ASA closed claims database, awareness represents almost 2% of 4183 total claims. The profile of the patient who suffered awareness was that of a healthy (ASA I or II) woman undergoing elective surgery. Awake paralysis, the most severe form of awareness, was caused by errors in administration or labeling of anesthetic drugs in 94% of cases. Other risk factors for the development of awareness were the intraoperative use of muscle relaxants and techniques that used little or no potent inhaled anesthetic (75).

A monitor designed to measure the sedative and amnesic effects of anesthetics in the central nervous system has been developed. The Bispectral Index (BIS) monitor is a processed electroencephalogram (EEG) with advanced algorithms derived from a database of thousands of patients undergoing multiple regimens of general anesthesia. The result is displayed on a scale of 0 (complete EEG inactivity) to 100 (awake), with 60 or lower representing unconsciousness associated with no recall (76).

The BIS monitor has been reported to decrease the total dose of anesthetics used over time (77), and to increase the number of patients who are able to bypass the first phase of the postanesthesia-care unit (78). However, the BIS monitor is not 100% foolproof, and awareness even with numbers below 60 has been reported (79).

COMPLICATIONS OF REGIONAL ANESTHESIA
Post–Dural Puncture Headache

Post–dural puncture headache (PDPH) is a known complication of spinal anesthesia, where the duramater is intentionally penetrated, and can also occur in epidural anesthesia, when the duramater is unintentionally perforated. Studies using small-gauge noncutting needles for spinal anesthesia have shown that the incidence of this complication is about 1%. When using a large 17-gauge epidural needle, the incidence can be as high as 75% (80).

The pathophysiology of PDPH is related to the loss of cerebrospinal fluid through the dural puncture, resulting in a downward traction of the meninges and intracranial vessels. Pain is characteristically described as frontal, radiating to the occiput, but can also extend to the posterior cervical region; with an increase in severity, it becomes circumferential and can be associated with blurred vision, diplopia, and tinnitus. It is worsened by sitting upright and improved by bed rest. PDPH usually occurs 12 to 24 hours postoperatively, but it can be immediate if the leak is significant.

Risk factors for developing PDPH can be mechanical or patient-related. Mechanical factors include needle size, with the incidence being directly proportional to the diameter of the needle, and design of the needle tip. Pencil-tipped (Whitacre) needles have a dramatically reduced incidence of causing PDPH compared with cutting-tipped (Quincke) needles of equal diameter. Pencil-tipped needles divide rather than cut fibers as they traverse the dura. Patients at risk of developing PDPH are young females. Old age seems to be protective.

Conservative management for PDPH, including bed rest, encouragement of oral or intravenous hydration, and use of caffeine-containing beverages or caffeine benzoide infusion is effective in 50% of the cases.

A more invasive form of treatment is the performing of an epidural blood patch. This consists of an injection of 10 to 20 mL of the patient's own blood into the epidural space with the purpose of sealing the dural hole and preventing further cerebrospinal fluid leakage. This method is effective in over 90% of the cases (81). The choice of conservative measures or epidural blood patch largely depends on the severity of the headache, the risk and/or potential difficulty for performing the procedure, and the patient's wishes. At our institution, epidural blood patch is offered prophylactically to all parturients who have suffered a dural puncture with an epidural needle ("wet tap"). This approach has been reported by others to decrease the incidence of PDPH by 58% (82).

Spinal Hematoma

This is an extremely rare, but potentially devastating complication that may develop from the accumulation of blood in the subarachnoid, subdural, or epidural space. Hematoma can occur after spinal or epidural anesthesia has been attempted or performed. Neurologic damage results from cord compression. The epidural space is rich in venous plexuses and is the most common site for blood accumulation.

The incidence of this complication is so small that it would require an enormous number of patients to define it with certainty; however, two large series reported an estimate of the incidence in 1:200,000 procedures (83,84).

The main risk factor for the development of epidural hematoma is the presence of coagulopathy, either native or acquired. Special care must be taken to ascertain whether there is a patient or family history of bleeding problems or use of anticoagulant drugs (85).

The initial diagnosis of an epidural hematoma is clinical and includes the presence of severe back pain at the site of the injection in association with a block that is not receding. Late signs include bowel and bladder dysfunction. Usually, signs and symptoms occur within 24 hours of the blockade. Because time is of the essence, as soon as an epidural hematoma is suspected, a neurosurgical consultation should be obtained.

Once diagnosis is confirmed, the treatment of choice is a surgical laminectomy; complete recovery is enhanced when the spinal cord is decompressed within eight hours of diagnosis (83).

COMPLICATIONS OF SPECIFIC NERVE BLOCKS

When performing a nerve block for any surgical procedure, the benefits of the technique must outweigh the risks inherent to the procedure. In the case of nerve blocks, advantages clearly relate to the fact that all the complications associated with airway manipulation are avoided and there is decreased interference with pulmonary and circulatory responses. However, nerve blocks also carry complications that occur as the result of four main mechanisms: local toxicity of the anesthetic, systemic toxicity of the local anesthetic, mechanical or direct nerve damage, and damage or injection to adjacent structures.

Local anesthetics are cytotoxic to neural tissue, an effect that is directly related to the concentration used. The effects of a concentrated solution of local anesthetic in close proximity to large trunks or nerves in the spinal cord has recently stirred a controversy regarding the safety of the most widely used local anesthetic, lidocaine (86,87).

Mechanical damage by direct trauma to the nerve is possible when using a technique that deliberately elicits paresthesias for identifying the location of a nerve. The risk of nerve damage is greater when using a cutting-edge needle than a blunt-tipped one. When the paresthesia technique was compared to the transarterial technique for upper arm blockades, the incidence of neuropathy postblock was not very different (88). Common sense, however, dictates that procedures should be stopped and the needle repositioned if paresthesia or pain increases during injection.

In sufficient concentrations, all local anesthetics have systemic toxic effects. The neurologic and cardiovascular effects are of particular concern. Toxic reactions correlate with the concentration of the anesthetic at the end organ, which usually correlates with the blood concentration of the drug, except in those cases where the anesthetic is injected almost directly into the affected organ, such as in carotid injection, where less than 1 mL of lidocaine 2% can produce seizures.

Intercostal blocks are associated with the highest plasma concentration of local anesthetics because these blocks are usually performed several times, and the area is richly vascularized. If the same amount of the local anesthetic is deposited in a deep sheath such as the axillary or the femoral sheath, the risks of toxicity are less because the absorption is considerably less from these areas.

The addition of epinephrine to the solution of a local anesthetic significantly reduces its systemic absorption, allowing the use of higher doses for any given block. This effect of epinephrine is not seen with bupivacaine, presumably because of its own vasocontrictive properties.

Blocks performed in the neck area, such as in the stellate ganglion or the cervical plexus, or in the laryngeal or interscalene approach to the brachial plexus, have a risk of intravascular (carotid, vertebral, or jugular) injection. They can also be complicated with intrathecal injection, producing total spinal anesthesia. There are reports of spinal cord damage when using long needles after interscalene blocks were performed in anesthetized patients for postoperative pain (89).

Ipsilateral phrenic nerve paralysis is a common temporary side effect of interscalene and stellate ganglion blocks, but it can produce ventilatory complications in patients with decreased respiratory reserve. The performance of bilateral interscalene blocks is contraindicated even in healthy individuals.

Compartment syndrome with nerve ischemia can occur if local anesthesia is injected into a nondistensible space, such as the ulnar groove at the level of the elbow.

Perioperative Nerve Injury

Although patient positioning and lack of adequate vigilance is blamed frequently for the development of perioperative nerve injury, the mechanism remains one of the most difficult to explain. Peripheral nerve injuries are a significant source of claims against anesthesiologists. Settlements are frequent in these lawsuits, despite the fact that in a large proportion of these cases the standard of care was met.

Ulnar nerve and brachial plexus injuries comprise approximately half of all the claims filed for nerve damage, followed by lumbosacral nerve root and spinal cord injuries.

The final common pathway to nerve injury seems to be ischemia, resulting from either compression or stretching. The presence of comorbidities seems to play an important role in the development of peripheral nerve injuries.

Injuries to the ulnar nerve represent 28% of all the cases studied in the ASA Closed Claims Project (90). The characteristics of this neuropathy are particularly difficult to explain because the vast majority of cases (75%) occur in males; it has a particularly late onset, with a median delay of three days; and it has occurred even when extra padding has been applied to the humeral epycondile. Anatomic considerations that could explain this neuropathy are the shallow location of the nerve at the elbow and the fact that it is surrounded by a taut aponeurosis. The ulnar nerve can be compressed against the lateral surface of the operating room table when the arms are "tucked in," or when the arm is abducted and in the prone rather than supine position.

Many characteristics of ulnar neuropathy defy simplistic explanation. Although one would expect that an awake or lightly sedated patient would complain of compression of the ulnar nerve, the reported incidence of neuropathy is no different when comparing general versus regional anesthesia (91). Age is also an important factor, with a median age for this complication being 50 years and there being a total absence of it in the pediatric population (90). Based on the above, it is clear that the positioning and lack of padding cannot always explain the occurrence of ulnar neuropathy. Currently, there are no evidence-based strategies to prevent it, and the cause of the problem is most likely beyond the control of the anesthesiologist. Furthermore, electromyography studies have shown evidence of subclinical neuropathy in the contralateral side of the injury (92).

Brachial plexus injuries can be more easily traced to positioning problems, usually the result of overstretching the plexus, with exaggerated abduction of the arm, or sustained neck extension. The use of shoulder braces and the head-down position have also been implicated.

Spinal cord and lumbosacral root injuries are the third most common perioperative nerve injuries, and they are usually related to the performance of a regional anesthetic or pain management procedure. Epidural injection in the presence of anticoagulants poses a special risk (see above).

Sciatic nerve injuries can result from compression during hip surgery because the nerve passes between the ischial tuberosity and the greater trochanter of the femur. In the lithotomy position, the nerve can be overstretched, which leads to injury.

The superficial branch of the common peroneal nerve is susceptible to injury when compressed against the support brace during lithotomy position because it superficially wraps the fibular neck.

The clinical presentation of the peripheral nerve damage varies widely, ranging from abrupt postoperative loss of sensation or motor function to slowly progressive deficits over the course of days, or even weeks. The presence of pain is common. When this complication occurs, it is useful to consult a neurologist. Spinal cord injuries mandate an immediate CT or magnetic resonance imaging scan. An electromyogram should be ordered to differentiate acute from chronic damage. Denervation changes usually take approximately three weeks to develop, so, if present, the diagnosis of preexisting neuropathy is made. Electromyography studies also help delineate the exact site of injury.

With the probable exception of ulnar nerve injuries, most of these complications can be prevented by the combined effort of the anesthesiologist, the surgeon, and the operating room personnel. Careful positioning, padding, and frequent reassessing of pressure points at regular intervals throughout the procedure represent simple and inexpensive measures that can reduce morbidity in the postoperative period.

SYSTEMIC AND METABOLIC COMPLICATIONS
Malignant Hyperthermia

Malignant hyperthermia (MH) is probably, of all the complications discussed in this chapter, the only one attributable directly and exclusively to anesthetic agents. It is defined as an acute, potentially fatal disorder in which skeletal muscles unexpectedly increase their metabolic rate during general anesthesia (93,94). This hypermetabolic state increases the oxygen consumption significantly, sometimes above oxygen delivery, and causes increased CO_2 production, lactate and heat production, respiratory and metabolic acidosis, muscle rigidity, sympathetic stimulation, and increased cellular permeability.

The incidence of MH is about 1:75,000 in the adult population, whereas in children it is reported to be approximately 1:4,000. A review of the calls to the MH Hotline, a dedicated 24-hour response line, showed that during 1990 to 1994, there were 978 clinical cases: 25% occurred during ENT surgery, 25%

during orthopedic surgery, and 25% during emergency surgery. It is important to note that 43% of cases in the ENT group had previously undergone anesthesia without developing this complication (95).

When MH was first described in 1960, the mortality rate was close to 90%. The rate declined slowly over the next decade and a half, but it was not until dantrolene sodium was introduced in 1975 that the mortality rate decreased substantially to 7%. In 1995, data show a mortality rate below 2%.

MH is a genetic disease, and its pattern of transmission is in the mode of autosomal dominance with reduced penetrance and variable expression. Reduced penetrance is implied when fewer offspring than one would predict are affected, whereas variable expression accounts for different susceptibilities among family members. One of the most common chromosome defects observed is located in chromosome 19, associated with the ryanodine receptor. This receptor is involved with the pathway of calcium release from the sarcoplasmic reticulum to the cytoplasm (96).

The pathogenesis of MH lies in the inability of the sarcoplasmic reticulum to store calcium, with high levels of myoplasmic calcium even in the resting stage, and as much as 17 times normal after the triggering of a MH episode. The elevated myoplasmic calcium causes the activation of ATPase, thus accelerating the hydrolysis of ATP to adenosine diphosphate. It also inhibits troponin, eventually leading to muscle contraction, and activates phosphorylase kinase, with the production of ATP and heat. The decrease in venous blood oxygen saturation and the overloading of carbon dioxide and lactic acid are the accumulative results of the cellular demands of hypermetabolism.

All potent inhalation anesthetics have been implicated in the genesis of MH, including the newer agents sevoflurane and desflurane. Nitrous oxide is a safe agent to use in patients with a history of MH. Among the muscle relaxants, only succinylcholine has been implicated. All other nondepolarizing muscle relaxants have failed to trigger an episode of MH. Induction agents, including thiopental, propofol, and ketamine, as well as opioids and benzodiazepines, are nontriggering. Local anesthetics also appear to be safe.

It is important to differentiate this syndrome from other causes of fever and hypercarbia in the operating room, such as sepsis, neurologic injury, thyroid storm, pheochromocytoma, and acute cocaine intoxication.

Of all the standard monitors required during general anesthesia, $ETCO_2$ is the most sensitive and useful for the diagnosis of a hypermetabolic event; the $ETCO_2$ concentration is elevated before any evident change in pulse or respiration, and usually does not respond to vigorous hyperventilation. The rising temperature is a late sign of this syndrome.

Therapy for a MH episode should not be delayed, and it is aimed at discontinuing triggering agents and decreasing the hypermetabolic state while treating the hyperthermia. The patient should receive 100% oxygen, surgery should conclude as soon as possible, and hyperventilation and cooling measures should be instituted. A Foley catheter to monitor the urinary output is essential. An arterial line to monitor blood pressure and to follow the acid–base status is also highly desirable.

Dantrolene sodium should be started at doses of 2.5 to 3.0 mg/kg, followed in 45 minutes by a bolus dose of 10 mg/kg if all signs and symptoms of the syndrome have not resolved. The response to dantrolene takes 6 to 20 minutes, and by 45 minutes, the patient's condition should return to normal. In about 10% of patients, the syndrome redevelops after four to eight hours, a phenomenon that has been called recrudescence.

It has been suggested that dantrolene prevents the release of calcium from the sarcoplasmic reticulum or antagonizes its effect at the myofibril level, or both. At the usual dosages, it has significant muscle relaxant properties, but does not depress respiration even at doses of up to 30 mg/kg. Prophylactic treatment with dantrolene sodium for patients susceptible to MH is no longer recommended. However, avoidance of MH-triggering agents is essential when caring for these patients.

Acute mortality from MH is usually a result of malignant arrhythmias; after a few hours, it is more likely the result of pulmonary edema, coagulopathy, or acid–base imbalance. Late complications include hemolysis and hemoglobinuria, leading to renal failure.

In summary, MH is a serious disease, but with adequate vigilance, proper monitoring, and aggressive therapy, it should be a less threatening and curable entity.

Latex Allergy

Latex allergy is a common problem among a specific group of patients in whom there is production of an antibody of the immunoglobulin E class in response to the protein component of sap of the rubber tree, *Hevea brasilienses*. Patients at risk for this complication include all those who are frequently exposed to the product. These comprise children with a history of spina bifida or those who require chronic urinary catheterization. Health-care workers, because of their constant exposure to latex products, also represent a risk group.

Latex allergy should be suspected if unexpected anaphylaxis occurs after the start of the surgical procedure, without any temporal relationship to medication or blood product administration. Any history or symptoms suggestive of latex allergy (itching, hives, or wheezing) after contact with latex products should raise a red flag in the mind of all the personnel taking care of the patient. The only effective way to prevent an episode of latex allergy is to avoid exposure to the antigen. It is now common to have a "latex allergy" cart, where all the products that are safe to use in this population are stored and labeled. It is generally recommended that these cases be posted first in the daily schedule in order to avoid cross-contamination with the equipment used in nonsusceptible patients.

When a case of anaphylaxis to latex exposure does occur, treatment is no different than that administered with other causes of life-threatening allergic reactions. Contact with the antigen must be stopped as soon as possible, and the airway should be secured if an endotracheal tube is not already in place. Anaphylactic reactions promote capillary leakage with massive redistribution of fluids to the interstitial space. Therefore, a rapid administration of isotonic crystalloids is necessary to maintain an effective perfusion. The mainstay of pharmacologic treatment for an anaphylactic reaction is the use of intravenous epinephrine. Rather than a fixed dose, the drug should be titrated in 100-μg increments, until the blood pressure is restituted. An infusion may be needed in cases of protracted hypotension. Antihistamines and glucocorticoids may also be useful to stabilize the allergic response after the initial resuscitation has taken place.

CONCLUSIONS

In this chapter, we have discussed complications that are related to the administration of anesthesia. Many of these problems cannot be exclusively attributed to the anesthetic agent or the technique that is chosen, but rather, they are a result of the compounding effects of surgery, previous medical conditions, and the overall stress response that is imposed on the body by the surgical procedure.

Although we may never know with certainty the true incidence of many of these complications, it is clear that the identification of patients at risk and advanced preparation play a major role in preventing most of them.

Anesthesia is perhaps the safest medical specialty of all, when parameters of appropriate care and vigilance are met. Anesthesia care has evolved in great leaps since its first public demonstration in 1846. A more profound understanding of the disease processes, better patient selection, and intraoperative monitoring and advances in surgical techniques have made possible the realization of increasingly complex procedures on sicker patients. In today's world, the risk of dying in a car accident is greater than that of dying while under anesthesia (97).

REFERENCES

1. Beecher HK, Todd DP. A study of deaths associated with anesthesia and surgery. Ann Surg 1954; 140:2.
2. Dripps RD, Lamont A, Eckenhoff JE. The role of anesthesia in surgical mortality. JAMA 1961; 178:261.
3. Bodlander FMS. Deaths associated with anesthesia. Br J Anaesth 1975; 47:36.
4. Holland R. Anaesthetic mortality in New South Wales. Br J Anaesth 1987; 59(7):834–841.
5. Buck N, Devlin HB, Lunn JL. Report on the Confidential Enquiry into Perioperative Death. London: Nuffield Provincial Hospitals Trust, The Kings Fund Publishing House, 1987.
6. Lunn JN. The study of anesthetic-related mortality. Anaesthesia 1982; 37:856.
7. Lunn JN, Hunter AR, Scott DB. Anaesthesia-related surgical mortality. Anaesthesia 1983; 38:1090.
8. Caplan RA. The closed claims project: looking back, looking forward. ASA Newslett 1999; 63(6):7–9.
9. Caplan RA, Posner KL, Ward RJ, Cheney FW. Adverse respiratory events in anesthesia: a closed claims analysis. Anesthesiology 1990; 72(5):828–833.
10. Domino KB. Closed malpractice claims for airway trauma during anesthesia. ASA Newslett 1998; 62(6):10–11.
11. Martian CH, Picard E, Jonquet O, et al. Membranous tracheal rupture after intubation. Ann Thorac Surg 1995; 60:1367–1371.
12. Marquette CH, Bocquillon N, Roumilhac D, Neviere R, Mathieu D, Ramon P. Conservative treatment of tracheal rupture. J Thorac Cardiovasc Surg 1999; 117(2):399–401.
13. Zettl R, Waydhas C, Biberthaler P, et al. Nonsurgical treatment of a severe tracheal rupture after endotracheal intubation. Crit Care Med 1999; 27(3):661–663.
14. Warner MA, Warner ME, Weber JG. Clinical significance of pulmonary aspiration during the perioperative period. Anesthesiology 1993; 78(1):56–62.
15. Lakshmipathy N, Bokesch PM, Cowen DE, Lisman SR, Schmid CH. Environmental tobacco smoke: a risk factor for pediatric laryngospasm. Anesth Analg 1996; 82(4):724–727.
16. LeResche L. Epidemiology of temporo-mandibular disorder: implication for the investigation of etiologic factors. Crit Rev Oral Biol Med 1997; 8:291–305.
17. Risk management foundation. Anesthesia claims analysis shows frequency loss, losses high. Risk Manage Found Forum 1983; 4:1–2.
18. Aitkenhead AR. The pattern of litigations against anaesthetists. Br J Anaesth 1994; 73:10–21.
19. Gaiser RR, Castro AD. The level of anesthesia resident training does not affect the risk of dental injury. Anesth Analg 1998; 87:255–257.
20. Lockhart PB, Feldbau EV, Gabel RA, et al. Dental complications during and after tracheal intubation. J Am Dent Assoc 1986; 112:480–483.
21. Cronin M, Redfern PA, Utting JE. Psychometry and postoperative complaints in surgical patients. Br J Anaesth 1973; 45:879–886.
22. Macario A, Weinger M, Carney S, Kim A. Which clinical anesthesia outcomes are important to avoid? The perspective of patients. Anesth Analg 1999; 89(3):652–658.
23. Mylis PS, Hunt JO, Moloney JT. Postoperative "minor" complications: comparison between men and women. Anaesthesia 1997; 52(4):300–306.
24. Lipp M, Brandt L, Daublander M, Peter R, Barz L. Frequency and severity of throat complaints following general anesthesia with the insertion of various endotracheal tubes. Anaesthesist 1988; 37(12):758–766.

25. Joorgensen LN, Weber M, Pedersen A, Munster M. No increased incidence of postoperative sore throat after administration of suxamethonium in endotracheal anaesthesia. Acta Anaesthesiol Scand 1987; 31(8):768–770.

26. Capan LM, Bruce DL, Patel KP, Turndorf H. Succinylcholine-induced postoperative sore throat. Anesthesiology 1983; 59(3):202–206.

27. Porter NE, Sidou V, Husson J. Postoperative sore throat: incidence and severity after the use of lidocaine, saline, or air to inflate the endotracheal tube cuff. AANA J 1999; 67(1):49–52.

28. Navarro RM, Baughman VL. Lidocaine in the endotracheal tube cuff reduces postoperative sore throat. J Clin Anesth 1997; 9(5):394.

29. Gal TJ, Suratt PM. Resistance to breathing in healthy subjects following endotracheal intubation under topical anesthesia. Anesth Analg 1980; 59(4):270–274.

30. Tam S, Chung F, Campbell M. Intravenous lidocaine: optimal time of injection before tracheal intubation. Anesth Analg 1987; 66(10):1036–1038.

31. Eames WO, Rooke GA, Wu RS, Bishop MJ. Comparison of the effects of etomidate, propofol, and thiopental on respiratory resistance after tracheal intubation. Anesthesiology 1996; 84(6):1307–1311.

32. Brown RH, Greenber RS, Wagner EM. Efficacy of propofol to prevent bronchoconstriction. Anesthesiology 2001; 94:851–855.

33. Tarhan S, Moffitt EA, Taylor WF, Giuliani ER. Myocardial infarction after general anesthesia. JAMA 1972; 220(11):1451–1454.

34. Shah KB, Kleinman BS, Sami H, Patel J, Rao TL. Reevaluation of perioperative myocardial infarction in patients with prior myocardial infarction undergoing noncardiac operations. Anesth Analg 1990; 71(3):231–235.

35. Eagle KA, Brundage BH, Chaitman BR, et al. Guidelines for perioperative cardiovascular evaluation for noncardiac surgery: an abridged version of the report of the American College of Cardiology/American Heart Association Task Force on Practice Guidelines. Mayo Clin Proc 1997; 72(6):524–531.

36. Badner NH, Knill RL, Brown JE, Novick TV, Gelb AW. Myocardial infarction after noncardiac surgery. Anesthesiology 1998; 88(3):572–578.

37. Poldermans D, Boersma E, Bax J, et al. The effect of bisoprolol on perioperative mortality and myocardial infarction in high-risk patients undergoing vascular surgery. The Dutch Echocardiographic Cardiac Risk Evaluation Applying Stress Echocardiography Study Group. N Engl J Med 1999; 341:1789–1794.

38. Johnston RR, Eger EI II, Wilson C. A comparative interaction of epinephrine with enflurane, isoflurane, and halothane in man. Anesth Analg 1976; 55(5):709–712.

39. Kasten GW, Martin ST. Bupivacaine cardiovascular toxicity: comparison of treatment with bretylium and lidocaine. Anesth Analg 1985; 64(9):911–916.

40. Mazze RI, Calverley RK, Smith NT. Inorganic fluoride nephrotoxicity: prolonged enflurane and halothane anesthesia in volunteers. Anesthesiology 1977; 46(4):265–271.

41. Mazze RI, Cousins MJ, Barr GA. Renal effects and metabolism of isoflurane in man. Anesthesiology 1974; 40(6):536–542.

42. Sutton TS, Koblin DD, Gruenke LD, et al. Fluoride metabolites after prolonged exposure of volunteers and patients to desflurane. Anesth Analg 1991; 73(2):180–185.

43. Frink EJ Jr., Ghantous H, Malan TP, et al. Plasma inorganic fluoride with sevoflurane anesthesia: correlation with indices of hepatic and renal function. Anesth Analg 1992; 74(2):231–235.

44. Gonsowski CT, Laster MJ, Eger EI II, Ferrell LD, Kerschmann RL. Toxicity of compound A in rats. Effect of a 3-hour administration. Anesthesiology 1994; 80(3):556–565.

45. Eger EI II, Koblin DD, Bowland T, et al. Nephrotoxicity of sevoflurane versus desflurane anesthesia in volunteers. Anesth Analg 1997; 84:160–168.

46. Campbell JAH, Corrigall AV, Guy A, Kirsch RE. Immunohistologic localization of alpha, mu, and pi class glutathione-s-transferase in human tissues. Cancer 1991; 67:1608–1613.

47. Kharasch ED, Frink EJ Jr., Zager R, Bowdle TA, Artu A, Nogami WM. Assessment of low-flow sevoflurane and isoflurane effects on renal function using sensitive markers of tubular toxicity. Anesthesiology 1997; 86:1238–1254.

48. Bito H, Ikeuchi Y, Ikeda K. Effects of low-flow sevoflurane anesthesia on renal function: comparison with high-flow sevoflurane anesthesia and low-flow isoflurane anesthesia. Anesthesiology 1997; 86:1231–1237.

49. Brezis M, Rosen S. Hypoxia of the renal medulla—its implications for disease. N Engl J Med 1995; 332(10):647–655.

50. Koning HM, Koning AJ, Leusink JA. Serious acute renal failure following open heart surgery. Thorac Cardiovasc Surgeon 1985; 33(5):283–287.

51. Mangano CM, Diamondstone LS, Ramsay JG, Aggarwal A, Herskowitz A, Mangano DT. Renal dysfunction after myocardial revascularization: risk factors, adverse outcomes, and hospital resource utilization. The Multicenter Study of Perioperative Ischemia Research Group. Ann Intern Med 1998; 128(3):194–203.

52. Kazmers A, Jacobs L, Perkins A. The impact of complications after vascular surgery in Veterans Affairs Medical Centers. J Surg Res 1997; 67(1):62–66.

53. Gornick CC Jr., Kjellstrand CM. Acute renal failure complicating aortic aneurysm surgery. Nephron 1983; 35(3):145–157.

54. Chawla SK, Najafi H, Ing TS, et al. Acute renal failure complicating ruptured abdominal aortic aneurysm. Arch Surg 1975; 110(5):521–526.

55. Morris JA Jr., Mucha P Jr., Ross SE, et al. Acute post-traumatic renal failure: a multicenter perspective. J Trauma-Injury Infect Crit Care 1991; 31(12):1584–1590.

56. Solomon R, Werner C, Mann D, D'Elia J, Silva P. Effects of saline, mannitol, and furosemide to prevent acute decreases in renal function induced by radiocontrast agents. N Engl J Med 1994; 331(21):1416–1420.

57. Tepel M, van der Giet M, Schwarzfeld C, Laufer U, Liermann D, Zidek W. Prevention of radiographic-contrast-agent-induced reductions in renal function by acetylcysteine. N Engl J Med 2000; 343(3):210–212.

58. Perdue PW, Balser JR, Lipsett PA, Breslow MJ. "Renal dose" dopamine in surgical patients: dogma or science. Ann Surg 1998; 227(4):470–473.

59. Bellomo R, Chapman M, Finfer S, Hickling K, Myburgh J. Low-dose dopamine in patients with early renal dysfunction: a placebo-controlled randomised trial. Australian and New Zealand Intensive Care Society

(ANZICS) Clinical Trials Group. Lancet 2000; 356(9248): 2139–2143.

60. Kellum JA, Decker JM. Use of dopamine in acute renal failure: a meta-analysis. Crit Care Med 2001; 29(8): 1526–1531.

61. MacGregor DA, Smith TE, Prielipp RC, Butterworth JF, James RL, Scuderi PE. Pharmacokinetics of dopamine in healthy male subjects. Anesthesiology 2000; 92(2): 338–346.

62. Mathur VS, Swan SK, Lambrecht LJ, et al. The effects of fenoldopam, a selective dopamine receptor agonist, on systemic and renal hemodynamics in normotensive subjects. Crit Care Med 1999; 27(9):1832–1837.

63. Warner MA, Shields SE, Chute CG. Major morbidity and mortality within 1 month of ambulatory surgery and anesthesia. JAMA 1993; 270(12):1437–1441.

64. Hart R, Hindman B. Mechanisms of perioperative cerebral infarction. Stroke 1982; 13(6):766–773.

65. Ropper AH, Wechsler LR, Wilson LS. Carotid bruit and the risk of stroke in elective surgery. N Engl J Med 1982; 307(22):1388–1390.

66. Korttila K, Tammisto T, Ertama P, Pfaffli P, Blomgren E, Hakkinen S. Recovery, psychomotor skills, and simulated driving after brief inhalational anesthesia with halothane or enflurane combined with nitrous oxide and oxygen. Anesthesiology 1977; 46(1):20–27.

67. Davison LA, Steinhelber JC, Eger EI II, Stevens WC. Psychological effects of halothane and isoflurane anesthesia. Anesthesiology 1975; 43(3):313–324.

68. Williams-Russo P, Sharrock NE, Mattis S, Szatrowski TP, Charlson ME. Cognitive effects after epidural versus general anesthesia in older adults. A randomized trial. JAMA 1995; 274(1):44–50.

69. Newman MF, Kirchner JL, Phillips-Bute B, et al. Longitudinal assessment of neurocognitive function after coronary-artery bypass surgery. N Engl J Med 2001; 344(6):395–402.

70. Lee LA. Post-operative visual loss data gathered and analyzed. ASA Newslett 2000; 64(9):25–27.

71. Williams EL, Hart WM, Tempelhoff R. Postoperative ischemic optic neuropathy. Anesth Analg 1995; 80(5): 1018–1029.

72. Liu WH, Thorp TA, Graham SG, Aitkenhead AR. Incidence of awareness with recall during general anaesthesia. Anaesthesia 1991; 46(6):435–437.

73. Juul J, Lie B, Friberg Nielsen S. Epidural analgesia versus general anesthesia for cesarean section. Acta Obstet Gynecol Scand 1988; 67(3):203–206.

74. Moerman N, Bonke B, Oosting J. Awareness and recall during general anesthesia. Facts and feelings. Anesthesiology 1993; 79(3):454–464.

75. Domino KB, Postner KL, Caplan RA, Cheney FW. Awareness during anesthesia: a closed claims analysis. Anesthesiology 1999; 90:1053–1061.

76. Glass PS, Bloom M, Kearse L, Rosow C, Sebel P, Manberg P. Bispectral analysis measures sedation and memory effects of propofol, midazolam, isoflurane, and alfentanil in healthy volunteers. Anesthesiology 1997; 86(4):836–847.

77. Song D, Joshi GP, White PF. Titration of volatile anesthetics using bispectral index facilitates recovery after ambulatory anesthesia. Anesthesiology 1997; 87(4): 842–848.

78. Sebel PS, Payne FB, Gan TJ, Rosow CE, Greenwald S. Bispectral analysis (BIS) monitoring improves PACU recovery from propofol/alfentanil/nitrous oxide anesthesia. Anesthesiology 1996; 85:A468.

79. Mychaskiw G II, Horowitz M, Sachdev V, Heath BJ. Explicit intraoperative recall at a Bispectral Index of 47. Anesth Analg 2001; 92(4):808–809.

80. Lambert DH, Hurley RJ, Hertwig L, Datta S. Role of needle gauge and tip configuration in the production of lumbar puncture headache. Region Anesth 1997; 22(1):66–72.

81. Molnar R. Spinal, Epidural and Caudal Anesthesia: Clinical Anesthesia Procedures of the Massachusetts General Hospital. 5th ed. Boston: Little, Brown and Company, 1993:206–225.

82. Colonna-Romano P, Shapiro B. Prophylactic epidural blood patch in obstetrics. Anesthesiology 1988; 69:A665.

83. Vandermeulen EP, Van Aken H, Vermylen J. Anticoagulants and spinal-epidural anesthesia. Anesth Analg 1994; 79(6):1165–1177.

84. Tryba M. Epidural regional anesthesia and low molecular heparin. Anasthesiologie, Intensivmedizin, Notfallmedizin, Schmerztherapie 1993; 28(3):179–181.

85. Cobas M. Preoperative assessment of coagulation disorders. Int Anesthesiol Clin 2001; 39(1):1–15.

86. Rigler ML, Drasner K, Krejcie TC, et al. Cauda equina syndrome after continuous spinal anesthesia. Anesth Analg 1991; 72(3):275–281.

87. Schell RM, Brauer FS, Cole DJ, Applegate RL II. Persistent sacral nerve root deficits after continuous spinal anaesthesia. Canadian J Anaesth 1991; 38(7): 908–911.

88. Selander D, Edshage S, Wolff T. Paresthesiae or no paresthesiae? Nerve lesions after axillary blocks. Acta Anaesthesiol Scand 1979; 23(1):27–33.

89. Benumof JL. Permanent loss of cervical spinal cord function associated with interscalene block performed under general anesthesia. Anesthesiology 2000; 93:1541–1544.

90. Cheney FW, Domino KB, Caplan RA, Posner KL. Nerve injury associated with anesthesia: a closed claims analysis. Anesthesiology 1999; 90(4):1062–1069.

91. Warner MA, Warner ME, Martin JT. Ulnar neuropathy. Incidence, outcome, and risk factors in sedated or anesthetized patients. Anesthesiology 1994; 81(6): 1332–1340.

92. Alvine FG, Schurrer ME. Postoperative ulnar-nerve palsy. Are there predisposing factors? J Bone Joint Surg—Am Vol 1987; 69(2):255–259.

93. Britt BA, Kalow W. Malignant hyperthermia: a statistical review. Can Anaesth Soc J 1970; 17(4):293–315.

94. Britt BA. Etiology and pathophysiology of malignant hyperthermia. Fed Proc 1979; 38(1):44–48.

95. Greenberg C, Hall S, Karan S. Malignant hyperthermia (MH) during outpatient pediatric ENT surgery—an anesthesia concern. Anesthesiology 1995; 83:A1004.

96. Ohnishi ST, Taylor S, Gronert GA. Calcium-induced CA2+ release from sarcoplasmic reticulum of pigs susceptible to malignant hyperthermia. The effects of halothane and dantrolene. FEBS Lett 1983; 161(1):103–107.

97. National Highway Traffic Safety Administration. National Center for Statistics and Analysis U.S. Department of Transportation. Traffic Safety Facts 1999: A Compilation of Motor Vehicle Crash Data from the Fatality Analysis Reporting System and the General Estimates System, December 2000:88.

2

Complications of Acute Fluid Loss and Replacement

Juan Carlos Puyana

Surgical/Trauma Intensive Care Unit, University of Pittsburgh Medical Center, Pittsburgh, Pennsylvania, U.S.A.

During the past 100 years, fluids have been given intravenously for the management of fluid deficits. In 1883, Sidney Ringer discovered that calcium-containing tap water was better than distilled water for resuscitation. The understanding of the circulatory system and the importance of maintaining the circulatory volume were realized long ago. Furthermore, many years ago, researchers discovered the desired elements and their approximate concentrations in fluids that serve as intravenous plasma substitutes. However, the search for the optimal resuscitation fluid has been uneventful for a notable period of time.

The first known intravenous infusions occurred in 1492. Blood from three youngsters was given to the dying pope by a vein-to-vein anastomosis in a desperate attempt to save him. The patient and the three donors died as a result of this transfusion. As early as 1667, the first known successful animal-to-animal transfusion was performed. In 1818, Dr. James Blundell performed the first successful transfusion of fluid into a human: the blood was given to a patient who was hemorrhaging during childbirth. In 1830, the gold-plated steel needle for intravenous use was invented. As Cosnett (1) reports, in 1831, a paper published by O'Shaughnessy described the effective use of salts and water to treat patients with cholera—an idea that was put into practice by Thomas Latta soon thereafter. During the 1930s, Baxter and Abbot produced the first commercial saline solutions. Two decades later, plastic intravenous tubing replaced rubber tubing, and soon thereafter, the central venous approach was described by a French military surgeon. This approach was a breakthrough in the estimation of the state of hydration [central venous pressure (CVP) measurements] and the application of volume support.

Perhaps the most serious complications of intravenous fluid therapy are those related to bloodstream infections and septicemia (discussed in a later chapter). Blalock's fundamental study of shock clearly showed that injury precipitates obligatory local and regional fluid losses, the effects of which can be ameliorated by vigorous restoration of intravascular volume. This concept became central to the understanding of the pathophysiology of shock, and provided new insight into the theory of shock

and a fundamental rationale for fluid-based therapy for hemorrhage and hypovolemia.

As a result of noteworthy contributions made by surgeons during World War I and World War II, the introduction of blood transfusions dramatically changed the outcome of patients experiencing severe hemorrhage and traumatic shock. During the Korean Conflict, fluid overload became a common and lethal side effect because little was known about how infusates are dispersed and eliminated during trauma. In the period between the Korean Conflict and the Vietnam War, researchers discovered that there are tremendous fluid shifts into cells after severe hemorrhagic shock. As a consequence, the treatment of patients with shock was altered during the Vietnam War; these changes resulted in better outcomes and fewer cases of renal failure.

Improved prehospital care, trauma system development, and emergency room management of shock have resulted in new issues related to the consequences of fluid loss, fluid replacement, and resuscitation. The understanding of shock today extends to a wide series of events that result from impaired cellular perfusion and compromised oxygen delivery with associated inflammatory and contrainflammatory responses, all of which ultimately result in severe organ dysfunction and failure if hypoperfusion is not promptly recognized and treated.

This chapter will review some basic concepts of fluid physiology and theoretical concepts of fluid therapy in several clinical conditions associated with fluid loss and fluid deficit. After a brief review of the literature on resuscitation, a summary of the current concepts about the adequacy of resuscitation and end points of fluid replacement therapy will be presented.

THEORETICAL BASIS OF FLUID DISTRIBUTION

Physicians' comprehension of the effectiveness of resuscitative fluid therapy can be greatly enhanced if they understand several basic principles of fluid dynamics, body compartments, and membrane behavior. These concepts not only are necessary for an understanding of the effects of volume expanders on the circulation, but also are required for an appropriate interpretation of the conflicting results frequently seen in studies of fluid replacement therapy. Recognition of these principles and their application to circulation can result in accurate predictions in real-life situations of what has been observed theoretically and also in anticipating the physiologic effects of a specific fluid-based therapeutic intervention in the trauma room, the operating room, the intensive care unit (ICU), or the surgical ward.

Severe fluid loss, fluid deficit, or both may result from a variety of clinical scenarios. Furthermore, a myriad of surgical conditions that are characterized by circulatory failure may trigger a complex inflammatory response that has been associated with the start of multiple organ dysfunction and death. Therefore, a fundamental knowledge of the physiologic basis of fluid therapy is necessary for preventing and minimizing the consequences of severe fluid losses and shock.

Body Fluid Compartments

There are three body fluid compartments: the intravascular or plasma volume, the interstitial volume, and the intracellular volume. Under normal conditions, the interstitial volume is three times greater than the intravascular volume, and the intracellular volume is about two and one-half to three times greater than the interstitial volume. Thus, the intracellular volume is seven to nine times greater than the intravascular volume (Fig. 1). The intravascular volume is extraordinarily well defended by the body. Significant changes in the intravascular volume are not well tolerated. Loss of 30% to 40% of the intravascular volume will lead to severe hypovolemia and profound hypotension. Cardiac arrest usually occurs after 50% to 60% of the blood volume has been lost. In contrast, a 20% to 30% increase in volume leads to pulmonary edema (2). Sophisticated homeostatic mechanisms are therefore in charge of maintaining the intravascular volume.

All reflexive defense mechanisms in the body that maintain intravascular volume do so very efficiently: specifically, the renovascular response is designed to use the kidney to conserve fluid, and the neurovascular responses, the chemoreceptor response, the baroreceptor response, and the angiotensin response are aimed at maintaining a constant intravascular volume.

Fluid Maintenance and Regulation

The interstitial volume is in continuous equilibrium with the intravascular volume, and, in fact, the interstitial volume acts like a large electrical capacitor that either absorbs fluid from the intravascular space when it is overhydrated, or fills the intravascular space when it is underhydrated. This constant equilibrium provides the flexibility necessary to withstand acute volume changes in the intravascular compartment. The interstitial volume has two very interesting properties. First, it is not extensively maintained by any of the reflexive mechanisms that exist to maintain the intravascular volume; therefore, the interstitial volume fluctuates widely during a particular disease course. Second, the interstitial volume has an impressive ability to expand. The compliance of the interstitial compartment is extraordinarily high, and until the interstitial compartment is filled to approximately three times its normal volume, the interstitial pressure remains low (3).

Understanding the properties of the membranes that separate the body fluid compartments is crucial to predicting the effects of a specific volume expander. These membranes are quite different, and the events that regulate fluid exchange also differ in each compartment. The intravascular space and the interstitial space are separated by the capillary endothelium; therefore, all properties of the capillary endothelium are relevant. The capillary endothelium, however, functions differently in different organs of the body. For example, the capillary endothelium is much more permeable in the lung and the liver than it is in peripheral tissues such as muscle, skin, and subcutaneous fat (4). This difference in permeability gives rise to dramatically different effects in the response of organs to hemodilution. The greater the permeability is in a capillary bed, the less the capillary bed is affected by hemodilution because the interstitial concentration of protein is already higher. This characteristic is intrinsic to the lung (5). The membrane that separates the interstitial space from the cells is the cell surface membrane (Fig. 2), which functions differently than the capillary endothelium. The permeability of the capillary endothelium allows small molecules to pass through essentially unhindered. Water and bicarbonate molecules and sodium, potassium, and chloride ions all move freely through the capillary endothelium. Larger molecules, however, are restricted at the capillary endothelium.

This restriction is apparent when the effect of albumin is analyzed. Albumin is a relatively large

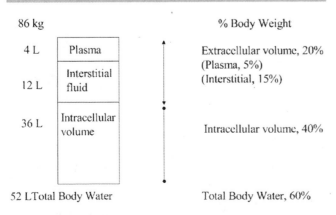

Figure 1 Body composition.

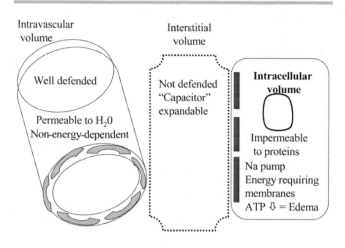

Figure 2 Membrane characteristics of body water compartments.

molecule that cannot readily pass through the pores of the capillary endothelium. However, substantial albumin leakage occurs through other membranes of the body, and this leakage can vary substantially depending on the endothelial characteristics of a specific organ. For example, albumin leakage from the lungs under normal circumstances is so high that the interstitial concentration is approximately 70% to 80% of the serum concentration. Therefore, the relative albumin concentration gradient across the pulmonary capillary membrane is relatively minor. The permeability of the liver endothelium to albumin is only slightly less than that of the lung; the interstitial concentration is approximately 60% of the serum concentration. In contrast, much less albumin leaks through peripheral tissues, specifically muscle and fat, than through the liver or the lung; therefore, the interstitial concentration is approximately 20% to 30% of the serum concentration.

Unlike the capillary endothelium and other membranes of the body, the cell surface membrane is impermeable to proteins. The entry of proteins into cells is accomplished by active transport; therefore, oncotic pressure has a minimal effect at the cell surface membrane. The sodium pump is the active mechanism that operates at the cell surface, ejecting sodium from the cells while potassium is exchanged or diffuses passively to maintain charge equilibrium on both sides of the cell membrane. Bicarbonate molecules and chloride ions cross the cell membrane relatively easily, and because the membrane is permeable to water, this fluid crosses readily to maintain osmotic equilibrium.

There are two crucial differences between the capillary endothelium and the cell surface membrane. First, the capillary endothelium is a passive membrane that does not require energy: it functions for an extended period of time independently of the delivery of oxygen and adenosine triphosphate (ATP). In contrast, the cell surface membrane requires energy. As soon as the production of ATP is impaired, as it is, for example, during severe shock, the sodium pump stops working. At that point, the passive diffusion of sodium into the cells increases their osmotic pressure, and water immediately follows. This influx of water causes increased cellular edema. This phenomenon was described by Shires et al. (6) in animal models of severe irreversible shock. During severe shock, the amount of energy delivery to the cell membrane decreases, the cell surface membrane is immediately affected, and the cellular exchange of fluid is immediately impaired. The capillary endothelium is much more resilient to these changes than is the cell membrane.

The second important difference between the capillary endothelium and the cell surface membrane is that large molecules that dictate the oncotic pressure or the differential gradient across the capillary endothelium do not play a crucial role at the cell membrane. The small molecules that pass through the cell surface membrane produce the total gradient. Osmotic pressure is the gradient that causes water to move across the cell membrane. Oncotic pressure and hydrostatic pressure across the capillary endothelium influence water movement.

VOLUME EXPANSION
Theoretical Models of Fluid Replacement

On the basis of the principles explained above, a theoretical model aimed at predicting the distribution of volume expanders can be constructed. These predictions result not from the findings of animal studies, but rather from theoretical calculations based on the rules that dictate membrane behavior and fluid exchange across biological membranes.

Resuscitation with Crystalloid Solutions

Multiple effects on the intravascular, interstitial, and intracellular volumes can be observed when 2 L of a balanced salt solution (such as Ringer's lactate solution) is infused. Thirty minutes after infusion, this crystalloid solution has equilibrated into the intravascular and interstitial space. Because all components of a balanced salt solution freely cross the capillary endothelium, the capillary endothelium in no way restricts the movement of a balanced salt solution. Therefore, when this salt solution is administered, in effect, it acts as though there is no boundary between the intravascular space and the interstitial space. The solution immediately crosses from one space to the other and is distributed between the two compartments in exact proportion to their starting volumes (Fig. 3). For example, if the starting volume of the interstitial space is three times that of the intravascular volume, as is normally the case in a healthy person, then the balanced salt solution will be distributed in

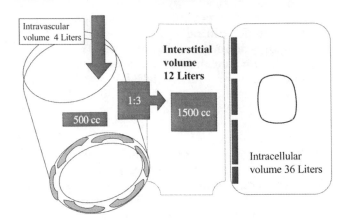

Figure 3 Infusion of 2 L of Ringer's lactate solution.

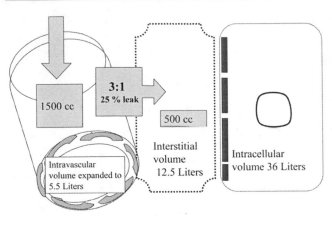

Figure 4 Infusion of 2 L of 5% albumin.

the same 1:3 ratio (Fig. 1). If 2 L of solution is given, then 500 mL will remain in the intravascular volume, and 1500 mL will move into the interstitial volume. Because a balanced salt solution is iso-osmotic, no gradient in osmolarity is produced; therefore, there is no net movement across the cell surface membrane, which responds only to osmotic pressures. The volume of the intracellular compartment is therefore unchanged. This effect is crucial, but it has never been adequately emphasized in the literature.

Resuscitation with Colloid Solutions

If a colloid solution such as 5% albumin is introduced into the intravascular volume, the relative leakage of the albumin solution will be proportional to the net albumin leakage in the entire body, i.e., approximately 25% to 35% depending on permeability. There is a reason that the net albumin leakage is much closer to the leakage of muscle, skin, and fat. The organs that are highly permeable to albumin (e.g., the liver and the lungs) make up a relatively small fraction of the body mass. The tissues that are not as permeable to albumin (e.g., muscle, skin, and fat) make up most of the body mass. As a result of this effect, an iso-oncotic solution administered into the intravascular compartment will leak in rough proportion to the total leakage of albumin in the body, i.e., approximately 25% to 35%. For example, if 2 L of a 5% albumin solution (colloid) is administered, the volume would be distributed as follows: 500 mL (25%) would leak into the interstitium, and 1500 mL would be retained in the intravascular volume. Because the albumin solution is iso-osmotic, there would be no net gradient into cells. Therefore, the cellular volume would not change (Fig. 4). When the net effect of volume expansion resulting from the administration of 2 L of Ringer's lactate is compared with that resulting from the administration of 2 L of albumin, the results show that one-fourth of the balanced solution (500 mL) would remain in

the vascular space and three-fourths of the colloid solution (1500 mL) would remain in the intravascular space. Therefore, the ratio of intravascular filling with a colloid solution to intervascular filling with a crystalloid solution is 3:1. Almost every study in which the effects of crystalloid and colloid solutions have been compared has found that this ratio of intravascular expansion is consistent at approximately 3:1. This ratio fits the proposed theoretical model; it is what is measured hemodynamically, and it is predictable. Unfortunately, analyzing the results of published studies is difficult because most studies of crystalloid and colloid solutions have been based on protocols that did not consider this physiologic reality. Achieving the same effect on intravascular volume expansion requires the administration of three times as much crystalloid solution as colloid solution because only one-fourth of the balanced crystalloid solution will remain in the vascular space (the rest of the crystalloid solution will end up in the interstitial space). Administering a crystalloid solution therefore may induce significant interstitial edema.

The concept of leakage or intravascular retention of a crystalloid solution is based on studies of shock in animal models using incomplete or inadequate resuscitation. When a volume deficit is created and then replaced with inadequate volume, even though the volume is similar to what has been lost, one may conclude that fluid has leaked. In a stable replacement model that includes the theoretical considerations explained above, the volume of distribution will be considered. Once full equilibration has been achieved, the relative volumes of distribution should remain the same. Depending on the volume used and the deficit replaced, the effects of volume resuscitation can therefore be predicted and anticipated on the basis of these three basic axioms: (i) one-fourth of the amount of balanced salt solutions administered remains in the vascular space; (ii) three-fourths of the amount of colloid solutions administered remains in the intravascular space; and (iii) the ratio of intra-vascular filling with crystalloid solutions to that with colloid solutions is 3:1.

Resuscitation with Hypertonic Saline Solution

Hypertonic saline solution has been the topic of con-siderable discussion in recent years because of its potential for use as a prehospital fluid. When a 7.5% saline solution is administered, its hypertonic effect immediately exerts eight times the normal osmotic pressure of the body. Therefore, infusing this solution increases the osmotic pressure in the intravascular space, and this increase in pressure immediately pulls water from the intracellular space. Again because all of the ions that produce the osmotic gradient move freely across the capillary endothelium, there are no osmotic gradients across the capillary endothelium. Only the cell membrane restricts them; therefore, the gradient is acutely generated only across the cell membrane (Fig. 5).

The osmotic pressures created by 7.5% saline infusions can be hundreds of millimeters of mercury, even when relatively small volumes of 7.5% saline solution are infused. As a result, fluid is pulled to the intravascular space with extraordinary rapidity. Whereas colloid equilibrium typically develops within 10 to 30 minutes of infusion, development of hypertonic saline equilibrium requires less than 60 seconds. In fact, this latter type of equilibration occurs so rapidly that it cannot be measured by any available technique. The best evidence indicates that the equilibration occurs within approximately three to five seconds after administration of the solution. Therefore, when a hypertonic solution is given, the pull of fluid into the vascular space is effectively instantaneously. The net effect, however, has a direct repercussion on the intravascular volume. Adminis-tering hypertonic solution forces equilibrium between the intracellular osmotic pressure and the intravascu-lar osmotic pressure; because the saline solution is eight times more concentrated than the normal osmotic pressure, the solution pulls seven times its volume and dilutes itself by a factor of eight in the vascular space. For example, an intravenous infusion of 250 mL of a 7.5% saline solution pulls 1750 mL from the cellular space, thus resulting in an initial net increase in the intravascular volume of 2 L. Therefore, the volume reexpansion achieved by the administration of 250 mL of 7.5% saline solution is equivalent to that achieved by the administration of 2 L of an isotonic salt solution. Once the 7.5% saline solution has forced 1750 mL of fluid into the vascular space (from the intra-cellular space), redistribution occurs between the intravascular space and the interstitial space. Again, the now balanced salt solution is distributed in propor-tion to the sizes of the spaces. Therefore, of the 2 L of fluid pulled from the cellular space, 500 mL ends up in the intravascular space and 1500 mL ends up in the interstitial space. The only difference is that the net deficit occurs at the expense of the cells; therefore, the cellular compartment now contains 1750 mL less fluid. In contrast, this compartment is unaffected by the administration of Ringer's lactate solution.

VOLUME REPLACEMENT AFTER ACUTE BLOOD LOSS

The objective of fluid replacement therapy is to restore isovolemia. However, in the case of hemorrhage, the following question should be asked: "What amount of fluid do we have to administer to compensate for a given volume of blood loss?" The answer can be cal-culated on the basis of the previous observations for each particular type of fluid. Because albumin leakage is equal to approximately one-fourth of the adminis-tered volume of colloid solution, we would have to administer 133 mL of colloid solution to achieve effec-tive volume reexpansion after the loss of 1 L of blood (Fig. 6). To compensate for the same amount of blood loss, we would have to administer 4 L of a balanced salt solution or 500 mL of a hypertonic salt solution (Fig. 6). Unfortunately, patients would not be able to tolerate the administration of that volume of hypertonic saline because it would induce severe hypernatremia and could cause seizures. The maxi-mum volume of hypertonic saline that can be safely administered is approximately 250 mL.

In 1967, Shires and his group (7) demonstrated the need for volume reexpansion in a classic model of hemorrhagic shock in dogs. The lowest survi-val rate occurred among animals whose lost fluid was replaced with blood alone; the survival rate was higher for the group treated with blood and plasma. The survival rate was highest for the group resusci-tated with blood plasma and crystalloid solution (lactated Ringer's): these dogs remained alive for as long as 14 days after the onset of hemorrhagic shock.

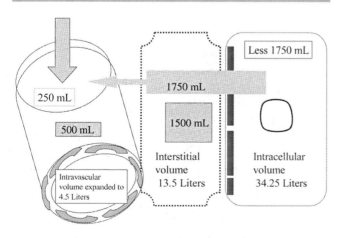

Figure 5 Infusion of 250 mL of 7.5% hypertonic saline.

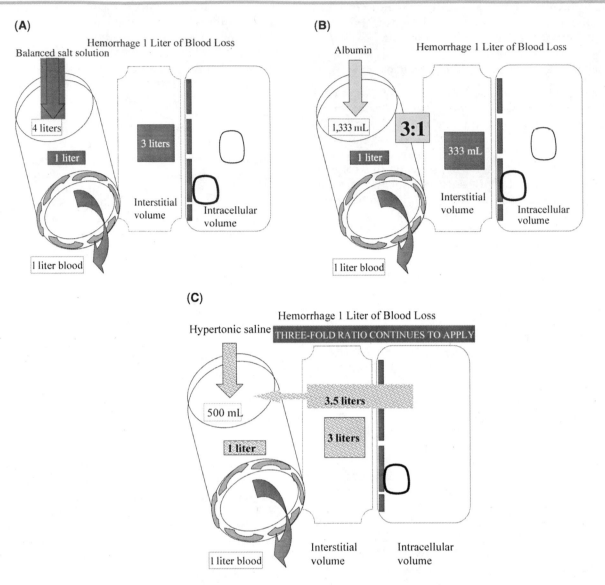

Figure 6 (A-C) Examples of volume replacement after acute blood loss.

In their original report, Shires and his colleagues (7) reported that the extracellular fluid volume (ECV) was severely contracted after the hemorrhagic insult. A 10% blood loss was well tolerated, with no evidence of hypotension. When 25% of the total blood volume was lost, the animals experienced severe hypotension associated with a reduction of 18% to 26% in the functional ECV. Further losses of ECV paralleled increases in the amount of blood lost. Shires and colleagues proposed that intracellular swelling occurs as a result of shock (7,8). It is likely that the cellular swelling is a phenomenon that occurs during the shock period and is most probably related to a failure of the sodium pump. The finding that there is an expansion of the intracellular volume, which in some patients is believed to last for several days, has not been observed in milder or reversible models of shock. Indeed, the findings of Shires and coworkers showed

that the cellular volume returned to normal in subjects whose period of shock did not last for more than two hours (8).

Cellular edema probably results from damage to the energetic machine of the membrane. In some patients, there may be an unrecognized, subclinical, ongoing energy deficit despite normal or near-normal values for clinical measures such as blood pressure, heart rate, and urinary output. These circumstances may occur more often than expected and may eventually generate a more protracted form of cellular dysfunction that ultimately will manifest itself as multiple organ failure.

In clinical practice, we often find that patients who require massive volume resuscitation will ultimately exhibit the effects of massive expansion of interstitial space. In these patients, the interstitial space may have increased by a factor of two or three on the second or third day after surgery; thus, the normal 3:1 ratio explained above is no longer applicable. These patients may exhibit a ratio of 4:1, 5:1, or even 6:1. At this point, any additional crystalloid solution administered to the patient will be distributed in the interstitial space in proportion to these size ratios; therefore, the intravascular filling will become progressively less effective. The efficiency of volume expansion by crystalloid solution is reduced; instead of retaining one-fourth of the volume in the intravascular space, the patient may retain no more than one-fifth or one-sixth of the volume administered (Fig. 7). There is a point at which the efficiency of volume expansion becomes so low that administering a colloid solution rather than a crystalloid solution may be a better option because the colloid solution causes more intravascular filling.

GOALS OF FLUID REPLACEMENT AND END POINTS OF RESUSCITATION

Porter and Ivatury (9) recently reviewed the available findings regarding end points for the resuscitation of patients with traumatic injury. Although their study focused only on the acute resuscitation of victims of trauma, their conclusions are probably also applicable to critically ill and high-risk patients in general. Most clinicians would agree that heart rate, systemic arterial blood pressure, skin temperature, and urine flow (i.e., the primary end points of resuscitation used by clinicians before the era of invasive hemodynamic monitoring) provide relatively little information about the adequacy of oxygen delivery to tissues. Accordingly, reliance on these simple indices of perfusion may result in failure to recognize ongoing anaerobiosis (cryptic shock).

With the introduction of central venous and Swan–Ganz catheterization, clinicians sought to titrate

resuscitation therapy to achieve "adequate" indices of ventricular preload, cardiac output, and systemic oxygen delivery. On the basis of extensive analyses of the hemodynamic profiles of survivors and nonsurvivors of critical illness, Shoemaker et al. (10) proposed that patients suffering from trauma and shock develop an oxygen "debt" and therefore require supranormal levels of oxygen delivery to reestablish homeostasis. Tuchschmidt et al. (11) later reported similar findings from a study of patients with sepsis. Subsequently, in three prospective, randomized trials (12–14), Shoemaker and coworkers obtained evidence that survival is improved by titrating resuscitative measures to achieve the target values established in earlier observational studies (specifically, a cardiac index greater than 4.5 L/min/m^2 of body area, a systemic oxygen delivery index greater than 600 mL/min/m^2, and systemic oxygen consumption greater than 170 mL/min/m^2). In another trial (15), a significant improvement in survival rates was achieved when high-risk surgical patients were treated with dopexamine, an inotrope and vasodilator that increases cardiac output during the perioperative period. No significant differences in systemic oxygen consumption or blood lactate concentration were found between patients who were and were not treated with dopexamine; this finding suggests that dopexamine has beneficial effects, independent of its hemodynamic actions. To complicate the picture, several subsequent clinical studies (16–19) have failed to demonstrate that survival rates improve when resuscitation therapy is titrated to achieve supranormal values for oxygen delivery or cardiac output.

Resuscitation therapy can also be adjusted to achieve certain biochemical end points, such as arterial base deficit or blood lactate concentration. These end points can be used because tissue hypoperfusion leads to increased anaerobic metabolism. During anaerobic metabolism, large quantities of pyruvate are converted to lactate, and thus do not enter the tricarboxylic acid cycle. Meanwhile because of the stoichiometry of substrate-level (rather than oxidative) phosphorylation of adenosine diphosphate to ATP, there is a net accumulation of protons (20). Accordingly, increases in arterial base deficit, blood lactate concentration, or both are evidence of an increase in the rate of anaerobic metabolism. Numerous studies (21–24) have documented that high concentrations of blood lactate portend an unfavorable outcome for patients with shock, but it has not been proven that survival is improved when therapy is titrated by using blood lactate concentration as an end point.

Base deficit is the amount of base (in millimoles) required to titrate 1 L of whole blood to a pH of 7.40 while the sample is maintained at 37°C, fully saturated with oxygen, and equilibrated with an atmosphere containing carbon dioxide at a PCO$_2$ of 40 mmHg. Base deficit is calculated by arterial blood gas analyzers that use a nomogram developed by Astrup et al. (25). Base deficit is more quickly and

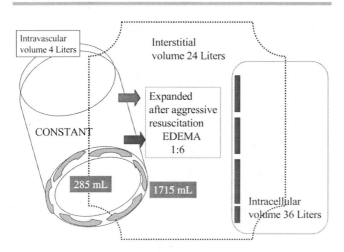

Figure 7 Effect of infusing 2L of Ringer's lactate solution in a patient with severe edema.

easily measured than is lactate concentration, and it has prognostic value for patients with shock (26–29). Although titrating therapy to a base deficit end point is intuitively reasonable, whether it improves survival rates remains unproven.

Until recently, a randomized clinical trial of gastric tonometry (30), a form of tissue capnometry, was the only source of published findings demonstrating that the use of a monitoring tool to guide resuscitation can improve the outcome of critically ill patients. However, Rivers et al. (31) recently published the results of a partially blinded, randomized trial of goal-directed therapy initiated in the emergency ward for patients with septic shock. An algorithm was developed to adjust CVP to 8 to 12 mmHg, mean arterial pressure to 65 to 90 mmHg, and central venous oxygen saturation to more than 70%. A central venous oximetry catheter was used to titrate resuscitative therapy in an attempt to balance systemic oxygen supply with oxygen demand. Unlike similar studies carried out in an ICU setting, this study initiated goal-directed therapy at an earlier point after injury. The findings showed that early institution of goal-directed hemodynamic support prevented cardiovascular collapse in high-risk patients, and reduced hospital mortality rates from 46.5% to 30.5% ($p = 0.009$) (31,32).

Perhaps the most rational way to titrate resuscitative therapy is to use a measure of the adequacy of regional tissue perfusion. Several highly complex approaches can achieve this goal, such as using near-infrared spectroscopy to assess the redox state of cytochrome α, α_3 (the terminal enzyme complex in the mitochondrial respiratory chain). However, tissue capnometry offers the promise of being inexpensive, reliable, and minimally invasive.

COMPLICATIONS OF FLUID LOSSES IN SURGICAL PATIENTS

Many surgical complications are associated with fluid losses and electrolyte disturbances that result from conditions other than hemorrhage. These conditions may have a broader but less acute impact on all of the body fluid compartments, and may be associated with severe electrolyte derangements. Therefore, therapy must be directed at restoring homeostasis and minimizing iatrogenic complications.

Because sodium and water are the primary determinants of the adequacy of volume status, the surgeon must have a clear understanding of the interactions of these two important components of the internal milieu.

External losses or internal shifts of fluids are commonly associated with surgical patients and may initially be indicated by signs of inadequate volume and perfusion, without marked changes in plasma sodium concentrations. The most common cause of hyponatremia is inappropriate therapy, and the most common conditions associated with hypernatremia are excessive diuresis and unrecognized or miscalculated

losses of free water. The plasma sodium concentration is an index of the relative proportions of sodium and water in the extracellular fluid (ECF). The constant redistribution of fluid across all body fluid compartments is ruled by the laws of tonicity. The combined depletion of sodium and water is a common occurrence among patients with volume depletion resulting from excessive fluid losses. In a similar fashion, the loss of gastrointestinal fluid, which may occur as the result of vomiting, diarrhea, fistulas, or prolonged nasogastric suction, is also typically characterized by combined deficits of water and sodium. Third spacing or sequestration of fluid in patients with severe peritonitis, pancreatitis, or other local inflammatory conditions in the abdominal cavity is also associated with combined losses of sodium and water.

Hyponatremia

Hyponatremia occurs when there is an excess of total body water relative to total body sodium content. Hyponatremia may be associated with decreased, increased, or near-normal amounts of total body sodium. In general, hyponatremia occurs as a disorder of the kidneys' ability to dilute urine. The approach to therapy for the hyponatremic patient can be simplified by establishing first whether the patient's ECV is reduced (depletion) or increased (edema). Renal losses, which include diuretic excess, mineralocorticoid deficiency, salt-losing nephritis, renal tubular acidosis, and osmotic diuresis, are characterized by volume depletion and a urinary sodium concentration greater than 20 mmol/L. When the urinary sodium concentration is less than 10 mmol/L, the hyponatremic state is usually the result of extrarenal losses, a common condition among surgical patients. Those with extrarenal losses usually have a history of vomiting or nasogastric suction, third spacing of fluid, pancreatitis, burns, or soft-tissue trauma. Both types of hyponatremic conditions (renal and extrarenal losses) respond to fluid replacement with isotonic solution (33). Patients with normal or mildly diminished ECV, abnormally low sodium concentration, and no edema are not commonly seen by surgery services. Such patients often have a glucocorticoid deficiency or inappropriate antidiuretic hormone secretion. These conditions usually respond to water restriction. Finally, hyponatremia can occur in patients with edema and enhanced ECF; these patients typically have conditions associated with impaired renal perfusion, such as congestive heart failure, cirrhosis, or nephrotic syndrome. In these patients, a urinary sodium concentration of less than 10 mmol/L is common. If the urinary sodium concentration is greater than 20 mmol/L in patients with edema, then a component of acute or chronic renal failure is also present.

Hypernatremia

The renal concentrating mechanism is the first defense against water depletion and hyperosmolality. When this mechanism is impaired, thirst becomes a very effective mechanism for preventing further increases in serum sodium concentration. Unfortunately, most clinical conditions experienced by surgical patients are also associated with an impairment in water intake. The most practical approach to treating the patient with an elevated serum sodium concentration relies on a basic assessment to determine whether the patient is experiencing hypernatremia with sodium and water losses, hypernatremia with mostly water losses, or hypernatremia with mostly increased sodium intake.

Again, identifying the site of sodium or water losses is crucial; for example, patients receiving diuretic therapy (osmotic or loop diuretics) or having postobstruction or intrinsic renal disease will produce isotonic or hypotonic urine, their urinary sodium concentration will be greater than 20 mEq/L, and their total body sodium concentration will be low (33). If the urinary sodium concentration is less than 10 mEq/L, the most likely cause of hypernatremia will be extrarenal losses (sweating, heat exposure, burns, diarrhea, or fistula). If most of the losses are free water, then the total body sodium concentration must be close to normal values. These patients' urinary sodium concentration will vary, and their clinical symptoms will resemble those of patients with diabetes insipidus syndromes, or those with insensible water losses that are purely respiratory and dermal. If hypernatremia is present and an increase in total body sodium concentration is suspected, the patient usually has primary hyperaldosteronism, Cushing syndrome, or hypertonic dialysis; alternatively, the patient may chronically ingest large amounts of sodium bicarbonate or sodium chloride tablets. The urinary sodium concentration usually exceeds 20 mEq/L. Management consists of the replacement of free water and the initiation of diuretic therapy.

INHERENT COMPLICATIONS OF COMMONLY USED FLUID REPLACEMENT SOLUTIONS

During the past 10 years, we have seen the publication of a plethora of reports presenting more specific findings about the many physiological and biochemical effects of several solutions used for fluid replacement therapy. Furthermore, new and intriguing findings concerning such solutions have been obtained from recent animal model studies, evidence-based medicine studies, meta-analyses, and clinical trials. The following is a summary of these recent findings.

Complications Associated with the Use of Albumin Solutions

Recently, a Cochrane report on the use of albumin as treatment for critically ill patients was published (34). The authors carried out a systematic review of 30 randomized controlled trials comparing the effects of administering albumin or plasma protein fraction

with the effects of not administering this protein fraction or administering crystalloid solution to 1419 critically ill patients with hypovolemia, burns, or hypoalbuminemia. For each patient category, the risk of death in the albumin-treated group was higher than that in the comparison group. The relative risk of death after albumin administration was 1.46 (95% confidence interval, 0.97–2.22) for hypovolemic patients, 2.40 (1.11–5.19) for patients with burns, and 1.69 (1.07–2.67) for patients with hypoalbuminemia. However because this review was based on relatively small trials in which the number of deaths was small, these results must be interpreted with caution. The analyses suggest that the use of human albumin to treat critically ill patients should be reconsidered. Interestingly, a recent abstract submitted to the Society of Critical Care Medicine reported the results of a study of the effectiveness and safety of plasbumin-5 in resuscitating adults with shock. In this open-label, randomized, multicenter, controlled trial, 19 patients were treated with albumin, and 23 were given Ringer's lactate solution. Baseline multiple organ dysfunction scores for the two groups were equivalent. There were no statistically significant differences between groups with respect to days on mechanical ventilation, oxygenation failure, length of stay in the ICU, or 28-day mortality rates. The incidence of bacteremia was significantly lower in the group treated with albumin ($p = 0.023$). The authors requested access to the Cochrane database, and added the results of their trial to the meta-analyses of the subgroup of critically ill patients with burns (34,35). When the data from the recent trial were added to the data considered in the Cochrane review, there was no longer a statistically significant difference in the relative risk of death between burn patients who received albumin and those who received crystalloid solution (35).

In summary, the benefit of administering albumin to critically ill patients is unproven. Epidemiologic evidence suggests that using human albumin solution to treat patients with burns, hypoalbuminemia, and hypotension is associated with an increased risk of death. In the face of critical illness, hypoalbuminemia results from transcapillary leak, decreased synthesis, large-volume body fluid losses, and dilution caused by fluid resuscitation. When treating patients with hypoalbuminemia, physicians must focus their efforts on correcting the underlying disorder rather than on reversing the hypoalbuminemia (36).

Complications Associated with the Use of Ringer's Lactate Solution

It is somewhat surprising that although Ringer's lactate solution has been used as a volume expander and resuscitation fluid for nearly 100 years, only recently have we begun to elucidate the immunologic and proinflammatory effects of the solution on neutrophils and other cells involved in host defense mechanisms. In one study using a swine model of shock, Rhee et al. (37) compared the effects of different methods of fluid resuscitation in three groups of patients: group I received Ringer's lactate solution; group II, shed blood; and group III, 7.5% hypertonic saline solution. Neutrophil activation in whole blood was measured by flow cytometry, which detected intracellular superoxide burst activity. Neutrophil activation increased significantly immediately after hemorrhage in all three groups, but the increase was greatest after resuscitation with Ringer's lactate. Neutrophil activity in animals that received shed blood or 7.5% hypertonic saline solution returned to the baseline state after resuscitation (37). Another study by the same research group (38) found that different resuscitative fluids may immediately affect the degree of apoptosis after hemorrhagic shock in rats. Fluid resuscitation with Ringer's lactate solution significantly increased apoptosis of cells in the small intestine and liver. Administering Ringer's lactate solution to rats in a sham hemorrhage group increased apoptosis of cells in the intestinal mucosa and muscularis externa. Animals that underwent sham hemorrhage, resuscitation with blood or hypertonic saline solution, or sham resuscitation experienced no increase in apoptosis in either the liver or the small intestine.

CONCLUSIONS

The use of intravenous fluids is one of the main pillars of resuscitative therapy for surgical patients. Many conditions, such as acute hemorrhage, burn injuries, and intra-abdominal inflammatory catastrophes, require aggressive fluid resuscitation. The clinician must be very familiar with the type and proper dosage of the many available solutions. Clear objectives and end points of resuscitation strategies must be determined in advance, and the possible side effects and complications need to be predicted and identified early in the course of treatment if the best possible outcome is to be achieved. Unfortunately, fluid therapy is not always seen as a pharmacologic intervention, but we must realize that fluids, like any other drug, may be indicated or contraindicated in specific situations.

Finally, we should note that, in contrast to the pace of new drug development, the pace of innovation in fluid therapy has been remarkably slow. For example, most studies of antisepsis drugs date only to the early 1980s, and new trials are reported every two to three months. The use of mechanical ventilation devices has been widespread since the 1960s, and a new model of ventilator appears every 22 months. Antibiotics have been in use since the 1940s, and a new agent is approved every six months. In contrast, intravenous fluid therapy has been used for resuscitation since the 1800s, and we still use these fluids today. After a century of Ringer's lactate use, the development of a new product is overdue (Kellum JA. Personal communication, 2003).

REFERENCES

1. Cosnett JE. The origins of intravenous fluid therapy. Lancet 1989; 333:768–771.
2. Tranbaugh RF, Lewis FR. Mechanisms and etiologic factors of pulmonary edema. Surg Gynecol Obstet 1984; 158:193–206.
3. Manning RD Jr, Guyton AC. Dynamics of fluid distribution between the blood and interstitium during overhydration. Am J Physiol 1980; 238:H645–H651.
4. Baldwin AL, Thurston G. Mechanics of endothelial cell architecture and vascular permeability. Crit Rev Biomed Eng 2001; 29:247–278.
5. Tranbaugh RF, Elings VB, Christensen J, Lewis FR. Determinants of pulmonary interstitial fluid accumulation after trauma. J Trauma 1982; 22:820–826.
6. Shires GT, Cunningham JN, Backer CR, et al. Alterations in cellular membrane function during hemorrhagic shock in primates. Ann Surg 1972; 176:288–295.
7. McClelland RN, Shires GT, Baxter CR, Coln CD, Carrico J. Balanced salt solution in the treatment of hemorrhagic shock. Studies in dogs. JAMA 1967; 199:830–834.
8. Illner HP, Cunningham JN Jr, Shires GT. Red blood cell sodium content and permeability changes in hemorrhagic shock. Am J Surg 1982; 143:349–355.
9. Porter JM, Ivatury RR. In search of the optimal end points of resuscitation in trauma patients: a review. J Trauma 1998; 44:908–914.
10. Shoemaker WC, Montgomery ES, Kaplan E, Elwyn DH. Physiologic patterns in surviving and nonsurviving shock patients. Use of sequential cardiorespiratory variables in defining criteria for therapeutic goals and early warning of death. Arch Surg 1973; 106:630–636.
11. Tuchschmidt J, Fried J, Swinney R, Sharma OP. Early hemodynamic correlates of survival in patients with septic shock. Crit Care Med 1989; 17:719–723.
12. Fleming A, Bishop M, Shoemaker W, et al. Prospective trial of supranormal values as goals of resuscitation in severe trauma. Arch Surg 1992; 127:1175–1179; discussion 1179–1181.
13. Shoemaker WC, Appel PL, Kram HB, Waxman K, Lee TS. Prospective trial of supranormal values of survivors as therapeutic goals in high-risk surgical patients. Chest 1988; 94:1176–1186.
14. Bishop MH, Shoemaker WC, Appel PL, et al. Prospective, randomized trial of survivor values of cardiac index, oxygen delivery, and oxygen consumption as resuscitation end points in severe trauma. J Trauma 1995; 38:780–787.
15. Boyd O, Grounds RM, Bennett ED. A randomized clinical trial of the effect of deliberate perioperative increase of oxygen delivery on mortality in high-risk surgical patients. JAMA 1993; 270:2699–2707.
16. Hayes MA, Timmins AC, Yau EH, Palazzo M, Hinds CJ, Watson D. Elevation of systemic oxygen delivery in the treatment of critically ill patients. N Engl J Med 1994; 330:1717–1722.
17. Tuchschmidt J, Fried J, Astiz M, Rackow E. Elevation of cardiac output and oxygen delivery improves outcome in septic shock. Chest 1992; 102:216–220.
18. Yu M, Levy MM, Smith P, Takiguchi SA, Miyasaki A, Myers SA. Effect of maximizing oxygen delivery on morbidity and mortality rates in critically ill patients: a prospective, randomized, controlled study. Crit Care Med 1993; 21:830–838.

19. Gattinoni L, Brazzi L, Pelosi P, et al. A trial of goal-oriented hemodynamic therapy in critically ill patients. SvO2 Collaborative Group. N Engl J Med 1995; 333: 1025–1032.
20. Hochachka PW, Mommsen TP. Protons and anaerobiosis. Science 1983; 219:1391–1397.
21. Marecaux G, Pinsky MR, Dupont E, Kahn RJ, Vincent JL. Blood lactate levels are better prognostic indicators than TNF and IL-6 levels in patients with septic shock. Intensive Care Med 1996; 22:404–408.
22. Bernardin G, Pradier C, Tiger F, Deloffre P, Mattei M. Blood pressure and arterial lactate level are early indicators of short-term survival in human septic shock. Intensive Care Med 1996; 22:17–25.
23. Broder G, Weil MH. Excess lactate: an index of reversibility of shock in human patients. Science 1964; 143:1457–1459.
24. Bakker J, Gris P, Coffernils M, Kahn RJ, Vincent JL. Serial blood lactate levels can predict the development of multiple organ failure following septic shock. Am J Surg 1996; 171:221–226.
25. Astrup P, Engel K, Jorgensen K, Siggaard-Andersen O. Definitions and terminology in blood acid-base chemistry. Ann N Y Acad Sci 1966; 133:59–65.
26. Siegel JH, Rivkind AI, Dalal S, Goodarzi S. Early physiologic predictors of injury severity and death in blunt multiple trauma. Arch Surg 1990; 125:498–508.
27. Davis JW, Parks SN, Kaups KL, Gladen HE, O'Donnell-Nicol S. Admission base deficit predicts transfusion requirements and risk of complications. J Trauma 1996; 41:769–774.
28. Davis JW, Kaups KL, Parks SN. Base deficit is superior to pH in evaluating clearance of acidosis after traumatic shock. J Trauma 1998; 44:114–118.
29. Rutherford EJ, Morris JA Jr, Reed GW, Hall KS. Base deficit stratifies mortality and determines therapy. J Trauma 1992; 33:417–423.
30. Gutierrez G, Palizas F, Doglio G, et al. Gastric intramucosal pH as a therapeutic index of tissue oxygenation in critically ill patients. Lancet 1992; 339:195–199.
31. Rivers E, Nguyen B, Havstad S, et al. Early Goal-Directed Therapy Collaborative Group. Early goal-directed therapy in the treatment of severe sepsis and septic shock. N Engl J Med 2001; 345:1368–1377.
32. Rivers EP, Ander DS, Powell D. Central venous oxygen saturation monitoring in the critically ill patient. Curr Opin Crit Care 2001; 7:204–211.
33. Berl T, Anderson RJ, McDonald KM, Schrier RW. Clinical disorders of water metabolism. Kidney Int 1976; 10:117–132.
34. Alderson P, Bunn F, Lefebvre C, et al. Human albumin solution for resuscitation and volume expansion in critically ill patients. Cochrane Database Syst Rev 2004; (4):CD001208.
35. Cooper A. Efficacy and safety of Plasbumin-5 for adult burn shock resuscitation. Crit Care Med, Suppl 2003; 31(2) (abstract 71).
36. Pulimood TB, Park GR. Debate: albumin administration should be avoided in the critically ill. Crit Care 2000; 4:151–155.
37. Rhee P, Burris D, Kaufmann C, et al. Lactated Ringer's solution resuscitation causes neutrophil activation after hemorrhagic shock. J Trauma 1998; 44:313–319.
38. Deb S, Martin B, Sun L, et al. Resuscitation with lactated Ringer's solution in rats with hemorrhagic shock induces immediate apoptosis. J Trauma 1999; 46:582–588; discussion 588–589.

3

Complications of Antibiotic Therapy

Mohamed Fahim
Anesthesia Critical Care, Davis Memorial Hospital, Elkins, West Virginia, U.S.A.

Nicholas Namias
Miller School of Medicine at the University of Miami, Miami, Florida, U.S.A.

Antibiotics are frequently used as an adjunct to the surgical therapy of infections. All antibiotics are potentially harmful, and various benefit-to-risk factors must be considered whenever they are used (1). Antimicrobial chemotherapy used in association with surgery may be complicated by failure of therapy or unwanted side effects. Most antibiotic-related adverse reactions are predictable and are often dose-dependent. Unpredictable reactions occur independently of the dose and route of administration and are due to drug intolerance, allergy, and other idiosyncratic responses (2). Other reactions occur rarely and are unique to the compound administered; one such example is toxic epidermal necrolysis (Stevens–Johnson Syndrome) induced by sulfonamides (1).

The problems encountered in the use of antimicrobial chemotherapeutic agents can be conveniently divided into general complications (e.g., those associated with the route of administration, hypersensitivity reactions, failure of therapy, induction of resistance, antagonism, and effects on immune response) and specific complications related to each individual antimicrobial agent.

GENERAL COMPLICATIONS

Complications Associated with the Route of Administration

Oral administration of an antimicrobial agent may cause complications involving the gastrointestinal tract, such as nausea, vomiting, diarrhea, gastritis, and pseudomembranous colitis (PMC). Parenteral administration of antimicrobial agents can result in reactions at the injection site, such as pain, inflammation, abscess, necrosis, edema, hemorrhage, cellulitis, hypersensitivity, atrophy, ecchymosis, and skin ulcer. Parenteral administration of antibiotics may also result in neurovascular reactions, including warmth, vasospasm, pallor, mottling, gangrene, numbness of the extremities, cyanosis of the extremities, and neurovascular damage. Intravenous administration of

antibiotics may cause thrombophlebitis. It is well known that intramuscular injection of antibiotics such as penicillin G may result in sciatic nerve injury (3).

Hypersensitivity Reactions

Anaphylaxis

Anaphylaxis is the most severe reaction experienced by patients treated with antibiotics. It is most frequently encountered after parenteral injection of penicillin or one of its synthetic analogs (4). Anaphylaxis occurs when certain pharmacologically active mediators are rapidly released in response to interactions between an antigen (the antimicrobial compound) and immunoglobulin E (IgE) antibody. These mediators, which are released from basophils and mast cells, include histamine, a slowly reacting substance of anaphylaxis, and, perhaps, serotonin and bradykinin (5).

Clinically, the reaction may develop within minutes to hours of drug administration. Patients may experience primary vascular collapse with hypotension, as well as bronchospasm and laryngeal edema. Dermal manifestations include eruption and hives. Angioedema may also occur. The drug of choice for the treatment of anaphylaxis is epinephrine, diluted 1:1000, given intramuscularly in a volume of 0.3 mL. However, when anaphylaxis is very severe, intravenous administration of epinephrine may be required if a clinical response is to be to achieved. Progression of the laryngeal edema may even require immediate tracheostomy or emergent cricothyroidotomy because endotracheal intubation may not be possible. Persistent hypotension that does not respond to epinephrine may be treated with volume expanders and vasoconstrictors (6).

Prevention of anaphylaxis depends on eliciting a thorough drug history before antibiotics are administered. The most reliable way to assess a patient's risk for a type I IgE-mediated reaction is to administer a skin test to measure the response to the "major" and "minor" skin determinants. Unfortunately, only the major skin-testing determinant is commercially available (7).

Cutaneous Eruptions

Cutaneous (dermal) eruptions, the most common manifestation of hypersensitivity to antibiotics, are due to delayed hypersensitivity mediated by the cellular immune system (8). Such eruptions may be morbilliform, petechial, maculopapular, or bullous. Stevens–Johnson syndrome, exfoliative dermatitis, and erythema nodosum may also occur. When a dermal reaction appears, the best course of action is to discontinue the administration of the drug (4).

Taking a careful drug history and avoiding drugs to which the patient has a history of hypersensitivity can prevent a reaction. An agent can be selected from another class of antibiotics that would be unlikely to cross-react with the drug to which the patient is allergic. Penicillins and cephalosporins both possess the beta-lactam ring, and cross-reactivity may occur, but this event probably occurs in no more than 5% to 10% of patients allergic to one of these types of antibiotics (9). Cephalosporins are usually safe for patients allergic to penicillins, but not for those who have had an immediate or anaphylactic reaction to the penicillins (4).

Drug Fever

Drug fever is presumably a hypersensitivity reaction, and may be the most difficult complication to diagnose because of its similarity to fever due to the infection. Also, other drugs administered simultaneously must be considered as possible causes of fever. Drug fever may be associated with the use of any antimicrobial agent (4) and may be accompanied by eosinophilia or cutaneous eruption. Diagnosis of drug fever should always be considered when fever is sustained or recurs despite the apparent effectiveness of antimicrobial therapy (10). Drug fever usually cannot be prevented; it is treated with prompt withdrawal of the antibiotic suspected of being responsible for causing it.

Failure of Antimicrobial Therapy

Antimicrobial therapy alone is invariably ineffective in treating abscesses because antibiotics cannot penetrate the abscess and thus cannot reach effective concentrations in the purulent exudates (4). Also, some antibiotics appear to be inactivated by constituents of the exudate in the abscess (11).

Induction of Resistance to Antimicrobial Agents

One of the most difficult problems in dealing with infectious diseases is microbial resistance to antimicrobial agents (12–14). In response to the specific and well-defined needs of the clinician, a number of procedures have been developed to guide the selection of antibiotic agents and their dosages for the treatment and eradication of a given bacterial infection. Among the procedures available, the most useful have been those that yield the qualitative antibiotic susceptibility profile and the quantitative minimum inhibitory concentration (MIC) of the clinically indicated antibiotics (15). The MIC is the concentration of the antibiotic that inhibits the growth of a standardized concentration of bacteria. In contrast, the minimum bactericidal concentration (MBC) is the concentration of a drug that kills 99.9% of a bacterial population after exposure to the antibiotic for 24 hours. Therefore, the MBC is often used to treat life-threatening infections such as endocarditis. The MBC, with a few exceptions, is greater than the MIC. Comparing the MIC with the MBC provides an estimate of the drug's potency: a small difference between the two indicates that the antibiotic is potent; a large difference indicates that the bacterium is tolerant of the antimicrobial compound (15).

Acquired resistance arises from the microbe's acquisition of genetic material or its mutation. Genetic exchange can arise from conjugation, transformation, phage transduction, or mutations within the genome of the bacterium. Plasmids and transposons can carry determinants that confer resistance in many ways; for example, enzymatic inactivation, decreased uptake, cell surface alterations, and efflux properties have all been reported to be transferable by plasmids. Mutation can also result in the loss of outer membrane proteins, or the alteration of target site (16,17).

Worldwide, many strains of *Staphylococcus aureus* are already resistant to all antibiotics except vancomycin. Methicillin-resistant *Staphylococcus aureus* (MRSA) was first detected in England (18), and constituted 46.7% of all *S. aureus* isolates collected in 1998 by the National Nosocomial Infections Surveillance Program of the Centers for Disease Control and Prevention; this percentage represented a 31% increase over the previous reported value for the years 1993 to 1997 (19).

Beta-lactamase production is also an important mechanism of resistance in gram-negative organisms. There is now an extended spectrum of organisms whose beta-lactamase will hydrolyze the beta-lactam ring of multiple beta-lactam drugs (20). Vancomycin-intermediate and vancomycin-resistant strains of *S. aureus* have been isolated, although they have not yet become widespread (21). Resistance to vancomycin has also become common in the enterococci (19), and there have been case reports of patients infected with vancomycin-dependent enterococci (22).

Antagonism

"Antibiotic synergy" connotes a greater-than-additive treatment effect that occurs when more than one antibiotic is used. Strictly defined, "antagonism" means a less-than-additive effect, but it is more often taken to mean that the effect produced by a group of antibiotics is less than that caused by the most active drug in the group (23). Synergy and antagonism can be categorized into five major groups: direct effects on the bacteria (e.g., interaction between the mechanisms responsible for antibiotics' specific antibacterial activity); indirect effects on the bacteria (e.g., drug inactivation, emergence of resistance, or environmental changes that modify antibiotic action); pharmacological effects (e.g., inactivation, bioconversion, or both; absorption, elimination, or both; and diffusion, binding, or both); modification of host defenses that enhance or adversely affect the antibiotic action (e.g., phagocytosis or immunologic response); and effects that cause toxicity (24).

The synergy or antagonism between antimicrobial drugs is a direct consequence of combining the agents used. There are at least five major reasons for using combinations of antimicrobial agents (25). First, such combinations may be used as initial therapy for serious infections. Empiric therapy for severely ill patients or for compromised hosts should involve a combination of antimicrobial drugs. No single drug can be reasonably expected to provide sufficient coverage against gram-positive and gram-negative bacteria that cause serious infections.

Second, combinations of antibiotics may be used to treat infections caused by multiple organisms. Mixed infections are a reasonable justification for the use of antimicrobial combinations because not all the pathogens may be susceptible to a single agent. The best examples of infections requiring treatment with multiple antibiotics are the mixed aerobic–anaerobic infections, which arise from the gastrointestinal or genital tracts.

Third, combinations of antibiotics may be used to decrease the emergence of antibiotic-resistant microbes. This rationale has been the basis for the use of combinations of antituberculous drugs.

Fourth, the use of antibiotic combinations may lessen the dose-related toxicity of treatment. This reason for using combinations is rarely advocated; most clinicians prescribe the maximum tolerated dose of a single drug and do not rely on synergy. Finally, combinations of antibiotics may be used to eradicate infections that cannot be successfully treated with a single active drug (synergism). The concept of synergy and its clinical relevance is the most controversial aspect of the use of antimicrobial combinations.

In some situations, antimicrobial agents may act synergistically on a given microorganism through their different binding to receptors in the cell membrane. Another mechanism is the sequential blockade of successive steps in a metabolic pathway in a given organism, such as that accomplished through the synergism achieved by the combined use of the combination of sulfamethoxazole and trimethoprim. Finally, synergism can result from the combined use of an antimicrobial agent that inhibits the synthesis of the bacterial cell wall and another agent that is otherwise unable to penetrate cells with an intact wall. For example, penicillins and various aminoglycosides exhibit this synergism against infections caused by enterococci and other microorganisms.

Many mechanisms may explain antagonism. Drugs that are capable of impairing cell division may antagonize the activity of antibiotics that alter the cell wall, such as the penicillins. However, the mechanisms of antagonism resulting from combination of drugs that act within the bacterial cell appear to be more complex.

Effects of Antimicrobial Agents on the Immune Response

Life-threatening bacterial, fungal, and opportunistic infections that occur among patients whose immune response is altered has led to the prolonged use of intensive prophylactic and therapeutic antimicrobial regimens, which often are administered concomitantly with corticosteroids, cytotoxic chemotherapy, or both. Because some antimicrobial agents at therapeutic concentrations can affect humoral or cellular immune responses, there is a need for a better understanding of the possible beneficial and deleterious effects of antibiotic therapy on the immune response, especially in the immunocompromised patient.

The impetus to evaluate the effect of antimicrobials on the immune response stems largely from observations of the toxic or allergic reactions to commonly used antimicrobial agents (26–31); the similarity between the structures of certain antibiotics and chemical structure of various antimetabolites and cytotoxic drugs (32,33); and the ability of certain antimicrobials to enter mammalian cells, especially phagocytes, thus raising the possibility of untoward effects on cellular function (34–41). Various detailed reviews of the literature on this subject have generally found that a large number of antimicrobial agents can affect various immune functions (42–47). However, the meaning, clinical relevance, and significance of the observed changes are unclear: the results of different studies have been conflicting, the effects of antibiotics in vitro have been incorrectly assumed to occur in vivo, the mechanisms by which antibiotics affect immune responses remain unknown, and few controlled clinical studies have been carried out to determine the effect of antimicrobials on the immune response in humans. Because of these limitations in interpreting the currently available data, we selectively review some of the more commonly used antimicrobial agents, specifically focusing on their effects on cell-mediated and humoral immunity, as well as on polymorphonuclear leukocyte function as determined by in vitro and in vivo investigations.

Lymphocyte Transformation

Lymphocyte transformation in vitro is the metabolic activation of lymphocytes with antigens or mitogens. Thus, lymphocyte transformation reflects the ability of lymphocytes to proliferate after exposure to such antigens or mitogens (48). This effect occurs in response to treatment with various antibiotics. For example, acyclovir appears to delay the development of and diminish the peak of in vitro lymphocyte transformation responses to inactivated herpes simplex virus antigens in patients with genital herpes (49).

Delayed-Type Hypersensitivity

Delayed-type hypersensitivity (DTH) is a cell-mediated immune reaction that can be elicited by intracutaneous injection of antigen; the subsequent cellular infiltrate and edema reach their peak between 24 and 48 hours after antigenic challenge (50). DTH can be thought of as an in vivo model of cell-mediated immune responses that are modulated by specifically sensitized thymus-derived lymphocytes (T-lymphocytes). In attempts to evaluate the effect of antibiotics on cell-mediated immune function in vivo, several investigators have studied DTH skin tests with a variety of antigens.

A significant reduction of DTH occurred in groups of mice treated with doxycycline and tetra-cycline. The fact that suppressive effects were more pronounced on the manifestation phase than the induction phase of DTH suggests that these antibiotics may have untoward effects on sensitized lymphocytes and on macrophages. This hypothesis is supported by the finding that the drugs inhibit mitogen-induced lymphocyte transformation in vivo.

Antibody Production

Several studies of humans have evaluated the effect of rifampin on the antibody response to vaccination. Seroconversion following vaccinia vaccination was suppressed in normal volunteers whose vaccination site was treated with a cream containing 15% rifampin (51).

Polymorphonuclear Leukocyte Function

Chemotaxis is the process by which phagocytes are attracted to the vicinity of pathogenic microorganisms by such factors as bacterial products, tissue proteases, and complement. A number of pharmacologic agents including tetracyclines and amphotericin B inhibit chemotaxis in vitro. The inhibitory effect of tetracyclines may be related to their ability to chelate calcium (52).

Miscellaneous Effects

Natural killer (NK) cells compose a lymphoid subpopulation that is cytotoxic for a variety of targeted tumor cells (53). Hauser et al. (54) demonstrated that murine NK cell cytotoxicity for the murine lymphoma YAC-1 is significantly augmented during acute toxoplasma infection. Amphotericin B inhibited toxoplasma-induced murine NK cell activity against YAC-1; this antibiotic may adversely affect NK cell activity in other hosts as well (55).

SPECIFIC ANTIBIOTICS AND THEIR ASSOCIATED COMPLICATIONS
Penicillins
Natural Penicillins
Penicillin G (Procaine Penicillin G and Benzathine Penicillin G)

Hypersensitivity to penicillin G is common; symptoms include skin eruptions that range from maculopapular to exfoliative dermatitis, urticaria, laryngeal edema, fever, and eosinophilia. Other serum sickness–like reactions (including chills, fever, edema, arthralgia, and prostration) may be controlled with antihistamines

and, if necessary, systemic corticosteroid therapy. Anaphylaxis including shock and death may also occur. Whenever hypersensitivity occurs, penicillin G should be discontinued. Anaphylactic reactions require immediate emergency treatment with epinephrine. Steroids should be administered intravenously, oxygen should be given, and airway management, including intubation, should also be conducted when indicated. Hemolytic anemia is an uncommon complication, and pancytopenia, though rare, can occur. Nephropathy in the form of interstitial nephritis can complicate intravenous administration of large doses of penicillin G. Most patients recover from this complication when administration of the drug is stopped. An overdose of penicillin can cause neuromuscular hyperirritability or convulsive seizures. Penicillin neurotoxicity can be prevented by determining the proper dose for patients with impaired renal function.

The Jarisch–Herxheimer reaction has been observed among patients treated for syphilis. The reaction is the possible result of exacerbation of an existing syphilitic lesion. It is apparent that it is mediated by the action of cytokines released into the circulation (56), causing malaise, chills, fever, sore throat, myalgia, headache, and tachycardia. This reaction usually occurs six to eight hours after penicillin G is administered; it subsides within 24 hours (57).

Aminopenicillin

Ampicillin, a semisynthetic antibiotic, and amoxicillin, an analog of ampicillin, have been associated with hypersensitivity reactions such as urticaria and anaphylaxis. Rashes associated with ampicillin are not always urticarial (58). Macular rashes appear to be ampicillin specific and do not indicate true hypersensitivity to penicillin (59). Orally or, less commonly, parenterally administered ampicillin therapy can cause nausea and diarrhea (60).

Penicillins with Beta-Lactamase Inhibitor
Amoxicillin–Clavulanate

Amoxicillin–clavulanate is an orally administered antibacterial combination consisting of the semisynthetic antibiotic amoxicillin and the beta-lactamase inhibitor clavulanate potassium. Clavulanic acid results from the fermentation of *Streptomyces clavuligerus* (61). Structurally related to the penicillins, this beta-lactam can inactivate a wide variety of beta-lactamases (62) by blocking the active sites of these enzymes. Side effects associated with the use of amoxicillin–clavulanate include gastrointestinal problems such as diarrhea, nausea, vomiting, indigestion, gastritis, stomatitis, glossitis, black "hairy" tongue, mucocutaneous candidiasis, enterocolitis, and PMC.

Ticarcillin–Clavulanate

Ticarcillin–clavulanate is a combination of the semisynthetic ticarcillin disodium and clavulanate potassium.

The administration of clavulanic acid has been associated with positive results on the direct Coomb's test, but hemolysis has not been observed (63).

Ampicillin–Sulbactam

Ampicillin–sulbactam consists of the semisynthetic antibiotic ampicillin sodium and the beta-lactamase inhibitor sulbactam sodium. Intramuscular administration of sulbactam causes pain at the site of injection, but no unexpected side effects have been seen after intravenous administration of ampicillin alone (64).

Piperacillin–Tazobactam

Piperacillin–tazobactam is a combination consisting of the semisynthetic antibiotic piperacillin sodium and the beta-lactamase inhibitor tazobactam sodium. Diarrhea was the only side effect reported more often after treatment with piperacillin–tazobactam than with piperacillin alone (65).

Antipseudomonal Penicillins

Antipseudomonal penicillins such as carbenicillin and ticarcillin can adversely affect platelets. Although almost all penicillins can cause platelet dysfunction (66), the effect is most severe with carbenicillin and ticarcillin. The penicillins disturb platelet membrane function by interfering with adenosine diphosphate receptors and leaving them unavailable to agonists that induce aggregation (67). The newer antipseudomonal penicillins (3) such as mezlocillin and piperacillin can disturb platelet function, but not as severely as carbenicillin and ticarcillin at an equivalent dosage (68).

Cephalosporins

Some patients who are allergic to penicillin are also allergic to cephalosporins (69). Therefore, it is best to avoid the use of cephalosporins to treat patients with a history of anaphylaxis to penicillin (70). Despite the possibility of this adverse cross-reactivity, it appears that 93% to 97% of patients with a history of penicillin allergy do not react to cephalosporins (71,72).

First-Generation Cephalosporins (Cefazolin)

Eosinophilia commonly occurs with cefazolin therapy (73). Nephrotoxicity is rare, mild, and reversible (74). Moreover, a transient rise in aspartate aminotransferase (AST) and alkaline phosphatase concentrations has been observed without clinical evidence of hepatic impairment (73).

Second-Generation Cephalosporins (Cefuroxime)

Second-generation cephalosporins are active against many gram-negative organisms that are resistant to the first-generation cephalosporins (75). Cefuroxime is associated with relatively few side effects (3), although high doses may interfere with platelet function (76) and may cause diarrhea (77). Reversible rises in AST concentrations may occur (78). Also, cefuroxime may exert an immunosuppressive effect that has no known clinical significance (79). The cephamycins, such as cefoxitin and cefotetan, are frequently included in discussions of second-generation cephalosporins. Frequently used in surgery, the cephamycins act against a spectrum of bacteria that include the facultative aerobic *Enterobacteriaceae* spp. and anaerobes. Cefotetan has been associated with hypoprothrombinemia and bleeding in patients with preexisting impaired coagulation, or in patients receiving anticoagulant therapy (80).

Third-Generation Cephalosporins

Third-generation cephalosporins are extended-spectrum compounds that are stable to the presence of beta-lactamases produced by gram-negative bacteria and are highly potent against most *Enterobacteriaceae* spp. (81). These drugs can be separated into groups with poor antipseudomonal activity (e.g., ceftizoxime), and those with good antipseudomonal activity (e.g., cefoperazone). Their side effects are similar to those of other cephalosporins.

Monobactams (Aztreonam)

The antibacterial spectrum of aztreonam somewhat resembles that of aminoglycosides and is not as wide as that of the third-generation cephalosporins (82). In patients with impaired hepatic or renal function, appropriate monitoring is recommended during therapy (83,84). Cross-reactivity with penicillins and cephalosporins seems to be rare.

Carbapenems (Imipenem–Cilastatin and Meropenem)

Imipenem has high activity against aerobic and anaerobic bacteria. Adverse effects on the central nervous system (CNS), such as confusion, myoclonic activity, and seizures, have been observed during treatment with imipenem, especially when recommended dosages were exceeded. These experiences have occurred most commonly in patients with CNS disorders (e.g., brain lesions or history of seizures), compromised renal function, or both (85).

Meropenem, which is similar to imipenem, but is relatively stable to human renal dehydropeptidase-1, may be less likely to induce convulsions (86). The most common side effects observed in one study were diarrhea and elevated liver enzymes (87).

Aminoglycosides (Amikacin, Gentamicin, Tobramycin, Netilmicin, and Streptomycin)

All aminoglycosides have the potential to induce auditory, vestibular, and renal toxicity, and neuromuscular blockade. These events are most common among patients with a history of renal impairment, those receiving other ototoxic or nephrotoxic drugs, and those treated for periods longer than recommended or given doses higher than recommended (85).

Neurotoxicity, appearing as vestibular and permanent bilateral auditory ototoxicity, may be a side effect of treatment with aminoglycosides. Vertigo may be an indication of vestibular injury. Damage to the vestibular system occurs more frequently with gentamicin administration, and cochlear damage is more common with amikacin therapy (88,89). Prolonged neuromuscular blockade and respiratory paralysis have been reported with the use of aminoglycosides, especially in patients receiving anesthetics and neuromuscular blocking agents (85,90). Other effects of neurotoxicity may include numbness, skin tingling, muscle twitching, and convulsions.

Patients who suffer cochlear damage during therapy may not experience symptoms to warn them of developing cranial nerve–eight toxicity. Total or partial irreversible bilateral deafness may occur after the drug has been discontinued. Aminoglycoside-induced ototoxicity is usually irreversible (85).

The most common clinical manifestation of gentamicin nephrotoxicity is nonoliguric renal failure with proteinuria and increased concentrations of serum creatinine and blood urea. Renal function changes are usually reversible when administration of the drug is discontinued (3). Although less common, an acute oliguric renal failure and a subsequent diuretic phase may occur (91). Avoiding this and other forms of toxicity requires careful monitoring of serum concentrations of aminoglycosides, when feasible, to ensure that drug concentrations are adequate, but are not at potentially toxic levels (85).

Macrolides
Erythromycin

Erythromycin is produced by a strain of *Streptomyces erythraeus* and belongs to the macrolide group of antibiotics. The most frequent side effects of orally administered erythromycin preparations are gastrointestinal and dose related. They include nausea, vomiting, abdominal pain, diarrhea, and anorexia (85). Intravenous administration of the drug can also cause these side effects (92).

Clarithromycin

The most frequently reported side effects experienced by adults taking clarithromycin (Biaxin® tablets) were diarrhea, nausea, abnormal taste, dyspepsia, and abdominal pain or discomfort (85).

Azithromycin

Overall, the most common side effects of azithromycin involved the gastrointestinal system. One study found that these side effects were more common in patients receiving a single-dose regimen of 1 g of azithromycin than among those receiving the multiple-dose regimen (85). Among patients with AIDS,

diarrhea is the principal side effect of azithromycin, but treatment cessation is not usually necessary (93).

Tetracyclines (Doxycycline, Oxytetracycline, and Minocycline)

The use of drugs of the tetracycline class during tooth development (last half of pregnancy, infancy, and childhood to the age of eight years) may cause permanent discoloration of the teeth (yellow, gray, or brown) (85). Nausea, heartburn, epigastric pain, vomiting, and diarrhea are more commonly associated with tetracyclines than with most other orally administered antibiotics (3).

Fluoroquinolones

Some patients treated with ciprofloxacin have experienced nausea, vomiting, diarrhea, abnormalities of the hepatic enzymes, and eosinophilia (3). Headache, restlessness, and rash were also observed among more than 1% of patients treated with the most common doses of ciprofloxacin (85). Moreover, ciprofloxacin may also cause CNS events (94), including dizziness, confusion, tremors, hallucinations, depression, and, rarely, suicidal thoughts or acts. Convulsions, increased intracranial pressure, and toxic psychosis have been observed among patients receiving quinolones, including ciprofloxacin (85). Like ciprofloxacin, ofloxacin is associated with multiple side effects: nausea, insomnia, headache, dizziness, diarrhea, vomiting, rash, and pruritus (95). Some quinolones have been associated with prolongation of the QT interval, as revealed by electrocardiography, and, infrequently, with cases of arrhythmia. Rare cases of torsades de pointes have reportedly occurred in patients taking levofloxacin (85). Temafloxacin was withdrawn from the market after five months of clinical use because of the "temafloxacin syndrome," which is characterized by fever, chills, hemolysis, and jaundice, and is frequently associated with renal failure, hepatic dysfunction, and coagulopathy (96). Because trovafloxacin was found to be associated with death due to hepatic failure, it is now used only to treat critically ill patients.

Antifolate Agents

The most serious type of adverse reaction to sulfonamides (trimethoprim and sulfamethoxazole) is the Steven–Johnson syndrome (97). This syndrome consists of erythema multiforme and ulceration of the mucous membranes of the mouth, eyes, and urethra, and it can sometimes be fatal. Acute agranulocytosis can occur, although it is more commonly associated with the use of older sulfonamides (3).

Miscellaneous
Vancomycin

Vancomycin, when administered rapidly (i.e., over several minutes) as a bolus, may be associated with exaggerated hypotension (98) and, rarely, cardiac arrest (99). During or soon after rapid infusion of vancomycin, patients sometimes experience anaphylactoid reactions such as hypotension, wheezing, dyspnea, urticaria, or pruritus (85). Rapid infusion may also cause flushing of the upper body ("Red Man syndrome") (100) or pain and spasms in the muscles of the chest and back. Although such events usually resolve within 20 minutes, they are infrequent if vancomycin is infused slowly over a 60-minute period (85). Ototoxicity has been reported in association with vancomycin. One study found that most patients who experienced ototoxicity had kidney dysfunction or were receiving an ototoxic drug such as aminoglycoside (101). Nephrotoxicity has occurred among patients who were given vancomycin and aminoglycosides concomitantly, or who had preexisting kidney dysfunction (85).

Clindamycin

Because clindamycin therapy has been associated with severe or even fatal colitis, the use of this agent should be reserved for serious infections for which less-toxic antimicrobial agents are inappropriate. Treatment with antibacterial agents alters the normal flora of the colon and may permit overgrowth of *Clostridium* spp. Studies have indicated that a toxin produced by *Clostridium difficile* is one primary cause of "antibiotic-associated colitis" and can be detected by tissue culture assay. Among some patients, diarrhea, colitis, and PMC occurred several weeks after the cessation of clindamycin therapy (85).

The most serious side effect of clindamycin therapy is PMC. The clinical manifestations of PMC include diarrhea (sometimes watery), cramping, abdominal pain, and fever. Manifestations that occur less frequently include abdominal tenderness with rebound and leukocytosis. The risk of PMC is apparently greater among patients who receive the drug orally than among those who receive it parenterally (4).

PMC is diagnosed by proctoscopy, which reveals raised yellow-whitish plaques on mucosa that is often erythematous or edematous and sometimes friable. The most important treatment for PMC is prompt withdrawal of clindamycin (or other inciting antibiotic). Fluid replacement is important. Among patients with prolonged diarrhea after discontinuation of antimicrobial therapy, several studies conducted (102,103) indicate that vancomycin or metronidazole given by mouth is effective in eliminating *C. difficile* from the colon and subsequently relieving diarrhea. For adults, vancomycin is given orally at a dosage of 500 mg every six hours for 7 to 14 days. There is no effective way to prevent PMC other than the judicious use of antimicrobial agents (4).

Quinpristin–Dalfopristin

One approved indication for the use of quinpristin–dalfopristin is the treatment of patients with serious or life-threatening infections associated with vancomycin-resistant *Enterococcus faecium* bacteremia. Quinpristin–dalfopristin is bacteriostatic against *E. faecium* and bactericidal against strains of methicillin-susceptible and methicillin-resistant *Staphylococcus* spp. The most common adverse reactions that are thought to be related to quinpristin–dalfopristin use are myalgia and arthralgia. Quinpristin–dalfopristin significantly inhibits cytochrome P450 3A4 metabolism of cyclosporine A, midazolam, nifedipine, and terfenadine. The concomitant administration of quinpristin–dalfopristin and other drugs primarily metabolized by the cytochrome P450 3A4 enzyme system may result in increased plasma concentrations of these drugs, which could increase or prolong their therapeutic effect, increase the number or severity of adverse reactions, or both (85).

Linezolid

Linezolid is a member of the oxazolidinone class of antibiotics. It is effective against *Enterococcus faecalis* and *E. faecium* infections and also against MRSA infections. Because myelosuppression has been reported with the use of linezolid, complete blood count should be monitored weekly while patients are taking this drug (104).

Metronidazole

Metronidazole has been shown to be carcinogenic in rodents (105). Convulsive seizures (106) and peripheral neuropathy (107) have been observed among patients treated with metronidazole. Metronidazole (intravenously administered Flagyl®) should be used with care in treating patients with evidence of or history of blood dyscrasia (85) because neutropenia, which is reversible, has been observed during its administration (108).

Chloramphenicol

Hematologic toxicity is the most important adverse effect that complicates the administration of chloramphenicol (3). Adults may experience two types of toxicity involving the hematopoietic system. The first type, which is reversible and dose dependent (3,4), is maturation arrest of bone marrow. This toxicity manifests itself as anemia, leukopenia, thrombocytopenia, and reticulocytopenia. Chloramphenicol is metabolized in the liver, and the inactive metabolites are not toxic. No change in dosage is needed in patients with severe renal failure (4). The second type of hematologic toxicity experienced by adults is bone marrow aplasia, which is very rare and usually irreversible (4). This form of toxicity may appear during the first two weeks of therapy or after a latent period of weeks or months (109). Bone marrow transplantation is the only effective treatment (110). This toxicity is best prevented by limiting the use of chloramphenicol to serious infections that could not be more effectively treated with other drugs. Chloramphenicol should not be administered to patients who have or may have preexisting marrow damage.

Gray baby syndrome is a type of circulatory collapse that can occur among premature and newborn infants who were given chloramphenicol (111).

Antifungal Agents
Azoles

Fluconazole, a synthetic triazole antifungal agent, can cause hepatic reactions that range from mild transient elevations in transaminases to clinical hepatitis, cholestasis and fulminant hepatic failure, and eventually death (85). Fatal hepatic reactions have occurred primarily among patients with serious underlying medical conditions, predominantly AIDS (112).

Polyenes

Amphotericin B is produced by *Streptomyces nodosus* and is one of the drugs of choice for the systemic treatment of invasive fungal infections. The most important side effect of amphotericin B is nephrotoxicity, which results from a reduction in renal blood flow and the glomerular filtration rate. This toxicity may be attenuated by the use of liposomal or lipid emulsion preparations. Renal acidosis occurs more frequently among patients who have received a total dose of 0.5 to 1.0 g or more, and is usually reversible after therapy has been discontinued (3). Although rare, anaphylaxis has been associated with both amphotericin–deoxycholate and liposomal amphotericin B (113).

Antiviral Drugs
Ganciclovir

Ganciclovir should not be administered if the absolute neutrophil count is less than 500, or the platelet count is less than 25,000 (3). Granulocytopenia (neutropenia), anemia, and thrombocytopenia have been observed in patients treated with ganciclovir (Cytovene®). The frequency and severity of these adverse events vary widely among different patient populations. Cell counts usually begin to recover within three to seven days of cessation of drug therapy (85). Colony-stimulating factors have been shown to increase neutrophil and white blood cell counts among patients receiving ganciclovir for the treatment of cytomegalovirus retinitis (114).

Acyclovir

Precipitation of acyclovir crystals in renal tubules can occur if the drug is administered by bolus injection (115). The abnormal renal function that can result from acyclovir administration depends on the state of the patient's hydration, other treatments, and the rate of drug administration. Concomitant use of other nephrotoxic drugs, preexisting renal disease, and dehydration make further renal impairment with acyclovir more likely (85).

Intravenous administration of acyclovir has been associated with neurologic symptoms such as lethargy, obtundation, tremors, confusion, hallucinations, agitation, seizures, or transient hemiparesis (116). Therefore, acyclovir should be used with caution in treating patients who have underlying neurologic abnormalities, and those who have significant hypoxia or serious renal, hepatic, or electrolyte abnormalities (85).

CONCLUSION

In conclusion, despite the medical advances that have been made due to the development of antibiotics, significant complications can occur from their use. Practitioners must remain abreast of the literature regarding the potential complications of the prescribed therapy.

REFERENCES

1. Gleckman RA, Borrego F. Adverse reactions to antibiotics. Clues for recognizing, understanding, and avoiding them. Postgrad Med 1997; 101:97–98, 101–104, 107–108.
2. Rieder MJ. Mechanisms of unpredictable adverse drug reactions. Drug Saf 1994; 11(3):196–212.
3. Kuckers A. Penicillin G. In: Kuckers A, Crowe SM, Grayson ML, Hoy JF, eds. The Use of Antibiotics. A Clinical Review of Antibacterial, Antifungal and Antiviral Drugs. 5th ed. Oxford: Butterworth-Heinemann, 1997:3–70.
4. Mayhall GG. Complications of antibiotic administration. In: Greenfield LG, ed. Complications in Surgery and Trauma. Philadelphia: J.B. Lippincott Company, 1984:193–214.
5. Austen KF. Systemic anaphylaxis in the human being. N Engl J Med 1974; 291:661.
6. Kelly JF, Patterson R. Anaphylaxis. Course, mechanisms and treatment. JAMA 1974; 227:1431.
7. Lin RY. A perspective on penicillin allergy. Arch Intern Med 1992; 152:930.
8. Weinstein L, Weinstein AJ. The pathophysiology and pathoanatomy of reactions to antimicrobial agents. Adv Intern Med 1974; 19:109–134.
9. Mandell GL. Cephalosporins. In: Mandell GL, Douglas RG, Bennett JE, eds. Anti-infective Therapy. New York: John Wiley & Sons, 1985:76–94.
10. Parker CW. Drug allergy. N Engl J Med 1975; 292: 511–514.
11. Vaudaux P, Waldvogel FA. Gentamicin inactivation in purulent exudates: role of cell lysis. J Infect Dis 1980; 142:586–593.
12. Finland M. Changing patterns of susceptibility of common bacterial pathogens to antimicrobial agents. Ann Intern Med 1972; 76:1009–1036.
13. Gross RJ, Ward LR, Threlfall EJ, King H, Rowe B. Drug resistance among infantile enteropathogenic *Escherichia coli* strains isolated in the United Kingdom. Br Med J 1982; 285:472–473.
14. Levy SB. Microbial resistance to antibiotics. An evolving and persistent problem. Lancet 1982; 2(8289):83–88.
15. Lorian V. The antibacterial range: an approach to the assessment of *in vitro* activity of antibiotics. In: Lorian V, ed. Significance of Medical Microbiology in

the Care of Patients. 2nd ed. Baltimore: Williams and Wilkins, 1982:370–382.

16. Fry D. Mechanisms of antibiotic resistance. In: Fry DE, ed. Surgical Infections. 1st ed. Boston: Little, Brown and Company, 1995:73–83.

17. Russell AD. Plasmids and bacterial resistance to biocides. J Appl Microbiol 1997; 83:155–165.

18. Jevons MP, Coe AW, Parker MT. Methicillin resistance staphylococci. Lancet 1963; 1:904–907.

19. National Nosocomial Infections Surveillance Antimicrobial Resistance Report. Atlanta: Centers for Disease Control and Prevention, 1998.

20. Medeiros AA. Beta-lactamases: quality and resistance.

21. Smith TL, Pearson ML, Wilcox KR, et al. Emergence of vancomycin resistance in *Staphylococcus aureus*. Glycopeptide-Intermediate *Staphylococcus aureus* Working Group. N Engl J Med 1999; 340(7):493–501.

22. Yowler CJ, Blinkhorn RJ, Fratianne RB. Vancomycin-dependent enterococcal strains: case report and review. J Trauma 2000; 48(4):783–785.

23. Klastersky J. Antibiotic synergy and antagonism. In: Ristuccia AM, Cunha BA, eds. Antimicrobial Therapy. New York: Raven Press, 1984:37–53.

24. Sabath LD. Theoretical basis of antibiotic: synergy and antagonism. In: Klastersky J, Staquet MJ, eds. Combination Antibiotic Therapy in the Compromised Host. Baltimore: Lippincott Williams & Wilkins, 1982:59–63.

25. Jawetz E. The use of combinations of antimicrobial drugs. Ann Rev Pharmacol 1968; 8:151–170.

26. Best WR. Drug-associated blood dyscrasias. Recent additions to the Registry. JAMA 1963; 185:286–290.

27. Caulfield JB, Burke JE. Inhibition of wound healing by chloramphenicol. Arch Pathol 1971; 92:119–125.

28. Di Berardino L, Giangostino P, Silvestri LG. Antibodies against rifampin patients with tuberculosis after discontinuation of daily treatment. Am Rev Respir Dis 1976; 114:1189–1190.

29. Koeffler HP, Golde DW. Amphotericin inhibition of hematopoiesis in vitro. Am J Hematol 1977; 3:57–62.

30. Spath P, Garratty G, Petz L. Studies on the immune response to penicillin and cephalothin in humans. II. Immunochematologic reactions to cephalothin administration. J Immunol 1971; 107:860–869.

31. Yunis AA. Chloramphenicol-induced bone marrow suppression. Semin Hematol 1973; 10:225–234.

32. Ghilchik MW, Morris AS, Reeves DS. Immunosuppressive powers of the antimicrobial agent trimethoprim. Nature 1970; 227:393–394.

33. Hartmann G, Honikel KO, Knusel J. The specific inhibition of the DNA-directed RNA synthesis by rifamycin. Biochim Biophys Acta 1967; 145:843–844.

34. Buss WC, Morgan R, Guttman J, Barela T, Stalter K. Rifampicin inhibition of protein synthesis in mammalian cells. Science 1978; 200:432–434.

35. Easmon CSF. The effect of antibiotics on the intracellular survival of *Staphylococcus aureus* in vitro. Br J Exp Pathol 1979; 60:24–28.

36. Johnson JD, Hand WL, Francis JB, King-Thompson N, Corwin RW. Antibiotic uptake by alveolar macrophages. J Lab Clin Med 1980; 95:429–439.

37. Klempner MS, Styrt B. Clindamycin uptake by human neutrophils. J Infect Dis 1981; 144:472–479.

38. Lobo MC, Mandell GL. The effect of antibiotics on *Escherichia coli* ingested by macrophages. Proc Soc Exp Biol Med 1973; 142:1048–1050.

39. Mandell GL. Interaction of intraleukocytic bacteria and antibiotics. J Clin Invest 1973; 52:1673–1679.

40. Mohindra JK, Rauth AW. Increased cell killing by metronidazole and nitrofurazone of phyoxic compared to aerobic mammalian cells. Cancer Res 1975; 36:930–936.

41. Pious DA, Hawley P. Effect of antibiotics on respiration in human cells. Pediatr Res 1972; 6:687–692.

42. Alexander JW. Antibiotic agents and the immune mechanisms of defense. Bull NY Acad Med 1975; 51: 1939–1945.

43. Finch R. Immunomodulating effects of antimicrobial agents. J Antimicrob Chemother 1980; 6:691–699.

44. Gillissen G. Antibiotika und immunantwortbegleiteffekte der chemotherapie. Immun Infekt 1980; 8:79–88.

45. Hauser WE Jr, Remington JS. Effect of antibiotics on the immune response. Am J Med 1982; 72:711–716.

46. Mandell LA. Effects of antimicrobial and antineoplastic drugs on the phagocytic and microbicidal function of the polymorphonuclear leukocyte. Rev Infect Dis 1982; 4:683–697.

47. Raeburn JA. Antibiotics and immunodeficiency. Lancet 1972; 2:954–955.

48. Stites DP. Clinical laboratory methods of detecting cellular immunity. In: Stites DP, Terr AI, Parslow TG, eds. Basic and Clinical Immunology. 8th ed. Norwalk, Connecticut: Appleton & Lange, 1994:195–215.

49. Lafferty WE, Brewer LA, Corey L. Alteration of lymphocyte transformation response to herpes simplex virus infection by acyclovir therapy. Antimicrob Ag Chemother 1984; 26:887.

50. Terr AI. Inflammation. In: Stites DP, Terr AI, Parslow TG, eds. Basic and Clinical Immunology. 8th ed. Norwalk, Connecticut: Appleton & Lange, 1994:137–150.

51. Moshkowitz A, Goldblum N, Heller E. Studies on the antiviral effect of rifampin in volunteers. Nature 1971; 229:422–424.

52. Desen P, Clark RA, Nauseef WM. Granulocytic phagocytes. In: Mandell GL, Bennett JE, Dolin R, eds. Mandell, Douglas and Bennett's Principles and Practice of Infectious Diseases. 4th ed. New York: Churchill Livingstone, 1995:78–101.

53. Herberman RB, Holden HT. Natural cell-mediated immunity. Adv Cancer Res 1978; 27:305–377.

54. Hauser WE Jr, Sharma SD, Remington JS. Natural killer cells induced by acute and chronic toxoplasma infection. Cell Immunol 1982; 69:330–346.

55. Hauser WE Jr, Remington JS. Effect of amphotericin B on natural killer cell activity *in vitro*. J Antimicrob Chemother 1983; 11:257–262.

56. Griffin GE. New insights into the pathophysiology of the Jarisch-Herxheimer reaction. J Antimicrob Chemother 1992; 29:613.

57. Gefland JA, Elin RJ, Berry FW Jr, Frank MM. Endotoxemia associated with the Jarisch-Herxheimer reaction. N Engl J Med 1976; 295:211.

58. Stevenson J, Mandal BK. Ampicillin and the fifth day rash. Br Med J 1966; 1:1359.

59. Prospective study of ampicillin rash. Report of a Collaborative Study Group. Br Med J 1973; 1(5844):7–9.

60. Bass JW, Crowley DM, Steele RW, et al. Adverse effects of orally administered ampicillin. J Pediatr 1973; 83: 106.

61. Reading C, Cole M. Calvulanic acid: a beta-lactamase inhibiting beta-lactam from *Streptomyces calvuligerus*. Antimicrob Ag Chemother 1977; 11:852.

62. Reading C, Farmer T, Cole M. The beta-lactamase stability of amoxycillin with b-lactamase inhibitor, calvulanic acid. J Antimicrob Chemother 1983; 11:27.

63. Williams ME, Thomas D, Harman CP, et al. Positive direct antiglobulin tests due to calvulanic acid. Antimicrob Ag Chemother 1985; 27:125.

64. Foulds G. Pharmacokinetics of sulbactam/ampicillin in humans: a review. Rev In Dis 1986; 8(suppl 5):503.

65. Kuye O, Teal J, De Vries VG, et al. Safety profile of piperacillin/tazobactam in phase I and III clinical studies. J Antimicrob Chemother 1993; 31(suppl A):113.

66. Fass RJ, Copelan EA, Brandt JT, et al. Platelet-mediated bleeding caused by broad-spectrum penicillins. J Infect Dis 1987; 155:1242.

67. Ferres H, Nunn B. Penicillin metabolites and platelet function. Lancet 1983; ii:226.

68. Gentry LO, Wood BA, Natelson EA. Effects of apalcillin on platelet function in normal volunteers. Antimicrob Ag Chemother 1985; 27:683.

69. Levine BB. Antigenecity and cross-reactivity of penicillins and cephalosporins. J Infect Dis 1973; 128(suppl):364.

70. Petz LD. Immunologic cross-reactivity between penicillins and cephalosporins: a review. J Infect Dis 1978; 137(suppl):74.

71. Dash CH. Penicillin allergy and the cephalosporins. J Anitmicrob Chemother 1975; 1(suppl):107.

72. Boguniewicz M, Leung DYM. Hypersensitivity reactions to antibiotics used commonly in children. Pediatr Inf Dis J 1995; 14:221.

73. Ries K, Levison ME, Kaye D. Clinical and in vitro evaluation of cefazolin, a new cephalosporins antibiotic. Antmicrob Ag Chemother 1973; 3:168.

74. Moellering RC Jr, Swartz MN. Drug therapy: the newer cephalosporins. N Engl J Med 1976; 294:24.

75. Turck M. Cephalosporins and related antibiotics: an overview. Rev Inf Dis 1982; 4(suppl):281.

76. Cazzola M, Matera MG, Santangelo G, et al. Effects of some cephalosporins and teicoplanin on platelet aggregation. Int J Clin Pharmacol Res 1993; 13(2):69–73.

77. Trollfors B, Alestig K, Norrby R. Local and gastrointestinal reactions to intravenously administered cefoxitin and cefuroxime Scan. J Infect Dis 1979; 11:315.

78. Norrby R, Foord RD, Hedlund P. Clinical and pharmacokinetic studies on cefuroxime. J Antimicrob Chemother 1977; 3:355.

79. Manzella JP, Clark JK. Effects of Moxalactam and cefuroxime on mitogen-stimulated human mononuclear leucocytes. Antimicrob Ag Chemother 1983; 23:360.

80. Kuckers A. Cefotetan. In: Kuckers A, Crowe SM, Grayson ML, Hoy JF, eds. The Use of Antibiotics. A Clinical Review of Antibacterial, Antifungal and Antiviral Drugs. 5th ed. Oxford: Butterworth-Heinemann, 1997:395–397.

81. Dunn GL. Ceftizoxime and other third generation cephalosporins: structure-activity relationships. J Antimicrob Chemother 1982; 10(suppl C):1.

82. Skyes RB, Bonner DP. Discovery and development of monobactams. Rev Infect Dis 1985; 7(suppl 4):279.

83. Tunkel AR, Scheld WM. Aztreonam. Infect Control Hosp Epidemiol 1990; 11:486.

84. El-Touny M, El Guinaidy M, Barry MA, et al. Pharmacokinetics of aztreonam in patients with liver cirrhosis and ascites. J Antimicrob Chemother 1992; 30:387.

85. The PDR® Electronic Library. Montvale, NJ: Medical Economics Company, Inc., 2001.

86. Patel JB, Giles RE. Meropenem: evidence of lack of proconvulsive tendency in mice. J Antimicrob Chemother 1989; 24(suppl A):307.

87. Bedikian A, Okamoto MP, Nkahiro RK, et al. Pharmacokinetics of meropenem in patients with intra-abdominal infections. Antimicrob Ag Chemother 1994; 38:151.

88. Appel GB, Neu HC. Gentamicin in 1978. Ann Intem Med 1978; 89:528.

89. Meyer RD. Amikacin. Ann Intern Med 1981; 95:328.

90. Hall DR, McGibbon DH, Evans CC, Meadows GA. Gentamicin, tubocurarine, lignocaine and neuromuscular blockade. Br J Anaesth 1972; 44:1329.

91. Khan T, Stein RM. Gentamycin and renal failure. Lancet 1972; I:498.

92. Itoh Z, Suzuki T, Nakaya M, et al. Gastrointestinal motor-stimulating activity of macrolide antibiotics and analysis of their side-effects on the canine gut. Antimicrob Ag Chemother 1984; 26:863.

93. Young LS, Wiviott L, Wu M, et al. Azithromycin for treatment of *Mycobacterium avium-intracellulare* complex infection in patients wit AIDS. Lancet 1991; 338:1107.

94. Christ W. Central nervous system toxicity of quinolones: human and animal findings. J Antimicrob Chemother 1990; 26(suppl B):219.

95. Tack KJ, Smith JA. The safety profile of ofloxacin. Am J Med 1989; 87:78S.

96. Blum MD, Graham DJ, McCloskey CA. Temafloxacin syndrome: review of 95 cases. Clin Infect Dis 1994; 18:946.

97. Claxton RC. A review of 31 cases of Steven-Johnson syndrome. Med J Aust 1963; 1:963.

98. Newfield P, Roizen MF. Hazards of rapid administration of vancomycin. Ann Intern Med 1979; 91:581.

99. Glicklich D, Figura I. Vancomycin and cardiac arrest. Ann Intern Med 1984; 101:808.

100. Polk RE, Healy DP, Schwartz LB, et al. Vancomycin and the red man syndrome: pharmacodynamics and histamine release. J Infect Dis 1988; 157:502.

101. Brummett RE, Fox KE, Jacobs F, et al. Augmented gentamicin ototoxicity induced by vancomycin in guinea pigs. Arch Otolaryngol Head Neck Surg 1990; 116:61.

102. Batts DH, Martin D, Holmes R. Treatment of antibiotic-associated *Clostridium difficile* diarrhea with oral vancomycin. J Pediatr 1980; 97:151.

103. Keighley MRB, Burdon DW, Arabi Y. Randomized controlled trial of vancomycin for pseudomembranous colitis and postoperative diarrhea. Br Med J 1978; 2:1667.

104. Zyvox Prescribing Information, Pharmacia Upjohn, 2002.

105. Rustia M, Shubik P. Induction of lung tumours and malignant lymphomas in mice by mitronidazole. J Natl Cancer Inst 1972; 48:721.

106. Frytak S, Moertel CG, Childs DS, Albers JW. Neurologic toxicity associated with high dose metronidazole therapy. Am Int Med 1978; 88:361.

107. Bradley WG, Karlsson IJ, Rassol CG. Metronidazole neuropathy. Br Med J 1977; 2:610.

108. Mckendrick MW, Geddes AM. Neutropenia associated with metronidazole. Br Med J 1979; 2:795.

109. Polak BCP, Wesseliny H, Dicu S. Blood dyscriasis attributed to Cholramphenicol. Acta Med Scan 1972; 192:409–418.

110. Storb R, Thomas ED, Buckner CD. Marrow transplantation in thirty "untransfused" patients with severe aplastic anemia. Am Int Med 1980; 92:30.

111. Sutherland JM. Fatal cardiovascular collapse of infants receiving large amounts of chloramphenicol. Am. J Dis Child 1959; 97:761.

112. Jacobson MA, Hanks DK, Ferrell LD. Fatal acute hepatic necrosis due to fluconazole. Am J Med 1994; 96:188.

113. Bates CM, Carey PB, Hind CR. Anaphylaxis due to liposomal amphotericin (AmBiosome). Genitourin Med 1995; 71:414.

114. Hardy D, Spector S, Polsky B, et al. Combination of gancylovir and granulocyte-macrophage colony stimulating factor in the treatment of cytomegalovirus retinitis in AIDS patients. The ACTG 073 team. Eur J Clin Microbiol Infect Dis 1994; 13:S34.

115. Tucker WE Jr. Preclinical toxicology of acyclovir: an overview. Am J Med 1982; 73:27.

116. Johnson GL, Limon L, Trikha G, Wall H. Acute renal failure and neurotoxicity following oral acyclovir. Ann Pharmacother 1994; 28:460.

4

Complications of Blood and Blood-Product Transfusion

Igor Jeroukhimov
Department of Surgery, Assaf Harophe Medical Center, Tel Aviv University, Zerifin, Israel

Mauricio Lynn
Division of Trauma and Surgical Critical Care, DeWitt Daughtry Family Department of Surgery, University of Miami, Miller School of Medicine, Miami, Florida, U.S.A.

Transfusion therapy continues to be widely discussed throughout all of medicine but particularly in surgery, where great regional and local variation in blood and blood product use can be documented (1).

Each year in the United States, approximately 11 million units of blood are transfused into about four million patients (2). The transfusion of blood products can cause numerous serious complications, even death, and therefore, blood products should be considered potentially dangerous substances. The main perceived risks of blood and blood products are primarily related to transmission of infectious diseases. Although these risks are actually decreasing steadily as newer screening tests are introduced and better antiviral processing and storage capabilities evolve, the risks of blood-related transmission of infectious disease continues to be a problem (3). In recent years, transfusion therapy has also been linked to serious adverse consequences of immune suppression, which involve postoperative infectious complications or tumor recurrence. Survival is decreased in patients with breast or colon cancer who received blood (4). Finally, it must be recognized that a blood-banking "system" is in large part dependent on human input for decisions and processing and thus subject to human error. In the case of fatal transfusion reactions— basically, transfusion of incompatible blood—"clerical error" continues to be the primary cause. Awareness of all these risks has forced the medical community to consider alternatives to transfusion, which frequently include a "transfusion avoidance strategy" (5).

HISTORICAL BACKGROUND

Since ancient times, blood has been regarded as synonymous with life. The ancients considered blood "the seat of the soul" and believed that it carried the physical and mental qualities of the person through whom it flowed (6).

In June 1667, Jean Baptiste Denis of Paris performed the first blood transfusion from animal to man. However, after the death of one of his patients, the French Parliament banned the practice of blood transfusion by issuing an edict on April 17, 1668 (7). This injunction halted the further development of blood transfusion for the next 150 years.

In 1818, a group of London obstetricians headed by James Blundell initiated direct man-to-man transfusion for acute hemorrhage. However, Blundell and later the German physician Landois discovered the undesirability of heterologous transfusion, primarily because of the high incidence of hemolysis and renal shutdown. Lindois' work from 1875 marked the end of any further heterogeneous transfusion.

In 1900, Karl Landsteiner from the University of Vienna discovered three blood groups (8), and two years later Von De Castello and Sturli identified the fourth and rarest one (9).

Clotting of blood during transfusion plagued all the early experiments and probably prevented many unfortunate outcomes of the procedure. In 1914, M. Hustin of Belgium introduced the use of citrate in collecting blood (10), and in 1916, Rous added glucose to lengthen the life span of the erythrocytes, thus permitting "delayed" transfusion (10). Many other improvements in blood storage and preservations were implemented before blood transfusion appeared to be relatively safe.

PHYSIOLOGY OF TRANSFUSION THERAPY

The indications for transfusion can be divided into two broad categories. The most common reason for transfusion is to enhance the oxygen-carrying capability of blood by expanding the red blood cell (RBC) mass. The second most common reason is to replace clotting factors that are lost, consumed, or not produced (11).

Enhancement of Oxygen-Carrying Capacity

Most oxygen atoms in arterial blood bind reversibly, which serve as a carrier for oxygen. If cardiac output is adequate, increasing the RBC mass will increase the oxygen-carrying capacity of the blood.

Nevertheless, the release of oxygen to the tissue is dependent on many factors. The most important is probably oxygen saturation of hemoglobin. As the degree of saturation increases, the binding affinity decreases and the release of oxygen to the tissues is enhanced.

Adequate tissue oxygenation depends not only on adequate delivery of oxygen, but also on the oxygen demands of the tissue. Under normal circumstances, the rate of oxygen delivery (1000 mL/min) is substantially greater than the rate of oxygen consumption (250 mL/min). Despite this large difference, clinical circumstances occur in which oxygen consumption exceeds delivery; one example of such a circumstance is massive multisystem injury and sepsis.

Traditionally, a hemoglobin concentration of 10 g/dL has been considered the lowest value acceptable before elective surgery. However, the limits of acceptability are currently being challenged. It is well known that hemoglobin concentration of 6 to 7 g/dL is well tolerated in patients with chronic renal failure. A hemoglobin concentration of 7 to 8 g/dL has been demonstrated to be adequate, except for patients with coronary artery disease or chronic obstructive pulmonary disease. Although there has been no widely accepted agreement on the lowest acceptable hemoglobin concentration before elective surgery, it is clear that the rate and magnitude of blood loss, the state of tissue perfusion, and the presence of cardiopulmonary disease affect patients' abilities to tolerate low concentrations of hemoglobin.

Decreased concentrations of 2,3-diphosphoglycerate increase the binding affinity between oxygen and hemoglobin. In fact, 2,3-DPG levels may decrease by 30% in blood stored for greater than two weeks, and by 60% to 70% in three weeks.

Enhancement of Hemostasis

The second most common reason for transfusion of blood products is to replace hemostatic agents. Surgeons should understand the pathophysiology of hemostasis before using replacement products. These products should be used only in preparation for elective surgery or for treating patients with clinically significant abnormalities in hemostasis, such as disorders of consumption or production of fibrinogen, extrinsic or intrinsic coagulation factor defects, and platelet dysfunction.

ROLE OF COMPONENT THERAPY

The primary indications for transfusion of packed RBCs, fresh frozen plasma (FFP), and platelets are

Table 1 Indications and Contraindications for Blood and Its Component Transfusion

Blood products	Major indications	Major contraindications
Whole blood	Acute blood loss	Chronic anemia
Packed RBCs	Symptomatic anemia	Anemia responsive to proper medication
Washed RBCs	Symptomatic anemia, febrile reaction to packed RBCs	Anemia responsive to proper medication
Frozen RBCs	Symptomatic anemia, RBC incompatibility	Anemia responsive to proper medication
Platelets concentrate	Thrombocytopenia	Presence of antiplatelet antibodies
Fresh frozen plasma	Deficiency of labile coagulation factors	Need for high-potency coagulation factors
Cryoprecipitate	Hemophilia A, von Willebrand's disease, Hypofibrinogenemia	Need for high-potency coagulation factors

Abbreviations: RBCs, red blood cells.

acute hemorrhage, coagulopathy, and thrombocytopenia, respectively. Contraindications for the use of these products are chronic anemia and anemia responsive to the other therapy. Indications and contraindications for other blood products are listed in Table 1.

PATHOPHYSIOLOGY OF BLOOD TRANSFUSION

Complications associated with blood transfusion can be serious and sometimes fatal. These complications can be categorized as immunologic reactions, metabolic disturbances, and infectious complications (Fig. 1).

Immunologic Complications

The immunologic consequences of receiving blood from donors are of great importance. Patients can become sensitized to antigens on transfused RBCs and other accompanying blood cells [platelets and white blood cells (WBC)]. Women can also become sensitized and form antibodies to these blood group antigens from exposure to blood cells carried by their babies during pregnancy. Because sensitization to red cell antigens can induce hemolytic disease of the newborn, transfusions of blood from blood banks should be avoided, whenever possible, by women who may later choose to bear children (12).

Immunologic complications of blood transfusion are characterized as hemolytic (red cell type) and nonhemolytic (non–red cell type). The nonhemolytic reactions are the most frequent and lead to the development of fever and urticaria, hives, or asthma after the administration of blood. The incidence of these reactions is approximately 2% to 10% (13). They may be related to leukocytes or proteins, and the incidence of these reactions may be reduced by the use of packed RBC or special filters for the removal of leukocytes from blood (14).

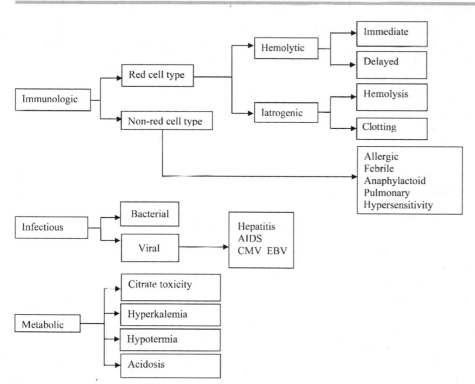

Figure 1 Complications of blood transfusion. *Abbreviations*: AIDS, acquired immunodeficiency syndrome; EBV, Epstein-Barr virus; CMV, Cytomegalovirus.

Febrile Reactions

Elevation in basal core temperature occurs in as many as 7% of transfusion recipients, but is usually self-limiting (11). Having undergone transfusions previously contributes to the development of fever-causing antibodies. The incidence of antileukocyte antibody development is high and increases with repeated exposure to blood and blood products.

Febrile reactions are diagnosed by exclusion. Therefore, when fever occurs during transfusion, the transfusion should be stopped and studies should be conducted to rule out hemolysis. If hemolysis is not a possibility, the patient may be given antipyretic agents (15). Patients may also develop hypotension, cyanosis, tachypnea, transient leucopoenia, or a syndrome of self-limiting fibrinolysis. A high level of leukoagglutinins in donor plasma may contribute to the reaction. The severity of the reaction depends on the magnitude of the antibody titer, the degree of increase in the number of leukocytes, and the rate at which the blood was transfused. The differential diagnosis includes red cell incompatibility, bacterial contamination, and unrelated disease process.

Antihistamines are not effective in the treatment of febrile reaction; therefore, premedication is not indicated with future transfusions (16).

Allergic Reaction

Two percent of transfusion reactions are classified as allergic reactions that result from the transfusion of antigen or immunoglobulin to which patient has pre-existing antibodies (17). A blood transfusion recipient can experience an allergic reaction to either medications or food ingested by the donor. The reaction can vary in severity from urticaria to anaphylaxis. Furthermore, allergic reaction can develop as a result of the passive transfer of sensitizing antibodies. When the recipient subsequently encounters the allergen to which the donor has produced antibodies, the recipient can experience an allergic reaction to that allergen. Unlike delayed hemolytic or febrile reactions, an allergic reaction does not require prior exposure to blood. The initial symptoms associated with allergic reactions are usually urticaria and pruritus. In mild cases, antihistamines may be used to decrease the number and severity of symptoms. Reactions of moderate severity have been described as "anaphylactoid." Less common is a full anaphylactic response characterized by hypotension, cutaneous flushing, and bronchospasm. In this situation, the transfusion should be stopped, and epinephrine may be required to support hemodynamics and relive bronchospasm (15). Reactions have been reported to be especially severe if anti-IgA antibodies are the cause of the crisis. IgA-associated reactions are also characterized by the initial symptoms of diarrhea and abdominal pain, in addition to hemodynamic instability and bronchospasm (18).

With future transfusions, the use of washed RBCs may decrease the incidence of anaphylactic reactions. Furthermore, the customary type and cross-match test should be supplemented with an assay for complement-activating activity.

Graft vs. Host Disease

Graft versus host disease (GVHD) occurs after the infusion of immunocompetent cells into a recipient whose immune system is incapable of rejecting the foreign cells (e.g., a patient with a deficiency in cell-mediated immunity). Consequently, the infused immunocompetent cells initiate rejection of the normal host tissues and thus cause GVHD. Acute GVHD also occurs in recipients of allogenic bone marrow transplants and in persons with primary immunodeficiencies who receive viable allogenic lymphocytes (19).

Blood products that place patients at risk of GVHD are whole blood, packed RBCs, fresh plasma, granulocytes, and platelets. GVHD has not been seen after transfusion of frozen blood, FFP, cryoprecipitate, or washed red cells. Irradiated blood products also may be given safely (20).

The initial signs and symptoms of GVHD involve many organ systems, including the skin, liver, gastrointestinal tract, and bone marrow. Fever occurs first; 24 to 48 hours later, a generalized erythroderma begins to appear on the face (frequently behind the ears), and then spreads to the trunk and extremities. Bullous formations can occur. Skin biopsy shows extensive lymphocytic infiltration. Other signs and symptoms that may occur are anorexia, nausea, vomiting, diarrhea, and hepatocellular dysfunction due to the increased activity of liver enzymes and pancytopenia.

GVHD usually occurs 2 to 30 days after transfusion (21). Fifty percent of patient with reported GVHD received a cationic drug before transfusion. The high mortality rate associated with GVHD results from severe bone marrow hypoplasia or aplasia, or from failure in bone marrow regeneration. Secondary infections occur as a result of agranulocytosis. There have been no reports of the occurrence of GVHD among immunologically competent persons or among those lacking only humoral immunity (22).

Posttransfusion Purpura

Posttransfusion purpura is a rare form of acute hemorrhagic thrombocytopenia that appears one week after transfusion and primarily affects multiparous women who lack the platelet-specific antigen (PLA) 1 [human platelet antigen (HPA) 1] (23). Anti-PLA1 antibodies are detected in the serum of most affected patients, but the precise mechanism of platelet destruction is unclear. Thrombocytopenia (platelet counts less than 50,000) results in bleeding from the skin and mucous membranes. Additional transfusions, even with platelets, accentuate the thrombocytopenia, but plasmapheresis and exchange transfusion have resulted in some benefit. The syndrome spontaneously abates in several days to months (16).

Transfusion-Related Acute Lung Injury

Transfusion-related acute lung injury is an acute respiratory distress syndrome that develops within four hours after transfusion of blood and is characterized by dyspnea and hypoxia due to noncardiogenic pulmonary edema. Although the actual incidence is not well known and its occurrence is almost certainly underreported, this injury has been estimated to occur once in approximately 5000 transfusions (24). This injury is most likely the result of several possible mechanisms. In some cases, blood donor's antibodies with specificity to human leucocyte antigen (HLA) or neutrophilic antigenics react with recipient's neutrophils; thus, this reaction leads to increased permeability of the pulmonary microcirculation.

Reactive lipid products that arise during storage of blood products have been recently been implicated in the pathophysiology of transfusion-related acute lung injury (25). Such substances are capable of neutrophil priming, with subsequent damage to pulmonary capillary endothelium in the recipient, particularly in the setting of sepsis. As in other cases of acute respiratory distress syndrome, therapy is indicated; at least 90% of the patients with transfusion-related acute lung injury recover (26).

Hemolytic Reaction

Hemolytic (RBC type) reactions occur as a result of the interaction between the antibodies in the plasma of the recipient and the antigens on the RBCs of the donor. These reactions can be acute (i.e., appear within minutes after beginning of the transfusion) or delayed (causing clinical symptoms 3 to 21 days after transfusion). Compared with other reactions, severe hemolytic reactions are associated with the highest morbidity and mortality rates.

Acute Hemolytic Reaction

Forty-five percent of acute hemolytic reactions are the result of errors in which blood samples were incorrectly identified, or the wrong type of blood was administered to the patient. Half of fatal hemolytic reactions occur among patients with O-negative blood and previously unidentified antibodies; the other half occur among patients with non–O blood who continued to receive type O blood and thus developed "admixture" blood types, which caused difficulty in subsequent crossmatching (14). To avoid these errors, the American Association of Blood Banks recommends that two unique identifiers (e.g., name and hospital identification number) always be used when linking blood products and blood samples to the intended patient (27).

Acute hemolytic reaction begins with the transfusion of as little as few milliliters of incompatible blood, and its severity is proportional to the volume of blood to which the recipient is exposed (28). This type of reaction is characterized by pain at the infusion site, fever, chills, back and substernal pain, mental status changes, dyspnea, hypotension, facial flashing, cyanosis, and a bleeding diathesis (11,28). During a surgical procedure, the only evidence of an acute hemolytic reaction may be hypertension and myoglobinuria. Most of these manifestations result from RBC–antibody complexes that activate complement and liberate anaphylatoxins, histamine, and serotonin (28). These complexes also activate Factor XII, with the release of bradykinin and activation of the extrinsic coagulation cascade, with resultant disseminated intravascular coagulation (DIC) (17).

Severe hemolytic reactions are also associated with renal cortical ischemia and subsequent redistribution of blood flow from the cortex to the medulla. Volume restoration corrects hypovolemia, but reperfusion induces oxygen free-radical formation, which further interfere with renal function (29).

By several mechanisms, hemoglobinuria decreases renal function. Acidosis and sluggish glomerular filtration (associated with shock) promote the precipitation of hemoglobin, with blockage of renal tubules. Filtered antigen–antibody complexes may activate compliment and induce a local inflammatory response. In addition, ferric ions associated with hemoglobin promote the oxygen free radical (Huber–Weiss reaction); such free-radical formation may account for the synergistic deterioration in renal function that occurs with hypotension and concomitant hemoglobinuria (30). When acute hemolytic reaction is suspected, the transfusion should be stopped immediately. The free hemoglobin and haptoglobin concentrations in the patient's serum should be assessed, and a direct Coombs' test should be performed. Serum haptoglobin concentration decreases markedly after hemolysis because the protein binds to free hemoglobin to augment its clearance through the reticuloendothelial system. The direct Coombs' test, in which antiglobulin antibodies are mixed with the patient's RBCs, detects RBC–antibody complexes. The blood product in question should be returned to the blood bank for repeated type- and cross-match tests (16).

Patients who are experiencing an acute hemolytic reaction characterized by urticaria or other allergic phenomena should receive diphenhydramine (Benadryl® 50 mg) intramuscularly or intravenously immediately and every six hours as needed. In addition, Ringer's lactate solution should be administered intravenously with 12.5 to 25 mg of mannitol to ensure copious output of urine (100 to 200 mL/hour). One to two ampules of sodium bicarbonate can be added to each liter of fluid to alkalinize the urine to a pH of at least 6.5. If shock occurs, hydrocortisone and additional fluids should be administered (14).

Delayed Hemolytic Reaction

Delayed hemolytic reactions are usually mild and appear 3 to 21 days after transfusion. The incidence of this type of reaction is 1 per 4000 transfusions. Delayed hemolytic reactions affect patients who have previously been exposed to blood products (e.g., patients who have been pregnant or have received transfusions) and have experienced a quick anamnestic response as a result of the previous sensitization. Several days after transfusion, patients experience hemolysis, which is characterized by jaundice, hemoglobinuria, and decreased hematocrit. However, as many as 35% of patients experience no symptoms (31).

The diagnosis is confirmed by an elevation in the serum concentration of indirect bilirubin, hemoglobinuria, and a decrease in the serum concentration of haptoglobin. Repeated type and screen tests of the donor's blood often detect previously unrecognized serum antibody to Kidd (JK^a and JK^b), Rh (D, E, and C), Duffy (Fy^a and Fy^b), or Kell (K) antigens (32). Furthermore, a repeated cross-match test using the patient's current serum often shows transfusion to be incompatible. Delayed hemolytic reactions are self-limiting, require no specific treatment, and do not affect the patient's compatibility in relation to future transfusions (16).

Iatrogenic Complications

Two other forms of red cell reactions are worth mentioning. Iatrogenic hemolysis is induced if blood is administered with 5% glucose and water, rather than with saline. These patients will display signs and symptoms of immediate massive hemolysis. Iatrogenic clotting will occur if blood is administered with a calcium-containing solution such as Ringer's lactate solution. If these clots are pushed into the circulation, massive pulmonary emboli will result (11).

Immune Suppression

The association between blood transfusion and immune suppression is receiving increased attention. Nonviable RBC and particulate matter found in blood products before transfusions may impede the reticuloendothelial system's ability to clear bacteria; such a block thereby predisposes the recipient to sepsis (33).

Tumor Recurrence

The fact that patients who received allogenic blood transfusions are at increased risk of postoperative infection and cancer recurrence suggests that such transfusions are associated with clinically significant immunomodulatory effects (34,35). Indeed, numerous reports have suggested an increase in tumor recurrence and a decrease in survival for transfusion recipients who have colorectal, breast, cervical, lung, prostate, or head and neck tumors. Because allogenic transfusions increase humoral immune responses and decrease cell-mediated responses, the mechanism of allogenic transfusion-induced immunomodulation may involve altered cytokine regulation that results in shift toward a type 2 (Th_2) immune response (36–38).

Septic Complications

Transfusions of RBCs are associated with an increase in septic complications among patients undergoing surgical procedures for carcinoma of the colon (38,39) and among patients who have suffered from multiple trauma (40). Among patients undergoing hip replacement or spine surgery, the postoperative infection rate with allogenic blood transfusion appears to be 7 to 10 times higher than that associated with autologous blood or absence of transfusion.

Infectious Complications

The primary perceived risks associated with the transfusion of blood and blood products are related to the transmission of infectious diseases. Although these risks are steadily decreasing as newer screening tests are introduced and better antiviral processing and storage capabilities evolve, such risks continue to be a problem (4,5). Recent estimates of the infectious risk per unit of blood are shown in (Table 2) (26).

Transmission of HIV

The first description of transfusion-associated human immunodeficiency virus (HIV) infection occurred in 1983 (41,42). After the implementation of HIV-antibody testing in 1985 (43), approximately five cases of transfusion-related HIV infection per year were recorded, whereas 714 cases were reported in 1984 (44). To decrease the risk of transfusion-transmitted HIV disease, blood banks began to test donors for p24 antigen in late 1995 (45). Nevertheless, the estimated risk of transfusion-associated HIV infection is now calculated as 1 per 200,000 to 2,000,000 units of blood transfused; thus, transfusion-associated HIV infection results in 0.5 to 5 deaths per million units of blood transfused (3).

Table 2   Risk of Blood Transfusion

Risk factor	Estimated per million units	Frequency per actual unit	No. of deaths per million units
Viral Infection			
Viral			
Hepatitis A	1	1/1,000,000	0
Hepatitis B	7–32	1/30,000– 1/250,000	0–0.14
Hepatitis C	4–36	1/30,000– 1/150,000	0.5–17
HIV	0.4–5	1/200,00– 1/2,000,000	0.5–5
HTLV types I and II	0.5–4	1/250,00– 1/2,000,000	0
Parvovirus B 19	100	1/10,000	0
Bacterial contamination			
Red cells	2	1/500,000	0.1–0.25
Platelets	83	1/12,000	21

Abbreviations: HIV, human immunodeficiency virus; HTLV, human T lymphotropic virus.

Transmission of Hepatitis B and C Viruses

In 1975, the implementation of third-generation screening tests for the surface antigens of hepatitis B virus (HBV) led to marked reduction in transfusion-transmitted HBV infection. Today, this infection accounts for approximately 10% of all cases of hepatitis after transfusion (46). Although an acute disease appeared in approximately 35% of infected persons, chronic infection develops in only 1% to 10% of patients. The estimated risk of transfusion-transmitted HBV infection is 7 to 32 per million units of blood transfused, or 1 case per 30,000 to 250,000 units transfused blood (3).

The estimated risk of transfusion-transmitted hepatitis C virus (HCV) is now in 103,000 transfusions (3). However, if one considers the unlikely possibility of chronic, immunologically silent state of infection, the risk of HCV may be as great as 1 in 30,000. Transfusion-transmitted HCV infection is important because the infection becomes chronic in 85% of cases, leads to cirrhosis in 20%, and results in hepatocellular carcinoma in 1% to 5% of cases (47).

Transmission of Other Viruses

The incidence of hepatitis G viremia in donors in the United States is 1% to 2%. Although the virus can be transmitted by transfusion, there is no evidence that it is particularly hepatotrophic or causes disease (48).

Transmission of hepatitis A virus by blood transfusion has been estimated to occur in one case per one million units of blood transfused (49). Hepatitis A infection is not commonly associated with blood transfusion because the absence of chronic carrier state and the presence of the symptoms that would eliminate the infected person as a potential donor during the brief viremic phase of the illness.

The risk of transfusion-related transmission of parvovirus B 19 is highly variable from year to year (50,51). Infection is usually not clinically significant except in certain populations such as pregnant women (in whom the virus can cause hydrops fetalis), patients with hemolytic anemia (in whom aplastic crisis may develop), and immunocompromised patients (in whom chronic aplastic anemia may develop).

Infection will develop in 20% to 60% of recipients of blood infected by human T-lymphotropic virus-I (HTLV-I) or HTLV-II (3). The rate of transmission is affected by the length of time that blood has been stored and by the number of WBCs in the unit. Blood that has been stored for more than 14 days and noncellular blood products such as cryoprecipitate and FFP do not appear to be infectious (52). The estimated risk of transfusion-related HTLV-I or HTLV-II infection is 0.5 to 4 cases per 1,000,000 units (53). Myelopathy can occur in persons infected with HTLV-I or HTLV-II (54).

Bacterial Contamination

The organism most commonly implicated in bacterial contamination of red cells is *Yersinia enterocolitica* (3).

Bacterial contamination of blood units is directly related to the length of storage, but *Yersinia* sp. RBC sepsis has been observed after transfusion of RBCs that had been stored as few as 7 to 14 days. In the United States, fewer than one per one million RBC units is contaminated.

Grossly contaminated units of RBCs can sometimes be identified by comparing the color of the blood bag with the color of the blood in the attached tubing; contaminated blood in the bag will appear darker as a result of hemolysis and decreased oxygen content (55).

The risk of platelet-related sepsis is estimated to be 1 case per 12,000 units transfused, but it is greater with transfusion of pooled platelet concentrates from multiple donors than for transfusion of platelet units obtained by aphaeresis from the single donor (56). Because of the risk of bacterial overgrowth with time, the shelf life of platelets stored at 20°C to 24°C is five days. In descending order, the organisms most commonly implicated in death due to bacterial contamination are *Staphylococcus aureus*, *Klebsiella pneumonia*, *Serratia marcescens*, and *Staphylococcus epidermidis* (57). The initial clinical signs associated with platelet-related sepsis vary more than those associated with transfusion of bacterially contaminated RBCs do and can range from mild fever (which can be undistinguishable from that seen with nonhemolytic febrile transfusion reactions) to acute sepsis, hypotension, and death. The overall mortality rate associated with platelet-associated sepsis is 26% (56).

To date, there is no widely accepted test method or device that can identify bacterially contaminated blood products. A promising approach is the use of psoralens and ultraviolet light to produce not only nonimmunogenic but also sterile blood products (58). In any patient in whom fever develops within six hours after platelet transfusion, the possibility of bacterial contamination should be examined, and empiric antibiotic therapy should be considered.

COMPLICATION OF MASSIVE TRANSFUSION

Massive transfusion is arbitrarily defined as the replacement of a patient's total blood volume in less than 24 hours, or as the acute administration of more than half the patient's estimated blood volume per hour. The complications of massive transfusion are the same as those associated with any blood transfusion and also include acidosis, abnormal hemostasis, changes in oxygen affinity, citrate toxicity, hyperkalemia, and hypothermia.

Acidosis

In traumatic shock, the severity of metabolic acidosis and the rapidity of its correction are correlated with the likelihood of survival. The predominant cause of acidosis is inadequate tissue perfusion, and the occurrence of this complication indicates a need for further

resuscitation. Stored red cells are acidotic, but the metabolism of citrate produces alkalosis. Therefore, a pH imbalance to RBC transfusion itself is rare.

Hemostasis Abnormality

Hemostasis may already be impaired in transfusion recipients because of an underlying condition. During massive transfusion of red cells, the number of platelets decreases because few functioning platelets exist in blood that has been stored more than 48 hours. The concentrations of factors V and VIII are reduced after storage for a few days, and the remaining concentration can be diluted if large volumes of crystalloid or colloid are given. In addition, DIC can be initiated by the release of thromboplastin-like material from platelets, WBCs, and RBCs broken down during storage and by the partial activation of coagulation factors. The extent of hemostatic derangement varies widely and is not predictable in relation to the volume of red cells transfused. Therefore, the use of prophylactic replacement formulas (e.g., administration of platelets and FFP after the transfusion of every eight units of red cells) is not recommended. It is preferable to monitor hemostasis and use FFP when abnormalities of the coagulation system appear. The use of cryoprecipitate is indicated for patients with DIC, when fibrinogen concentration is below 0.8 g/L. Thrombocytopenia below $50 \times 10^3/L$ contributes to microvascular bleeding from mucosal surfaces, wounds, and puncture sites. A standard adult dose of platelets is usually six to eight units, which equals approximately one unit of platelets per 10 kg body weight (59).

Changes in Oxygen Affinity

Stored hemoglobin has a high affinity for oxygen. Therefore, massive transfusion of stored RBCs with high oxygen affinity adversely affects oxygen delivery to the tissues. It seems wise to use fairly fresh red cell transfusions (less than one week old), but evidence supporting this practice has not been reported. Using fresh (less than 24 hours old) blood is not indicated. The concentration of 2,3-DPG rises rapidly after transfusion, and normal oxygen affinity is usually restored in a few hours.

Citrate Toxicity

Coagulation and normal cardiac function require that serum contain ionized calcium. Each unit of blood contains approximately 3 g of citrate, which binds the ionized calcium.

Because citrate is commonly used as an anticoagulant for blood storage, rapid infusion of blood may induce hypocalcemia if excess citrate binds with serum calcium.

Normothermic patients can metabolize citrate from stored blood when it is transfused at a rate of 150 mL/70 kg/min (i.e., one unit given every five minutes) (60).

However, the metabolism of citrate is decreased in patients with hypothermia, liver dysfunction, shock states, or hypocarbia (17). All of these conditions that may be present in the exsanguinating patient significantly increase the patient's risk of hypocalcemia. Abnormal calcium concentrations are more closely related to the rate of blood transfusion than to the total volume transfused (61). Empiric calcium administration of 1 g of calcium gluconate repletion for every four to six units of blood transfused has been suggested for rapid transfusion. However, calcium-related hemostasis must be judiciously maintained because of the risk of poor contractility due to hypocalcemia and arrhythmia due to hypercalcemia (62,63). Serum calcium concentration should be measured prospectively. The effect of treatment is gauged by ionized calcium concentration rather than by total serum calcium concentrations because more than half of serum calcium is protein bound. Therefore, a low total serum calcium concentration may reflect only hypoalbuminemia due to dilution and not a physiologic hypocalcemia.

Hyperkalemia

Hyperkalemia is an often discussed but rarely documented complication of blood transfusion (64). Potassium escapes from RBCs during storage: the plasma potassium concentration can reach 70 mEq/L in a stored unit of packed RBCs. However, this is usually clinically insignificant because each unit of packed red cells contains only 10 to 20 mL of plasma (1 mEq of potassium), and red cells resorb much of this leaked cation upon transfusion. Even so, death due to hyperkalemia has been associated with massive transfusion; therefore, the serum potassium concentration should be closely monitored (65).

Hypothermia

The infusion of room-temperature crystalloid solutions decreases the patient's core temperature. Transfusions with blood received from the blood bank at 4°C to 5°C can decrease the core temperature from 0.5°C to 1°C per unit transfused (17). Hypothermia leads to a reduction in citrate and lactate metabolism (leading to hypocalcemia and metabolic acidosis), an increased affinity of hemoglobin for oxygen, an impairment of red cell deformability, platelet dysfunction, and an increased tendency to cardiac dysrhythmias. Hypothermia can be avoided or at least minimized by warming all fluids, particularly blood, before they are infused. If transfusion-related hypothermia occurs, rapid infusion of warmed blood will help alleviate its deleterious effects.

VOLUME OVERLOAD

Overload of circulatory system occurs when blood, especially whole blood and plasma, is infused in too large a quantity or at too fast a rate. Elderly and neonatal patients are most sensitive to rapid volume shifts and constitute the largest groups in which this condition commonly develops. Also, patients with impaired cardiac function require careful monitoring so as to prevent circulatory overload during transfusion.

Initially, volume overload is indicated clinically by labored respiration, but pulmonary edema can rapidly occur if the necessary measurements are not promptly undertaken. In mild cases of volume overload, decreasing the rate of transfusion or stopping the transfusion will allow equilibration of circulatory system. In more severe instances, oxygen may be required to prevent hypoxemia, and aggressive diuresis should be provided.

DIFFERENTIAL DIAGNOSIS AND ROLE OF LABORATORY TESTS

The main purpose in evaluating a possible transfusion reaction is to recognize the early manifestations of life-threatening complications such as anaphylactic or endotoxic shock or acute hemolysis. These complications may be accompanied by apparently insignificant signs and symptoms rather than by those more commonly attributed to the reaction. Therefore, even minimal signs and symptoms have to be evaluated promptly, so that the blood transfusion can be terminated if necessary and appropriate management can be started.

The first step in evaluating any transfusion reaction is a clerical check of all identifying information on the unit of blood, laboratory slips, and the patient's chart. Next, the most crucial laboratory tests, i.e., those that can quickly provide evidence that supports or rules out a lethal transfusion reaction, should be performed.

Examination of a clotted or anticoagulated blood sample drawn at the time of the suspected reaction may provide the earliest evidence of a hemolytic transfusion reaction. Hemolysis of as little as 10 mL to 20 mL of blood may be visually apparent in the blood sample at the bedside, but the blood sample should be centrifuged and the plasma or serum compared to a suitable pretransfusion sample from the patient, so that the occurrence of hemolysis can be ascertained. Finding of hemolysis does not necessarily confirm immunologic destruction; instead hemolysis may have been produced by physical agents. A direct Coombs' test, which can be readily performed at the time that blood sample is examined visually, can rapidly determine whether the hemolysis is due to an immunologic process. When sequential negative results from pretransfusion direct Coombs' tests are followed by a positive result after transfusion, the presence of RBC incompatibility is strongly suggested. The possibility of false-positive result from a Coombs' test should be considered if the patient has a history of long-term treatment with Aldomet® (Merck & Co., Inc., New Jersey, U.S.A.) or other drugs. False-negative results from a Coombs' test can occur when incompatible RBCs are completely destroyed; such destruction is not uncommon in samples from recipients of ABO-incompatible transfusion.

If a clerical error is discovered or if the results of a direct Coombs' test performed on the reaction sample obtained after the transfusion are positive, crossmatching tests of blood samples obtained before and after transfusion should be repeated.

When clerical checks and laboratory tests fail to identify the cause of the suspected transfusion reaction, the possibility that the blood or blood product is contaminated by bacteria should be evaluated. This evaluation can be made quickly by performing a gram stain of a dried blood smear or, even better, of the plasma supernatant from the unit of blood or blood product. The presence of bacteria should be presumptive evidence of contamination; however, units containing *Clostridium* spp. may be rarely found.

Examination of urine for hemoglobinuria may be useful in documenting the presence of significant hemolysis, but this is usually delayed because filtration of hemoglobin occurs only after the plasma haptoglobin is saturated (about 100 mg hemoglobin/dL of plasma) and the level of free hemoglobin exceeds approximately 150 mg/dL.

Quantitative determination of hemoglobin and haptoglobin requires additional time and testing facilities and is usually not a useful initial study. Furthermore, both levels can be elevated or decreased as a result of the patient's state of nutrition, the presence of inflammatory process, and the effect of recent blood transfusions. Serum bilirubin levels reach their maximum five to seven hours following acute hemolysis. Most often they provide evidence supporting hemolysis, although there are many other intrahepatic and extrahepatic causes for hyperbilirubinemia (66).

The laboratory assessment including prothrombin time (PT), partial thromboplastin time (PTT), fibrinogen, bleeding time, and platelet count should provide useful information for guiding therapeutic intervention (67), but provide no information about ongoing hemolysis.

PREVENTION OF TRANSFUSION COMPLICATIONS
Preoperative Autologous Donation

Preoperative autologous donation was rarely used before the recognition that HIV could be transmitted via blood transfusion. Both autologous blood donation and transfusion are associated with risks (Table 3). In one study (68), 1 in 16,783 autologous donations was associated with an adverse reaction severe enough to require hospitalization; this risk is 12 times as high as the risk associated with voluntary donations by healthy persons. Myocardial ischemia events have also been reported in association with, but not necessarily

Table 3 Advantages and Disadvantages of Autologous Blood Donation

Advantages	Disadvantages
Prevents transfusion-transmitted disease	Does not eliminate the risk of bacterial contamination and volume overload
Avoids red cell alloimmunization	Does not eliminate the risk of administrative error, resulting in ABO incompatibility
Supplements the blood supply	Costs more than allogenic blood donation
Provides compatible blood for patients with alloantibodies	Results in discarding of blood that is not transfused
Prevents some adverse transfusion reactions	Causes perioperative anemia and increases the likelihood of transfusion

as a result of, autologous blood transfusion (69,70). The transfusion of autologous blood has many of the same complications as transfusion of allogenic units (Table 3). Published guidelines have been considered on the types of patients for whom autologous donation is most appropriate (71). Most commonly, the number of units of autologous blood obtained preoperatively is based on the number of units that would be crossmatched before surgery if allogenic blood were being used (72). However, even for such procedures as joint replacement or radical prostatectomy, as much as 50% of autologous blood goes unused (73,74). When autologous blood is collected for procedures that seldom require transfusion, such as hysterectomy, vaginal delivery, and transuretheral resection of prostate, up to 90% of the units collected before these procedures go unused (75). A recent British consensus conference on autologous transfusion stated that autologous blood donation should be considered only if the likelihood of transfusion exceeds 50% (76).

Acute Normovolemic Hemodilution

Acute normovolemic hemodilution entails the removal of whole blood from a patient immediately before surgery and simultaneous replacement with acellular fluid such as crystalloid or colloid to maintain normovolemia. Blood is collected in standard blood bags containing anticoagulants, remains in operating room, and is reinfused after major loss of blood has ceased, or sooner if indicated. Recent guidelines state that acute normovolemic hemodilution should be considered when the potential surgical blood loss is likely to exceed 20% of the blood volume in patients who have a preoperative hemoglobin level of more than 10 g/dL and who do not have severe myocardial disease, such as moderate-to-severe left ventricular impairment, unstable angina, severe aortic stenosis, or critical left main coronary artery disease (77). Acute normovolemic hemodilution has several advantages over autologous blood donation. First, the units procured by hemodilution require no testing, so that the costs are substantially lower than those of autologous blood donation (78). Second because the units of blood are not removed from the operating room, the possibility of administrative error that could lead to ABO-incompatible blood transfusion is theoretically eliminated, as is the risk of bacterial contamination. Third, blood obtained by hemodilution does not require an additional investment of time by the patient because it is done at the time of surgery, nor does it prolong the duration of surgery or anesthesia (79).

Intraoperative Recovery of Blood

Intraoperative recovery of blood involves collection and reinfusion of autologous red cells lost by patient during the surgery. A cell-washing device can provide the equivalent of 10 units of banked blood per hour to a patient with massive bleeding. The length of survival of recovered red cells appears to be similar to that of transfused allogenic red cells (80). Relative contraindications include the potential to aspiration of malignant cells, the presence of infection, and presence of other contaminants as amniotic or ascitic fluid in the operative field. Because washing does not completely remove bacteria from the recovered blood, intraoperative recovery should not be used if operative field has gross bacterial contamination (71).

Inactivation of Microbes in Platelet Units

The inactivation of viruses in a unit of platelets while retaining the viability and hemostatic properties of these blood cells has proved to be a formidable challenge. Viral inactivation in a unit of platelets by means of exposure to psoralen derivatives followed by exposure to ultraviolet A has been intensively investigated and can greatly reduce the levels of HIV and hepatitis viruses. This treatment appears to inactivate any contaminating bacteria (81) and reduce or eliminate immunomodulation due to lymphocytes.

Use of Plasma with Reduced Viral Infectivity

Treatment of plasma with a solvent-detergent process provides a means to inactivate all the viruses with lipid envelopes, including HIV, HBV, and HCV (82). The contents of plasma appear to be unchanged except for the procoagulant activity, which is reduced by about 15%, and the levels of large multimers von Willebrand factor and some other factors, including protein S, are decreased by over 50%. The pooling of plasma from so many donors as part of the solvent-detergent process has aroused concern about the possible transmission of nonenveloped viruses (e.g., hepatitis A and parvovirus B19) that are not inactivated by the process. Transmission of parvovirus B19 is a potential problem for some transfusion recipients such as patients with sickle-cell disease or thalassemia (71). Clinicians are also concerned that the pooled product may transmit viruses that are yet undiscovered. Furthermore, the high cost of the product has slowed widespread acceptance. Other

improvement to the product, such as screening for parvovirus infectivity by PCR testing and removal of ABO system antibodies, are in progress (83).

Viral Inactivation

Because donor testing and screening will never be perfect, viral inactivation has been pursued and is becoming available. Leukodepletion can limit the transmission of cell-borne viruses such as cytomegalovirus. Data have been obtained in bone marrow transplant recipients, which shows that removing white cells from transfused blood components is equivalent to providing blood components from donors who are seronegative to cytomegalovirus (84). To accomplish this degree of viral safety, it is necessary to decrease the concentration of contaminating white cells below 5×10^6; this represents a 1000-fold reduction, which is best accomplished by new filters that can be applied in blood centers to provide prestorage leukocyte-depleted blood products. Because the removal of white cells to this concentration also reduces the risk of alloimmunization to HLA factors and reduces the rate of other immunologic transfusion reactions in blood recipients, the implementation of universal leukodepletion is progressing in transfusion medicine practice (85).

Pharmacologic Agents

In addition to the autologous option, other transfusion alternatives have been pursued. Physicians are now encroached to use drugs without biohazardous risks in favor of blood components. Patients with von Willebrand disease are given 1-desamino-8-D-arginine-vasopressin (DDAVP) rather than cryoprecipitate to improve hemostasis (86); aprotinin and other fibrinolytic inhibitors have been used in high-blood loss surgeries (87), and hematopoetic growth factors such as erythropoietin are advocated for dialysis patients or for patients undergoing elective surgery (88). Recombinant factor VIIa was successfully used for the treatment of acute bleeding episodes in hemophilia patients, as well in patients with liver cirrhosis, who underwent major surgery (89,90).

Use of Red Cell Substitute

A number of blood substitutes have completed safety trials and are now undergoing efficacy evaluation. There are numerous potential advantages to the use of these solutions compared to RBCs. They are readily available and have a long shelf life, do not require type- and crossmatching, are free of viral or bacterial contamination, have a much lower viscosity than blood, and may lack the immunosuppressive effect of blood.

These products appear to be safe and have potential for extensive use, particularly in the surgical patient. Optimization of oxygen delivery to individuals suffering from organ ischemia may ultimately represent the greatest potential use of these solutions, but a short circulation time may limit their utility in emergent resuscitation (91,92).

TREATMENT AXIOMS

- Major hemolytic transfusion reaction generally appears clinically before 50 to 100 mL of blood has been infused. Nonhemolytic febrile or allergic reactions may not occur until all units of blood have been administrated.
- Most allergic or febrile reactions occur in spite of a satisfactory type and crossmatch.
- If a major transfusion reaction is suspected, the transfusion should be stopped immediately, and the remainder of the stored blood and the sample of the patient's blood should be sent to the blood bank for repeated crossmatch and analysis.

REFERENCES

1. Sirchia G, Giovanetti AM, eds. Safe and Good Use of Blood in Surgery (Sanguis): Use of Blood Products and Artificial Colloids in 43 European Hospitals. Vol. 153. Luxembourg: The European Commission, 1994.
2. Wallace EL, Churchill WH, Surgenor DM, Cho GS, McGurk S. Collection and transfusion of blood and blood components in the United States, 1994. Transfusion. 1998; 38(7):625–636.
3. Schreider GB, Busch MP, Kleinman SH, Korelitz JJ. The risk of transfusion-transmitted viral infection. The Retrovirus Epidemiology Donor Study. N. Engl J Med 1996; 334(26):1685–1690.
4. Klein HG. Allogeneic transfusion risks in the surgical patient. Am J Surg. 1995; 170(suppl 6A):21S–26S.
5. Greenburg AG. New transfusion strategies volume. Am J Surg 1997; 173:49–52.
6. Hutchin P. History of blood transfusion: a tercentennial look. Surgery 1967; 64(3):685–700.
7. Hoff HE, Guillemin R. The first experiments on transfusion in France. J Hist Med 1963; 18:103.
8. Mollison PL, Engelfriet CP. Marcelo contreras immunology of red cells. In: Mollison PL, Engelfriet CP, eds. Marcelo Contreras Blood Transfusion in Clinical Medicine. 9th ed. Oxford: Oxford Publication, 1993: 76–147.
9. Race RR, Sanger R. The ABO blood groups. In: Race RR, Sanger R, eds. Blood Groups in Men. 5th ed. Oxford, Edinburgh: Blackwell Scientific Publication, 1968:9–63.
10. Rossi EC, Simon TL, Moss GS, Gould SA. Transfusion into the next millennium. In: Rossi EC, Simon TL, Moss GS, Gould SA, eds. Principles of Transfusion Therapy. 6th ed. Baltimore: Williams & Wilkins, 1996:1–11.
11. Rotondo MF. Physiology of transfusion therapy. In: Savage EB, Fishman SJ, Miller LD, eds. Essentials of Basic Science in Surgery. Philadelphia: JB Lippincott, 1993:61–67.
12. Ness PM. Transfusion medicine: an overview and update. Clin Chem 2000; 46:1270–1276.
13. Barnes A. Transfusion of universal donor and uncrossmatched blood. Bibl Haematol 1980; (46):132–142.
14. Wilson RF, ed. Handbook of Trauma: Pitfalls and Pearls. Vol. 4. Philadelphia: JB Lippincott, Williams & Wilkins, 1999:32–33.
15. Barton JC. Nonhemolytic, noninfectious transfusion reactions. Semin Hematol 1981; 18(2):95–121.
16. Phillips G, Rotondo M, Schwab CW. Transfusion therapy. In: Maull KI, Rodrigez A, Wiles CE III, eds. Complications in Trauma and Critical Care. Philadelphia: WB, Saunders, 1996: 73–79.
17. Edelman B, Heyman MR. Blood component therapy for trauma patients. In: Stene JK, Grande CM, eds. Trauma Anesthesia. Baltimore: Williams and Wilkins, 1991: 133–176.
18. Miller WV, Holland PV, Sugarbaker E, Strober W, Waldman TA, Neil SY. Anaphylactic reactions to IgA: a difficult transfusion problem. Am J Clin Pathol 1970; 54(4):618–621.
19. Dennis RC, Clas D, Niehoff JM, et al. Transfusion therapy. In: Civetta JM, Taylor RW, Kirby R, eds. Critical Care. Philadelphia: Lippincott Williams & Wilkins, 1997:653–654.
20. Brubaker DB. Human posttransfusion graft-versus-host disease. Vox Sang 1983; 45(6):401–420.
21. Brubaker DB. Immunopathogenic mechanism of posttransfusion graft-vs-host disease. Proc Soc Exp Biol Med 1993; 202(2):122–147.
22. Hong M, Gatti RA, Good RA. Hazards and potential benefits of blood transfusion in immunologic deficiency. Lancet 1968; 2:388–389.
23. Nauck MS, Gierens H, Nauck MA, Marz W, Wieland H. Rapid genotyping of human platelet antigen 1 (HPA-1) with fluorophore-labelled hybridization probes on the LightCycler. Br J Haematol 1999; 105(3): 803–810.
24. Popovsky MA, Moore SB. Diagnostic and pathogenetic considerations in transfusion-related acute lung injury. Transfusion 1985; 25(6):573–577.
25. Silliman CC, Paterson AJ, Dickey WO, et al. The association of biologically active lipids with the development of transfusion-related acute lung injury: a retrospective study. Transfusion 1997; 37(7):719–726.
26. Goodnough LT, Brecher ME, Kanter MH, AuBuchon JP. Transfusion medicine. First of two parts – blood transfusion. N Eng J Med 1999; 340(6):438–447.
27. Standards for Blood Banks and Transfusion Services. 15th ed. Bethesda: American Association of Blood Banks, 1993:23.
28. Greenwalt TJ. Pathogenesis and management of hemolytic transfusion reactions. Semin Hematol 1981; 18(2): 84–94.
29. Paller MS, Hoidal JR, Ferris TF. Oxygen free radicals in ischemic acute renal failure in the rat. J Clin Invest 1984; 74:1156–1164.
30. Paller MS. Hemoglobin- and myoglobin-induced acute renal failure in rats: role of iron in nephrotoxicity. Am J Physiol 1988; 255:F539–F544.
31. Moore SB, Taswell HF, Pineda AA, Sonnenberg CL. Delayed hemolytic transfusion reaction: evidence of the need for an improved pre-transfusion compatibility test. Am J Clin Pathol 1980; 74:94–97.
32. Pineda AA, Taswell HF, Brzica SM Jr. Transfusion reaction: an immunologic hazard of blood transfusion. Transfusion 1978; 18(1):1–7.
33. Rutledge R, Sheldon GF, Collins ML. Massive transfusion. Criti Care Clinics 1986; 2(4):791–805.
34. Blumberg N. Allogeneic transfusion and infection: economic and clinical implications. Seminars in Hematology 1997; 34(3 suppl 2):34–40.

35. Wu HS, Little AG. Perioperative blood transfusion and cancer recurrence. J Clin Oncol 1988; 6(8):1348–1354.

36. van Aken WG. Does perioperative blood transfusion promote tumor growth? Transfus Med Rev 1989; 3(4):243–252.

37. Tartter PI. The association of perioperative blood transfusion with colorectal cancer recurrence. Ann Surg 1992; 216(6):633–638.

38. Blumberg N, Heal JM. Transfusion and host defenses against cancer recurrence and infection. Transfusion 1989; 29(3):236–245.

39. Tartter PI. Blood transfusion and infectious complications following colorectal cancer surgery. Br J Surg 1988; 75(8):789–792.

40. Nichols RL, Smith JW, Klein DB, et al. Risk of infection after penetrating abdominal trauma. N Eng J Med 1984; 311(17):1065–1070.

41. Joint statement on acquired immune deficiency syndrome (AIDS) related to transfusion. Transfusion 1983; 23:87–88.

42. Provisional Public Health Service inter-agency recommendations for screening donated blood and plasma for antibody to the virus causing acquired immunodeficiency syndrome. Morb Mortal Wkly Rep 1985; 34:1–5.

43. Selik RM, Ward JW, Buehler JW. Trends in transfusion-associated acquired immune deficiency syndrome in the United States, 1982 through 1991. Transfusion 1993; 33(11):890–893.

44. Stramer SL, Aberle-Grasse J, Brodsky JP, Busch MP, Lackritz EM. US blood donor screening with p24 antigen (Ag): one year experience [abs.]. Transfusion 1997; 37 (suppl):1S.

45. Domen RE. Paid-versus-volunteer blood donation in the United States: a historical review. Transfus Med Rev 1995; 9(1):53–59.

46. Conry-Cantilena C, VanRaden M, Gibble J, et al. Routes of infection, viremia, and liver disease in blood donors found to have hepatitis C virus infection. N Eng J Med 1996; 334(26):1691–1696.

47. Tong MJ, el-Farra NS, Reikes AR, Co RL. Clinical outcomes after transfusion-associated hepatitis C. N Eng J Med 1995; 332(22):1463–1466.

48. Alter HJ, Nakatsuji Y, Melpolder J, et al. The incidence of transfusion-associated hepatitis G virus infection and its relation to liver disease. N Eng J Med 1997; 336(11):747–754.

49. Dodd RY. Adverse consequences of blood transfusion: quantitative risk estimates. In: Nance ST, ed. Blood Supply: Risk Perceptions, and Prospects for the Future. Bethesda, MD: American Association of Blood Banks, 1994:1–24.

50. Risk associated with human parvovirus B 19 infection. Morb Mortal Wkly Rep 1989; 38:81–88, 93–97.

51. Luban NL. Human parvoviruses: implication for transfusion medicine. Transfusion 1994; 34:821–827.

52. Guidelines for counseling persons infected with human T-lymphotropic virus type-I (HTLV-I) and type II (HTLV-II). Centers for Disease Control and Prevention and the U.S.P.H.S Working Group. Ann Intern Med 1993; 118:448–454.

53. Manns A, Wilks RJ, Murphy EL, et al. A prospective study of transmission by transfusion of HTLV-I and risk factors associated with seroconversion. Int J Cancer 1992; 51(6):886–891.

54. Gout O, Baulac M, Gessain A, et al. The Rapid development of myelopathy after HTLV-I infection acquired by transfusion during cardiac transplantation. N Eng J Med 1990; 322(6):383–388.

55. Kim DM, Brecher ME, Bland LA, Estes TJ, Carmen RA, Nelson EJ. Visual identification of bacterially contaminated red cells. Transfusion 1992; 32(3):221–225.

56. Chiu EK, Yuen KY, Lie AK, et al. A prospective study of symptomatic bacteremia following platelet transfusion and of its management. Transfusion 1994; 34(11):950–954.

57. Goldman M, Blajchman MA. Blood product-associated bacterial sepsis. Transfus Med Rev 1991; 5(1):73–83.

58. Lin L, Cook DN, Wiesehahn GP, Alfonso R, et al. Photochemical inactivation of viruses and bacteria in platelets concentrates by use of a novel psoralen and long-wavelength ultraviolet light. Transfusion 1997; 37(4):423–435.

59. Hewitt P, Regan F. Blood transfusion. In: Webb AR, Shapiro MJ, Singer M, Sater PM, eds. Oxford Textbook of Critical Care. Oxford: Oxford University Press, 1999:691–694.

60. Rudowski WJ. Blood transfusion: yesterday, today and tomorrow. World J Surg 1987; 11(1):86–93.

61. Denlinger JK, Nahrwold ML, Gibbs PS, Lecky JH. Hypocalcemia during rapid blood transfusion in anaesthetized man. Br J Anesthes 1976; 48(10):995–1000.

62. Denlinger JK, Nahrwold ML. Cardiac failure associated with hypocalcemia. Anesthesia Analgesia 1976; 55(1):34–36.

63. Olinger GN, Hottenrott C, Mulder DG, et al. Acute clinical hypocalcemic myocardial depression during rapid blood transfusion and postoperative hemodialysis: a preventable complication. J Thorac Cardiovasc Surg 1976; 72(4):503–511.

64. Wilson RF, Binkley LE, Sabo FM Jr, et al. Electrolyte and acid-base changes with massive blood transfusions. Am Surg 1992; 58(9):535–544.

65. Jameson LC, Popic PM, Harms BA. Hypercalcemic death during use of high capacity fluid warmer for massive transfusion. Anesthesiology 1990; 73(5):1050–1052.

66. Sharp DE. Complication of blood and blood-product transfusion. In: Greenfeld LJ, ed. Complications in Surgery and Trauma. Philadelphia: JB Lippincot, 1984:148–152.

67. Mannucci PM, Federici AB, Sirchia G. Hemostasis testing during massive blood replacement. A study of 172 cases. Vox Sanguinis 1982; 42(3):113–123.

68. Popovsky MA, Whitaker B, Arnold NL. Severe outcomes of allogenic and autologous blood donation: frequency and characterization. Transfusion 1995; 35(9):734–737.

69. Goodnough LT, Monk TG. Evolving concepts in autologous blood procurement and transfusion: case reports of perisurgical anemia complicated by myocardial infarction. Am J Med 1996; 101(2A):33S–37S.

70. Kasper SM, Ellering J, Stachwitz P, Lynch J, Grunenberg R, Buzello W. All adverse events in autologous blood donors with cardiac disease are not necessarily caused by blood donation. Transfusion 1998; 38(7):669–673.

71. Goodnough LT, Brecher ME, Kanter MH, AuBuchon JP. Transfusion medicine. Second of two parts – blood conservation. N Eng J Med 1999; 340(7):525–533.

72. Axelrod FB, Pepkowitz SH, Goldfinger D. Establishment of a schedule of optimal preoperative collection of autologous blood. Transfusion 1989; 29(8):677–680.

73. Renner SW, Howanitz PJ, Bachner P. Preoperative autologous blood donation in 612 hospitals. A College of American Pathologists' Q-Probes study of quality issues in transfusion practice. Arch Pathol Laboratory Med 1992; 116(6):613–619.

74. Goodnough LT, Saha P, Hirschler NV, Yomtovian R. Autologous blood donation in nonorthopaedic surgical procedures as a blood conservation strategy. Vox Sanguinis 1992; 63(2):96–101.

75. AuBuchon JP, Gettinger A, Littenberg B. Determinants of physician ordering of preoperative autologous donations. Vox Sanguinis 1994; 66(3):176–181.

76. Thomas MJ, Gillon J, Desmond MJ. Consensus conference on autologous transfusion. Preoperative autologous donation. Transfusion 1996; 36(7):633–639.

77. Napier JA, Bruce M, Chapman J, et al. Guidelines for autologous transfusion II. Perioperative hemodilution and cell salvage. British Committee for Standards in Hematology Blood Transfusion Task Force. Autologous Transfusion Working Party. Br J Anesth 1997; 78(6): 768–771.

78. Monk TG, Goodnough LT, Birkmeyer JD, Brecher ME, Catalona WJ. Acute normovolemic hemodilution is a cost-effective alternative to preoperative autologous blood donation by patients undergoing radical retropubic prostatectomy. Transfusion 1995; 35(7):559–565.

79. Goodnough LT, Despotis GJ, Merkel K, Monk TG. A randomized trial comparing acute normovolemic hemodilution and preoperative autologous blood donation in total hip arthroplasty. Transfusion 2000; 40(9):1054–1057.

80. Williamson KR, Taswell HF. Intraoperative blood salvage: a review. Transfusion 1991; 31(7):662–675.

81. Grass JA, Hei DJ, Metchette K, et al. Inactivation of leukocytes in platelets concentrates by photochemical treatment with psoralen plus UVA. Blood 1998; 91(6): 2180–2188.

82. Klein HG, Dodd RY, Dzik WH, et al. Current status of solvent/detergent-treated frozen plasma. Transfusion 1998; 38(1):102–107.

83. Judd WJ, Davenport RD, Downs T, Hammond DJ, Chin S, Pehta JC. Isohemagglutinin-depleted solvent detergent plasma: a universal viral-inactivated plasma for patients of any ABO type. Blood 1999; 94:375a.

84. Bowden RA, Slichter SJ, Sayers MH, Mori M, Cays M, Meyers JD. Use of leukocyte-depleted platelets and cytomegaloviruses-seronegative red blood cell store prevention of primary cytomegalovirus infection after marrow transplant. Blood 1991; 78(1): 246–250.

85. Blajchman MA. Transfusion-associated immunomodulation and universal white cell reduction: are we putting the cart before the horse? Transfusion 1999; 39(7):665–670.

86. Mannucci PM, Canciani MT, Rota L, Donovan B. Response of factor VIII/von Willebrand factor to DDAVP in healthy subjects and patients with haemophilia A and von Willebrand disease. Br J Haematol 1981;47(2):283–293.100.

87. Salzman EW, Weinstein MJ, Weintraub RM, et al. Treatment with desmopressin acetate to reduce blood loss after cardiac surgery. A double blind randomized trial. N Eng J Med 1986; 314(22):1402–1406.

88. Eschbach JW, Egrie JC, Downing MR, Browne JK, Adamson JW. Correction of the anemia of end-stage renal disease with recombinant human erythropoetin. Results of combined phase I and II clinical trial. N Eng J Med 1987; 316(2):73–78.

89. Negrier C, Lienhart A. Overall experience with Novo-Seven. Blood Coagul Fibrinolysis 2000; 11(suppl 1): 19–24.

90. Papatheodoridis GV, Chung S, Keshav S, et al. Correction of both prothrombin time and primary hemostasis by recombinant factor VII during therapeutic alcohol injection of hepatocellular cancer in liver cirrhosis. J Hepatol 1999; (31):747–750.

91. Cohn S. Blood substitutes in surgery. Surgery 2000; 127(6):599–602.

92. Goodnough LT, Monk TG, Brecher ME. Autologous blood procurement in surgical setting: lessons learned in the last 10 years. Vox Sanguinis 1996; 71(3): 133–141.

5

Hypovolemic and Septic Shock

Matthew O. Dolich
*Division of Trauma and Surgical Critical Care, University of California,
Irvine School of Medicine, Irvine, California, U.S.A.*

Don H. Van Boerum
*Section of Trauma Surgery, Department of Surgery, Sutter Roseville Medical Center,
Roseville, California, U.S.A.*

Shock is a term used to broadly categorize a group of physiologic states, which, if left untreated, ultimately result in cardiovascular failure and death. Credit for the earliest use of this term goes to the French surgeon, Le Dran, in 1737. In his manuscript "A Treatise of Reflections Drawn from Experience with Gunshot Wounds," the word "choc" was used to describe a severe jolt or impact (1). Over a century later, Gross eloquently described shock as "a rude unhinging of the machinery of life" (2), a sentiment shared by many who followed him, frustrated at the difficulty of resuscitating a patient from severe shock. At the end of the 19th century, shock was referred to as "a momentary pause in the act of death" by Warren (3). At approximately the same time, Crile noted a decrease in central venous pressure in response to hemorrhage, as well as a survival benefit associated with saline resuscitation (4). Blalock, in one of the first "modern" descriptions, defined shock as "peripheral circulatory failure, from a discrepancy between the size of the vascular bed and the volume of intravascular fluid" (5). Blalock's description of shock has served as a starting point toward our current understanding of shock, which is characterized by the presence of inadequate tissue perfusion and oxygenation.

As mentioned previously, shock is a very broad term that necessitates further subclassification. Four types of shock that are generally described are hypovolemic, distributive, cardiogenic, and obstructive. Hypovolemic shock most commonly results from hemorrhage, but may also be caused by any process that results in dehydration or volume loss. Distributive shock, resulting from alterations in vasomotor tone, is most commonly caused by sepsis. Less common causes of distributive shock include spinal cord injury, anaphylaxis, and adrenocortical insufficiency. Cardiogenic shock may be caused by any process that results in decreased myocardial contractility (e.g., myocardial infarction, cardiomyopathy, and blunt cardiac injury), and obstructive shock results from mechanical etiologies such as pericardial tamponade, tension pneumothorax, constrictive pericarditis, and ventricular outflow obstruction. The remainder of this chapter will specifically address the diagnosis, management, and complications of hypovolemic and septic shock.

HYPOVOLEMIC SHOCK

Hypovolemic shock may be caused by any process that ultimately results in depletion of intravascular volume. Most commonly, hypovolemic shock is related to hemorrhage, but it may also result from fluid sequestration in the extravascular space, which occurs in the setting of severe pancreatitis or burns. Insensible losses and volume loss via the gastrointestinal or urinary tract may also produce hypovolemic shock. Hypovolemic shock and, in particular, hemorrhagic shock are further classified by the percentage of lost intravascular volume (Table 1). It is particularly important to note that normal blood pressure may be maintained despite intravascular volume losses of up to 30%.

Diagnosis

Uncompensated hypovolemic shock, comprising class III and class IV fluid loss, is usually diagnosed readily by alterations in blood pressure, heart rate, and urinary output. This determination is especially straightforward when an obvious source of hemorrhage is present. Compensated shock, which may be present despite significant intravascular volume depletion, requires a much higher index of suspicion because the diagnosis may be masked by relatively normal vital signs and urinary output. In compensated shock, regional alterations in blood flow occur because the body attempts to maintain perfusion of the brain and heart. While teleologically adaptive for short-term survival, this response occurs at the expense of other organ systems, in particular, the mesenteric circulation. As regional perfusion decreases, aerobic glycolysis is replaced at the cellular level by anaerobic metabolism.

Table 1 Classification of Volume Loss in Hypovolemic Shock

	Class I	Class II	Class III	Class IV
Percentage volume loss	≤15%	15–30%	30–40%	>40%
Blood pressure	Normal	Normal	↓	↓↓
Heart rate	Normal	↑	↑↑	↑↑↑
Urinary output	Normal	↓	↓↓	↓↓↓

Source: From Ref. 6.

During this process, pyruvate is hydrolyzed into lactate, with a resultant rise in serum lactate levels. Excess H^+ ions generated during this reaction contribute to a metabolic lactic acidosis, which is one of the clinical hallmarks of hypovolemic shock. A complete description of the physiologic alterations associated with hypovolemic shock falls outside the scope of this chapter and the reader is directed to one of the many excellent texts on this subject.

The incidence of compensated hemorrhagic shock is high in victims of trauma, as much as 85% in some studies (7,8). Early diagnosis is crucial because persistence of malperfusion associated with compensated shock has been shown to be highly associated with multiple organ dysfunction syndrome (MODS) and death (9). Because vital signs and urinary output may be normal despite derangements in perfusion, other modalities must be utilized to establish an early diagnosis of compensated shock.

Among the simplest diagnostic measures are determination of biochemical parameters including serum lactate and arterial base deficit. Serum lactate levels provide a global estimate of anaerobic metabolism. Many studies have shown that high initial or maximal serum lactate levels correlate with severity of hypovolemic shock and subsequent mortality (10–12). Additionally, the duration of time for normalization of lactate levels after resuscitation has been directly associated with mortality. Failure to achieve a normal serum lactate level within 48 hours has been associated with mortality rates as high as 86% in some studies (12). Lactic acidosis resulting from hypovolemic shock may also be measured indirectly by arterial blood gas analysis. The arterial base deficit, as calculated by the Siggard–Anderson nomogram, is defined as the amount of additional base required to titrate 1 L of blood to a pH of 7.40, assuming a partial pressure of CO_2 of 40 mmHg and a temperature of 37°C. In the absence of preexisting metabolic derangements, the arterial base deficit will vary directly with the level of lactic acidemia. Several studies have verified the clinical utility of arterial base deficit determinations in establishing the severity of hypovolemic shock, as well as assessing the adequacy of resuscitation (13,14). Thus, lactate and arterial base deficit determination represent simple, global diagnostic modalities in suspected hypovolemic shock.

Invasive hemodynamic monitoring provides another avenue for establishing the presence of compensated hypovolemic shock. Pulmonary artery catheterization is an effective diagnostic maneuver

that is easily performed percutaneously at the bedside in most intensive care units (ICUs) today. Although some recent evidence (15) has associated pulmonary artery catheterization with increased mortality rates, the results of another large study suggest that pulmonary artery catheter-directed therapy significantly improves outcome (16). Despite some controversy in the literature, most intensivists consider the pulmonary artery catheter to be an indispensable tool in the clinical management of critically ill patients. Although pulmonary artery catheterization does not definitively establish the presence or absence of compensated hypovolemic shock, several parameters may lead the clinician to consider this diagnosis. Typically, hypovolemic shock is associated with low pulmonary artery pressures and central venous pressure. Pulmonary artery occlusion pressure (PAOP), measured distal to a balloon "wedged" in a proximal pulmonary vessel, provides a close approximation of left atrial pressure, a surrogate for ventricular end-diastolic volume (EDV) traditionally referred to as preload. Thus, in hypovolemia, PAOP is typically low. Cardiac output, easily measured by thermodilution, is secondarily low due to decreased preload, although compensatory sinus tachycardia may mitigate this finding. Systemic vascular resistance (SVR) is usually increased in an attempt to maintain central circulatory volume and pressure. Current pulmonary artery catheters also have the ability to continuously measure mixed venous oxygen saturation (SvO_2) by reflectance oximetry. Decreased SvO_2 levels generally indicate inadequate oxygen delivery, and thus may be associated with hypovolemia prior to changes in vital signs or urinary output. Newer pulmonary artery catheters also provide continuous measurement of right ventricular EDV and right ventricular ejection fraction. While the measured EDV of the right ventricle typically overestimates the left ventricular EDV, it may in fact be a more accurate predictor of preload than PAOP. Normal cardiovascular pressures are listed in Table 2. Normal hemodynamic parameters and their derivations are outlined in Table 3.

In addition to global markers of hypoperfusion associated with hypovolemic shock, several newer modalities have emerged that allow better assessment of regional perfusion. Because gut perfusion decreases in the early stages of compensated hypovolemia and is restored relatively late during resuscitation,

Table 2 Normal Cardiovascular Pressures

Parameter	Normal range (mmHg)
Systolic blood pressure	100–140
Diastolic blood pressure	60–90
Mean arterial pressure	70–100
Central venous pressure	0–6
Pulmonary artery systolic	15–30
Pulmonary artery diastolic	6–12
Mean pulmonary arterial pressure	10–18
Pulmonary artery occlusion pressure	6–12

Table 3 Normal Hemodynamic Parameters

Parameter	Derivation	Normal value
CO	Stroke volume × heart rate	4–8 L/min
CI	CO/body surface area	2.5–4 L/min/m²
SVR	(MAP − CVP)/CO × 80	800–1400 dyne/sec/cm⁻⁵
SVR index	(MAP − CVP)/CI × 80	1200–2500 dyne/sec/cm⁻⁵/m²
PVR	(MPAP − PAOP)/CO × 80	80–200 dyne/sec/cm⁻⁵
PVR index	(MPAP − PAOP)/CI × 80	200–400 dyne/sec/cm⁻⁵/m²
Mixed venous oxygen saturation	Direct or oximetric measurement	68–72%
RVEF	Thermodilution	35–60%
RVEDV	Stroke volume/RVEF	150–225 mL
RVEDV index	Stroke volume index/RVEF	80–110 mL

Abbreviations: CO, cardiac output; CI, cardiac index; SVR, systemic vascular resistance; PVR, pulmonary vascular resistance; RVEF, right ventricular ejection fraction; RVEDV, right ventricular end-diastolic volume; MAP, mean arterial pressure; CVP, central venous pressure; PAOP, pulmonary artery occlusion pressure; MPAP, mean pulmonary artery pressure.

recent attention has been directed toward assessment of this parameter.

One technique that has shown some promise involves measurement of gastric intramucosal pH (pHi) by method of gastric tonometry. This is accomplished by insertion of a specialized nasogastric tube constructed with a semipermeable membrane balloon tip. Carbon dioxide is able to equilibrate across this membrane, allowing determination of the regional CO_2 concentration within the gastric mucosa. During periods of hypoperfusion, the regional mucosal CO_2 rises with a resultant decrease in pHi, as calculated by the Henderson–Hasselbalch equation:

$$pHi = 6.1 + \log(HCO_3^- / PCO_2 \times 0.03)$$

It is important to note that gastric tonometry, by detecting changes in regional CO_2 concentration, measures pHi (which is related to perfusion), as opposed to "intraluminal" pH (which is related to gastric acid secretion). Thus, gastric tonometry can be used as a window through which the perfusion status of the foregut can be assessed. Studies in animals and humans have verified that gastric tonometry provides an accurate assessment of mucosal perfusion in hypovolemia and shock. However, controlled trials of pHi-directed interventions have, in general, failed to demonstrate improved outcomes in most studies to date (17,18).

Another modality by which regional perfusion can be estimated is near-infrared spectroscopy (NIRS). This technique relies on differential absorption and reflectance patterns of mitochondrial cytochrome a and cytochrome a_3 that vary depending on the state of cellular respiration. As photons in the near-infrared spectrum pass through bone and soft tissue, NIRS transducers have been designed to noninvasively assess various tissue beds ranging from gastric mucosa to the brain. NIRS has been shown to reflect alterations in mesenteric blood flow associated with hemorrhagic shock (19);

however, at this time it is unclear whether NIRS-directed therapy will result in improved outcomes.

Treatment

Therapy for hypovolemic shock is both deceptively simple and frustratingly controversial. The two mainstays of treatment are correcting the source of intravascular fluid loss (e.g., hemorrhage) and restoration of adequate circulating volume. Once a source of hypovolemia is identified, rectification is usually straightforward and may involve surgical or angiographic hemostasis, medical intervention to decrease gastrointestinal or urinary losses, or measures to combat insensible fluid loss. However, controversies persist regarding the appropriate intravenous fluid for resuscitation, as well as the timing and volume of fluid to be given.

Four basic categories of resuscitative fluid may be utilized in hypovolemic shock: crystalloids, colloids, hypertonic solutions, and oxygen-carrying solutions such as blood products. Each has relative advantages and disadvantages; the past four decades have witnessed fervent debate regarding the appropriate choice for treating hypovolemic shock. Resuscitative efforts should be toward achieving two main goals: restoration of adequate circulating volume, and maintenance of adequate oxygen delivery.

Crystalloid Solutions

Isotonic crystalloid solutions such as lactated Ringer's (LR) and normal saline (NS) comprise the initial mainstay of therapy for hypovolemic shock. These solutions are cheap, safe, and readily available. In hemorrhagic shock, both are equally effective as resuscitative fluids when given in a ratio of three-volume units of crystalloid solution per unit volume of shed blood. However, each fluid does have certain advantages and disadvantages. LR infusion may ameliorate the metabolic acidosis associated with hypovolemic shock, as the lactate it contains is rapidly metabolized to bicarbonate by the liver. Unfortunately, infusion of large volumes of LR also appears to have a negative immunologic effect, in particular, the activation of neutrophils in the blood stream. This neutrophil priming effect may be associated with development of systemic inflammatory response syndrome (SIRS) and MODS (20). Additionally, because LR is mildly hypotonic (Na = 130), infusion of large volumes of this fluid in the setting of traumatic brain injury may be deleterious due to worsening cerebral edema, intracranial pressure, and secondary brain injury. Thus NS, due to its mild hypertonicity (Na = 154 mmol/L), may be superior to LR in this setting. An additional advantage of NS is that it may be safely infused with banked blood, whereas the calcium content of LR overwhelms the chelating ability of citrate in stored blood. This may result in clot formation; thus, infusion of blood and LR together is relatively contraindicated. Conversely, administration of large volumes of NS may result in a hyperchloremic metabolic acidosis, an undesirable side effect in the hypovolemic, acidemic patient.

Colloid Solutions

Colloid solutions, including human serum albumin, modified starches, and dextrans, have provided alternatives to crystalloids for over half a century. They offer, at least theoretically, the advantage of increased intravascular colloid oncotic pressure, resulting in a net influx of fluid from the interstitium into the vascular space. Multiple studies have shown that resuscitation with colloid entails significantly less total volume infusion when compared with isotonic crystalloid. A secondary benefit of decreased volume requirement is decreased resuscitation time. Hundreds of studies comparing crystalloid with colloid have been performed over the last 25 years; however, most large reviews and meta-analyses of the available prospective data fail to show any survival benefit favoring colloid solutions in the setting of hypovolemic shock (21). In fact, albumin administration in hypovolemic shock may increase mortality rate (22). Colloid resuscitation is extremely expensive when compared with crystalloid; thus, in the absence of clear benefit, it is difficult to recommend the routine use of colloids in hypovolemic shock.

Hypertonic Solutions

Because resuscitation with isotonic crystalloid inherently involves relatively large volumes of fluid, recent interest has focused on hypertonic solutions, which have the benefit of requiring much smaller volume infusion. Decreased infusion volumes may provide significant advantage in prehospital and military settings, where carriage of large volumes of intravenous fluid is impractical. The best studied of these fluids are 7.5% NaCl hypertonic saline (HTS) and 7.5% NaCl/6% dextran 70 solution (HTS-D). Hypertonic solutions may provide additional benefits in patients with traumatic brain injury, as the high osmolarity of these solutions may ameliorate the cerebral edema and decreased cerebral perfusion that accompany large-volume fluid resuscitation (23). In addition, HTS causes less neutrophil activation and adhesion when compared with LR (20). Thus, it is possible that large-volume resuscitation with HTS or HTS-D may reduce the inflammatory response that accompanies LR infusion, but human data are lacking at this time.

Blood and Blood Substitutes

In hypovolemic shock due to significant hemorrhage, the asanguinous fluids mentioned in the previous paragraphs may be inadequate for complete resuscitation. In this circumstance, oxygen delivery must be augmented with an oxygen-carrying solution. Most commonly, this is accomplished by allogenic blood transfusion, typically in the form of packed red blood cells (RBC). Although RBC transfusion is frequently life saving, it is also associated with many pitfalls and complications. Despite improvements in screening techniques, small but finite risks of infectious complications, including infections with human immunodeficiency virus, human T-lymphotrophic virus, hepatitis C, and hepatitis B, persist. Blood transfusion is also associated with immunosuppression and increased frequency of wound infection, and has been shown to increase the risk of developing MODS (24). Perhaps most importantly, blood is an extremely limited and costly resource.

In light of the limitations of RBC transfusion, recent efforts have focused on other oxygen-carrying blood substitutes. The goal has been to identify a blood substitute that has a long shelf life, is universally compatible, has no potential for disease transmission, and has oxygen-carrying and dissociation characteristics similar to blood. Although initially promising, perfluorocarbon-based blood substitutes have had disappointing results, and most current efforts center on the clinical utility of hemoglobin-based oxygen carriers (HBOC). Early stroma-free hemoglobin solutions contained significant amounts of monomeric and dimeric hemoglobin, which led to nephrotoxicity. Subsequent formulations included cross-linking of hemoglobin, reducing the incidence of this complication. However, pulmonary and systemic hypertension, thought secondary to binding of nitric oxide by hemoglobin, continued to be undesirable side effects. More recently, this effect has been addressed by creation of polymerized hemoglobin solutions, which appear to have decreased affinity for nitric oxide and fewer undesirable vasoactive effects, while maintaining oxygen affinity. Currently, three HBOCs are undergoing phase III clinical trials: human glutaraldehyde polymerized hemoglobin, human o-raffinose polymerized hemoglobin, and ultrapurified polymerized bovine hemoglobin.

Delayed Fluid Resuscitation

For most of the last half century, immediate administration of large volumes of resuscitative fluid has been the mainstay of treatment in hypovolemic shock. Upon further reflection, this practice may be questionable in the setting of uncontrolled hemorrhage. In theory, hemorrhagic shock is teleologically adaptive in the short term, as blood is directed to the brain and heart, and lower blood pressure allows hemostasis at the site of hemorrhage. Standard treatment with large volumes of crystalloid results in a dilutional coagulopathy, hypothermia, decreased blood viscosity, and elevated blood pressure, all of which may favor recurrent hemorrhage from an unsecured vessel. This has proven to be the case in animal studies, where immediate resuscitation with LR resulted in an increased blood loss following aortotomy (25). A recent prospective clinical trial has supported this hypothesis; overall survival and hospital stay were improved in penetrating truncal trauma victims receiving delayed fluid resuscitation after surgical hemostasis, as compared with patients receiving immediate fluid resuscitation in the prehospital setting (26).

SEPTIC SHOCK

Septic shock is a state of complete homeostatic deterioration resulting from a host's response to infection. It is a form of distributive shock, characterized by inadequate tissue perfusion due to microcirculatory alterations in the blood flow. Severe sepsis is estimated to affect 750,000 patients in the United States annually, with an associated mortality rate of approximately 30%. By comparison, a similar number of people in the United States die of acute myocardial infarction each year. Despite advances in critical care, the incidence of sepsis is not declining, and may indeed be on the rise. As the average age in industrialized nations increases, so does the number of sepsis-related ICU admissions. The average length of stay for septic patients is nearly three weeks, consuming an estimated total of $16.7 billion each year in the United States (27).

Definitions

To adequately address the diagnosis, pathophysiology, and management of sepsis-related disorders, appropriate terminology must be defined. The term sepsis is broad and has been traditionally used to describe a vast spectrum of disease. Over the last 20 years, attempts have been made to apply more uniform diagnostic criteria to better define specific disease entities. Fairly specific criteria now define the terms sepsis, severe sepsis, septic shock, and SIRS (28,29). "Sepsis" refers to the systemic response to infection, including altered temperature, heart rate, respiratory rate, and leukocyte count. "Severe sepsis" adds the criterion of associated end-organ dysfunction to the above. Severe sepsis with hypotension or other evidence of hypoperfusion is referred to as "septic shock." "SIRS" is defined by the same criteria

as sepsis, only in the absence of documented or presumed infection. SIRS may occur in a variety of clinical circumstances, including trauma, burns, major surgery, and massive blood transfusion. Generally accepted diagnostic criteria are listed in Table 4, although considerable variability persists within the literature. Medications such as vasopressors or beta-blockers may alter physiologic parameters used in the definitions. This, in part, explains the inconsistency found in published reports. The remainder of this section will address the pathophysiology and management of septic shock.

Pathophysiology

A complete understanding as to the pathophysiology of septic shock remains elusive. One major theory holds that sepsis represents an uncontrolled overstimulation of the inflammatory response. This theory has been challenged many times, and alternate hypotheses demonstrate evidence of immune failure. It is likely that both theories are at least partially correct. Early in the course of sepsis, the immune system appears to become activated, with high levels of circulating tumor necrosis factor (TNF)-α and interleukin (IL)-1. Increased levels of these cytokines are associated with the clinical hyperdynamic state. Later in the course of septic illnesses, there is a shift toward anti-inflammatory mediator production. Patients may eventually become anergic and more susceptible to nosocomial infections. Much research has been done, beyond the scope of this chapter, attempting to clarify the complex interaction of bacteria and their byproducts with the host production of cytokines and other inflammatory mediators. While inflammatory cytokines have long been felt to be generally deleterious in sepsis, it is also known that TNF-α plays an important role in combating infection. Studies in both animals and humans have shown worse outcomes when TNF-α was blocked (30–33). More recently, a strong association between the inflammatory response of sepsis and perturbations of coagulation has been established. Specifically, sepsis-associated alterations in conversion of protein C into its activated form may lead to microvascular thrombosis, which may, in

Table 4 Sepsis: Definitions

Systemic inflammatory response syndrome (SIRS)	The generalized inflammatory response to a variety of clinical insults. The response is manifested by two or more of the following conditions: (i) temperature $>38°C$ or $<36°C$; (ii) heart rate >90 beats/min; (iii) respiratory rate >20 breaths/min or $PaCO_2$ <32 mmHg; and (iv) white blood cell count $>12,000/mm^3$, $<4000/mm^3$, or $>10\%$ band forms.
Sepsis	SIRS as described above with a presumed or confirmed infection.
Severe sepsis	Sepsis as described above with associated organ dysfunction, hypoperfusion, or hypotension. Perfusion abnormalities may include, but are not limited to, lactic acidosis, oliguria, or an acute alteration in mental status.
Septic shock	Severe sepsis as described above with associated hypotension despite adequate fluid resuscitation. Patients on inotropic or vasopressor agents may not be hypotensive at the time perfusion abnormalities are measured.

Abbreviation: $PaCO_2$, arterial pressure of carbon dioxide.
Source: From Ref. 28.

turn, be at least partially responsible for end-organ dysfunction. Ongoing research will hopefully allow a more thorough understanding of this complex disease process.

Treatment

There are five crucial components in the management of septic shock: fluid resuscitation, septic source control, appropriate use of vasopressor agents, appropriate use of inotropic agents, and rational utilization of antimicrobials. More recently, control of the perturbation of coagulation inherent in septic shock is emerging as a promising adjunctive measure that will be discussed in a later section. Once septic shock is suspected, rapid institution of these steps is necessary to avoid MODS and death. Early intervention has clearly been shown to improve outcomes and suggests that invasive hemodynamic monitoring and goal-directed therapy be initiated as early as possible (34).

Fluid Resuscitation

The initial treatment of septic shock such as hypovolemic shock involves intravenous fluid administration. Accompanying the systemic vasodilation of septic shock is disruption of microvascular endothelial integrity. Although the exact mechanism has not clearly been elucidated, the result is a net egress of intravascular fluid and protein into the interstitial space. This phenomenon of fluid sequestration is commonly referred to as a "capillary leak syndrome." Vasodilation and capillary leak conspire to decrease the central circulating blood volume and result in relative hypovolemia. Maintenance of adequate perfusion requires careful and repeated assessment of volume status, with fluid resuscitation guided by hemodynamic parameters. In most instances, an isotonic crystalloid such as LR solution is the preferred initial resuscitative fluid. Blood products may be required if cardiac ischemia is present or if anemia precludes adequate oxygen delivery. Transfusion of blood products should be based on physiologic variables rather than the predetermined notion of an "optimal" hematocrit of 30%. Inappropriate blood transfusion may actually increase the incidence of infectious complications, cardiac events, and mortality (35,36). Fluid management in septic shock mandates frequent and repeated assessments of intravascular volume. Total body weight or running totals of net fluid balance are not effective surrogates for intravascular volume status. In most instances, pulmonary artery catheter-guided fluid administration is invaluable, as fluid shifts may occur quite rapidly. Diuretic administration based on oliguria in septic shock is frequently detrimental and may increase the likelihood of death. Aggressive fluid replacement should be continued until endothelial integrity is reestablished. Onset of recovery is generally heralded by fluid mobilization and diminished volume requirements.

Septic Source Control

In an ICU population, numerous potential sources for infection exist. An adequate history and careful examination of the patient coupled with appropriate use of diagnostic studies is essential to accurately localize an infectious focus serving to fuel septic shock. The process of accurately localizing a source of infection can frequently be quite challenging. In many instances, the septic source is a site of previous intervention. It is essential that all surgical and traumatic wounds be carefully examined for evidence of superficial or deep infection. Implanted prosthetic devices should always be considered as possible sources of infection. Peripheral intravenous catheters, central venous lines, prosthetic meshes, and implanted orthopedic hardware may all become infected and lead to an episode of septic shock. Because many ICU patients have undergone recent abdominal surgery, consideration of intra-abdominal abscess, anastamotic leak, bowel ischemia, or iatrogenesis should prompt appropriate diagnostic workup. Computed tomography has proven invaluable in this regard, and modern high-resolution helical scanners are extremely accurate in detecting intra-abdominal sources of sepsis. Abscesses should be drained after initiating fluid resuscitation, so as to avoid cardiovascular collapse, which may result from the cytokine surge accompanying a drainage procedure. The importance of abscess drainage should not be underestimated because it is very rare for antibiotics alone to control an abscess. Drainage also facilitates culture-directed, narrow-spectrum antibiotic therapy, with the important secondary goal of prevention of antibiotic resistance.

Overwhelmingly, the most common site of infection in patients in modern ICUs is the respiratory tract. Ventilator-associated pneumonia and aspiration pneumonia are unfortunately common. Endotracheal intubation and mechanical ventilation for greater than 24 hours significantly increases the risk of developing pneumonia. Despite their frequency, however, respiratory infections are not common causes of septic shock. As a general rule, septic shock should not be attributed to an infiltrate on chest X ray without first giving adequate consideration to other possible sources. A common pitfall is the delayed diagnosis of severe intra-abdominal pathology in a patient being treated for presumed pneumonia, often with disastrous consequences.

Infections related to central venous catheterization represent another relatively common source of septic shock. It is estimated that over five million central venous catheters are utilized yearly in the United States alone, and most critically ill patients will require central venous catheterization at some point. The advent of central venous catheterization has truly been a double-edged sword. Central venous catheterization provides an avenue for monitoring and treatment of critically ill patients, while at the same time serving as an intravascular prosthetic nidus for bacteria. The risk of catheter-related infection is directly proportional to both the number of catheter lumens and the duration of catheter dwelling time. Catheters may become colonized by hematogenous seeding from other septic foci or, more commonly, via direct transcutaneous colonization at the insertion site. Catheters with 15 or more colony-forming units of bacteria, as described by Maki et al., are associated with higher relative risk of bacteremia and sepsis and should be removed (37). Further management depends on the organism isolated and the patient's clinical status. Uncomplicated gram-positive catheter-related bacteremia in the minimally symptomatic patient may only require removal of the offending device. Gram-negative organisms, resistant microbes, or gram-positive infections with persistent systemic symptoms usually require adjuvant antibiotic therapy. Prevention is the best method of treatment. Sterile technique at the time of insertion as well as at any time of manipulation is mandatory. Catheters should be removed when no longer needed, so as to limit the number of catheter days for any given patient.

Occasionally, the source of septic shock remains unclear despite aggressive evaluation. Careful consideration of less common etiologies should be given to avoid unnecessary delays in diagnosis. Sinusitis, perirectal abscess, meningitis, acalculous cholecystitis, ischemic colitis, and infected decubitus ulcer may all result in a septic picture. A high index of suspicion is crucial so that infectious foci can be drained or removed.

Vasopressors

Persistent hypotension despite adequate ongoing fluid administration may be an indication for vasopressor administration (38). Dopamine, epinephrine, norepinephrine, phenylephrine, and vasopressin are potential agents for use in this setting. The goal of vasopressor administration is to provide enough mean arterial pressure to maintain organ perfusion. This may be accomplished by counteracting the vasodilatory effects of circulating mediators released during SIRS. Vasoactive agents are appropriately administered after adequate volume resuscitation has been effected because failure to do so may increase morbidity and mortality by vasoconstriction of already ischemic capillary beds. Because shock, by definition, results in inadequate perfusion at the cellular level, global pharmacologic vasoconstriction in an effort to raise SVR and blood pressure also has the potential for reduction in end-organ blood flow. Teleologically, one might expect that the ability to autoregulate perfusion to ischemic tissues would give the most vital organs priority and protection. This occurs in hypovolemic or hemorrhagic shock, where blood flow is redirected from the periphery in order to maintain cerebral and cardiac perfusion. In sepsis, as well as some chronic disease states, the ability to autoregulate blood flow may be impaired. Recently

it has been suggested that sepsis is associated with subphysiologic levels of circulating vasopressin (39). Replacement therapy with extremely low-dose vasopressin (0.01–0.04 units/min) has resulted in hemodynamic improvement without the detrimental effects of vasoconstriction (40,41).

Exogenous vasopressors must be administered with great caution because the potential for serious adverse effect exists. Cardiac, mesenteric, and digital ischemia with infarction are well-described complications of vasopressor therapy, and a potential for worsening renal insufficiency exists as well. Tachycardia is frequently observed and may be mild, or, in certain circumstances, may be severe and limit therapeutic use of these drugs. In addition to unintended local consequences, global deleterious effects may also be observed. By increasing afterload, vasopressors have the potential to lower cardiac output and thereby exacerbate tissue oxygen debt. In general, the adage of "less is more" is well applied here. These agents should only be used in doses required to achieve the lowest acceptable blood pressure required to maintain cerebral and coronary perfusion. Continuous mixed SvO_2 combined with continuous cardiac output monitoring is often extremely helpful in titration of this therapy.

Inotropes

Septic shock is frequently characterized by a hyperdynamic state, with hypotension, low SVR, and a cardiac index that is normal or elevated (42). It should be noted, however, that an elevated cardiac index does not ensure adequate oxygen delivery; thus, inotropic agents are occasionally required to augment oxygen delivery in the septic patient (43). Retrospective studies (44–46) have repeatedly shown that septic patients who were able to mount a hyperdynamic cardiovascular response have lower mortality than patients with normal or subnormal cardiac indexes. Extending the concept that supranormal cardiac performance was associated with improved outcome, Shoemaker and coworkers popularized the concept of flow-dependent oxygen consumption and suggested that resuscitation should be directed to push cardiac performance to a state of flow-independent oxygen consumption (47,48). However, randomized prospective trials that employed inotropic agents to increase cardiac indices to predetermined levels have had mixed results (49–52). Thus, the goal should be to provide enough cardiac output to meet the metabolic demands of the patient. This assessment should be made using serial lactate measurements, arterial blood gas analysis, and establishment of acceptable mixed SvO_2.

Complications of inotropic support are most frequently cardiac in origin. Improved inotropy comes at a cost of increased myocardial oxygen consumption. Although inotropic support is usually well tolerated in young patients, elderly patients with coronary artery disease may experience myocardial ischemia or infarction. Dobutamine, one of the most commonly used inotropes, is frequently associated with hypotension due to associated vasodilation. This effect can frequently be overcome by additional fluid administration. In instances where severe hypotension persists, dobutamine may require concomitant infusion of a vasopressor. Occasionally, hypotension or tachyarrhythmia may limit or preclude dobutamine administration. In these circumstances, second-line inotropic agents such as amrinone or milrinone may be utilized.

Antibiotics

After adequate resuscitation of a patient with apparent sepsis or SIRS, two challenges remain: whether to administer antibiotics, and, if so, which antibiotic to administer. As mentioned previously, it can be quite difficult to differentiate between sepsis and SIRS, as SIRS is frequently a diagnosis of exclusion. This pursuit is an important one, however, because antibiotics provide no therapeutic benefit in the patient with SIRS in the absence of infection. Patients with presumed septic shock should receive empiric antibiotic therapy directed at likely pathogens while the search for a septic focus occurs and microbiologic data are gathered. When feasible, cultures should be taken prior to administration of antibiotics. Depending on the clinical circumstance, broad-spectrum agents may be required initially. Empiric therapy may be guided by the institution's antibiogram. When available, culture-directed antibiotic therapy should be the standard. The antibiotic spectrum should be narrowed to specifically cover the pathogens known or believed to be responsible for the infection. It is crucial that antibiotic therapy does not overshadow the need for surgical source control, if indicated. If infection is ruled out, empiric antibiotics should be discontinued.

Coagulation In Sepsis

As our understanding of cellular and molecular pathophysiology has progressed, many mediators involved in the inflammatory response of septic shock have been identified. Many investigators have put forth great efforts to identify an agent capable of attenuating or enhancing these mediators in the hope of favorably altering the inflammatory response present in septic patients. The search for a "magic bullet" antisepsis drug has, for the most part, had disappointing results. Anti-TNF antibodies, endotoxin-binding antibodies, IL-1 antagonists, and tissue factor pathway inhibitors are a few examples of sepsis drugs that have failed to improve the outcomes (53–62). This is likely the effect of a system with many inherent redundancies, as well as the fact that the inflammatory response is exceedingly complex and, at best, only partially understood.

Recent attention has turned toward the role of coagulation in sepsis, specifically regarding the role of protein C. Protein C is best known for its anticoagulant role in maintaining microcirculatory homeostasis. Protein C is activated by the thrombin–thrombomodulin complex, which is formed by the binding of thrombin to thrombomodulin. Activated protein C then in turn limits thrombin formation and downregulates coagulation activation by inactivating factor VIIIa and factor Va, which are cofactors for factor IXa-induced factor X activation and factor Xa–induced prothrombin activation, respectively (63–65). There exists significant overlap and interaction between mediators of the coagulation cascade and promoters of inflammation (66,67). The exact mechanism by which protein C interferes with the propagation of the inflammatory response in sepsis has not yet been fully elucidated. It may be that the conversion of protein C to its activated form may be impaired during sepsis due to downregulation of thrombomodulin by inflammatory cytokines (68). Protein C has been shown to interfere with cytokine production by monocytes.

In light of the above observations, a new agent that has shown promise in recent studies is recombinant human activated protein C (rHAPC). In a recent randomized, prospective, double-blind, placebo-controlled, multicenter trial (69) of nearly 1700 subjects, septic patients with evidence of end-organ dysfunction were randomized to receive a course of rHAPC or placebo. A significant mortality benefit was observed in the rHAPC-treated group. The beneficial effect of rHAPC may be secondary to an anticoagulant effect ameliorating microvascular thrombosis induced organ damage; alternately, there may be a direct anti-inflammatory effect as well. The anticoagulant effect of rHAPC can result in significant morbidity and mortality, however. Bleeding complications may severely limit the use of this agent in trauma victims or surgical patients. Additional clinical trials of rHAPC in sepsis are underway.

SPECIFIC COMPLICATIONS OF HYPOVOLEMIC AND SEPTIC SHOCK
Abdominal Compartment Syndrome

Compartment syndrome is defined as increasing pressure within an unyielding body cavity or compartment, resulting in organ injury, ischemia, or other undesirable physiologic effects. Commonly seen in the lower extremity following crush injury of muscle, it may also develop in the abdomen following injury, shock, or resuscitation. In abdominal compartment syndrome (ACS), visceral edema within the bony, fascial, and muscular confines of the abdominal cavity leads to rising intra-abdominal pressure. Visceral swelling may occur in directly injured tissues, or may follow large-volume resuscitation of various shock states. Elevated intra-abdominal pressure results in respiratory impairment secondary to cephalad displacement of both hemidiaphragms. Increased pressure on renal capillaries diminishes kidney perfusion, resulting in renal insufficiency. Impaired splanchnic venous return may worsen visceral edema, creating a vicious cycle that, if left untreated, frequently results in MODS and death. Additionally, ACS may increase intracranial pressure in head-injured patients (70).

ACS is most frequently encountered in the setting of major abdominal injury or ruptured abdominal aortic aneurysm. It may occur postoperatively or intraoperatively, as an unsuspecting surgeon struggles to close a laparotomy incision over particularly distended or edematous abdominal contents. However, ACS may occur even in the absence of abdominal injury or surgery, and has been described in burns, isolated orthopedic injuries, and septic shock from non-abdominal sources. Overall incidence in ICU patients is estimated to be between 2% and 5%, but the mortality rate of ACS is approximately 50% (71,72).

Intra-abdominal hypertension leading to ACS may be diagnosed with relative ease by manometric transduction of urinary bladder pressure. Because the dome of a partially filled urinary bladder acts as a passive diaphragm to the abdominal cavity, the pressure within the bladder serves as an accurate surrogate for intra-abdominal pressure. Pressures above 20 mmHg may be associated with the physiologic derangements of ACS; treatment involves decompressive laparotomy with temporary silo closure.

Adrenocortical Insufficiency

The response to shock typically involves activation of the hypothalamic-pituitary-adrenal (HPA) axis by neural and systemic pathways. Septic shock, in particular, results in HPA stimulation due to circulating cytokines such as TNF-α, IL-1, and IL-6. However, in up to 50% of septic patients, blunted HPA response may occur, resulting in relative adrenocortical insufficiency. Most commonly, this phenomenon is observed in vasopressor-dependent septic shock.

Early studies of steroid administration in septic shock utilized large doses of glucocorticoids aimed at ameliorating the inflammatory cascade. The underlying hypothesis at the time was that high-dose steroid-induced interruption of inflammation might decrease the incidence of MODS. However, the results of these early trials of high-dose steroids in sepsis were uniformly disappointing, and mortality increases were even noted. However, in light of the frequent observation of HPA suppression in vasopressor-dependent sepsis, there has been renewed interest in low-dose steroid replacement. In a recent randomized, prospective study (73), low-dose hydrocortisone and fludrocortisone administration significantly decreased both mortality and duration of vasopressor therapy in septic patients. At the very least, septic patients with exogenous catecholamine dependency should receive a cosyntropin stimulation test; nonresponders should be considered for corticosteroid replacement therapy.

REFERENCES

1. Le Dran HF. A Treatise, or Reflections Drawn from Practice on Gun-Shot Wounds. Avignon: Jean Chaillot, 1790.
2. Gross SD. A System of Surgery: Pathological, Diagnostic, Therapeutique, and Operative. 4th ed. Philadelphia: H.C. Lea, 1866.
3. Warren JC. Surgical Pathology and Therapeutics. Philadelphia: WB Saunders, 1895.
4. Crile GW. An Experimental Research into Surgical Shock. Philadelphia: JB Lippincott, 1899.
5. Blalock A. Principles of Surgical Care, Shock, and Other Problems. St. Louis: CV Mosby, 1940.
6. Advanced Trauma Life Support Manual. Chicago, Illinois: American College of Surgeons, 1997.
7. Abou-Khalil B, Scalea TM, Trooskin SZ, Henry SM, Hitchcock R. Hemodynamic responses to shock in young trauma patients: need for invasive monitoring. Crit Care Med 1994; 22(4):633–639.
8. Scalea TM, Maltz S, Yelon J, Trooskin SZ, Duncan AO, Sclafani SJ. Resuscitation of multiple trauma and head injury: role of crystalloid fluids and inotropes. Crit Care Med 1994; 22(10):1610–1615.
9. Manikis P, Jankowski S, Zhang H, Kahn RJ, Vincent JL. Correlation of serial blood lactate levels to organ failure and mortality after trauma. Am J Emer Med 1995; 13(6):619–622.
10. Dunham CM, Siegel JH, Weireter L, et al. Oxygen debt and metabolic acidemia as quantitative predictors of mortality and the severity of the ischemic insult in hemorrhagic shock. Crit Care Med 1991; 19(2):231–243.
11. Vincent JL, Dufaye P, Berre J, Leeman M, Degaute JP, Kahn RJ. Serial lactate determinations during circulatory shock. Crit Care Med 1983 11(6):449–451.
12. Abramson D, Scalea TM, Hitchcock R, Trooskin SZ, Henry SM, Greenspan J. Lactate clearance and survival following injury. J Trauma 1993; 35:584–589.
13. Davis JW, Kaups K. Base deficit in the elderly: a marker of severe injury and death. J Trauma 1998; 45(5):873–877.
14. Davis JW, Shackford SR, Mackersie RC, Hoyt DB. Base deficit as a guide to volume resuscitation. J Trauma 1988; 28(10):1464–1467.
15. Connors AF Jr, Speroff T, Dawson NV, et al. The effectiveness of right heart catheterization in the initial care of critically ill patients. SUPPORT Investigators. JAMA 1996; 276(11):889–897.
16. Mimoz O, Rauss A, Rekik N, Brun-Buisson C, Lemaire F, Brochard L. Pulmonary artery catheterization in critically ill patients: a prospective analysis of outcome changes associated with catheter-prompted changes in therapy. Crit Care Med 1994; 22:573.
17. Gomersall CD, Joynt GM, Freebairn RC, Hung V, Buckley TA, Oh TE. Resuscitation of critically ill patients based on the results of gastric tonometry: a prospective, randomized, controlled trial. Crit Care Med 2000; 28(3):607–614.
18. Ivatury RR, Simon RJ, Islam S, Fueg A, Rohman M, Stahl WM. A prospective randomized study of end points of resuscitation after major trauma: global oxygen transport indices versus organ-specific gastric mucosal pH. J Am Coll Surg 1996; 183(2):145–154.
19. Cohn SM, Varela JE, Giannotti G, et al. Splanchnic perfusion evaluation during hemorrhage and resuscitation with gastric near-infrared spectroscopy. J Trauma 2001; 50(4):629–634.

20. Rhee P, Wang D, Ruff P, et al. Human neutrophil activation and increased adhesion by various resuscitation fluids. Crit Care Med 2000; 28(1):264–265.

21. Alderson P, Schierhout G, Roberts I, Bunn F. Colloids versus crystalloids for fluid resuscitation in critically ill patients. Cochrane Database Syst Rev 2000; (2).

22. Alderson P, Bunn F, Lefebvre C, et al. Human albumin solution for resuscitation and volume expansion in critically ill patients. Cochrane Database Syst Rev 2002; (1).

23. Wade CE, Grady JJ, Kramer GC, et al. Individual patient cohort analysis of the efficacy of hypertonic saline/dextran in patients with traumatic brain injury and hypotension. J Trauma 1997; 42:S61–S65.

24. Sauaia A, Moore FA, Moore EE, Haenel JB, Read RA, Lezotte DC. Early predictors of postinjury multiple organ failure. Arch Surg 1994; 129(1):39–45.

25. Holmes JF, Sakles JC, Lewis G, Wisner DH. Effects of delaying fluid resuscitation on an injury to the systemic arterial vasculature. Acad Emerg Med 2002; 9(4):267–274.

26. Bickell WH, Wall MJ, Pepe PE, et al. Immediate versus delayed fluid resuscitation for hypotensive patients with penetrating truncal injuries. N Engl J Med 1994; 331(17):1105–1109.

27. Angus DC, Linde-Zwirble WT, Lidicker J, Clermont G, Carcillo J, Pinsky MR. Epidemiology of severe sepsis in the United States: analysis of incidence, outcome and associated costs of care. Crit Care Med 2001; 29(7): 1303–1310.

28. Bone RC, Balk RA, Cerra FB, et al. Definitions for sepsis and organ failure and guidelines for the use of innovative therapies in sepsis. The ACCP/SCCM Consensus Conference Committee. American College of Chest Physicians/Society of Critical Care Medicine. Chest 1992; 101(6):1644–1655.

29. Balk RA. Severe sepsis and septic shock: definitions, epidemiology, and clinical manifestations. Crit Care Clin 2000; 16(2):179–192.

30. Echtenacher B, Weigl K, Lehn N, Mannel DN. Tumor necrosis factor-dependent adhesions as a major protective mechanism early in septic peritonitis in mice. Infect Immun 2001; 69(6):3550–3555.

31. Eskandari MK, Bolgos G, Miller C, Nguyen DT, DeForge LE, Remick DG. Anti-tumor necrosis factor antibody therapy fails to prevent lethality after cecal ligation and puncture or endotoxemia. J Immunol 1992; 148(9):2724–2730.

32. Opal SM, Cross AS, Jhung JW, et al. Potential hazards of combination immunotherapy in the treatment of experimental septic shock. J Infect Dis 1996; 173(6):1415–1421.

33. Fisher CJ, Agosti JM, Opal SM, et al. Treatment of septic shock with the tumor necrosis factor receptor: Fc fusion protein. N Engl J Med 1996; 334(26):1697–1702.

34. Rivers E, Nguyen B, Havstad S, et al. Early goal-directed therapy in the treatment of severe sepsis and septic shock. N Engl J Med 2001; 345(19):1368–1377.

35. Hebert PC, Wells G, Blajchman MA, et al. A multicenter randomized, controlled clinical trial of transfusion requirements in critical care. Transfusion Requirements in Critical Care Investigators, Canadian Critical Care Trials Group. NEJM 1999; 340(6):409–417.

36. Hebert PC, Yetisir E, Martin C, et al. Is a low transfusion threshold safe in critically ill patients with cardiovascular diseases? Crit Care Med 2001; 29(2): 227–234.

37. Maki DG, Weise CE, Sarafin HW. A semiquantitative culture method for identifying intravenous-catheter-related infection. N Engl J Med 1977; 296(23):1305–1309.

38. Rudis MI, Basha MA, Zarowitz BJ. Is it time to reposition vasopressors and inotropes in sepsis? Crit Care Med 1996; 24(3):525–537.

39. Landry DW, Levin HR, Gallant EM, et al. Vasopressin deficiency contributes to the vasodilation of septic shock. Circulation 1997; 95(5):1122–1125.

40. Malay MB, Ashton RC Jr, Landry DW, Townsend RN. Low-dose vasopressin in the treatment of vasodilatory septic shock. J Trauma 1999; 47(4):699–703.

41. Landry DW, Levin HR, Gallant EM, et al. Vasopressin pressor hypersensitivity in vasodilatory septic shock. Crit Care Med 1997; 25(8):1279–1282.

42. Parrillo JE, Parker MM, Natanson C, et al. Septic shock in humans: advances in the understanding of pathogenesis, cardiovascular dysfunction, and therapy. Ann Intern Med 1990; 113(3):227–242.

43. Parker MM, Shelhamer JH, Bacharach SL, et al. Profound but reversible myocardial depression in patients with septic shock. Ann Intern Med 1984; 100(4):483–490.

44. Edwards JD, Brown GCS, Nightingale P, Slater RM, Faragher EB. Use of survivors' cardiorespiratory values as therapeutic goals in septic shock. Crit Care Med 1989; 17(11):1098–1103.

45. Gilbert EM, Haupt MT, Mandanas RY, Huaringa AJ, Carlson RW. The effect of fluid loading, blood transfusion, and catecholamine infusion on oxygen delivery and consumption in patients with sepsis. Am Rev Respir Dis 1986; 134(5):873–878.

46. Shoemaker WC, Appel PL, Kram HB. Hemodynamic and oxygen transport responses in survivors and nonsurvivors of high-risk surgery. Crit Care Med 1993; 21(7):977–1090.

47. Shoemaker WC, Appel PL, Kram HB, Waxman K, Lee TS. Prospective trial of supranormal values of survivors as therapeutic goals in high-risk surgical patients. Chest 1988; 94(6):1176–1186.

48. Bishop MH, Shoemaker WC, Appel PL, et al. Prospective, randomized trial of survivor values of cardiac index, oxygen delivery, and oxygen consumption as resuscitation endpoints in severe trauma. J Trauma 1995; 38(5):780–787.

49. Boyd O, Grounds RM, Bennett ED. A randomized clinical trial of the effect of deliberate perioperative increase of oxygen delivery on mortality in high risk surgical patients. JAMA 1993; 270(22):2699–2707.

50. Hayes MA, Timmins AC, Yau EHS, Palazzo M, Hinds CJ, Watson D. Elevation of systemic oxygen delivery in the treatment of critically ill patients. N Engl J Med 1994; 330(24):1717–1722.

51. Gattinoni L, Brazzi L, Pelosi P, et al. A trial of goal-oriented hemodynamic therapy in critically ill patients. SVO$_2$ Collaborative Group. N Engl J Med 1995; 333(16):1025–1032.

52. Tuchschmidt J, Fried J, Astiz M, Rackow E. Elevation of cardiac output and oxygen delivery improves outcome in septic shock. Chest 1992; 102(1):216–220.

53. Ziegler EJ, McCutchan JA, Fierer J, et al. Treatment of Gram-negative bacteremia and shock with human antiserum to a mutant Escherichia coli. N Engl J Med 1982; 307(20):1225–1230.

54. Calandra T, Glauser MP, Schellekens J, Verhoef J. Treatment of Gram-negative septic shock with human IgG antibody to Escherichia coli J5: a prospective, double-blind, randomized trial. J Infect Dis 1988; 158(2):312–318.

55. Ziegler EJ, Fisher CJ Jr, Sprung CL, et al. Treatment of Gram-negative bacteremia and septic shock with HA-1A human monoclonal antibody against endotoxin. N Engl J Med 1991; 324(7):429–436.

56. Abraham E, Anzueto A, Gutierrez G, et al. Double-blind, randomized, controlled trial of monoclonal antibody to human tumor necrosis factor in treatment of septic shock. NORASEPT II Study Group. Lancet 1998; 351(9107):929–933.

57. Abraham E, Wunderink R, Silverman H, et al. Efficacy and safety of monoclonal antibody to human tumor necrosis factor-alpha in patients with sepsis syndrome: a randomized, controlled, double-blind multicenter clinical trial. TNF-alpha MAb Sepsis Study Group. JAMA 1995; 273(12):934–941.

58. Cohen J, Carlet J. INTERSEPT: an international, multicenter, placebo-controlled trial of monoclonal antibody to human tumor necrosis factor-alpha in patients with sepsis. International Sepsis Trial Study Group. Crit Care Med 1996; 24(9):1431–1440.

59. Abraham E, Glauser MP, Butler T, et al. p55 tumor necrosis factor receptor fusion protein in the treatment of patients with severe sepsis and septic shock. JAMA 1977; 277(19):1531–1538.

60. Opal SM, Fisher CJ Jr, Khainaut Jf, et al. Confirmatory interleukin-1 receptor antagonist trial in severe sepsis: a phase III, randomized, double-blind, placebo-controlled, multicenter trial. The Interleukin-1 Receptor Antagonist Sepsis Investigator Group. Crit Care Med 1997; 25(7):1115–1124.

61. Abraham E. Tissue factor inhibition and clinical trial results of tissue factor pathway inhibitor in sepsis. Crit Care Med 2000; 28(suppl 9):S31–S33.

62. De Jonge E, Dekkers PE, Creasey AA, et al. Tissue factor pathway inhibitor does not influence inflammatory pathways during human endotoxemia. J Infect Dis 2001; 183(12):1815–1818.

63. Gruber A, Mori E, del Zoppo GJ, Waxman L, Griffin JH. Alteration of fibrin network by activated protein C. Blood 1994; 83(9):2541–2548.

64. De Fouw NJ, van Hinsbergh VW, de Jong YF, Haverkate F, Bertina RM. The interaction of activated protein C and thrombin with the plasminogen activator inhibitor released from human endothelial cells. Thromb Haemost 1987; 57(2):176–182.

65. Esmon CT. The roles of protein C and thrombomodulin in the regulation of blood coagulation. J Biol Chem 1989; 264(9):4743–4746.

66. Esmon CT, Taylor FB Jr, Snow TR. Inflammation and coagulation: linked processes potentially regulated through a common pathway mediated by protein C. Thromb Haemost 1991; 66(1):160–165.

67. Stouthard JM, Levi M, Hack CE, et al. Interleukin-6 stimulates coagulation, not fibrinolysis, in humans. Thromb Haemost 1996; 76(5):738–742.

68. Boehme MW, Deng Y, Raeth U, et al. Release of thrombomodulin from endothelial cells by concerted action of TNF-alpha and neutrophils: in vivo and in vitro studies. Immunology 1996; 87(1):134–140.

69. Bernard GR, Vincent JL, Laterre PF, et al. Efficacy and safety of recombinant human activated protein C for severe sepsis. N Engl J Med 2001; 344(10):699–709.

70. Citero G, Vascotto E, Villa F, Celotti S, Pesenti A. Induced abdominal compartment syndrome increases intracranial pressure in neurotrauma patients: a prospective study. Crit Care Med 2001; 29(7):1466–1471.

71. Hong JJ, Cohn SM, Perez JM, Dolich MO, Brown M, McKenney MG. Incidence and outcome of intra-abdominal hypertension and the abdominal compartment syndrome. Br J Surg 2002; 89(5):591–596.

72. Tremblay LN, Feliciano DV, Schmidt J, et al. Skin only or silo closure in the critically ill patient with an open abdomen. Am J Surg 2001; 182(6):670–675.

73. Annane D, Sébille V, Charpentier C, et al. Effect of treatment with low doses of hydrocortisone and fludrocortisone on mortality in patients with septic shock. JAMA 2002; 288(7):862–871.

6

Complications Associated with the Use of Invasive Devices in the Intensive Care Unit

Victor Cruz
Department of Surgery, Stony Brook University Hospital, Stony Brook, New York, U.S.A.

J. Martin Perez
Robert Wood Johnson University Hospital, New Brunswick, New Jersey, U.S.A.

The ability of the practitioner to care for the critically ill patient is closely associated with the types and functions of the many invasive and noninvasive devices that can be used. Because the use of central venous catheterization in the intensive care unit (ICU) permits more intensive monitoring and directed interventions, improvements have been achieved in hemodynamic and metabolic assessment, administration of total parental nutrition, chemotherapies, and the performance of hemodialysis. Despite the low incidence of complications associated with these invasive and noninvasive devices, if mortality and morbidity rates are to be reduced even further, the practitioner must be aware of the many complications that may accompany the use of each type of device. Knowledge of these complications will enable the practitioner to not only implement preventive measures but also rapidly recognize and treat complications that may arise. This chapter will discuss the preventive measures and the treatment of complications associated with the use of central venous lines, arterial lines, intracerebral pressure monitors, gastric tubes, and thoracostomy tubes.

CENTRAL VENOUS ACCESS

The increasing complexity of the ICU has paralleled the development and increased use of central venous catheterization. Central venous access has become a mainstay in the ICU; several million devices are used annually (1). Unlike the catheters introduced by Broviac et al. (2) and Hickman et al. (3), the catheters used in the ICU lack cuffs and do not require tunneling. Thus, they can be easily placed at the bedside with the Seldinger method or other percutaneous techniques. Although central venous lines are technically less challenging to use and care for than are the Broviac et al. (2) and Hickman et al. (3) catheters, central venous lines are associated with their own set of complications.

Venous Air Embolus

The complication of venous air embolism is rare; in fact, the occasional case report represents the majority of the literature about this entity. However, this complication should be suspected if a patient becomes dyspneic on insertion of a central venous line. Venous air embolism can lead to hypotension, acute pulmonary edema, and cardiac arrest. If the foramen ovale is patent, the risk of an ischemic stroke also exists. During the physical examination of a patient with a venous air embolism, a murmur with a characteristic mill wheel may be heard over the right side of the heart. Because a small pressure gradient of 4 mmHg can cause enough air to enter in one second to cause a fatal air embolus (4), prevention techniques should include attempts to increase intrathoracic pressure. Such an increase can be accomplished by placing the patient in Trendelenberg position or by asking the patient to perform a Valsalva maneuver or to hum during placement of a central venous line. Intrathoracic pressure can also increase during exchange over a guide wire. Once venous air embolism occurs, the patient should be placed in the left lateral decubitus position; a syringe should be used to aspirate fluid, air, or both from the line; and a pericardiocentesis can be performed, if necessary, by inserting a needle into the right ventricle in an attempt to aspirate air.

Pneumothorax

A pneumothorax from central venous lines occurs when the needle injures lung parenchyma and air escapes into the pleural space. This type of complication occurs in approximately 1% to 4% of all central venous line attempts. Symptoms such as coughing, wheezing, chest pain, and dyspnea may be evident; however, in approximately 0.5% of cases, the appearance of symptoms may be delayed (5). Regardless of when the symptoms appear, a pneumothorax may develop into a tension pneumothorax, and patients who are on a ventilator may be at increased risk (5). In a study of patients with cancer for whom central venous access was established through the subclavian approach, older patients with a body mass index of less than 19 were more likely to experience pneumothorax (6). Pneumothoraces may occur with the same frequency whether the subclavian approach is used or the internal jugular approach is used (7). A relatively high rate of pneumothorax development is also associated with a difficulty in obtaining central venous access, such as repeated attempts at cannulation (6).

The diagnosis of pneumothorax is facilitated by an expiratory chest radiograph of the upright patient; however, most chest X rays taken in the ICU are performed with the patient in the supine position. When patients are supine, air usually presents along the lung base and mediastinum, and this makes the diagnosis of a pneumothorax by X-ray relatively more difficult.

The risk of a pneumothorax can be reduced if the patient lies on a rolled towel placed under the thoracic spine and between the scapulae during cannulation of the vessel. If the risk of a pneumothorax is to be eliminated, a cut-down of the cephalic vein can be performed.

Rates of pneumothorax are lower if experienced physicians perform the central venous access procedure (7). Management of this complication may include observation if pneumothoraces are less than 30% and placement of a pigtail catheter or chest tube if the pneumothorax is larger than 30% or expands after initial observation, or if the patient is on a ventilator.

Hemorrhage and Hemothorax

Hemorrhage resulting from central line catheterization can be categorized as either localized or regional. Localized hemorrhage is confined to the site of access, whereas regional hemorrhage occurs in the soft tissue of the neck or extends to the thoracic and mediastinal spaces. Localized hemorrhage due to central line access is uncommon, even if coagulopathy or thrombocytopenia is present (8).

Carotid artery puncture, a complication that occurs during approximately 2% to 10% of attempts at internal jugular line placement (9), usually manifests itself as a hematoma when the needle is removed from the artery. Insertion of a needle into the carotid artery may be indicated by bright red, pulsatile blood that fills the hub of the syringe. Removing the needle and applying pressure usually suffices in arresting the bleeding. Close follow-up of the patient who has experienced carotid artery puncture is prudent because acute airway obstruction has been reported from a large cervical hematoma (10). Complications have also resulted from cannulation of the carotid artery (11); these complications include hematoma, arteriovenous fistula, stroke, and death (12). If cannulation of the carotid artery is suspected but the chest X-ray does not reveal it or is inconclusive, an arterial

blood gas can be obtained or catheter pressures can be transduced to confirm a venous wave form.

Hemorrhage that results in a hemothorax is not commonly reported. A hemothorax can be caused by an injury to the subclavian artery or vein at the time of insertion or by the gradual erosion of the superior vena cava (SVC). A hemothorax can occur ipsilaterally or contralaterally to the insertion site. Reports of hemothorax caused by the internal jugular approach are rare.

Diagnosis of hemothorax can be based on the results of plain-film radiography. However, a substantial hemothorax can cause tachycardia and hypotension. Hemothorax resulting from erosion of the SVC can be prevented by careful placement of the catheter tip so that it does not press against the SVC when placed from left side (13). Once the SVC has been injured, conservative measures are recommended for maintaining the volume and treating any coagulopathy. However, surgical intervention is usually required for both adults (14) and children (15).

Bleeding into the mediastinum can occur when a vein is injured or the catheter penetrates the mediastinum. This complication most commonly appears initially on chest radiographs as a widened mediastinum, but it can also cause chest pain after line insertion. When the mediastinum is widened after the placement of a central line, additional chest radiographs should be obtained with the injection of contrast material through the central catheter. If extravasation of the contrast agent occurs and the catheter is in the mediastinum, it should be withdrawn quickly; however, if the catheter is in the vein, it can be left in place, with careful observation of the patient's condition. According to Whitman (14), most mediastinal hematomas are self-limiting, and the venous injury will resolve without intervention. This is unlike a hemorrhage into the pleural space, which usually requires further intervention. Mediastinal hematomas occur in less than 1% of patients who undergo line placement (14). The unrecognized presence of a catheter in the mediastinum, regardless of the type of fluid being administered, is associated with high morbidity and mortality rates (16).

Cardiac Tamponade

According to the 1989 Food and Drug Administration (FDA) drug bulletin, cardiac tamponade is the most commonly reported lethal complication associated with central venous access. Cardiac tamponade occurs when the catheter tip penetrates the pericardium. Cardiac tamponade is signaled by an acute onset of tachycardia, hypotension, jugular venous distention, and pulsus paradoxus. However, the symptoms of tamponade may also be delayed.

Cardiac tamponade can be prevented by careful placement of the catheter tip. The FDA has stated that placing the tip into the atrium is associated with a higher risk of tamponade. There have also been reports of cardiac tamponade when the catheter tip is placed in the SVC (17). Cardiac tamponade is treated by rapidly increasing intravenous volume followed by subxiphoid pericardiocentesis to stabilize the patient's condition. Surgical intervention may be warranted to repair lacerations of the atria or the SVC, as well as the need for a pericardial window as a more definitive measure.

Central Venous Device and Infection

Central venous access devices are a common source for bacterial nosocomial infections in the ICU setting. In fact, catheter-related bloodstream infection (CRBSI) is the most frequently occurring type of bloodstream infection in the ICU (18,19). Approximately 250,000 patients develop CRBSI each year (18). According to one study (20), nosocomial bloodstream infection occurs in 2.7 of every 100 patients admitted to a surgical ICU. A case control analysis found that such infections are associated with a 35% increase in mortality, a 24-day increase in median length of stay, and a $40,000 increase in expense per survivor. The National Nosocomial Infections Surveillance (NNIS) System reported that a median range of bloodstream infections associated with central lines was 2.4 to 7.8 central line–patient days (21).

The pathogenesis of CRBSI involves colonization of the catheter by microorganisms that inhabit the skin surface at the site of catheter insertion (18). Other important sources of catheter colonization are contaminated infusates, distant sites of infection, and hub contamination. Microorganisms migrate along the transcutaneous tract and adhere to the catheter's biofilm. The exact sequence of events leading from biofilm colonization to bloodstream infection is poorly defined, as are the factors that determine establishment of infection. According to the NNIS, the most commonly reported organisms involved in CRBSI, in decreasing order of frequency, are coagulase-negative *Staphylococcus* spp. (39.3%), *Staphylococcus aureus* (10.7%), *Enterococcus* spp. (10.3%), *Candida albicans* (4.9%), and other gram-negative organisms.

The Centers for Disease Control and Prevention define catheter colonization as growth of 15 or more colony-forming units isolated from a catheter segment and cultured by the roll-plate method. CRBSI is defined as an infection in which the same organism with a similar drug susceptibility pattern is isolated from a catheter segment and simultaneously from peripheral blood in a patient with clinical manifestations of sepsis and no other apparent source of blood stream infection (22). If signs of local infection, such as erythema, induration, tenderness, or purulent drainage, develop at the site of catheter insertion, the catheter should be removed and the catheter segment submitted for culture. If CRBSI is established, in addition to catheter removal, systemic antibiotics are usually indicated. Currently, a lack of consensus exists regarding antibiotic selection and duration of therapy;

however, with the increasing emergence of methicillin-resistant strains, vancomycin is commonly used as first-line therapy. Most clinicians will develop a treatment plan according to the isolate, known susceptibility patterns, and response to therapy; this response is indicated by clinical variables such as fever and leukocytosis. Persistent fever, leukocytosis, and bacteremia may warrant further investigation of a deep-seated infection such as suppurative thrombophlebitis. In patients who are febrile but have no obvious clinical source of infection and no clinical signs of infection at the site of catheter insertion, the catheter segment may be submitted for quantitative culture. If the culture of the catheter segment demonstrates significant microbial growth, the replacement catheter should be removed and a new catheter should be inserted at a different site.

Multiple methods have been studied for preventing CRBSI. Ruesch et al. (23) have reviewed several prospective studies demonstrating that the subclavian site of insertion is associated with a lower risk of infection than is the jugular or femoral sites. Another review (24) has shown that chlorhexidine gluconate is superior to 10% povidone iodone for skin preparation in the prevention of CRBSI. A prospective observational study (25) showed that full-barrier precautions, including sterilized gloves, gown, cap, mask, and barrier drape that covers the entire patient, reduces the incidence of CRBSI associated with the insertion of central venous devices. Several studies have demonstrated that the use of transparent occlusive dressings increases the risk of clinically significant catheter colonization. The use of antibiotic ointments at the catheter insertion site appears to increase catheter colonization with fungi. Using chlorhexidine-impregnated sponges as a dressing for central venous, pulmonary artery, and arterial catheters have been shown to significantly decrease catheter colonization and CRBSI (26). Minocycline- or rifampin-impregnated catheters are associated with lower rates of catheter colonization and CRBSI than are catheters impregnated with chlorhexidine/silver sulfadiazine (27). Patients should be asked about potential allergic reactions to the components of the catheter before it is placed. The emergence of resistant organisms in response to the use of antibiotic-impregnated catheter may have an impact on future clinical use.

Preventative measures that have been proven to reduce catheter colonization and CRBSI should be implemented and adhered to as a part of an overall effort to reduce nosocomial infection rates associated with the use of central venous access devices.

Thrombosis

Central venous thrombosis after placement of a central line appears to be related to several factors. Larger catheters, which are more likely to obstruct flow, have been shown to be associated with higher thrombosis rates (28). Moreover, the location of the catheter tip may be a factor. An analysis of several retrospective studies has shown a correlation between placement of catheter tips high in the SVC and higher rates of thrombosis (29).

Patients with bone marrow transplants, malignancies, sickle cell disease, and renal failure are more likely to experience thrombosis (30). Other factors that play a role in thrombosis are hypercoagulable states secondary to illness and endothelial injury from catheter insertion.

Venous thrombosis can be diagnosed by duplex ultrasonography. However, duplex ultrasound is unable to adequately visualize the subclavian vein deep to the clavicle. This limitation is partially overcome by the fact that the presence of subclavian thrombosis can be predicted by a lack of flow in the internal jugular or axillary vein. This observation of a lack of flow may be adequate for the diagnosis of thrombosis. However, if a patient exhibits symptoms such as superficial venous engorgement, unilateral arm swelling, pain, and discoloration, contrast venography should be performed even if the findings of venous duplex ultrasonography are negative.

Management of thrombosis depends on the patient's symptoms and on whether the catheter is functioning properly. If a patient has no symptoms, a functional catheter can safely be left in place while anticoagulation therapy is started to prevent clot propagation, or to prevent the formation of a pulmonary embolism from an upper-extremity thrombosis (the risk of such an embolism is less than 10%) (31). If the catheter is clotted or if the patient's symptoms worsen, the catheter should be removed.

Prevention of thrombosis should take into account the location of the catheter, with the optimal placement being just proximal to the right atrium. Anticoagulation has also been useful in preventing the formation of thrombosis. Both heparin (32) and low doses of Coumadin® (warfarin sodium; 1 mg/day) (33) have been shown to effectively reduce the rate of thrombosis formation. However, no studies have compared the effectiveness of heparin with that of Coumadin in preventing thrombosis.

The incidence of complications such as fracture of the catheter, loss of the guide wire, and arteriovenous fistula is unknown. However, when fracture or loss of the guide wire has occurred, the catheter can be safely removed via interventional radiologic techniques (34).

ARTERIAL LINES

The radial, brachial, dorsal pedal, and femoral arteries can be safely cannulated for invasive blood pressure monitoring and frequent blood draws. The complications commonly associated with these catheters are those associated with central venous lines—infection, bleeding, and thrombosis. The most common complication associated with these catheters, however, is not infection, as is the case with central venous lines. In a

study of more than 2000 patients (35), the most common complications were vascular insufficiency (4%), bleeding (2%), and infection (0.5%).

Arterial thrombosis due to catheterization can occur in as many as 25% of patients with radial arterial lines, but the occurrence of this complication is lower among patients with femoral arterial lines (36). Fortunately, thrombosis of the radial or femoral artery rarely causes ischemia to the distal extremity. Flushing the catheter with heparin has been shown to decrease the rate of thrombosis in both femoral and radial arterial lines (37).

The incidence of infection is similar with femoral and radial arterial lines. *Staphylococcal* species continue to be the most common organism associated with catheter-related infections. Although many ICUs routinely change arterial line tubing and solution in an attempt to decrease infection rates, O'Malley and colleagues (38) demonstrated in a prospective study that routinely changing the tubing increases the likelihood of introducing contamination into the pressure-monitoring system.

Preventing arterial catheter infections requires methods similar to those used to prevent infection of central venous lines. Sterile techniques should be used during catheter placement, and hygienic manipulation should be employed when the line is accessed.

GASTROSTOMY TUBES

The popularity of gastrostomy tubes has increased over the years. Although their use for gastrointestinal decompression has been widely accepted for some time, it was not until the late 1970s that their usefulness in providing enteral access for nutritional support was appreciated. Kudsk et al. (39) first demonstrated the benefits of enteral nutrition over parenteral nutrition in rats. Alexander (40) reported that the outcome of children with burns to 60% of their total body surface area was improved when enteral nutrition rather than parenteral nutrition was used. Several subsequent studies continued to report the benefits of enteral nutrition over parenteral nutrition in reducing the rates of nosocomial infection.

Although gastrointestinal intubation has improved clinical outcome by providing enteral nutrition and gastric decompression, the placement of nasogastric tubes (NGTs) has it own set of complications—aspiration pneumonia, esophageal perforation, sinusitis, malposition, and arterial esophageal fistula.

Aspiration Pneumonia

The incidence of aspiration pneumonia increases among patients with certain risk factors (Table 1). Mullan and Roubenoff (41) have stated that the incidence of aspiration ranges from 1% to 30%. This variation is most likely due to the variety of patient populations included and the different methods used in the diagnosis of aspiration pneumonia. In one

Table 1   Risk Factors for Aspiration Pneumonia

Delayed gastric emptying
Decreased gag, cough, or swallow reflexes
Mechanical ventilation
Large bore feeding tubes
Neurologic injury

study, the incidence of aspiration among patients receiving enteral nutrition was approximately 5%, and mortality from aspiration in this population was less than 5%. A retrospective analysis using national medical claims has reported the mortality of aspiration pneumonia to be as high as 23.9%. Mortality is correlated with the amount of aspiration, acidity of aspirate, number of lobes involved, and the overall condition of the patient.

A dramatic change in the appearance of the chest on radiograph can suggest the diagnosis of aspiration pneumonia; however, such changes may not be evident until 24 hours after aspiration has occurred. The diagnosis of aspiration may be aided by testing the pulmonary aspirate for glucose. Previously, Food Drug and Cosmetic Blue No. 1 dye was added to enteral nutrition formulas in order to facilitate the detection of gastric aspirate in tracheal secretions. However, reports (42) of systemic blue dye absorption and associated adverse outcomes are emerging. This has caused many hospitals to withdraw the practice of adding dye to their enteral formulas. Bronchoscopy is a helpful tool that can be used to diagnose aspiration in addition to providing immediate lavage for removing aspirate.

Aspiration can be prevented by correctly placing the NGT and closely monitoring gastric residuals. Other preventive measures include elevating the head of a patient's bed to an angle of 30° to 45° so the patient is not supine. Using small-bore NGTs has also been suggested as a means of decreasing aspiration pneumonia and reflux. Conversely, the incidence of pneumothorax and tracheal intubation with insertion of a feeding tube is increased with small-bore nasoenteral tubes (less than 5 mm diameter). Aspiration should be treated by removing the aspirate with nasotracheal suction or bronchoscopy when necessary. Antibiotics, intubation, and ventilator support may be indicated. Other treatments such as corticosteroids therapy have not proven to be beneficial.

Esophageal Perforation

Esophageal perforation is a rare complication of nasogastric intubation; however, its occurrence may be fatal. One study of hospitalized patients with esophageal perforation showed that the most common cause of this complication is iatrogenic (43).

The most common site of iatrogenic perforation is the thoracic esophagus. The mortality rates associated with esophageal perforation range from 16% to 30% (44), but the mortality rate is lower when

the cause of perforation is iatrogenic or when the injury is promptly recognized and treatment is not delayed. The risk of esophageal perforation is higher among patients with carcinoma, stricture, or altered mental status, as well as among those who have undergone tracheal intubation or have undergone multiple attempts at nasogastric intubation (45).

In the critically ill, the diagnosis of esophageal perforation may be difficult and requires a high level of clinical suspicion. The most common clinical features are neck and substernal pain, fever, and subcutaneous or mediastinal emphysema that may cause nuchal crepitus or xiphisternal crepitus (also known as Hamman's sign). Radiography of the chest or abdomen with the patient in the upright position is diagnostic in most cases. However, when the results are negative and the level of clinical suspicion remains high, esophageal study using Gastrografin® as a contrast agent should be performed. The prognosis of esophageal perforation is dependent upon early diagnosis and treatment and the site and size of the perforation. Medical management includes the use of broad-spectrum antibiotics and nasogastric decompression. These treatments may be adequate for patients with cervical perforation, who are asymptomatic and whose condition is hemodynamically stable (44). Surgical management, if necessary, involves drainage alone, drainage and repair, or drainage and diversion.

Sinusitis

The use of a NGT with tracheal intubation has been associated with an increase risk of sinusitis. In these cases, sinusitis occurs because the NGT obstructs the ostial meatal complex and impairs the drainage of mucous. According to Fasqualle et al. (46), nosocomial sinusitis occurs most commonly in the ICU. The most commonly involved organism is *Pseudomonas aeruginosa*, *Streptococcal pneumonia*, and *Hemophilus influenza*.

Pain and pressure over the cheeks are the most common symptoms of sinusitis, but may be difficult to assess among ICU patients. Purulent nasal discharge may not be present, but if it is, the likelihood of sinusitis is increased. Often patients initially present with fever of unknown etiology. Once the most common causes of fever have been ruled out, further evaluation of the sinuses is warranted if intubation and an NGT are in use. Westergren et al. (47) have advocated the use of ultrasonography as a sensitive test for the presence of fluid and edema in the sinuses of critically ill patients. For improved diagnostic accuracy, computer tomography of the sinuses (coronal view) can be performed. Sinoscopy can aid in the diagnosis by yielding a culture specimen that can be tested for the purpose of directing antibiotic therapy; sinoscopy can also be used to treat sinusitis by creating an ostium to allow drainage of sinus secretions. Treatment consists of antibiotic therapy targeted at specific bacteria, removal of any foreign objects from the nose, using nasal decongestants, and if necessary, sinoscopy drainage.

Malposition

Retrospective case review of complications associated with NGTs have indicated that approximately 0.5% to 1% of NGTs are malpositioned (48). The most common location of malpositioning is the tracheal bronchial tree, especially the bronchi of the right lower lobe; misplacement in the pleural space, intracranial space, and internal jugular vein is rarely reported. The types of complication of malpositioned NGTs are based on location (Table 2).

NGTs are contraindicated for patients with basal skull injuries because such injuries increase the likelihood of intracerebral placement of the tube. However, this type of malpositioning has also been observed in patients without basal skull fractures (49). Diagnosis of malpositioning has been based on several commonly acceptable clinical guidelines. Proper placement of the NGT can be performed by insufflation of air in the tube with auscultation over the stomach or by aspiration of gastric contents. Aspiration prior to insufflation is preferred, in order to prevent a fatal air embolus, in the rare case of NGT malposition in a vascular structure. However, malpositioning of the NGT in the left lung base can also be detected by auscultation over the stomach, and secretions can also be suctioned from the bronchial tree, the esophagus and stomach, or the brain. Bankier et al. (48) have demonstrated that the clinical signs of NGT malpositioning may not accurately indicate the tube's location. A chest radiograph taken with the patient in the supine position can accurately detect malpositioning. Prevention lies in the use of clinical guidelines described above and of chest radiographs when there is any doubt about the position of the NGT.

Arterial Esophageal Fistula

Arterial esophageal fistula is a rare complication of gastric esophageal intubation and can involve the aorta and other great vessels in the chest. Symptoms are similar to those of aortic enteric fistulas. Sentinel bleeding, which first alerts the practitioner to the presence of this complication, is followed by a symptom-free period that precedes exsanguinations. Reports

(50) suggest that anomalies of the aortic arch predispose patients to this complication.

THORACOSTOMY TUBES

Thoracostomy tubes have been used since the time of Hippocrates but were not popularized until the Korean War. Indications for chest tube placement are pneumothorax, tension pneumothorax, penetrating chest injury, hemothorax, empyema, chylothorax, post–thoracic surgery, and bronchopleural fistula. Thoracostomy tubes can be placed via sharp cut down, by the trochar method (the use of a sharp metal rod), or by a percutaneous Seldinger techniques. The percutaneous technique using the Seldinger method is employed when smaller pigtail-type chest tubes are used. Complications associated with chest tubes can be separated into three categories (Table 3).

Empyema

Empyema occurs in 1% to 16% of patients; the higher incidence occurs among trauma patients (51). Chest tubes placed for pleural effusions are associated with higher rates of empyema. This complication is indicated by purulent exudative fluid with a low pH, low glucose concentrations, and a high white blood cell count. Empyema is treated with intravenously administered antibiotics, chest tube drainage, and, possibly, open thoracotomy.

Prevention of empyema begins with the use of appropriate sterile technique. The use of antibiotics remains controversial, with early studies demonstrating no benefit or only minimal benefit in association

Table 2 Nasogastric Tube Malpositioning and Associated Complications

Location of malposition	Complications
Tracheobronchial tree	Loss of tidal volume
	Pneumonia
Pleural space	Pneumothorax
	Tension pneumothorax
Internal jugular vein	Hypotension
	Anemia
Intracranial	Death

Table 3 Thoracostomy Tube Complications

Infectious
    Chest tube site wound infection
    Tracheitis[a]
    Pneumonia
    Empyema
Anatomic
    Subcutaneous emphysema
    Pneumothorax
        Residual
        Iatrogenic
    Hemothorax/pleural effusion
        Residual
        Iatrogenic
    Arteriovenous fistula[a]
    Malposition
        Subcutaneous
        Intrathoracic
            With or without visceral injury[a]
        Intra-abdominal
            With or without visceral injury[a]
Physiologic
    Re-expansion pulmonary edema
    Myocardial ischemia[a]
    Horner's syndrome[a]

[a]Rare complications only illustrated by the rare case report.

with their use. However, more recent studies and a meta-analysis by Evan et al. (52) of six prospective, randomized studies found that a beneficial effect was associated with the use of antibiotics effective against *Staphylococcus* spp.

Pneumothorax and Hemothorax

Pneumothorax and hemothorax are the most common indications for chest tube placement; however, these complications may also occur in association with thoracostomy tube placement and use. Thoracostomy tube placement may fail as an effective treatment for these conditions, and pneumothorax and hemothorax may recur after the tube has been removed or may be an iatrogenic sequela of removal. A study of chest radiographs after thoracostomy tube insertion demonstrated that the most common complications were tube malposition and unresolved pneumothorax and hemothorax (53). Recurrence of a pneumothorax after thoracostomy tube removal is most likely caused by the entry of air through the wound or by reaccumulation from a small air leak. To prevent such pneumothoraces, the thoracostomy tube should be pulled out quickly while the patient is exhaling, so that intrapleural pressure is positive, thus decreasing the risk of air entry. When placing chest tubes, some practitioners place a second stitch through the site of chest tube insertion; this stitch is left untied. When the chest tube is removed, a second person places tension on this stitch to close the incision as the chest tube is being removed.

To decrease the likelihood of a recurrent pneumothorax caused by an undetected small air leak, it is best to convert the tube to water seal before the tube is removed. In a randomized trial, Martino et al. demonstrated that converting thoracostomy tubes to water seal before removing them reduces the number of pneumothoraces that occur after tube removal and also reduces the need for chest tube replacement (54). There have also been reports of ipsilateral or contralateral pneumothoraces in association with the placement of chest tubes for effusion (55).

Pneumothorax associated with thoracostomy tube placement can be treated in several ways. The pneumothorax can be carefully observed and may resolve even if it is not adequately drained by the tube. Increasing the suction of the thoracostomy tube, by increasing the column of fluid in a wet hemovac system or simply turning the pressure dial on a dry hemovac system, can resolve a persistent pneumothorax. A second thoracostomy tube can also be placed to resolve the pneumothorax or hemothorax. Pleurodesis may be necessary to resolve a persistent leak or effusion, but a thoracotomy is rarely necessary for adequate resolution of a pneumothorax.

Malpositioning

In one radiologic evaluation of thoracostomy tubes placed in the emergency room, tube malpositioning was the reason for as many as 26% of inadequate tube placements and was the most common complication (53). Malpositioned chest tubes can be located in the subcutaneous tissue of the chest wall or in incorrect locations in the intrathoracic and intra-abdominal regions. A malpositioned thoracostomy tube may cause injury to the visceral organs and may even result in death. One study (53) suggests that chest tube placement by clinicians other than surgeons is associated with a higher rate of complications, but another study (56) refuted this finding. The use of trochars for insertion is also associated with a high rate of complications; thus, this method of tube insertion has largely been replaced by blunt dissection.

Re-expansion Pulmonary Edema

Re-expansion pulmonary edema (RPE) can occur after pulmonary re-expansion by thoracostomy tube for pneumothorax, pleural effusion, or atelectasis. One retrospective review of the placement of thoracostomy tubes for pneumothorax in Japan (57) suggested that RPE occurs in approximately 14% of cases. However, in the United States, RPE is generally considered a rare complication; the mortality rate associated with RPE may be as high as 20% (58). Although the cause of RPE is unknown, certain risk factors such as young age, a large pneumothorax, and long duration of collapse are associated with RPE (59). Some patients with RPE may exhibit no symptoms other than radiographic findings; others may experience severe tachypnea, tachycardia, hypoxemia, or chest pain. The two most common symptoms are dyspnea and chest pain, which usually occur within minutes to hours of re-expansion.

Diagnosis of RPE is based on chest radiography, which shows pulmonary edema in a previously collapsed lung. Cases of contralateral RPE have also been reported (58). Treatment involves supportive care, which may include hemodynamic and ventilatory support; most cases are self-limiting and resolve within a week.

INTRACRANIAL PRESSURE MONITORING

Intracranial pressure (ICP) monitoring plays a key role in the management of increased ICP. ICP monitoring is frequently used for patients with brain injuries and those undergoing elective neurosurgery. Complications associated with ICP monitoring include infection and hemorrhage, as well as malfunction, obstruction, and malpositioning of the tube. Long-term morbidity and mortality associated with complications of ICP monitoring appear to be rare.

Infection

Infection related to ICP monitoring is characterized by positive results from either a culture of cerebrospinal fluid or a culture of material on the intracranial portion of the catheter, along with clinical signs of infection. No semiquantitative or quantitative methods exist for distinguishing infections of the ICP-monitoring device from colonization of the device, and clinical signs of infection are needed to establish the diagnosis of infection. Colonization of ICP monitors has been associated with either implantation for more than five days or irrigation of fluid-coupled devices. In one study, the incidence of bacterial colonization increases from 6% to 19% when irrigation was employed (60). Differences in the rates of colonization of ICP devices appear to be related to the type of device used. Parenchymal devices are associated with the highest average rates of colonization (14%; range 11.7–16.6%); the other types of devices associated with colonization are subdural devices (4%; range 1–10%), subarachnoid devices (5%; range, 0–10%), and ventricular devices (5%; range, 0–9.5%) (61). For all types of devices, the rates of colonization increased as time of implantation increased. A retrospective cohort study (62) yielded similar results in a pediatric subgroup of patients; the infection rate associated with Camino® fiberoptic monitors was 0.3%. There is no evidence-based consensus regarding antibiotic prophylaxis for various classes of devices or for duration of implantation.

Hemorrhage

Hemorrhage associated with ICP monitoring has not been clearly defined in many reports but appears to occur infrequently; the overall incidence of hematoma is 1.4%. In two studies, substantial hematomas requiring evacuation occurred in 0.5% of patients who required ICP monitoring (63,64).

Malfunctioning and Malpositioning of Intracranial Pressure Monitors

Malfunctioning and displacement of ICP monitors are the most frequently reported complications associated with the use of these devices. Malfunction or obstruction has been observed in association with 6.3% of fluid-coupled ventricular devices, 16% of subarachnoid bolts, and 10.5% of subdural catheters (65,66). In a pediatric population, Camino fiberoptic monitors malfunctioned in 2.6% of cases and were displaced in 1% (62). The implications of malfunction and displacement include inaccurate ICP readings, potential morbidity associated with reinsertion, and additional cost.

CONCLUSION

Invasive devices, such as lines and tubes, have increased the ability of the practitioner to care for critically ill patients in the ICU. However, although such devices can be invaluable tools in caring for patients, their use is also associated with significant morbidity and mortality. Understanding the potential pitfalls associated with these devices will increase the clinician's ability to diagnose and treat such complications and to implement strategies that may prevent the occurrence of such complications in the future.

REFERENCES

1. Mansfield PF, Hohn DC, Fornage BD, Gregurich MA, Ota DM. Complication and failures of subclavian-vein catheterization. N Eng J Med 1994; 331:1735–1738.
2. Broviac JW, Cole JJ, Scibner BH. A silicone rubber atrial catheter for prolonged parenteral alimentation. Surg Gynecol Obstet 1973; 136:602.
3. Hickman RO, Buckner CD, Cliftra, et al. A modified right atrial catheter for access to the venous system in marrow transplant recipients. Surg Gynecol Obstet 1979; 148:871.
4. Sladen A. Complications of invasive hemodynamic monitoring in the intensive care unit. Curr Probl Surg 1988; 25:69–145.
5. Plewa MC, Ledrich D, Sferra JJ. Delayed tension pneumothorax complicating central venous catheterization and positive pressure ventilation. Am J Emerg Med 1995; 13(5):532–535.
6. Harrington KJ, Pandha HS, et al. Risk factors for pneumothorax during percutaneous Hickman line insertion in patients with solid and hematologic tumors. Clin Oncol 1995; 7(6):373–376.
7. Broadwater JR, Henderson MA, Bell JL, et al. Outpatient percutaneous central venous access in cancer patients. Am J Surg 1990; 160:676–680.
8. Foster PF, Moore LR, Sankay HN, et al. Central venous catheterization in patients with coagulopathy. Arch Surg 1992; 127:273–275.
9. Seneff MG. Central venous catheterization: a comprehensive review. Intensive Care Med 1987; 2:163–175, 218–232.
10. Wiemann J, Frass M, Traindl O. Acute upper airway obstruction caused by cervical hematoma as a complication of internal jugular venous catheterization. Acta Med Aust 1990; 17(4):77–79.
11. Silverman JM, Olson KW. Avoiding unintentional arterial cannulation. Crit Care Med 1990; 18(4):460.
12. Heffner JE. A 49 year-old man with tachypnea and a rapidly enlarging pleural effusion. J Crit Illness 1994; 9:101–109.
13. Harrer J, Brtico M, Zacek P, Knap J. Hemothorax—a complication of subclavian vein cannulation. Acta Med 1997; 40(1):21–23.
14. Whitman E. Complication associated with the use of central venous access devices. Curr Probl Surg 1996; 312–317.
15. Bagwell CE, Salzbery AM, Sourrcio RE, Haynes JH. Potentially lethal complication of central venous catheter placement. J Pediatr Surg 2000; 35(5):709–713.
16. Sheep RE, Guiney WB. Fatal cardiac tamponade occurrence with other complications after left internal jugular vein catheterization. JAMA 1982; 248:1632–1635.
17. Karnauchow PN. Cardiac tamponade from central venous catheterization. J Can Med Assoc 1986; 135: 1145–1147.
18. Maki DG. Infection caused by intravascular devices used for infusion therapy: pathogenesis, prevention, and management. Infections Associated with Indwelling Medical Devices. 2nd ed. Washington, DC: ASM Press, 1994:155–205.

19. Taynes R, Culver D, Emori T, et al. The National Noso-comial Infections Surveillance System: plans for the 1990's and beyond. Am J Med 1991; 91(3B):116S–120S.

20. Pittet D, Tarara D, Wenzel RP. Nosocomial bloodstream infections in critically ill patients: excess length of stay, extra costs, and attributable mortality. JAMA 1994; 271:598–601.

21. National Nosocomial Infections Surveillance (NNIS) System. December 2000. Available at http://www.cdc.gov/ncidod/dhqp/pdf/nnis/DEC2000sar.PDF. Accessed June 16, 2006.

22. Pearson ML. Hospital Infection Control Advisory Committee. Guidelines for prevention on vascular device-related infections. Am J Infect Control 1996; 23: 262–277.

23. Ruesch S, Walder B, Tramer MR. Complications of Cen-tral venous catheters: internal jugular versus subcla-vian access—a systemic review. Crit Care Med 2002; 30(2):454–460.

24. Chaiyakunapruk N, Veenstra DL, Lipsky BA, Saint S. Chlorhexadine compared with povidone-iodine solu-tion for vascular catheter site care: a meta-analysis. Ann Intern Med 2002; 136(11):792–801.

25. Raad II, Hohn DC, Gilbraith BJ. Prevention of central venous catheter-related infections by using maximal sterile barrier precautions during insertion. Infect Con-trol Hosp Epidemiol 1994; 15:231–238.

26. Maki DG, Ringer M, Alvarado CJ. Prospective rando-mized trial of povidone-iodone, alcohol, and chlorhex-idine for prevention of infection associated with central venous and arterial catheters. Lancet 1991; 338:339–343.

27. Veenstra DL, Lipsky BA, Saint S. The cost effectiveness of minocycline/rifampin versus chlorhexidine/silver sulfadiazine central venous catheters. 10th Annual Meeting for the Society for Hospital Epidemiology of America, Atlanta, GA, March 5–9, 2000.

28. Puel V, Candry M, LeMetayer P, et al. Superior vena cava thrombosis related to catheter malposition in can-cer chemotherapy. Cancer 1993; 72:2248–2252.

29. Dierks MM, Whitman ED. Catheter tip position in the analysis of central venous access device outcome. J Can Intra Nurses Association 1997; 13(3):7–10.

30. Whitman ED. Complications with the use of central venous access devices. Curr Probl Surg 1996; 33(4): 309–378.

31. Becker DM, Philbrick JT, Walker FB. Axillary and sub-clavian venous thrombosis. Arch Intern Med 1991; 151:1934–1943.

32. Randolph AG, Cook DJ, Gonzalez CA, Andrew M. Benefit of heparin in central venous and pulmonary artery catheters: a meta-analysis of randomized control trials. Chest 1998; 113(1):165–171.

33. Bern MM, Lokich JJ, Wallach SR, Bothe A, Benotti PN. Very low dose of warfarin can prevent thrombosis in central venous catheters. A randomized prospective trial. Ann Intern Med 1990; 112(6):423–428.

34. Coles CE, Whitear WP, Levay JH. Spontaneous fracture and embolization of central venous catheter: prevent-ion and early detection. Clin Oncol 1998; 10(6):412–414.

35. Frezza EE, Mezghebe H. Indications and complications of arterial catheter use in surgical and medical inten-sive care units. Am Surg 1998; 64(2):127–131.

36. Sfeir R, Khoury S, Khoury G, Rustum J, Ghabash M. Ischemia of the hand after radial artery monitoring. Cardiovasc Surg 1996; 4(4):456–458.

37. Zevola DR, Dioso J, Maggio R. Comparison of hepar-inized and nonheparinized solutions for maintaining patency of arterial and pulmonary artery catheters. Am J Crit Care 1997; 6(1):52–55.

38. Omalley MK, Rhames FS, Cerra FB, McLomb RC. Value of routine pressure monitoring system changes after 72 hours of continuous use. Crit Care Med 1994; 22(9): 1424–1430.

39. Kudsk KA, Stone JM, Carpenter G, Sheldon GF. Effects of enteral versus parenteral feeding of malnourished rats on body composition. Curr Surg 1981; 38(5): 322–323.

40. Alexander JW. Nutrition and infection. New per-spective for an old problem. Arch Surg 1986; 121(8): 966–972.

41. Mullan H, Roubenoff RA, Roubenoff R. Risk of pul-monary aspiration among patients receiving enteral nutrition. J Parenteral Enteral Nutr 1992; 16(2): 160–164.

42. Lucarelli MR, Shirk MB, Julian MW, Crouser ED. Toxi-city of Food Drug and Cosmetic Blue No. 1 dye in critically ill patients. Chest 2004; 125(2):793–795.

43. Norman EA, Sosis M. Iatrogenic esophageal perfora-tion due to tracheal or nasogastric intubation. J Can Anaesth Soc 1986; 33:222–226.

44. Michael L, Grillo HC, Malt RA. Operative and non-operative management of esophageal perforations. Ann Surg 1981; 194:57–63.

45. Jackson RH, Payne DK, Bacon BR. Esophageal perfora-tion due to nasogastric intubation. Am J Gastroenterol 1990; 37:439–442.

46. Fasqualle D, Alami M, Dumas G, Fockenier F, Sibille JP. Epidemiology of sinusitis seen in hospitalized patients. Pathologie Biologie 1998; 46(10):751–759.

47. Westergren U, Berg S, Lundreg J. Ultrasonographic bedside evaluation of maxillary sinus disease in mechanically ventilated patients. Intensive Care Med 1997; 23(4):393–398.

48. Bankier AA, Wiesmayr MN, Henk C, et al. Radiographic detection of intrabronchial malposi-tions of nasogastric tubes and subsequent complication in ICU patients. Intensive Care Med 1997; 23: 406–410.

49. Frei RM, Mullet ST. Inadvertent intracranial insertion of a nasogastric tube in a non trauma patient. Emerg Med J 1997; 14(1):45–47.

50. Minyard AN, Smith DM. Arterial-esophageal fistulae in patients requiring nasogastric esophageal intubation. Am J Forensic Med Pathol 2000; 21(1):74–78.

51. Etoch SW, Bar-Natam MF, Miller FB, Richardson JD. Tube thoracostomy. Factors related to complications. Arch Surg 1995; 130(5):521–525.

52. Evan JT, Green JD, Carlin PE, Barrett LO. Meta-analysis of antibiotics in tube thoracostomy. Am Surg 1995; 61(3):215–219.

53. Baldt MM, Bankier AA, Germann PS, et al. Complica-tions after emergency tube thoracostomy: assessment with CT. Radiology 1995; 195(2):539–543.

54. Martino K, Merrit S, Sernas T, et al. Prospective of randomized trial of thoracostomy removal algo-rithms. J Trauma Injury Infect Crit Care 1999; 46(3): 369–373.

55. Gerard PS, Kaldarvi E, Litani V, Lenora RA, Tessler S. Right-sided pneumothorax as a result of left-sided chest tube. Chest 1993; 103(5):1602–1603.

56. Chan L, Reilly KM, Henderson C, Kahn F, Salluzzo RF. Complication rates of tube thoracostomy. Am J Emerg Med 1997; 15(4):368–370.

57. Matsura Y, Nomimura T, Murakami H, et al. Clinical analysis of reexpansion pulmonary edema. Chest 1991; 100(6):1562–1566.

58. Heller BJ, Grathwohl MK. Contralateral reexpansion pulmonary edema. Southern Med J 2000; 17(3):234.

59. Murat A, Arslan A, Balci AE. Re-expansion pulmonary Edema. Acta Radiol 2004; 45(4):431–433.

60. Aucoin PJ, Kotilainen HR, Gantz NM, et al. Intracranial pressure monitors. Epidemiologic study of risk factors and infections. Am J Med 1986; 80:369–376.

61. Bullock R, Chestnut RM, Clifton G, et al. Guidelines for the Management of Severe Head Injury. New York, NY: Brain Trauma Foundation, 1995.

62. Pople IK, Muhlbauer MS, Sanford RA, et al. Results and complications of intracranial pressure monitoring in 303 children. Pediatr Neurosurg 1995; 23(2): 64–67.

63. Narayan RK, Kishore P RS, Becker DP, et al. Intracranial pressure: to monitor or not to monitor? J Neurosurg 1982; 56:650–659.

64. Paramore CG, Turner DA. Relative risks of ventriculostomy infection and morbidity. Acta Neurochir (Wien) 1994; 127:79–84.

65. Barlow P, Mendelow AD, Lawrence AE, et al. Clinical evaluation of two methods of subdural pressure monitoring. J Neurosurg 1985; 63:578–582.

66. North B, Reilly P. Comparison among three methods of intracranial pressure recording. Neurosurgery 1986; 18:730.

7

Complications of Abdominal Wall Surgery and Hernia Repair

James C. Doherty
*Division of Trauma Surgery, Advocate Christ Medical Center, Oak Lawn, and Department of
Surgery, University of Illinois College of Medicine at Chicago, Chicago, Illinois, U.S.A.*

Robert W. Bailey
*Division of Laparoscopic and Bariatric Surgery, Daughtry Family Department of Surgery,
Miller School of Medicine, University of Miami, Miami, Florida, U.S.A.*

*Abdominal wall closure, including ventral and inguinal
hernia repair, are among the most frequently performed of
all procedures in general surgery. Although the complication rates associated with these procedures are relatively
low, the number of procedures performed renders their
associated surgical complications among the most common
encountered in clinical practice.*

COMPLICATIONS OF ABDOMINAL WOUND CLOSURE

The complications associated with abdominal wound
closure can be broadly classified as infection (superficial or deep), acute wound failure (dehiscence or
evisceration), and incisional hernia.

Wound Infection

The infection rate for laparotomy wounds has been
reported to range from 1.5% to 40% (1). Well-described
factors contributing to abdominal wound infection
include the degree of bacterial wound contamination,
host immune status, lack of adequate antiseptic skin preparation, and lack of appropriate antimicrobial prophylaxis. Additional factors are length of operation, hair
removal, tissue trauma, and break in sterile technique.
Wounds are classified into distinct classes based on the
degree of potential bacterial contamination. The individual classes with their respective infection rates are as
follows: Class I, clean (1.5%); Class II, contaminated
(7.5%); Class III, clean/contaminated (15%); and Class
IV, dirty (40%) (1). The diagnosis of wound infection is
usually made on the basis of signs and symptoms of
inflammation locally (erythema, warmth, swelling, tenderness, and purulence) and systemically (fever and sepsis). Infections occurring during the first 48 hours of the

postoperative period must raise concern for infection
with *Clostridium perfringens* or B-hemolytic streptococci.
Such infections can rapidly progress to life-threatening
necrotizing soft-tissue infections requiring aggressive
surgical debridement. Fortunately, most postoperative
wound infections are uncomplicated infections of the
skin, the superficial subcutaneous tissue, or both. Such
infections are usually controlled by opening, draining,
debriding, and observing the wound. In most cases,
neither antibiotics nor wound cultures are necessary.

Acute Wound Failure

The incidence of dehiscence of laparotomy wounds has
been reported to be 0.2% to 2.3% (2). In most cases, acute
wound failure is preceded by acute drainage of serosanguineous fluid from the incision site. In rare cases, the
first sign of dehiscence is acute evisceration. The timing
of evisceration is quite variable, but the average time of
occurrence is the seventh postoperative day. A number
of patient factors have been associated with abdominal
wound dehiscence. These are: age greater than 65 years,
anemia, emergency procedure, pulmonary disease,
hypoproteinemia, hemodynamic instability, sepsis, obesity, uremia, malignancy, ascites, steroid therapy, and
hypertension (2,3). The same studies have also identified postoperative risk factors for dehiscence, such as
vomiting, prolonged ileus, urinary retention, and cough.
Despite the presence of these patient factors and postoperative factors, the most common cause of acute
wound failure is the technical failure of suture material
tearing through the fascia. Sutures tied too tightly,
sutures placed too close together or too far apart,
and sutures placed with inadequate fascial bites are all
at risk of tearing through the fascia with subsequent
fascial dehiscence (4).

The management of acute wound failure is
immediate wound exploration with reduction of

evisceration, wound irrigation, and primary closure if possible. Retention sutures are frequently necessary. Occasionally, fascial dehiscence occurs in only a short segment of the fascial closure, with no evidence of evisceration. Acutely, this so-called "controlled dehiscence" can be managed nonoperatively with careful local wound care and observation. However, if bowel is exposed, there is a risk of fistula. The bowel must be protected either by closing the fascia, using adhesive packs, or by applying a split-thickness skin graft. The surgeon who uses such an approach must recognize that the wound will almost always progress to form a clinically evident incisional hernia that may require repair at a later date.

The prognostic importance of fascial dehiscence cannot be overemphasized. Reported mortality rates range from 18% to 36% (2); cardiorespiratory failure and peritonitis are the most common direct causes of mortality. Other complications of dehiscence are recurrent dehiscence (2–5%), incisional hernia (14–48%), infection (14%), fistula (6%), and intra-abdominal abscess (4%).

Incisional Hernia

Incisional hernia is the best studied of the complications of abdominal wound closure. The incidence of incisional hernia after laparotomy has been reported to be 4% to 20%. In 5.9% of cases, the hernia becomes evident within one year of surgery; in 78% of cases, it becomes evident within two years; and in 90% of cases, within three years (5). The key risk factor for the development of incisional hernia is infection (5). Additional nontechnical factors that increase the risk of hernia are similar to those associated with dehiscence: advanced age, poor nutrition, obesity, jaundice, early reoperation, pulmonary disease, abdominal distension, emergency surgery, and midline laparotomy.

A number of prospective studies, retrospective studies, and meta-analyses have found that several technical factors are associated with an increased risk of incisional hernia (6,7). These studies demonstrate that the incidence of hernia is higher when absorbable suture materials are used than when nonabsorbable materials are used, as well as when layered closure rather than mass closure is performed. The studies have not found that the use of interrupted closure rather than continuous closure substantially reduces the risk of hernia (6,7). Other studies have associated incisional hernia with factors such as the ratio of suture length to wound length (SL/WL), a measure of suture tension and size of tissue bites, and with stitch length (ratio of SL to number of stitches), another measure of wound tension. Specifically, an SL/WL ratio less than four has been associated with an increased risk of incisional hernia, and a stitch length of five or greater has been associated with an increased risk of wound infection (8,9). Excessive tension is believed to compromise local blood flow to the approximated fascial edges, and this reduction

in blood flow results in necrosis and inadequate healing. Fascial bites of inadequate size are thought to be more prone to tearing, especially with changes in intra-abdominal pressure. Techniques of incisional hernia repair and their respective complications are discussed later in this chapter.

The Difficult Abdominal Wound

Closing large abdominal wall defects after emergent surgery is particularly challenging. Massive resuscitation-induced visceral edema and substantial fascial loss are the most common clinical scenarios producing such difficult wounds. In addition to increasing the risk of dehiscence and hernia, closing wounds under excessive tension can cause intra-abdominal hypertension and the abdominal compartment syndrome. This syndrome is characterized by decreased blood flow to abdominal viscera, impaired venous return to the heart, renal dysfunction, and compromised diaphragmatic function, manifested as elevated airway pressures and impaired ventilation. The diagnosis of abdominal compartment syndrome is a clinical diagnosis and is based on the presence of the above-mentioned signs and symptoms in concert with intra-abdominal hypertension. Intra-abdominal hypertension is best measured by transduction of the bladder pressure via an indwelling bladder catheter. Urgent abdominal decompression is recommended if bladder pressure exceeds 25 mmHg (10).

Laparotomy wounds left open or those opened emergently to decompress an abdominal compartment syndrome present a difficult clinical problem. Because of the loss of abdominal wall integrity, such wounds are prone to infection and desiccation of abdominal viscera. A number of techniques for temporary wound closure have been advocated, such as towel clip skin closure, temporary silos, zippers, absorbable prosthetic mesh closure, and permanent mesh closure. In general, a staged approach to such wounds is best and often requires the application of temporary prosthetic meshes before definitive abdominal wall reconstruction. When absorbable mesh is used, it is only a temporary measure for restoring abdominal wall integrity, and hernia formation is an expected outcome. Complications of temporary prosthetic closure are mesh extrusion, wound sepsis, adhesions, and enterocutaneous fistula. The incidence of each of these complications depends on a number of factors, including the type of mesh used, the timing of mesh placement, and the degree of wound contamination.

Other Complications

Relatively minor, local complications of the incisional wound are hypertrophic scar formation, scar ossification, chronic incisional pain, peri-incisional numbness (resulting from cutaneous sensory nerve injury), and stitch abscesses or stitch fistulae. Other, less common complications are enterocutaneous fistulae and inadvertent visceral injury during closure. These complications are associated with potentially high morbidity and mortality rates and can present challenging management issues. Fortunately, these complications occur relatively infrequently and are mentioned here only for the sake of completeness.

COMPLICATIONS OF VENTRAL HERNIA REPAIR

The term "ventral hernia" refers to a heterogeneous group of ventral abdominal wall defects that range in size and complexity from the small, uncomplicated umbilical hernia to the large, complex incisional hernia. For the most part, the present discussion will focus on the latter group. In general, larger hernias are associated with increased atrophy of the abdominal musculature, increased trophic changes in the overlying skin, and greater alteration in pulmonary mechanics. As a result, repair of large ventral hernias often requires the use of prosthetic material and frequently mandates extensive preoperative preparation, so that the incidence of complications can be reduced. At present, two operative approaches to the repair of such hernias are available to the surgeon: open ventral herniorrhaphy and laparoscopic ventral herniorrhaphy.

Complications of Open Ventral Herniorrhaphy

The most common complication of open ventral hernia repair is hernia recurrence. The risk factors for recurrence after open ventral hernia repair are identical to the previously mentioned risk factors for hernia formation after laparotomy. These include patient factors, perioperative factors, and technical factors. Because infection is associated with the development of incisional hernias and substantially increases the rate of recurrence after repair, measures should be taken to minimize the risk of infection. Such measures include antimicrobial prophylaxis, avoidance of intraoperative wound contamination, and antiseptic skin preparation. In addition, host immune status must be optimized by correcting nutritional deficiencies, aggressively managing perioperative diabetes, and timing elective surgery to occur remotely from the administration of immunosuppressive drug therapies such as cancer chemotherapy and corticosteroids.

As is true of successful laparotomy closure, successful repair of large incisional hernias requires adherence to a number of basic technical principles. The fascia incorporated in the repair must be healthy and must be approximated with minimal tension. Fascial bites should incorporate healthy fascia approximately 1 cm from the fascial edge and should be placed approximately 1 cm apart. To further limit tension, the repair must be undertaken with anesthesia that provides sufficient relaxation of the abdominal wall. Before the availability of prosthetic mesh materials, the recurrence rates for incisional hernia repair were

reported to be as high as 30% to 50%, but after the use of prosthetic materials became widespread, the recurrence rates decreased to their current level of 0% to 10% in most studies (11). This decrease is directly attributable to the use of tension-free prosthetic repairs. Despite this dramatic reduction in recurrence rates, mesh repairs should not be employed indiscriminately. The use of mesh should be limited to instances in which primary closure cannot be performed without excessive wound tension. To avoid the complications associated with the use of mesh for ventral hernia repair, several modifications of primary closure have been advocated, such as using internal retention sutures, placing incisions to relax the anterior rectus sheath, and mobilizing the inferior aspect of the rectus musculature (11).

When mesh is needed, the ideal prosthetic material should exhibit two fundamental properties: retention of high-intrinsic tensile strength and allowance of external tissue ingrowth or incorporation. Prosthetic materials are classified as absorbable or nonabsorbable. The absorbable meshes are polyglyactin (Vicryl®, ETHICON, INC., Johnson & Johnson Corporation, New Brunswick, New Jersey, U.S.A.) and polyglycolic acid (Dexon®, Syneture, a division of United States Surgical Corporation, Norwalk, Conneticut, U.S.A.). The nonabsorbable meshes include two types of polypropylene mesh: Marlex®/Bard®, Murry Hill, New Jersey, U.S.A.; and Prolene®, ETHICON, INC., Johnson & Johnson Corporation, New Brunswick, New Jersey, U.S.A.). Other nonabsorbable meshes are polyester (Mersilene®, ETHICON, INC., Johnson & Johnson Corporation, New Brunswick, New Jersey, U.S.A.), and expanded polytetrafluoroethylene (ePTFE; Gore-Tex®, W.L. Gore & Associates, Inc., Newark, Delaware, U.S.A.). The nonabsorbable materials have the advantages of long-term retention of tensile strength and, with the notable exception of ePTFE, extensive tissue ingrowth. The absorbable materials have the advantage of being safer for use in the presence of contamination or active infection.

As mentioned previously, tension-free mesh repairs have the advantage of being associated with lower recurrence rates than primary closure under tension. On the other hand, both animal experiments and clinical trials have demonstrated that the use of prosthetic materials is associated with a higher incidence of local wound complications. In a recent large retrospective study, Leber et al. (12) reported a variety of early and late complications associated with the use of prosthetic mesh for incisional hernia repair. Early postoperative complications were ileus (8%), cellulitis (7%), wound drainage (4%), hematoma/seroma (3%), pneumonia (1%), pulmonary embolus (1%), and deep venous thrombosis (0.5%). Late complications were hernia recurrence (16.8%, occurring at a median of one year), chronic infection/sinus (6%, at a median of six months), small-bowel obstruction (5.5%, at a median of 18 months), and enterocutaneous fistulae. Other factors contributing to the increased risk of fistula were incarceration, obstruction, upper abdominal location of hernia, and history of previous wound infection.

The formation of enterocutaneous fistulae has also been associated with failure to interpose tissue between prosthetic mesh and underlying bowel. This risk of fistula and the related risk of adhesions between bowel and mesh have led many authors to recommend preserving a portion of the dissected hernia sac for use as an extra layer of the closure, which can isolate the abdominal contents from the mesh. When the hernia sac is not available, free peritoneal grafts and commercially available bioabsorbable membranes and dual-sided mesh products have been advocated for this purpose. The local wound complication rates associated with polypropylene and ePTFE nonabsorbable meshes are low (0–6% for each specific complication), as are the recurrence rates (0–10%), provided that these meshes are placed in uninfected and uncontaminated wounds. With ePTFE, an infection rate as low as 3% has been reported, but this rate triples when infection is present and quadruples when gross local purulence is present (13).

A number of studies have shown that the technique employed for mesh fixation does not affect complication rates. Nevertheless, onlay techniques in which mesh is placed anterior to a completed fascial closure are not recommended because of the risk of inadvertent bowel injury. An onlay technique in which an anteriorly placed mesh is sutured under direct vision before fascial approximation and is secured afterward is a safe alternative. The mesh position can be extrafascial, subfascial, or intraperitoneal, with no significant difference in recurrence rates. Low risk of recurrence depends more on secure suturing and generous (4 to 8 cm) overlapping of the mesh and fascia than on position.

Complications of Laparoscopic Ventral Herniorrhaphy

In recent years, a laparoscopic alternative to open ventral herniorrhaphy has emerged. Although several variations of the procedure exist, the basic approach involves laparoscopic reduction of the hernia contents, intraperitoneal placement of prosthetic mesh, and fixation of the mesh to the anterior abdominal wall. Although small defects can occasionally be repaired primarily by using laparoscopic intracorporeal suturing techniques, laparoscopic ventral hernia repair usually requires intraperitoneal mesh placement. To limit the potential for complications arising from inflammatory reactions between the mesh and the abdominal contents (adhesions and fistulae), the least reactive prosthetic material, ePTFE, is usually used for laparoscopic repair.

A large number of retrospective and prospective studies (14–18) have demonstrated complication rates of 5% to 20% for the laparoscopic approach. Intraoperative complications are subcutaneous emphysema

and hypercarbia from abdominal insufflation (0.7%), respiratory failure (0.7%), and inadvertent enterotomy (0–4.8%). Postoperative complications are seroma (1.2–16%), mesh infection (0–3.6%), trocar site infection (0–3.3%), ileus (2–10%), small-bowel obstruction (0–4.8%), pulmonary compromise (0–4.8%), and chronic pain (0–3.6%). Excluding the complications unique to the laparoscopic approach, nearly all of these complications occur at lower rates than those reported for open herniorrhaphy. The exception is seroma, which appears to be related to the use of nonreactive ePTFE mesh. Some surgeons advocate the use of dual-sided (smooth inner surface and rough outer surface) ePTFE mesh to reduce the high incidence of seroma.

The rates of recurrence for laparoscopic ventral herniorrhaphy are also quite low (1–4%), much lower than the rates generally reported for open repair. Laparoscopic ventral hernia repair also has the advantages of decreased hospital length of stay, decreased postoperative pain, and more rapid return to baseline level of physical activity (14–18).

Complications of Ventral Hernia Repair for Patients with Cirrhosis

Although preoperative control of ascites is strongly recommended, patients with cirrhosis can usually safely undergo inguinal herniorrhaphy without a substantial increase in the rates of local wound complications or recurrence (19). For patients with uncontrolled cirrhosis, however, ventral herniorrhaphy is associated with high morbidity and mortality rates; the rates increase to 15% in association with rupture and to 26% is association with strangulation (20). The most common intraoperative complication is bleeding; it occurs as the result of the coagulopathy, thrombocytopenia, and periumbilical hypervascularity often associated with cirrhosis. When ascites is present, postoperative complications usually relate to ascites leak. These complications are impaired wound healing, wound infection, and peritonitis. These complications and the large amount of tension placed on the repair by massive ascites result in recurrence rates as high as 50% to 60%. Therefore, ascites should be aggressively corrected preoperatively. In cases of intractable ascites, herniorrhaphy may be delayed until after peritoneovenous shunting, portasystemic shunting, transjugular intrahepatic portacaval shunting, or liver transplantation has been performed. If a patient with ascites requires emergent herniorrhaphy and no intra-abdominal infection or contamination is present, simultaneous peritoneovenous shunt placement can be performed. The hernia repair itself should include separate closure of the peritoneum and primary approximation of the fascial edges with absorbable suture, and tight closure of the skin with a continuous nylon suture or a subcuticular suture. Afterwards, the wound should be carefully observed for any signs of infection or leakage; such findings mandate immediate wound exploration.

Loss of Domain

Large, chronic incisional and inguinal hernias can cause the abdominal viscera to lose the "right of domain" in the abdominal cavity. Under such circumstances, reduction of the hernia contents into the abdomen and subsequent repair of the hernia defect may cause intra-abdominal hypertension and may precipitate abdominal compartment syndrome. Several maneuvers can limit the risk of this highly morbid complication. One such maneuver is progressive preoperative pneumoperitoneum, the gradual enlargement of the peritoneal cavity by repetitive air insufflation over a period of two to three weeks (21). The goal of therapy is to expand the capacity of the abdominal cavity, so that it can accommodate the hernia contents and allow a safe reduction and repair of the hernia. Another technique often used in conjunction with progressive pneumoperitoneum for repair of large inguinal and incisional hernias is the placement of a large sheet of mesh that extends well beyond the edges of the defect. This technique (the "Stoppa repair") provides wide adhesion of the mesh to the abdominal wall and renders the visceral sac indistensible (22).

Regardless of the technique used to repair such large hernias, whenever loss of domain is suspected the patient should undergo preoperative pulmonary function testing and preoperative optimization of pulmonary status. Aggressive respiratory physiotherapy, cardiovascular conditioning, and smoking cessation can improve pulmonary function and thus limit adverse pulmonary sequelae of postoperative intra-abdominal hypertension and diaphragmatic embarrassment.

COMPLICATIONS OF INGUINAL HERNIA REPAIR

Despite the fact that it is one of the most commonly performed procedures in general surgery, inguinal herniorrhaphy presents the surgeon with a unique set of challenges. Because of the complex anatomical relationships in the inguinal region, a number of important structures are susceptible to injury, and the surgeon will be faced with a variety of technical options for repair. The present discussion is intended to outline the main complications of open and laparoscopic inguinal herniorrhaphy. Specific approaches and techniques are discussed only with reference to their association with specific complications and to the differences in their rates of recurrence.

Complications of Open Inguinal Herniorrhaphy

Complications of open inguinal herniorrhaphy can be either intraoperative or postoperative. In general, both intraoperative and postoperative complications are technical in nature and can be avoided by precise knowledge of inguinal anatomy, the experience of the surgeon, and keen attention to detail during the performance of the operation.

Intraoperative Complications

Intraoperative complications are injury to vascular structures, spermatic cord transection, injury to the vas deferens, nerve injury, testicular devascularization, and injury to the viscera (23). As will be discussed below, these complications are often not recognized at the time of surgery and may occur as complications during the postoperative period. Nevertheless, they are discussed here as intraoperative complications because the initial technical error occurs during the surgical procedure itself.

Hemorrhage can result from injury to any of multiple vascular structures in the inguinal region: the pubic branch of the obturator artery, the cremasteric artery, the inferior, deep epigastric vessels, the deep circumflex iliac vessels, the external iliac vessels, and the femoral vessels. Injuries to the epigastric, pubic, and cremasteric vessels can usually be managed safely and effectively with direct ligation of the bleeding vessel. Injuries to the deep circumflex iliac, external iliac, and femoral vessels usually result from careless suture placement and are best managed by removing the offending suture and applying direct pressure. If direct pressure fails to provide adequate hemostasis, wide exploration of the femoral sheath is necessary for providing access for more effective manual compression or for future suture repair when necessary.

When a vascular injury occurs intraoperatively, careful postoperative observation is necessary so that arterial or venous thrombosis or thromboembolic events can be detected. Perioperative venous thrombosis has been associated with thrombophlebitis of the dorsal vein of the penis, a complication with an incidence as high as 0.65% (23). Delayed complications of vascular injury are arterial or venous stenosis, pseudoaneurysm, and arteriovenous fistula. Failure to detect or adequately address small vascular injuries at the time of surgery often results in the formation of postoperative hematomas in the wound or in the scrotum. These hematomas usually resolve spontaneously and rarely require exploration, but they can cause substantial discomfort for the patient and can become secondarily infected.

Hernia repair may occasionally require intentional sacrifice of the spermatic cord. This maneuver is usually reserved for particularly difficult large or recurrent inguinal hernias in elderly men. After inguinal herniorrhaphy, inadvertent cord transection usually causes fever and testicular swelling and tenderness; it may cause the long-term complications of testicular atrophy or hydrocele formation. These complications are discussed in detail below.

The nerves at risk of injury during open inguinal hernia repair are the ilioinguinal nerve, the iliohypogastric nerve, and the genital and femoral branches of the genitofemoral nerve. The ilioinguinal nerve lies beneath the external oblique aponeurosis along the surface of the spermatic cord. Injury most commonly occurs when the external oblique is opened for exposure of the inguinal canal; it results in loss of sensation to the base of the penis, upper scrotum, and inner thigh. The iliohypogastric nerve can be injured by relaxing incisions in the rectus sheath or by medial dissection during preperitoneal hernia repair. Such injury usually causes sensory loss to the suprapubic area. The genitofemoral nerve perforates the internal oblique muscle at the origin of the cremaster muscle. Injury to this nerve causes motor weakness of the cremaster muscle and cutaneous sensory loss in the penis and scrotum. The femoral branch of this nerve lies deep to the inguinal canal; injury to this branch causes sensory loss to the lateral thigh. Injury to any of these nerves usually produces only temporary symptoms that characteristically resolve within six months. Reports indicate that as many as 18% to 20% of patients with hernias experience neurapraxia and hyperesthesia (23). When nerve transection is recognized during surgery, the severed nerve end should be ligated so as to reduce the possibility of the formation of a painful neuroma.

Unlike nerve transection, nerve entrapment can result in the development of serious long-term pain syndromes. Chronic pain after herniorrhaphy has been reported to occur in as many as 5% of cases (23). Genitofemoral neuralgia is a well-described chronic pain syndrome associated with inguinal herniorrhaphy. Symptoms are hyperesthesia in the cutaneous distribution of the genitofemoral nerve and chronic inguinal pain extending to the genitalia and upper thigh. This pain is often exacerbated by walking, hip extension, and pubic tubercle pressure and can frequently be relieved by hip flexion at rest. Pain and paresthesias associated with nerve entrapment and neuroma formation can initially be managed with local nerve blocks. The iliohypogastric and ilioinguinal nerves can be blocked by using an L1 and L2 block. Persistent symptoms may require reexploration, with ligation and severance of the involved nerve. The presence of a short-lived response to a local block can help guide therapy toward a specific nerve, but in the absence of such evidence, therapy is best directed empirically at all three nerves. Occasionally, the condition does not respond to appropriate nonsurgical and surgical therapies; in such cases, patients should be referred to a chronic pain specialist.

The blood supply to the testis is primarily derived from the internal spermatic artery, which is part of the spermatic cord. In the event of any interruption of flow in the internal spermatic artery, collateral circulatory input provided by branches of the vesical, prostatic, and deferential arteries can prevent testicular ischemia. If the collateral circulation is also disrupted, acute testicular necrosis or testicular atrophy may result. Thus, care must be taken to preserve the collateral vessels and the internal spermatic artery during inguinal herniorrhaphy.

Because of its potential impact on fertility, injury to the vas deferens is a serious concern of all surgeons performing inguinal hernia surgery. When it occurs, transection of the vas deferens mandates immediate repair. Approximately 50% of such repairs yield a functional result. Improper handling of the vas deferens can cause injury in the absence of transection. Such injury may involve obstruction of the lumen of the vas, a lesion that can cause painful ejaculatory dysfunction.

Injury to abdominal viscera during inguinal herniorrhaphy usually occurs in association with sliding hernias involving bladder or bowel wall. The wall of the urinary bladder can participate as a sliding component of the medial aspect of a direct inguinal hernia. As such, it can be injured during the placement of medial sutures during the hernia repair. When recognized intraoperatively, injury to the urinary bladder should be repaired immediately, and the repair should be protected with bladder decompression via an external bladder catheter. Bowel injury can occur during high ligation of an indirect hernia sac, when the bowel wall is a component of the sac. The injury can be a simple enterotomy or a mesenteric injury with segmental vascular compromise. In either case, potential sequelae are bowel obstruction, fistula, and abscess formation. Enterotomies are best managed with primary repair, wound irrigation, and hernia repair without prosthetic material if possible. Devascularization of bowel may require resection, with or without laparotomy, and proximal diversion may occasionally be required for colon injures.

Postoperative Complications

In addition to the postoperative complications of scrotal ecchymosis, testicular atrophy, and neuroma mentioned in the preceding discussion, a number of other postoperative complications are associated with open inguinal herniorrhaphy. These are urinary retention, osteitis pubis, testicular swelling, hydrocele, infection, missed hernia, and recurrence.

Urinary retention can occur in association with as many as one-third of all open inguinal hernia repairs; it appears to be more common when bilateral hernia repair is performed. It also appears to be directly related to administration of increasing doses of postoperative narcotics. This complication is exacerbated by the presence of other conditions associated with urinary retention, such as benign prostatic enlargement. Initial management of postoperative urinary retention is intermittent bladder catheterization until the patient is able to void spontaneously. In some cases, long-term bladder catheterization and referral to a urologist may be necessary. To avoid this complication, urology referral and treatment of known or suspected prostatic disease may be advisable prior to elective hernia repair (24).

The placement of suture material in the periosteum of the pubic bone during inguinal herniorrhaphy has been associated with persistent inflammation of the periosteal layer, a condition known as osteitis pubis. This painful syndrome is usually self-limiting and responds to the administration of nonsteroidal anti-inflammatory agents. Although osteitis pubis was once a well-described complication of inguinal hernia repair, modern techniques of inguinal herniorrhaphy have rendered this complication exceedingly rare.

A swollen testis after inguinal hernia repair is usually caused by tight closure of the tissues around the spermatic cord. Occasionally, such swelling results from lymphatic injury, venous injury, or venous thrombosis induced during the surgical dissection of the cord; other causes are hematoma or seroma. Regardless of its cause, postoperative testicular swelling is usually self-limiting; the management involves scrotal support and pain control until swelling resolves. Postoperative swelling associated with severe testicular pain and fever indicates ischemic orchitis. In the absence of obvious arterial injury, ischemic orchitis may result from venous thrombosis of the cord vessels. In severe cases, the pain may last for as long as six weeks, and the condition may progress to testicular atrophy. The incidence of testicular atrophy has been estimated to be 0.036% after primary repairs and 0.46% after repair of recurrent hernias (23).

The development of fluid collections along the course of the spermatic cord is not uncommon after inguinal hernia repair; it occurs with an incidence of 0.7% (23). These collections are commonly referred to as hydroceles, but they actually result from a number of different causes such as retained distal hernia sac, impaired lymphatic or venous drainage, and inflammatory fluid accumulations in proximity to mesh. Postoperative formation of seromas has been associated with the degree of tissue trauma and the use of prosthetic mesh material; its incidence ranges from 0% to 17.6% (23). Hydroceles and seromas rarely require operative intervention unless they become infected. Those that persist for more than six to eight weeks may require aspiration, open drainage, or both.

The incidence of wound infection after open inguinal herniorrhaphy is approximately 1%. Factors that increase infection rates are advanced age (3.2-fold increase), female sex (2.1-fold increase), presence of a drain (9-fold increase), duration of operation (increased infection risk from 2.7% to 9.9% with increased duration from 30–90 minutes), incarceration (7.8% infection rate), and recurrent hernia (10.8% infection rate) (23). The use of prosthetic mesh does not appear to increase these rates, but it has been associated with the phenomenon of delayed infection months to years after herniorrhaphy. Moreover, the presence of infection or contamination preludes the use of mesh. Wound infections are managed with drainage and local wound care. Antibiotics are rarely indicated. The presence of deep infections after inguinal herniorrhaphy increases the risk of hernia recurrence.

Occasionally, a new hernia will be noted after an apparently successful inguinal hernia repair. Such cases usually involve a small indirect or femoral hernia not appreciated at the time of direct inguinal herniorrhaphy. A second hernia is present in at least

13% of cases (23). This complication is entirely preventable and can be avoided by careful palpation for other hernias at the time of repair and by complete opening of the floor of the inguinal canal, a maneuver not performed by a large number of surgeons.

Although fascial weakness may contribute to some hernia recurrences, the cause of recurrence is almost always a technical error. The primary technical factor influencing hernia recurrence is the degree of tension on the repair. Tension causes impaired healing and renders the repair susceptible to disruption and subsequent recurrence. The differences in recurrence rates among the various techniques of open inguinal hernia repair probably reflect differences in the degree of intrinsic tension of the repair. A summary of these recurrence rates appears in Table 1 (23). As this table demonstrates, the recurrence and rerecurrence rates associated with the two techniques of open inguinal hernia repair most commonly used today, the tension-free mesh technique and the mesh plug technique, are similarly low. The widespread acceptance of these two tension-free approaches to inguinal herniorrhaphy is due primarily to the widespread recognition of the important relationship between tension and recurrence.

Complications of Laparoscopic Inguinal Herniorrhaphy

Laparoscopic inguinal hernia repair recently entered its second decade of existence, and substantial improvements in techniques and instrumentation continue to advance the field. The three main techniques of laparoscopic inguinal herniorrhaphy are the intraperitoneal onlay method (IPOM), the transabdominal preperitoneal repair (TAPP), and the total extraperitoneal repair (TEP). The evolution of laparoscopic inguinal herniorrhaphy from IPOM to TAPP to TEP has been driven by the desire to maintain low

Table 1 Rates of Recurrence and Re-recurrence of Hernia for Various Techniques of Open Inguinal Hernia Repair

Technique	Recurrence rate (%)	Re-recurrence rate (%)
Bassini	2.9–25	6.5–13.4
Shouldice	0.2–2.7	2.9–6.4
McVay	1.5–15.55	2.4–5.5
Nyhus	3.2–21.0	9.5–27.0
Nyhus mesh buttress	0–1.7	0–1.7
Rives mesh	0–9.9	1.7–3.2
Stoppa mesh	0–7	0–8
Tension-free mesh (Lichtenstein)	0–1.7	0–3.4
Mesh plug repairs	0–1.6	0.5–1.6
Bassini femoral	2.3	–
Bassini-Kushner femoral	2–6.5	–
Moschowitz femoral	0.9	–
Nyhus femoral	0–0.95	–
McVay femoral	0–3.1	–
Mesh femoral (Stoppa, Wantz, Bendavid, Lichtenstein, Rutkow)	0–1.1	–

Source: From Ref. 23.

recurrence rates while reducing operative time, cost, complications, and anesthetic risk. The IPOM technique involves placing an intra-abdominal sheet of mesh directly over the hernia defect. Although IPOM remains important from a historical perspective, the TAPP and TEP repairs have become the favored approaches of nearly all laparoscopic surgeons. The TAPP repair involves transabdominal laparoscopic dissection of the anterior abdominal wall and secure coverage of the mesh with peritoneum. This approach has the advantage of preperitoneal mesh placement, but it has the disadvantage of requiring entry into the peritoneal cavity and the use of general anesthesia. The TEP repair involves extraperitoneal dissection to separate the peritoneum from the inguinal area, laparoscopic dissection and reduction of the hernia, and placement of mesh between the peritoneum and the transversalis fascia defect.

Because laparoscopic inguinal herniorrhaphy is a relatively new procedure and is subject to continual modification and refinement, the complication rates associated with it have steadily declined over the past decade. The reported overall complication rates for both TAPP and TEP range from 5% to 32%, and the recurrence rates range from 0% to 2% (25). The complications of laparoscopic inguinal herniorrhaphy can be classified as those related to patient selection, those related to laparoscopy, those common to both TAPP and TEP, and those unique to each specific technique.

Complications Related to Patient Selection

With respect to patient selection, the European Association for Endoscopic Surgery approves the use of laparoscopic inguinal hernia repair for Nyhus Type IIIA to IIIC and Type IV inguinal hernias. For these types of hernias, the laparoscopic approach is a safe and reasonable alternative to traditional open approaches. Contraindications to the laparoscopic approach are based on the potential for complications arising from difficult laparoscopic dissections and from the mandatory use of mesh. Relative contraindications to the laparoscopic approach are prior ipsilateral laparoscopic repair, prior groin irradiation or inflammation, large scrotal hernia, small congenital hernia not requiring mesh, and morbid obesity. Absolute contraindications are contraindication to general anesthesia, contraindication to the use of mesh (i.e., infection), and incarceration.

Complications Related to Laparoscopy

The complications related to laparoscopy itself are those related to the access technique and those related to pneumoperitoneum. Those related to access technique are Veress needle or trocar injuries to abdominal viscera with the TEP approach. Complications related to CO_2 insufflation are pneumothorax, hypercarbia, and subcutaneous emphysema.

Complications Related to Transabdominal Preperitoneal Repair

Complications unique to the TAPP approach are those related to the administration of general anesthesia and those related to mesh placement and fixation. The TAPP approach requires general anesthesia to allow pneumoperitoneum and adequate operative exposure. Thus, unlike open inguinal herniorrhaphy and the laparoscopic TEP approach, TAPP cannot be performed with local or regional anesthesia alone. Although most patients tolerate general anesthesia without serious adverse sequelae, the use of general anesthesia for high-risk patients, such as those with severe cardiac and pulmonary disease, is associated with considerable risk. The TAPP approach may therefore expose such patients to substantial risk for perioperative cardiac and pulmonary complications. The TAPP approach also requires that the mesh prosthesis be adequately secured and isolated from the abdominal contents by the peritoneum. Failure to achieve adequate fixation or coverage may result in fistula, internal hernia, bowel obstruction, or hernia recurrence.

Complications Related to Total Extraperitoneal Repair

Complications related to the TEP approach are primarily those associated with extraperitoneal dissection and exposure of the inguinal area. Injury to the epigastric vessels can be avoided by midline port placement and preservation of the vessel's location on the abdominal wall. Peritoneal injury can cause loss of exposure due to the leakage of insufflated CO_2 into the peritoneal cavity. Although this loss of exposure may precipitate conversion to TAPP or open repair, restoration of the operative exposure may be possible by venting the pneumoperitoneum with a Veress needle and repairing the peritoneal defect laparoscopically.

Complications Common to Transabdominal Preperitoneal Repair and Total Extraperitoneal Repair

In general, the complications common to TAPP and TEP are also shared with open techniques of inguinal herniorrhaphy. These are vascular injury, visceral injury, testicular atrophy, nerve injury, and complications related to the use of mesh. Vascular structures at particular risk of injury during laparoscopic hernia repair are the iliac, iliopubic, and accessory obturator vessels. Bladder injury can occur with either TAPP or TEP, but is more common with TAPP. Bladder injury during TAPP can be avoided by limiting dissection to the area lateral to the medial umbilical ligament. The management principles for bladder injuries sustained during laparoscopic herniorrhaphy are the same as those for bladder injuries that occur during open inguinal herniorrhaphy. The bladder should be repaired primarily by using laparoscopic techniques, and bladder decompression should be maintained postoperatively via an indwelling bladder catheter. Although ischemic orchitis and testicular atrophy are relatively common complications of open inguinal herniorrhaphy, these complications are rarely seen after laparoscopic repair. The low incidence of these complications is mainly due to the fact that both TAPP and TEP laparoscopic techniques use preperitoneal approaches and avoid excessive cord dissection, thus limiting the risk of testicular devascularization.

The overall incidence of nerve injuries in association with laparoscopic inguinal hernia repair has been reported to be 0% to 5.1%. The specific nerves at risk of injury are the genitofemoral nerve (40% of laparoscopic nerve injuries) and the lateral femoral cutaneous nerve (26.7% of injuries); the remaining one-third of nerve injuries are not attributable to a specific nerve (26). In general, nerve injuries can be avoided by leaving the distal sac in place, avoiding dissection in the area of the iliacus fascia, and placing all lateral staples above the iliopubic tract and medial to the anterior superior iliac spine. As is true of nerve injuries after open hernia repair, those that occur after laparoscopic repair usually resolve spontaneously, but nerve blocks, surgical reexploration, or both will be required. As is also true of open hernia repair, with laparoscopic repair mesh complications such as infection and erosion into adjacent structures (i.e., bowel or urinary bladder) are quite rare.

Overall Complication Rates

A number of prospective and retrospective studies (27–33) have determined the rates of specific complications after laparoscopic herniorrhaphy. These complication rates are presented in Table 2.

Table 2 Rates of Specific Complications After Laparoscopic Herniorrhaphy

Type of complication	Rate of occurrence (%)
Intraoperative	
Inadvertent enterotomy	0–1
Bladder injury	0–3.3
Bleeding	1–4
Conversion to open approach or transabdominal preperitoneal repair	0–5
Injury to vas deferens	<1
Equipment for extra trocars	<1
Intraoperative cardiac events	<1
Postoperative	
Seroma	0–7.6
Hematoma	2–8
Wound infection	0–8
Urinary retention	0–11.6
Persistent pain or paresthesias	0–9.6
Pneumoscrotum	0–1
Scrotal hematoma	0–3
Hydrocele	1–2
Epididymitis	0–2
Internal hernia	0–2
Unplanned admission	0–28

Source: From Refs. 26–32.

Recurrence

As mentioned previously, the recurrence rate for laparoscopic herniorrhaphy is reported to range from 0% to 3% (34–36). Technical factors contributing to recurrence include inadequate mesh size, incomplete pelvic dissection, missed hernias, and clips pulling through tissue. Inadequate experience on the part of the surgeon also contributes to recurrence. The importance of this factor is underscored by the fact that most published studies (25,34,36) have found that the recurrence rates for both TEP and TAPP have decreased to less than 1%, probably because of the increased experience gained as these techniques have become more widespread.

Comparison of Transabdominal Preperitoneal Repair and Total Extraperitoneal Repair

A number of retrospective and prospective studies (33,34,37) have compared the results achieved by TAPP with those achieved by TEP. These studies consistently demonstrate that both techniques are associated with low complication and recurrence rates, but conclude that TEP is the favored laparoscopic approach because of its substantially lower risk of intraperitoneal complications and its superior recurrence rates. Because of the contraindications to TEP, many surgeons favor TAPP (33,34).

CONCLUSION

Complications of abdominal wall surgery and hernia repair are some of the most common complications encountered by general surgeons. Therefore, a thorough knowledge of the causes and implications of these complications and of their management is essential to the successful practice of general surgery.

REFERENCES

1. Cruse PJ, Foord R. The epidemiology of wound infection. Symposium of surgical infections. Surg Clin North Am 1980; 60(1):27–40.
2. Riou JP, Cohen JR, Johnson H Jr. Factors influencing wound dehiscence. Am J Surg 1992; 163:324–330.
3. Makela JT, Kiviniemi H, Juvonen T, Laitinen S. Factors influencing wound dehiscence after midline laparotomy. Am J Surg 1995; 170:387–390.
4. Carlson MA. Acute wound failure. Surg Clin North Am 1997; 77(3):607–633.
5. Carlson MA, Ludwig KA, Condon RE. Ventral hernia and other complications of 1,000 midline incisions. South Med J 1995; 88(4):450–453.
6. Weiland DE, Bay RC, Del Sordi S. Choosing the best abdominal closure by meta-analysis. Am J Surg 1998; 176(6):666–670.
7. Hodgson NC, Malthaner RA, Ostbye T. The search for the ideal method of abdominal fascial closure: a meta-analysis. Ann Surg 2000; 231(3):436–442.

8. Israelsson LA, Jonsson T, Knutsson A. Suture technique and wound healing in midline laparotomy incisions. Eur J Surg 1996; 162(8):605–609.

9. Israelsson LA, Jonsson T. Overweight and healing of midline incisions: the importance of suture technique. Eur J Surg 1997; 163(3):175–180.

10. Meldrum DR, Moore FA, Moore EE, Franciose RJ, Sauaia A, Burch JM. Prospective characterization and selective management of the abdominal compartment syndrome. Am J Surg 1997; 174:667–673.

11. Santora TA, Roslyn JJ. Incisional hernia. Surg Clin North Am 1993; 73(3):557–570.

12. Leber GE, Garb JL, Alexander AI, Reed WP. Long-term complications associated with prosthetic repair of incisional hernias. Arch Surg 1998; 133:378–382.

13. Gillion JF, Begin GF, Marecos C, Fourtanier G. Expanded polytetrafluoroethylene patches used in the intraperitoneal or extraperitoneal position for repair of incisional hernias of the anterolateral abdominal wall. Am J Surg 1997; 174:16–19.

14. Park A, Gagner A, Pomp A. Laparoscopic repair of large incisional hernias. Surg Laparosc Endosc 1996; 6(2):123–128.

15. Holzman MD, Purut CM, Reintgen K, Eubanks S, Pappas TN. Laparoscopic ventral and incisional hernioplasty. Surg Endosc 1997; 11(1):32–35.

16. Park A, Birch DW, Lovrics P. Laparoscopic and open incisional hernia repair: a comparison study. Surgery 1998; 124:816–822.

17. Toy FK, Bailey RV, Carey S, et al. Prospective multicenter study of laparoscopic ventral hernioplasty. Preliminary results. Surg Endosc 1998; 12:955–959.

18. Franklin ME, Dorman JP, Glass JL, Balli E, Gonzalez JJ. Laparoscopic ventral and incisional hernia repair. Surg Laparosc Endosc 1998; 8(4):294–299.

19. Hurst RD, Butler BN, Soybel DI, Wright HK. Management of groin hernias in patients with ascites. Ann Surg 1992; 216(6):696–700.

20. Belghiti J, Durand F. Abdominal wall hernias in the setting of cirrhosis. Semin Liver Dis 1997; 17(3):219–226.

21. Raynor RW, Del Guerico LR. The place for pneumoperitoneum in the repair of massive hernia. World J Surg 1989; 13:581–585.

22. Stoppa RE. The treatment of complicated groin and incisional hernias. World J Surg 1989; 13:545–554.

23. Bendavid R. Complications of groin hernia surgery. Surg Clin North Am 1998; 78(6):1089–1103.

24. Cramer SO, Malangoni MA, Schulte WJ, Condon RE. Inguinal hernia repair before and after prostatic resection. Surgery 1983; 94:627.

25. Payne JH Jr, Grininger LM, Izawa MT, Podoll EF, Lindahl PJ, Balfour J. Laparoscopic or open inguinal herniorrhaphy? A randomized prospective trial. Arch Surg 1994; 129:973–981.

26. Rosser JC Jr. Commentary on Corbitt JD: laparoscopic herniorrhaphy. In: Bailey RW, Flowers JL, Zucker KA, eds. Complications of Laparoscopic Surgery. Philadelphia: Lippincott, 1995:205–217.

27. Brooks DC. A prospective comparison of laparoscopic and tension-free open herniorrhaphy. Arch Surg 1994; 129:361–366.

28. Vogt DM, Curet MJ, Pitcher DE, Martin DT, Zucker KA. Preliminary results of a prospective randomized trial of laparoscopic onlay versus conventional inguinal herniorrhaphy. Am J Surg 1995; 169:84–90.

29. Wright DM, Kennedy A, Baxter JN, et al. Early outcome after open versus extraperitoneal endoscopic tension-free hernioplasty: a randomized clinical trial. Surgery 1996; 119(5):552–557.

30. Liem MS, van der Graaf Y, van Steensel CJ, et al. Comparison of conventional anterior surgery and laparoscopic surgery for inguinal-hernia repair. N Engl J Med 1997; 336(22):1541–1547.

31. Paganini AM, Lezoche E, Carle F, et al. A randomized, controlled clinical study of laparoscopic vs open tension-free inguinal hernia repair. Surg Endosc 1998; 12:979–986.

32. Zieren J, Zieren HU, Jacobi CA, Wegner FA, Muller JM. Prospective randomized study comparing laparoscopic and open tension-free inguinal hernia repair with Shouldice's operation. Am J Surg 1998; 175:330–333.

33. Felix EL, Michas CA, Gonzales MH Jr. Laparoscopic hernioplasty. TAPP vs TEP. Surg Endosc 1995; 9:984–989.

34. Ramshaw BJ, Tucker JG, Conner T, Mason EM, Duncan TD, Lucas GW. A comparison of the approaches to laparoscopic herniorrhaphy. Surg Endosc 1996; 10(1):29–32.

35. Swanstrom LL. Laparoscopic herniorrhaphy. Surg Clin North Am 1996; 76(3):483–491.

36. Heithhold DL, Ramshaw BJ, Mason EM, et al. 500 total extraperitoneal approach laparoscopic herniorrhaphies: a single-institution review. Am Surg 1997; 63:299–301.

37. Kald A, Anderberg B, Smedh K, Karlsson M. Transperitoneal or totally extraperitoneal approach in laparoscopic hernia repair: results of 491 consecutive herinorrhaphies. Surg Laparosc Endosc 1997; 7(2):86–89.

8

Complications of Biliary Tract Surgery and Trauma

Akpofure Peter Ekeh and James B. Peoples[a]

*Department of Surgery, Wright State University School of Medicine,
Dayton, Ohio, U.S.A.*

Gallbladder and biliary tract operations are among the most common abdominal procedures performed in the United States. Approximately 800,000 new cases of cholelithiasis are diagnosed annually, half of which are symptomatic. Gallstones are present in approximately 10% of the adult population of the United States. The recent advent of minimally invasive surgery for cholecystectomy has added a new dimension to biliary surgery and its resulting complications. Laparoscopic techniques have produced shorter hospital stays, less postoperative pain, and earlier return to full activity. These gains have been accompanied, however, by an increased rate of injuries to the biliary ducts. Timely recognition of injuries, prompt referral, and a multidisciplinary approach involving surgeons, interventional radiologists, and gastroenterologists are imperative for the proper management of these complications.

Patients undergoing biliary procedures are prone to the usual complications that may occur after any major abdominal procedure. Elderly patients are at highest risk of morbidity and mortality (1).

COMMON BILIARY OPERATIONS

It is estimated that 500,000 to 700,000 cholecystectomies are performed annually in the United States. This procedure, first performed by Karl Langenbuch in 1882 (2,3), has been the gold standard for treatment of gallbladder disease for more than 100 years. Alternative treatments such as shockwave lithotripsy and gallstone dissolution have been demonstrated to be inferior to surgical therapy (4,5). Currently, approximately 85% to 90% of cholecystectomies in the United States are performed laparoscopically. The most usual indication is symptomatic cholelithiasis. The overall complication rate associated with laparoscopic cholecystectomy (LC) is 5% (6), whereas that with open cholecystectomy (OC) is 14% (1). However, the incidence of bile duct injury is twice as high after LC than after OC.

Operations on the common bile duct (CBD), such as common bile duct explorations (CBDEs) for biliary calculi, are now performed less frequently because of the widespread use of endoscopic retrograde cholangiopancreatography (ERCP). This procedure has been very successful in effecting stone removal, both preoperatively and postoperatively; thus, CBDE can be avoided in many cases.

PREVENTION OF POTENTIAL PITFALLS DURING ELECTIVE BILIARY SURGERY

Since it was first successfully performed in France by Mouret in 1987 (7), LC has very rapidly emerged as the most popular treatment method for cholelithiasis. Unfortunately, its widespread use has been accompanied by an increase in biliary tract complications. The rate of bile duct injury in association with LC is 0.3% to 0.6% (6,8–10). In contrast, the rate of such injuries in association with OC is 0.2% to 0.3% (1–11). The complication rate associated with LC appears to decrease as the surgeon's experience with the procedure increases. The overall injury rate, however, has remained relatively high, even in the current "steady state" (12).

Conversion to OC should occur when LC cannot be performed safely or when injury is suspected. The conversion rate from LC to OC is reported to be 5% to 10% (6,8,12). Common reasons for conversion are acute inflammation, severe chronic inflammation, adhesions from previous surgery, aberrant anatomy, equipment problems, stone spillage, bile duct laceration, and bowel injury. Other frequently cited reasons are the need for common duct exploration, gallbladder carcinoma, and obesity.

Several studies have found that certain factors are associated with an increased propensity for injury during LC. These are acute inflammation, chronic scarring or fibrosis of the gallbladder and biliary tree, fat in the porta hepatis, bleeding during the procedure, and aberrant anatomy (6,13–18).

Other common complications that may occur after LC are wound infection (usually at the site of

---

[a] James B. Peoples is deceased

the umbilical trocar), bleeding due to trocar insertion, bowel injury, retained stones, and subcutaneous emphysema. Serious complications can generally be prevented during LC and OC by simple attention to detail. Certain safeguards and tips for the performance of LC are highlighted in the following sections.

Trocar Placement During Laparoscopic Cholecystectomy

Serious injuries have occurred with the establishment of access into the abdominal cavity, including bowel perforation, retroperitoneal hematoma, and omental injuries. Vascular injuries, such as lacerations of the aorta, the inferior vena cava, and the iliac vessels, although rare, have been reported (19). The Hasson open technique is associated with the fewest complications (20–22). This technique eliminates all vascular injuries; however, it does not decrease the rate of bowel injuries and thus is not an absolute safeguard against injuries (23,24). Whatever method is used, the surgeon must take care when establishing access and should promptly perform laparotomy in cases of suspected injury. Subcutaneous emphysema, pneumothorax, and gas embolism are rarely reported complications of the creation of pneumoperitoneum.

Gallbladder Dissection and Retraction

Cephalad and lateral traction to the gallbladder tends to align the cystic duct in parallel with the CBD. In the face of severe inflammation, scarring, or bleeding, the CBD can be confused with the cystic duct. Chronic inflammation may result in fusion of the cystic duct and the common hepatic duct (CHD), and this fusion may lead to CHD injury. Conversion to an open procedure should be performed without hesitation in the face of severe scarring or inability to properly retract or grasp the gallbladder. Decompressing a distended gallbladder may make it easier to handle, particularly in cases of acute inflammation.

The Use of Intraoperative Cholangiography

The debate about whether intraoperative cholangiography should be routinely used preceded the laparoscopic era. Several authors currently advocate cholangiography in all cases for delineating the anatomy and improving the surgeon's laparoscopic skills (13,25–27). Other authors have argued for selective use of this procedure (28–31). When it is used, cholangiography should be performed dynamically under fluoroscopic guidance rather than statically. Proper interpretation of the findings is very important (32). Intraoperative cholangiography aids in identifying injuries, minimizing the extent of injury, and directing the course of management in cases of retained common duct stones. Cholangiography should always be used in cases of uncertain anatomy.

Hunter has proposed five specific technical steps aimed at preventing bile duct injuries during LC. These are (i) the liberal use of the 30-degree laparoscope, (ii) firm cephalad-fundal retraction, (iii) lateral infundibular retraction, (iv) dissection of the cystic duct continuously into the gallbladder, and (v) conversion to OC whenever bleeding is more than a minor problem (33).

Cholecystectomy for Patients with Cirrhosis

The morbidity and mortality rates associated with cholecystectomy are higher for patients with liver disease than for the general population. Complication rates as high as 40% and mortality rates of 14% to 27% have been reported after major abdominal operations (34,35). Bleeding, both intraoperatively and postoperatively, is a serious concern. Factors contributing to tendency for bleeding among patients with cirrhosis include portal hypertension with portosystemic shunting, thrombocytopenia, and coagulopathy. Some authors (36) have proposed that leaving the posterior wall of the gallbladder adherent to the liver will aid in preventing intraoperative and postoperative bleeding from the liver bed. Fulguration of the retained mucosa with electrocautery or the argon beam coagulator is advised in these instances.

LC, once considered to be contraindicated in patients with cirrhosis and symptomatic cholelithiasis, is currently accepted as the procedure of choice for patients with early or well-compensated cirrhosis (37–39). Overall, for patients with cirrhosis, preoperative optimization of liver function is imperative. Only patients with symptoms clearly indicative of cholecystitis should undergo cholecystectomy. The simplest and most expeditious procedure is recommended. Tube cholecystostomy should be considered as an option to surgery when the operative risk is very high.

Preoperative Administration of Antibiotics

Most patients are given a single dose of preoperative antibiotics just before undergoing cholecystectomy. However, this routine use of prophylactic antibiotics has not been shown to confer any added benefit in cases of uncomplicated elective gallbladder surgery; thus, antibiotics should not be administered in such cases (40,41). For patients with risk factors such as age of more than 65 years, jaundice, acute cholecystitis, choledocholithiasis, cholangitis, obesity, or diabetes mellitus, antibiotics have demonstrated value in decreasing the incidence of wound and intra-abdominal infections (42).

DIAGNOSIS OF BILIARY COMPLICATIONS

Postoperative bile leaks after cholecystectomy may occur from any portion of the biliary tract. The Luschka ducts, which arise from the gallbladder bed, are occasionally a source. Leaks from these accessory ducts are usually self-limited and do not require surgical intervention (43). Biliary leaks may also arise from the cystic duct stump, the CBD, hepatic duct lacerations or transections, or small bowel injury.

Presentation

Patients with postoperative biliary leaks exhibit a wide range of clinical symptoms and signs. After biliary leaks, the common symptoms are abdominal pain, distension, nausea, vomiting, fever, and jaundice. Other symptoms include prolonged ileus and failure to thrive. Presentation can occur in the immediate postoperative period or as late as several weeks postoperatively.

Physical examination may reveal jaundice, abdominal tenderness, or both. Tenderness may be localized to the right upper quadrant or generalized. Fever and other signs of sepsis may accompany these findings in cases of infected bile.

Laboratory findings may be nonspecific. Leukocytosis and hyperbilirubinemia may be present. There is not usually a consistent pattern of direct or indirect hyperbilirubinemia in cases of free bile leakage into the abdomen. Direct bilirubinemia, however, predominates in cases of retained stones or a clipped common duct. Elevations in the activities of hepatic transaminase, alkaline phosphatase, and gamma-glutaryl transpeptidase may also be pertinent findings in cases of biliary obstruction.

Diagnostic Methods
Ultrasonography

Ultrasonography (US) is a fast, inexpensive, and noninvasive method of confirming suspected injuries to the biliary tract. Findings of intrahepatic ductal dilatation indicate obstruction of the distal common duct. US easily detects fluid collections. However, this procedure cannot characterize the fluid as a bile collection, a hematoma, a seroma, or a lymphocele. The effectiveness of US is limited by abundant bowel gas, which may accompany cases of ileus. Obesity can also present technical difficulties. US can be used as a guide for percutaneous drainage of bilomas.

Computed Axial Tomography

Computed axial tomography (CT) also easily detects and localizes fluid collections but cannot characterize them. CT scanning should not be the first choice for diagnosing bile duct injuries because CT does not demonstrate details of the biliary tree as well as US does. CT can also be used for guided percutaneous aspiration and drainage.

Hepatobiliary Scintigraphy

Hepatobiliary scintigraphy is a safe, highly sensitive, and noninvasive detector of biliary leaks (44–46). It is accurate in 83% to 87% of cases and is more sensitive

and specific than CT or US for ongoing biliary leaks (47). When imaging is delayed to 90 minutes, the sensitivity of this diagnostic method is further increased. Imaging is performed with technetium 99m–labeled iminodiacetic acid contrast agents. This procedure can be performed in cases of hyperbilirubinemia. The entry of the agent into the duodenum is an indication of the continuity of the biliary tract. Although good at detecting bile leaks, hepatobiliary scintigraphy cannot precisely determine the anatomical location of leaks. Therefore because injury may occur anywhere in the biliary tree or even in the small bowel, hepatobiliary scintigraphy is not regularly used to detect injuries. Other diagnostic studies are needed to pinpoint the exact location of a leak (48).

Endoscopic Retrograde Cholangiopancreatography

ERCP can be either a diagnostic or a therapeutic procedure in cases of bile duct injury. Cholangiography can easily pinpoint the exact location of injury to the biliary tree. Therapeutic maneuvers such as sphincterotomy, stone extraction, and biliary stent placement may be performed when appropriate. ERCP can easily detect cystic duct leaks and lacerations to the common duct. In cases of transections of the biliary tree, however, ERCP may not allow visualization of proximal anatomy, and complete delineation of the injury may not be possible. In 5% of cases, ERCP is associated with the serious complication of pancreatitis, hemorrhage, cholangitis, and perforation (49).

Percutaneous Transhepatic Cholangiography

Percutaneous transhepatic cholangiography (PTC) is an excellent method for illustrating the anatomy of the proximal biliary tree. A complete picture of the injury can often be obtained solely by using this method. Furthermore, temporary therapeutic procedures, such as placing drainage catheters and stents, can be performed using this approach as a bridge before definitive repair. PTC allows adequate decompression of the bile ducts. Catheters placed by PTC can serve as guides during operative dissection for definitive repair procedures.

Magnetic Resonance Cholangiopancreatography

Magnetic resonance cholangiopancreatography (MRCP) has played an increasingly important role in the diagnosis of gallbladder disease in recent years. MRCP can reduce the indications for and the frequency of use of ERCP. It has consistently demonstrated high sensitivity, specificity, and accuracy in detecting common duct stones, and it allows visualization of the proximal and distal anatomy of the bile duct (50–52). Because MRCP is noninvasive, it has a unique advantage over ERCP and PTC; in fact, MRCP may render ERCP and PTC useful only as therapeutic tools (53). MRCP has also been used to diagnose postoperative biliary leaks (54).

MANAGEMENT OF SPECIFIC COMPLICATIONS
Leaks from the Stump of the Cystic Duct

Cystic duct leaks generally occur after inadequate ligature of the cystic duct or slippage of clips, although they can also be caused by retained stones. Another cause of such leaks is injury to the cystic duct distal to the clips or ligature applied during cholecystectomy. Accumulation of free bile from this source usually occurs in the subhepatic space. Depending on the severity and rate of the leak and the length of time before it is detected, bile may spread freely throughout the peritoneal cavity or may be loculated. The symptoms of cystic duct leaks are abdominal pain, fever, and jaundice.

The definitive diagnosis is usually made by either ERCP or PTC. Treatment usually involves reducing the pressure on the proximal duct by placing an endoscopic stent in the common duct through the ampulla of Vater. Equalization of pressures in the biliary tree and the duodenum by stent placement is believed to be sufficient to allow the healing of these minor leaks (44). These stents typically remain in place for six to eight weeks; surgical intervention is rarely necessary. The type of stent used (long, short, or nasobiliary) does not appear to influence the outcome. Cystic duct leaks can be managed with or without sphincterotomy, but sphincterotomy alone without stent placement can result in prolonged bile leakage and delayed healing (55). Any residual stone can be extracted when ERCP is performed.

Injuries to the Common Bile Duct

As stated earlier, the incidence of injuries to the CHD and the CBD has increased in the laparoscopic era. These injuries can result in long-term morbidity, recurrent hospital admissions, multiple radiological and surgical interventions, costly litigation, and mortality. Branum et al. (56) and Strasberg et al. (11) have developed classification systems for these injuries.

The classic injury associated with LC is caused by misidentification of the common duct as the cystic duct followed by resection of parts of the common bile and hepatic ducts. These injuries are detected during the original procedure in 50% of cases, although they may be detected as late as postoperative day 9. Although the precise location of the leak can be determined by either PTC or ERCP, PTC has the distinct advantage of revealing the intrahepatic system and the bifurcation of the hepatic ducts. When the common duct has been transected, the procedure of choice for repair is hepaticojejunostomy (57). Primary anastomosis and repair of common duct injuries over a T-tube is associated with a high failure rate and is not recommended for the repair of biliary injuries (58,59).

Stewart and Way (60) reported that several factors are associated with the successful repair of common duct injuries after biliary surgery. These factors are preoperative cholangiography, the choice of surgical repair, the details of the surgical repair, and the experience of the surgeon performing the repair. These authors demonstrated that 96% of repair procedures for bile duct injury were unsuccessful without preoperative cholangiography. When complete cholangiography was performed preoperatively, 84% of the initial repair procedures were successful. Primary end-to-end anastomosis led to unsuccessful outcomes in all cases, whereas Roux-en-Y hepaticojejunostomy led to success in 63% of cases. The success rate was 94% if the first repair was performed by a tertiary care biliary surgeon but only 17% if the initial repair was performed by the primary surgeon.

The timing of the repair appears to be crucial. If the injury is detected during the original cholecystectomy, the repair should be performed at that time, provided that the primary surgeon's expertise and experience are sufficient for tackling the problem. For injuries that are not detected until the postoperative period, operative repair can be delayed for days to weeks to allow abatement of inflammation and infection. If a bile leak persists, repair can be postponed for four to six weeks, provided that adequate drainage has been obtained (57). Percutaneous transhepatic catheters may be adequate for controlling an ongoing leak, but separate percutaneous catheters may be necessary for draining bile collections. Some surgeons routinely perform the hepaticojejunostomy repair over a stent. This externalized stent is used for postoperative studies and also for measurement of biliary pressures (61–64). These stents are maintained postoperatively for variable lengths of time. One advantage of these stents is that they allow access to the anastomosis for radiological intervention in the event of stricture formation. Other surgeons remove stents shortly after the repair has been performed or do not use them at all (59,65,66).

Anastomosis of the small intestine to the CBD, when it is present (choledochojejunostomy), yields poorer results than anastomosis of the intestine to the CHD (hepaticojejunostomy). Initial repair of proximal injury is even more successful, probably because the bile duct closer to the bifurcation has a better blood supply (67–69). Long-term results after serious bile duct injury are good when the injury is appropriately managed. The results of repair after laparoscopic injury compare favorably with the results of repair after open injuries if the surgeon has sufficient experience. Five-year success rates of more than 90% have been reported (57,67,70–72).

Biliary Strictures

Strictures arising from biliary surgery typically manifest themselves months to years after the initial procedure. Most benign biliary strictures occur after cholecystectomy. The patient generally experiences an insidious onset of jaundice that is usually complicated by cholangitis. The definitive diagnosis of biliary stricture is made by cholangiography, which can be achieved under the guidance of ERCP, PTC, or MRCP. Benign biliary strictures should be managed operatively. Surgery is the gold standard against which all other methods are measured (59,73,74). The area of stricture is resected and reconstructed with a Roux-en-Y hepaticojejunostomy.

Some surgeons repair benign biliary strictures by using endoscopic dilatational techniques (75–77). The use of dilation and stent placement is not recommended as the first line of definitive management of benign strictures. Metallic stents have been used to treat benign biliary strictures, but they should be considered only when the patient is a poor candidate for surgery, when intrahepatic biliary strictures have occurred, or when attempts at surgical repair have failed. Most patients treated with metallic stents will experience recurrent cholangitis or stent obstruction and will require repeated intervention (78–81). Hutson and coworkers (82,83) have described the subfascial placement of the jejunal Roux limb to provide easy access for the dilation of postoperative biliary strictures. The limb may be marked with surgical clips that will facilitate its easy identification by the interventional radiologist. Balloon dilation of strictures after the completion of biliary anastomoses is also frequently used as a first line of treatment for patients who have undergone orthotopic liver transplantation (84,85).

Retained Common Duct Stones

Gallstones can be dislodged into the common duct in the course of dissection during cholecystectomy. Smaller stones will pass through uneventfully into the duodenum. Larger stones, however, can be retained and can cause complications.

Common duct stones will be missed in approximately 1% to 2% of cases after cholecystectomy. Most of these stones will be asymptomatic. Retained common duct stones can cause biliary stasis, which enhances bacterial replication and can result in postoperative cholangitis.

Patients with suspected retained stones should be treated with broad-spectrum antibiotics for the prophylaxis or treatment of cholangitis. US may demonstrate dilated proximal bile ducts. ERCP is a definitive diagnostic method in this setting. When ERCP is combined with sphincterotomy and stone extraction, successful CBD clearance can be achieved in 95% of cases. Failure of ERCP to achieve stone clearance is an indication for common duct exploration.

Pancreatitis

Pancreatitis can occur as a complication of many abdominal procedures. Biliary surgery particularly tends to precipitate this complication. Pancreatitis may occur after the passage of common duct stones originating from the gallbladder. Pancreatitis can also result from direct instrumentation with probes,

catheters, choledoscopes, and other instruments used for CBDE. An analysis of more than 10,000 LCs performed in Switzerland found that the postoperative incidence of pancreatitis was 0.34% (86). Rates of 1% to 4% have been reported after OC (87,88).

The treatment of postoperative pancreatitis involves bowel rest, fluid resuscitation, and nutritional support as indicated. Pancreatitis can be complicated by the development of pancreatic abscesses, pseudocysts, or pancreatic ascites. Antibiotics are used only for severe cases and for cases of documented infectious complications.

Infectious Complications

The wound infection rate after LC has been reported to be 0.9%; the overall postoperative infection rate is 1.1% (6). Biliary microorganisms, most frequently *Escherichia coli*, are usually responsible for wound infection. Wound infection rates are higher after bouts of acute cholecystitis and cholangitis.

Retained common duct stones may lead to cholangitis. Postoperative bile collections may also become infected.

BILIARY TRAUMA
Introduction

In general, iatrogenic injuries to the biliary tree occur more frequently than injuries that result from blunt or penetrating trauma. Moreover, only approximately 3% to 5% of victims of abdominal trauma sustain injuries to the biliary tract. Most traumatic injuries to the biliary system are the result of penetrating trauma and occur in association with more severe injuries to other organs. Most traumatic injuries to the biliary system involve the gallbladder (89,90).

Presentation and Diagnosis

The diagnosis of biliary system injury is most frequently made intraoperatively. Such injuries are usually found in conjunction with other injuries, most often hepatic, major vascular, duodenal, and splenic injuries (90–92). Accurate preoperative diagnosis of traumatic biliary injuries is difficult. Bile leakage may occasionally elicit clinical signs of bile peritonitis. The presence of bile-stained fluid in the effluent from diagnostic peritoneal lavage may indicate liver or small bowel injury; this finding is not specific for injury to the bile ducts or gallbladder.

Abdominal CT scanning and US are not often useful in detecting isolated biliary tract injuries. Neither of these imaging methods can distinguish biliary collections from collections of blood or other fluids (93). Radionuclide scanning may be useful for confirming the suspicion of a disruption in the biliary tree. ERCP is also a method of diagnosing biliary tract lacerations with subsequent leakage. The usefulness of these two diagnostic studies is limited, however, because they cannot be performed on trauma patients in unstable condition.

Gallbladder injuries range from simple disruptions (laceration) to avulsions, contusions, or hemobilia. Bile duct injuries can be simple lacerations or more complex injuries involving transections of more than 50% of the lumen of the duct.

Management

Treatment of traumatic injury to the biliary system follows the same principles as management of injuries produced by iatrogenic mishaps. In the operating room, all immediately life-threatening injuries, such as liver and vascular lesions, should be addressed first. Abbreviated laparotomies without the definitive repair of biliary injuries may be necessary to achieve correction of acidosis, coagulopathy, and hypothermia. Thorough external drainage of extravasated bile is necessary. Definitive repair of injuries can be undertaken if the patient is stable.

Gallbladder injuries are treated by simple cholecystectomy. Ductal injuries are approached as addressed previously. Intraoperative cholangiography should be used liberally when the surgeon is uncertain about the presence or extent of injury. Patients may require Roux-en-Y hepaticojejunostomy. As is true for elective procedures, emergent procedures involving primary duct-to-duct anastomosis over a T-tube do not yield very good long-term results.

SUMMARY

Biliary tract trauma and its associated complications can present difficult challenges in management. Important points for surgeons are attention to detail during common gallbladder procedures, discretion during difficult dissections, prompt conversion of laparoscopic procedures to open procedures when indicated, and early identification and prompt management of complications.

The laparoscopic era has added a new dimension to the treatment of biliary disease. This new era in treatment has been accompanied by an increase in ductal injuries and the continued evolution of techniques for biliary tract management.

REFERENCES

1. Roslyn JJ, Binns GS, Hughes EF, Saunders-Kirkwood K, Zinner MJ, Cates JA. Open cholecystectomy. A contemporary analysis of 42,474 patients. Ann Surg 1993; 218:129–137.
2. Langenbuch CJA. Ein Fall von Exstirpation der Gallenblase wegen chronischer Cholelithiasis. Berliner Klin Wochenschr 1882; 19:725–727.
3. Glenn F, Grafe WR Jr. Historical events in biliary tract surgery. Arch Surg 1966; 93:848–852.
4. Magnuson TH, Lillemoe KD, Pitt HA. How many Americans will be eligible for biliary lithotripsy? Arch Surg 1989; 124:1195–1200.
5. Sackmann M, Ippisch E, Sauerbruch T, Holl J, Brendel W, Paumgartner G. Early gallstone recurrence rate after successful shock-wave therapy. Gastroenterology 1990; 98:392–396.
6. A prospective analysis of 1518 laparoscopic cholecystectomies. The Southern Surgeons Club. N Engl J Med 1991; 324:1073–1078.
7. Dubois F, Icard P, Berthelot G, Levard H. Coelioscopic cholecystectomy. Preliminary report of 36 cases. Ann Surg 1990; 211:60–62.
8. Orlando R III, Russell JC, Lynch J, Mattie A. Laparoscopic cholecystectomy. A statewide experience. The Connecticut Laparoscopic Cholecystectomy Registry. Arch Surg 1993; 128:494–499.
9. Deziel DJ, Millikan KW, Economou SG, Doolas A, Ko ST, Airan MC. Complications of laparoscopic cholecystectomy: a national survey of 4,292 hospitals and an analysis of 77,604 cases. Am J Surg 1993; 165:9–14.
10. Bernard HR, Hartman TW. Complications after laparoscopic cholecystectomy. Am J Surg 1993; 165: 533–535.
11. Strasberg SM, Hertl M, Soper NJ. An analysis of the problem of biliary injury during laparoscopic cholecystectomy. J Am Coll Surg 1995; 180:101–125.
12. Wherry DC, Marohn MR, Malanoski MP, Hetz SP, Rich NM. An external audit of laparoscopic cholecystectomy in the steady state performed in medical treatment facilities of the Department of Defense. Ann Surg 1996; 224:145–154.
13. Asbun HJ, Rossi RL, Lowell JA, Munson JL. Bile duct injury during laparoscopic cholecystectomy: mechanism of injury, prevention, and management. World J Surg 1993; 17:547–552.
14. Adams DB, Borowicz MR, Wootton FT III, Cunningham JT. Bile duct complications after laparoscopic cholecystectomy. Surg Endosc 1993; 7:79–83.
15. Soper NJ, Flye MW, Brunt LM, et al. Diagnosis and management of biliary complications of laparoscopic cholecystectomy. Am J Surg 1993; 165:663–669.
16. Roy AF, Passi RB, Lapointe RW, McAlister VC, Dagenias MH, Wall WJ. Bile duct injury during laparoscopic cholecystectomy. Can J Surg 1993; 36:509–516.
17. Rantis PC Jr, Greenlee HB, Pickleman J, Prinz RA. Laparoscopic cholecystectomy bile duct injuries: more than meets the eye. Am Surg 1993; 59:533–540.
18. Christensen RA, vanSonnenberg E, Nemcek AA Jr, D'Agostino HB. Inadvertent ligation of the aberrant right hepatic duct at cholecystectomy: radiologic diagnosis and therapy. Radiology 1992; 183:549–553.
19. Schafer M, Lauper M, Krahenbuhl L. Trocar and Veress needle injuries during laparoscopy. Surg Endosc 2001; 15:275–280.
20. Sigman HH, Fried GM, Garzon J, et al. Risks of blind versus open approach to celiotomy for laparoscopic surgery. Surg Laparosc Endosc 1993; 3:296–299.
21. Ballem RV, Rudomanski J. Techniques of pneumoperitoneum. Surg Laparosc Endosc 1993; 3:42–43.
22. Mayol J, Garcia-Aguilar J, Ortiz-Oshiro E, De-Diego Carmona JA, Fernandez-Represa JA. Risks of the minimal access approach for laparoscopic surgery: multivariate analysis of morbidity related to umbilical trocar insertion. World J Surg 1997; 21:529–533.

23. Woolcott R. The safety of laparoscopy performed by direct trocar insertion and carbon dioxide insufflation under vision. Aust N Z J Obstet Gynaecol 1997; 37: 216–219.

24. Kornfield EA, Sant GR, O'Leary MP. Minilaparotomy for laparoscopy: not a foolproof procedure. J Endourol 1994; 8:353–355.

25. Rossi RL, Schirmer WJ, Braasch JW, Sanders LB, Munson JL. Laparoscopic bile duct injuries. Risk factors, recognition, and repair. Arch Surg 1992; 127: 596–602.

26. Moossa AR, Easter DW, Van Sonnenberg E, Casola G, D'Agostino H. Laparoscopic injuries to the bile duct. A cause for concern. Ann Surg 1992; 215:203–208.

27. Stuart SA, Simpson TI, Alvord LA, Williams MD. Routine intraoperative laparoscopic cholangiography. Am J Surg 1998; 176:632–637.

28. Snow LL, Weinstein LS, Hannon JK, Lane DR. Evaluation of operative cholangiography in 2043 patients undergoing laparoscopic cholecystectomy: a case for the selective operative cholangiogram. Surg Endosc 2001; 15:14–20.

29. Borjeson J, Liu SK, Jones S, Matolo NM. Selective intraoperative cholangiography during laparoscopic cholecystectomy: how selective? Am Surg 2000; 66: 616–618.

30. Braghetto I, Debandi A, Korn O, Bastias J. Long-term follow-up after laparoscopic cholecystectomy without routine intraoperative cholangiography. Surg Laparosc Endosc 1998; 8:349–352.

31. Silverstein JC, Wavak E, Millikan KW. A prospective experience with selective cholangiography. Am Surg 1998; 64:654–658.

32. Olsen D. Bile duct injuries during laparoscopic cholecystectomy. Surg Endosc 1997; 11:133–138.

33. Hunter JG. Avoidance of bile duct injury during laparoscopic cholecystectomy. Am J Surg 1991; 162:71–76.

34. Doberneck RC, Sterling WA Jr, Allison DC. Morbidity and mortality after operation in nonbleeding cirrhotic patients. Am J Surg 1983; 146:306–309.

35. Aranha GV, Kruss D, Greenlee HB. Therapeutic options for biliary tract disease in advanced cirrhosis. Am J Surg 1988; 155:374–377.

36. Bornman PC, Terblanche J. Subtotal cholecystectomy: for the difficult gallbladder in portal hypertension and cholocystitis. Surgery 1985; 98:1–6.

37. Sleeman D, Namias N, Levi D, et al. Laparoscopic cholecystectomy in cirrhotic patients. J Am Coll Surg 1998; 187:400–403.

38. Poggio JL, Rowland CM, Gores GJ, Nagorney DM, Donohue JH. A comparison of laparoscopic and open cholecystectomy in patients with compensated cirrhosis and symptomatic gallstone disease. Surgery 2000; 127:405–411.

39. Fernandes NF, Schwesinger WH, Hilsenbeck SG, et al. Laparoscopic cholecystectomy and cirrhosis: a case-control study of outcomes. Liver Transpl 2000; 6: 340–344.

40. Tocchi A, Lepre L, Costa G, Liotta G, Mazzoni G, Maggiolini F. The need for antibiotic prophylaxis in elective laparoscopic cholecystectomy: a prospective randomized study. Arch Surg 2000; 135:67–70.

41. Watkin DS, Wainwright AM, Thompson MH, Leaper DJ. Infection after laparoscopic cholecystectomy: are antibiotics really necessary?. Eur J Surg 1995; 161:509–511.

42. Dobay KJ, Freier DT, Albear P. The absent role of prophylactic antibiotics in low-risk patients undergoing cholecystectomy. Am Surg 1999; 65:226–228.

43. Bjorkman DJ, Carr-Locke DL, Lichtenstein DR, et al. Postsurgical bile leaks: endoscopic obliteration of the transpapillary pressure gradient is enough. Am J Gastroenterol 1995; 90:2128–2133.

44. Pasmans HL, Go PM, Gouma DJ, Heidendal GA, van Engelshoven JM, van Kroonenburgh MJ. Scintigraphic diagnosis of bile leakage after laparoscopic cholecystectomy. A prospective study. Clin Nucl Med 1992; 17:697–700.

45. Kulber DA, Berci G, Paz-Partlow M, Ashok G, Hiatt JR. Value of early cholescintigraphy in detection of biliary complications after laparoscopic cholecystectomy. Am Surg 1994; 60:190–193.

46. Estrada WN, Zanzi I, Ward R, Negrin JA, Margouleff D. Scintigraphic evaluation of postoperative complications of laparoscopic cholecystectomy. J Nucl Med 1991; 32:1910–1911.

47. Brugge WR, Rosenberg DJ, Alavi A. Diagnosis of postoperative bile leaks. Am J Gastroenterol 1994; 89:2178–2183.

48. Walker AT, Shapiro AW, Brooks DC, Braver JM, Tumeh SS. Bile duct disruption and biloma after laparoscopic cholecystectomy: imaging evaluation. Am J Roentgenol 1992; 158:785–789.

49. Masci E, Toti G, Mariani A, et al. Complications of diagnostic and therapeutic ERCP: a prospective multicenter study. Am J Gastroenterol 2001; 96:417–423.

50. Liu TH, Consorti ET, Kawashima A, et al. The efficacy of magnetic resonance cholangiography for the evaluation of patients with suspected choledocholithiasis before laparoscopic cholecystectomy. Am J Surg 1999; 178:480–484.

51. Varghese JC, Farrell MA, Courtney G, Osborne H, Murray FE, Lee MJ. A prospective comparison of magnetic resonance cholangiopancreatography with endoscopic retrograde cholangiopancreatography in the evaluation of patients with suspected biliary tract disease. Clin Radiol 1999; 54:513–520.

52. Magnuson TH, Bender JS, Duncan MD, Ahrendt SA, Harmon JW, Regan F. Utility of magnetic resonance cholangiography in the evaluation of biliary obstruction. J Am Coll Surg 1999; 189:63–72.

53. Raval B, Kramer LA. Advances in the imaging of common duct stones using magnetic resonance cholangiography, endoscopic ultrasonography, and laparoscopic ultrasonography. Semin Laparosc Surg 2000; 7:232–236.

54. Vitellas KM, El-Dieb A, Vaswani K, et al. Detection of bile duct leaks using MR cholangiography with mangfodipir trisodium (Teslascan). J Comput Assist Tomogr 2001; 25:102–105.

55. Barton FR, Russell RC, Hatfield AR. Management of bile leaks after laparoscopic cholecystectomy. Br J Surg 1995; 82:980–984.

56. Branum G, Schmitt C, Baillie J, et al. Management of major biliary complications after laparoscopic cholecystectomy. Ann Surg 1993; 217:532–541.

57. Lilemoe KD, Melton GM, Cameron JL, et al. Postoperative bile duct strictures: management and outcome in the 1990s. Ann Surg 2000; 232:430–441.

58. Csendes A, Diaz JC, Burdiles P, Maluenda F. Late results of immediate primary end to end repair of

accidental section of the common bile duct. Surg Gynecol Obstet 1989; 168:125–130.

59. Pellegrini CA, Thomas MJ, Way LW. Recurrent biliary stricture. Patterns of recurrence and outcome of surgical therapy. Am J Surg 1984; 147:175–180.

60. Stewart L, Way LW. Bile duct injuries during laparoscopic cholecystectomy. Factors that influence the results of treatment. Arch Surg 1995; 130:1123–1129.

61. Savader SJ, Cameron JL, Lillemoe KD, Lund GB, Mitchell SE, Venbrux AC. The biliary manometric perfusion test and clinical trial—long-term predictive value of success after treatment of bile duct strictures: 10-year experience. J Vasc Interv Radiol 1998; 9: 976–985.

62. vanSonnenberg E, Ferrucci JT Jr, Neff CC, Mueller PR, Simeone JF, Wittenberg J. Biliary pressure: manometric and perfusion studies at percutaneous transhepatic cholangiography and percutaneous biliary drainage. Radiology 1983; 148:41–50.

63. Pitt HA, Miyamoto T, Parapatis SK, Tompkins RK, Longmire WP Jr. Factors influencing outcome in patients with postoperative biliary strictures. Am J Surg 1982; 144:14–21.

64. Cameron JL, Gayler BW, Zuidema GD. The use of silastic transhepatic stents in benign and malignant biliary strictures. Ann Surg 1978; 188:552–561.

65. Sutherland F, Launois B, Stanescu M, Campion JP, Spiliopoulos Y, Stasik C. A refined approach to the repair of postcholecystectomy bile duct strictures. Arch Surg 1999; 134:299–302.

66. Innes JT, Ferrara JJ, Carey LC. Biliary reconstruction without transanastomotic stent. Am Surg 1988; 54:27–30.

67. Tocchi A, Costa G, Lepre L, Liotta G, Mazzoni G, Sita A. The long-term outcome of hepaticojejunostomy in the treatment of benign bile duct strictures. Ann Surg 1996; 224:162–167.

68. Terblanche J, Worthley CS, Spence RA, Krige JE. High or low hepaticojejunostomy for bile duct strictures? Surgery 1990; 108:828–834.

69. Terblanche J, Allison HF, Northover JM. An ischemic basis for biliary strictures. Surgery 1983; 94:52–57.

70. Johnson SR, Koehler A, Pennington LK, Hanto DW. Long-term results of surgical repair of bile duct injuries following laparoscopic cholecystectomy. Surgery 2000; 128:668–677.

71. Murr MM, Gigot JF, Nagorney DM, Harmsen WS, Ilstrup DM, Farnell MB. Long-term results of biliary reconstruction after laparoscopic bile duct injuries. Arch Surg 1999; 134:604–609.

72. Rothlin MA, Lopfe M, Schlumpf R, Largiader F. Long-term results of hepaticojejunostomy for benign lesions of the bile ducts. Am J Surg 1998; 175:22–26.

73. Tocchi A, Mazzoni G, Liotta G, et al. Management of benign biliary strictures: biliary enteric anastomosis vs. endoscopic stenting. Arch Surg 2000; 135: 153–157.

74. Millis JM, Tompkins RK, Zinner MJ, Longmire WP Jr, Roslyn JJ. Management of bile duct strictures. An evolving strategy. Arch Surg 1992; 127:1077–1084.

75. Cheng YF, Lee TY, Sheen-Chen SM, Huang TL, Chen TY. Treatment of complicated hepatolithiasis with intrahepatic biliary stricture by ductal dilatation and stenting: long-term results. World J Surg 2000; 24: 712–716.

76. Born P, Rosch T, Bruhl K, et al. Long-term results of endoscopic and percutaneous transhepatic treatment of benign biliary strictures. Endoscopy 1999; 31: 725–731.

77. Morrison MC, Lee MJ, Saini S, Brink JA, Mueller PR. Percutaneous balloon dilatation of benign biliary strictures. Radiol Clin North Am 1990; 28:1191–1201.

78. Lopez RR Jr, Cosenza CA, Lois J, et al. Long-term results of metallic stents for benign biliary strictures. Arch Surg 2001; 136:664–669.

79. Yoon HK, Sung KB, Song HY, et al. Benign biliary strictures associated with recurrent pyogenic cholangitis: treatment with expandable metallic stents. Am J Roentgenol 1997; 169:1523–1527.

80. Bonnel DH, Liguory CL, Lefebvre JF, Cornud FE. Placement of metallic stents for treatment of postoperative biliary strictures: long-term outcome in 25 patients. Am J Roentgenol 1997; 169:1517–1522.

81. Hausegger KA, Kugler C, Uggowitzer M, et al. Benign biliary obstruction: is treatment with the Wallstent advisable? Radiology 1996; 200:437–441.

82. Hutson DG, Russell E, Yrizarry J, et al. Percutaneous dilatation of biliary strictures through the afferent limb of a modified Roux-en-Y choledochojejunostomy or hepaticojejunostomy. Am J Surg 1998; 175:108–113.

83. Russell E, Yrizarry JM, Huber JS, et al. Percutaneous transjejunal biliary dilatation: alternate management for benign strictures. Radiology 1986; 159:209–214.

84. Schwartz DA, Petersen BT, Poterucha JJ, Gostout CJ. Endoscopic therapy of anastomotic bile duct strictures occurring after liver transplantation. Gastrointest Endosc 2000; 51:169–174.

85. Davidson BR, Rai R, Nandy A, Doctor N, Burroughs A, Rolles K. Results of choledochojejunostomy in the treatment of biliary complications after liver transplantation in the era of nonsurgical therapies. Liver Transpl 2000; 6:201–206.

86. Z'graggen K, Aronsky D, Maurer CA, Klaiber C, Baer HU. Acute postoperative pancreatitis after laparoscopic cholecystectomy. Results of the Prospective Swiss Association of Laparoscopic and Thoracoscopic Surgery Study. Arch Surg 1997; 132:1026–1031.

87. Bardenheier JA, Kaminiski DL, Willman VL. Pancreatitis after biliary tract surgery. Am J Surg 1968; 116: 773–776.

88. Vernava A, Andrus C, Herrmann VM, Kaminski DL. Pancreatitis after biliary tract surgery. Arch Surg 1987; 122:575–580.

89. Posner MC, Moore EE. Extrahepatic biliary tract injury: operative management plan. J Trauma 1985; 25: 833–837.

90. Bade PG, Thomson SR, Hirschberg A, Robbs JV. Surgical options in traumatic injury to the extrahepatic biliary tract. Br J Surg 1989; 76:256–258.

91. Soderstrom CA, Maekawa K, DuPriest RW Jr, Cowley RA. Gallbladder injuries resulting from blunt abdominal trauma: an experience and review. Ann Surg 1981; 193:60–66.

92. Ivatury RR, Rohman M, Nallathambi M, Pas PM, Gunduz Y, Stahl WM. The morbidity of injuries of the extra-hepatic biliary system. J Trauma 1985; 25:967–973.

93. Gottesman L, Marks RA, Khoury PT, Moallem AG, Wichern WA Jr. Diagnosis of isolated perforation of the gallbladder following blunt trauma using sonography and CT scan. J Trauma 1984; 24:280–281.

9

Complications of Intestinal Surgery

John J. Hong
*Robert Wood Johnson Medical School, University of Medicine and Dentistry of New Jersey,
New Brunswick, New Jersey, U.S.A.*

Sapoora Manshaii
St. Louis University School of Medicine, St. Louis, Missouri, U.S.A.

Postoperative ileus, fever, and incisional pain have traditionally been viewed as the unavoidable, and in many ways related, consequences of laparotomy and intestinal surgery. Although all patients inevitably experience some degree of physiologic derangement after intestinal surgery, the optimal diagnostic and therapeutic treatment of the postoperative patient depends on the surgeon's (and the patient's) understanding of what is considered normal and acceptable during postoperative convalescence as opposed to what may be viewed as a complication. Although the extremes—routine postoperative course in contrast with multiple, unexpected complications and death—are easy to define, it is the gray middle of the spectrum of postoperative recovery that may be difficult for the surgeon to evaluate. At what point is postoperative ileus a complication? How much pain can be considered acceptable as normal incisional pain?

GENERAL COMPLICATIONS OF INTESTINAL SURGERY
Postoperative Ileus and Pain

Any violation of the peritoneal cavity causes a cascade of physiologic events, some of which may result in the inhibition of gastrointestinal function. Physical manipulation of the viscera further impairs gut motility as the result of inhibition of the splanchnic sympathetic reflex and stimulation of local inflammatory mediators (1). Although gross motor function of the small bowel is commonly observed during laparotomy, such motility may not be a part of effective, coordinated peristalsis (2). Depending on the site and degree of visceral manipulation, the underlying disease process, and patient characteristics, paralytic ileus may last from hours to days. Ileus has been recognized as an inevitable consequence of intestinal surgery. Postoperative ileus is further exacerbated by

the use of opioids for analgesia. The high density of μ-opioid receptors throughout the gastrointestinal tract as the result of endogenous release and exogenous administration of opioids results in prolonged transit time after surgical stress (3–5).

Traditionally, postoperative ileus has been treated with bowel rest, nasogastric suction, and early mobilization. Despite what we commonly tell our patients, early mobilization does not appear to hasten recovery from ileus (6); more likely, it is a marker of adequate postoperative pain control, which may decrease other postoperative complications. A variety of promotility agents have been used with mixed results (7–10). Nasogastric suction and early enteral feeding have been studied, and small but statistically significant improvements in the resolution of postoperative ileus have been associated with early resumption of enteral nutrition (11,12). The use of regional analgesic agents has also been shown to decrease the duration of postoperative ileus (13,14). The use of minimally invasive rather than open surgical techniques appears to decrease the duration of postoperative ileus (15,16). Selective μ-opioid receptor antagonists that may reduce the gastrointestinal effects of opioids without impairing analgesia are currently being investigated (17,18).

To date, none of these studies have involved patients undergoing extensive small-intestinal surgery. Patients undergoing extensive small-bowel manipulation are at greatest risk of prolonged postoperative ileus, probably because an extensive local inflammatory response is superimposed on neural reflexes (19). Prolonged paralytic ileus in these patients may rightfully be considered as an expected consequence of the disease. Conversely, prolonged ileus in a patient who has undergone an elective colorectal procedure or gynecologic procedure may be considered a surgical complication. Factors that may contribute to a delay in the return of bowel function are inappropriate use of nasogastric tubes, excessive use of opioid analgesics, the presence of intra-abdominal or systemic infection, and postoperative mechanical small-bowel obstruction (SBO).

Postoperative Obstruction and Adhesion Formation

Prolonged postoperative ileus may be difficult to distinguish from partial mechanical SBO, and both may be present to a degree among patients who have undergone extensive intestinal surgery. Patients who have undergone gynecologic or colorectal procedures are at higher risk of SBO during the postoperative period. Postoperative partial SBO usually resolves with nonoperative management: nasogastric suction, parenteral fluid, and nutritional support.

Peritoneal adhesions are the most common cause of postoperative mechanical obstructions; they are responsible for more than 90% of cases (20). Adhesion formation is a generalized response to tissue injury and, as such, is essentially universal (21); it has been considered as an unavoidable consequence of laparotomy. However, there is clearly individual variation in the amount, severity, and duration of peritoneal adhesions that are found at the time of re-operation. Some of the factors that may contribute to adhesion formation may be preventable.

Means of preventing peritoneal adhesions have traditionally been the same as measures designed to reduce the likelihood of postoperative ileus and minimize the inflammatory peritoneal reaction to laparotomy: gentle tissue handling, meticulous hemostasis, avoidance of contamination with enteric contents and tissue desiccation, and minimization of exposure to foreign bodies, for example, by washing powder from surgical gloves before peritoneal exposure. In theory, strict attention to surgical technique should minimize the effects of preventable causes of adhesion formation (22).

Additional "adjuvant" preventative measures have been studied, all aimed at modulating various points of the wound healing or inflammatory process. Nonsteroidal anti-inflammatory drugs (23), calcium-channel blockers (24), corticosteroids (25), colloid solutions (26), heparinized solutions (27), fibrinolytic agents (28), cellulose (29), and hyaluronic acid–based barrier agents and solutions (30,31) have been studied, and all have various degrees of effectiveness. Investigation has been limited by the lack of an experimental animal model that correlates with human peritoneum and the lack of a standardized clinical model. Currently, no means of reducing peritoneal adhesions is routinely used during laparotomy, and adhesion formation continues to be viewed as an unavoidable consequence of abdominal surgery.

COMPLICATIONS OF SPECIFIC INTESTINAL OPERATIONS
Lysis of Adhesions

Inadvertent bowel injury is the most common complication of adhesiolysis. The bowel is most commonly injured upon initial entry into the peritoneal cavity, when recognition of dense adhesions of bowel to a previous laparotomy incision is most difficult. Inadvertent enterotomy with spillage of enteric contents is associated with substantially increased morbidity rates (32): increased likelihood of wound and intra-abdominal infection, increased likelihood of further postoperative adhesions, increased duration of postoperative ileus, increased likelihood of intensive care unit admission, and increased duration of hospital stay. Full-thickness bowel injuries should be immediately repaired with care to minimize contamination. No studies have obtained definitive findings regarding the necessity for repair of bowel from which the serosa has been lost.

A missed enterotomy is a potentially catastrophic injury. Both small and large bowel should be meticulously examined after any extensive adhesiolysis so that injuries, if any, can be detected.

Bowel Resection and Repair

Bowel resection is performed to remove nonviable or severely diseased bowel. Considerable surgical judgment may be necessary for properly executing this seemingly simple objective. We can divide the surgical decision-making process into three phases: (i) diagnosis, or identification and determination of the severity of disease in the bowel; (ii) debridement, or resection, drainage, and lavage; and (iii) reconstruction, or anastomosis, diversion, or both. Each step involves potential complications.

Inadequate or Excessive Resection

Inadequate resection is caused by failure of diagnosis. In the setting of bowel infarction, residual nonviable bowel will cause unrelenting abdominal sepsis in the postoperative period, thereby further complicating a typically complex clinical picture. Evidence of ongoing inflammatory response after bowel resection may indicate inadequate resection. Intraoperatively, questionable segments of bowel may be evaluated by the use of a Wood's lamp and the intravenous administration of fluorescein. A staged laparotomy, with initial exploration and resection followed by aggressive fluid resuscitation and medical optimization, and then a planned "second-look" laparotomy, may also allow for preservation of additional viable intestine. In the setting of inflammatory or neoplastic disease, adequate resection requires removal of all diseased tissue; gross or histologic identification of healthy, nondiseased margins of intestine must be available for anastomosis.

Crohn's disease may pose a difficult clinical problem because the need for resection may be outweighed by the need for preserving intestinal length in anticipation of future progression of disease. A variety of surgical techniques have been described for preserving intestinal length among patients with Crohn's disease. A desirable length of resection of inflamed bowel in a patient with, for example, a perforated Meckel's diverticulitis may constitute excessive resection in a patient with Crohn's ileitis and a comparable degree of inflammation.

Excessive intestinal resection may cause a spectrum of disease, from clinically inconsequential removal of nondiseased bowel, to diarrhea, to debilitating, even lethal, short-bowel syndrome. Loss of the ileocecal valve and the terminal ileum is particularly debilitating. The loss of more than 100 cm of terminal ileum may cause macrocytic anemia due to inadequate B12 absorption and may also cause diarrhea due to impaired enterohepatic recycling of bile salts.

Short-bowel syndrome may be unavoidable. It is most commonly the result of the emergency resection of a large length of nonviable intestine as treatment for mesenteric occlusion or midgut volvulus; it is also seen among patients with Crohn's disease who have undergone multiple enterectomies and among infants after extensive resections for enterocolitis or intestinal atresia. Loss of 80% of intestinal length results in short-bowel syndrome, which cannot be improved with intestinal adaptation. Short-bowel syndrome is caused by a remnant of viable bowel whose length is not compatible with adequate enteral nutrition; this condition results in malabsorption of nutrients, vitamins, and water. Current therapy is directed first at managing the early fluid and electrolyte abnormalities and maintaining adequate nutritional support; later, attempts are made to optimize intestinal adaptation through the use of enteral nutrition and gut trophic agents (33). Surgical techniques range from intestinal lengthening techniques to small-bowel transplantation (34–36).

Debridement

Adequate debridement involves removal of nonviable tissue, drainage of areas of questionable viability, and removal and avoidance of further gross contamination. Areas of perforation should be quickly closed so that ongoing contamination can be prevented. Spillage during bowel resection can be minimized by placing intestinal clamps proximal and distal to the segment before resection. The abdomen and the surgical wound should be protected during bowel resection and anastomosis by drapes consisting of moist laparotomy pads or towels. Peritoneal irrigation should be used to remove the gross contamination and particulate matter. The benefit of adding antibiotics to the lavage solution has not been conclusively demonstrated (37–39).

Reconstruction

Complications after primary small-bowel anastomosis are usually the consequences of technical error. Obstruction at the anastomotic site may be caused by incorporating too much tissue into a handsewn anastomosis, transient edema, hematoma, or improper suture placement that catches the back wall. Meticulous attention to technique is necessary if these potential errors are to be avoided. Studies have found no difference in the complication rates between hand-sewn anastomoses and stapled anastomoses for elective bowel resection (40–43).

Bleeding at the anastomosis site is usually self-limited and resolves without the need for reoperation. Substantial hemorrhage may be associated with a preexistent bleeding diathesis or excessive iatrogenic anticoagulation.

Leaks are a common but serious complication after intestinal anastomosis, although the exact frequency of this complication has not yet been determined (44). Ischemia at the site of anastomosis may be caused by ligation of the blood supply too close to the bowel end, by accidental ligation of mesenteric vessels, or by rotation of the ends of the bowel limbs, which causes arterial or venous insufficiency (45). Anastomotic leaks, as mentioned above, may also be the result of inadequate resection of the diseased bowel. Patients' characteristics also influence the risk of leaks (46). Clinical manifestations of anastomotic leak range from florid postoperative sepsis to asymptomatic leakage, which is apparent only radiographically. Given the variable presentation and severity of anastomotic leak, the ideal method of management has not yet been determined. If the leak is small, it may result in localized phlegmon or abscess that may be amenable to diagnosis with computed tomography (CT) scanning of the abdomen and nonoperative treatment with systemic antibiotics and percutaneous drainage if necessary. Larger leaks may require reoperation.

Nonoperative management of an anastomotic leak may result in fistula formation. Enterocutaneous fistulas may also occur when the intestine is incorporated into the sutures that are used to close the abdominal wall, or they may be caused by an unrecognized injury. A fistulogram, a CT scan, or both may demonstrate the site of the defect and may detect any associated abscess. Most fistulas close without surgical intervention, especially if the daily output is less than 500 mL. The initial management is bowel rest with parenteral nutritional support (47), management of fluid and electrolyte losses, and skin protection. The benefit of octreotide is controversial (48,49). Enteral nutrition may be resumed if it does not cause worsening of the fistula output. Fistulas with a distal obstruction, very short tracts, complete epithelialization of the tract, the presence of a foreign body, cancer, or inflammatory bowel disease may not heal without surgical intervention (50). The mortality rate associated with enterocutaneous fistulas has decreased to 10% to 20% (51).

Blind-loop syndrome is a rare complication of intestinal surgery that is characterized by abdominal pain, diarrhea, steatorrhea, macrocytic anemia, and vitamin disorders. Creation of an antiperistaltic or blind loop of bowel, with resultant stasis and bacterial overgrowth, causes derangements in the metabolism of carbohydrate, fat, bile acid, and vitamins. A D-xylose breath test definitively diagnoses bacterial overgrowth of the small intestine. Antibiotic therapy may reduce the bacterial load enough to improve some symptoms; however, definitive treatment requires operative reconstruction or resection of the involved loop of bowel (52).

COMPLICATIONS OF INTESTINAL SURGERY FOR TRAUMA

The principles of intestinal surgery for trauma are the same as those of elective surgery, with the additional need for the immediate control of hemorrhage. Once adequate hemostasis has been obtained, rapid identification of injuries is carried out by "running" the small bowel from the ligament of Treitz to the ileocecal valve. Temporary control of contamination before definitive repair or resection may be obtained by placing bowel clamps proximal and distal to the site of injury or by placing Allis clamps on multiple enterotomies. With control of ongoing contamination, gross enteric contents and fecal contamination may be lavaged from the peritoneal cavity, and the bowel may be carefully inspected for areas of injury or questionable viability. When patients with severe injuries require staged or "damage control" laparotomies, definitive intestinal reconstruction may be delayed until the second or even the third laparotomy. Patients with injuries that involve mesenteric vessels may also require reexploration for evaluation of the extent of associated ischemic injury to the bowel (53). Some findings indicate that handsewn anastomoses are superior to stapled anastomoses for trauma patients (54).

The complication of missed small-bowel injury after blunt abdominal trauma is occurring with increasing frequency, especially with the widespread use of CT scanning and ultrasonography for evaluating trauma and the increasing frequency of nonoperative management of intra-abdominal injuries. The finding of free intraperitoneal fluid in a patient in hemodynamically stable condition after blunt abdominal trauma may indicate a small-bowel injury. This finding may be especially confounding when it is associated with small lacerations of the liver or spleen. Some reports suggest that, in such cases, diagnostic peritoneal lavage may be useful in detecting occult injury to the small intestine and in differentiating it from the otherwise nonoperative abdominal injuries (55–57).

COMPLICATIONS OF APPENDECTOMY

Complications of appendicitis may be categorized as preoperative, intraoperative, or postoperative.

Preoperative Complications: Misdiagnosis

Errors in diagnosis result in either a false-positive (unnecessary) appendectomy or a false-negative or missed (or perforated or gangrenous) case of appendicitis. Traditionally, surgeons have accepted a certain number of appendectomies performed for a normal appendix as not only inevitable, but also desirable because they indicate sufficient clinical suspicion in light of the increased morbidity associated with a false-negative diagnosis of acute appendicitis. The acceptable number of normal appendices removed has traditionally been between 10% and 25%, with higher or lower rates depending on patient demographics (58–61). Some reports suggest that CT scanning or a variety of nuclear medicine studies, may improve diagnostic accuracy (62–64). There is as yet no consensus about the acceptable rate of negative appendectomy or about the appropriate diagnostic work-up for suspected appendicitis (65).

Intraoperative Complications: Complicated Appendicitis

Findings suggest that most cases of complicated appendicitis are due not to physicians' delay in performing surgery, but rather to patients' delay in presenting for treatment (66). Patients with a diagnosis of phlegmon or abscess before surgery are often initially treated with a trial of nonoperative management with antibiotics and eventually with interval appendectomy. This approach may yield complication rates lower than those associated with primary appendectomy in the setting of a necrotic appendiceal stump or cecum, a setting associated with an increased risk of fecal fistula formation (67,68). The necessity of interval appendectomy is controversial; some authors advocate simple observation without surgery after nonoperative management of perforated appendicitis (69,70). However, studies examining cases of acute appendicitis treated with antibiotics alone found a high rate of recurrent appendicitis (71). Despite the intensity of opinion, no large, prospective studies with long-term follow-up have been performed to determine the best type of care.

Surgeons confronting advanced, complicated appendicitis in the operating room must balance the security of the appendiceal stump and the viability of adjacent inflamed cecum with the morbidity associated with the resection of additional large and small bowel so that viable margins can be obtained (72). Typically, this problem occurs when patients have presented for treatment late in the course of neglected disease or when nonoperative management has failed. Adequate debridement and drainage notwithstanding, the development of fecal fistula, intra-abdominal abscess, or both in these patients with severe advanced disease may be unavoidable or even anticipated complications. Some findings suggest that laparoscopic appendectomy may be associated with fewer postoperative complications (73).

Postoperative Complications: Infection

Wound infection and intra-abdominal infection are the most common types of morbidity after appendectomy. Gangrenous appendicitis and perforation appear to be important independent risk factors for the development of intra-abdominal abscess after appendectomy (74,75). Whether laparoscopic (rather than open) appendectomy increases the risk of intra-abdominal abscess is controversial (76,77).

Regardless of the method of appendectomy, wounds at high risk of becoming infected should be left open. Primary closure of dirty wounds has been associated with a substantially higher incidence of wound infection than delayed primary closure or a decision not to close abdominal wounds (78).

COMPLICATIONS OF COLORECTAL SURGERY
General Complications

With the availability of new antibiotics, meticulous preoperative preparation of the patient, and improvements in surgical techniques and postoperative critical care management, the safety of colorectal surgery has improved greatly over the past 50 years. The morbidity rates associated with elective colorectal surgery have decreased substantially (79). Age, obesity, diabetes, and cardiopulmonary disorders increase postoperative morbidity and mortality rates. Emergency colorectal surgery continues to be associated with considerable morbidity and mortality because of the nature of the disease and the limited time available for preoperative preparation.

Infection

Infection is the most common postoperative complication after colorectal surgery. Postoperative infection can range from a minor wound infection to septicemia, with shock and organ failure. The determining factors are age, associated disorders such as diabetes, and duration and degree of contamination (80). The incidence of postoperative sepsis can be minimized with good bowel preparation, proper use of antibiotics, meticulous surgical technique, and good judgment.

Wound infections are more common after emergency colorectal surgery than after elective procedures; an infection rate as high as 50% has been reported (81). As stated above, wounds at high risk of becoming infected should be left open, with the possibility of delayed primary closure as an option on postoperative days 4 through 6. If a wound that has been closed shows evidence of erythema, tenderness, or drainage, the wound should be opened and packed with saline-soaked gauze. There is controversy about the use of antiseptic solutions for infected wounds because in vivo animal studies have shown that these solutions are toxic to fibroblast cultures (82,83). If diffuse erythema surrounds the wound, treatment with a parenteral antibiotic effective against streptococci is justified. Necrotizing soft-tissue infections are uncommon but carry very high rates of morbidity and must be recognized and treated promptly. Possible symptoms are erythema,

edema, severe incisional pain, and crepitus. If a necrotizing soft-tissue infection is suspected, the incision must be promptly opened, subjected to surgical debridement, and treated with broad-spectrum parenteral antibiotics (84).

Mechanical bowel preparations, which are usually not possible before emergency colorectal surgery, decrease the fecal mass and may decrease the incidence of wound infections. Usually, there is no time to administer oral antibiotics before emergency colorectal procedures. However, multiple studies have demonstrated the effectiveness of oral antibiotics in reducing the risk of wound infections (85,86). Studies have failed to demonstrate the effectiveness of plastic wound drapes in preventing wound infections (87).

When patients demonstrate systemic signs of infection with no evidence of wound infection, an intra-abdominal infection should be suspected. CT of the abdominal and pelvic cavity has demonstrated the greatest sensitivity in detecting an intra-abdominal abscess; several authors report that its sensitivity exceeds 90% (88). Gallium- or indium-labeled white blood cell scans are less accurate, but may be useful (89).

CT-guided or, less commonly, ultrasound-guided percutaneous drainage is often used to drain postoperative abscesses. Clinical signs of sepsis should improve within 48 hours after drainage. If they do not, the CT scan should be repeated with possible manipulation or reinsertion of drains. If percutaneous drainage fails to fully drain the intra-abdominal abscess, surgical drainage of the abscess may be necessary (90). Percutaneous drainage of an abscess is less likely to be successful if the abscess is located between loops of bowel, is multilocular, is due to a fungal infection, contains a large solid component (such as an infected hematoma or a necrotic tumor), or is associated with a fistula (91). The presence of an intra-abdominal abscess also mandates the use of parenteral antibiotics. Multiple studies in the literature do not demonstrate any advantage for using several antibiotics rather than single broad-spectrum agents (92).

Anastomotic Leak

Postoperative intra-abdominal infection may be the result of an anastomotic leak. Colonic anastomoses pose a greater risk of leakage than small-intestinal anastomoses. Anastomoses below the peritoneal reflection carry a substantially higher risk of leakage (93). Other risk factors involved in the development of an anastomotic leak include local tissue ischemia, edema, tension, generalized ischemia (shock), sepsis, malnutrition, steroid therapy, previous irradiation, inflammatory bowel disease (94), inadequate bowel preparation, and obstruction distal to the anastomosis (95). When an anastomotic leak is suspected, an abdominal CT scan should be performed with intravenous, oral, and rectal contrast agents.

Management of an anastomotic leak depends on the degree and location of leakage and the patient's clinical condition. The main priority in management is control of the ongoing contamination. An asymptomatic leak demonstrated only on routine radiographic surveillance typically requires no surgical intervention. Patients with such leaks may be treated with broad-spectrum parenteral antibiotics and bowel rest. Patients with clinical evidence of anastomotic leak may demonstrate a spectrum of signs and symptoms ranging from mild "failure to thrive" to septic shock. Lack of clinical improvement after nonoperative management mandates surgery for obtaining adequate debridement, drainage, and diversion of the fecal stream. Nonoperative management should not be attempted when patients have diffuse peritonitis.

Colocutaneous Fistula

A colocutaneous fistula is usually the late manifestation of an unrecognized anastomotic leak or injury to the bowel. Colonic fistulas are more likely to have a low output than are small-bowel fistulas; they are also more likely to close without operative intervention. Fistulas are managed as described above.

Injuries to Adjacent Organs

Vital structures that can be injured during colorectal surgery include the spleen, ureters, bladder, kidneys, duodenum, gallbladder, pancreas, stomach, ovaries, and fallopian tubes, as well as the iliac and superior mesenteric vessels (96).

The reported incidence of operative ureteral injury varies from 1.5% to 12% (97). This injury is the most common intraoperative urological complication. The ureters are most vulnerable to injury at the pelvic brim and at the site of insertion into the bladder. When the ureters are injured, treatment depends on the severity of the injury and the site of injury along the course of the ureter. The different types of ureteral injury are devascularization, crush injury, transection, and avulsion. Intraoperatively, the diagnosis of ureteral injury can be made by intravenous injection of methylene blue dye or by intravenous pyelography. Postoperatively, the diagnosis is made by intravenous pyelography. The procedure of choice for injuries to the lower third of the ureter is ureteroneocystostomy. The preferred technique for injuries to the mid-ureter is ureteroureterostomy. Injuries to the proximal third of the ureter are the most challenging and sometimes require replacement with ileum. If ureteral injury is undetected, uncontrolled urinary leakage may lead to the development of sepsis, cutaneous urinary fistula, or both, as well as to metabolic derangements associated with resorption of urine in the peritoneal cavity.

The incidence of bladder injuries is less than 5% (98). Intraoperatively recognized injuries may be closed primarily and drained with a Foley catheter. If injuries are not detected immediately, they may result in substantial morbidity and enterovesical fistula or persistent perineal drainage, as well as in the same metabolic derangements that are associated with ureteral injury.

Injury to the spleen most commonly occurs during left hemicolectomy or subtotal colectomy (99). Traction on the peritoneum and omentum, typically during resection or dissection of the splenic flexure, leads to avulsion of a portion of the splenic capsule. Adequate visualization is crucial to preventing this complication. The proximal descending colon and the distal transverse colon should be mobilized concomitantly so that excessive traction on the omentum and the splenocolic ligament can be avoided. Injured vessels in the splenocolic ligament and the splenic hilum are managed by clamping and ligatures. Direct pressure and the application of Avitene® (Davol, Cranston, Rhode Island, U.S.A.), Surgicell® (Johnson & Johnson, New Brunswick, New Jersey, U.S.A.), or fibrin glue can be used to treat capsular tears. Occasionally, splenorrhaphy or even splenectomy may be necessary.

Complications of Stomas

The overall incidence of stoma construction is decreasing (100). However, the creation of stomas is still required during many operations for inflammatory bowel disease, colorectal tumors, trauma, and diverticulitis. When a stoma is required, every effort should be made to create a stoma that functions well and interferes only minimally with the patient's lifestyle. The creation of a stoma should not be regarded as a minor surgical procedure. Complications are relatively frequent; emergency stoma formation seems to be associated with the highest complication rates (101–103). Elderly patients experience more complications, and obese patients are at a higher risk of early complications (104). Improper positioning of the stoma also affects the incidence of complications. Many complications are preventable with careful surgical technique. Ideally, the location of the stoma should be chosen and marked preoperatively. When a complication does arise, it should be recognized promptly and dealt with appropriately. Stoma complications are classified by stoma type and the time of occurrence (105).

Ileostomy

Various types of ileostomies can be constructed. As the number of sphincter-preserving procedures increases, the number of permanent ileostomies will continue to decrease and the number of protective loop ileostomies will increase. Before the 1950s, ileostomy dysfunction was common as the result of serositis, which led to partial SBO. It was not until the technique of Brooke and Turnbull was popularized that the problem of ileostomy dysfunction was resolved. Ileostomies have been associated with the highest morbidity rates of any type of stoma; loop ileostomies are associated with the largest number of complications (106–108). The output of ileostomies can exceed 1000 mL in a 24-hour period; this large output may lead to severe dehydration and sodium loss, which will require fluid replacement and correction of electrolyte imbalance. Chronic dehydration and acidic urine can lead to the formation of uric acid renal calculi. The ileostomy effluent is also rich in proteolytic enzymes that cause skin irritation.

Skin Problems

Skin problems are the most common early and late complications after the creation of the stoma (109). These problems usually result from poor adherence of the appliance and exposure of the skin to the stoma effluent. Predisposing conditions are an improperly placed stoma, inadequate care of a stoma, and allergy to adhesive materials. This most common complication of an ileostomy is also the most preventable. Proper stoma placement and maintenance can usually eliminate this complication.

Necrosis

Necrosis is most frequently a result of devascularization of the ileum during stoma placement (110). It can also result from a small, inadequate abdominal wall opening. Necrosis above the fascia can usually be treated conservatively with bowel rest and total parenteral nutrition until the stoma can be revised. Necrosis below the fascia usually requires exploratory laparotomy, resection of nonviable bowel, and revision of the ileostomy.

Retraction

Retraction occurs in as many as 15% of cases (111). Predisposing factors are tension on the stoma, ischemia, obesity, and improper placement of the stoma. Retraction may require surgical intervention because it is often associated with severe excoriation of the skin.

Obstruction

Obstruction within six months after construction of a stoma is usually caused by impacted enteric contents. This condition is usually managed by gentle irrigation of the stoma or by injection of Hypaque® material into the stoma. Obstruction for more than six months after construction of a stoma is usually caused by adhesions or stenosis, which can be due to recurrent inflammatory bowel disease. In these situations, a Hypaque study can bring relief. If this procedure is unsuccessful, stenoses are best treated with local revision or repositioning of the stoma.

Stenosis

Stenosis of ileostomies is usually caused by inflammatory bowel disease (112), ischemic necrosis, or exposure of ileal serosa to fecal irritants. This complication usually causes a partial SBO. Management of this problem consists of decompression with a nasogastric tube and local revision or relocation of the stoma. Usually the problem can be prevented by adequate preservation of the mesentery, preferably to within 2 cm of the bowel end, and by eliminating serosal exposure by turning 2 cm of ileum back onto itself.

Prolapse and Parastomal Hernia

Ileostomy prolapse is an uncommon complication, which is usually associated with a parastomal hernia. Predisposing factors are obesity and placement of the stoma outside the rectus sheath. This complication can be prevented by placing the stoma in the rectus sheath, by fixing the distal ileum to the lateral abdominal wall, or by suspending the ileum mesentery from the abdominal wall along the cut edge of the mesentery. Fixation of the distal ileum can be accomplished either by tunneling the ileum beneath the peritoneum or by suturing the ileum to the abdominal wall with interrupted sutures. Repair of the prolapse usually involves repair of the associated parastomal hernia. Initially, local revision may be attempted, although it is rarely successful over the long term. Repair consists of prolapse reduction, repair of the abdominal wall hernia, and revision of the stoma in a different location on the abdominal wall (113).

Parastomal hernias are more common after colostomies and are quite rare after ileostomies (114). Predisposing factors are previous repair, obesity, and chronic obstructive pulmonary disease. Local repair of the fascia is rarely successful (115). The ultimate management is the relocation of the stoma. When relocation is not possible, repair of the fascia with Marlex® (Bard, Cranston, Rhode Island, U.S.A.) mesh may be necessary.

Colostomy

Colostomy is typically not associated with the physiologic changes associated with ileostomy.

Skin Problems

Skin irritation is less common around a colostomy than around an ileostomy. Stool from a right-sided or transverse colostomy can cause local skin irritation. A predisposing factor may be malpositioning of the stoma, which may require relocation. Skin irritation is rarely due to fungal or bacterial skin infection.

Ischemia and Necrosis

The incidence of colostomy necrosis ranges from 2% to 17% (101,116). Factors predisposing patients to this complication are devascularization of the bowel, obesity, and a tight opening in the abdominal wall. Other contributing factors are shock and arteriosclerosis. If the necrosis is above the fascia, conservative management is justified, but may lead to long-term stenosis of the colostomy. Necrosis below the fascia necessitates laparotomy, resection of necrotic colon, and revision of the colostomy.

Retraction

The incidence of retraction ranges from 1.5% to 10% (101,116). The main predisposing factor for retraction is tension. When the stoma separates and releases into the peritoneum, immediate wound exploration with stoma revision is required. If this procedure is unsuccessful, laparotomy and further mobilization of colon are necessary for preventing fecal spillage and development of late stoma stenosis.

Obstruction

Obstruction early after surgery is rare and usually results from a parastomal hernia or stenosis at the skin level. Fecal impaction can usually be managed with injection of water-soluble contrast material into the stoma; this material acts as a laxative.

Prolapse

The incidence of colostomy prolapse is 2% to 5% (101,116). Occurring early in the postoperative period, prolapse is usually due to improper construction and is usually associated with a parastomal hernia. It is most commonly associated with a transverse loop colostomy. The treatment of this problem is usually not urgent; it requires excision of the redundant segment and lateral fixation of the colon. Recurrence of the prolapse is common. The best treatment, however, remains the reversal of the colostomy. If the prolapse recurs, relocating the stoma or colectomy may be necessary.

Stenosis and Stricture

The incidence of stenosis and stricture is 2% to 9% (101,116); this complication is usually due to early ischemia or separation at the skin. This complication can usually be prevented by suturing the full thickness of the colon to skin at the time of initial surgery. For urgent relief, the stoma can be dilated, although this procedure often leads to recurrent contraction. In most cases, local excision is successful.

Parastomal Hernia

Parastomal hernia is the most common complication after colostomy placement. The incidence of this complication ranges from 1% to 58% (101,116). Parastomal hernia most commonly occurs within the first two years after surgery. The risk factors for this complication are obesity, chronic obstructive pulmonary disease, and the existence of other hernias. There is controversy about the effect of the stoma site on hernia development. Parastomal hernia causes pain, inability to maintain an ostomy appliance, intestinal obstruction, and incarceration. Surgical repair of a parastomal hernia often yields disappointing results

and should be considered only if the patient's symptoms are bothersome. It is acceptable to attempt local repair with or without mesh. If local repair is unsuccessful, the stoma should be relocated.

Complications of Specific Procedures
Abdominoperineal Resection

Today, with our ability to perform low anastomoses and coloanal procedures, abdominoperineal resection (APR) is typically reserved only for rectal carcinomas involving the pelvic floor or the upper anal canal and for anal cancers that do not respond to chemoradiation therapy. APR is associated with a morbidity rate as high as 59%; the highest morbidity rates occur among patients who have undergone irradiation (117–120). The most common complications are urinary retention and impotence. Although the morbidity rates associated with this procedure can be quite high, most of the complications are treatable and resolve without serious sequelae. Intraoperatively, the two primary complications are ureteral injury and presacral hemorrhage. The incidence of ureteral injury during APR ranges from 0.3% to 6% (121). The diagnosis, treatment, and prevention of this complication have been discussed in the section "General Complications." The incidence of bladder injury during APR ranges from 0% to 5% (121). Most of these injuries respond to prolonged bladder drainage; surgical repair is rarely necessary. Urethral injuries occur in 0.7% to 6.7% of cases (121) and direct repair is recommended (27).

During APR, bleeding may occur at a number of sites, including the pelvic sidewalls, the iliac veins, and the middle sacral artery. Presacral hemorrhage can sometimes not be prevented and can be difficult to control. Methods of control are packing, suture ligation, cautery, and clips. A bleeding basivertebral vein can be controlled with sterile thumbtacks (122).

Other possible intraoperative complications include extremity compartment syndromes and peripheral neuropathies (123). The mechanism of injury is compression, which leads to local ischemia. Contributing factors are the stirrups, poor positioning of retractors, long operative time, and leaning on the patient's legs. The nerves at risk of positioning injuries are the sciatic, femoral, tibial, common peroneal, sural, obturator, genitofemoral, and lateral cutaneous nerves. Prevention of injury consists of careful positioning, with adequate padding and avoidance of long operative times.

Common postoperative complications after APR involve perineal wound complications and bladder and sexual dysfunction resulting from nerve injury. Perineal wound complications consist of hemorrhage, abscess, and formation of perineal sinus and perineal hernia. Several methods of perineal wound closure have been described, including partial closure, primary closure, and closure with continuous irrigation and omental plugging. In 1908, when Miles originally described this procedure, he recommended open packing of the perineal wound (124). The incidence of perineal hemorrhage is higher when open packing is used and ranges from 0% to 4% (125). Usually, packing the wound for 48 to 72 hours leads to cessation of bleeding.

Perineal abscess is almost always associated with primary closure of the perineal wound. The incidence of abscess ranges from 11% to 16% (126). The main risk factor is fecal contamination. Rectal injury during dissection is another factor predictive of abscess (127). Superficial subcutaneous abscesses are managed by opening the wound and performing local wound care. Deeper perineal or presacral abscesses may require percutaneous drainage. A perineal wound that has not healed within six months is called a perineal sinus. This complication is quite common, with an incidence ranging from 14% to 40%, especially among patients with inflammatory bowel disease (128). Risk factors for perineal sinus are inflammatory bowel disease, radiation therapy, and fecal contamination. Curettage and primary closure can be performed. However, large and persistent perineal sinuses usually require debridement and a gracilis or gluteus myocutaneous flap.

Perineal hernias are uncommon. Evisceration requires immediate surgery with reduction and packing. Symptoms of a perineal hernia are a perineal bulge, pain, and, possibly, voiding problems. Indications for surgery are discomfort refractory to conservative management, impending skin loss, and bowel obstruction. Various techniques have been proposed in order to repair these perineal hernias, such as primary repair, with or without transperitoneal prosthetic material, and tensor fascia lata grafts (129).

Urinary retention, urinary tract infection, and sexual dysfunction are common complications after APR. They are more common among male patients, especially if the procedure is performed for cancer rather than for inflammatory bowel disease. Voiding problems after APR are due to malalignment of the bladder, neurologic injury, or aggravation of a preexisting outlet obstruction. Sympathetic denervation can lead to urgency or incontinence, and parasympathetic denervation results in decreased bladder emptying and high postvoid residuals. Goldman et al. have recommended the prophylactic use of alpha-adrenergic blockers before surgery for preventing postoperative urinary retention and infection (130).

Sexual dysfunction is common and has been reported to occur with a frequency of 33% to 75% in these patients (131,132). Sympathetic injury results in ejaculatory difficulty, and parasympathetic injury leads to erectile difficulty. The incidence of sexual dysfunction increases with patient age and is higher after resections for cancer than after resections for inflammatory bowel disease. These injuries can be temporary or permanent, and partial or complete.

Restorative Proctocolectomy with Ileal Pouch Anal Anastomosis

Restorative proctocolectomy with ileal pouch anal anastomosis (IPAA) has become an established procedure for patients with ulcerative colitis and familial adenomatous polyposis. The overall mortality rate is approximately 1%; however, the morbidity rate is substantial and may be as high as 62.7% (133,134). Despite this high complication rate, functional results are good and patient satisfaction is high (135,136). Early complications are vascular compromise, bleeding, sepsis, and SBO. Vascular compromise may lead to anastomotic leak, sepsis, or stricture formation. Patients undergoing this procedure may be taking steroids, may be immunocompromised, and may have inflammatory bowel changes, which make the tissues especially fragile and make bleeding very likely. Therefore, extra caution is necessary if hemorrhage is to be prevented. Bleeding at the suture or staple line rarely requires surgical intervention.

The incidence of pelvic sepsis in association with IPAA ranges from 5% to 15% (137). This complication usually results from leakage at the suture line or, less commonly, from fecal contamination. The diagnosis is usually made by abdominal CT scanning. Some abscesses may be amenable to percutaneous drainage. If conservative management with parenteral antibiotics does not lead to improvement, then laparotomy is indicated. Pelvic sepsis is also possible after ileostomy closure. Therefore, a pouchogram is necessary for detecting leaks or fistulas before the stoma is closed. If pelvic sepsis does occur after ileostomy closure, then reestablishment of fecal diversion is necessary. Pelvic sepsis can lead to pelvic fibrosis and decreased pouch compliance; it can also affect the anal sphincter mechanism and result in incontinence. The incidence of this complication has been decreasing as surgeons gain more experience with IPAA. The incidence of SBO after this procedure ranges from 7% to 30% (138). This relatively high incidence is partially due to the fact that two procedures are being performed and a temporary diverting ileostomy is being created. Fewer than 50% of patients who experience SBO require laparotomy. Initial nonoperative management is justified.

Fistula and stricture formation and pouchitis are the most common late complications of an IPAA. The incidence of fistula formation ranges from 2% to 16% (139). These fistulas can arise at various locations. Predisposing factors include ischemia with anastomotic breakdown, entrapment of adjacent organs, and postoperative sepsis. In these situations, Crohn's disease must be ruled out. The most common type of fistula is the pouch vaginal fistula. The technique of repair depends on the site and complexity of the fistula. Pouch excision is rarely required.

Anastomotic strictures are the most common anastomotic complication after IPAA, with an incidence ranging from 5% to 20% (140). Strictures may develop as a result of disuse during fecal diversion. Whether surgical technique (handsewn anastomoses rather than stapled anastomoses) plays a role in stricture formation is debatable. Stricture formation is often due to tension or ischemia at the site of the anastomosis. The presence of an abscess also contributes to stricture development. Treatment consists of anal dilatation and, rarely, pouch revision or permanent fecal diversion.

Pouchitis is the most common late complication of IPAA; the incidence ranges from 10% to 30% (141). Pouchitis causes cramps, diarrhea, urgency, incontinence, malaise, and fever. Pouchitis is more common among patients with ulcerative colitis than among those with familial adenomatous polyposis. Oxygen free radicals, stasis, and bacterial overgrowth may play a role in the development of pouchitis (142). Patients with pouchitis must undergo anal examination so that a stricture leading to stasis can be ruled out. Usually, pouchitis responds well to a five- to seven-day course of metronidazole. If this treatment is ineffective, then treatment with ciprofloxacin should be attempted. In very rare cases of recurrence and persistent pouchitis, treatment with diversion, pouch excision, or both will be necessary.

COMPLICATIONS OF ANAL SURGERY

The most common postoperative complications of anal surgery are urinary retention, pain, infection, and bleeding. Urinary retention can occur in as many as 30% of cases. The cause is neural because the anal sphincter and the urethral sphincter share the same innervation. Risk factors for this complication are pain, anxiety, male sex, and the use of spinal anesthesia. The appropriate treatment for this problem is intermittent sterile catheterization. Preventive measures include adequate pain control and limitation of intravenous fluids to less than 250 mL perioperatively (143). Persistent pain after surgery is usually due to inadequate analgesia; however, persistent pain may be associated with infection or fecal impaction. Appropriate use of analgesics, local injection of long-acting anesthetic agents, and prevention of constipation are necessary for avoiding this complication. Infectious complications after anal surgery are rare because there is a good local blood supply and drainage is usually spontaneous. Symptoms of local infection are fever, persistent pain, and difficulty in urinating. A thorough examination should be performed, and broad-spectrum parenteral antibiotics and debridement should be used when perianal infection is present. Patients should be forewarned and reassured that a small amount of bleeding during the postoperative period is quite common and is usually of no consequence. However, massive bleeding is typically caused by a technical error and requires prompt surgical repair.

Complications of Anorectal Abscesses and Fistulas

An understanding of the anatomy of the anal canal is particularly important for diagnosing and properly managing anal abscesses and fistulas. In more than 95% of cases, anorectal infection arises in the anal glands to form an intersphincteric abscess between the internal and external sphincters. The abscess can then extend in either direction, and the direction of extension determines the anatomical classification of the abscess. The chronic stage is recognized as an anal fistula. The management of an abscess consists of incision and drainage; catheter drainage may be necessary. Therapeutic options for fistulas are fistulotomy, fistulectomy, advancement flaps, and placement of a seton. In addition to the possible general complications discussed above, the main complications of these procedures are incontinence and recurrence.

Incontinence is usually due to iatrogenic damage of the sphincter or to inappropriate wound care, especially if continence was borderline preoperatively. Prolonged wound packing can lead to the formation of excess scar tissue and to incontinence. After fistulotomy, continence disorders have been reported in as many as 52% of cases (144). Risk factors for this complication are age, anterior fistulas, complicated fistulas with high internal openings, and Crohn's disease. Fistulotomy should be avoided at the time of abscess drainage because it increases the risk of incontinence. Fistulectomy is associated with an unacceptably high risk of incontinence and is therefore not the procedure of choice. In contrast, rectal advancement flaps have demonstrated excellent results with an incidence of continence problems of only approximately 6% to 7% (145). Setons are extremely useful in treating high anterior fistulas for which a fistulotomy would lead to frank incontinence. The incontinence rate associated with the seton procedure has been reported to be 6.7% (146).

Recurrence of anal sepsis may be caused by incomplete drainage of an abscess because of a small, inadequate incision or because a fistula is missed. Intersphincteric and ischiorectal abscesses are associated with a recurrence rate as high as 89% in certain cases (147). During abscess drainage, one must be diligent to not overlook an associated fistula. If a fistula is detected during abscess drainage, fistulotomy should be reserved for a second elective procedure because it is associated with a high rate of incontinence if it is performed simultaneously with abscess drainage. Recurrent fistulas are rare if treated appropriately; in such cases, cancer, Crohn's disease, and tuberculosis should be ruled out.

Complications of Hemorrhoidectomy

The general complications of anal surgery discussed earlier also apply to hemorrhoidectomy. Possible late complications of hemorrhoidectomy are fecal incontinence and anal stenosis (148). Incontinence is due to damage to the internal anal sphincter. This injury can be prevented by lifting the hemorrhoid tissue off the sphincter and then excising it. Repairing a damaged internal sphincter may be very difficult. Treatment includes slowing and bulking agents and, possibly, biofeedback therapy.

Anal stenosis is usually due to excessive removal of anal mucosa. It can usually be managed with anal dilatation. Rarely, surgery with the use of skin flaps may be required. The most common of these is the Y-V advancement flap. Prolapsed thrombosed hemorrhoids may require emergency surgery that can result in anal stenosis. However, there is no statistically significant difference in the incidence of complications in association with elective or emergency hemorrhoidal surgery (149).

COMPLICATIONS OF COLORECTAL TRAUMA

Colorectal trauma is typically categorized as blunt or penetrating. Iatrogenic injury may also be considered a type of colon injury (150). Blunt trauma accounts for only 4% of colorectal trauma; motor vehicle accidents are the most common cause. Anorectal injuries are rarely associated with blunt trauma; when they are present, they are usually associated with pelvic fractures.

Most colorectal injuries are due to penetrating trauma. Penetrating injuries to the colon and rectum are usually due to projectile injury. Projectiles can cause injury by direct penetration, blast effect, or secondary penetration from fragmented bone. Other common causes of penetrating colorectal trauma are stab wounds, impalements, and falls onto a penetrating object.

Injuries to the rectum should be ruled out during the initial assessment of trauma because they may not be apparent during exploratory laparotomy. The detection of gross blood by digital rectal examination may indicate injury to the colon or rectum.

The treatment of colonic injuries continues to be controversial. In general, primary closure is the procedure of choice if it is feasible. Relative contraindications to primary repair include more than eight hours of delay between the injury and the repair, shock, multiple organ system injuries, significant colonic damage or contamination, and multiple colonic injuries. Other management options are exteriorization, repair with proximal diversion, and resection with or without anastomosis (151). Currently, exteriorization is seldom used because it is associated with a risk of leakage or obstruction as high as 50%. Rectal injuries may be difficult to diagnose. Intraperitoneal rectal injuries must be repaired. Extraperitoneal injuries, if they are extensive, may require proximal diversion and presacral drainage. The need for presacral drainage, especially for low-velocity injuries, is debatable (152).

For all types of injuries, debridement of nonviable tissues and removal of gross contamination are crucial. The perioperative use of systemic antibiotics provides an important adjunct to therapy. In the presence of significant contamination, skin should be left open because the incidence of wound infection is 29–65% (153).

The most common cause of death among patients with colorectal injuries is exsanguination; the second most common cause is sepsis. In general, the postoperative complications associated with surgery for treating colorectal trauma are similar to those associated with other types of colorectal surgery: anastomotic leakage, infection, abscess, fistulas, and stoma complications. Intra-abdominal abscess is the most frequent septic complication, with an incidence of 5% to 15%. If not recognized promptly and managed appropriately, colorectal injury is associated with substantial morbidity. A systematic approach is necessary for reducing the incidence of complications. Priorities for the management of colorectal trauma are cessation of exsanguinating hemorrhage, followed by removal of ongoing contamination and nonviable tissues, and, finally, reconstruction.

REFERENCES

1. Kehlet H, Holte K. Review of postoperative ileus. Am J Surg 2001; 182:3S–10S.
2. Holte K, Kehlet H. Postoperative ileus: a preventable event. Br J Surg 2000; 87:1480–1493.
3. Yoshida S, Ohta J, Yamasaki K, et al. Effect of surgical stress on endogenous morphine and cytokine levels in the plasma after laparoscopic or open cholecystectomy. Surg Endosc 2000; 14:137–140.
4. Kaufman PN, Krevsky B, Malmud LS, et al. Role of opiate receptors in the regulation of colonic transit. Gastroenterology 1988; 94:1351–1356.
5. Manara L, Bianchetti A. The central and peripheral influence of opioids on gastrointestinal propulsion. Annu Rev Pharmacol Toxicol 1985; 25:249–273.
6. Waldhausen JH, Schirmer BD. The effect of ambulation on recovery from postoperative ileus. Ann Surg 1990; 212:671–677.
7. Jepsen S, Klaerke A, Nielsen PH, Simonsen O. Negative effect of metoclopramide in postoperative adynamic ileus. A prospective, randomized, double blind study. Br J Surg 1986; 73:290–291.
8. Brown TA, McDonald J, Williard W. A prospective, randomized, double-blinded, placebo-controlled trial of cisapride after colorectal surgery. Am J Surg 1999; 177:399–401.
9. Tollesson PO, Cassuto J, Rimback G, Faxen A, Bergman L, Mattsson E. Treatment of postoperative paralytic ileus with cisapride. Scand J Gastroenterol 1991; 26:477–482.
10. Bonacini M, Quiason S, Reynolds M, Gaddis M, Pemberton B, Smith O. Effect of intravenous erythromycin on postoperative ileus. Am J Gastroenterol 1993; 88:208–211.
11. Cutillo G, Maneschi F, Franchi M, Giannice R, Scanbia G, Benedetti-Panici P. Early feeding compared with nasogastric decompression after major oncologic gynecologic surgery: a randomized study. Obstet Gynecol 1999; 93:41–45.

12. Reissman P, Teoh TA, Cohen SM, Weiss EG, Nogueras JJ, Wexner SD. Is early oral feeding safe after elective colorectal surgery? A prospective randomized trial. Ann Surg 1995; 222:73–77.

13. Neudecker J, Schwenk W, Junghans T, Pietsch S, Bohm B, Muller JM. Randomized controlled trial to examine the influence of thoracic epidural analgesia on postoperative ileus after laparoscopic sigmoid resection. Br J Surg 1999; 86:1292–1295.

14. Liu SS, Carpenter RL, Mackey DC, et al. Effects of perioperative analgesic technique on rate of recovery after colon surgery. Anesthesiology 1995; 83:757–765.

15. Schwenk W, Bohm B, Haase O, Junghans T, Muller JM. Laparoscopic versus conventional colorectal resection: a prospective randomised study of postoperative ileus and early postoperative feeding. Langenbecks Arch Surg 1998; 383:49–55.

16. Lacy AM, Garcia-Valdecasas JC, Pique JM, et al. Short-term outcome analysis of a randomized study comparing laparoscopic vs open colectomy for colon cancer. Surg Endosc 1995; 9:1101–1105.

17. Liu SS, Hodgson PS, Carpenter RL, Fricke JR Jr. ADL 8–2698, a trans-3,4-dimethyl-4-(3-hydroxyphenyl) piperidine, prevents gastrointestinal effects of intravenous morphine without affecting analgesia. Clin Pharmacol Ther 2001; 69:66–71.

18. Schmidt WK. Alvimopan (ADL 8–2698) is a novel peripheral opioid antagonist. Am J Surg 2001; 182 (suppl 5A):27S–38S.

19. Kalff JC, Schraut WH, Simmons RL, Bauer AJ. Surgical manipulation of the gut elicits an intestinal muscularis inflammatory response resulting in postsurgical ileus. Ann Surg 1998; 228:652–663.

20. Stewart RM, Page CP, Brender J, Schwesinger W, Eisenhut D. The incidence and risk of early postoperative small bowel obstruction. A cohort study. Am J Surg 1987; 154:643–647.

21. Luijendijk RW, de Lange DC, Wauters CC, et al. Foreign material in postoperative adhesions. Ann Surg 1996; 223:242–248.

22. Risberg B. Adhesions: preventive strategies. Eur J Surg Suppl 1997(577):32–39.

23. Rodgers K, Girgis W, diZerega GS, Johns D. Intraperitoneal tolmetin prevents postsurgical adhesion formation in rabbits. Int J Fertil 1990; 35:40–45.

24. Steinleitner A, Lambert H, Montoro L, Kelly E, Swanson J, Sueldo C. The use of calcium channel blockade for the prevention of postoperative adhesion formation. Fertil Steril 1988; 50:818–821.

25. Avsar FM, Sahin M, Aksoy F, et al. Effects of diphenhydramine HCl and methylprednisolone in the prevention of abdominal adhesions. Am J Surg 2001; 181(6):512–515.

26. Larsson B, Lalos O, Marsk L, et al. Effect of intraperitoneal instillation of 32% dextran 70 on postoperative adhesion formation after tubal surgery. Acta Obstet Gynecol Scand 1985; 64:437–441.

27. Jansen RP. Failure of peritoneal irrigation with heparin during pelvic operations upon young women to reduce adhesions. Surg Gynecol Obstet 1988; 166:154–160.

28. Vipond MN, Whawell SA, Scott-Coombes DM, Thompson JN, Dudley HA. Experimental adhesion prophylaxis with recombinant tissue plasminogen activator. Ann R Coll Surg Engl 1994; 76(6):412–415.

29. The efficacy of Interceed(TC7) for prevention of reformation of postoperative adhesions on ovaries, fallopian tubes, and fimbriae in microsurgical operations for fertility: a multicenter trial. Nordic Adhesion Prevention Study Group. Fertil Steril 1995; 63:709–714.

30. Becker JM, Dayton MT, Fazio VW, et al. Prevention of postoperative abdominal adhesions by a sodium hyaluronate-based bioresorbable membrane: a prospective, randomized, double-blind, multicenter study. J Am Coll Surg 1996; 183:296–306.

31. Johns DB, Keyport GM, Hoehler F, diZerega GS; Intergel Adhesion Prevention Study Group. Reduction of postsurgical adhesions with Intergel adhesion prevention solution: a multicenter study of safety and efficacy after conservative gynecologic surgery. Fertil Steril 2001; 76(3):595–604.

32. Van Der Krabben AA, Dijkstra FR, Nieuwenhuijzen M, Reijnen MM, Schaapveld M, Van Goor H. Morbidity and mortality of inadvertent enterotomy during adhesiotomy. Br J Surg 2000; 87(4):467–471.

33. Platell CF, Coster J, McCauley RD, Hall JC. The management of patients with the short bowel syndrome. World J Gastroenterol 2002; 8(1):13–20.

34. Figueroa-Colon R, Harris PR, Birdsong E, Franklin FA, Georgeson KE. Impact of intestinal lengthening on the nutritional outcome for children with short bowel syndrome. J Pediatr Surg 1996; 31(7):912–916.

35. Thompson JS, Langnas AN, Pinch LW, Kaufman S, Quigley EM, Vanderhoof JA. Surgical approach to short-bowel syndrome. Experience in a population of 160 patients. Ann Surg 1995; 222(4):600–607.

36. Kaufman SS. Small bowel transplantation: selection criteria, operative techniques, advances in specific immunosuppression, prognosis. Curr Opin Pediatr 2001; 13(5):425–428.

37. Bondar VM, Rago C, Cottone FJ, Wilkerson DK, Riggs J. Chlorhexidine lavage in the treatment of experimental intra-abdominal infection. Arch Surg 2000; 135:309–314.

38. Schein M, Gecelter G, Freinkel W, Geerding H, Becker PJ. Peritoneal lavage in abdominal sepsis. A controlled clinical study. Arch Surg 1990; 125: 1132–1135.

39. Schein M, Saadia R, Decker G. Intraoperative peritoneal lavage. Surg Gynecol Obstet 1988; 166:187–195.

40. Reiling RB, Reiling WA Jr., Bernie WA, Huffer AB, Perkins NC, Elliott DW. Prospective controlled study of gastrointestinal stapled anastomoses. Am J Surg 1980; 139:147–152.

41. Lowdon IM, Gear MW, Kilby JO. Stapling instruments in upper gastrointestinal surgery: a retrospective study of 362 cases. Br J Surg 1982; 69:333–335.

42. Suturing or stapling in gastrointestinal surgery: a prospective randomized study. West of Scotland and Highland Anastomosis Study Group. Br J Surg 1991; 78:337–341.

43. MacRae HM, McLeod RS. Handsewn vs. stapled anastomoses in colon and rectal surgery: a meta-analysis. Dis Colon Rectum 1998; 41:180–189.

44. Bruce J, Krukowski ZH, Al-Khairy G, Russell EM, Park KG. Systematic review of the definition and measurement of anastomotic leak after gastrointestinal surgery. Br J Surg 2001; 88(9):1157–1168.

45. Jex RK, van Heerden JA, Wolff BG, Ready RL, Ilstrup DM. Gastrointestinal anastomoses. Factors

affecting early complications. Ann Surg 1987; 206: 138–141.

46. Golub R, Golub RW, Cantu R Jr., Stein HD. A multivariate analysis of factors contributing to leakage of intestinal anastomoses. J Am Coll Surg 1997; 184(4): 364–372.

47. Rose D, Yarborough MF, Canizaro PC, Lowry SF. One hundred and fourteen fistulas of the gastrointestinal tract treated with total parenteral nutrition. Surg Gynecol Obstet 1986; 163:345–350.

48. Spiliotis J, Briand D, Gouttebel MC, et al. Treatment of fistulas of the gastrointestinal tract with total parenteral nutrition and octreotide in patients with carcinoma. Surg Gynecol Obstet 1993; 176:575–580.

49. Dorta G. Role of octreotide and somatostatin in the treatment of intestinal fistulae. Digestion 1999; 60 (suppl 2):53–56.

50. Rubelowsky J, Machiedo GW. Reoperative versus conservative management for gastrointestinal fistulas. Surg Clin North Am 1991; 71:147–157.

51. Borison DI, Bloom AD, Pritchard TJ. Treatment of enterocutaneous and colocutaneous fistulas with early surgery or somatostatin analog. Dis Colon Rectum 1992; 35:635–639.

52. Isaacs PE, Kim YS. Blind loop syndrome and small bowel bacterial contamination. Clin Gastroenterol 1983; 12(2):395–414.

53. Stevens SL, Maull KI. Small bowel injuries. Surg Clin North Am 1990; 70(3):541–560.

54. Brundage SI, Jurkovich GJ, Hoyt DB, et al. WTA Multi-institutional Study Group. Western Trauma Association. Stapled versus sutured gastrointestinal anastomoses in the trauma patient: a multicenter trial. J Trauma 2001; 51(6):1054–1061.

55. Jaffin JH, Ochsner MG, Cole FJ, Rozycki GS, Kass M, Champion HR. Alkaline phosphatase levels in diagnostic peritoneal lavage fluid as a predictor of hollow visceral injury. J Trauma 1993; 34(6):829–833.

56. Otomo Y, Henmi H, Mashiko K, et al. New diagnostic peritoneal lavage criteria for diagnosis of intestinal injury. J Trauma 1998; 44(6):991–997.

57. Fang JF, Chen RJ, Lin BC. Cell count ratio: new criterion of diagnostic peritoneal lavage for detection of hollow organ perforation. J Trauma 1998; 45(3): 540–544.

58. Velanovich V, Satava R. Balancing the normal appendectomy rate with the perforated appendicitis rate: implications for quality assurance. Am Surg 1992; 58:264–269.

59. Hale DA, Molloy M, Pearl RH, Schutt DC, Jaques DP. Appendectomy: a contemporary appraisal. Ann Surg 1997; 225(3):252–261.

60. Bergeron E, Richer B, Gharib R, Giard A. Appendicitis is a place for clinical judgement. Am J Surg 1999; 177:460–462.

61. Styrud J, Eriksson S, Segelman J, Granstrom L. Diagnostic accuracy in 2,351 patients undergoing appendicectomy for suspected acute appendicitis: a retrospective study 1986–1993. Dig Surg 1999; 16:39–44.

62. Rao PM, Rhea JT, Novelline RA, Mostafavi AA, McCabe CJ. Effect of computed tomography of the appendix on treatment of patients and use of hospital resources. N Engl J Med 1998; 338:141–146.

63. Balthazar EJ, Rofsky NM, Zucker R. Appendicitis: the impact of computed tomography imaging on negative appendectomy and perforation rates. Am J Gastroenterol 1998; 93:768–771.

64. Rypins EB, Evans DG, Hinrichs W, Kipper SL. Tc-99m-HMPAO white blood cell scan for diagnosis of acute appendicitis in patients with equivocal clinical presentation. Ann Surg 1997; 226(1):58–65.

65. Weyant MJ, Eachempati SR, Maluccio MA, et al. Interpretation of computed tomography does not correlate with laboratory or pathologic findings in surgically confirmed acute appendicitis. Surgery 2000; 128:145–152.

66. Pittman-Waller VA, Myers JG, Stewart RM, et al. Appendicitis: why so complicated? Analysis of 5755 consecutive appendectomies. Am Surg 2000; 66(6): 548–554.

67. Friedell ML, Perez-Izquierdo M. Is there a role for interval appendectomy in the management of acute appendicitis? Am Surg 2000; 66(12):1158–1162.

68. Vargas HI, Averbook A, Stamos MJ. Appendiceal mass: conservative therapy followed by interval laparoscopic appendectomy. Am Surg 1994; 60(10): 753–758.

69. Oliak D, Yamini D, Udani VM, et al. Nonoperative management of perforated appendicitis without periappendiceal mass. Am J Surg 2000; 179(3):177–181.

70. Ein SH, Shandling B. Is interval appendectomy necessary after rupture of an appendiceal mass? J Pediatr Surg 1996; 31(6):849–850.

71. Eriksson S, Granstrom L. Randomized controlled trial of appendicectomy versus antibiotic therapy for acute appendicitis. Br J Surg 1995; 82(2):166–169.

72. Lane JS, Schmit PJ, Chandler CF, Bennion RS, Thompson JE Jr. Ileocecectomy is definitive treatment for advanced appendicitis. Am Surg 2001; 67(12):1117–1122.

73. Wullstein C, Barkhausen S, Gross E. Results of laparoscopic vs. conventional appendectomy in complicated appendicitis. Dis Colon Rectum 2001; 44(11): 1700–1705.

74. Andersen BR, Kallehave FL, Andersen HK. Antibiotics versus placebo for prevention of postoperative infection after appendicectomy. Cochrane Database Syst Rev 2001(3):CD001439.

75. Schmit PJ, Hiyama DT, Swisher SG, Bennion RS, Thompson JE Jr. Analysis of risk factors of postappendectomy intra-abdominal abscess. J Am Coll Surg 1994; 179(6):721–726.

76. Hellberg A, Rudberg C, Kullman E, et al. Prospective randomized multicentre study of laparoscopic versus open appendicectomy. Br J Surg 1999; 86(1):48–53.

77. Paik PS, Towson JA, Anthone GJ, Ortega AE, Simons AJ, Beart RW Jr. Intra-abdominal abscesses following laparoscopic and open appendectomies. J Gastrointest Surg 1997; 1(2):188–193.

78. Cohn SM, Giannotti G, Ong AW, et al. Prospective randomized trial of two wound management strategies for dirty abdominal wounds. Ann Surg 2001; 233(3):409–413.

79. Nwiloh J, Dardik H, Dardik M, Aneke L, Ibrahim IM. Changing patterns in the morbidity and mortality of colorectal surgery. Am J Surg 1991; 162:83–85.

80. Haley RW, Culver DH, Morgan WM, White JW, Emori TG, Hooton TM. Identifying patients at high risk of surgical wound infection. A simple multivariate index of patient susceptibility and wound contamination. Am J Epidemiol 1985; 121:206–215.

81. Cruse PJ, Foord R. The epidemiology of wound infection. A 10-year prospective study of 62,939 wounds. Surg Clin North Am 1980; 60:27–40.

82. Kjolseth D, Frank JM, Barker JH, et al. Comparison of the effects of commonly used wound agents on epithelialization and neovascularization. J Am Coll Surg 1994; 179:305–312.

83. McKenna PJ, Lehr GS, Leist P, Welling RE. Antiseptic effectiveness with fibroblast preservation. Ann Plast Surg 1991; 27:265–268.

84. Lewis RT. Necrotizing soft-tissue infections. Infect Dis Clin North Am 1992; 6:693–702.

85. Bartlett JG, Condon RE, Gorbach SL, Clarke JS, Nichols RL, Ochi S. Veterans Administration Cooperative Study on Bowel Preparation for Elective Colorectal Operations. Impact of oral antibiotic regimen on colonic flora, wound irrigation cultures, and bacteriology of septic complications. Ann Surg 1978; 188(2): 249–254.

86. Condon RE, Bartlett JG, Greenlee H, et al. Efficacy of oral and systemic antibiotic prophylaxis in colorectal operations. Arch Surg 1983; 118:496–502.

87. Psaila JV, Wheeler MH, Crosby DL. The role of plastic wound drapes in the prevention of wound infection following abdominal surgery. Br J Surg 1977; 64: 729–732.

88. Koehler PR, Moss AA. Diagnosis of intra-abdominal and pelvic abscesses by computerized tomography. JAMA 1980; 244:49–52.

89. Goldman M, Ambrose NS, Drolc Z, Hawker RJ, McCollum C. Indium-111-labelled leucocytes in the diagnosis of abdominal abscess. Br J Surg 1987; 74: 184–186.

90. Hemming A, Davis NL, Robins RE. Surgical versus percutaneous drainage of intra-abdominal abscesses. Am J Surg 1991; 161:593–595.

91. Malangoni MA, Shumate CR, Thomas HA, Richardson JD. Factors influencing the treatment of intra-abdominal abscesses. Am J Surg 1990; 159:167–171.

92. Malangoni MA, Condon RE, Spiegel CA. Treatment of intra-abdominal infections is appropriate with single-agent or combination antibiotic therapy. Surgery 1985; 98:648–655.

93. Moran B, Heald R. Anastomotic leakage after colorectal anastomosis. Semin Surg Oncol 2000; 18(3): 244–248.

94. Post S, Betzler M, von Ditfurth B, Shurmann G, Kuppers P, Herfarth C. Risks of intestinal anastomoses in Crohn's disease. Ann Surg 1991; 213:37–42.

95. Schrock TR, Deveney CW, Dunphy JE. Factors contributing to leakage of colonic anastomoses. Ann Surg 1973; 177:513–518.

96. Daly JM, DeCosse JJ. Complications in surgery of the colon and rectum. Surg Clin North Am 1983; 63(6): 1215–1231.

97. Bright TC III, Peters PC. Ureteral injuries secondary to operative procedures. Report of 24 cases. Urology 1977; 9:22–26.

98. Lapides J, Tank ES. Urinary complications following abdominal perineal resection. Cancer 1971; 28: 230–235.

99. Langevin JM, Rothenberger DA, Goldberg SM. Accidental splenic injury during surgical treatment of the colon and rectum. Surg Gynecol Obstet 1984; 159(2):139–144.

100. Shellito PC. Complications of abdominal stoma surgery. Dis Colon Rectum 1998; 41:1562–1572.

101. Park JJ, Del Pino A, Orsay CP, et al. Stoma complications: the Cook County Hospital experience. Dis Colon Rectum 1999; 42:1575–1580.

102. Stothert JC Jr., Brubacher L, Simonowitz DA. Complications of emergency stoma formation. Arch Surg 1982; 117(3):307–309.

103. Fleshman JW, Lewis MG. Complications and quality of life after stoma surgery: a review of 16,470 patients in the UOA data registry. Semin Colon Rectal Surg 1991; 2:66–72.

104. Leenen LP, Kuypers JH. Some factors influencing the outcome of stoma surgery. Dis Colon Rectum 1989; 32:500–504.

105. Londono-Schimmer EE, Leong AP, Phillips RK. Life table analysis of stomal complications following colostomy. Dis Colon Rectum 1994; 37:916–920.

106. Fazio VW, Tjandra JJ. Prevention and management of ileostomy complications. J ET Nurs 1992; 19:48–53.

107. Brooke BN. The management of an ileostomy including its complications, 1952. Dis Colon Rectum 1993; 36:512–516.

108. Carlsen E, Bergan AB. Loop ileostomy: technical aspects and complications. Eur J Surg 1999; 165(2): 140–144.

109. Porter JA, Salvati EP, Rubin RJ, Eisenstat TE. Complications of colostomies. Dis Colon Rectum 1989; 32:299–303.

110. Pearl RK, Prasad LM, Orsay CP, Abcarian H, Tan AB, Melzl MT. Early local complications from intestinal stomas. Arch Surg 1985; 120:1145–1147.

111. Cheung MT. Complications of an abdominal stoma: an analysis of 322 stomas. Aust N Z J Surg 1995; 65(11):808–811.

112. Carlstedt A, Fasth S, Hulten L, Nordgren S, Palselius I. Long-term ileostomy complications in patients with ulcerative colitis and Crohn's disease. Int J Colorectal Dis 1987; 2:22–25.

113. Cheung MT, Chia NH, Chiu WY. Surgical treatment of parastomal hernia complicating sigmoid colostomies. Dis Colon Rectum 2001; 44(2):266–270.

114. Pearl RK. Parastomal hernias. World J Surg 1989; 13:569–572.

115. Rubin MS, Schoetz DJ Jr., Matthews JB. Parastomal hernia. Is stoma relocation superior to fascial repair? Arch Surg 1994; 129:413–419.

116. Phillips R, Pringle W, Evans C, Keighley MR. Analysis of a hospital-based stomatherapy service. Ann R Coll Surg Engl 1985; 67(1):37–40.

117. Colcock BP, Jarpa S. Complications of abdominoperineal resection. Dis Colon Rectum 1958; 1:90–96.

118. Pollard CW, Nivatvongs S, Rojanasakul A, Ilstrup DM. Carcinoma of the rectum. Profiles of intraoperative and early postoperative complications. Dis Colon Rectum 1994; 37(9):866–874.

119. Farid H, O'Connell TX. Methods to decrease the morbidity of abdominoperineal resection. Am Surg 1995; 61(12):1061–1064.

120. Schoetz DJ Jr. Complications of surgical excision of rectum. Surg Clin North Am 1991; 71(6):1271–1281.

121. Enker WE, Merchant N, Cohen AM, et al. Safety and efficacy of low anterior resection for rectal cancer: 681 consecutive cases from a specialty service. Ann Surg 1999; 230(4):544–552; discussion 552.

122. Stolpi VM, Milsom JW, Lavery IC, Oakley JR, Church JM, Fazio VW. Newly designed occluder pin for presacral hemorrhage. Dis Colon Rectum 1992; 35: 166–169.

123. Petrelli NJ, Nagel S, Rodriguez-Bigas M, Piedmonte M, Herrera L. Morbidity and mortality following abdominoperineal resection for rectal adenocarcinoma. Am Surg 1993; 59(7):400–404.

124. Miles WE. A method of performing abdominoperineal excision for carcinoma of the rectum and of the terminal portion of the pelvic colon. Lancet 1908; 2:1812–1813.

125. Robles Campos R, Garcia Ayllon J, Parrila Paricio P, et al. Management of the perineal wound following abdominoperineal resection: prospective study of three methods. Br J Surg 1992; 79:29–31.

126. Tompkins RG, Warshaw Al. Improved management of the perineal wound after proctectomy. Ann Surg 1985; 202:760–765.

127. Porter GA, O'Keefe GE, Yakimets WW. Inadvertent perforation of the rectum during abdominoperineal resection. Am J Surg 1996; 172(4):324–327.

128. Rosen L, Veidenheimer MC, Coller JA, Corman ML. Mortality, morbidity, and patterns of recurrence after abdominoperineal resection for cancer of the rectum. Dis Colon Rectum 1982; 25:202–208.

129. So JB, Palmer MT, Shellito PC. Postoperative perineal hernia. Dis Colon Rectum 1997; 40(8):954–957.

130. Goldman G, Kahn PJ, Kashtan H, Stadler J, Wiznitzer T. Prevention and treatment of urinary retention and infection after surgical treatment of the colon and rectum with alpha adrenergic blockers. Surg Gynecol Obstet 1988; 166:447–450.

131. Aboseif SR, Matzel KE, Lue TE. Sexual dysfunction after rectal surgery. Perspect Colon Rectal Surg 1990; 3:157–172.

132. Cunsolo A, Bragaglia RB, Manara G, Poggioli G, Gozzetti G. Urogenital dysfunction after abominoperineal resection for carcinoma of the rectum. Dis Colon Rectum 1990; 33:918–922.

133. Fazio VW, Ziv Y, Church JM, et al. Ileal pouch-anal anastomoses complications and function in 1005 patients. Ann Surg 1995; 222(2):120–127.

134. Meagher AP, Farouk R, Dozois RR, Kelly KA, Pemberton JH. J ileal pouch-anal anastomosis for chronic ulcerative colitis: complications and long-term outcome in 1310 patients. Br J Surg 1998; 85(6):800–803.

135. Mikkola K, Luukkonen P, Jarvinen HJ. Long-term results of restorative proctocolectomy for ulcerative colitis. Int J Colorectal Dis 1995; 10(1):10–14.

136. Scott NA, Dozois RR, Beart RW Jr., Pemberton JH, Wolff BG, Ilstrup DM. Postoperative intra-abdominal and pelvic sepsis complicating ileal pouch-anal anastomosis. Int J Colorectal Dis 1988; 3:149–152.

137. Marcello PW, Roberts PL, Schoetz DJ Jr., Coller JA, Murray JJ, Veidenheimer MC. Obstruction after ileal pouch-anal anastomosis: a preventable complication? Dis Colon Rectum 1993, 36:1105–1111.

138. Keighley MR, Grobler SP. Fistula complicating restorative proctocolectomy. Br J Surg 1993; 80:1065–1067.

139. McMullen K, Hicks TC, Ray JE, Gathright JB, Timmcke AE. Complications associated with ileal pouch-anal anastomosis. World J Surg 1991; 15: 763–777.

140. Heuschen UA, Autschbach F, Allemeyer EH, et al. Long-term follow-up after ileoanal pouch procedure: algorithm for diagnosis, classification, and management of pouchitis. Dis Colon Rectum 2001; 44(4): 487–499.

141. Levin KE, Pemberton JH, Phillips SF, Zinsmeister AR, Pezim ME. Role of oxygen free radicals in the etiology of pouchitis. Dis Colon Rectum 1992; 35:452–456.

142. Hoff SD, Bailey HR, Butts DR, et al. Ambulatory surgical hemorrhoidectomy—a solution to postoperative urinary retention? Dis Colon Rectum 1994; 37: 1242–1244.

143. van Tets WF, Kuijpers HC. Continence disorders after anal fistulotomy. Dis Colon Rectum 1994; 37: 1194–1197.

144. Aguilar PS, Plasencia G, Hardy TJ Jr., Hartmann RF, Stewart WR. Mucosal advancement in the treatment of anal fistula. Dis Colon Rectum 1985; 28:496–498.

145. Pearl RK, Andrews JR, Orsay CP, et al. Role of the seton in the management of anorectal fistulas. Dis Colon Rectum 1993; 36:573–579.

146. Vasilevsky CA, Gordon PH. The incidence of recurrent abscesses or fistula-in-ano following anorectal suppuration. Dis Colon Rectum 1984; 27:126–130.

147. Bleday R, Pena JP, Rothenberger DA, Goldberg SM, Buls JG. Symptomatic hemorrhoids: current incidence and complications of operative therapy. Dis Colon Rectum 1992; 35:477–481.

148. Eu KW, Seow-Choen F, Goh HS. Comparison of emergency and elective haemorrhoidectomy. Br J Surg 1994; 81:308–310.

149. Gedebou TM, Wong RA, Rappaport WD, Jaffe P, Kahsai D, Hunter GC. Clinical presentation and management of iatrogenic colon perforations. Am J Surg 1996; 172(5):454–458.

150. Falcone RE, Carey LC. Colorectal trauma. Surg Clin North Am 1988; 68(6):1307–1318.

151. Levine JH, Longo WE, Pruitt C, Mazuski JE, Shapiro MJ, Durham RM. Management of selected rectal injuries by primary repair. Am J Surg 1996; 172(5):575–579.

152. Orsay CP, Merlotti G, Abcarian H, Pearl RK, Nanda M, Barrett J. Colorectal trauma. Dis Colon Rectum 1989; 32(3):188–190.

153. Velmahos GC, Vassiliu P, Demetriades D, et al. Wound management after colon injury: open or closed? A prospective randomized trial. Am Surg 2002; 68(9): 795–801.

10

Complications of Gastric Surgery

Dory Jewelewicz
Department of Anesthesiology, University of Miami/Jackson Memorial Hospital, Miami, Florida, U.S.A.

Dean Goldberg
Department of Surgery, Lee Memorial Hospital, Fort Myers, Florida, U.S.A.

Erik Barquist
Ryder Trauma Center, Department of Surgery, University of Miami, Miller School of Medicine, Miami, Florida, U.S.A.

Gastric surgery, once a common procedure in general surgery, is now performed much less frequently. Changes in our understanding of the pathophysiology of ulcer disease have shifted treatment from surgery to medical therapy. In addition, the incidence of gastric cancer has decreased dramatically in Western countries. However, skill and knowledge in this field are still required, particularly in light of the increasing numbers of antireflux and bariatric procedures that are being performed today. Younger surgeons do not approach gastric surgery with the same comfort and familiarity that were once common. Although the development of endoscopic, radiographic, and laparoscopic equipment allows less-invasive procedures, morbidity and mortality rates remain high.

ANATOMY

Because of its rich vascular supply, the stomach is difficult to devascularize. The blood supply comes from the left gastric artery; the right gastric and gastroepiploic arteries, which originate from the hepatic artery; and the left gastroepiploic and short gastric arteries, which originate from the splenic artery. Parasympathetic innervation comes from the terminal branches of the left and right vagi. Sympathetic fibers of the celiac plexus are distributed along the stomach.

DIAGNOSTIC PROCEDURES

In the diagnosis of gastric disease, visualization of pathology in the stomach's mucosa is essential. Contrast barium studies may detect defects in gastric anatomy, but they do not add therapeutic capability. Endoscopy, although associated with higher costs, more patient discomfort, and increased morbidity rates, is far superior. An esophagogastroduodenoscopy (EGD) allows for mucosal biopsy, polypectomy, sclerosing of vessels, and placement of feeding tubes, as well as direct visualization of the mucosa. Complications associated with EGD are rare, but include perforation, aspiration, and oversedation. The endoscope is passed from the oropharynx to the esophagus and into the stomach, and perforation may occur at any point along this path. Most perforations are caused by passing the scope without visualization of a patent lumen or by using excessive force in passing a barrier; perforations occur most frequently after therapeutic procedures such as biopsy, cautery, or dilation.

PEPTIC ULCER DISEASE

The discovery that an infectious agent, *Helicobacter pylori*, may be the cause of most duodenal and gastric ulcers has changed our understanding of the pathogenesis of peptic ulcer disease. Coupling this understanding with the introduction of H2 blockers and proton pump inhibitors has dramatically shifted our approach to the treatment of ulcers. In the past, patients underwent various surgical procedures as definitive treatment designed to reduce gastric acid secretion. Although this treatment was effective in most cases, patients were subjected to the risks of surgery, and many experienced postgastrectomy syndrome, postvagotomy syndrome, or both.

Today, medical management is the mainstay of therapy. Elective peptic ulcer surgery is infrequent even at large centers. The number of elective operations decreased by more than 70% in the 1980s, and emergent operations accounted for more than 80% of cases (1). Most procedures are now performed to treat the complications of peptic ulcer, such as bleeding, perforation, and gastric outlet obstruction. Despite these advances, the annual incidence of emergency surgery and the mortality rates associated with peptic ulcer disease have not decreased since the introduction of H2 blockers (1–4). Therefore, the treatment of complications of gastric surgery is still an important topic.

Operative Treatment of Duodenal Ulcer

Operative therapy is reserved for complications of duodenal ulcer disease. Intractability, hemorrhage, perforation, and obstruction are the most common causes. Goals of surgery are safety, repair, removal of underlying causes, and prevention of postoperative side effects. The three procedures most commonly used to treat duodenal ulcer disease today are truncal vagotomy and pyloroplasty, truncal vagotomy and antrectomy, and highly selective vagotomy (HSV). Truncal vagotomy requires transection of the left and right vagus nerves at the esophageal hiatus. This transection removes parasympathetic innervation of the abdominal viscera to the level of the transverse colon. Denervation of the pylorus necessitates a pyloroplasty so that subsequent gastric stasis and retention of solids and liquids can be avoided. The Heineke–Mikulicz pyloroplasty is the most common variant; others are the Finney and Jaboulay procedures. Truncal vagotomy combined with antrectomy ensures an even greater reduction in acid production by removing the source of gastrin production. Gastrointestinal (GI) continuity is achieved by gastroduodenostomy (Billroth I anastomosis) or gastrojejunostomy (Billroth II anastomosis). HSV involves division of vagal fibers to the acid-secreting regions of the stomach, with sparing of fibers to the distal antrum and pylorus.

Intractability is the primary indication for elective surgery to treat duodenal ulcers. Intractable ulcers may be defined as those that do not heal after three months of medical therapy, those that recur within one year despite medical therapy, or those that are characterized by cycles of prolonged activity with brief or absent remissions so that lifestyle is severely affected. Pain is generally controlled by medical therapy and is rarely a reason for surgery. Elective surgery also should be considered for ulcers associated with a history of hemorrhage or perforation. Because these elective procedures are associated with a low mortality rate, the procedure of choice is a HSV, which carries a slightly higher risk of recurrence but a lower incidence of side effects than procedures involving truncal vagotomy.

Hemorrhage is the leading cause of death associated with duodenal ulcer and is the reason for approximately one-third of emergent procedures for peptic ulcer disease (5). The incidence of bleeding has not decreased since the introduction of H2 blockers (2). The associated mortality rate has remained constant at 10%, although this consistency is due in part to the increasing age of patients and their associated comorbid conditions (6). When required, emergency surgery for bleeding duodenal ulcer aims to control

hemorrhage. The necessity of performing a definitive antiulcer procedure is a point of controversy, but such procedures are commonly performed. Control of hemorrhage usually requires a duodenotomy and direct suturing of the bleeding site. The gastroduodenal artery should always be ligated. If a definitive procedure is chosen, HSV is preferred for patients in stable condition; vagotomy and pyloroplasty are recommended when a short procedure is advisable.

The overall incidence of perforation, like that of hemorrhage, has remained stable, although evidence indicates that older patients with more comorbid conditions are increasingly affected (7). Approximately two-thirds of operations for complicated peptic ulcer disease are performed because of perforations with ensuing peritonitis (5). There is an ongoing debate about whether perforated duodenal ulcers generally need to be treated surgically. If the ulcer spontaneously seals, it may not always need surgical treatment. When surgery is required for perforated duodenal ulcer, its goals are safety, cleansing, and repair. The need for a definitive ulcer operation is controversial, but several recent studies provide evidence suggesting that such surgery is no longer required (8–10). The procedure of choice is thorough peritoneal irrigation followed by omental patch closure. Operative risk factors are concurrent medical illness, preoperative shock, and perforations of more than 48 hours duration. For patients without these risk factors, a definitive ulcer procedure may be added if desired; HSV is the preferred procedure.

Gastric outlet obstruction, usually the result of recurrent ulceration, is the least common complication of duodenal ulcer disease. Approximately 1% to 2% of patients are affected, and approximately 80% of obstructions due to peptic ulcer disease are caused by duodenal ulcers (11,12). Endoscopic balloon dilation is a safe treatment but provides only temporary relief. Because of extensive scarring, pyloroplasty is rarely feasible. Antrectomy is frequently performed; if this procedure is impossible, truncal vagotomy and gastrojejunostomy are carried out. In most instances, however, truncal vagotomy and pyloroplasty or truncal vagotomy and antrectomy can be safely performed. HSV with pyloroduodenal dilation should not be used because it is associated with high rates of ulcer recurrence and with restenosis in more than 40% of cases (11,13).

Operative Treatment of Gastric Ulcer

Indications for elective surgical treatment of gastric ulcer include failure of a newly diagnosed ulcer to heal after 12 weeks of medical therapy, failure of a recurrent ulcer to respond to therapy, or recurrence after two initial courses of successful treatment. When gastric ulcers fail to heal completely, malignancy must be ruled out; inability to do so qualifies as an indication for surgery. Treatment differs according to anatomic location, presence of a coexisting duodenal ulcer, and acid secretory status. Numerous procedures have been described for each type of ulcer; however, the goal should be complete excision of the ulcer for histologic examination. As is true for duodenal ulcer, the need for a definitive acid-reducing measure to treat gastric ulcer is currently a point of contention.

Hemorrhage, perforation, and obstruction are the three most common complications of gastric ulcer. Emergent operations for hemorrhage carry higher mortality rates for gastric ulcer than for duodenal ulcer because patients tend to be older with more comorbid conditions. For ulcers located in the prepyloric region or in the body of the stomach, the preferred operation is antrectomy with Billroth I anastomosis. A truncal vagotomy usually is added for prepyloric ulcers or for gastric ulcers associated with a duodenal ulcer. If the ulcer is located proximally on the lesser curvature, antrectomy with extension of the lesser curvature to include the ulcer is preferred. If the ulcer lies too close to the esophagogastric junction to allow resection, it is treated by vessel transfixion and ulcer oversewing. A HSV is usually added. Truncal vagotomy and pyloroplasty after ulcer oversewing is a secondary option. In the presence of life-threatening hemorrhage, suture ligation of the ulcer followed by vagotomy and pyloroplasty is an acceptable alternative. Multiple biopsies of the ulcer should be performed whenever possible; this procedure is associated with high rates of rebleeding.

A perforated gastric ulcer is associated with a mortality rate twice that of a perforated duodenal ulcer. Operative treatment is accomplished by distal gastrectomy that includes the site of perforation. For patients in an unstable condition, excision of the ulcer with patch closure is an acceptable alternative. Gastric outlet obstruction is most commonly associated with prepyloric ulcers but can occur when ulcers of the stomach body are associated with duodenal ulcers. It is rarely seen in solitary ulcers of the body, and its occurrence in this situation is suggestive of malignancy. The procedure of choice is antrectomy and Billroth I anastomosis. Gastrojejunostomy is an acceptable alternative in the presence of severe scarring, although such scarring is rare.

GASTRIC CARCINOMA

Fifty years ago, gastric cancer was the leading cause of cancer death in men in the United States. Today, only 3% of cancer deaths in men, and even fewer in women, are due to this disease (14). The reasons for this decline remain unclear despite intensive study. Gastric cancer is a serious health problem in other countries, including Japan, Russia, Costa Rica, and Chile.

The mainstay of therapy for gastric cancer is surgery, which provides the only hope of cure. In the United States, however, most patients are not seen until the disease is already advanced; thus, curative resection is precluded. The goals of surgery, therefore, are to maximize the chances for cure among patients with localized disease and to provide adequate palliation for those with advanced disease. In the United States, the overall five-year survival rate of patients undergoing gastrectomy for cancer is 15% to 20%. In Western countries, although no recent improvement in surgical cure rates have been observed, the operative risks associated with gastrectomy for gastric cancer have decreased substantially. Before 1970, overall operative mortality for gastrectomy for gastric cancer was 16%; it has since decreased to 5% (15).

If preoperative evaluation does not suggest metastatic disease, exploratory laparotomy should be undertaken. At the time of operation, if no gross metastases are found, a curative resection should be attempted. The goal is to completely remove the primary tumor and the associated lymph nodes. However, the extent of gastric resection required and the role of radical lymphadenectomy in achieving cure have been controversial. Some patients will have occult metastases at the time of exploration. In most cases, these patients benefit from a palliative resection, with the goal of removing the primary tumor but leaving gross metastases behind. Patients known to have advanced disease preoperatively must be treated on a case-by-case basis. Factors such as the overall condition of the patient, the extent of metastases, and the presence of bleeding or obstruction due to the primary tumor must be weighed before palliative resection is undertaken.

When planning a curative resection, surgeons should remember that microscopic tumor extension is common in gastric cancer. Margins of 4 to 6 cm around the primary tumor are required. For distal lesions, subtotal gastrectomy with a Billroth II anastomosis is the most frequently used procedure (16,17). Some centers advocate total gastrectomy, but evidence indicates that this procedure does not confer improved survival rates and is actually associated with slightly higher morbidity and mortality rates (18). Lesions of the midbody or the fundus require total gastrectomy. Other indications for total gastrectomy include gastric stump cancer after distal resection for benign disease, linitus-plastica lesions, and cancer associated with multiple polyps. En bloc splenectomy also is performed for lesions of the greater curvature. Reconstruction is usually through an end-to-side Roux-en-Y esophagojejunostomy. Cardiac lesions near the gastroesophageal junction require esophagogastrectomy. Proximally, at least 10 cm of esophagus should be resected, with frozen section to ensure adequate margins. The distal margin should include 6 cm of stomach.

All patients undergoing curative resection should also undergo en bloc resection of lymph nodes draining the region of the primary tumor. This resection should include at least omental, pyloric, and lesser-curvature nodes; splenic hilar nodes should be added for lesions of the greater curvature. In Japan, radical lymphadenectomy is routinely performed, and improved outcomes have been attributed to this procedure. However, this benefit has not been confirmed in Western countries, perhaps because in Japan, a higher proportion of patients have good prognostic factors, such as early gastric cancer and intestinal-type histology.

GASTRIC LYMPHOMA

Primary gastric lymphoma is the second most common malignant gastric tumor. Approximately 2% to 5% of all gastric malignancies are lymphomas; however, their incidence appears to be increasing (19,20). Treatment is controversial because of the absence of controlled clinical trials comparing treatment options. A multimodality approach is most often used, with treatment directed by the stage of the disease. The strategy for management of early stage lymphoma is clearance of all gross disease. Such clearance is usually accomplished by distal gastrectomy with en bloc resection of primary nodal drainage groups. Biopsies of the liver and of any suspicious lymph nodes are performed; splenectomy is performed only if the spleen is involved by direct extension. Surgery for patients with advanced disease is primarily aimed at treating complications such as perforation, hemorrhage, or obstruction.

GASTROINTESTINAL MOTILITY

Gastric surgery inherently has adverse effects on GI motility. As a result of the improved understanding of the origin and control of GI motility, a scientific approach to the diagnosis and treatment of motility disorders has evolved. Movement of ingested food from the mouth to the anus is based on coordinated digestive tract motility. The nervous system modulates motility through extrinsic and intrinsic neurons. The extrinsic nervous system coordinates the voluntary actions at either end of the GI system: the esophagus and the anus. Between the stomach and the rectum, where all movement is involuntary, control is exerted by the intrinsic nervous system. The extrinsic system fine-tunes the intrinsic nervous system through its sympathetic and parasympathetic inputs.

The stomach functions to receive and store food, to mix it with gastric juice and begin the process of digestion, and to propel the prepared chyme into the duodenum at a rate optimal for digestion and absorption by the small intestine. The organ achieves this function through careful regulation of motility and emptying. Unfortunately, gastric surgery disrupts this finely tuned process and can cause one of several postgastrectomy syndromes. Understanding the alterations caused by disease requires an understanding of the mechanisms that control gastric motility and emptying in a healthy human.

The stomach can be thought of as having two distinct areas: the proximal region, consisting of the fundus and the proximal corpus, and the distal region, consisting of the distal corpus, the antrum, and the pylorus. The proximal stomach is relatively silent electrically and functions primarily to receive and store food and to transfer liquids to the duodenum. The distal stomach, in contrast, is electrically active and functions to reduce the size of ingested solids, to control their emptying into the duodenum, and to prevent duodenogastric reflux.

The proximal stomach receives and stores food from the esophagus. This region is capable of sustained alteration in tension via two vagally mediated reflexes: accommodation and receptive relaxation. Receptive relaxation refers to the anticipatory relaxation of the proximal stomach to accept a food bolus from the esophagus. Accommodation describes the stomach's ability to adapt to large changes in volume with only minimal increases in intragastric pressure. A number of hormones also regulate the contractions of the proximal stomach. Because of its ability to regulate intragastric pressure, the proximal stomach plays a pivotal role in the emptying of liquids. If accommodation is impaired, proximal gastric tone increases markedly during distension, and this increase leads to increased intragastric pressure and rapid emptying of liquids (21–23).

Control of gastric emptying of solids is a function of the distal stomach; the proximal stomach plays only a minor role. Solids are retained in the distal stomach, where they are mixed with gastric juice and broken down to particles no larger than approximately 0.1 mm before they are allowed to pass into the duodenum. Indigestible solids are retained to be emptied later. Contraction of the distal stomach and the pylorus is regulated by neural and hormonal control. The pylorus coordinates with the rest of the distal stomach to retain gastric solids and to prevent reflux of duodenal contents.

EFFECT OF SURGICAL PROCEDURES ON GASTRIC MOTOR PHYSIOLOGY

Procedures performed on the stomach include resection, vagotomy, and drainage procedures. Each has specific effects on gastric motility and emptying. Combining vagotomy with a distal gastric resection or a drainage procedure produces alterations in gastric motor physiology that are the net result of the two procedures. These disruptions may cause a variety of symptoms, termed *postgastrectomy syndromes*, which occur after 5% to 50% of gastric operations (24,25).

Vagotomy

As discussed previously, two types of vagotomy are currently performed: truncal vagotomy and HSV. Selective gastric vagotomy is rarely used. Truncal vagotomy abolishes innervation to the stomach and the entire abdominal viscera, whereas HSV removes vagal innervation to the fundus and corpus, leaving branches to the antrum and pylorus intact. Truncal vagotomy must be combined with a drainage procedure; HSV does not require such a combination. However, both procedures remove vagal innervation to the proximal stomach, and this removal severely impairs accommodation and reflexive relaxation. The stomach's ability to store food is altered so that distension leads to larger increases in intragastric pressure than would normally be the case. This increase in pressure speeds emptying of liquids during the postprandial period; however, this increase is limited when the pylorus is left intact. Patients also may experience dysphagia and feelings of early satiety.

HSV does not disturb the gastric pacemaker or the distal propagation of these potentials (26,27). More important, the strength (antral contractions, gastric trituration, and gastric emptying) of solids is not altered (28,29). The function of the pylorus in preventing duodenogastric reflux also is maintained. Truncal vagotomy, however, has profound effects on distal gastric motor physiology. Gastric peristalsis is weakened, trituration is impaired, and emptying of digestible and indigestible solids is slowed (30–32). Gastric emptying must be facilitated by a drainage procedure.

Drainage Procedures

The two most common drainage procedures are pyloroplasty and gastrojejunostomy with either a Billroth II or a Roux-en-Y anastomosis. Pyloroplasty has little effect on the functions of the proximal stomach; however, its disruption impairs trituration, causes rapid emptying of solids, and increases duodenogastric reflux. Emptying of liquids is unchanged or slightly increased. Gastrojejunostomy also has little effect on the function of the proximal stomach. Its effect on gastric emptying is variable. Generally, liquids tend to empty faster, but emptying of solids may be hastened or delayed.

Gastric Resection

The effect of gastric resection on proximal gastric motor physiology depends on the extent of resection. The most common gastric resection is a distal resection of the antrum and pylorus with a Billroth I or II anastomosis. Receptive relaxation, accommodation, and storage are minimally affected. Emptying of liquids is slightly faster, probably because of decreased resistance to outflow (33,34). As resections become more extensive, the functions of the proximal stomach become increasingly impaired, and this impairment results in faster emptying of liquids. Distal resection abolishes antral trituration, removes the barrier to duodenal gastric reflux, and results in rapid emptying of solids (34–36). Proximal gastrectomy results in rapid emptying of liquids (37).

The effect on distal function depends on the extent of resection. If the region of the gastric pacemaker is included, a new pacemaker appears in the distal stomach. When compared with the natural pacemaker, the new pacemaker cycles at a slower frequency and with a less regular rhythm (27). This alteration in cycling may weaken antral peristalsis, thereby impairing trituration and emptying of solids.

ACUTE COMPLICATIONS OF GASTRIC SURGERY
Rebleeding

Early recurrence of bleeding is more likely after surgery for peptic ulcer disease than after surgery for gastric neoplasm. Bleeding may be intraluminal or intra-abdominal. Intraluminal bleeding most commonly occurs among patients with multiple comorbid conditions who have undergone a simple oversewing of an ulcer without an associated ulcer operation (38). Overall, intraluminal bleeding occurs among 5% of all postgastrectomy patients; one-third bleed from the source that prompted the original operation, one-third bleed from an anastomotic line, and one-third bleed from an unknown source. Bleeding substantial enough to cause signs of shock warrants aggressive resuscitative and corrective measures, followed by endoscopy. If endoscopic therapeutic measures cannot control the bleeding, open surgery is indicated. Intraoperatively, a proximal gastrotomy is performed above any anastomosis or stoma.

Bleeding from a lesser-curvature closure or an anastomotic line may be controlled by suture ligation. Alternatively, re-resection and a second anastomosis may be required. Blood coming from the duodenum (in the case of a Billroth I anastomosis) or the afferent limb (in the case of a Billroth II anastomosis) suggests a recurrent bleeding ulcer. Control may require opening the duodenal stump (Billroth II) or gastroduodenostomy (Billroth I). The esophagus and cardia should be examined for any ulcers, tears, or varices, and any bleeding should be controlled by suture ligation.

Intra-abdominal bleeding presents symptoms similar to those of intraluminal bleeding, but nasogastric aspirates will contain little or no blood, and there may be signs of peritoneal irritation. Ultrasonography or computed tomography (CT) scanning may show evidence of an intra-abdominal fluid collection. Endoscopy may be helpful by excluding an intraluminal source of bleeding. Sources of bleeding include splenic tear, anastomotic line, excluded ulcer crater, bleeding mesenteric vessel, hemorrhagic pancreatitis, or the vagotomy site on the esophagus.

Management is similar to that of intraluminal bleeding. Aggressive supportive measures are instituted and are followed by endoscopy. If endoscopy points toward an intra-abdominal source and the patient is in stable condition, the next step may be CT scanning or ultrasonography. Radiologic embolization of bleeding vessels is a therapeutic option. A patient in unstable condition should undergo immediate exploration. Splenic tears may be controlled by hemostatic agents or splenorrhaphy; splenectomy may be required. Anastomotic lines, any excluded ulcers, and all mesenteric margins should be examined, and any bleeding should be controlled by suture ligation. The esophagus should be examined for active bleeding, which is controlled by suture ligation or hemoclips.

Gastroparesis

Gastroparesis is most commonly seen after surgery for gastric outlet obstruction, particularly if this condition was managed with vagotomy and pyloroplasty. Patients with a history of diabetes mellitus, scleroderma, or a collagen vascular disorder are at high risk of postoperative gastroparesis. Overall, 4% of patients undergoing a gastric procedure will experience delayed gastric emptying (39). The cause is probably multifactorial, involving metabolic, mechanical, and functional factors.

Appropriate laboratory tests or CT scanning must exclude concurrent illness, infections, metabolic disturbances, or other treatable causes, including leaks or abscesses. Once these conditions have been excluded, prolonged conservative management is advised and should consist of gastric decompression, correction of electrolyte abnormalities, nutritional support, and weaning from potentially exacerbating drugs. Prokinetic agents may be useful in a few cases, but usually observation is all that is required. If no other cause is discovered and gastroparesis continues for more than 7 to 14 days after surgery, evaluation with barium, a radioisotope, or the endoscope is indicated. Among patients with gastroparesis, 95% will pass some contrast agent by day 14, whereas 95% of patients who pass no contrast agent will have a mechanical obstruction (40). Endoscopy can be used when radiographic findings are equivocal. Surgical intervention is reserved for patients with early marginal ulcers that are unresponsive to medical therapy, for those with anatomic abnormalities of the gastric outlet, and for those without abnormalities whose stomach fails to empty by one month after the operation.

Duodenal Stump Blowout

The incidence of duodenal stump leak is approximately 3%; the associated mortality rate, although often reported to be as high as 50%, is probably closer to 10% (38). A blown duodenal stump is usually the result of an overzealous dissection of the duodenum in the setting of chronic scarring; such a dissection disrupts the organ's blood supply. The duodenum should be mobilized only enough to ensure an adequate closure. Another common cause of a blown duodenal stump is acute afferent limb obstruction, caused by kinking or retroanastomotic hernia. Patients with this condition usually exhibit an acute exacerbation of abdominal pain on the fifth to seventh postoperative day. Occasionally, the leak is confined to the right upper quadrant and appears with signs of localized sepsis. CT scanning or ultrasonography may show an abscess cavity; an upper GI series or a dimethyl iminodiacetic acid [hepatobiliary iminodiacetic acid (HIDA)]

scan may show a leak. Patients with this type of leak may respond to percutaneous drainage. The more common presentations are severe abdominal sepsis and an acute abdomen. Patients with these signs require exploration, drainage of the right upper quadrant, and closure of the duodenum around a tube, along with the initiation of hyperalimentation. If the fistula has not closed after six weeks, it should be treated operatively.

Gastric Perforation

Gastric perforation after HSV is rare. It is caused by devascularization of the lesser curvature, which results in ischemic perforation. Patients with this condition exhibit severe sepsis and require laparotomy, debridement, and closure of the perforation. Gastric resection may be needed to ensure adequate closure.

Anastomotic Leak

Excluding esophageal anastomoses after total gastrectomy, the overall incidence of anastomotic leak is less than 2% after gastric operations. Presentation may be severe but is commonly more subtle. Contained leaks may be controlled by percutaneous drainage, hyperalimentation, nasogastric decompression, and broadspectrum antibiotics. Unless there is distal obstruction or carcinoma of the suture line, the fistula tract should close. For patients with peritonitis and shock, or those in whom drainage is inadequate, an operation is needed. Small anastomotic defects may be closed primarily and covered with omentum. Commonly, revision of the anastomosis is required. Operations for anastomotic dehiscence should be supplemented with wide abdominal drainage, gastrostomy, broadspectrum antibiotics, and hyperalimentation.

The incidence of leak in a pyloroplasty after an ulcer operation is 5% (38). If there is minimal contamination, the anastomotic margins can be trimmed, and a new pyloroplasty can be performed. Large defects may require revision of the anastomosis. A Heineke–Mikulicz pyloroplasty may be converted to a Finney pyloroplasty, or, alternatively, a Billroth II anastomosis may be fashioned. This type of reconstruction avoids the risk of postoperative gastric outlet obstruction. For patients in unstable condition, the area should be widely drained, and a gastrostomy should be placed for gastric decompression. Similar treatment is used for a leaking gastroduodenostomy after a Billroth I anastomosis. Leaks along the reconstructed lesser curvature usually require additional resection and conversion to a Billroth II anastomosis. A leaking gastrojejunostomy after a Billroth II anastomosis also requires resection and reconstruction.

Pancreatitis

The incidence of pancreatitis after gastric surgery is 1% to 2%; the associated mortality rate may be as high as 50%. Usually, pancreatitis is induced by excessive trauma to the pancreas during dissection of a duodenal ulcer or closure of a duodenal stump. The symptoms may be mild, with epigastric pain, vomiting, prolonged ileus, leukocytosis, oliguria, and icterus, or they may be severe, with fever, hypotension, a decreasing hematocrit, and an epigastric mass. Diagnosing this complication is made more difficult by the fact that modest elevations of amylase activity are common after gastric surgery. The diagnosis is even further obscured because symptoms of severe pancreatitis are similar to those of other complications that require emergent operation, such as duodenal stump leak, acute afferent loop syndrome, or anastomotic dehiscence. Diagnosis is usually made on the basis of the results of CT scanning and laboratory tests. CT scanning or ultrasonography may be helpful by showing pancreatic inflammation, phlegmon, or pseudocyst. Pancreatitis should be treated with parenteral nutrition, aggressive fluid resuscitation, nasogastric decompression, and antibiotics. Endoscopic retrograde cholangiopancreatography may be performed to ensure patency of and drainage through the common duct.

LONG-TERM COMPLICATIONS OF GASTRIC SURGERY

Any operation on the stomach, especially one that destroys or bypasses the pylorus or involves vagotomy, may cause substantial impairment of gastric motility. Although such impairment is common, adaptation usually occurs by six months after surgery. A small but meaningful number of patients, however, experience bothersome and, at times, debilitating symptoms. These constellations of signs and symptoms have been termed *postgastrectomy syndromes* and include dumping, alkaline reflux gastritis, postvagotomy diarrhea, roux stasis, afferent/efferent loop obstruction, chronic gastric atony, and small gastric remnant syndromes. These signs and symptoms can be divided into conditions in which gastric emptying is delayed and those in which it is accelerated. Other long-term complications—including recurrent ulcer, gastric remnant carcinoma, and malabsorption—are not as clearly related to disturbances in gastric motor function.

Dumping Syndrome

The dumping syndrome is one of the most common causes of morbidity after gastric surgery. Symptoms develop after the ingestion of food, and patients are free of symptoms under fasting conditions. The syndrome is characterized by both GI and vasomotor symptoms. GI symptoms include crampy abdominal pain, bloating, nausea, vomiting, and explosive diarrhea. Vasomotor symptoms include diaphoresis, dizziness, palpitations, weakness, flushing, and an overwhelming desire to lie down. The reported incidences of dumping are highly variable and depend on the type of surgery performed and the diligence

with which symptoms are observed. Overall, an estimated 25% to 50% of patients experience some symptoms of dumping after gastric surgery; however, only 1% to 5% experience severe, disabling symptoms (41,42). Severe dumping is reported to occur among 3% to 5% of patients after HSV, 6% to 14% of patients after truncal vagotomy and drainage, and 14% to 20% of patients after partial gastrectomy (43,44).

Dumping is classified as early or late on the basis of the timing of onset of symptoms. Early dumping starts 10 to 30 minutes after eating. Patients with this condition usually experience a mixture of GI and vasomotor symptoms. Late dumping starts two to three hours after eating and usually involves only vasomotor symptoms. Approximately 75% of patients experience early dumping and 25% experience late dumping; a small number of patients experience both. Symptoms usually start during the first few weeks after surgery when patients resume their normal diets. Liquid foods and meals rich in carbohydrates are particularly poorly tolerated. Severely affected patients may lose weight because of fear of eating.

It is widely accepted that an important mechanism leading to early dumping is accelerated gastric emptying. Four surgical factors lead to this rapid emptying: the loss of accommodation and receptive relaxation that accompanies vagotomy, the loss of gastric capacity that accompanies resection, the loss of control of emptying by destruction or bypass of the pylorus, and the loss of duodenal feedback mechanisms by bypass with a gastrojejunostomy. Several studies have provided evidence indicating that symptoms of dumping are provoked in healthy control subjects by the rapid infusion of glucose directly into the duodenum or jejunum (45,46). The accelerated entry of hyperosmolar chyme into the intestine causes large fluid shifts from the intravascular space to the intestinal lumen. The resulting bowel distension causes increases in the amplitude and the frequency of contractions, and these increases may be responsible for GI symptoms (47). Fluid sequestration results in a relative hypovolemia, which may be the cause of the vasomotor symptoms.

Some evidence suggests, however, that factors other than gastric emptying are relevant. Several studies show a considerable overlap in gastric emptying times between patients with and without dumping after gastric surgery (48–50); others fail to show differences between patients with dumping syndrome and surgical control subjects (51,52). One study, which measured the degree of dilution in the jejunum of a hyperosmolar glucose solution, found no difference in this variable between postgastrectomy patients with or without symptoms. This finding casts doubt on hyperosmolarity as the cause of symptoms (53). Furthermore, the magnitude of these fluid shifts was moderate, only 300 to 700 mL, an amount that is usually well tolerated.

Hypovolemia should be accompanied by an increase in heart rate, and, indeed, such an increase is seen in patients with early dumping. The increased heart rate should be accompanied by peripheral vasoconstriction; however, several studies report a paradoxical peripheral vasodilation among patients with symptoms during dumping provocation with oral glucose (54,55). Other studies document an increase in superior mesenteric artery flow after dumping provocation in patients with early dumping (56). Splanchnic vasodilation and pooling of blood may be an additional factor predisposing these patients to vasomotor symptoms. Finally, a study involving patients with early dumping after total gastrectomy found that the blood volume and the extracellular space volume of these patients were smaller than those of patients without symptoms (57).

Humoral factors also play a role in the pathogenesis of early dumping. The release of numerous enteric hormones is enhanced among patients with symptoms. These hormones include vasoactive intestinal peptide, pancreatic polypeptide, neurotensin, enteroglucagon, serotonin, peptide YY, motilin, and glucose-dependent insulinotropic peptide (GIP). However, the significance of elevated levels of these enteropeptides in the development of dumping symptoms remains unclear (58).

Rapid gastric emptying is also believed to play a role in the pathogenesis of late dumping. Fast delivery of food to the small intestine and rapid glucose absorption cause an initial hyperglycemia, leading to a hyperinsulinemic response. This response causes a reactive hypoglycemia two to three hours postprandially. The symptoms are relieved by the ingestion of carbohydrates, whereas in early dumping, they are made worse by carbohydrate ingestion. The pathophysiology behind this enhanced insulin release is complex. It has been shown that gut administration of glucose causes higher insulin release than intravenous administration; this has been termed the *incretin effect*. Thus, hyperinsulinemia could be due to enhanced absorption of glucose, an enhanced incretin effect, or both. Gut hormones mediating the enteroinsular axis include cholecystokinin, enteroglucagon, GIP, and glucagon-like peptide-1 (GLP1). After gastric surgery, the GIP responses among patients with late dumping were found to be dampened or less powerful than those among patients without symptoms (59,60). In one small series, more GLP1 was released after gastrectomy in patients with symptoms than in patients without symptoms (50).

The diagnosis of dumping is based on a thorough medical history and the provocation of signs and symptoms by an oral glucose challenge. The Sigstad scoring system, which is based on weighted factors allocated to symptoms, may be helpful in diagnosing the condition and judging the success of therapy (60). Gastric-emptying studies using radionuclide markers in both liquid and solid phase may be used to document accelerated gastric emptying. Endoscopy and barium radiography are helpful in precisely defining the anatomy and in diagnosing other postgastrectomy syndromes that may be present.

When treatment options are considered, the severity and duration of symptoms must be kept in mind; most patients have mild-to-moderate symptoms that improve with time. Dietary modification is the mainstay of therapy. Patients should be instructed to eat small, frequent meals that are low in carbohydrate and high in protein. It is often helpful to postpone drinking for at least half an hour after eating. In addition, patients should add fiber and a modest amount of fat to their diets and should substitute complex carbohydrates (e.g., raw vegetables) for simple sugars. If symptoms are severe, patients can be told to lie down for half an hour after eating. Many patients have intuitively already made many of these changes.

Most patients are adequately treated by dietary changes, but a small number may need additional therapy. The addition of dietary fibers is effective because these fibers form gels with carbohydrates, thereby delaying glucose absorption and lengthening bowel transit time; however, the palatability of these fibers is low. Acarbose, an alpha-glycoside hydrolase inhibitor, interferes with the digestion and subsequent absorption of carbohydrate. It is effective in preventing late dumping, but its use is limited by the occurrence of diarrhea and flatulence as the result of fermentation of unabsorbed carbohydrates.

Octreotide, a long-acting somatostatin analogue given by subcutaneous injection, has been used with some success to treat severe symptoms of early and late dumping. Its effectiveness is due to its actions at several different levels in the pathophysiology of dumping. Gastric emptying and small-bowel transit time are delayed, probably because of the induction of a fasting intestinal motility pattern and the inhibition of the release of enteric peptides known to stimulate bowel motility (61). Octreotide also inhibits the release of insulin, the absorption of glucose, and the secretion of jejunal fluid (62,63). Furthermore, food-induced vasodilation in the peripheral and splanchnic circulations is inhibited (64,65). Long-term complications of octreotide therapy are unknown. The need for self-administered injections may limit patient compliance. Octreotide-induced diabetes, possibly caused by the inhibition of glucagon release, has rarely been reported but can usually be adequately treated with an oral hypoglycemic agent (66). Steatorrhea resulting from the inhibition of pancreatic secretions is more common but responds well to enzyme replacement therapy (67). Cholelithiasis, probably due to the inhibition of gallbladder contraction, is another rarely reported side effect (68).

Multiple surgical procedures have been advocated for the treatment of dumping, including pyloric reconstruction, narrowing of the gastrojejunal stoma, conversion of a Billroth II anastomosis to a Billroth I anastomosis, jejunal interposition, and conversion to a Roux-en-Y anastomosis. Although initial success rates vary, long-term results are generally disappointing. Surgery should be the very last resort for treating patients with severe dumping that is unresponsive to dietary and medical therapy.

For patients who have previously undergone pyloroplasty, pyloric reconstruction is a viable option. The pyloroplasty is opened, the sphincter muscle is reapproximated, and the incision is closed longitudinally. This procedure is simple and carries few risks, but reported success rates vary widely (69–71). Although simple in concept, stomal revision has largely been discarded. It is difficult to judge exactly the size of stoma that will prevent recurrence of symptoms and also minimize the risk of gastric outlet obstruction. Furthermore, stricture or dilation of the stoma may occur with time. Conversion of a Billroth II anastomosis to a Billroth I anastomosis reestablishes the gastroduodenal flow of food, is associated with low rates of complication, and improves the symptoms of approximately 75% of patients. However, 25% of patients, for reasons unknown, do not benefit from this procedure (72). Many types of jejunal interpositions, both isoperistaltic and antiperistaltic, have been described. The most successful has been the 10-cm antiperistaltic jejunal segment, which may be interposed between the stomach and the duodenum, in the efferent limb of a gastrojejunostomy, or in a Roux-en-Y limb. Several authors report good results with this procedure (73,74), but others report a serious risk of gastric outlet obstruction (75,76). For patients with a previous Billroth I or II anastomosis, conversion to a Roux-en-Y gastrojejunostomy has provided the most consistent results (76–78). Transection of the jejunum during construction of the limb leads to the formation of ectopic pacemakers. These pacemakers result in retrograde contractions within the limb, thereby increasing the resistance to the transit of chyme and slowing gastric emptying (79). However, this procedure may lead to the development of roux stasis syndrome, to be discussed later.

Postvagotomy Diarrhea

Although diarrhea is not uncommon after gastric surgery, its incidence is higher among patients who have undergone vagotomy. The incidence is highest after truncal vagotomy at 20%; the incidence after selective vagotomy is 5%, and the incidence after HSV is 4% (80,81). Severe symptoms are characterized by frequent, watery stools, often nocturnal, and are usually not associated with ingestion of a meal. Attacks may be episodic, lasting a few days and then not recurring for several months. Symptoms generally improve over the first year, and the problem rarely remains debilitating or constant.

The diagnosis of postvagotomy diarrhea is made on clinical grounds, with care taken to distinguish other postgastrectomy syndromes that can occur concomitantly. Other causes of diarrhea should be excluded; appropriate initial diagnostic tests are stool culture, *Clostridium difficile* titer, fecal white blood cell count, and fecal fat quantification. Patients with persistent symptoms may require upper GI series, barium enema, colonoscopy, or endoscopy with small-bowel biopsies so that other causes of diarrhea can be adequately excluded.

The pathophysiology of postvagotomy diarrhea is unclear but is probably multifactorial. Rapid gastric emptying is often associated with the diarrhea, but surgical correction often does not improve the problem. Changes in the rate of flow and pathway of chyme may lead to malabsorption of nutrients normally digested by mucosal enzymes; in this manner, for example, a subclinical lactase deficiency may be unmasked and may lead to diarrhea. As the vagotomy performed becomes more selective, the incidence of postvagotomy diarrhea decreases; this fact suggests that one cause of the problem may be vagal denervation of the small bowel or the biliary tree. One theory points to impaired gallbladder emptying and increased excretion of bile salts as the cause. Supporting evidence includes studies showing that patients with postvagotomy diarrhea have higher levels of fecal bile salts than do normal control subjects, and the fact that the administration of cholestyramine, a bile acid–binding agent, substantially improves symptoms (82,83). Disruption of extrinsic control of GI motility by vagotomy is another leading theory.

Medical treatment for postvagotomy diarrhea is similar to that for dumping; dietary measures are the mainstay of therapy. Antidiarrheal agents such as loperamide, diphenoxylate, and opiates are useful. Cholestyramine, as discussed above, improves diarrhea for most patients. For patients unresponsive to these measures, octreotide has been used with mixed success. It may actually worsen symptoms by inhibiting pancreatic secretions, thereby exacerbating malabsorption (75,77,84).

Surgical options should be reserved for the minority of patients with chronic, debilitating symptoms unresponsive to other therapies. As discussed above, although rapid gastric emptying is associated with diarrhea, surgical correction does not improve symptoms. The strategy, therefore, is a slowing of small-bowel transit time. The most frequently used procedure is the construction of a 10- to 15-cm antiperistaltic jejunal segment 100 cm distal to a gastroenterostomy or the Treitz ligament. The results achieved by this procedure, however, have been mixed (85,86). The distal-onlay reversed-ileal graft has also been used (87). This procedure involves isolating a 10-cm ileal segment 20 to 30 cm from the ileocecal valve; continuity is achieved by an end-to-end anastomosis. The isolated segment is opened along the antimesenteric border, rotated so that it is antiperistaltic, and sutured as an onlay just proximal to the prior anastomosis.

Alkaline Reflux Gastritis

Five to fifteen percent of patients undergoing gastric surgery will experience alkaline reflux gastritis (88). The symptoms include burning epigastric pain, which is unrelieved by antacids and frequently made worse by eating or lying down, nausea, and bilious vomiting. In an effort to avoid these symptoms, patients often decrease their food intake, and this action results in weight loss and anemia. Alkaline reflux gastritis requires surgical treatment more often than does any other postgastrectomy syndrome.

The presence of symptoms means that bilious intestinal contents are coming into contact with the gastric mucosa. For such contact to occur, the pylorus must be destroyed, resected, or bypassed. The incidence of alkaline reflux gastritis is highest after a Billroth II anastomosis and is much less frequent after a Billroth I anastomosis or after truncal vagotomy and drainage. It is important to note, however, that the magnitude of reflux has not been demonstrated to be any greater after gastrojejunostomy than after gastroduodenostomy. Almost no cases of reflux have been reported after HSV.

Although the exact mechanisms of the production of alkaline reflux gastritis are unknown, the unifying concept is that the gastric mucosa must contact bilious intestinal material. Several mechanisms, acting alone or in combination, may result in excessive volume of refluxate, altered composition of refluxate, inadequate clearance of refluxate, or impairment in gastric mucosal defense mechanisms. Several studies have demonstrated that the magnitude of reflux is greater for postgastrectomy patients with symptoms than for those without symptoms (89–91). Studies analyzing the concentration and composition of bile salts have shown that patients with symptoms have a higher total bile acid concentration and a higher concentration of deoxycholic acid than patients without symptoms (92,93). Studies of gastric emptying have yielded inconsistent results.

The components of upper intestinal content that have received the most attention are the bile acids. Colic acid and chenodeoxycholic acid, the primary bile acids, are synthesized in the liver, whereas deoxycholic and lithocolic acid, the secondary bile acids, are formed in the colon by the action of colonic bacteria. These bacteria can also deconjugate both primary and secondary bile acids. Bile acids are toxic to the gastric mucosa: secondary acids are more toxic than primary and deconjugated acids are more toxic than conjugated. This fact is important because, after operations for peptic ulcer disease, patients commonly experience hypoacidity and gastric stasis, which permit bacterial overgrowth (94). These bacteria then produce deconjugated, secondary bile acids, which are most injurious to the gastric mucosa. Pancreatic secretions have been less well investigated. Studies have shown that lysolecithin and phospholipase A2 cause severe mucosal damage in vitro; others have shown that the combination of bile and pancreatic juice is more toxic than bile alone (95,96).

The diagnosis of alkaline reflux gastritis is made by exclusion. Recurrent ulcer, gastroparesis, afferent or efferent loop obstruction, and diseases of the gallbladder and pancreas must be ruled out. Endoscopic examination with biopsy of the mucosa is the most useful diagnostic procedure. It can rule out recurrent ulcer and afferent loop syndrome, both of which are included in the differential diagnosis of bilious vomiting. Grossly, the gastric mucosa is characterized by marked hyperemia and bile staining. Superficial gastritis and ulcerations usually involve the entire gastric remnant, but these findings are most profound along the lesser curvature. Histologically, the characteristic changes observed include a decrease in the number of or the complete absence of both parietal cells and chief cells, along with an increase in the number of mucin-secreting cells; ulcerations and atrophic changes of the superficial mucosa; accumulation of chronic inflammatory cells in the submucosa of the gastric glands; distorted gland anatomy; and intestinal metaplasia. The severity of symptoms does not correlate with the extent of histologic change, however. An upper GI barium study is often performed, but it is rarely helpful in making the diagnosis. It is useful in defining postoperative anatomy and in excluding other causes of symptoms, including recurrent ulcer and obstruction.

Documentation and quantification of reflux into the stomach may be assessed by HIDA scan with cholecystokinin administration. The patient is given a radiolabeled hepatocystic agent; when radioactivity is maximal over the hepatobiliary tree, the patient is given cholecystokinin, and radioactivity is monitored over the liver, gallbladder, biliary tree, small bowel, and gastric remnant. Additionally, intragastric infusion of alkaline solution as a provocative test appears to be helpful both in diagnosis and in determining which patients may benefit from surgery. The test consists of blind, sequential instillation into the stomach of standardized volumes of saline, 0.1 N HCl, and 0.1 N NaOH. A positive response is defined as a reproduction of symptoms by NaOH but not by the other solutions. In one series of 147 patients, a four-year follow-up showed that a positive response to the test was associated with benefit from surgery and that a negative response to the test was associated with a lack of benefit from surgery; the predictive accuracy was 75% to 85% (97).

Medical management generally has been ineffective. Nonetheless, a trial of medical therapy is warranted, and the occasional patient may be adequately treated. Cholestyramine has been used because of the assumption that bile acids are the cause of the gastritis. Antacids containing aluminum hydroxide have also been used because they bind bile acids and lysolecithin. Sucralfate has been shown to protect rat gastric mucosa from bile acids; in one human study, it substantially decreased gastric inflammation. However, this finding was not associated with any improvement in symptoms (98). Various promotility agents and antibiotics have been tried without much effect. In contrast, adding the bile acid ursodeoxycholic acid to a patient's diet has shown some success in relieving mild symptoms. The concentration of "nontoxic" ursodeoxycholic acid increased by 40%, whereas the concentrations of "toxic" cholic, deoxycholic, chenodeoxycholic, and lithocholic acids decreased by 25% to 50% (99).

The goal of surgical treatment is to divert duodenal contents away from the gastric remnant. The procedure most often used is the Roux-en-Y gastrojejunostomy, which creates a 45-cm roux limb. If vagotomy has not been previously performed, it should be performed at the time of the roux operation so that the formation of a marginal ulcer can be prevented. Other alternatives are the interposition of an isoperistaltic jejunal segment between the residual stomach and intestine, and the Roux-en-Y Tanner-19 gastrojejunostomy, in which the proximal end of the afferent limb is anastomosed to the roux limb, thereby forming a small, circular route for the passage of chyme. No advantages have been shown with any these procedures, however. Each is effective in virtually eliminating reflux into the gastric remnant, and all yield good short-term results. Unfortunately, longer follow-up shows that bilious emesis is the only symptom that is consistently relieved. Epigastric pain can recur in as many as 30% of cases, and nausea and vomiting can recur in as many as 50% (91). The causes of such recurrences are unknown.

A potential problem is the development of delayed gastric emptying of solids; this problem causes early satiety, epigastric pain, and nonbilious vomiting, a constellation of symptoms that has been termed the *roux stasis syndrome* (discussed later). There is evidence that patients with delayed gastric emptying preoperatively may be at increased risk of this syndrome. Preoperative assessment of gastric emptying may be helpful in determining which patients are at high risk; the addition of subtotal gastrectomy to the reconstruction procedure may speed gastric emptying during the postoperative period.

Loop Syndromes

The loop syndromes require the presence of an afferent or efferent limb and can occur only after a Billroth II or a Roux-en-Y anastomosis. Either the afferent or the efferent limb may become obstructed, and both types of obstruction can present with either an acute and complete obstruction or a chronic partial obstruction. Afferent limb obstruction is more common and is usually due to anatomic factors. Known causes are internal herniation of the small intestine, volvulus of the loop, and kinking at the anastomosis. Each is thought to occur more frequently when the anastomosis is antecolic or is positioned along the lesser curvature or when the afferent limb is too long (>10–15 cm). Because surgeons have become more cognizant of underlying causes, the loop syndromes, once more common, now occur among fewer than 1% of patients (100).

Acute afferent limb obstruction is the most common cause of duodenal stump blowout and constitutes a surgical emergency. It most commonly appears within the first or second postoperative week and results from complete obstruction of the afferent limb. Biliary and pancreatic secretions accumulate within the limb. As the pressure rises, the pancreatic and biliary ducts are obstructed, and necrosis of the intestinal wall may occur. Patients complain of severe epigastric or left upper quadrant pain that increases in severity and is followed by nausea and vomiting. Serum amylase activity is typically elevated, and physical examination, radiography, or ultrasonography may indicate an abdominal mass. An intraoperative finding may be necrosis of the limb. If only the distal portion is involved, the limb may be resected and a Roux-en-Y anastomosis fashioned. Involvement of the duodenal portion of the limb necessitates a pancreaticoduodenectomy. Volvulus is prone to recurrence, and any redundancy in the limb should be resected. The retroanastomotic space and all mesenteric defects should be closed so that recurrence of hernias can be avoided.

Chronic afferent limb obstruction results from partial obstruction of the limb. Additional anatomic factors are anastomotic stricture, extrinsic compression by adhesions or carcinoma, recurrent ulceration, gastric remnant carcinoma, scarring of the opening of the mesocolon after a retrocolic anastomosis, or jejunogastric intussusception (although this is rare). Symptoms include nausea, right upper quadrant pain brought on by meals, and bilious vomiting, possibly projectile, which is not mixed with food and which quickly relieves the pain. Stasis in the loop may result in a "blind loop syndrome," with bacterial overgrowth, bile salt deconjugation, steatorrhea, vitamin B12 deficiency, and diarrhea. Patients consciously or unconsciously avoid food and typically lose weight.

Clinical history is extremely helpful in diagnosing afferent loop obstruction; however, alkaline reflux gastritis must be ruled out. The results of routine radiologic studies are usually normal because the limb generally obstructs only as it distends. CT scanning and ultrasonography are helpful, but endoscopy is the method of choice. Endoscopy allows direct visualization of the anastomosis and biopsy of any pathologic lesions. Once the diagnosis has been made, surgery is warranted. A Billroth II anastomosis may be converted to a Billroth I or, alternatively, a Roux-en-Y anastomosis.

Obstruction of the efferent loop is less common and is most frequently caused by a retroanastomotic hernia. Other causes of obstruction are adhesions, fibrotic stenosis, and jejunogastric intussusception. Efferent loop obstruction also exists in acute and chronic forms, but the acute form is more common. Symptoms consist of colicky abdominal pain, nausea, and bilious vomiting (with food). A diagnosis of chronic efferent loop obstruction is confirmed by radiography, which shows delayed emptying across a point of obstruction in the efferent limb. Surgical treatment is mandated. The specific therapy depends on the cause and may include lysis of adhesions, reduction of hernias, closure of anatomic defects, revision of the anastomosis, or conversion to a Billroth I or Roux-en-Y anastomosis.

Chronic Gastric Atony and the Roux Stasis Syndrome

Chronic gastric atony is characterized by nausea, vomiting, epigastric pain, postprandial bloating, and frequent bezoar formation. Patients cannot tolerate solids but can usually tolerate liquids, and they intuitively change their diets. The cause is believed to be a loss of gastric vagal innervation, and the incidence depends on the type of vagotomy performed. The incidence of delayed gastric emptying is higher after less selective vagotomies (101). Both the postprandial peristaltic antral contractions and the tonic contractions of the proximal stomach in the late phases of gastric emptying are under vagal control.

The assessment of the patient with chronic gastric atony must exclude mechanical causes of obstruction. The results of upper GI series are most often read as normal but may show a distended, flaccid gastric remnant. Endoscopic examination confirms the absence of any obstruction. Scintigraphic testing reveals severe, delayed gastric emptying of solids. Medical treatment is based on the use of prokinetic drugs. Intermittent or chronic gastric decompression may be necessary, in conjunction with nutritional support and weaning from exacerbating drugs. Prokinetic agents used include bethanechol, metaclopramide, domperidone, cisapride, and erythromycin. Reported success rates vary widely, but, overall, roughly 30% to 40% of patients experience limited relief of symptoms. Surgical therapy aims at decreasing the reservoir capacity of the stomach; the most common procedure is near-total gastrectomy with a Roux-en-Y gastrojejunostomy (with a 45-cm roux limb).

Distinguishing the elements of the roux stasis syndrome from those of gastric atony is extremely difficult; the symptoms are equivalent. In fact, the existence of roux stasis syndrome as an entity separate from gastric atony has been questioned. However, the fact that the roux stasis syndrome has been documented after total gastrectomy and esophagojejunostomy provides evidence that the creation of a roux limb does increase the risk of delayed gastric emptying. Additionally, transit through the roux limb itself has been measured scintigraphically and found to be slowed (102). Although their relative contributions to stasis are unclear, both the vagotomized gastric remnant and the roux limb play a role. Although prior studies have reported incidences ranging from 10% to 50%, two more recent reviews have placed the incidence at 27% to 33% (103). Several subsets of patients appear to be at particular risk of this condition: those with substantial delays in gastric emptying preoperatively, those with a large residual pouch, and those in whom a long roux limb is created.

Investigations into the cause of the roux syndrome have revealed several possible mechanisms by which the roux limb may delay gastric emptying. However, they have yielded conflicting data on the relative role of vagotomy or intrinsic myoelectric abnormalities in causing this delay. The most important finding was the reversal of the pacemaker potential within the limb, a reversal that results in retrograde contractions (104,105). Furthermore, the interdigestive migrating motor complexes, periodic peristaltic contractions that normally perform a "housekeeping" function by sweeping the bowel clear of residual foodstuff, occur at a higher frequency, are irregular, and do not propagate normally within the limb (106,107).

Another abnormality noted in the roux limb is the lack of conversion from a fasting to a fed pattern after the ingestion of food (102,108). It has been hypothesized that transection of the jejunum, required in constructing the roux limb, disturbs the normal conduction of pacemaker potentials from the duodenum distally. This disturbance leads to the development of ectopic pacemakers within the limb, and these pacemakers cause the observed myoelectric abnormalities. Alternatively, vagal denervation may be the underlying cause. Strong evidence for this alternative cause is provided by the study of patients who have undergone gastric bypass, in which a roux limb is constructed with preservation of vagal input. In these patients, the jejunal pacesetter potential is normal and is propagated in an aboral direction, and the interdigestive migrating myoelectric complex activity is normal.

Evaluation and medical treatment of the patient with possible roux stasis are the same as those of the patient with gastric atony. The most important issue is ruling out mechanical causes of obstruction. Upper GI series and endoscopy are helpful in this regard, and *scintigraphic* studies can document delayed emptying in the gastric remnant, in the roux limb, or in both. Medical therapy is seldom successful. Surgical therapy usually involves a near-total gastrectomy and adjustment of the limb length to 40 cm; this procedure is successful in 70% to 80% of patients (109). The fact that further gastric resection often relieves symptoms is the strongest evidence that the primary component of this syndrome is gastric atony.

As a means of preventing the roux stasis syndrome, the "uncut roux" gastroenterostomy has been developed (110). A loop gastrojejunostomy is formed, and the afferent limb is occluded with staples. The staples prevent the flow of pancreatic and biliary secretions across the gastrojejunostomy but allow normal propagation of pacemaker potentials. Proximal to the staple line, the afferent and efferent limbs are anastomosed; this anastomosis allows the flow of chyme. Canine studies have been promising, but postoperative staple line dehiscence remains a problem (111). Several canine studies examining the use of GI pacing in the treatment of dumping (to slow emptying) and roux stasis (to speed emptying) showed promising results (112,113). However, the results of human trials have been disappointing.

Small Gastric Remnant Syndrome

The small gastric remnant syndrome is also characterized by early satiety, bloating, epigastric pain soon after eating, and vomiting. It is caused by loss of the reservoir function of the stomach as the result of resection, vagotomy, or both. This syndrome is most prevalent after operations that remove 80% or more of the stomach (114). Symptoms are usually mild but can be severe enough to cause weight loss, malnutrition, and anemia.

Diagnosis is based primarily on clinical history, but mechanical obstruction must be ruled out. Dietary management consisting of frequent, small meals and the addition of vitamins, iron, and pancreatic enzymes is successful in most patients. Some patients may benefit from antispasmodic agents. Surgery is reserved for patients with severe symptoms who are resistant to dietary and medical management. Several complicated pouches have been devised in an attempt to restore the reservoir function of the gastric remnant. The Tanner Roux-19 pouch and the Hunt-Lawrence pouch are used most frequently; both involve creation of a Roux-en-Y gastrojejunostomy. In the Tanner-19 pouch procedure, the end of the afferent limb is anastomosed to the roux limb to form a loop reservoir. In the Hunt-Lawrence pouch procedure, the afferent and efferent limbs are anastomosed side-to-side just distal to the gastrojejunostomy to form a pouch. Although these procedures yield satisfactory results for approximately 50% of patients, they may be complicated by the development of stasis, dilation, and ulceration in the limbs and pouches, and they should be used only as a last resort.

Recurrent Ulcer

Duodenal, gastric, or jejunal ulcers that occur after corrective surgery for peptic ulcer disease are known as recurrent ulcers, stomal ulcers, or marginal ulcers. Together with alkaline reflux gastritis, they are the leading cause of unsatisfactory long-term postoperative results. The most common symptom of recurrent ulcer is pain, usually similar to the original ulcer pain, which is reported by 80% to 95% of patients (115,116). However, it is difficult to distinguish this pain from the pain that accompanies several other postgastrectomy syndromes. GI blood loss is common; it occurs among 40% to 60% of patients and is more than twice as common than the blood loss that occurs among patients who initially present with peptic ulcer disease and do not undergo surgery (117,118). The bleeding usually is occult, but massive bleeding is not rare. Perforation is uncommon; recurrent ulcers at a gastrojejunostomy site may penetrate into the colon and form a gastrojejunocolic fistula. Patients experience diarrhea, weight loss, and feculent vomiting but usually have little pain. Weight loss, nausea, and vomiting are other frequent findings. Recurrent ulcer, once a common complication, is extremely rare now that most anastomoses are retrocolic. Recurrence in the pyloric channel, in the duodenum, or at a gastrojejunal anastomosis can lead to gastric outlet obstruction.

The first diagnostic test for evaluating a patient's symptoms is endoscopy. A barium upper GI series is useful in defining anatomic relations and in assessing the adequacy of gastric drainage, but the results of this study are unreliable in the diagnosis of ulcer. Normal postoperative changes are frequently misinterpreted as ulcers, and, conversely, many recurrent ulcers are missed. Most ulcers occur within 2 cm of the GI anastomosis and are seen on endoscopy; the accuracy rate of endoscopy in the diagnosis of this condition approaches 90% (115,116). When a recurrent ulcer has been diagnosed, the underlying cause must be determined. Most recurrent ulcers will respond to standard medical therapy. Some rare causes, however, prevent such a response and require specific treatments; these causes must be excluded before therapy is initiated.

The leading cause of recurrent ulcer in nearly 60% of cases is an inadequate or inappropriate operation; no identifiable cause is found in the remaining cases (116). Inadequate vagotomy is the most common identified cause and is found in as many as one-third of cases. Vagal anatomy is highly variable, and nearly 12% of persons have more than two vagal trunks (119). Most intact vagal fibers that are found at reoperation are on the right side of the esophagus or in the posterior paraesophageal tissues, including those supplying the upper fundus (the criminal nerve of Grassi) (115,120). In the past, inadequate gastric resection was a common cause of recurrent ulcer, but gastric resection without a vagotomy is rarely performed today. Inadequate resection of antral tissue, which can extend one or more centimeters into the duodenum, can result in the retained antrum syndrome, a rare but highly ulcerogenic cause of recurrence. The retained antral tissue is constantly exposed to an alkaline pH because an absence of gastric acid in the duodenal stump results in continuous hypersecretion of gastrin from the mucosa. Other rare causes are antral G-cell hyperplasia, Zollinger–Ellison syndrome, foreign body (stitch) ulcer, and gastric cancer. Contributing factors include ulcerogenic drugs, smoking, delayed gastric emptying, enterogastric reflux, bezoar, and primary hyperparathyroidism.

Three diagnostic tests establish the cause of recurrent ulcer in most cases: endoscopy, determination of the serum calcium concentration, and determination of the serum gastrin concentration. For patients with gastric ulcer, aspirin concentrations should be determined so that aspirin abuse can be ruled out. Initial endoscopy, in addition to visualizing the ulcer, may exclude causes such as gastric outlet obstruction, gastric bezoar, silk suture, and enterogastric reflux. If a gastric ulcer is present, biopsy may be able to exclude gastric cancer. Furthermore, if an afferent limb is present, biopsy of the duodenal stump may exclude retained antral tissue. Because patients with hyperparathyroidism are at increased risk of peptic ulcer, the calcium concentration should be determined for all patients with recurrent ulcer.

The serum gastrin concentration should be determined for all patients with recurrent ulcer. A concentration greater than 1000 pg/mL is virtually diagnostic of Zollinger–Ellison syndrome, whereas a normal serum concentration excludes the diagnosis except in rare cases (121). The fasting serum gastrin concentrations of patients with retained antrum syndrome are typically two to four times above the normal range (122). Delayed gastric emptying caused by obstruction or gastric atony may result in hypergastrinemia due to retained food; gastrin concentrations should decrease after the evacuation of the stomach, thus excluding this cause. Elevated gastrin concentrations due to H2 or proton pump blockers should decrease within 24 hours of discontinuing the drug.

The differential diagnosis for a modest elevation of gastrin concentration also includes Zollinger–Ellison syndrome, retained antrum, postvagotomy hypergastrinemia, and antral G-cell hyperplasia. Postvagotomy hypergastrinemia results in modest elevations of the gastrin concentration; such elevated concentrations, usually less than twice the normal limit, occur among 30% to 40% of patients postoperatively. Antral G-cell hyperplasia, also called antral G-cell hyperfunction and pseudo–Zollinger–Ellison syndrome, is an extremely rare condition causing fasting hypergastrinemia and acid hypersecretion in the absence of gastrinoma (123). Provocative gastrin testing with secretin is indicated for these patients. For patients with Zollinger–Ellison syndrome, the injection of secretin will cause an increase of more than 100 pg/mL in the gastrin concentration (124,125), whereas gastrin concentrations among postvagotomy patients usually remain at baseline or increase minimally. Gastrin concentrations among patients with retained antrum and G-cell hyperplasia may increase after the injection of secretin but usually increase by less than 100 pg/mL. For patients with equivocal results of secretin stimulation, meal stimulation may be indicated. A standard high-protein meal results in marked increases in the gastrin concentration among patients with retained antrum or G-cell hyperplasia. Technetium pertechnetate antral scans may aid in diagnosing retained antrum among patients with recurrent ulcer who have undergone antrectomy (126,127). Although studies have reported that the specificity of these scans is as high as 100%, assessing these results is difficult because the diagnosis is very rare.

If one of these diagnoses is made, the therapy specific to the diagnosis is instituted. The stitch is removed from a stitch ulcer. Retained antrum can be cured by resecting the cuff of antral tissue at the end of the afferent limb. Antral G-cell hyperplasia responds to antrectomy. A diagnosis of hyperparathyroidism requires parathyroidectomy; multiple endocrine neoplasia (MEN) syndromes should also be excluded. Therapy for gastric cancer depends on its stage. If Zollinger–Ellison syndrome is diagnosed, the patient must undergo additional tests aimed at determining whether operative intervention is required. Operation is indicated for patients with sporadic, nonmetastatic gastrinoma and for those who have gastrinoma and cannot tolerate or are resistant to medical management. Medical therapy alone is indicated for patients who have gastrinoma associated with MEN syndrome and for patients with metastatic gastrinoma.

This initial evaluation will exclude most rare causes of recurrent ulcer that require specific treatment. Most of the remaining cases are probably due to incomplete vagotomy, and most can be successfully treated with medical therapy. Tests of vagal integrity measure acid secretion. At this point, these tests do not provide useful findings because most ulcers respond to medical therapy regardless of the result. These tests should be reserved for use when medical treatment fails and surgery is anticipated. In such cases, tests are helpful in documenting persistent vagal innervation and may aid the surgeon in selecting the type of reoperation to be performed.

Several tests can measure gastric acid secretion. The first is measurement of basal acid output, followed by stimulation with gastrin or pentagastrin and measurement of peak acid output. This test determines parietal cell function rather than vagal innervation; aside from excluding achlorydia, it provides little information about the cause of recurrence and hence is not the test of choice. The Hollander test uses hypoglycemia to test the completeness of vagotomy. Central nervous system hypoglycemia activates vagal nuclei, which stimulate acid secretion by vagal pathways. However, the acid secretion stimulated by the Hollander test is not solely vagally mediated. Furthermore, hypoglycemia among the elderly or among patients with coronary artery disease may cause arrhythmia, myocardial infarction, or even death. The Hollander test is rarely used today because of its inaccuracy and associated morbidity.

Several studies have found that sham feeding, which stimulates acid secretion solely via vagal pathways, is a reproducible test of vagal function (115,128). It involves measurement of basal acid output, followed by sham feeding and measurement of sham acid output. The patient chews the food but then expectorates it into a basin. After sham feeding, pentagastrin is administered and peak acid output is measured. The residual vagal innervation of the stomach can be determined by calculating the ratio of sham acid output to peak acid output. As can be imagined, patient compliance with this test is low. Furthermore, the test is prone to false positives when the peak output is very low or when a hypergastrinemic state is present; false-negative results are common in the presence of alkaline reflux. Measurement of pancreatic polypeptide combined with sham feeding has also been used as a test of vagal integrity. Congo red, a nontoxic, inexpensive azine dye that turns from red to black at a pH below 3, may also be used to determine vagal innervation of the stomach (129,130). Congo red may be used preoperatively, intraoperatively, or postoperatively; vagally innervated mucosa stains black, whereas vagotomized tissue remains red. Because excessive sedation may produce false-negative results, the test should be performed with as little sedation as possible; this requirement limits patient acceptance. Furthermore, hypergastrinemia invalidates results.

Medical therapy is indicated for patients with uncomplicated recurrent ulcers who have no evidence of hypersecretory state or gastric outlet obstruction. Studies show that standard doses of H2 blockers will heal approximately 80% of recurrent ulcers (131,132). A typical regimen involves treatment with proton pump inhibitors until healing is documented endoscopically. Maintenance therapy, consisting of a nocturnal dose of H2 blockers, is then instituted. Discontinuation of antiulcer therapy is usually associated with rapid recurrence, and lifetime maintenance is generally required. It is also mandatory that ulcerogenic drugs, cigarette smoking, and perhaps even alcohol use be discontinued.

Surgery is indicated if the recurrent ulcer does not heal after three months of medical therapy; if the ulcer recurs within one year despite maintenance therapy; if the ulcer disease is characterized by cycles of prolonged activity with brief or absent remissions, so that lifestyle is severely affected; or if the patient cannot comply with medical therapy. When decisions are made about which procedure to use, factors such as the original surgery, the overall health status of the patient, and the underlying cause should be taken into account. To this end, all patients should undergo preoperative vagotomy testing. Gastric emptying studies also are helpful in determining whether impaired motility is part of the cause.

If test results demonstrate an incomplete vagotomy with adequate drainage, revagotomy is indicated. Most surgeons also recommend gastric resection if it was not part of the original procedure. If impaired motility is demonstrated, the resection should be generous, leaving a small gastric remnant. However, if excessive morbidity is anticipated, transthoracic revagotomy alone provides good results. If alkaline reflux is believed to be the underlying cause, the Roux-en-Y gastrojejunostomy may be used. If gastric emptying studies show delay, a generous gastric resection should be employed, and a complete vagotomy should be ensured so that stomal ulceration can be avoided.

Gastric Remnant Carcinoma

It has been postulated that gastric surgery for benign disease increases the risk of subsequent gastric cancer. Although the relationship remains tenuous, evidence suggests that the risk of cancer is increased approximately two- to fourfold after a latency period of 15 years. The association has been noted in all types of gastric surgery, including those that do not include a gastric resection, e.g., truncal vagotomy with drainage (133). Some studies suggest that the risk of gastric remnant carcinoma is even higher after a Billroth II anastomosis (134,135).

The most frequent symptoms of this carcinoma are epigastric pain, fullness, vomiting, dysphagia, weight loss, upper GI bleeding, weakness, obstruction, and diarrhea. Because these are similar to the symptoms produced by recurrent ulcer or by several other postgastrectomy syndromes, the diagnosis of carcinoma is difficult. Given the long latency period of gastric cancer, the diagnosis should be strongly suspected when new GI complaints occur among patients who have experienced years with no symptoms. Frequently, patients will be seen with nonspecific complaints and physical findings that respond to medical treatment, presumably because of partial healing of the malignant ulceration. The diagnosis usually is made on the basis of endoscopy with biopsy. Surgical treatment is mandated; however, the results are not as good as those for patients who have not undergone prior gastric surgery.

NUTRITIONAL CONSEQUENCES OF GASTRIC SURGERY

Nutritional deficiencies are common after gastric surgery. These deficiencies are aggravated by the postprandial symptoms often experienced by patients who have undergone gastric surgery. Failure to sustain an adequate intake of food because of the desire to avoid these symptoms worsens the malnutrition that arises from disturbances of digestion. Furthermore, these disturbances in digestion may enhance satiety, which also decreases food intake. Commonly encountered nutritional impairments are maldigestion and malabsorption of polymeric foods, sustained underweight, abnormal satiety, iron deficiency, and osteomalacia.

Postgastrectomy malabsorption is caused primarily by maldigestion in the intestinal lumen. The function of the intestinal mucosa is normal. Absorption of salt, water, and monomeric nutrients such as glucose and fatty acids is not impaired (136). This maldigestion is caused by alterations in digestive balance resulting from gastric operations. The term *digestive balance* refers to the optimal ratio of substrate and enzyme required to maximize digestion and absorption within the available length of bowel. The main factors involved in this balance are entry of enzymes, duodenal entry of substrate, and time or distance of contact with absorptive mechanisms along the intestinal length (137). Gastric operations commonly affect the first two of these factors.

The secretion of pancreatic enzymes is maximal during the first postcibal hour and then declines over the next several hours. Billroth I and II anastomoses and total gastrectomies, although they do not substantially reduce the overall secretion of pancreatic enzymes, eliminate this early peak, presumably through disruption of a gastropancreatic reflex (138). In addition, total gastrectomies and Billroth II anastomoses delay contact between enzyme and substrate because the initial secretion is held in an afferent loop. Truncal vagotomy with pyloroplasty reduces pancreatic secretions by 30% to 50%, whereas truncal vagotomy with antrectomy reduces them by 50% to 70% (138–140). Pancreatic secretion is normal after HSV (141).

Gastric procedures have a much larger effect on the duodenal entry of substrates than on the secretion of pancreatic enzymes. Gastric emptying of liquids is consistently accelerated because of the mechanisms previously discussed. Gastric emptying of solids is more variable. However, the problem is not only the abnormal transit of food but also the impaired trituration and defective sieving that often accompany gastric procedures. These problems allow abnormally large, poorly digestible foodstuff to enter the duodenum. However, these observations alone do not fully account for the patterns of malabsorption that are seen after various procedures. Steatorrhea follows any procedure that destroys or bypasses the pylorus or resects all or part of the stomach. On the other hand, malabsorption of nitrogen (azotorrhea) is rare. This selective malabsorption of fat may be explained by the fact that the half-life of pancreatic lipase is shorter than that of protease. This shorter half-life allows for greater digestion and absorption of protein during intestinal transit. In addition, steatorrhea is aggravated in the presence of an afferent loop or a Roux-en-Y anastomosis because of the initial sequestration of pancreatic output.

All operations for ulcer disease, with the notable exception of HSV, lead to substantial underweight among patients. Underweight occurs whether or not a gastric resection has been performed, and the amount of weight loss is similar whether patients have undergone a resective operation or nonresective therapy with a truncal vagotomy (142,143). The amount of weight loss correlates most closely with reduced intake of food rather than with malabsorption, as measured by steatorrhea (144,145). This reduced intake of food may be due to inappropriate satiety after gastric operations. Loss of gastric volume through resection, the *small stomach syndrome*, is not sufficient to account for increased satiety. The extent of resection correlates poorly with satiety and with weight loss. Studies have shown that a reduction in volume of more than 90% is needed to produce a high level of satiety.

It is known that nutrient sensors in the stomach and small intestine can induce feelings of satiety. It is possible that, as increasing lengths of small intestine are used for digestion because of the maldigestive mechanisms discussed above, more of these sensors come into contact with digestive products, thereby causing enhanced satiety. This theory is controversial; however, evidence supporting it is provided by the fact that HSV, which does not produce alterations in pancreatic secretion, emptying of solids, or gastric sieving, rarely produces increased satiety (146,147). Additional evidence is provided by comparing the outcomes of gastroplasty with those of gastric bypass.

Although gastroplasty produces a greater loss of gastric volume, gastric bypass, which causes defects similar to those found in resective gastric therapies, is more successful in causing decreased food intake and weight loss (148). In patients experiencing postcibal symptoms, aversive conditioning to avoid these uncomfortable symptoms also probably contributes to diminished food intake. Weight loss and diminished intake are difficult to treat. Patients are advised to eat small, frequent meals, which serve to keep pancreatic secretions flowing and to limit the speed of gastric emptying.

Mild-to-moderate anemias are common after gastric surgery. Iron deficiency is the most common cause; it results in a hypochromic, microcytic anemia. This condition is seen after both resective and nonresective therapies. Folate and vitamin B12 concentrations may also decrease after gastric operations; such decreases cause a mixed anemia (hypochromic, microcytic with a macrocytic component). Pure macrocytic anemias are rare except after total gastrectomy. Because of complete loss of intrinsic factor, vitamin B12 deficiency follows total gastrectomy. Parenteral administration of vitamin B12 is required so that pernicious anemia can be avoided. Because intrinsic factor is produced in great excess, resections less than a total gastrectomy rarely cause decreases in vitamin B12 concentrations that are severe enough to cause clinical symptoms.

Folate deficiency occasionally contributes to a mixed anemia. The primary dietary sources of folate are high-fiber vegetables and organ meats, foods typically avoided by postsurgical patients who experience increased satiety. Folate is primarily absorbed in the proximal small intestine, and this absorption is highly dependent on an acidic pH. Thus, folate absorption is impaired among patients with hypochloremia. Dietary iron is consumed primarily as ferric compounds within solid food or as ferrous iron complexed with heme. Ferric iron must be dissolved in gastric acid and reduced to ferrous iron if it is to be efficiently absorbed. All surgical procedures used to treat peptic ulceration reduce gastric acid secretion and impair iron absorption. However because the absorption of heme iron increases as the pH increases, this process acts as a complementary pathway for iron absorption. Absorption is most efficient in the duodenum; however, at times of deficiency, more distal segments of bowel may increase their iron absorption efficiency. Deficiencies in iron, folate, or vitamin B12 respond well to replacement. Iron should be given in the ferrous form, and tablets should be crushed so that they can be better absorbed.

Gastric resection accelerates the process of osteoporosis, and this acceleration becomes more pronounced with time after surgery (149,150). This process is faster after total gastrectomy than after subtotal gastrectomy, and it is only minimally affected after vagotomies without resection (151,152). There appear to be no differences in the speed of this process after Billroth I or II anastomoses (153). Patients with osteoporosis also often experience osteomalacia. Postoperative concentrations of vitamin D are usually within the normal range, as is the absorption of calcium. The principal dietary source of calcium is dairy products. An inadequate intake of calcium because of a desire to avoid the symptoms of postoperative lactose intolerance may play a role in bone disease; however, this factor does not explain the absence of bone disease after nonresective therapies. At this time, the cause is unknown. Calcium and vitamin D supplements have been prescribed to prevent postoperative bone disease; however, their effectiveness has not been documented.

GASTROESOPHAGEAL REFLUX DISEASE

Gastroesophageal reflux is a normal physiologic occurrence. However, when these episodes cause symptoms or histologic changes within the esophagus, the diagnosis of gastroesophageal reflux disease (GERD) is made. The most common symptom is heartburn, usually made worse by lying down. Atypical symptoms include noncardiac chest pain, asthma, hoarseness, dysphagia, or odynophagia. Hematemesis and melena may be seen with severe disease.

In the diagnostic workup of GERD, radiology is helpful in defining the anatomy and may diagnose the presence of a hiatal hernia. Although barium studies may be able to document gastric and esophageal abnormalities, such abnormalities are not usually present unless the disease is moderate or severe. In addition, the reflux of barium into the esophagus does not diagnose the disease because such reflux is often seen among persons without GERD. Endoscopy has become the gold standard for biopsy and diagnosis because it allows direct visualization of ulcers, strictures, and metaplasia. Motility studies are used to document the presence and degree of esophageal dysmotility. Twenty-four–hour pH monitoring will precisely measure the amount, timing, and frequency of reflux, and will allow correlation of these episodes with the presence of symptoms. Bile reflux also may be measured by using the same technique.

For patients with mild or occasional symptoms, symptomatic treatment and lifestyle changes are often successful in alleviating the problem. Patients are encouraged to avoid foods known to decrease the tone of the lower esophageal sphincter, as well as to avoid cigarettes and alcohol. Sleeping with the head elevated helps gravity to clear any refluxate. Antacids will often provide immediate relief of symptoms but do not address the underlying cause. For more severe disease, initial medical therapy is warranted. H2 blockers are effective in relieving symptoms and healing esophagitis among more than 50% of patients after 6 to 12 weeks of treatment (154). For more severe disease that is unresponsive to treatment with H2 blockers, proton pump inhibitors are effective. However, these medications do not address the underlying cause of the disease, and lifelong therapy is required.

Laparoscopic surgery has added a new dimension to the treatment of GERD. Previously, surgery was deemed necessary only when medical intervention failed. Today, although most patients are adequately treated by medical therapy, laparoscopic antireflux surgery is often performed because it avoids the need for and cost of lifelong therapy and the unknown effects of lifelong acid suppression. Open surgery for GERD has been well characterized since being first described by Nissen in 1956. This technique has undergone many modifications since its introduction, and the debate continues as to which procedure yields the best outcome with the lowest rates of morbidity and mortality. The aim of all of these procedures is to restore normal anatomy by restoring an intra-abdominal segment of the esophagus, recreating an appropriate high-pressure zone at the esophagogastric junction, and maintaining this repair in a normal position (154). Most of the debate centers on the use of a full or a partial fundoplication. The Nissan procedure uses a full fundoplication, whereas the Belsey Mark IV fundoplication and Toupet, Dor, Hill, and Lind procedures use a partial fundoplication. Good to excellent results have been reported for all of these procedures. The decision about which procedure to use should be tailored to the individual patient's underlying pathophysiology.

In cases of severe disease, the esophagus is often shortened by stricture or periesophageal inflammation. This shortening may preclude the restoration of an adequate length of intra-abdominal esophagus without undue tension. In such cases, standard antireflux procedures have an unacceptably high failure rate. The Collis gastroplasty involves fashioning the lesser curvature into a tube that is used to elongate the esophagus. A full or partial fundoplication is then added to complete the procedure.

The laparoscopic Nissan fundoplication is the most commonly performed antireflux procedure. The fundamental benefits of laparoscopy are the reduction of postoperative morbidity and the shortening of hospital stay. In particular, these benefits relate to the smaller incisions made possible by laparoscopy, which lead to less splinting and fewer respiratory complications, and to the reduced retraction and manipulation of abdominal viscera, which result in earlier return of function. However, minimal access does not mean minimal risk. Most of the risks associated with antireflux surgery are the same whether the procedure is open or laparoscopic. Intraoperative complications common to both include splenic tears from excessive traction, esophageal injury from excessive dissection at the hiatus or from passage of a large bougie used to calibrate the fundoplication, and GI perforation. However, some risks are unique to the laparoscopic procedure. For example, CO_2 pneumoperitoneum causes hemodynamic and pulmonary effects, probably because of increased intra-abdominal pressure and the physiologic effects of absorbed CO_2. These effects are transient and are unlikely to affect patients with normal or minimally disturbed cardiac and pulmonary function. However, these effects must be kept in mind when patients have cardiac or lung disease. In addition, the pressure of CO_2 insufflation may cause self-dissection of planes, resulting in the risk of pneumothorax or pneumomediastinum and increasing the risk of stomach migrating into the thorax. Other inherent features of laparoscopy that may precipitate complications include altered visibility, reduced tactile sensation, and limited instrument movement. Specifically, laparoscopic repair is associated with a higher incidence of paraesophageal hiatus hernia, dysphagia, GI perforation, and unrecognized complications (155).

The increased incidence of paraesophageal herniation may be caused by a tendency to extend esophageal dissection further into the thorax than would be done in an open procedure or by the self-dissecting effects of CO_2 insufflation (these also increase the risk of pneumothorax) (155). Other factors that can cause paraesophageal herniation include breaches of the left pleural membrane during dissection behind the esophagus, which allow the stomach to more easily slide into the left hemithorax; the concomitant presence of a hiatal hernia; and the reduction in postoperative pain, which leads to earlier and more forceful coughing and an earlier return to physical activity. Risks may be reduced by narrowing and reinforcing the hiatus with sutures. In addition, excessive strain during the postoperative period can be avoided by the use of antiemetics and antitussives and by restrictions on lifting and straining for one month.

Dysphagia is common during the early postoperative period, but usually subsides by postoperative week six. The higher incidence of dysphagia in association with the laparoscopic approach may be caused by the decrease in tactile feedback, which can lead to excessive tightening of either the hiatus or the fundoplication. There may be a tendency to create a tighter wrap if the short gastric vessels are not taken down (156). If dysphagia persists, patients should undergo a barium swallow followed by endoscopy. The most important factor predictive of dysphagia is the integrity of the fundoplication (157). The fundoplication should be short, parallel to the diaphragm, and at the top of the stomach (157). If the fundoplication is intact, esophageal dilation may be helpful but often produces only short-term results. If the fundoplication is not intact, is too long, or is twisted, or if gastric folds are seen above the wrap (because the wrap has been mistakenly placed around the upper stomach or the esophagus, thereby pulling the stomach through the wrap; this problem is called a *slipped Nissan*), revision is usually necessary (157). For patients who require reoperation, a laparoscopic approach is usually feasible. A large bougie is used to distend the esophagus and to aid in the assessment of the fundoplication and hiatus. If the fundoplication is loose and the hiatus is tight around the bougie, widening of the hiatus alone is usually sufficient. Alternatively, if the hiatal ring is loose around the distended esophagus, revision of the fundoplication is necessary.

Gastric perforation may be due to excessive traction on the cardia by the surgical assistant or due to the use of inappropriate graspers (157). Posterior perforation of the esophagus usually occurs during dissection, whereas anterior perforation usually occurs during placement of a bougie during calibration. Both types of perforation can be treated with minimal morbidity if they are recognized at the time of the operation. Hemorrhage is particularly worrisome in association with the laparoscopic approach because blood tends to pool at the hiatus, thereby obscuring the view. It has been reported that the incidence of hemorrhage due to splenic injury is substantially lower in association with the laparoscopic approach, but an increase in liver injury has been seen because of the use of laparoscopic instruments and retractors (157).

The inability to belch and the gas bloat syndrome are late complications of antireflux surgery. Patients feel full of gas and bloated, especially after a meal. They develop discomfort because of their inability to belch and expel the gas. They not only develop abdominal cramps but may also pass large amounts of flatus, which can result in socially embarrassing situations. This syndrome occurs among 25% to 50% of patients after fundoplication surgery, but symptoms resolve over time in most cases. Dietary modifications are successful in most patients, and extreme cases are rare. Although the exact mechanisms of this syndrome are unknown, it is postulated that vagal injury during esophageal dissection may play a role. Vagal injury may also be involved in some of the other rare complications, such as prolonged diarrhea or nausea. Prokinetic agents may be helpful for some patients if dietary changes prove unsuccessful. Revision surgery may occasionally be needed to correct the problem.

INFANTILE HYPERTROPHIC PYLORIC STENOSIS

Infantile hypertrophic pyloric stenosis occurs in approximately two to three of every 1000 live births. Extramucosal pyloromyotomy, performed either as an open procedure or laparoscopically, is the standard treatment for this condition. The laparoscopic procedure begins with the insertion of an umbilical trocar. The abdomen is insufflated to a pressure of 8 mmHg, and a trocar is inserted into each upper abdominal quadrant. The duodenum is grasped distal to the pyloric vein, and a sheathed blade is used to make a seromuscular incision over the hypertrophied muscle. A spreader is used to gently separate the muscle fibers until the underlying mucosa is exposed. Mucosal integrity is assessed by insufflating air through a nasogastric tube. The open procedure begins with an incision in the supraumbilical fold, followed by a vertical incision along the linea alba. The pylorus is delivered through this incision, and the pyloromyotomy is performed as described above. It is important to avoid pushing the scalpel in too deeply and to avoid extending the incision too far proximally toward the stomach. Once the incision has been made, the muscle must be retracted slowly and gradually. The repeated use of the scalpel should be avoided.

The proposed advantages of the laparoscopic approach are improved cosmesis, earlier postoperative recovery, and shorter hospitalization. One randomized study showed significant decreases in time to full feeding, incidence of postoperative emesis, and mean length of stay when the procedure was performed laparoscopically (158). Intraoperative complications include gastric or duodenal perforation, which can be treated with minimal morbidity when recognized intraoperatively. Persistent vomiting is the most common postoperative complication; in most cases, it resolves with bowel rest. Radiologic studies are indicated if emesis continues for more than five days. The causes of continued emesis may include incomplete pyloromyotomy, gastroesophageal reflux, or unrecognized perforations requiring reoperation (159).

REFERENCES

1. Rockall TA, Logan RF, Devlin HB, Northfield TC. Incidence of and mortality from acute upper gastrointestinal haemorrhage in the United Kingdom. Steering Committee and members of the National Audit of Acute Upper Gastrointestinal Haemorrhage. BMJ 1995; 311:222–226.
2. Paimela H, Tuompo PK, Perakyl T, Saario I, Hockerstedt K, Kirilaakso E. Peptic ulcer surgery during the H2-receptor antagonist era: a population-based epidemiological study of ulcer surgery in Helsinki from 1972 to 1987. Br J Surg 1991; 78:28–31.
3. Christensen A, Bousfield R, Christiansen J. Incidence of perforated and bleeding peptic ulcers before and after the introduction of H2-receptor antagonists. Ann Surg 1988; 207:4–6.
4. Taylor TV. Current indications for elective peptic ulcer surgery. Br J Surg 1989; 76:427–428.
5. Bukhave K, Rask-Madsen J, Hogan DL, Koss MA, Isenberg JI. Proximal duodenal prostaglandin E2 release and mucosal bicarbonate secretion are altered in patients with duodenal ulcer. Gastroenterology 1990; 99:951–955.
6. Bulut OB, Rasmussen C, Fischer A. Acute surgical treatment of complicated peptic ulcer with special reference to the elderly. World J Surg 1996; 20:574–577.
7. Gilinsky NH. Peptic ulcer disease in the elderly. Gastroenterol Clin North Am 1990; 19:255–271.
8. Gunshefski L, Flancbaum L, Brolin RE, Frankel A. Changing patterns in perforated peptic ulcer disease. Am Surg 1990; 56:270–274.
9. Hentschel E, Brandstatter G, Dragosics B, et al. Effect of ranitidine and amoxicillin plus metronidazole on the eradication of *Helicobacter pylori* and the recurrence of duodenal ulcer. N Engl J Med 1993: 328:308–312.
10. Van der Hulst RW, Rauws EA, Koycu B, et al. Prevention of ulcer recurrence after eradication of *Helicobacter pylori*: a prospective long-term follow-up study. Gastroenterology 1997; 113:1082–1086.
11. Blomgren LG. Perforated peptic ulcer: long term study after simple closure in the elderly. World J Surg 1997; 21:412–417.
12. Makela JT, Kiviniemi H, Laitinen S. Gastric outlet obstruction caused by peptic ulcer disease. Analysis of 99 patients. Hepatogastroenterology 1996; 43:547–552.
13. Khullar SK, DiSario JA. Gastric outlet obstruction. Gastrointest Endosc Clin North Am 1996; 6:585–603.
14. Boring CC, Squires TS, Tong T. Cancer statistics, 1993. CA Cancer J Clin 1993; 43:7–12.
15. Macintyre IM, Akoh JA. Improving survival in gastric cancer: review of operative mortality in English language publications from 1970. Br J Surg 1991; 78:773–776.
16. Heberer G, Teichmann RK, Kramling HJ, Gunther B. Results of gastric resection for carcinoma of the stomach: the European experience. World J Surg 1988; 12:374–381.
17. Wanebo HJ, Kennedy BJ, Chmiel J, Steele G Jr, Winchester D, Osteen R. Cancer of the stomach. A patient care study by the American College of Surgeons. Ann Surg 1993; 218:583–592.
18. Gouzi JL, Huguier M, Fagniez PL, et al. Total versus subtotal gastrectomy for adenocarcinoma of the antrum. A French prospective controlled study. Ann Surg 1989; 209:162–166.
19. Hayes J, Dunn E. Has the incidence of primary gastric lymphoma increased? Cancer 1989; 63:2073–2076.
20. Severson RK, Davis S. Increasing incidence of primary gastric lymphoma. Cancer 1990; 66:1283–1287.
21. Chey WY, Hitanant S, Hendricks J, Lorber SH. Effect of secretin and cholecystokinin on gastric emptying and gastric secretion in man. Gastroenterology 1970; 58:820–827.
22. Dozois RR, Kelly KA. Effect of gastrin pentapeptide on canine gastric emptying of liquids. Am J Physiol 1971; 221:113–117.
23. Wilbur BG, Kelly KA. Effect of proximal gastric, complete gastric, and truncal vagotomy on canine gastric electric activity, motility, and emptying. Ann Surg 1973; 178:295–303.
24. Johnston D, Blackett RL. A new look at selective vagotomies. Am J Surg 1988; 156:416–427.
25. Thompson JC, Weiner I. Evaluation of surgical treatment of duodenal ulcer. Short- and long-term effects. Clin Gastroenterol 1984; 13:569–600.
26. Hinder RA, Kelly KA. Human gastric pacesetter potential. Site of origin, spread, and response to gastric transection and proximal gastric vagotomy. Am J Surg 1977; 133:29–33.
27. Weber J Jr, Koatsu S. Pacemaker localization and electrical conduction patterns in the canine stomach. Gastroenterology 1970; 59:717–726.

28. Lopasso FP, Meneguetti JC, Bruno de Mello J, Gama-Rodrigues J, Raia AA. Study of gastric emptying in duodenal ulcer patients before and after proximal gastric vagotomy. Use of solid, digestible particles labeled with 99mTc. AMB Rev Assoc Med Bras 1983; 29:10–13.

29. Wilkinson AR, Johnston D. Effect of truncal, selective and highly selective vagotomy on gastric emptying and transit of a food-barium meal in man. Ann Surg 1973; 178:190–193.

30. Dozois RR, Kelly KA. Gastric secretion and motility in duodenal ulcer: effect of current vagotomies. Surg Clin North Am 1976; 56:1267–1276.

31. Kelly KA, Code CF. Effect of transthoracic vagotomy on canine gastric electrical activity. Gastroenterology 1969; 57:51–58.

32. Mroz CT, Kelly KA. The role of the extrinsic antral nerves in the regulation of gastric emptying. Surg Gynecol Obstet 1977; 145:369–377.

33. Berger T. Studies on the gastric emptying mechanisms in healthy persons and patients after partial gastrectomy. Acta Chir Scand Suppl 1969; 404:1–51.

34. Dozois RR, Kelly KA, Code CF. Effect of distal gastrectomy on gastric emptying of solids and liquids. Gastroenterology 1971; 61:675–681.

35. MacGregor IL, Martin P, Meyer JH. Gastric emptying of solid food in normal man and after subtotal gastrectomy and truncal vagotomy with pyloroplasty. Gastroenterology 1977; 72:206–211.

36. Meyer JH, Thompson JB, Cohen MD, Shadchehr A, Mandiola SA. Sieving of solid food by the canine stomach and sieving after gastric surgery. Gastroenterology 1979; 76:804–813.

37. Wilbur BG, Kelly KA, Code CF. Effect of gastric fundectomy on canine gastric electrical and motor activity. Am J Physiol 1974; 226:1445–1449.

38. Pappas TN. Historical aspects, anatomy, pathology, physiology, and peptic ulcer disease. In: Sabiston DC Jr, Bralow L, eds. Textbook of Surgery: The Biological Basis of Modern Surgical Practice. Philadelphia: Saunders, 1997:847–868.

39. Bushkin FL, Woodward ER. Delayed gastric emptying. In: Bushkin FL, Woodward ER, eds. Major Problems in Clinical Surgery. Vol. XX. Postgastrectomy Syndromes. Philadelphia: Saunders, 1976:72–79.

40. Hermann G, Johnson V. Management of prolonged gastric retention after vagotomy and drainage. Surg Gynecol Obstet 1970; 130:1044–1048.

41. Lamers CB, Bijlstra AM, Harris AG. Octreotide, a long-acting somatostatin analog, in the management of postoperative dumping syndrome. An update. Dig Dis Sci 1993; 38:359–364.

42. Sawyers JL. Management of postgastrectomy syndromes. Am J Surg 1990; 159:8–14.

43. Eisenberg MM, Woodward ER, Carson TJ, Dragstedt LR. Vagotomy and drainage procedure for duodenal ulcer: the results of ten years' experience. Ann Surg 1969; 170:317–328.

44. Hoffmann J, Jensen HE, Christiansen J, Olesen A, Loud FB, Hauch O. Prospective controlled vagotomy trial for duodenal ulcer. Results after 11–15 years. Ann Surg 1989; 209:40–45.

45. Fenger HJ. The dumping disposition in normal persons. Acta Chir Scand 1965; 129:201–210.

46. Sessions RT, Reynolds VH, Ferguson JL, Sctt HW Jr. Correlation between intraduodenal osmotic pressure changes and Cr51 blood volumes during induced dumping in men with normal stomachs. Surgery 1962; 52:266–279.

47. Jordan GL Jr, Overton RC, De Bakey ME. The postgastrectomy syndrome: studies on pathogenesis. Ann Surg 1957; 145:471–478.

48. Ralphs DN, Thomson JP, Haynes S, Lawson-Smith C, Hobsley M, Le Quesne LP. The relationship between the rate of gastric emptying and the dumping syndrome. Br J Surg 1978; 65:637–641.

49. Kaushik SP, Ralphs DN, Hobsley M, Le Quesne LP. Use of a provocation test for objective assessment of dumping syndrome in patients undergoing surgery for duodenal ulcer. Am J Gastroenterol 1980; 74:251–257.

50. Miholic J, Orksov C, Holst JJ, Koetzerke J, Meyer HJ. Emptying of the gastric substitute, glucagon-like peptide 1 (GLP-1), and reactive hypoglycemia after total gastrectomy. Dig Dis Sci 1991; 36:1361–1370.

51. Sigstad H. Post-gastrectomy radiology with a physiologic contrast medium: comparison between dumpers and non-dumpers. Br J Radiol 1971; 44:37–43.

52. Palermo F, Boccaletto F, Magalini M, Chiara G, Tommaseo T, Dapporto L. Radioisotope evidence of varying transit of solid food in gastrectomized patients with and without dumping syndrome. Nuklearmedizin 1988; 27:195–199.

53. Kalser MH, Cohen R. Correlation of jejunal transfer of water and electrolytes with blood volume in postgastrectomy patients: response to hypertonic glucose meal. Ann Surg 1966; 164:821–829.

54. Hinshaw DB, Joergenson EJ, Davis HA, Stafford CE. Peripheral blood flow and blood volume studies in the dumping syndrome. Arch Surg 1957; 74:686–693.

55. Huse WM, Hinshaw DB. Blood flow studies in the experimental dumping syndrome. Surg Forum 1960; 11:316–317.

56. Aldoori MI, Qamar MI, Read AE, Williamson RC. Increased flow in the superior mesenteric artery in dumping syndrome. Br J Surg 1985; 72:389–390.

57. Miholic J, Reilmann L, Meyer HJ, Korber H, Kotzerke J, Hecker H. Extracellular space, blood volume, and the early dumping syndrome after total gastrectomy. Gastroenterology 1990; 99:923–929.

58. Blackburn AM, Christofides ND, Ghatei MA, et al. Elevation of plasma neurotensin in the dumping syndrome. Clin Sci (Lond) 1980; 59:237–243.

59. Lawaetz O, Blackburn AM, Bloom SR, Aritas Y, Ralphs DN. Gut hormone profile and gastric emptying in the dumping syndrome. A hypothesis concerning the pathogenesis. Scan J Gastroenterol 1983; 18:73–80.

60. Sigstad H. A clinical diagnostic index in the diagnosis of the dumping syndrome. Changes in plasma volume and blood sugar after a test meal. Acta Med Scand 1970; 188:479–486.

61. Richards WO, Geer R, O'Dorosio TM, et al. Octreotide acetate induces fasting small bowel motility in patients with dumping syndrome. J Surg Res 1990; 49:483–487.

62. Dharmsathaphorn K, Sherwin RS, Dobbins JW. Somatostatin inhibits fluid secretion in the rat jejunum. Gastroenterology 1980; 78:1554–1558.

63. Krejs GJ, Browne R, Raskin P. Effect of intravenous somatostatin on jejunal absorption of glucose, amino acids, water, and electrolytes. Gastroenterology 1980; 78:26–31.

64. Kooner JS, Peart WS, Mathias CJ. The peptide release inhibitor, Octreotide (SMS 201 995), prevents the haemodynamic changes following food ingestion in normal human subjects. Q J Exp Physiol 1989; 74: 569–572.

65. Cooper AM, Braatvedt GD, Qamar MI, et al. Fasting and post-prandial splanchnic blood flow is reduced by a somatostatin analogue (octreotide) in man. Clin Sci (Lond) 1991; 81:169–175.

66. Wass JA, Popovic V, Chayvialle JA. Proceedings of the discussion, "Tolerability and safety of Sandostatin." Metabolism 1992; 41:80–82.

67. Witt K, Pedersen NT. The long-acting somatostatin analogue SMS 201–995 causes malabsorption. Scan J Gastroenterol 1989; 24:1248–1252.

68. Dowling RH, Hussaini SH, Murphy GM, Besser GM, Wass JA. Gallstones during octreotide therapy. Metabolism 1992; 41:22–33.

69. Cheadle WG, Baker PR, Cuschieri A. Pyloric reconstruction for severe vasomotor dumping after vagotomy and pyloroplasty. Ann Surg 1985; 202:568–572.

70. Koruth NM, Krukowski ZH, Matheson NA. Pyloric reconstruction. Br J Surg 1985; 72:808–810.

71. Kelly KA, Becker JM, van Heerden JA. Reconstructive gastric surgery. Br J Surg 1981; 68:687–691.

72. Woodward ER, Desser PL, Gasster M. Surgical treatment of the postgastrectomy dumping syndrome. West J Surg Obstet Gynecol 1955; 63:567–573.

73. Jordan GL Jr, Angel RT, McIlhaney JS Jr, Williams RK. Treatment of the postgastrectomy dumping syndrome with a reversed jejunal segment interposed between the gastric remnant and the jejunum. Am J Surg 1963; 106:451–459.

74. Sanders GB. Interposed jejunal segments in ulcer surgery. J Ky Med Assoc 1965; 63:855–860.

75. Sawyers JL, Herrington JL Jr. Superiority of antiperistaltic jejunal segments in management of severe dumping syndrome. Ann Surg 1973; 178:311–321.

76. Miranda R, Steffes B, O'Leary JP, Woodward ER. Surgical treatment of the postgastrectomy dumping syndrome. Am J Surg 1980; 139:40–43.

77. Lygidakis NJ. A new method for the surgical treatment of the dumping syndrome. Ann R Coll Surg Engl 1981; 63:411–414.

78. Vogel SB, Hocking MP, Woodward ER. Clinical and radionuclide evaluation of Roux-Y diversion for postgastrectomy dumping. Am J Surg 1988; 155:57–62.

79. Karlstrom L, Kelly KA. Ectopic jejunal pacemakers and gastric emptying after Roux gastrectomy: effect of intestinal pacing. Surgery 1989; 106:867–871.

80. Emas S, Fernstrom M. Prospective, randomized trial of selective vagotomy with pyloroplasty and selective proximal vagotomy with and without pyloroplasty in the treatment of duodenal, pyloric, and prepyloric ulcers. Am J Surg 1985; 149:236–243.

81. Storer EH. Postvagotomy diarrhea. Surg Clin North Am 1976; 56:1461–1468.

82. Allan JG, Gerskowitch VP, Russell RI. The role of bile acids in the pathogenesis of postvagotomy diarrhoea. Br J Surg 1974; 61:516–518.

83. Allan JG, Russell RI. Proceedings: double-blind controlled trial of cholestyramine in the treatment of post-vagotomy diarrhoea. Gut 1975; 16:830.

84. Mackie CR, Jenkins SA, Hartley MN. Treatment of severe postvagotomy/postgastrectomy symptoms with the somatostatin analogue octreotide. Br J Surg 1991; 78:1338–1343.

85. Cuschieri A. Postvagotomy diarrhoea: is there a place for surgical management? Gut 1990; 31:245–246.

86. Herrington JL Jr, Edwards WH, Carter JH, Sawyers JL. Treatment of postvagotomy diarrhea by reversed jejunal segment. Ann Surg 1968; 168:522–541.

87. Cuschieri A. Surgical management of severe intractable postvagotomy diarrhoea. Br J Surg 1986; 73:981–984.

88. Stabile BE, Passaro E Jr. Sequelae of surgery for peptic ulcer. In: Berk JE, Kalser MH, Haubrich WS, eds. Bockus Gastroenterology. Vol. 7. 4th ed. Philadelphia: Saunders, 1985:1225–1242.

89. Hoare AM, Keighley MR, Starkey B, Alexander-Williams J. Measurement of bile acids in fasting gastric aspirates: an objective test for bile reflux after gastric surgery. Gut 1978; 19:166–169.

90. Malagelada JR, Phillips SF, Shorter RG, et al. Postoperative reflux gastritis: pathophysiology and long-term outcome after Roux-en-Y diversion. Ann Intern Med 1985; 103:178–183.

91. Ritchie WP Jr. Alkaline reflux gastritis. Late results on a controlled clinical trial of diagnosis and treatment. Ann Surg 1986; 203:537–544.

92. Drapanas T, Bethea M. Reflux gastritis following gastric surgery. Ann Surg 1974; 179:618–627.

93. Harmon JW, Lewis CD, Gadacz T. Bile salt composition and concentration as determinants of canine gastric mucosal injury. Surgery 1981; 89:348–354.

94. Brooks WS, Wenger J, Hersh T. Bile reflux gastritis. Analysis of fasting and postprandial gastric aspirates. Am J Gastroenterol 1975; 64:286–291.

95. Davenport HW. Effect of lysolecithin, digitonin, and phospholipase A upon the dog's gastric mucosal barrier. Gastroenterology 1970; 59:505–509.

96. Lawson HH. Effects of duodenal contents on the gastric mucosa under experimental conditions. Lancet 1964; 18:469–472.

97. Rutledge PL, Warshaw AL. Diagnosis of symptomatic alkaline reflux gastritis and prediction of response to bile diversion operation by intragastric alkali provocation. Am J Surg 1988; 155:82–87.

98. Romano M, Razandi M, Ivey KJ. Effect of sucralfate and its components on taurocholate-induced damage to rat gastric mucosal cells in tissue culture. Dig Dis Sci 1990; 35:467–476.

99. Stefaniwsky AB, Tint GS, Speck J, Shefer S, Salen G. Ursodeoxycholic acid treatment of bile reflux gastritis. Gastroenterology 1985; 89:1000–1004.

100. Herrington JL Jr, Sawyers JL. Complications following gastric operation. In: Schwartz SI, Ellis H, eds. Maingot's Abdominal Operations. Norwalk, Connecticut: Appleton & Lange, 1990:701–712.

101. Hom S, Sarr MG, Kelly KA, Hench V. Postoperative gastric atony after vagotomy for obstructing peptic ulcer. Am J Surg 1989; 157:282–286.

102. Perino LE, Adcock KA, Goff JS. Gastrointestinal symptoms, motility, and transit after Roux-en-Y operation. Am J Gastroenterol 1988; 83:380–385.

103. McAlhany JC Jr, Hanover TM, Taylor SM, Sticca RP, Ashmore JD Jr. Long-term follow-up of patients with Roux-en-Y gastrojejunostomy for gastric disease. Ann Surg 1994; 219:451–457.

104. Karlstrom L, Soper NJ, Kelly KA, Phillips SF. Ectopic jejunal pacemakers and enterogastric reflux after Roux

gastrectomy: effect of intestinal pacing. Surgery 1989; 106:486–495.

105. Miedema BW, Kelly KA. The Roux stasis syndrome. Treatment by pacing and prevention by use of an 'uncut' Roux limb. Arch Surg 1992; 127:295–300.

106. Fich A, Neri M, Camilleri M, Kelly KA, Phillips SF. Stasis syndromes following gastric surgery: clinical and motility features of 60 symptomatic patients. J Clin Gastroenterol 1990; 12:505–512.

107. Mathias JR, Fernandez A, Sninsky CA, Clench MH, Davis RH. Nausea, vomiting, and abdominal pain after Roux-en-Y anastomosis: motility of the jejunal limb. Gastroenterology 1985; 88:101–107.

108. Hall EK, el-Sharkawy TY, Diamant NE. Vagal control of canine postprandial upper gastrointestinal motility. Am J Physiol 1986; 250:G501–G510.

109. Hinder RA, Esser J, DeMeester TR. Management of gastric emptying disorders following the Roux-en-Y procedure. Surgery 1988; 104:765–772.

110. Van Stiegmann G, Gott JS. An alternative to Roux-en-Y for treatment of bile reflux gastritis. Surg Gynecol Obstet 1988; 166:69–70.

111. Mulholland MW, Magellanes F, Quigley TM, Delaney JP. In-continuity gastrointestinal stapling. Dis Colon Rectum 1983; 26:586–589.

112. Becker JM, Sava P, Kelly KA, Shturman L. Intestinal pacing for canine postgastrectomy dumping. Gastroenterology 1983; 84:383–387.

113. Cranley B, Kelly KA, Go VL, McNichols LA. Enhancing the anti-dumping effect of Roux gastrojejunostomy with intestinal pacing. Ann Surg 1983; 198:516–524.

114. Delcore R, Cheung LY. Surgical options in postgastrectomy syndromes. Surg Clin North Am 1991; 71:57–75.

115. Zinner MJ, McFadden DW. Surgery for recurrent peptic ulcer disease. In: Fry DE, ed. Reoperative Surgery of the Abdomen. New York: Marcel Dekker, 1986:53–58.

116. Stabile BE, Passaro E Jr. Duodenal ulcer: a disease in evolution. Curr Probl Surg 1984; 21:1–79.

117. Schirmer BD, Meyers WC, Hanks JB, Kortz WJ, Jones RS, Postlethwait RW. Marginal ulcer. A difficult surgical problem. Ann Surg 1982; 195:653–661.

118. Wychulis AR, Priestley JT, Foulk WT. A study of 360 patients with gastrojejunal ulceration. Surg Gynecol Obstet 1966; 122:89–99.

119. Skandelakis JE, Rowe JS Jr, Gray SW, Androulakis JA. Identification of vagal structures at the esophageal hiatus. Surgery 1974; 75:233–237.

120. Grassi G, Orecchia CA. Comparison of intraoperative tests of completeness of vagal section. Surgery 1974; 75:155–160.

121. Wolfe MM, Jain DK, Edgerton JR. Zollinger-Ellison syndrome associated with persistently normal fasting serum gastrin concentrations. Ann Intern Med 1985; 103:215–217.

122. Stremple JF, Elliot DW. Gastrin determinations in symptomatic patients before and after standard ulcer operations. Arch Surg 1975; 110:875–878.

123. Friesen SR, Tomita T. Pseudo-Zollinger-Ellison syndrome: hypergastrinemia, hyperchlorhydia without tumor. Ann Surg 1981; 194:481–493.

124. Metz DC, Pisegna JR, Fishbeyn VA, Benya RV, Jensen RT. Control of gastric acid hypersecretion in the management of patients with Zollinger-Ellison syndrome. World J Surg 1993; 17:468–480.

125. Primrose JN, Ratcliffe JG, Joffe SN. Assessment of the secretin provocation test in the diagnosis of gastrinoma. Br J Surg 1980; 67:744–746.

126. Cortot A, Fleming CR, Brown ML, Go VL, Malagelada JR. Isolated retained antrum diagnosis by gastrin challenge tests and radioscintillation scanning. Dig Dis Sci 1981; 26:748–751.

127. Lee CH, P'eng FK, Yeh PH. Sodium pertechnetate Tc 99m antral scan in the diagnosis of retained gastric antrum. Arch Surg 1984; 119:309–311.

128. Athow AC, Lewin MR, Sewerniak AT, Clark CG. Gastric secretory responses to modified sham feeding (MSF) and insulin after vagotomy. Br J Surg 1986; 73:132–135.

129. Thirlby RC, Patterson DJ, Kozarek RA. Prospective comparison of Congo red and sham feeding testing to determine vagal innervation of the stomach. Am J Surg 1992; 163:533–536.

130. Saik RP, Greenburg AG, Farris JM, Peskin GW. The practicality of the Congo Red test, or is your vagotomy complete? Am J Surg 1976; 132:144–149.

131. Gugler R, Lindstaedt H, Miederer S, et al. Cimetidine for anastomotic ulcers after partial gastrectomy. A randomized controlled trial. N Engl J Med 1979; 301:1077–1080.

132. Kennedy T, Spencer A. Cimetidine for recurrent ulcer after vagotomy or gastrectomy: a randomised controlled trial. Br Med J 1978; 1:1242–1243.

133. Caygill CP, Hill MJ, Kirkham JS, Northfield TC. Mortality from gastric cancer following gastric surgery for peptic ulcer. Lancet 1986; 1:929–931.

134. Viste A, Bjornestad E, Opheim P, et al. Risk of carcinoma following gastric operations for benign disease. A historical cohort study of 3470 patients. Lancet 1986; 2:502–505.

135. Lundegardh G, Adami HO, Helmick C, Zach M, Meirik O. Stomach cancer after partial gastrectomy for benign ulcer disease. N Engl J Med 1988; 319:195–200.

136. Johnson JH, Horswell RR, Tyor MP, Owen EE, Ruffin JM. Effect of intestinal hormones on I-131-triolein absorption in subtotal gastrectomy patients and intubated normal persons. Gastroenterology 1961; 41:215–219.

137. Meyer JH. Nutritional outcomes of gastric operations. Gastroenterol Clin North Am 1994; 23:227–260.

138. MacGregor I, Parent J, Meyer JH. Gastric emptying of liquid meals and pancreatic and biliary secretion after subtotal gastrectomy or truncal vagotomy and pyloroplasty in man. Gastroenterology 1977; 72:195–205.

139. Mayer EA, Thompson JB, Jehn D, Reedy T, Elashoff J, Meyer JH. Gastric emptying and sieving of solid food and pancreatic and biliary secretion after solid meals in patients with truncal vagotomy and antrectomy. Gastroenterology 1982; 83:184–192.

140. Mayer EA, Thomson JB, Jehn D, et al. Gastric emptying and sieving of solid food and pancreatic and biliary secretion after solid meals in patients with nonresective ulcer surgery. Gastroenterology 1984; 87:1264–1271.

141. Lavigne ME, Wiley ZD, Martin P, et al. Gastric, pancreatic, and biliary secretion and the rate of emptying after parietal cell vagotomy. Am J Surg 1979; 138:644–651.

142. Johnson HD, Khan TA, Srivatsa R, Doyle FH. The late nutritional and haematological effects of vagal section. Br J Surg 1969; 56:4–9.

143. Postlethwait RW, Shingleton WW, Dillon ML, Willis MT. Nutrition after gastric resection for peptic ulcer. Gastroenterology 1961; 40:491–496.

144. Johnston ID, Welbourn R, Acheson K. Gastrectomy and loss of weight. Lancet 1958; 1:1242–1245.

145. McIntosh HW, Robertson R, Robins RE. Fecal fat and nitrogen studies in postgastrectomy patients: the relationship of fat and nitrogen excretion to weight loss and a comparison between Billroth I and Billroth II subtotal gastrectomies. Surgery 1957; 41:248–253.

146. Fraser AG, Brunt PW, Matheson NA. A comparison of highly selective vagotomy with truncal vagotomy and pyloroplasty—one surgeon's results after 5 years. Br J Surg 1983; 70:485–488.

147. Koo H, Lam SK, Chan P, et al. Proximal gastric vagotomy, truncal vagotomy with drainage, and truncal vagotomy with antrectomy for chronic duodenal ulcer. A prospective, randomized and controlled trial. Ann Surg 1983; 197:265–271.

148. Naslund I. Gastric bypass versus gastroplasty. A prospective study of differences in two surgical procedures for morbid obesity. Acta Chir Scand Suppl 1987; 536:1–60.

149. Aukee S, Alhava EM, Karjalainen P. Bone mineral after partial gastrectomy II. Scand J Gastroenterol 1975; 10:165–169.

150. Bisballe S, Eriksen EF, Melsen F, Mosekilde L, Sorensen OH, Hessov I. Osteopenia and osteomalacia after gastrectomy: interrelations between biochemical markers of bone remodeling, vitamin D metabolites, and bone histomorphometry. Gut 1991; 32:1303–1307.

151. Blichert-Toft M, Beck A, Christiansen C, Transbol I. Effects of gastric resection and vagotomy on blood and bone mineral content. World J Surg 1979; 3: 99–102, 133–135.

152. Wastell C. Long-term clinical and metabolic effects of vagotomy with either partial gastrojejunostomy or pyloroplasty. Ann R Coll Surg Engl 1969; 45:193–211.

153. Paakkonen M, Alhava EM, Karjalainen P, Korhonen R, Savolainen K, Syrjanen K. Long-term follow-up after Billroth I and II partial gastrectomy. Gastrointestinal tract function and changes in bone metabolism. Acta Chir Scand 1984; 150:485–488.

154. Eubanks TR, Pellegrini CA. Hiatal hernia and gastroesophageal reflux disease. In: Sabiston DC Jr, Townsend CM Jr, eds. Textbook of Surgery. The Biological Basis of Modern Surgical Practice. Philadelphia: Saunders, 2001:755–768.

155. Watson DI, de Beaux AC. Complications of laparoscopic antireflux surgery. Surg Endosc 2001; 15:344–352.

156. Carlson MA, Frantzides CT. Complications and results of primary minimally invasive antireflux procedures: a review of 10,735 reported cases. J Am Coll Surg 2001; 193:428–439.

157. Waring JP. Postfundoplication complications. Prevention and management. Gastroenterol Clin North Am 1999; 28(4):1007–1019.

158. Fujimoto T, Lane GJ, Segawa O, Esaki S, Miyano T. Laparoscopic extramucosal pyloromyotomy versus open pyloromyotomy for infantile hypertrophic pyloric stenosis: which is better? J Pediatr Surg 1999; 34:370–372.

159. Hulka F, Harrison MW, Campbell TJ, Campbell JR. Complications of pyloromyotomy for infantile hypertrophic pyloric stenosis. Am J Surg 1997; 173:450–452.

11

Complications of Hepatic Surgery and Trauma

Adrian W. Ong
*Department of Surgery, Allegheny General Hospital, Drexel University College of Medicine,
Pittsburgh, Pennsylvania, U.S.A.*

Danny Sleeman
*DeWitt Daughtry Family Department of Surgery, Miller School of Medicine,
University of Miami, Miami, Florida, U.S.A.*

The liver is divided into two lobes along a plane from the inferior vena cava posteriorly to the gallbladder fossa anteroinferiorly (Cantlie's line); the plane defined by the middle hepatic vein demarcates the division of the lobes. The umbilical fissure, lying to the left of Cantlie's line, marks the point of attachment of the ligamentum teres that continues into the falciform ligament anteriorly. The widely accepted numbering system of Couinaud (1), that divides the liver into functional segments on the basis of hepatic venous drainage, is the most useful classification. The three main hepatic veins divide the liver into four sectors, and each of these sectors receives its blood supply from independent portal pedicles. The sectors are further subdivided into segments, each supplied by a branch from a portal pedicle.

The right lobe contains segments V, VI, VII, and VIII. The left lobe contains segments II, III, and IV. Segment I (caudate lobe) is located just anterior to the inferior vena cava, inferior to the entrance of the main hepatic veins into the vena cava, and posterior to the hilum. This segment may receive branches from both the right and the left portal systems, and the bile ducts may enter the left or the right ducts or the duct confluence. Hepatic veins from segment I may enter the left or middle hepatic veins or drain directly into the vena cava (2).

The hepatic arteries carry oxygenated blood and account for approximately 25% of blood flow to the liver. The portal vein accounts for the remainder of the blood flow. The right and left hepatic arteries usually arise from the proper hepatic artery. In about 20% of patients, the right hepatic artery originates from the superior mesenteric artery. The left hepatic artery arises from the left gastric artery in as many as 30% of patients.

The portal vein is formed behind the pancreas at the confluence of the superior mesenteric vein, the splenic vein, and sometimes the inferior mesenteric vein. The left portal vein is longer than the right; it courses through the hilar plate to the left and turns to enter the liver in the umbilical fissure. This portion of the left portal vein has branches

supplying the medial sector of the left lobe (segments IVa and IVb), the lateral sector (segments II and III), and the caudate lobe. These branches should be noted when the resection margin involves the umbilical fissure. The branches of the left hepatic artery, however, do not parallel those of the left portal vein in this area.

Because the liver occupies most of the right upper quadrant of the abdomen and extends across the midline, any blunt or penetrating trauma to the lower chest or upper abdomen places the liver at risk of injury. For patients undergoing surgery, the incidence of liver injury is approximately 35% in cases of blunt trauma and as high as 60% in cases of penetrating trauma. The American Association for the Surgery of Trauma liver injury scale is commonly used to grade liver injury; its grading system is based on findings from operative procedures, radiologic imaging, or autopsy (Table 1) (3).

OPERATIVE TECHNIQUES FOR HEPATIC SURGERY AND TRAUMA SURGERY
Elective Liver Resection

The most commonly used incision is the bilateral subcostal incision. Major liver resection, defined as removal of three or more Couinaud segments, is usually carried out by isolating the vessels supplying the area to be removed. Intraoperative ultrasonography is commonly used to determine the size and location of a tumor in relation to the hepatic and portal venous systems and to identify the presence of tumor thrombus. For the purpose of minimizing blood loss, the Pringle maneuver may be used safely for more than 60 minutes, even for patients with cirrhosis (4,5). In a prospective, randomized trial, use of the Pringle maneuver was shown to reduce blood loss and transfusion requirements during hepatic resection for liver tumors (6). The relevant structures in the porta hepatis are usually dissected extrahepatically or

Table 1 American Association for the Surgery of Trauma Liver Injury Classification

Grade		Injury description
I	Hematoma	Subcapsular, less than 10% surface area
	Laceration	Capsular tear, less than 1 cm parenchymal depth
II	Hematoma	Subcapsular, 10–50% surface area; intraparenchymal, less than 10 cm in length
	Laceration	1–3 cm parenchymal depth, less than 10 cm in length
III	Hematoma	Subcapsular, more than 50% surface area or expanding; ruptured subcapsular or parenchymal hematoma; intraparenchymal hematoma
	Laceration	More than 3 cm parenchymal depth
IV	Laceration	Parenchymal disruption involving 25–75% of hepatic lobe or 1–3 Couinaud segments within a single lobe
V	Laceration	Parenchymal disruption involving more than 75% of hepatic lobe or more than three Couinaud segments within a single lobe
	Vascular	Juxtahepatic venous injuries
VI	Vascular	Hepatic avulsion

Source: From Ref. 3.

controlled and ligated individually; alternatively, the entire pedicle as a unit may be ligated (7). Demarcation of the liver before division of the portal structures indicates a correctly placed clamp. The hepatic veins are usually approached by extrahepatic dissection along the retrohepatic cava and are divided before parenchymal transection. The liver parenchyma is divided by various methods, such as crushing with a Kelly clamp, finger fracture technique, or ultrasonic dissection. Vessels and biliary radicals are ligated and divided with sutures or clips.

Total vascular isolation of the liver, or interruption of both inflow and vena caval flow by placing suprahepatic and infrahepatic clamps on the inferior vena cava, is used rarely, most often for tumors involving the hepatic vein confluence, the inferior vena cava, or both (8). However, this maneuver may cause hemodynamic instability for some patients in spite of good preloading in these elective cases. An alternative is vascular isolation without vena caval clamping; this isolation is achieved by controlling the hepatic veins individually (9). Extracorporeal venous bypass is another alternative. In extremely difficult cases, transection of the hepatic veins (ex situ in vivo) or removal of the liver from the abdomen (ex vivo) combined with hypothermic perfusion have been attempted with success (10).

Liver Trauma

Management of liver trauma involves a multimodal approach incorporating close observation, interventional and endoscopic techniques, and surgery. The majority (50–80%) of patients who arrive at the emergency room with blunt liver trauma may be treated nonoperatively. Criteria for nonoperative management of liver injuries include hemodynamic stability, absence of peritonitis, and absence of associated

intra-abdominal injuries requiring laparotomy. In one large study (11), a nonoperative initial approach eventually failed in only 7.5% of cases. Although computed tomography (CT) grading of hepatic injury is seldom a factor in determining the need for operation, and although most higher-grade injuries can be managed without surgical intervention, most patients for whom nonoperative treatment fails will have higher-grade liver injuries.

When surgery is contemplated, an autologous blood recovery system is prepared. Once the abdomen has been entered, blood and clot are quickly evacuated, and the four quadrants of the abdomen are packed. After removal of the perihepatic packing, the liver injury is inspected. The need for further treatment depends on the severity of the liver injury and whether there is active bleeding; if necessary, such treatment may consist of direct pressure, suturing, topical hemostatic agents, electrocautery, or laser coagulation for minor injuries. More severe injuries, if they are actively bleeding, may require full mobilization of the liver to the midline. If simple packing has failed to control the hemorrhage, the Pringle maneuver is used, followed by controlled hepatotomy using finger fracture to expose and ligate the bleeding vessels. The Pringle maneuver can then be released, and further assessment of bleeding can be performed.

When large lacerations involve anatomic segments of the liver, removal of injured liver peripheral to the line of fracture may control bleeding. Formal lobectomy is rarely required for control of bleeding. Although some centers can achieve a mortality rate as low as 10% (12,13), most experience a high mortality rate (50%) when emergent formal resection is performed during the initial laparotomy (14,15). Selective hepatic artery ligation (16), although almost always safe, does not stop bleeding of hepatic venous or portal venous origin. It may be a useful technique for controlling arterial bleeding when portal occlusion is released and direct suture of vessels is impossible.

When bleeding occurs from hepatic veins or the retrohepatic vena cava, packing with tamponade may be sufficient for some cases (17,18), but most will require further maneuvers for controlling bleeding. Finger fracture of the parenchyma with venorrhaphy has been used successfully. Otherwise, total vascular isolation coupled with either atriocaval shunting (19–21) or extracorporeal venovenous bypass, aided through a median sternotomy or right anterolateral thoracotomy, may be necessary.

In cases of severe liver injury, abbreviating the laparotomy after control of surgical bleeding may be necessary. The abdomen is packed and temporarily closed, and the patient is taken to the intensive care unit, where rewarming, correction of acidosis, and coagulopathy are carried out. Once the patient's condition has been optimized, early planned reoperation with removal of packing is performed.

Angiography may also be performed immediately after surgery if intraoperative hemostasis has not been satisfactory and embolization can be used as an adjunct to control hemorrhage. Rarely, for severe liver injuries with ongoing active bleeding despite conventional operative and angiographic techniques, total hepatectomy with liver transplantation as a two-step procedure has been attempted with some success (22,23).

COMPLICATIONS
Liver Dysfunction

Hyperbilirubinemia is seen infrequently after elective liver resection. More commonly, parenchymal liver enzyme activity shows a transient elevation that peaks during the first day or two after surgery and returns to normal in approximately one week (4,24). Serious liver failure (development of encephalopathy or the hepatorenal syndrome) is also uncommon (Table 2). However, when liver failure occurs, the mortality rate is quite high and approaches 100% (45). In a large study of 1803 patients, the overall incidence of hyper-bilirubinemia, ascites, and liver failure was 5.5% (46).

Cirrhosis is an important risk factor contributing to poor outcome after hepatic resection. Therefore, preoperative evaluation should include assessment of liver function and of any known complications due to cirrhosis. The Child-Turcotte-Pugh classification remains a widely used model to predict outcome after liver resection in these patients. Several authors have used the indocyanine green retention rate at 15 minutes (ICGR-15) as an indicator of the extent of hepatic resection that can be safely performed. In fact, some have proposed using the degree of ascites, the serum

bilirubin concentration, and the ICGR-15 to guide the extent of liver resection (25). Others have found that, in the absence of uncontrollable ascites and when the serum bilirubin was less than 1.9 mg/dL, an ICGR-15 of less than 10% allowed major liver resection to proceed safely with low rates of postoperative liver failure (26,27). A recently developed scoring system, the "model for end stage liver disease" (MELD) score, may also be of value in predicting outcome after liver resection in cirrhotic patients (67).

Intraoperative blood loss and operating time have also been recognized as independent factors that influence morbidity rates (25,45,47). The length of the period of inflow occlusion during liver resection does not appear to influence postoperative morbidity rates for normal or cirrhotic patients, as long as the ischemic time does not exceed 60 to 80 minutes (4,5,9). This finding may be attributed to careful patient selection for liver resection and to the fact that inflow occlusion minimizes intraoperative blood loss. Late development of liver failure has been reported for trauma patients who required surgery for liver injury; the liver failure was managed with liver transplantation (48).

Bleeding

The extent of intraoperative bleeding depends on the technique of resection, the extent of resection, and whether the liver is diseased. Intraoperative exsanguination is rare during elective liver resection, occurring in fewer than 1% of patients in a large series (38) because surgeons are becoming increasingly familiar with techniques of vascular isolation. Hemorrhage arises most commonly from the major hepatic veins and the vena cava. Therefore, controlling the hepatic veins is usually necessary before parenchymal transection. The central venous pressure can be kept low (less than 5 mmHg) intraoperatively so as to minimize bleeding during transection of the hepatic tissue (49). Blood transfusions are required for 10% to 60% of patients; cirrhotic patients tend to need a greater amount of blood (38). However, bleeding requiring reoperation is uncommon even for patients with cirrhosis (Table 2). This finding could again be due to patient selection bias because poor-risk cirrhotic patients are generally not candidates for major liver resection.

For trauma patients in a hemodynamically stable condition and who are initially managed nonoperatively, delayed bleeding requiring intervention is relatively uncommon, occurring among fewer than 5% of patients in a large series (11). If delayed bleeding occurs but the patient is in a hemodynamically stable condition, a CT scan should be obtained to assess the amount of hemoperitoneum and the presence or absence of a hepatic artery pseudoaneurysm that may benefit from angioembolization.

When surgery is required for a liver injury, postoperative bleeding requiring intervention is more

Table 2 Incidence of Complications of Liver Surgery and Trauma

Complication	Incidence and setting	References
Hepatic failure	Elective liver resection: 0–8%	25–28
Intra-abdominal abscess	Trauma: 5–10% (operative management)	29–32
	0–2% (nonoperative management)	32–34
	Elective surgery: 1–28%	28,35
Biloma/bile fistula	Trauma: 0.5–14% (nonoperative management)	33
	4–6% (operative management)	36,37
	Elective liver resection: 5–12%	26,28,38,39
Hemobilia	Trauma: 0.5–1%	40,41
	Percutaneous transhepatic procedures: 4–15%	42,43
Biliary stricture	Trauma (after repair of bile duct injury): 3–55%	44
	Elective surgery: 5% or more	25,28
Bleeding requiring operation	Elective surgery: 0–3%	26,28
	Trauma: less than 5% (initial nonoperative management)	11,33
Mortality	Elective liver resection: 0–7% (operative mortality)	25,26,28,38
	Trauma: liver-related mortality: 0.3–0.5% (initially planned nonoperative management)	11,33
	16–23% (urgent operation at admission)	11

commonly encountered, probably because of the severity of the liver injury and the fact that temporary hemostatic measures (e.g., packing) are needed during the initial laparotomy to staunch the bleeding. If initial packing is unsuccessful, the mortality rate is extremely high (50). If packing is successful and the patient can be optimally resuscitated, removal of packs during a planned second procedure is usually possible. A few patients will require further surgical hemostasis, repacking, or both.

Biloma and Biliary Fistula

Biloma and biliary fistula are usually the result of injury to a small intrahepatic biliary radical with leakage of bile. They are relatively uncommon complications of liver surgery and injury, occurring in 0.5% of cases in a multicenter study of trauma patients managed nonoperatively (33) and in about 5% of patients undergoing operative treatment for liver injuries (36). These complications are generally associated with higher grades of liver injury (37), and their incidence is similar after elective liver resection (Table 2). Sites of biliary leakage after liver resection include the hepatic duct stump, the bilioenteric anastomosis, the common hepatic duct, and the raw surface of the liver (39).

Patients may have no symptoms or may exhibit right upper quadrant fullness or tenderness, fever, or jaundice one to four weeks after the initial operation or injury. Some will have persistent biliary drainage from drains placed intraoperatively. CT scans may show a loculated fluid collection within the hepatic parenchyma or in the peritoneal cavity, findings consistent with a diagnosis of biloma (Fig. 1). CT-guided drainage is the treatment of choice if the patient exhibits symptoms, fever, or leukocytosis. Asymptomatic collections may resolve spontaneously. If percutaneous drainage is not successful, operative drainage is performed.

A biliary fistula is commonly defined as persistent drainage of bile for more than two weeks after injury or operation. Biliary fistulas will usually close spontaneously with drainage (36,37). However, endoscopic retrograde cholangiopancreatography (ERCP) is necessary if a fistula is persistent. The findings of this test may reveal a peripheral or main bile duct as the source of drainage. Sphincterotomy during ERCP with placement of a biliary stent or a nasobiliary drain may result in spontaneous fistula closure when the fistula arises from the biliary radicals of the second order or higher (51–53). Reoperation may be necessary when leakage originates from the common bile duct or the main hepatic ducts. Outcome in these cases is usually poor. Percutaneous transhepatic biliary drainage may be useful if surgical or endoscopic methods are unsuccessful.

Resection of the left side of the liver has been reported as a risk factor for the occurrence of bile leak during elective liver resections (39), probably because the right posterior segmental duct and the caudate lobe ducts may drain into the left duct. Cholangiography is recommended before resections of the left side of the liver are performed. This test would show the anomaly and allow the surgeon to resect the duct away from the bifurcation, thereby minimizing the potential for injury.

Occasionally, bile leakage results in generalized ascites with bile peritonitis. This may be seen with non-operative management of liver injuries, when the patient presents with fever, abdominal pain, jaundice and ileus several days after the injury. Repeat CT will reveal generalized free fluid. Diagnosis is usually made during open or laparoscopic exploration. We favor a laparoscopic approach with placement of perihepatic drains and subsequent ERCP with bile duct stenting (54,55).

Intra-abdominal Abscess

A perihepatic abscess can form as a postoperative complication or as a complication of nonoperative management of a liver injury. Reports of large series (29–32) of patients undergoing operative treatment of liver injuries have shown a 5% to 10% incidence of abscess formation. The rate of abscess formation is lower when liver injuries are managed nonoperatively (0–2%) (Table 2) (32–34). Abscess formation is associated with the severity of intra-abdominal injury, the use and the number of blood transfusions, and the type of drainage used (closed or sump) (17,29,30). When complex liver injuries require perihepatic packing for hemorrhage control, the rate of abscess formation approaches 40% to 50% among patients who survive the perioperative period (56). After elective hepatic resection, the overall incidence of infected collections ranges from less than 1% to 28%

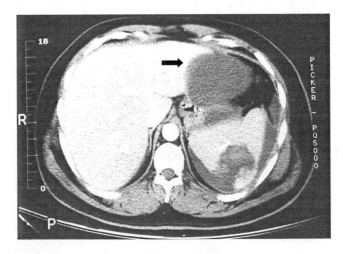

Figure 1 Biloma (*arrow*) after blunt injury to the liver. A concomitant splenic injury is also present.

AVOIDING COMPLICATIONS IN LIVER SURGERY AND TRAUMA

■ Perform careful selection of cirrhotic patients for liver resection
■ Biliary–enteric anastomosis should be used for complete or near-complete traumatic transection of the bile ducts
■ Avoiding a high central venous pressure may lessen blood loss during major liver resections
■ Hepatotomy with the finger fracture technique is a quick and effective way of controlling hemorrhage deep in the hepatic parenchyma
■ Preparation for total hepatic vascular isolation with or without bypass is important for major liver resection and trauma
■ A contrast "blush" in the liver parenchyma on CT scans usually mandates angiography with possible embolization or operative intervention for liver trauma
■ Hemodynamic stability is a more important factor than grade of injury or degree of hemoperitoneum during the planning stages for nonoperative management of liver injury

---

(Table 2). In particular, hepatic resection for cholangiocarcinoma has been associated with a rate of abscess formation as high as 50% in one study (35).

A CT scan of the abdomen aids in the diagnosis of perihepatic or intra-abdominal abscess. Treatment with percutaneous drainage and adjunctive broad-spectrum antibiotics is usually adequate.

The need for routine drainage after elective liver resection is controversial. Prospective randomized trials found that, whether or not drains were placed intraoperatively, approximately 10% to 30% of patients required delayed drainage of an abscess or fluid collection, and there were no statistically significant differences in the incidence of abscess formation (57,58). These studies, however, excluded patients who underwent simultaneous biliary–enteric anastomosis. One randomized study (59) found that, for patients who underwent laparotomy for traumatic liver injuries and for whom no bile leak was detected on a dry laparotomy pad before abdominal closure, there were no differences in the rates of subsequent abscess formation with or without drains.

Hemobilia

Hemobilia is a rare complication after trauma or iatrogenic injury (e.g., liver biopsy and invasive transhepatic procedures). This complication is often associated with a hepatic artery pseudoaneurysm and can occur days to months or even years after injury. The patient may experience right upper quadrant pain, fever, gastrointestinal bleeding, and even shock (60,61). The incidence of hemobilia is not well documented after liver surgery, but open biliary tract surgery, in particular, has been associated with this complication (62). In two large series of liver injuries, the incidence of hemobilia ranged from 0.5% to 1% (40,41). On the other hand, this complication has been well recognized in association with percutaneous transhepatic procedures (Table 2) (42,43). Cases of arteriovenous or arterioduodenal fistulas have been

reported (40,63). Other nontraumatic causes of hemobilia include tumors, cholangitis, coagulopathy, and parasitic disorders (64).

Endoscopy of the upper gastrointestinal tract is usually nondiagnostic because the bleeding is often intermittent, but this procedure should be performed to rule out other sources of gastrointestinal bleeding. Jaundice with radiographic evidence of a dilated common bile duct due to blood clots in the biliary tract may suggest the diagnosis (65). A CT scan performed with the use of intravenous contrast material may reveal a "blush" in the liver parenchyma (Fig. 2). The management of choice is hepatic arteriography with selective embolization of the feeding artery (Fig. 3). Rarely, patients with evidence of sepsis and

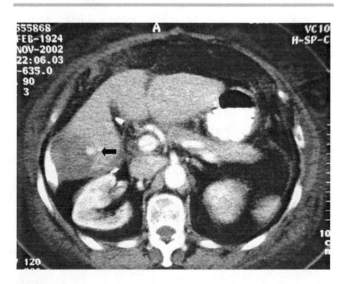

Figure 2 This patient experienced intermittent gastrointestinal bleeding one week after blunt liver injury. Computed tomography scan of the abdomen depicts a contrast "blush" (*arrow*) consistent with a hepatic artery pseudoaneurysm at the site of injury.

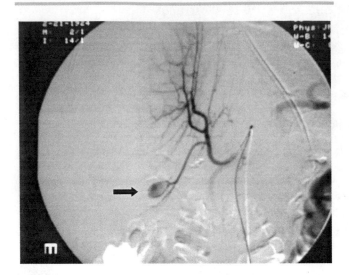

Figure 3 The same patient underwent hepatic angiography, which confirmed the presence of the pseudoaneurysm (*arrow*). The pseudoaneurysm was successfully embolized with resolution of hemobilia.

angiographic evidence of a large cavity have been treated with formal lobectomy (41). Severe jaundice may also be a consequence of injuries to the central portion of the liver with disruption of the hepatic veins. In this case, the jaundice is due to communication between the bile duct and the hepatic vein in a cavity of necrotic liver tissue and blood (66).

Biliary Stricture

The incidence of biliary stricture after elective liver resection is less than 5% (28,46). It is an uncommon late complication that is probably related to intraoperative injury to bile ducts, devascularization, or tumor recurrence. A distal biliary stricture may be responsible for a persistent biliary fistula. Reoperation with hepaticojejunostomy is usually necessary.

Biliary stricture among trauma patients may develop after operative repair of injury to the extraparenchymal bile ducts; such injuries are usually due to penetrating wounds. The incidence of stricture depends on the nature of the injury and the method of repair. For complete transection of the bile duct, repair with a biliobiliary anastomosis has been associated with higher rates of stricture than repair with a biliary–enteric anastomosis. For a tangential laceration of the bile duct, primary repair with or without a T tube is usually successful (44).

Mortality

Mortality after elective liver surgery is usually related to liver failure or multisystem organ failure. Exsanguination during the surgical procedure is an uncommon cause of death. Jarnagin et al. (46) found that factors affecting mortality rates in association with elective liver resection included blood loss, preoperative hyperbilirubinemia or thrombocytopenia, advanced age, and complex hepatectomy. In this study, the subgroup of patients with extrahepatic biliary tumors experienced the highest rates of mortality and morbidity. For patients who have suffered trauma, the mortality rates associated with initially planned nonoperative management are much lower than those associated with urgent operation at the time of admission because hemodynamic instability is the main indication for emergent procedures (Table 2). Currently, approximately 25% of deaths among patients admitted with liver injuries are liver related; other causes of death are multisystem organ failure and associated injuries, including head trauma (11,14).

REFERENCES

1. Couinaud C. Lobes et segments hepatiques. Notes sur l'architecture anatomique et chirurgicale du foie. Presse Med 1954; 62:709–712.
2. Filipponi F, Romagnoli P, Mosca F, Couinaud C. The dorsal sector of the human liver: embryological, anatomical and clinical relevance. Hepatogastroenterology 2000; 47:1726–1731.
3. Moore EE, Cogbill TH, Jurkovich GJ, Shackford SR, Malangoni MA, Champion HR. Organ injury scaling: spleen and liver (1994 revision). J Trauma 1995; 38: 323–324.
4. Huguet C, Gavelli A, Chieco PA, et al. Liver ischemia for hepatic resection: where is the limit? Surgery 1992; 111:251–259.
5. Wu CC, Hwang CR, Liu TJ, P'eng FK. Effects and limitations of prolonged intermittent ischaemia for hepatic resection of the cirrhotic liver. Br J Surg 1996; 83: 121–124.
6. Man K, Fan ST, Ng IO, Lo CM, Liu CL, Wong J. Prospective evaluation of Pringle maneuver in hepatectomy for liver tumors by a randomized study. Ann Surg 1997; 226:704–713.
7. Blumgart LH, Fong Y, Jarnagin WR. Major hepatic resection for primary and metastatic tumors. In: Baker RJ, Lillemoe KL, Fischer JE, eds. Mastery of Surgery. 4th. Philadelphia: Lippincott Williams and Wilkins, 2000: 1108–1127.
8. Grazi GL, Mazziotti A, Jovine E, et al. Total vascular exclusion of the liver during hepatic surgery. Selective use, extensive use, or abuse? Arch Surg 1997; 132: 1104–1109.
9. Elias D, Dube P, Bonvalot S, Debanne B, Plaud B, Lasser P. Intermittent complete vascular exclusion of the liver during hepatectomy: technique and indications. Hepatogastroenterology 1998; 45:389–395.
10. Vaillant JC, Borie DC, Hannoun L. Hepatectomy with hypothermic perfusion of the liver. Hepatogastroenterology 1998; 45:381–388.
11. Malhotra AK, Fabian TC, Croce MA, et al. Blunt hepatic injury: a paradigm shift from operative to nonoperative management in the 1990s. Ann Surg 2000; 231:804–813.
12. Strong RW, Lynch SV, Wall DR, Liu CL. Anatomic resection for severe liver trauma. Surgery 1998; 123:251–257.

13. Balasegaram M, Joishy SK. Hepatic resection: the logical approach to surgical management of major trauma to the liver. Am J Surg 1981; 142:580–583.

14. Fang JF, Chen RJ, Liu BC, Hsu YB, Kao JL, Chen MF. Blunt hepatic injury: minimal intervention is the policy of treatment. J Trauma 2000; 49:722–728.

15. Cox EF, Flancbaum L, Dauterive AH, Paulson RL. Blunt trauma to the liver. Analysis of management and mortality in 323 consecutive patients. Ann Surg 1988; 207:126–134.

16. Flint LM, Mays ET, Aaron WS, Fulton RL, Polk HC. Selectivity in the management of hepatic trauma. Ann Surg 1977; 185:613–618.

17. Cue JI, Cryer HG, Miller FB, Richardson JD, Polk HC Jr. Packing and planned reexploration for hepatic and retroperitoneal hemorrhage: critical refinements of a useful technique. J Trauma 1990; 30:1007–1013.

18. Beal SL. Fatal hepatic hemorrhage: an unresolved problem in the management of complex liver injuries. J Trauma 1990; 30:163–169.

19. Schrock T, Blaisdell W, Mathewson C Jr. Management of blunt trauma to the liver and hepatic veins. Arch Surg 1968; 96:698–704.

20. Misra B, Wagner R, Boneval H. Injuries of hepatic veins and retrohepatic vena cava. Am Surg 1983; 49:55–60.

21. Kudsk KA, Sheldon GF, Lim RC Jr. Atrial-caval shunting (ACS) after trauma. J Trauma 1982; 22:81–85.

22. Ringe B, Pichlmayr R. Total hepatectomy and liver transplantation: a life-saving procedure in patients with severe hepatic trauma. Br J Surg 1995; 82:837–839.

23. Fernandez DE, Lange K, Lange R, Eigler FW. Relevance of two-stage total hepatectomy and liver transplantation in acute liver failure and severe liver trauma. Transpl Int 2001; 14:184–190.

24. Takayama T, Makuuchi M, Inoue K, Sakamoto Y, Kubota K, Harihara Y. Selective and unselective clamping in cirrhotic liver. Hepatogastroenterology 1998; 45:376–380.

25. Miyagawa S, Makuuchi M, Kawasaki S, Kakazu T. Criteria for safe hepatic resection. Am J Surg 1995; 169:589–594.

26. Midorikawa Y, Kubota K, Takayama T, et al. A comparative study of postoperative complications after hepatectomy in patients with and without chronic liver disease. Surgery 1999; 126:484–491.

27. Wu CC, Yeh DC, Lin MC, Liu TJ, P'Eng FK. Improving operative safety for cirrhotic liver resection. Br J Surg 2001; 88:210–215.

28. Finch MD, Crosbie JL, Currie E, Garden OJ. An 8-year experience of hepatic resection: indications and outcome. Br J Surg 1998; 85:315–319.

29. Fabian TC, Croce MA, Stanford GG, et al. Factors affecting morbidity following hepatic trauma. A prospective analysis of 482 injuries. Ann Surg 1991; 213:540–548.

30. Bender JS, Geller ER, Wilson RF. Intra-abdominal sepsis following liver trauma. J Trauma 1989; 29:1140–1145.

31. Feliciano DV, Mattox KL, Jordan GL Jr, Burch JM, Bitondo CG, Cruse PA. Management of 1000 consecutive cases of hepatic trauma (1979–1984). Ann Surg 1986; 204:438–445.

32. Hsieh CH. Comparison of hepatic abscess after operative and nonoperative management of isolated blunt liver trauma. Int Surg 2002; 87:178–184.

33. Pachter HL, Knudson MM, Esrig B, et al. Status of nonoperative management of blunt hepatic injuries in 1995: a multicenter experience with 404 patients. J Trauma 1996; 40:31–38.

34. Farnell MB, Spencer MP, Thompson E, Williams HJ Jr, Mucha P Jr, Ilstrup DM. Nonoperative management of blunt hepatic trauma in adults. Surgery 1988; 104:748–756.

35. Pace RF, Blenkharn JI, Edwards WJ, Orloff M, Blumgart LH, Benjamin IS. Intra-abdominal sepsis after hepatic resection. Ann Surg 1989; 209:302–306.

36. Hollands MJ, Little JM. Post-traumatic bile fistulae. J Trauma 1991; 31:117–120.

37. Howdieshell TR, Purvis J, Bates WB, Teeslink CR. Biloma and biliary fistula following hepatorrhaphy for liver trauma: incidence, natural history, and management. Am Surg 1995; 61:165–168.

38. Capussotti L, Polastri R. Operative risks of major hepatic resections. Hepatogastroenterology 1998; 45:184–190.

39. Lo CM, Fan ST, Liu CL, Lai EC, Wong J. Biliary complications after hepatic resection: risk factors, management, and outcome. Arch Surg 1998; 133:156–161.

40. Olsen WR. Late complications of central liver injuries. Surgery 1982; 92:733–743.

41. Croce MA, Fabian TC, Spiers JP, Kudsk KA. Traumatic hepatic artery pseudoaneurysm with hemobilia. Am J Surg 1994; 168:235–238.

42. Savader SJ, Trerotola SO, Merine DS, Venbrux AC, Osterman FA. Hemobilia after percutaneous transhepatic biliary drainage: treatment with transcatheter embolotherapy. J Vasc Interv Radiol 1992; 3:345–352.

43. Jeng KS, Sheen IS, Yang FS. Are modified procedures significantly better than conventional procedures in percutaneous transhepatic treatment for complicated right hepatolithiasis with intrahepatic biliary strictures? Scand J Gastroenterol 2002; 37:597–601.

44. Ivatury RR, Rohman M, Nallathambi M, Rao PM, Gunduz Y, Stahl WM. The morbidity of injuries of the extra-hepatic biliary system. J Trauma 1985; 25:967–973.

45. Nonami T, Nakao A, Kurokawa T, et al. Blood loss and ICG clearance as best prognostic markers of post-hepatectomy liver failure. Hepatogastroenterology 1999; 46:1669–1672.

46. Jarnagin WR, Gonen M, Fong Y, et al. Improvement in perioperative outcome after hepatic resection: analysis of 1803 consecutive cases over the past decade. Ann Surg 2002; 236:397–407.

47. Shimada M, Takenaka K, Fujiwara Y, et al. Risk factors linked to postoperative morbidity in patients with hepatocellular carcinoma. Br J Surg 1998; 85:195–198.

48. Ginzburg E, Shatz D, Lynn M, et al. The role of liver transplantation in the subacute trauma patients. Am Surg 1998; 64:363–364.

49. Johnson M, Mannar R, Wu AV. Correlation between blood loss and inferior vena caval pressure during liver resection. Br J Surg 1998; 85:188–190.

50. Feliciano DV, Mattox KL, Burch JM, Bitondo CG, Jordan GL Jr. Packing for control of hepatic hemorrhage. J Trauma 1986; 26:738–743.

51. Binmoeller KF, Katon RM, Shneidman R. Endoscopic management of postoperative biliary leaks: review of 77 cases and report of two cases with biloma formation. Am J Gastroenterol 1991; 86:227–231.

52. Sugiyama M, Atomi Y, Matsuoka T, Yamaguchi Y. Endoscopic biliary stenting for treatment of persistent

biliary fistula after blunt hepatic injury. Gastrointest Endosc 2000; 51:42–44.

53. Sugimoto K, Asari Y, Sakaguchi T, Owada T, Maekawa K. Endoscopic retrograde cholangiography in the nonsurgical management of blunt liver injury. J Trauma 1993; 35:192–199.

54. Carrillo EH, Reed DN Jr, Gordon L, Spain DA, Richardson JD. Delayed laparoscopy facilitates the management of biliary peritonitis in patients with complex liver injuries. Surg Endosc 2001; 15:319–322.

55. Griffen M, Ochoa J, Boulanger BR. A minimally invasive approach to bile peritonitis after blunt liver injury. Am Surg 2000; 66:309–312.

56. Krige JE, Bornman PC, Terblanche J. Therapeutic perihepatic packing in complex liver trauma. Br J Surg 1992; 79:43–46.

57. Fong Y, Brennan MF, Brown K, Heffernan N, Blumgart LH. Drainage is unnecessary after elective liver resection. Am J Surg 1996; 171:158–162.

58. Belghiti J, Kabbej M, Sauvanet A, Vilgrain V, Panis Y, Fekete F. Drainage after elective hepatic resection. A randomized trial. Ann Surg 1993; 218:748–753.

59. Mullins RJ, Stone HH, Dunlop W, Strom PR. Hepatic trauma: evaluation of routine drainage. South Med J 1985; 78:259–261.

60. Inoguchi H, Mii S, Sakata H, Orita H, Yamashita S. Intrahepatic pseudoaneurysm after surgical hemostasis for a delayed hemorrhage due to blunt liver injury: report of a case. Surg Today 2001; 31:367–370.

61. Basile KE, Sivit CJ, Sachs PB, Stallion A. Hepatic arterial pseudoaneurysm: a rare complication of blunt abdominal trauma in children. Pediatr Radiol 1999; 29:306–308.

62. Hsu KL, Ko SF, Chou FF, Sheen-Chen SM, Lee TY. Massive hemobilia. Hepatogastroenterology 2002; 49:306–310.

63. Aboujaoude M, Noel B, Beaudoin M, et al. Pseudoaneurysm of the proper hepatic artery with duodenal fistula appearing as a late complication of blunt abdominal trauma. J Trauma 1996; 40:123–125.

64. Sandblom P, Saegesser F, Mirkovitch V. Hepatic hemobilia: hemorrhage from the intrahepatic biliary tract, a review. World J Surg 1984; 8:41–50.

65. Clancy TE, Warren RL. Endoscopic treatment of biliary colic resulting from hemobilia after nonoperative management of blunt hepatic injury: case report and review of the literature. J Trauma 1997; 43: 527–529.

66. Carrillo EH, Wohltmann C, Richardson JD, Polk HC Jr. Evolution in the treatment of complex blunt liver injuries. Curr Probl Surg 2001; 38:1–60.

67. Teh SH, Christein J, Donohue J, et al. Hepatic resection of hepatocellular carcinoma on patients with cirrhosis: Model of end-stage Liver Disease (MELD) score predicts perioperative mortality. J Gastrointest Surg 2005; 9:1207–1215.

12

Complications of Pancreatic Surgery and Trauma

Christopher K. Senkowski

Mercer University School of Medicine, Memorial Health University Medical Center, Savannah, Georgia, U.S.A.

Pancreatic surgery has undergone a number of changes during the past few decades. The trend is toward an increase in the incidence of pancreatic adenocarcinoma but a decrease in the incidence of periampullary tumors. The mortality and morbidity rates associated with major pancreatic resection have decreased dramatically because diagnostic and treatment methods have been refined. The increased survival rates of patients with multisystem trauma, coupled with advances in imaging techniques, have increased the frequency with which pancreatic injury is diagnosed. For the trauma surgeon, resident, or student who performs pancreatic surgery only occasionally, it is crucial to study the pancreas and its response to surgery, so that the potential complications of pancreatic surgery can be recognized and pancreatic injury can be managed.

ANATOMY

The pancreas is situated in a relatively fixed position in the retroperitoneum and is surrounded by crucial structures. It is divided into a head, a neck, a body, and a tail (Fig. 1). The gland lies across the second lumbar vertebra; thus, it is commonly injured by blunt trauma. Penetrating injury can affect any area of the gland and is associated with a high mortality rate, before the injured patient even reaches the hospital. The intricate involvement of the pancreas with the duodenum, the mesenteric vessels, and the portal venous system makes elective surgery on the pancreas technically challenging (Fig. 2).

It is helpful to conceptualize the pancreas as having both exocrine and endocrine functions. Obviously, the production of insulin is an endocrine function, and the potential complications of resection or injury include diabetes mellitus. The exocrine pancreas consists of the acinar cells with their ductal system that delivers the enzymes to the duodenum. The average human produces 750 to 1500 mL of pancreatic fluid daily. The enzymes secreted in this fluid include proteases, amylase, nucleases, elastases, collagenases, and lecithinases. These proteolytic enzymes are the most potentially damaging, but fortunately they are secreted in their inactive form as zymogens. However, when these enzymes are activated in the interstitium of the gland or in the retroperitoneum, or when they leak from an anastomosis, severe inflammation and necrosis occur. As a result of this mechanism, the exocrine pancreas causes most pancreatic complications. Controlling the exocrine pancreas is crucial to managing complications associated with pancreatic surgery.

Knowledge of the anatomy of the pancreatic ducts is important for any pancreatic or trauma surgeon. The main pancreatic duct, the Wirsung duct, traverses the entire gland, lies slightly superior in the gland, and ends by joining the common bile duct and emptying into the duodenum. The accessory duct, the Santorini duct, drains the superior proximal portion of the gland through an accessory opening directly into the duodenum about 2 to 2.5 cm above the papilla. A substantial number of pancreatic ductal anomalies exist (Fig. 3). In approximately 20% of cases, the minor duct drains directly into the main pancreatic duct, and in 5% to 8% of cases, it is the

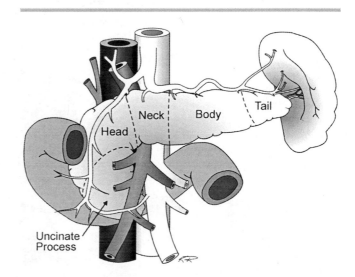

Figure 1 Anatomy of pancreas.

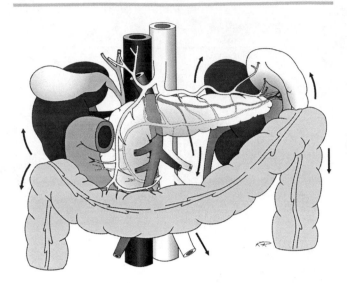

Figure 2 Pancreas with surrounding anatomy. Arrows indicate planes of dissection for blood, infection, etc.

only duct for the entire pancreas. The common bile duct and the pancreatic duct may have separate openings into a combined papilla or they may share a common channel.

The arterial and venous anatomies are relatively constant in the pancreas; however, knowledge of the main vascular branches is important when the gland is to be dissected and particularly when such dissection occurs near the portal triad. The common hepatic artery traverses the superior border of the pancreas toward the portal triad. It divides to form the proper hepatic artery and the gastroduodenal artery. The gastroduodenal artery descends retrograde and within

the gland itself. In about 15% of cases, there is an aberrant right hepatic artery directly off the superior mesenteric artery. Whether this artery is replaced or aberrant is difficult to determine at the time of surgery; therefore, the artery must be carefully preserved. The venous drainage system includes the splenic vein and the portal vein. This anatomy is familiar to any surgeon who performs pancreatic surgery.

GENERAL COMPLICATIONS ASSOCIATED WITH PANCREATIC SURGERY

All elective and emergent pancreatic surgery procedures as well as pancreatic trauma are associated with a commonly occurring set of complications. This statement largely applies to the complications associated with acute pancreatitis. Later sections of this chapter address these issues as a group with specific nuances.

Whenever the pancreas is injured, incised, or inflamed, the pancreatic ducts are disrupted. When pancreatic secretions leak into the retroperitoneal space or into the true peritoneal cavity, as occasionally occurs, complications will include fluid collections, abscess, or fistula (Fig. 2). If the enzymes erode into blood vessels, the complication is hemorrhage. The other main difficulty occurs with repeated insult, which results in scar formation within the pancreas; this scarring causes biliary obstruction, obstruction of the pancreatic duct, or both.

Fluid Collections

Understanding fluid collections is particularly important because the simple nomenclature can be confusing. Too often, the term "pseudocyst" is applied to a

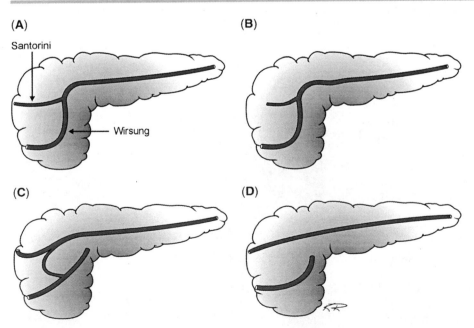

Figure 3 Pancreatic ductal variants. **(A)** Normal (60%). **(B)** Regression dorsal duct (<10%). **(C)** Functional divisum (<10%). **(D)** Divisum (15%).

peripancreatic fluid collection. It is crucial to remember that any cystic lesion of the pancreas must be suspected to be a cystic neoplasm before it is erroneously labeled a pseudocyst. Many peripancreatic fluid collections result simply from manipulation, injury, or inflammation and will resolve. Not all of these are pseudocysts. Approximately 40% to 50% of patients who undergo computed tomography (CT) scans for the assessment of acute pancreatitis have a fluid collection. Sixty percent of these cases resolve with observation alone (1). A more accurate definition of a pseudocyst is a cyst that has been present for four to six weeks and has a well-defined wall (Fig. 4).

In 1992, a group of pancreatic experts convened the Atlanta Symposium to define appropriate terms for various peripancreatic fluid collections (2). These definitions are very important in discussions of treatment. A pseudocyst, as defined by this group, "is a collection of pancreatic juice enclosed by a wall of fibrous or granulation tissue, which arises as a consequence of acute pancreatitis, pancreatic trauma, or chronic pancreatitis" (2). Importantly, the Atlanta Symposium defines pancreatic abscess as a purulent collection. Not uncommonly, a pseudocyst with clear fluid will exhibit a positive result on Gram staining. Such a pseudocyst is not an abscess and is inconsequential. For these reasons, surgeons should not use the terms "infected pseudocyst" or "acute pseudocyst."

If the fluid collection is clinically associated with acute pancreatitis, the appropriate initial therapy is observation because many of these fluid collections will resolve. Aspiration or CT-guided drainage is not recommended. If the fluid collection persists, a wall will form over a period of four to six weeks; at that time the collection can be classified as a pseudocyst. The fluid in these cysts is rich in pancreatic enzymes

and is usually sterile. Endoscopic or surgical therapy should be considered for collections that have a definite wall, that have been present for more than six weeks, and that are larger than 6 cm in diameter. However, observation, even in these cases, is often a successful treatment strategy. Yeo et al. (3) retrospectively reviewed the outcome of expectant management of 76 asymptomatic pseudocysts as large as 10 cm in diameter; 60% of these pseudocysts resolved over a period of one year with only one complication. In Bradley's classic study of pseudocysts (4), he found in pseudocysts that had been present for less than six weeks, 40% of the cysts resolved with a complication rate of 20%, whereas pseudocysts that had been present for more than 12 weeks did not resolve and were associated with a complication rate of 67%.

Pancreatic Abscess

Pancreatic abscesses occur in 2% to 9% of cases of acute pancreatitis (5). Abscesses are more common among patients with pancreatitis resulting from gallstones or trauma; the incidence of abscess formation in association with alcoholic pancreatitis is much lower (6,7). It is important to understand that pancreatic abscess and infected pancreatic necrosis are two separate entities. Both conditions will be associated with symptoms such as fever, leukocytosis, and intestinal ileus; however, a pancreatic abscess will be seen on CT scans as a fluid collection with air (Fig. 5). In select cases, when abscesses are localized and accessible, percutaneous drainage can be performed, but most cases will require operative exploration and drainage of the abscess. A review by Widdison and Karanjia (6) found that 60% of patients had a single abscess and 38% had multiple abscesses. The mortality rate associated with this condition is approximately 5% to 10%, a rate lower than that associated with pancreatic necrosis (8). In such cases, the

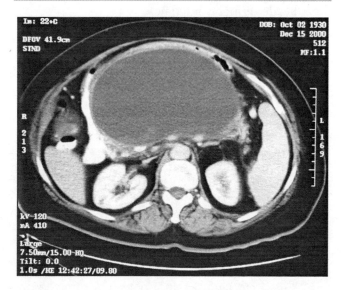

Figure 4 CT scan of patient with giant pancreatic pseudocyst as a late sequelea of pancreatitis. Stomach is compressed anteriorly.

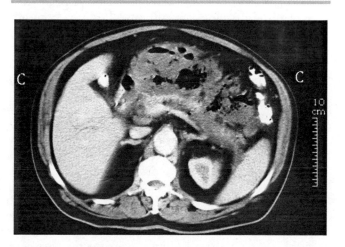

Figure 5 Pancreatic abscess with obvious air in a patient with stone impacted at ampulla.

fluid in the abscess should be cultured, and treatment with appropriate antibiotics should be initiated.

Unlike pancreatic abscesses, which are usually localized, pancreatic necrosis is usually associated with inflammation that spreads throughout the retroperitoneum and with massive release of cytokines. Pancreatic necrosis runs a more indolent course than pancreatic abscess. The agents typically responsible for the condition include, in the order of frequency, *Escherichia coli*, *Staphylococcus aureus*, *Pseudomonas aeruginosa*, and *Enterobacter* species (8). Carefully selected patients with a single-localized abscess are treated with percutaneous drainage (9).

Hemorrhage

The pancreas is intimately associated with the superior mesenteric vein (SMV), the portal vein, the vena cava, the aorta, the superior mesenteric artery, and the celiac trunk. Penetrating injury to the pancreas alone carries an estimated mortality rate of 5% (10); however, isolated injury is an exception, and the mortality rate increases to 34% when the injury is associated with vascular injury (11). Blunt pancreatic injury requires a substantial kinetic force. At times, this force can result in an isolated injury, but it is more often associated with multiple injuries, and such injuries are related to the risk of hemorrhage.

After major elective procedures for resection, 2% to 4% of patients experience hemorrhage. In this situation, either a technical error in hemostasis or an erosion of a vessel resulting from leakage of pancreatic enzymes has occurred (12). Both situations require prompt operative intervention; when vessel erosion is involved, it is crucial to rule out anastomotic leak as the cause of the hemorrhage.

Hemorrhage resulting from pancreatitis is rare but lethal. The term "hemorrhagic pancreatitis" is rarely used; instead, the term "severe necrotizing pancreatitis" is standard. With this condition, hemorrhage occurs as the result of erosion of a major vessel or rupture of a pseudoaneurysm, although it is most common after the formation of a pseudocyst. The incidence of hemorrhage associated with pseudocyst is 1% to 2.5%, and approximately 10% of patients who experience such hemorrhage will have chronic pancreatitis with angiographic evidence of pseudoaneurysms (12). The splenic artery or its branches are the most common sites of bleeding (Table 1) (13,14). Angiographic embolization is the key tool in the management of this problem; it identifies the source of bleeding in 90% of cases. Prompt recognition and action are crucial to outcome. Most cases are controlled with resuscitation and angiographic embolization. In the few cases in which operation is required, the surgery is difficult because of inflammation. Isolating the vessel is generally not possible; instead, the bleeding site is directly oversewn. Resection is exceptionally difficult in the acute situation. A review of the literature shows that embolization is successful in 70% to 80% of cases and that the

Table 1 Vessel Sites of Bleeding in Patients with Hemorrhagic Complications of Pancreatitis and Pancreatic Pseudocyst

Vessel	Percent
Splenic artery	37
Pancreaticoduodenal artery	19
Gastroduodenal artery	18
Dorsal pancreatic artery	7
Transverse pancreatic artery	3.5
Left gastric artery	2.6
Hepatic artery	2.6
Superior mesenteric artery	2.6

Source: From Refs. 13,14.

mortality rate is half that associated with operative control of hemorrhage.

Angiography with embolization is the best choice if bleeding is into or involves a pseudocyst. If this procedure fails, the best operative approach is resection. If the cyst is associated with the distal pancreas, ligation of the artery with angiographic guidance is a successful approach. Attempting to control bleeding with direct suturing inside the pseudocyst usually results in failure. Resection, although difficult, carries the best chance for success.

When hemorrhage occurs among patients with chronic pancreatitis, the presentation is usually less dramatic, but is nonetheless extremely serious. The typical presentation includes gastrointestinal bleeding caused by erosion of the pseudoaneurysm into the stomach or duodenum. If it erodes into the pancreatic ductal system, the result is a condition known as "hemosuccus pancreaticus," which causes blood to drain from the ampulla, as shown by endoscopic retrograde cholangiopancreatography (ERCP). In such cases, initial diagnosis and treatment require angiography and embolization. Performing a surgical procedure without preoperative angiography because of hemodynamic instability is a dire situation and leads to a decidedly poor outcome.

Jaundice

Jaundice is a common complication of pancreatic surgery, trauma, or acute pancreatitis. However, after resection of the head of the pancreas, jaundice is uncommon and suggests a technical problem with the biliary–enteric anastomosis. Careful attention to detail when the procedure is performed can prevent this problem.

Among patients with chronic pancreatitis, biliary obstruction resulting from intrapancreatic scar tissue causes jaundice and often requires surgical correction by either a local resection of the pancreatic head or a biliary bypass procedure. Occasionally, a patient may have both a pseudocyst and a jaundice. Treatment of the pseudocyst relieves extrinsic biliary obstruction, but when the biliary obstruction is caused by chronic scarring, a drainage procedure is indicated (15).

Persistent jaundice in a patient with acute pancreatitis suggests the need for evaluating the ductal system with ERCP or magnetic resonance cholangiopancreatography (MRCP), so that choledocholithiasis or other causes of mechanical obstruction, such as tumor or stricture, can be ruled out. The technological advances in both diagnosis and management made possible by ERCP and MRCP make evaluation of these conditions easier; thus, these procedures have largely replaced transhepatic cholangiography (16,17). The importance of intraoperative cholangiography in guiding the surgical procedure cannot be overemphasized.

Fistula

Pancreatic fistulas can be internal or external and can be the result of unrecognized ductal injury, leakage, or rupture of a pseudocyst. Internal fistulas within the peritoneal cavity are classified as pancreatic ascites. This condition is uncommon but produces peritoneal fluid that is rich in amylase. Fistulas can also communicate to the pleural cavity (Fig. 6). Most fistulas are external and track along previous drain sites. The fluid they produce is clear, thin, and rich in amylase. It is relatively innocuous to the skin because the zymogens have not yet been activated. Pancreatic fistulas that coexist with biliary or gastric secretions are more caustic because the zymogens have been activated and cause more internal damage and greater excoriation of the skin.

Initial treatment involves controlling external drainage and treating the associated sepsis. ERCP documents the integrity of the ductal system. Generally, when the fistula is persistent, a ductal leak occurs. Performing a sphincterotomy, placing a pancreatic stent, or both will decrease the time required for healing (18). If the leak is distal or persistent, a distal resection is required.

After distal resection of the pancreas, the rate of ductal leakage is approximately 10% (19). As many as 90% of cases of ductal leakage heal with closed suction drainage (20). When the output is high or persistent, ERCP provides additional information. Reasons for failure to close include proximal stricture, stone, or plug; epithelialization of the tract; or super-infection of the pancreatic fluid. Leakage of a pancreatic anastomosis occurs in approximately 10% of cases and is controlled with prolonged drainage. With current techniques of percutaneous drainage, parenteral nutrition, sphincterotomy, and pancreatic stent, many of these fistulas heal without the need for operative management.

The use of octreotide for managing pancreatic fistulas has yielded mixed results. Administering octreotide can decrease the volume or output of the fistula, but such treatment does not shorten the time required for closing off the fistula (21).

The role of total parenteral nutrition (TPN) for patients with pancreatic fistulas is to provide protein and calories and to sustain the patient's nutritional status. Whenever possible, however, enteral feeding is preferred. Enteral feeding obviates the risks associated with line placement, pneumothorax, and line sepsis, and it also provides the benefits of gut immunoprotection. Optimally, a feeding tube distal to the ampulla is more desirable than gastric feeding. With the use of specialized modular elemental diets, the increase in the fistula's output should be inconsequential.

Exocrine Insufficiency

Loss of exocrine function is a common problem among patients with chronic pancreatitis. Forty percent of these patients have some exocrine insufficiency (22). Consequently, surgical procedures for chronic pancreatitis, especially resection, invariably result in some level of exocrine insufficiency. Patients who undergo these procedures are usually discharged from the hospital with pancreatic enzyme supplementation. Pancreaticoduodenectomy is associated with a 10% to 20% risk of symptomatic exocrine insufficiency (23). This risk is obviously higher after subtotal pancreatectomy and is 100% after total pancreatectomy. Symptoms of exocrine insufficiency are gas bloating, postprandial cramping, and foul, loose stools (steatorrhea). Acute pancreatitis, pancreatic trauma, and distal resection usually do not result in exocrine insufficiency. Fortunately, when this diagnosis is confirmed, the treatment is straightforward. Commercially available enzyme supplements, given orally and titrated to effect, are suggested.

Diabetes Mellitus

Approximately 80% to 90% of a normal pancreas can be resected without causing endocrine insufficiency (24). Diabetes mellitus develops spontaneously among 30% of patients with chronic pancreatitis (25). In these cases, the pancreas is atrophic and fibrotic; resection of 50% of the organ can result in diabetes. Acute pancreatitis and traumatic pancreatic injury rarely result in endocrine insufficiency.

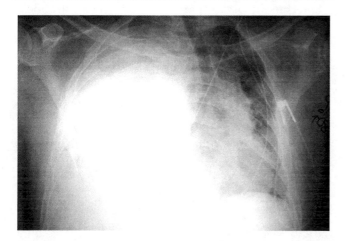

Figure 6 Massive pleural effusion secondary to pleuropancreatic fistula, years after gunshot wound to pancreas was treated by distal pancreatectomy.

Postresectional diabetes is difficult to manage. Younger patients fare better. The glucose swings are broad and severe hypoglycemic episodes are common (26). Some surgeons believe that preserving the duodenum and the duodenogastric axis during the operation helps smooth out the broad swings between hypoglycemia and hyperglycemia. This effect may be related to the larger meals ingested by patients with an intact stomach.

COMPLICATIONS OF OPERATIVE TREATMENT FOR ACUTE PANCREATITIS

When severe acute pancreatitis is treated surgically, the procedure is technically challenging and fraught with hazards. Generally, the procedure is undertaken to resolve one of the aforementioned complications. Necrosectomy is reserved for cases of infected pancreatic necrosis or significant sterile necrosis that is unresponsive to aggressive care and organ support in the intensive care unit (ICU), but the effectiveness of necrosectomy in sterile necrosis is still intensely debated (27). After the onset of symptoms, pancreatic necrosectomy is usually performed within two to four weeks of a severe episode. Earlier intervention is less beneficial because the pancreatic tissue is still formed and is impossible to debride. After a short period of time, ongoing injury, infection, and necrosis will soften and liquefy the gland. At this phase, operative debridement offers the best chance for improving the patient's condition.

Different approaches to pancreatic necrosectomy have been advocated: bilateral subcostal incision or midline incision, drainage through the gastrocolic omentum or through the transverse mesocolon, open packing or continuous lavage, and closed treatment (28,29). All of these options have merits, and their use must be tailored to the specific situation. The author advocates the bilateral subcostal incision because it affords wide exposure to all areas of the gland.

The main principles of the procedure are adequate first-time debridement, drainage of the lesser sac, and examination of all possible areas of spread, including perinephric, retrocolic gutter, and inframesocolic areas. The surgeon must also remember that catastrophic retroperitoneal sepsis can induce intestinal serosal infection and full-thickness intestinal gangrene. Adequate debridement includes intestinal resection if full-thickness gangrene is present. The gland must be fully evaluated and inspected, and full "kocherization" of the pancreatic head must be performed. Bleeding may be significant and diffuse, but is usually controlled with pressure. Occasionally, packing is required to control bleeding until ICU management can correct acidosis, hypothermia, and coagulopathy.

When pancreatic tissue is debrided, any vascular band–like structures are ligated. Judicious manipulation in the retrocolic and paraduodenal spaces is crucial because iatrogenic fistulas can result. The rate of fistula formation was 30% in one series (30).

Table 2 Complications of Pancreatic Debridement in Sterile Versus Infected Necrosis

Complication	Sterile ($N = 128$) (%)	Infected ($N = 93$) (%)
Fistula		
Pancreatic	20 (16)	21 (22)
Biliary	2 (2)	3 (3)
Bowel	12 (9)	18 (19)
Wound infection	19 (15)	12 (13)
Bleeding	20 (16)	12 (13)

Source: From Ref. 28.

Pancreatic debridement is a very complex situation, requiring aggressive ICU support and meticulous operative care. Various methods of draining and maintaining lavage of the lesser sac are beyond the scope of this chapter; however, crucial to any pancreatic debridement is placement of a jejunal feeding tube (27). Enteral nutrition is the preferred method of feeding; the findings of prospective randomized trials indicate that this type of feeding decreases the incidence of septic complications (31). Cholecystectomy with T-tube drainage is often difficult and is performed only if the pancreatitis is caused by gallstones. If the inflammation is too severe for the safe performance of cholecystectomy, then a cholecystostomy provides drainage and later access for interventional techniques. Gastrostomy, rather than a nasogastric tube, can be used selectively for decompression.

Octreotide has been studied as a treatment for severe necrotizing pancreatitis, but its effect is not yet clear. One study showed that treatment with octreotide is associated with a decrease in the incidence of acute respiratory distress syndrome (32). Octreotide also seems to decrease the output of fistulas.

A massive release of cytokines occurs in association with necrotizing pancreatitis, and various methods of blocking this release have been studied. A recent prospective randomized trial found that platelet-activating factor provides no improvement or change in mortality rates (33). Some studies champion the technique of continuous venous hyperfiltration as a method of cytokine clearance (34).

The mortality rate associated with infected pancreatic necrosis is 100% when the condition is not treated with surgery and approximately 30% to 50% when it is treated with surgery (28). The morbidity rate of operative management is 50% to 80%; 30% of patients require an additional surgical procedure, and 20% experience major organ failure (Table 2) (28). These complex cases test the surgeon's skills to the fullest.

COMPLICATIONS OF SURGERY FOR CHRONIC PANCREATITIS
Strictures of the Common Bile Duct or the Ampulla of Vater

Operations for stricture of the common bile duct have largely been replaced by the endoscopic technique of sphincterotomy and stent, but on occasion enterobiliary drainage, transduodenal sphincteroplasty, and pancreatic septoplasty are necessary. Unfortunately, today's surgical residents see few of these operative procedures. When patients require such surgical interventions, other techniques for repairing strictures have already failed, and the previous procedures make additional interventions more difficult. These interventions require meticulous attention to detail so that complete division of the sphincter can be ensured. If pancreatic divisum coexists with a distal stricture, the surgeon must perform a minor duct sphincteroplasty.

The worst complication, which occurs in 10% to 40% of cases, is failure to improve the patient's symptoms (35). The mortality rate associated with these procedures is less than 1%, and the morbidity rate is no higher than 10% (35). A leak from the duodenotomy or an unrecognized injury to the posterior wall of the common duct into the retroperitoneum is a rare complication. Routine closed suction drainage controls this complication. Postoperative pancreatitis can occur, but as long as the sphincter is widely patent and the septum is not inadvertently occluded, this complication should resolve spontaneously.

Debilitating Pain

Some patients experience debilitating pain after undergoing surgery for chronic pancreatitis. This complication is often treated with longitudinal pancreaticojejunostomy (LPJ). In such cases, the pancreas, after years of chronic inflammation, is fibrotic and scarred. As a result, incision, biopsy, and anastomosis are easier to perform, and the firm gland will hold a suture. During LPJ, the pancreatic duct is opened throughout its entire length. It is crucial to remove all stones and debris within the duct before anastomosis of the jejunum is performed. LPJ is a relatively safe procedure. Leaks are uncommon but can be controlled with closed suction drainage. Both single-layer and double-layer suturing techniques are effective. Because the gland is firm, there is little risk of exacerbation of pancreatitis.

Nevertheless, LPJ often fails to achieve 100% pain relief. Some surgeons believe that the clearance of the proximal duct in the head of the gland is important for pain control. Thus, they advocate resection in combination with LPJ (Fig. 7) (36). Others believe that the pancreatic head is the pacemaker for the pain associated with this disease. Newer techniques use ultrasonic lithotripsy to clear the proximal duct, and these procedures have resulted in improved pain relief (37).

When LPJ fails to relieve the pain associated with chronic pancreatitis, pancreaticoduodenectomy may be successful if the disease is mostly confined to the head of the gland. Although this is an extensive procedure to be undertaken for benign disease, the morbidity and mortality rates associated with this operation seem to be lower than those associated with

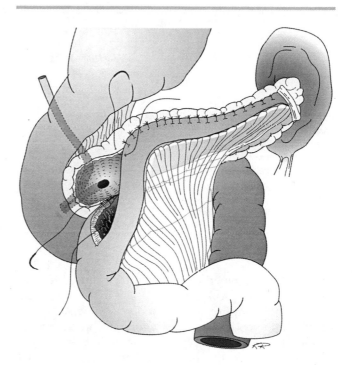

Figure 7 Local resection of pancreatic head combined with lateral pancreaticojejunostomy.

resection for cancer. A number of other procedures have also been used when LPJ fails. Local resection of the pancreatic head, as described by Frey and Smith (36), preserves the duodenum, cores out the head of the pancreas, and includes LPJ. The procedure described by Beger et al. (38) also preserves the duodenum but resects more of the head of the pancreas than the procedure described by Frey and colleagues (Fig. 7). Several reports indicate that resection of the pancreatic head achieves better pain relief than LPJ and is associated with lower morbidity and mortality rates than pancreaticoduodenectomy (Table 3) (39–42). Beger et al. (38) have also demonstrated that preserving the duodenogastric axis leads to less glucose instability. These operations are technically sophisticated; however because the gland is relatively firm, the sutures hold and the anastomoses are relatively sturdy. Additionally because the operation is used for benign disease, the principles of surgical oncology, such as wide excision, are not necessary.

COMPLICATIONS OF SURGERY FOR PANCREATIC PSEUDOCYST

Once surgical intervention is required for a patient with a persistent pseudocyst, the first decision to be made is whether an endoscopic or an open procedure will be performed. Excellent technological developments over the past 10 years allow internal drainage of most retrogastric and retroduodenal pseudocysts. With direct

Table 3 Results of Classic and Extended Resection for Chronic Pancreatitis

Results	Pylorus-preserving pancreatoduodenectomy Stapleton et al. (1996) ($n = 45$)	Partial pancreatoduodenectomy Saeger et al. (1993) ($n = 111$)	Longitudinal pancreaticojejunostomy combined with local pancreatic head excision Frey et al. (1994) ($n = 50$)	Duodenum-preserving resection of the head of the pancreas Buechler et al. (1997) ($n = 298$)
Pain relief or substantial alleviation (%)	80	79	75	88
Hospital morbidity rate (%)	47	10	22	29
Hospital mortality rate (%)	0	1	0	1
Late mortality rate (%)	7	10	4	9
Endocrine insufficiency rate (%)	37	39	11	2
Exocrine insufficiency rate (%)	80	40	11	–
Increase of body weight (%) >5 kg	100	77	64	81
Occupational rehabilitation rate (%)	–	66	32	63
Follow-up period (yr)	2–12	0.5–16.0	2–9	1–22

Source: From Refs. 39–42.

vision through the endoscope, cautery is used to enter the cyst. One or more stents are placed to create either a cystgastrostomy or a cystduodenostomy. A number of series have demonstrated good technical success (Table 4) (43–45). Complications include bleeding and leakage, particularly when the pseudocyst is not adherent to the viscera. Therefore, careful patient selection is crucial. As techniques are further refined, most pseudocysts will probably be treated endoscopically.

Cystjejunostomy and Cystgastrostomy

Cystgastrostomy is a useful procedure when retrogastric pseudocysts are adherent to the stomach wall, which they are in most cases. However, approximately 11% of these pseudocysts are not adherent to the stomach wall (4), and in such cases, the better option is to perform a Roux-en-Y cystjejunostomy.

The cystgastrostomy begins with an anterior gastrotomy. The posterior wall of the stomach is carefully palpated so that the thinnest area of the protruding cyst can be found. The cystgastrostomy is created in this area. Bleeding at the edges of the cystgastrostomy must be carefully controlled; some surgeons recommend using running interlocked sutures for hemostasis. The dilated aneurysmal vessels within the cyst can be easily damaged; thus, aggressive suctioning within the cavity of the cyst can cause massive bleeding. For this reason, great care must be exercised during palpation or suction inside the cyst. Once the fluid within the cyst has been drained, an opening is created in the posterior wall of the stomach. Because one complication of the operation is premature closure of the cyst and reoccurrence of the pseudocyst, this opening in the stomach must be 4 to 6 cm long. Postoperative bleeding can occur at site of anastomosis and may necessitate reoperation. Overall, the mortality rate associated with this procedure is less than 2%, and the rates of morbidity and recurrence are less than 5% (46).

Occasionally, the diagnosis of pseudocyst is erroneous (Fig. 8). For this reason, a biopsy of the cyst wall should be performed so that the frozen-section examination can determine whether the sample contains epithelium. A true pseudocyst consists of a fibrous wall but no epithelium. If the sample contains epithelium, the lesion is instead a cystic neoplasm, and it must be resected. If examination of the internal

Table 4 Comparison of Series for Endoscopic Treatment of Pancreatic Pseudocysts

References	Year	No. of patients	ECG size (mm)	Stent type (Fr)	Nasocystic drain	Technical failures	Bleeding	Other complications	Initial success	Recurrences	Long-term success	Follow-up (mo)
Endoscopic cystgastrostomy												
Smits et al.	1995	10	3–5	7/10	No	3	2 (1)	Two perforations	6	3	3	32
Cremer et al.	1989	11	10	No	All	0	1 (1)	Two infections	11	2	9	18
Dohmoto et al.	1994	10	5	7P	No	0	–	–	10	2	8	Not stated
Endoscopic cystduodenostomy												
Smits et al.	1995	7	3–5	7/10	No	0	0	0	7	0	7	32
Cremer et al.	1989	22	8	No	All	1	0	One perforation	21	2	19	35
Dohmoto et al.	1994	3	5	7P	1	0	0	0	3	0	3	Not stated

Abbreviation: ECG, endoscopic cystgastrostomy.
Source: From Refs. 43–45.

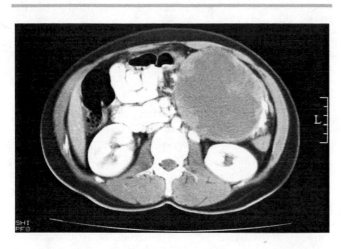

Figure 8 Papillary cystic tumor in a young female with no previous history of pancreatitis. Notice heterogenous frond-like projections into the cyst.

aspect of the pseudocyst reveals frond-like papillary projections, a cystic neoplasm must be suspected. In this case, the results of biopsy will indicate a tumor that must be resected.

If the pseudocyst is larger than 10 cm in diameter, cystjejunostomy should be performed even if the cyst is adherent to viscera. Cystjejunostomy is a widely applicable technique for all types of pseudocysts, including large pseudocysts, multiple pseudocysts, and pseudocysts not adherent to adjacent viscera. This procedure is a better choice than cystgastrostomy because it facilitates dependent drainage. Surgeons who perform procedures for pseudocyst should be comfortable with Roux-en-Y cystjejunostomy, a versatile procedure that should probably be the first choice for treating most pseudocysts. The opening created in the cyst should be 6 to 8 cm wide. The arrangement of the Roux limb provides excellent dependent drainage; the best drainage is achieved by retrocolic positioning. The Roux limb should be at least 60 cm long so that reflux of enteric contents into the cyst can be prevented. The procedure can be performed with either a one-layer or a two-layer anastomosis; both methods offer good results and good success. Closed suction drainage should be provided near the most dependent portion of the anastomosis. Again, biopsy of the wall is necessary.

One serious postoperative complication is hemorrhage, although it occurs more infrequently after this procedure than after cystgastrostomy. Massive hemorrhage suggests bleeding from vessels within the cyst, and angiography with possible embolization is indicated. If the patient's condition is unstable, emergent surgical examination of the anastomosis should be followed by examination of the cyst if necessary. A preoperative diagnostic angiogram will aid in identifying the vessel that is the source of bleeding. If bleeding arises from the cyst, either resection or ligation of the artery is a good

option. Placing sutures directly into the cyst is difficult because of poor exposure and friable tissues. Less severe bleeding probably indicates hemorrhage from the gastric wall, and endoscopy will be required to find the source of the bleeding. This complication occurs among fewer than 5% of patients (12). Leakage from the anastomosis may occur but can be prevented by good technique and closed suction drainage. Recurrence rates are less or equal to 5%.

Cystduodenostomy

Cystduodenostomy is infrequently performed to treat pseudocysts; it is indicated only for cysts that are clearly located in the head of the pancreas, where drainage through the posterior duodenal wall provides the best access. This procedure can be performed endoscopically, although cysts larger than 10 cm in diameter should be drained with a cystjejunostomy. When a patient with jaundice experiences a pseudocyst in the head of the pancreas, relieving the pseudocyst may or may not relieve the jaundice, and a biliary bypass procedure may be required. Liberal intraoperative use of cholangiography ensures relief of the obstruction.

Cystduodenostomy is performed by creating a duodenotomy; entrance into the cyst is made through the medial posterior wall of the duodenum. The ampulla must be carefully identified and avoided. Identifying the ampulla can be facilitated by passing a small catheter through the cystic duct or the common bile duct into the ampulla. At the most protuberant part of the cyst, a biopsy of the posterior duodenal wall should be performed, and a tissue sample should be sent for frozen-section studies that can determine whether the tissue contains epithelial cells. A 3- to 4-cm anastomosis should be created between the duodenal wall and the cyst. Whether absorbable or permanent sutures should be used is a topic of debate; however, silk sutures should be avoided. The author's preference is to use uninterrupted polydioxanone surgical sutures for obtaining hemostasis.

Complications of cystduodenostomy include injury to the bile duct, gastrointestinal bleeding, and duodenal leakage. The use of closed suction drainage is prudent in most cases, especially when the duodenal closure is difficult. Injuries to the bile duct can be prevented by carefully identifying the ampulla and placing a stent into that structure. If a bile duct injury persists, ERCP is the first step for diagnosis and biliary stenting; open surgery can usually be avoided.

Resection

Resection is the procedure of choice when distal pancreatic pseudocysts are small and are the result of focal pancreatitis in the tail of the gland. When pseudocysts accompany severe pancreatitis that involves the entire gland, inflammation is usually too severe to allow resection. Such resections are difficult because of inflammation and desmoplastic reaction. Preserving the spleen is normally very difficult; the surgeon contemplating distal resection of pseudocysts should plan to perform a splenectomy in conjunction with distal pancreatectomy. The most common intraoperative complication is bleeding from the multiple aneurysmal, dilated arteries, and veins. Careful hemostasis and ligation of the pancreatic duct at the margin of resection are crucial. Another serious complication of resection is postoperative leakage of the pancreatic duct. When distal resection is contemplated, preoperative ERCP is prudent because there may be strictures in the proximal duct.

The rate of leakage in association with distal resection is higher if the proximal duct is obstructed. In such cases, a stent should be placed preoperatively. Alternatively, the anastomosis of a Roux-en-Y jejunal limb to the distal resection margin (Duval procedure) may be performed. Should a postoperative pancreatic fistula develop, it will close spontaneously with closed suction drainage. If the fistula persists, ERCP may be helpful in defining proximal obstruction. Abscess or hematoma can occur; both are amenable to treatment with percutaneous drainage and antibiotics.

COMPLICATIONS OF SURGERY FOR PANCREATIC TRAUMA

Penetrating trauma from either a bullet or a blade can injure the pancreas. The mortality rate directly attributable to pancreatic injury is approximately 5%, but can be as high as 40% to 50% with concomitant vascular injuries. Blunt pancreatic trauma usually results from the application of blunt force to the mid-abdomen. Approximately 70% to 90% of patients with pancreatic trauma will have other injuries in the abdomen (47). Mortality rates associated with blunt trauma range from 10% to 30%, depending on associated injuries (48). It is particularly difficult to separate the mortality rates associated with duodenal injuries (Table 5) (49). The trauma surgeon who treats pancreatic injuries must be familiar with a few basic concepts. Foremost among these is the need to adhere to standard trauma principles and to manage life-threatening hemorrhage and intestinal contamination first because these problems are associated with the highest mortality rates. Because many of these injuries are found intraoperatively rather than by a preoperative workup, the surgeon must be very familiar with the pancreatic anatomy, so that any injury can be exposed and treated. Two important intraoperative questions must be answered: whether pancreatic injury is combined with duodenal injury and whether the pancreatic duct is disrupted. These factors are the key determinants of outcome for patients with pancreatic trauma.

In general, patients with pancreatic trauma have a 30% to 40% likelihood of experiencing hemodynamic instability; patients often require operative intervention without a preoperative workup. In this setting, careful assessment of the pancreas is important. In cases of penetrating trauma, simply following the trajectory of the missile leads to the diagnosis of a pancreatic injury. In the case of blunt trauma, examination of the pancreas includes complete opening of the lesser sac. If a contusion, hematoma, or swelling is seen, the pancreatic capsule must be opened because complete transection of the pancreatic tissue can occur even if the capsule is intact. Some surgeons hesitate to explore pancreatic hematomas that are not expanding or are not actively hemorrhaging; however, a thorough examination markedly decreases the morbidity rates associated with a missed pancreatic injury.

Intraoperative assessment of the integrity of the pancreatic duct is crucial when an injury to the gland is found. The surgeon must be confident in performing various maneuvers that help determine whether a ductal injury is present. A ductal injury is easier to see when direct inspection of the wound is accompanied by systemic injection of cholecystokinin or secretin to stimulate pancreatic enzyme secretion. Another radiologic technique that can aid in visualizing the pancreatic duct is transcholecystic cholangiography, with concomitant intravenous administration of morphine to cause ampullary contraction. Most surgeons are comfortable with this simple technique, which is a good first choice. Less commonly used is duodenotomy with injection through the ampulla. A more reasonable option is to transect the very distal tip of the pancreas and cannulate the duct distally. The trauma surgeon dealing with pancreatic trauma should be capable of performing all of these techniques.

Table 5   Pancreatic Organ Injury Scale

Grade	Type	Injury description	ICD-9	AIS-90
I	Hematoma	Minor contusion without ductal injury	863.81–863.84	2
	Laceration	Superficial laceration without ductal injury		2
II	Hematoma	Major contusion without ductal injury or tissue loss	863.81–863.84	2
	Laceration	Major laceration without ductal injury or tissue loss		3
III	Laceration	Distal transection or parenchymal injury with ductal injury	863.92–863.94	3
IV	Laceration	Proximal transection or parenchymal injury involving ampulla	863.91	4
V	Laceration	Massive disruption of the pancreatic head	863.91	5

Abbreviations: ICD-9, International Classification of Disease 9th Revision; AIS-90, Abbreviated Injury Scale.
Source: From Ref. 49.

Injuries to the Left Side of the Pancreas

Pancreatic injuries to the left side of the portal vein, including those to the neck, body, and tail, are more straightforward in their management than are proximal injuries. Usually the duodenum is not injured. In cases of penetrating trauma, gastric and colonic injuries are common. The main intraoperative decision is determining whether the duct is intact. If there is no ductal damage, simple drainage is appropriate. However, if there is any question of a ductal injury with penetrating trauma, a distal resection is necessary. Resections to the left of the portal vein include approximately 60% of the pancreas, and most patients who undergo such procedures will not experience postoperative endocrine or exocrine deficiencies. In a number of series, resection for ductal injury rather than drainage decreased the mortality and morbidity rates (50). Distal resection should be performed with direct ligation of the main pancreatic duct and closed suction drainage.

Complications associated with this procedure include pseudocyst formation, pancreatic leak from the resection line, and the rare hemorrhage or abscess. Closed suction drainage controls pancreatic leaks, 90% of which will heal. A pancreatic leak that persists for more than two weeks indicates a proximal problem; ERCP with sphincterotomy can be helpful in correcting or diagnosing the problem. Overall, most distal pancreatic ducts leaks will seal even if prolonged drainage is required.

Injuries to the Right Side of the Pancreas

Injuries to the head or the right side of the gland range from simple contusions to severe combined duodenal and pancreatic injuries requiring pancreaticoduodenectomy. In truth, a Whipple procedure is rare in trauma surgery because simpler techniques are usually adequate. More commonly, when both the duodenum and the pancreas are injured by penetrating trauma, the duodenal injuries can be managed with standard techniques of either primary pair or diversion, and the pancreatic injury can normally be drained. If the ampulla is available, i.e., if the duodenum is already lacerated by the injury, injection for pancreatic duct visualization is an important adjunct. Recent reports advocate drainage of any proximal pancreatic injury, with or without ductal injury because the magnitude of the resection is so large that delayed or staged operations can be performed should a leak persist (51). Closed suction drainage, anterior and posterior to the gland, is performed after "kocherization" of the duodenum (Fig. 9).

Delayed Presentation of Pancreatic Injuries

Patients who do not undergo emergent surgery may exhibit delayed presentation of pancreatic injury, particularly in cases of blunt trauma. Although patients with penetrating injuries invariably undergo exploratory surgery for injuries, patients with blunt

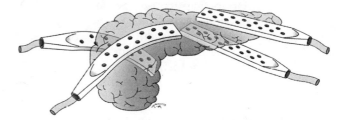

Figure 9 Complete drainage of pancreas for trauma or pancreatitis.

abdominal trauma, if their condition is stable, are evaluated with ultrasound for the presence of free fluid. If the results of the ultrasound are positive or if the patient experiences persistent tenderness, a CT scan is performed. Newer CT scanners with multiple detectors and multiphase ability have improved the sensitivity of detecting pancreatic injury to 80%; the sensitivity of older scanners may be as low as 50% (52).

Measurements of serum amylase activity are not very effective in diagnosing pancreatic trauma, except in one situation. If the serum amylase activity is normal when measured more than three hours after injury, the negative predictive value of this result is approximately 95% (53). An elevation in amylase activity is not a reliable indicator of injury. The findings of CT scans can indicate contusion, fluid, hematoma, or obvious fracture (Fig. 10). Once the diagnosis has been made, the patient should undergo a complete assessment. If the patient's condition seems to be improving, the injury is probably a contusion that can be treated by observation. A few such patients may later experience pseudocysts, but these problems can be managed later. If the patient's condition is not improving, the integrity of the duct must be

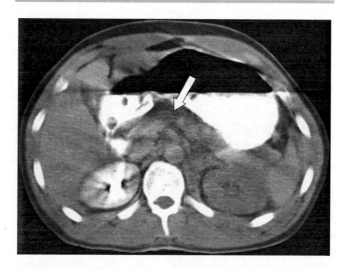

Figure 10 Pancreatic neck transection after blunt trauma (*arrow*). Also, the left kidney devascularized, with no contrast.

evaluated. In this situation, posttraumatic ERCP is indicated for diagnostic purposes. If the duct is intact, no therapy is needed. If the duct is injured, particularly distally, surgical intervention is advised and should include distal resection. Pancreatic stenting is not advised for the acute trauma patient, although some case reports have suggested limited success (54).

Surgical Complications

The complications associated with all of these procedures are similar to those associated with elective resection. The most severe complication is operating on a patient with trauma to the pancreas but failing to recognize the injury. Wide drainage should be instituted for all patients with pancreatic injuries, and appropriate resection should be performed for those with ductal injury. Postoperative problems include bleeding with hematoma formation, pseudocyst, and the rare abscess.

Pancreatitis sometimes occurs after blunt trauma and can be treated with supportive care, as is the case for acute pancreatitis. When a pancreatic injury goes unrecognized, the symptoms can mimic those of severe necrotizing pancreatitis: cytokine overload and multiple organ failure. Complications associated with surgical intervention for pancreatic injury occur in about 20% to 40% of patients. The higher end of this range includes those with combined pancreaticoduodenal injuries, and most deaths among these patients result from sepsis and multiorgan failure (50). When such reported cases are carefully examined, the general finding is that pancreatic duct injury was not well identified and may have led to the patient's death (55).

Pancreatic fistula occurs among approximately 10% to 20% of patients with insolated pancreatic trauma and among as many as 35% of those with associated duodenal trauma (51). With proper drainage, most fistulas will resolve. Nutritional support is crucial: the surgeon must realize that pancreatic injuries are associated with a large number of persistent problems, particularly fistula, and should treat all patients with such injuries with enteral feeding started at the time of the initial operation. Jejunal feeding with an elemental diet can be carried out without much increase in the pancreatic effluent from a pancreatic fistula. Many patients with such injuries will not tolerate oral or gastric feedings and will require the implementation of total parenteral hyperalimentation (TPN), if a jejunostomy is not in place. Jejunal feeding is by far preferable to TPN, but requires some foresight on the part of the surgeon. Administering octreotide to treat pancreatic fistulas decreases the amount of secretion, particularly in long-term fistulas, but does not decrease the interval to healing (21).

Abscess is also a complication of both the pancreatic trauma and the surgical procedures used to treat pancreatic trauma. The incidence of abscess is related to the number of concomitant injuries, particularly hollow visceral injuries. True pancreatic abscesses are unusual and result from inadequate debridement of necrotic glandular tissue. If a CT scan indicates necrosis or air in the gland, surgical debridement and drainage are appropriate because these complications will not respond to percutaneous drainage. Pseudocysts occur among some patients who are treated nonoperatively for pancreatic trauma. These cysts probably result from unsuspected or undocumented ductal injury and can be treated in the standard fashion.

COMPLICATIONS OF SURGERY FOR CANCER
Pancreatic Biopsy

Currently, pancreatic tissue obtained by biopsy can be examined with either radiologic or surgical techniques. Radiologic procedures include fine-needle aspiration (FNA), which uses a needle with a very small bore. Complications associated with this technique are uncommon. Biopsy material can also be obtained with FNA, with guidance by endoscopic ultrasonography Intraoperative techniques used to obtain pancreatic tissue include laparoscopic or open surgical biopsy, either directly into the pancreas by FNA or a core needle, or via a transduodenal route with a true-cut needle. With a 16- or 18-gauge needle, a biopsy is easily performed and is quite safe. The duodenum is kocherized to lift the head of the pancreas, and the true-cut needle is passed through the second portion of the duodenum into the pancreas. This technique allows any leakage from the pancreatic biopsy site to go into the duodenum; a single suture is placed at the site of duodenal penetration. When the lesion is in the body or tail of the pancreas, a direct biopsy should be performed. Again, the safest method is the use of a true-cut needle. Multiple passes are not necessary; they serve only to increase the morbidity rates and the possibility of postoperative leak or pancreatitis. Wedge biopsies should be avoided unless the lesion can be completely enucleated. Careful attention to the anatomy of the duct is necessary if serious ductal injury is to be avoided.

Complications after a biopsy are rare. The most feared complication of pancreatic biopsy is pancreatitis (56), which occurs in 1% of cases and can, at times, be severe. As in the treatment of acute pancreatitis, supportive care should be sufficient.

Distal Resection

Distal resections for pancreatic cancer are generally uncommon because tumors in the body and the tail of pancreas are usually found too late to allow curative resection. However, in these rare cases, distal resection with a good margin is the appropriate operation when possible. Tumors other than adenocarcinomas, such as slowly growing cystic neoplasms or neuroendocrine tumors, are good candidates for this procedure. As is the case with distal pancreatectomy, careful ligation of the main pancreatic duct is important for preventing leaks from the pancreatic duct. Several techniques are available for closing the pancreatic stump, including horizontal mattress sutures and staplers. Whichever method is chosen, independent ligation of the main pancreatic duct is crucial.

Operations that attempt splenic preservation are more time-consuming and more meticulous than distal resection because of the need for dissection of the small venous tributaries that come off the splenic vein. There are reports of ligating the splenic vein while still preserving the spleen and its blood supply via the short gastric arteries (57). This procedure is associated with a 10% rate of pancreatic abscess formation; most cases respond to treatment with antibiotics. Oncologically, for adenocarcinoma, the procedures of choice are distal pancreatectomy and splenectomy. Complications include pancreatic leakage (which can be controlled with closed suction drainage), bleeding, abscess, or pseudocyst formation.

Proximal Resection

A number of techniques may be used for resecting cancers of the pancreatic head, including the standard Whipple procedure, the pylorus-preserving procedure, and the various extended resections for wide clearance of lymph nodes. The proximal resection procedure has changed rapidly during the past 15 to 20 years; most of the improvement has occurred in perioperative, operative, and postoperative management. The mortality rate associated with this procedure, which was once 20% to 30%, is now routinely 2% to 5% for experienced surgeons (58). The morbidity rate, however, is still approximately 30%. Discussion of the intraoperative procedure can prevent some of the pitfalls of management. Thorough knowledge of the anatomy, including the vascular anatomy and particularly the anatomy of the superior mesenteric artery (SMA) and the SMV, is obviously very important.

Preoperative Considerations

Patients who are to undergo a large procedure such as cancer resection must be in good physiologic condition at the time of surgery. Routine bowel preparation should be performed because in rare cases the middle colic vessels are involved and may require ligation. The colon usually survives such intervention, but colonic resection is occasionally required. The patient's nutritional status is also important. The evidence indicates that preoperative treatment with octreotide does not decrease the incidence of postoperative pancreatic fistula. Preoperative biliary decompression neither decreases nor increases the rate of serious postoperative complications (59).

Intraoperative Therapy and Pitfalls

The details of pancreaticoduodenectomy will not be discussed here, but several pitfalls associated with this surgical procedure will be highlighted.

Inadvertent Ligation of Hepatic Blood Vessels

Hepatoduodenal dissection involves dissection of the hepatic artery from the common bile duct so that the posterior portal vein can be exposed. Such an exposure is achieved by dividing and ligating the gastroduodenal artery. Inadvertent ligation of the proper or common hepatic artery is lethal. Avoiding this complication requires dissecting the gastroduodenal artery to its origin. If the hepatic artery is transected, reanastomosis with good vascular technique is mandatory. In approximately 10% to 15% of patients, a right hepatic artery may originate from the SMA; this artery is seen in the posterior aspect of the portal triad, tracking posterior to the portal vein. This artery must be preserved; ligating it greatly increases the mortality rates associated with the surgical procedure. If the artery is inadvertently divided, it must be reanastomosed.

The presence of an anterior portal vein is very rare. However, this possibility must be considered when the hepatoduodenal ligament is dissected. Failure to recognize the anatomy will lead to injury to the portal vein.

Injury to the Superior Mesenteric Vein

The SMV is usually dissected from below the pancreatic neck. Injury to this vein during dissection can be lethal. Should such an injury occur, bimanual pressure should be applied while the pancreatic neck is divided so that the bleeding from the SMV below can be controlled.

Leaks from the Pancreatic Anastomosis

The most difficult and problematic anastomosis associated with pancreaticoduodenectomy is reconstructing the cut ends of the pancreas and the jejunum. This anastomosis is especially difficult among patients with a soft pancreas and a duct of normal size, as is most often the case for patients with periampullary tumors. These cases are very difficult to manage and are associated with a high rate of leakage. If the duct is small, an invaginating anastomosis is preferred (Fig. 11). Fibrin sealants may be used to further seal the anastomosis, but published reports do not demonstrate that this technique is beneficial for decreasing the rate of leakage.

The sutures used in a pancreatic anastomosis must be placed precisely; published reports differ with regard to the type of suture that should be used. The benefit of monofilament suture is the minimal reaction; however, multiple knots are required. Silk holds its strength with just a few knots, but it is associated with intense inflammation. When the gland is soft, buttress sutures help hold the distal resection margin together. One report suggests that pancreaticojejunostomy should not be performed when the gland is very soft but rather that the pancreatic ductal system should be injected with sterile neoprene,

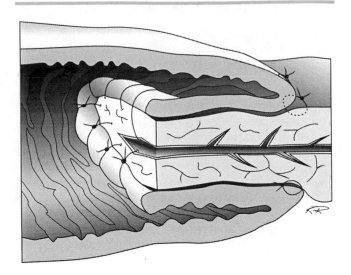

Figure 11 Invaginating two-layer "duct-to-mucosa" pancreaticojejunal anastomosis.

which solidifies and blocks off the entire exocrine system (60). This technique preserves endocrine function but not exocrine function; it also avoids the need for an anastomosis, which is prone to leakage and increased morbidity rates.

Postoperative Complications

A number of large series demonstrate substantial improvement in the mortality and morbidity rates associated with pancreatic resection. Two large series report a mortality rate of 2% and a morbidity rate of 30% (Table 6) (58,61).

The most feared complication of this procedure is pancreatic fistula resulting from leakage at the

anastomosis. This complication occurs in approximately 5% to 15% of cases, but can often be controlled with closed suction drainage. The problem is more difficult to treat if both enteric fluid and pancreatic fluid are draining; in such cases, a larger disruption of the pancreaticojejunostomy should be suspected, and a repeated operation is indicated. Additionally, if the fluid from a pancreatic fistula becomes bloody after initially being clear, a second operation should be strongly considered because this finding suggests inflammation and erosion of surrounding vessels. In two large series, the rate of reoperation was approximately 4%; the second procedure was performed largely because of bleeding.

Delayed gastric emptying (DGE) is a nuisance problem that occurs in approximately 15% to 30% of cases (61) and is the most commonly observed complication. The incidence of DGE may be improved by performing the duodenum-preserving pancreatectomy. Cameron and colleagues have demonstrated that routinely administering erythromycin postoperatively reduces the incidence of DGE from 30% to 19% (62). In addition, using nasogastric suction to treat DGE results in the resolution of more than 90% of cases with time and patience. Even if gastric atony persists for more than three weeks, reoperation is not recommended until a full six weeks have passed without improvement. Postoperative upper endoscopy shows a patent anastomosis. The problem is related to functional gastroparesis caused by disruption of the gastric pacemaker. When a patient requires delayed reoperation because of persistently poor gastric emptying, the gastrojejunostomy should be revised with a larger resection of the stomach and a Roux-en-Y reconstruction.

Another complication of pancreatic resection is bile leakage, which usually resolves within 48 hours postoperatively and is purely a technical problem. Cholangitis occurs in a small percentage of cases; wound infection and abdominal abscess occur in 3% to 5% of cases. Other complications include pneumonia, urinary tract infection, and line sepsis. The average length of stay for a large series of patients undergoing pancreatic resection was 10 to 15 days. Because of the number of problems that may occur, specifically DGE, placing a jejunal access tube is advocated by some surgeons. Other believe the enternal tube is unnecessary and can leads to delayed time to oral feeding. This tube prevents the need for central access and TPN and allows simpler management with enteral feedings.

Total Pancreatectomy

Total pancreatectomy is not commonly performed for adenocarcinoma, but patients with positive intraoperative pancreatic margins after a Whipple procedure may be candidates for such an operation. The most common indication for total pancreatectomy is probably intraductal papillary mucinous tumors.

Table 6 Complications of Pancreaticoduodenectomy

	Cameron et al. (61) (n = 564)	Warshaw et al. (58) (n = 489)
Perioperative mortality	2.3%	1%
Overall complications	31%	37%
Specific complications		
Reoperation	3%	2%
Delayed gastric emptying	14%	12%
Cholangitis	3%	0.6%
Bile leak	2%	0.8%
Wound infection	7%	5.1%
Pancreatic fistula	5%	11%
Intra-abdominal abscess	3%	1.6%
Pneumonia	1%	1.0%
Pancreatitis	1%	–
Postoperative length of stay		
Mean ± SE	14.0 ± 0.4 days	9.5 ± 0.4 days
Median	11 days	8 days

Source: From Refs. 58,61.

The incidence of these tumors has increased because of better diagnostic methods. Total pancreatectomy proceeds as with the Whipple procedure, but also includes resection of the spleen and the distal tail of the pancreas. Reconstruction includes a biliary jejunal anastomosis and a gastrojejunostomy or a duodenojejunostomy. The biggest difference between a total pancreatectomy and a Whipple procedure is that total pancreatectomy avoids the need for a pancreatic anastomosis and thus also avoids many of the postoperative complications associated with the Whipple procedure. However, the patient will now require insulin and pancreatic enzyme substitution. DGE complicates this procedure, as do biliary leaks, cholangitis, bleeding, sepsis, and wound infection. Pancreatic fistula is not an issue with pancreatectomy.

The most serious postoperative complications are exocrine and endocrine insufficiency. Exocrine insufficiency is readily controlled with pancreatic enzyme supplementation, but control of the endocrine problem is somewhat more difficult. Glucose concentrations are easier to control among patients who undergo a total pancreatectomy for tumor than among patients who undergo the procedure for chronic pancreatitis. Approximately 40% of patients with chronic pancreatitis are susceptible to postoperative episodes of hypoglycemia, and half of these require hospitalization (63). A few cases of fatal hypoglycemia have been documented and may be related to the relationship between caloric intake and insulin dosages. Patients who undergo duodenum-preserving pancreatectomy require more insulin because they eat a more normal diet and larger meals (64). Some physicians believe that glucagon secretion is more balanced when the duodenogastric axis is left intact (65). With good compliance, most issues related to diabetes are controllable after total pancreatectomy.

The rate of postoperative abscess is somewhat higher among patients who undergo total pancreatectomy than among those who undergo a Whipple procedure. These patients also experience a slightly higher rate of left subdiapragmatic hematoma and abscess. These collections are amenable to percutaneous drainage, and repeated operation is seldom required.

REFERENCES

1. Clavien PA, Hauser H, Meyer P, Rohner A. Value of contrast-enhanced computerized tomography in the early diagnosis and prognosis of acute pancreatitis. A prospective study of 202 patients. Am J Surg 1988; 155(3):457–466.
2. Bradley EL III. A clinically based classification system for acute pancreatitis. Summary of the International Symposium on Acute Pancreatitis, Atlanta, GA, September 11–13, 1992. Arch Surg 1993; 128(5):586–590.
3. Yeo CJ, Bastidas JA, Lynch-Nyhan A, Fishman EK, Zinner MJ, Cameron JL. A natural history of pancreatic pseudocysts documented by computed tomography. Surg Gynecol Obstet 1990; 170(5):411–417.
4. Bradley EL, Clements JL Jr, Gonzales AC. The natural history of pancreatic pseudocysts: a unified concept of management. Am J Surg 1979; 137(1):135–141.
5. Bassi C, Vesentini S, Nifosi F, et al. Pancreatic abscess and other pus-harboring collections related to pancreatitis: a review of 108 cases. World J Surg 1990; 14(4):505–512.
6. Widdison AL, Karanjia ND. Pancreatic infection complicating acute pancreatitis. Br J Surg 1993; 80: 148–154.
7. Howard TJ, Wiebke EA, Mogavero G, et al. Classification and treatment of local septic complications in acute pancreatitis. Am J Surg 1995; 170(1):44–50.
8. Uhl W, Isenmann R, Buchler MW. Infections complicating pancreatitis: diagnosing, treating, preventing. New Horiz 1998; 6(2 suppl):S72–S79.
9. Rotman N, Mathieu D, Anglade MC, Fagniez PL. Failure of percutaneous drainage of pancreatic abscesses complicating severe acute pancreatitis. Surg Gynecol Obstet 1992; 174(2):141–144.
10. Wilson RH, Moorehead RJ. Current management of trauma to the pancreas. Br J Surg 1991; 78(10): 1196–1202.
11. Jordan GL Jr. Pancreatic resection for pancreatic cancer. Surg Clin North Am 1989; 69(3):569–597.
12. Waltman AC, Luers PR, Athanasoulis CA, Warshaw AL. Massive arterial hemorrhage in patients with pancreatitis. Complementary roles of surgery and transcatheter occlusive techniques. Arch Surg 1986; 121(4): 439–443.
13. Stabile BE, Wilson SE, Debas HT. Reduced mortality from bleeding pseudocysts and pseudoaneursyms caused by pancreatitis. Arch Surg 1983; 118(1):45–51.
14. Boudghene F, L'Hermine C, Bigot JM. Arterial complications of pancreatitis: diagnostic and therapeutic aspects in 104 cases. J Vasc Interv Radiol 1993; 4(4):551–558.
15. Warshaw AL, Rattner DW. Fact and fallacies of common bile duct obstruction by pancreatic pseudocysts. Ann Surg 1980; 192(1):33–37.
16. Cotton PB. ERCP. Gut 1977; 18(4):316–341.
17. Reinhold C, Bret PM. MR cholangiopancreatography. Abdom Imaging 1996; 21(2):105–116.
18. Kozarek RA. Endoscopic therapy of complete and partial pancreatic duct disruptions. Gastrointest Endosc Clin N Am 1998; 8(1):39–53.
19. Martin FM, Rossi RL, Munson JL, ReMine SG, Braasch JW. Management of pancreatic fistulas. Arch Surg 1989; 124(5):571–573.
20. Pederzoli P, Bassi C, Vesentini S, eds. Pancreatic Fistulas. New York: Springer, 1992.
21. Li-Ling J, Irving M. Somatostatin and octreotide in the prevention of postoperative pancreatic complications and the treatment of enterocutaneous pancreatic fistula: a systematic review of randomized controlled trials. Br J Surg 2001; 88(2):190–199.
22. Lankisch PG, Lohr-Happe A, Otto J, Creutzfeldt W. Natural course in chronic pancreatitis. Pain, exocrine and endocrine pancreatic insufficiency and prognosis of the disease. Digestion 1993; 54(3):148–155.
23. Doty JE, Fink AS, Meyer JH. Alterations in digestive function caused by pancreatic disease. Surg Clin North Am 1989; 69(3):447–465.
24. Cogbill TH, Moore EE, Morris JA Jr, et al. Distal pancreatectomy for trauma: a multicenter experience. J Trauma 1991; 31(12):1600–1606.

25. Layer P, Yamamoto H, Kalthoff L, Clain JE, Bakken LJ, DiMagno EP. The different courses of early- and late-onset idiopathic and alcoholic chronic pancreatitis. Gastroenterology 1994; 107(5):1481–1487.

26. Trede M, Schwall G. The complications of pancreatectomy. Ann Surg 1988; 207(1):39–47.

27. Bradley EL III, Allen K. A prospective longitudinal study of observation versus surgical intervention in the management of necrotizing pancreatitis. Am J Surg 1991; 161(1):19–25.

28. Beger HG, Isenmann R. Surgical management of necrotizing pancreatitis. Surg Clin North Am 1999; 79(4):783–800.

29. Orlando R III, Welch JP, Akbari CM, Bloom GP, Macaulay WP. Techniques and complications of open packing of infected pancreatic necrosis. Surg Gynecol Obstet 1993; 177(1):65–71.

30. Sarr MG, Nagorney DM, Mucha P Jr, Farnell MB, Johnson CD. Acute necrotizing pancreatitis: management by planned, staged pancreatic necrosectomy/debridement and delayed primary wound closure over drains. Br J Surg 1991; 78(5):576–581.

31. Kalfarentzos F, Kehagias N, Mead N, Kokkinis K, Gogos CA. Enteral nutrition is superior to parenteral nutrition in severe acute pancreatitis: results of a randomized prospective trial. Br J Surg 1997; 84(12): 1665–1669.

32. Fiedler F, Jauernig G, Keim V, Richter A, Bender HJ. Octreotide treatment in patients with necrotizing pancreatitis and pulmonary failure. Intensive Care Med 1996; 22(9):909–915.

33. Johnson CD, Kingsnorth AN, Imrie CW, et al. Double blind, randomised, placebo controlled study of a platelet activating factor antagonist, lexipafant, in the treatment and prevention of organ failure in predicted severe acute pancreatitis. Gut 2001; 48(1):62–69.

34. Cole L, Bellomo R, Journois D, Davenport P, Baldwin I, Tipping P. High-volume haemofiltration in human septic shock. Intensive Care Med 2001; 27(6):978–986.

35. Izbicki JR, Bloechle C, Knoefel WT, Rogiers X, Kuechler T. Surgical treatment of chronic pancreatitis and quality of life after operation. Surg Clin North Am 1999; 79(4):913–944.

36. Frey CF, Smith GJ. Description and rationale of a new operation for chronic pancreatitis. Pancreas 1987; 2(6):701–707.

37. Rios GA, Adams DB. Does intraoperative electrohydraulic lithotripsy improve outcome in the surgical management of chronic pancreatitis? Am Surg 2001; 67(6):533–538.

38. Beger HG, Buchler M, Bittner R, Uhl W. Duodenum-preserving resection of the head of the pancreas—an alternative to Whipples procedure in chronic pancreatitis. Hepatogastroenterology 1990; 37(3):283–289.

39. Stapleton GN, Williamson RC. Proximal pancreatoduodenectomy for chronic pancreatitis. Br J Surg 1996; 83(10):1433–1440.

40. Saeger HD, Schwall G, Trede M. Standard Whipple in pancreatitis. In: Beger HG, Buchler M, Malfertheiner P, eds. Standards in Pancreatic Surgery. New York: Springer, 1993:385–391.

41. Frey CF, Amikura K. Local resection of the head of the pancreas combined with longitudinal pancreaticojejunostomy in the management of patients with chronic pancreatitis. Ann Surg 1994; 220(4):492–507.

42. Buchler MW, Friess H, Bittner R, et al. Duodenum-preserving pancreatic head resection: long-term results. J Gastrointest Surg 1997; 1(1):13–19.

43. Smits ME, Rauws EA, Tygat GN, Huibregtse K. The efficacy of endoscopic treatment of pancreatic pseudocysts. Gastrointest Endosc 1995; 42(3):202–207.

44. Cremer M, Deviere J, Engelholm L. Endoscopic management of cysts and pseudocysts in chronic pancreatitis: long-term follow-up after 7 years of experience. Gastrointest Endosc 1989; 35(1):1–9.

45. Dohmoto M, Rupp KD. Endoscopic drainage of pancreatic pseudocysts. Surg Endosc 1992; 6(3):118–124.

46. Vitas GJ, Sarr MG. Selected management of pancreatic pseudocysts: operative versus expectant management. Surgery 1992; 111(2):123–130.

47. Stone HH, Fabian TC, Satiani B, Turkleson ML. Experiences in the management of pancreatic trauma. J Trauma 1981; 21(4):257–262.

48. Jones RC. Management of pancreatic trauma. Am J Surg 1985; 150(6):698–704.

49. Moore EE, Cogbill TH, Malangoni MA, et al. Organ injury scaling, II: Pancreas, duodenum, small bowel, colon, and rectum. J Trauma 1990; 30(11): 1427–1429.

50. Jurkovich GJ, Carrico CJ. Pancreatic trauma. Surg Clin North Am 1990; 70(3):575–593.

51. Patton JH Jr, Lyden SP, Croce MA, Pritchard FE, Minard G, Kudsk KA, Fabian TC. Pancreatic trauma: a simplified management guideline. J Trauma 1997; 43(2):234–241.

52. Peitzman AB, Makaraoun MS, Slasky BS, Ritter P. Prosepective study of computed tomography in initial management of blunt abdominal trauma. J Trauma 1986; 26(7):585–592.

53. Bouwman DL, Weaver DW, Walt AJ. Serum amylase and its isoenzymes: a clarification of their implications in trauma. J Trauma 1984; 24(7):573–578.

54. Kim HS, Lee DK, Kim IW, et al. The role of endoscopic retrograde pancreatography in the treatment of traumatic pancreatic duct injury. Gastrointest Endosc 2001; 54(1):49–55.

55. Leppaniemi A, Haapiainen R, Kiviluoto T, Lempinen M. Pancreatic trauma: acute and late manifestations. Br J Surg 1988; 75(2):165–167.

56. Buice WS, Walker LG Jr. The role of intra-operative biopsy in the treatment of resectable neoplasms of the pancreas and periampullary region. Am Surg 1989; 55(5):307–310.

57. Warshaw AL. Pancreatic necrosis: to debride or not to debride-that is the question. Ann Surg 2000; 232(5): 627–629.

58. Balcom JH IV, Rattner DW, Warshaw AL, Chang Y, Fernandez-del Castillo C. Ten-year experience with 733 pancreatic resections: changing indications, older patients, and decreasing length of hospitalization. Arch Surg 2001; 136(4):391–398.

59. Pisters PW, Hudec WA, Hess KR, et al. Effect of preoperative biliary decompression on pancreaticoduodenectomy-associated morbidity in 300 consecutive patients. Ann Surg 2001; 234(1):47–55.

60. Di Carlo V, Chiesa R, Pontiroli AE, et al. Pancreaticoduodenectomy with occlusion of the residual stump by Neoprene injection. World J Surg 1989; 13(1):105–111.

61. Sohn TA, Yeo CJ, Cameron JL, et al. Resected adenocarcinoma of the pancreas-616 patients: results, outcomes,

and prognostic indicators. J Gastrointest Surg 2000; 4(6):567–579.

62. Yeo CJ, Barry MK, Sauter PK, et al. Erythromycin accelerates gastric emptying after pancreaticoduodenectomy. A prospective, randomized, placebo-controlled trial. Ann Surg 1993; 218(3):229–238.

63. Pliam MB, ReMine WH. Further evaluation of total pancreatectomy. Arch Surg 1975; 110(5):506–512.

64. Linehan IP, Lambert MA, Brown DC, Kurtz AB, Cotton PB, Russell RC. Total pancreatectomy for chronic pancreatitis. Gut 1988; 29(3):358–365.

65. Izbicki JR, Bloechle C, Knoefel WT, Kuechler T, Binmoeller KF, Broelsch CE. Duodenum-preserving resection of the head of the pancreas in chronic pancreatitis. A prospective, randomized trial. Ann Surg 1995; 221(4):350–358.

13

Complications of Splenic Surgery and Splenic Injury

David S. Lasko
University of Miami School of Medicine/Jackson Memorial Hospital, Miami, Florida, U.S.A.

Louis R. Pizano
*DeWitt Daughtry Family Department of Surgery, University of Miami, Miller School of
Medicine, Miami, Florida, U.S.A.*

Surgery of the spleen has a rich history that reflects advances in the knowledge of this organ's role and function. Pean reported the first successful splenectomy in 1867; throughout the 20th century, the indications for elective and emergent splenectomy increased substantially (1). During the past two decades, improvements in diagnostic imaging and an increase in our understanding of the risks of asplenia have led to an increase in the popularity of splenic conservation surgery and nonoperative management of splenic injury when possible. Each therapeutic approach (e.g., splenectomy, splenic conservation surgery, and nonoperative management) is accompanied by a unique set of potential complications. One must examine the complications of splenic surgery, whether performed electively or for trauma, in light of the overall management approach.

CATEGORIES OF SPLENIC SURGERY

Two fundamental categories of splenic disease have emerged as surgical procedures involving this organ have become more common. Types of splenic disease that can lead to elective surgery include hematologic diseases and malignancies. Splenic injuries that can lead to emergent trauma surgery include blunt and penetrating trauma and iatrogenic damage.

COMPLICATIONS OF ELECTIVE SPLENIC SURGERY

A thorough assessment of the morbidity rates associated with elective splenic surgery is complicated by several factors. Many of the largest series of cases involving open elective splenectomy were collected several decades ago, and improvements in diagnosis, surgical technique, and perioperative care are likely to have decreased the complication rates reported by those studies (2). Conversely, many of the splenectomies reported in the older series were part of staging procedures performed on young, immunologically healthy patients with Hodgkin's disease (3), a patient group for which the rate of complications was probably low (2). Staging laparotomy has virtually disappeared as an indication for splenectomy (1); therefore, the published rates could be lower than those encountered in current practice.

The assessment of morbidity rates associated with elective splenic surgery is further complicated by the fact that there are numerous hematologic indications for splenectomy. In the larger reported series, several underlying disorders with various levels of preoperative disability were indications for open, elective splenectomy (3–7). Series large enough to identify specific complications associated with each of the various operative indications do not exist. When the specific indications are grouped into broader categories, however, elective splenectomy for myeloproliferative disorders is associated with a much higher complication rate (58%) than is splenectomy performed for lymphoproliferative disorders (26% complication rate) or idiopathic thrombocytopenic purpura (ITP) (17% morbidity rate) (2).

The overall complication rates associated with open, elective splenectomy range from approximately 20% to 25%, whereas the perioperative mortality rates range from 1% to 6% (2–4). Massive splenomegaly (defined as a spleen weighing more than 1500 g) uniformly increases morbidity rates to 35% to 40% (3,5,7). Other statistically significant independent risk factors leading to increases in the morbidity rates associated with open splenectomy include patient age greater than 65 years (40% complication rate), estimated blood loss of more than 500 mL (50% morbidity rate), and myelofibrosis as the operative indication (50% morbidity rate) (3).

The most common perioperative complication of open splenectomy is infection. Although overwhelming postsplenectomy infection (OPSI) has been reported as early as 24 days after splenectomy, this is a rare and usually late (several years after the procedure) postoperative complication (8,9). More common postoperative infections, including respiratory tract, wound, and urinary tract infections and intraabdominal abscesses, account for approximately 50% to 75% of the perioperative complications associated with open splenectomy (3,5,6). Postoperative bleeding requiring transfusion, reoperation, or both occurs with approximately 6% to 7% of open splenectomies (3,5,6). Surgeons should also be aware of a few rare but potentially devastating complications of open splenectomy. One such complication is gastric perforation, which is estimated to occur with fewer than 1% of open splenectomies, but is associated with a mortality rate as high as 25%, even with appropriate treatment (10). Splanchnic vein thrombosis has also been associated with splenectomy, occurring in 0.2% to 6% of cases with a widely varying mortality rate that can be as high as 75%. Other complications associated with upper abdominal surgery, such as deep venous thrombosis, small bowel obstruction, and pancreatitis, are also reported to have occurred in large series of open splenectomies, but their incidence varies widely (3,5,6).

The advent of the laparoscopic approach has changed both the complication rates and the specific morbidity rates associated with elective splenectomy. Some complications (such as physiologic alterations caused by insufflation and trocar injuries) arise from the use of laparoscopy in general, rather than from its application to splenectomy. The current chapter will address only the complications related specifically to laparoscopic splenectomy.

Direct comparisons of laparoscopic and open splenectomy for hematologic disorders almost uniformly show that the laparoscopic approach is associated with longer operative times, but with less operative blood loss; a more rapid return to a liquid diet; and shorter postoperative stays (4,11,12). Baccarani et al. (4) performed a meta-analysis of several such comparative studies and calculated that, in patients undergoing laparoscopic splenectomy, the average blood loss was 100 mL less and the hospital stay was 3.7 days shorter than for open splenectomy. Importantly, the frequency of detecting accessory splenic tissue was equal with the two approaches. The ability to identify accessory splenic tissue is especially important for elective splenic surgery because an important goal of the procedure is often the complete elimination of accessory splenic function.

Despite these advantages of laparoscopic splenectomy, the data are equivocal regarding whether the procedure is associated with a lower complication rate than is open splenectomy. Some studies report that laparoscopic splenectomy is associated with complication rates as high as 50% to 75% (4,11), whereas others indicate that the rates are equivalent (13–15). It is possible that the studies reporting lower complication rates for laparoscopic surgery were affected by selection bias. The previously mentioned meta-analysis of laparoscopic splenectomy series showed that the indication for 61% of the procedures was ITP (4), which is generally associated with a smaller spleen, less blood loss, and lower complication rates than are other

indications for splenectomy. ITP was the operative indication for only 25% to 50% of patients in the large reported series of open splenectomies (2,3,7).

COMPLICATIONS IN THE TREATMENT OF SPLENIC INJURY

Splenic rupture, especially when caused by blunt trauma, is associated with a mortality rate ranging from 10% to 15%, even in the modern era of highly advanced imaging methods and multiple therapeutic options (16). Treatment of splenic injury has changed substantially during the modern surgical era. Understanding the particular morbidity rates associated with each therapeutic approach is, therefore, very important for the modern surgeon.

For most of the 20th century, splenectomy was the treatment of choice for all splenic injuries. However, during the 1960s and 1970s, an increase in the recognition of OPSI made splenic salvage the preferred surgical treatment when possible (17–22). During the last decade, improved imaging methods and the demonstrated success of nonoperative treatment for children have increased the frequency of nonoperative management of blunt splenic trauma (23–25). Reports of large series now show that as many as 65% of adults undergo nonoperative management of blunt splenic injury, whereas only approximately 15% of such patients were treated without surgery during the late 1970s (16,26–29). Reports indicate that this approach is successful nearly 90% of the time, although failure rates increase with the severity of the injury (16,27,28).

Direct comparison of the various treatment approaches is difficult because the severity of injury differs greatly in patients undergoing nonoperative therapy and those undergoing splenorrhaphy or splenectomy. Nearly all studies have shown that patients undergoing nonoperative management experience splenic and systemic insults that are less severe, and this finding almost certainly contributes to the lower overall morbidity rates reported in patients undergoing treatment with this approach (23,6,30–34). As expected, the studies comparing various approaches to treating splenic trauma show that most of the patients who die are more severely injured and generally undergo splenectomy. Few of the deaths, however, can be directly linked to the operation.

Although mortality may be related more closely to the severity of injury than to the treatment approach, the various treatment methods are associated with unique complications. When making treatment decisions, surgeons must understand the unique types of morbidity and mortality rates associated with each of the three general treatment approaches.

Splenectomy

In recent years, the indications for splenectomy after splenic injury have decreased; thus, the most recent extensive data regarding the complications associated with this approach were gathered in the 1970s. At that time, splenectomy was the mainstay of therapy for splenic rupture and was associated with mortality rates ranging from 10% to 25% and with overall morbidity rates of nearly 40% on average (33,35–37). Again, few of the deaths were related directly to the splenectomy. Many of the complications, however, were probably directly related to the operation and must be appreciated by the surgeon if they are to be minimized. Pulmonary complications occur in as many as 48% of patients undergoing splenectomy for splenic injury. Venous thrombosis occurs in 11% of these patients (37), with rates of pulmonary embolus of 1% to 4% for splenectomy as compared to 0.5% for emergent laparotomy without splenectomy (37,38). The thromboembolic complications were associated with thrombocytosis greater than $500 \times 10^3/\mu L$.

Infectious complications are also relatively common after splenectomy for trauma. Patients who suffer traumatic injury and undergo splenectomy as a result experience postoperative subphrenic abscess at rates as high as 13% (30). Overall, infection rates among such patients range from 30% to 36%, as compared with 9% among patients who do not undergo splenectomy (30,38). Even when analyses are controlled for severity of injury, patients undergoing splenectomy experience higher rates of septic complications (23%) than do patients undergoing splenorrhaphy (11%), although this difference is not statistically significant (30).

The most feared complication of splenic trauma, OPSI, is uniquely associated with splenectomy. This complication is associated with a mortality rate of 50% to 75%. It begins with flu-like symptoms and, if not aggressively treated, rapidly progresses to cause pneumonia, meningitis, coma, and death (33,39). The causative agent is nearly always an encapsulated bacterium, usually pneumococcus, Haemophilus, meningococcus, or group A streptococcus (39). OPSI can occur from a few days to many years after splenectomy (33). The lifetime incidence of OPSI among patients who have undergone splenectomy for trauma is estimated to range from 0.4% to 2.5%; however, this is more than 50 times the rate among the general population. The severe morbidity and high mortality rates associated with OPSI, along with its greatly increased frequency among patients who undergo splenectomy for trauma, led to the search for spleen-conserving approaches to treating splenic trauma (17–22,40).

One potential method of decreasing the risk of OPSI in patients undergoing splenectomy for trauma is autotransplantation of splenic tissue at the time of the operation. Although various techniques exist for autotransplantation of splenic tissue, most involve the implantation of 5 to 10 small pieces of spleen within the omentum. Several studies have shown that autotransplantation can be accomplished safely during splenectomy for trauma (41–43). Both immunologic activity against encapsulated bacteria and reticuloendothelial function are better preserved by autotransplantation than by total splenectomy, even when only a small amount of splenic tissue is reimplanted (44–47). No studies, however, have demonstrated that autotransplantation at the time of splenectomy decreases postoperative infection rates or the risk of OPSI.

Splenorrhaphy

Splenic repair also prevents the increased risk of OPSI after splenectomy. In addition, splenorrhaphy has generally been found to be associated with lower morbidity rates than splenectomy for trauma. The overall complication rates associated with splenorrhaphy range from 5% to 12%, rates similar to those associated with laparotomy for trauma in general (18,20,22,48,49). Most of the complications, including pneumonia, atelectasis, bowel obstruction, and abdominal abscess, can be attributed to laparotomy rather than to splenorrhaphy. Most authors report a mortality rate of zero in association with splenorrhaphy.

One potential complication that might be expected after splenic repair is failure of the repair and renewed bleeding. In most reports, however, in nearly all cases, failure of splenic conservation is noted at the time of the operation, and the procedure is converted to splenectomy. Rates of renewed bleeding range from 0% to 3% (18,31,49,50).

Nonoperative Management

Although splenorrhaphy can be accomplished safely for appropriately selected patients, nonoperative management has emerged as the conservative treatment of choice over the past decade because it can avoid all of the complications associated with laparotomy, as well as those associated with splenectomy (16). Most patients who now undergo surgery for splenic trauma have severe injuries that are not amenable to repair (51). When nonoperative management was initially introduced in adult patients with splenic trauma, failure rates were as high as 73%; these high failure rates caused some authors to warn against the use of nonoperative management (52–54).

Two changes have resulted in much lower failure rates, now reported to be between 6% and 12%, and in widespread acceptance of selective nonoperative management by trauma surgeons (16,24,55–57). First, radiologic advances have enabled more specific diagnosis and management of splenic injuries. These advances include high-definition computed tomographic (CT) imaging and the addition of angiographic embolization to the treatment methods of splenic trauma. When expert interventional radiologists are available, the success rates of embolization have been reported to be as high as 90% in patients with CT-demonstrated "blush" and no active extravasation of contrast (25,58).

Second, improved success rates for nonoperative management of splenic injury have resulted from the development of more focused criteria for selecting patients for whom this treatment method is appropriate (16,19,28,33). A recent large multi-institutional trial (16) showed that approximately 80% of grade I and II splenic injuries can be successfully treated nonoperatively. Approximately 50% of grade III injuries, 80% of grade IV injuries, and 95% of grade V injuries will ultimately require laparotomy, however. Increased initial hemoperitoneum was also shown to be an independent risk factor for the failure of nonoperative management. Other reports (31,59,60) identified additional predictors of the success of nonoperative management of splenic injury; these predictors include absolute hemodynamic stability and the absence of peritoneal signs suggesting the need for laparotomy. Some studies (61,62) have suggested that the failure rates associated with nonoperative management of splenic injury are higher in patients over 55 years of age. However, other trials (16,63,64) have reported that nonoperative management is safe for older patients. At this time, nonoperative management should be undertaken with extra caution in patients over 55 years of age.

More than 90% of the failures of nonoperative management are attributed to renewed bleeding. Indeed, 1% to 6% of patients treated nonoperatively experience delayed splenic rupture more than five days or as long as two weeks after the initial injury (16,55). These occurrences are particularly worrisome because patients with isolated splenic trauma may have been discharged from the hospital by this time. Other complications associated with nonoperative management also result in the need for laparotomy or other invasive intervention. Although rare, instances of splenic artery pseudoaneurysm have been reported after nonoperative treatment of splenic injury (55,65,66). This condition may be one of the mechanisms of delayed rupture. In addition, case reports and small series have described the appearance of splenic abscesses, within as long as one month after injury, among patients treated nonoperatively (55,66,67). These cases have generally been treated with splenectomy.

REFERENCES

1. Lefor AT, Phillips EH. Spleen. In: Norton JA, Bollinger RR, Chang AE, eds. Surgery: Basic Science and Clinical Evidence. New York: Springer, 2000: 763–785.
2. MacRae HM, Yakimets WW, Reynolds T. Perioperative complications of splenectomy for hematologic disease. Can J Surg 1992; 35(4):432–436.
3. Arnoletti JP, Karam J, Brodsky J. Early postoperative complications of splenectomy for hematologic disease. Am J Clin Oncol 1999; 22(2):114–118.
4. Baccarani U, Terrosu G, Donini A, Bressdola F, Baccarani M. Splenectomy in hematology. Current practice and new perspectives. Haematologica 1999; 84(5):431–436.
5. Danforth DN Jr, Fraker DL. Splenectomy for the massively enlarged spleen. Am Surg 1991; 57(2):108–113.
6. O'Sullivan ST, Reardon CM, O'Donnell JA, Kirwan WD, Brady MP. "How safe is splenectomy?" Ir J Med Sci 1994; 163(8):374–378.
7. Wobbes T, van der Sluis RF, Lubbers EJ. Removal of the massive spleen: a surgical risk? Am J Surg 1984; 147(6):800–802.
8. Waghorn DJ. Overwhelming infection in asplenic patients: current best practice preventive measures are not being followed. J Clin Pathol 2001; 54(3):214–218.
9. Waghorn DJ, Mayon-White RT. A study of 42 episodes of overwhelming post-splenectomy infection: is current guidance for asplenic individuals being followed? J Infect 1997; 35(3):289–294.
10. McClenathan JH. Gastric perforation as a complication of splenectomy: report of five cases and review of the literature. Can J Surg 1991; 34(2):175–178.
11. Park A, Marcaccio M, Sternbach M, Witzke D, Fitzgerald P. Laparoscopic vs open splenectomy. Arch Surg 1999; 134(11):1263–1269.
12. Franciosi C, Caprotti R, Romano F, et al. Laparoscopic versus open splenectomy: a comparative study. Surg Laparosc Endosc Percutan Tech 2000; 10(5):291–295.
13. Friedman RL, Fallas MJ, Carroll BJ, Hiatt JR, Phillips EH. Laparoscopic splenectomy for ITP. The gold standard. Surg Endosc 1996; 10(10):991–995.
14. Decker G, Millat B, Guillen F, Atgei J, Linon M. Laparoscopic splenectomy for benign and malignant hematologic diseases: 35 consecutive cases. World J Surg 1998; 22(1):62–68.
15. Targarona EM, Espert JJ, Bombuy E, et al. Complications of laparoscopic splenectomy. Arch Surg 2000; 135(10):1137–1140.
16. Peitzman AB, Heil B, Rivera L, et al. Blunt splenic injury in adults. Multi-institutional Study of the Eastern Association for the Surgery of Trauma. J Trauma 2000; 49(2):177–189.
17. Buntain WL, Gould HR, Maull KI. Predictability of splenic salvage by computed tomography. J Trauma 1988; 28(1):24–34.
18. Pickhardt B, Moore EE, Moore FA, McCroskey BL, Moore GE. Operative splenic salvage in adults: a decade perspective. J Trauma 1989; 29(10):1386–1391.
19. Velanovich V, Tapper D. Decision analysis in children with blunt splenic trauma: the effects of observation, splenorrhaphy, or splenectomy on quality-adjusted life expectancy. J Pediatr Surg 1993; 28(2):179–185.

20. Norby II, Max MH. Splenorrhaphy in patients with abdominal trauma. South Med J 1986; 79(12):1503–1505.
21. O'Connor GS, Geelhoed GW. Splenic trauma and salvage. Am Surg 1986; 52(8):456–462.
22. Wetzig NR, Strong RW, Theile DE. Splenorrhaphy in the management of splenic injury. Aust N Z J Surg 1986; 56(10):781–784.
23. Delius RE, Frankel W, Coran AG. A comparison between operative and nonoperative management of blunt injuries to the liver and spleen in adult and pediatric patients. Surgery 1989; 106(4):788–793.
24. Myers JG, Dent DL, Stewart RM, et al. Blunt splenic injuries: dedicated trauma surgeons can achieve a high rate of nonoperative success in patients of all ages. J Trauma 2000; 48(5):801–806.
25. Sclafani SJ, Shaftan FW, Scalea TM, et al. Nonoperative salvage of computed tomography-diagnosed splenic injuries: utilization of angiography for triage and embolization for hemostasis. J Trauma 1995; 39(5): 818–827.
26. Powell M, Courcoulas A, Gardner M, et al. Management of blunt splenic trauma: significant differences between adults and children. Surgery 1997; 122(4):654–660.
27. Konstantakos AK, Barnoski AL, Plaisier BR, Yowler CJ, Fallon WF Jr, Malangoni MA. Optimizing the management of blunt splenic injury in adults and children. Surgery 1999; 126(4):805–813.
28. Pachter HL, Guth AA, Hofstetter SR, Spencer FC. Changing patterns in the management of splenic trauma: the impact of nonoperative management. Ann Surg 1998; 227(5):708–719.
29. Pachter HL, Grau J. The current status of splenic preservation. Adv Surg 2000; 34:137–174.
30. Hebeler RF, Ward RE, Miller PW, Ben-Menachem Y. The management of splenic injury. J Trauma 1982; 22(6):492–495.
31. Mucha P Jr, Daly RC, Farnell MB. Selective management of blunt splenic trauma. J Trauma 1986; 26(11): 970–979.
32. Rappaport W, McIntyre KE Jr, Carmona R. The management of splenic trauma in the adult patient with blunt multiple injuries. Surg Gynecol Obstet 1990; 170(3):204–208.
33. Wilson RH, Moorehead RJ. Management of splenic trauma. Injury 1992; 23(1):5–9.
34. Carlin AM, Tyburski JG, Wilson RF, Steffes C. Factors affecting the outcome of patients with splenic trauma. Am Surg 2002; 68(3):232–239.
35. Pitcher ME, Cade RJ, Mackay JR. Splenectomy for trauma: morbidity, mortality and associated abdominal injuries. Aust N Z J Surg 1989; 59(6):461–463.
36. Mustard RA Jr, Hanna SS, Blair G, et al. Blunt splenic trauma: diagnosis and management. Can J Surg 1984; 27(4):330–333.
37. Coltheart G, Little JM. Splenectomy: a review of morbidity. Aust N Z J Surg 1976; 46(1):32–36.
38. Steele M, Lim RC Jr. Advances in management of splenic injuries. Am J Surg 1975; 130(2):159–165.
39. Brigden ML, Pattullo AL. Prevention and management of overwhelming postsplenectomy infection—an update. Crit Care Med 1999; 27(4):836–842.
40. Shandling B. Conservative management of ruptured spleen. S Afr Med J 1980; 57(16):655–658.
41. Ludtke FE, Mack SC, Schuff P, Voth E. Splenic function after splenectomy for trauma. Role of autotransplantation and splenosis. Acta Chir Scand 1989; 155(10):533–539.
42. Moore FA, Moore EE, Moore GE, Millikan JS. Risk of splenic salvage after trauma. Analysis of 200 adults. Am J Surg 1984; 148(6):800–805.
43. Mizrahi S, Bickel A, Haj M, Lunski I, Shtamler B. Post-traumatic autotransplantation of spleen tissue. Arch Surg 1989; 124(7):863–865.
44. Zoli G, Corazza GR, D'Amato G, Bartoli R, Baldoni F, Gasbarrini G. Splenic autotransplantation after splenectomy: tuftsin activity correlates with residual splenic function. Br J Surg 1994; 81(5):716–718.
45. Szendroi T, Miko I, Hajdu A, et al. Splenic autotransplantation after abdominal trauma in childhood. Clinical and experimental data. Acta Chir Hung 1997; 36(1–4):349–351.
46. Moore FA, Moore EE, Moore GE, Erdoes L. Fivefold enlargement of implants in a splenic autotransplant recipient. Surgery 1993; 113(4):462–465.
47. Budihna N, Milcinski M, Heberle J. Long-term follow-up after heterotopic splenic autotransplantation for traumatic splenic rupture. J Nucl Med 1991; 32(2): 204–207.
48. Beal SL, Spisso JM. The risk of splenorrhaphy. Arch Surg 1988; 123(9):1158–1163.
49. Flancbaum L, Dauterive A, Cox EF. Splenic conservation after multiple trauma in adults. Surg Gynecol Obstet 1986; 162(5):469–473.
50. Chadwick SJ, Huizinga WZ, Baker LW. Management of splenic trauma: the Durban experience. Br J Surg 1985; 72(8):634–636.
51. Black JJ, Snow RM, Wilson SE, Williams RA. Subcapsular hematoma as a predictor of delayed splenic rupture. Am Surg 1992; 58(12):732–735.
52. Mahon PA, Sutton JE Jr. Nonoperative management of adult splenic injury due to blunt trauma: a warning. Am J Surg 1985; 149(6):716–721.
53. Malangoni MA, Levine AW, Froege EA, Aprahamian C, Condon RE. Management of injury to the spleen in adults. Results of early operation and observation. Ann Surg 1984; 200(6):702–705.
54. Bitseff EL, Adkins RB Jr. Splenic trauma: a trial at selective management. South Med J 1984; 77(10):1286–1290.
55. Cocanour CS, Moore FA, Ware DN, Marvin RG, Clark JM, Duke JH. Delayed complications of nonoperative management of blunt adult splenic trauma. Arch Surg 1998; 133(6):619–625.
56. Cogbill TH, Moore EE, Jurkovich GJ, et al. Nonoperative management of blunt splenic trauma: a multicenter experience. J Trauma 1989; 29(10):1312–1317.
57. Longo WE, Baker CC, McMillen MA, Modlin IM, Degutis LC, Zucker KA. Nonoperative management of adult blunt splenic trauma. Criteria for successful outcome. Ann Surg 1989; 210(5):626–629.
58. Davis KA, Fabian TC, Croce MA, et al. Improved success in nonoperative management of blunt splenic injuries: embolization of splenic artery pseudoaneurysms. J Trauma 1998; 44(6):1008–1015.
59. Jalovec LM, Boe BS, Wyffels PL. The advantages of early operation with splenorrhaphy versus nonoperative management for the blunt splenic trauma patient. Am Surg 1993; 59(10):698–705.
60. Falimirski ME, Provost D. Nonsurgical management of solid abdominal organ injury in patients over 55 years of age. Am Surg 2000; 66(7):631–635.

61. Harbrecht BG, Peitzman AB, Rivera L, et al. Contribution of age and gender to outcome of blunt splenic injury in adults. Multicenter Study of the Eastern Association for the Surgery of Trauma. J Trauma 2001; 51(5):887–895.

62. Smith JS Jr, Cooney RN, Mucha P Jr. Nonoperative management of the ruptured spleen: a revalidation of criteria. Surgery 1996; 120(4):745–751.

63. Albrecht RM, Schermer CR, Morris A. Nonoperative management of blunt splenic injuries: factors influencing success in age > 55 years. Am Surg 2002; 68(3):227–231.

64. Krause KR, Howells GA, Bair HA, et al. Nonoperative management of blunt splenic injury in adults 55 years and older: a twenty-year experience. Am Surg 2000; 66(7):636–640.

65. Sugg SL, Gerndt SJ, Hamilton BJ, Francis IR, Taheri PA, Rodriguez JL. Pseudoaneurysms of the intraparenchymal splenic artery after blunt abdominal trauma: a complication of nonoperative therapy and its management. J Trauma 1995; 39(3):593–595.

66. Frumiento C, Sartorelli K, Vane D. Complications of splenic injuries: expansion of the nonoperative theorem. J Pediatr Surg 2000; 35(5):788–791.

67. Sands M, Page D, Brown RB. Splenic abscess following nonoperative management of splenic rupture. J Pediatr Surg 1986; 21(10):900–901.

14

Complications of Laparoscopy in General Surgery

David S. Lasko
University of Miami School of Medicine/Jackson Memorial Hospital, Miami, Florida, U.S.A.

Robert W. Bailey
Division of Laparoscopic and Bariatric Surgery, Daughtry Family Department of Surgery, Miller School of Medicine, University of Miami, Miami, Florida, U.S.A.

The last 15 years have witnessed an unprecedented change in the manner in which general surgical procedures are performed. The technical approach to the surgical patient has been redefined. It is imperative, therefore, that all surgeons become conversant with the complications that might occur during minimally invasive surgery. In general, most complications occur with comparable frequency during both minimally invasive and open surgical procedures. However, a substantial proportion of laparoscopic complications are unique, in many respects, when compared with those encountered during open surgery. This chapter will focus primarily on this latter subset of problems.

Complications unique to laparoscopy stem from several sources. First, patients who undergo minimally invasive procedures experience distinct, observable, and, occasionally, clinically significant physiologic alterations. Second, specific complications are related to the technical aspects of gaining access to the peritoneal cavity so that laparoscopic surgery can be performed. Finally, the inherent limitations of a two-dimensional laparoscopic image present a substantial, although not insurmountable, obstacle that must be overcome by the laparoscopic surgeon. All of these factors contribute to the fourth potential source of complications, that of a clearly recognizable learning curve for surgeons attempting to become proficient in laparoscopic surgery.

PHYSIOLOGIC CHANGES

The establishment of pneumoperitoneum typically results in transient physiologic alterations involving the major organ systems, such as the heart, lung, kidney, and liver. Among these, hemodynamic and respiratory changes are the most clinically relevant and well studied. Fortunately, in otherwise healthy patients, these changes rarely result in a deleterious clinical outcome. However, in patients with preexisting cardiac, pulmonary, renal, or hepatic dysfunction, the establishment of pneumoperitoneum may lead to serious, life-threatening complications. It is important that the surgeon be aware of these potential events so that timely intervention may be instituted when necessary.

Pulmonary Effects

The establishment of pneumoperitoneum leads to changes both in ventilation parameters and in gas exchange. One of the most obvious and most common alterations in ventilation is an increase in airway pressures. These increases result from a decrease in diaphragmatic excursion and in lung and chest wall compliance as the result of the increase in intra-abdominal pressure (1–3). Clinically, both peak and end-inspiratory pressures are increased by as much as 30% to 40% above baseline when routine insufflation pressures of 10 to 15 mmHg are used (1,3–5). Measured respiratory compliance is decreased by approximately 35% as a result of these changes. For healthy patients with pulmonary reserve, the altered physiologic parameters are usually clinically inconsequential. Fortunately, airway pressures rapidly return to normal (preinsufflation) levels after the release of the pneumoperitoneum. Therefore, the surgeon should immediately discontinue the inflow of insufflation and evacuate the existing pneumoperitoneum whenever any untoward ventilatory or sudden hemodynamic changes occur during laparoscopic surgery.

Carbon dioxide is universally used to establish and maintain pneumoperitoneum. Hypercarbia, and subsequent respiratory acidosis, can result from abdominal insufflation and transperitoneal absorption of carbon dioxide. This increase in carbon dioxide absorption is reflected by an increase in arterial carbon dioxide levels. Arterial $p\text{CO}_2$ (partial pressure of carbon dioxide) commonly increases by approximately 8 to 12 mmHg above baseline, and pH dips to approximately 7.35 to 7.38 during routine laparoscopic cases (4–7). However, repetitive arterial $p\text{CO}_2$ monitoring requires an arterial line, which is not necessary or practical in most routine laparoscopic cases. Therefore, surgeons commonly use end-tidal carbon dioxide measurements to assess the adequacy of ventilation (8) because this value can be monitored noninvasively. End-tidal CO_2 levels normally increase by about 10% (4) at normal insufflation pressures. Fortunately, such alterations are generally well tolerated by otherwise healthy patients (4–7). Furthermore, the anesthesiologist can lower these elevated levels of carbon dioxide to a more normal range simply by increasing the rate of mechanical ventilation. It is important to remember, however, that changes in end-tidal carbon dioxide levels generally underestimate the actual increase in arterial pCO_2 (9). Therefore, surgeons should carefully consider using arterial line blood gas monitoring when performing laparoscopic surgery on patients with significant cardiovascular or pulmonary disease who may be more sensitive to respiratory alterations. For such patients, the differences between end-tidal and true arterial carbon dioxide levels are reported (9) to be greater than those for healthy persons. Fortunately, for all patients, abnormal carbon dioxide and pH values generally return to baseline within several minutes after the release of pneumoperitoneum (5–7). Once again, the appearance of any untoward, sudden clinical effects, such as arrhythmias, hypotension, or uncompensated acidemia, should lead to the immediate release of pneumoperitoneum and to hyperventilation of the patient so that respiratory acidosis can be reduced.

Hemodynamic Effects

Experimental and clinical studies have clearly demonstrated that several hemodynamic changes occur during abdominal insufflation. The increase in intra-abdominal pressure that accompanies pneumoperitoneum results in a decrease in the venous return to the heart via the inferior vena cava (10). This decrease, in turn, leads to a decrease in cardiac preload, which results in a global decrease in left ventricular (LV) function. From a pathophysiologic standpoint, the most striking and observable hemodynamic change is a decrease of 10% to 30% in cardiac output (5,11–16). This decrease in cardiac performance appears to lead to a neurohumoral cascade involving increases in the levels of renin, angiotensin, and aldosterone, increases that probably alter other hemodynamic values (17,18). These other changes include decreases in LV end-diastolic pressures and volumes, which are associated with increases of as much as 25% in systemic and pulmonary vascular resistances (5,19). The altered hemodynamic indices often contribute to other physiologic changes such as increases in the mean arterial pressure (7–15 mmHg) and decreases in renal blood flow and glomerular filtration rate (3,5,10,20).

In addition to altered cardiac function, arrhythmias may occur in as many as 47% of patients who undergo laparoscopic surgery (21). Tachycardia appears to be the most common type of arrhythmia and is believed to result from a decrease in cardiac output. Fortunately, such tachycardic events are usually well tolerated. However, on rare occasions, otherwise healthy patients may experience dangerous bradyarrhythmias during minimally invasive surgery (21–23). Several factors have been suggested to cause these bradyarrhythmias. However, the most likely cause is related to the hypercapnia that develops as a result of the increased afterload and the subsequent increase in myocardial workload resulting from pneumoperitoneum. Unlike tachycardia, these bradyarrhythmias are usually not well tolerated and should be treated aggressively with the immediate evacuation of pneumoperitoneum and the use of appropriate pharmacologic measures to restore normal rhythm.

The cardiovascular effects of pneumoperitoneum, like the pulmonary changes, are of minimal clinical importance for most patients undergoing elective laparoscopic surgery. This statement assumes, however, that insufflation pressure is maintained within the normal range of 10 to 15 mmHg. Surgeons should be careful to ensure that these levels are not exceeded throughout the operative procedure. Unrecognized and unusually high increases in the insufflation pressure can lead to very deleterious effects. Surgeons should also be aware that patients with compromised cardiac or respiratory function may not tolerate the impairments in cardiovascular function that are imposed by pneumoperitoneum. The surgical team should carefully consider the use of more invasive intraoperative monitoring, or even a different surgical approach, for patients with such preexisting conditions, especially elderly or obese patients whose respiratory or cardiac function may be subclinically compromised. Nonetheless, and despite all efforts, some patients will not tolerate even normal insufflation pressures.

COMPLICATIONS RELATED TO LAPAROSCOPIC ACCESS

Laparoscopic surgery, in general, is associated with an extremely low morbidity rate, between 2% and 10%, depending on the type of operation and the experience of the surgeon. When complications do arise in laparoscopic surgery, however, they are commonly related to methods of obtaining access to the peritoneal cavity. In fact, access-related complications compose as much as 38% of the morbidity related to minimally invasive surgery (24). The overall incidence of access-related injury during laparoscopic surgery is reported to range from 0.2% to 5% (25–30). However, further analysis of access-related morbidity is hindered by the fact that many reports do not differentiate between the various access techniques.

Injuries Caused by Needle or Trocar

Vascular injury to the abdominal wall and the retroperitoneal vessels is the most common access-related laparoscopic complication, accounting for approximately 65% of these injuries (28). Fortunately, the overwhelming majority of vascular injuries involve the epigastric vessels and not the major retroperitoneal vessels. The overall incidence of abdominal wall bleeding is reported to range from 0.5% to 2% (24,30,31). As would be expected, such injuries are usually of minimal clinical significance. Temporary control of abdominal wall bleeding can often be attained by one of several simple but effective methods: pressure against the bleeding site with the offending trocar; laparoscopic-guided, percutaneous suture ligation; or, when necessary on rare occasions, open suture ligation. Injury to small omental vessels may be easily controlled with laparoscopic clips (32). Interestingly, it is generally assumed that many more vascular injuries to the abdominal wall go unrecognized because they are often considered to be self-limiting and of minimal clinical importance.

Major retroperitoneal vascular injury occurs far less frequently (in 0.1–0.25% of all laparoscopic operations), but injury to these vessels accounts for 35% of all deaths during laparoscopic surgery (26,28,33). The major vessels most commonly injured are the iliac artery and vein (24–27% of injuries), followed by the aorta, the inferior vena cava, or both (10–15% of injuries), and the major visceral or mesenteric vessels (5–10% of injuries) (26,28). Earlier studies found that major vascular injuries were associated with extremely high mortality rates; in fact, combined aortocaval injuries were associated with mortality rates of 80% to 100%. However, more recent reports demonstrate that approximately 8% of all major vascular injuries result in mortality (34). In the face of a major vascular injury, temporary control of the hemorrhage should be achieved by any means necessary. In general, a midline laparotomy should be performed to allow for definitive proximal and distal control and repair of the injury. Depending on the laparoscopic surgeon's judgment and experience, a vascular surgeon should be called for intraoperative consultation.

Visceral injuries occur far less frequently during laparoscopic surgery than vascular complications; they reportedly occur during 0.1% to 0.2% of all laparoscopic procedures (24,27,29,30,33). Most large series indicate that small-bowel perforations account for nearly 90% of visceral injuries, followed, in decreasing frequency, by perforations of the liver, colon, and stomach (27–29,33). The overall mortality rate associated with intestinal injury during laparoscopy is approximately 3% to 5% (28,29,33). Importantly, and despite the surgical team's best efforts, as many as 69% of all access-related intestinal injuries go unrecognized intraoperatively (28,29). Failure to recognize such injuries is associated with a 10-fold increase in mortality rates, reported to be approximately 20% to 25% (26,28). A recent review of 182 access-related visceral injuries demonstrated that the mortality rate was zero if all injuries were identified intraoperatively. However, 21% of unrecognized bowel injuries resulted in death (28). This finding demonstrates the importance of performing a thorough diagnostic survey of the abdomen at the completion of each procedure,

especially if there is any suspicion of a visceral injury. Unfortunately, small, occult, or delayed injuries may not be detectable at the time of surgery. Therefore, despite a surgeon's best efforts, unrecognized injuries may still occur.

One rare but often lethal complication of laparoscopic access is gas embolism, which occurs in approximately one of every 100,000 laparoscopic cases (35,36). Gas embolism is nearly always associated with insertion of a Veress needle into a major vascular structure and subsequent insufflation (35). The associated mortality rate is reported to be more than 30% (35,36). Although only sporadic case reports exist, gas embolism is generally managed by deflating the pneumoperitoneum, placing the patient into a Trendelenburg and left lateral decubitus position, administering 100% oxygen, and instituting general supportive measures. Some surgeons have also advocated the emergent placement of a central line so that aspiration of the intravascular gas can be attempted. Unfortunately because of the sudden nature of the cardiovascular collapse, there is little time for deploying these management techniques; therefore, such measures have achieved only limited success (36,37).

One additional access-related complication that deserves mention is extraperitoneal dissection of carbon dioxide. This is generally a minor issue with little attendant morbidity. However, it can be alarming to the surgeon, the anesthesiologist, or the patient after he or she awakens. The anesthesiologist may be particularly concerned because subcutaneous emphysema, especially in and around the neck and chest, is also an indicator of a serious airway disruption. Subcutaneous emphysema can occur anywhere, from the lower extremities, as seen after hernia repair, to the head, neck, and chest, as can occur after mediastinal dissection during antireflux surgery. Patients should be made aware that the subcutaneous emphysema is generally harmless and usually resolves within 48 to 72 hours (34). Extraperitoneal insufflation is usually caused by improper angling of the Veress needle, which results in suprafascial or properitoneal positioning of its tip. Like many access-related complications, extraperitoneal insufflation can be avoided by the use of proper access techniques.

Because access-related injuries may be associated with morbidity and mortality, laparoscopic surgeons must have a good working knowledge of methods for preventing such injuries. Should the surgeon choose the Veress needle as the initial method of access, established techniques and principles should be followed. The needle should be inserted at a 15° to 30° angle to the abdominal wall, in the direction of the pelvis. This maneuver is believed to help prevent injury to the aorta; however, conclusive evidence supporting this theory is lacking. Once inserted, the needle should be stabilized so that inadvertent injury to the underlying viscera can be avoided (34). Established means of confirming proper positioning should be also used, including performing a saline drop test and ensuring low intra-abdominal pressure. When an open access technique is used, careful visualization and identification of all layers of the abdominal wall is paramount to safe entrance into the peritoneal cavity (34).

Choice of Access Technique

Most large series examining laparoscopic access injuries do not differentiate between the specific access techniques. Thus, the data remain equivocal as to the relative safety of open (Hasson) and closed (Veress needle) access techniques. On the one hand, several large series reporting access injuries and including as many as 20,000 patients demonstrate equivalent complication rates for the two access approaches (24,26,27). However, other reports demonstrate substantial decreases in morbidity rates in association with the open technique (30,35,38). A large meta-analysis encompassing nearly 500,000 patients (35) found that the rate of visceral injury associated with closed access with a Veress needle (0.08%) was nearly double that associated with open access (0.05%). Major retroperitoneal vascular injury was nearly nonexistent in association with open access (only two cases ever reported) but occurred at a rate of 0.08% with closed laparoscopy (35). A further potential advantage of the open technique is the increased likelihood of intraoperative recognition of an injury (24,30,35). Additionally, when the patient has had other abdominal surgery, especially near the site of intended entry, the open approach is clearly indicated. Therefore, although both Veress needle insufflation and the Hasson technique are established and generally safe methods of obtaining access, the evidence suggests that open laparoscopy is the safer approach.

Careful preoperative consideration of the proper choice for abdominal access and meticulous technique remain the mainstays of safe establishment of pneumoperitoneum. However, recent years have seen the emergence of new technologies that could prevent even more access-related morbidity. Of these technologies, optically equipped trocars and Veress needles may offer the most promise. These unique devices allow direct visualization of individual layers of the abdominal wall during entry into the peritoneum (39). Although optical trocars provide excellent visualization, the inferior optical resolution of the optical needles has limited their popularity and adaptation (28).

Trocar-Site Hernias

Sporadically published reports have addressed trocar-site incisional hernias. The largest studies cite an incidence of 0.2% (40,41). Leibl et al. demonstrated that the incidence of trocar-site incisional hernia is approximately nine times higher when cutting trocars are used (1.8%) instead of blunt or optical-type trocars (0.2%) (40). Trocar-site hernias have been reported at both 5- and 10-mm trocar sites and can result in incarcerated or strangulated viscera. However, more than 95% of all reported trocar-site hernias occur at incision sites involving trocars 10 mm or more in diameter. It is also recognized that trocar-site hernias tend to occur more commonly among obese patients for whom closure of the fascial defect poses the greatest challenge. Because these hernias are small, detecting them by physical examination is often difficult, especially among obese patients. Because the necks of trocar-site hernias are small, they are more subject to incarceration and subsequent strangulation. Many of these hernias may be caused by Richter-like hernias, in which a defect exists in the posterior fascia, but the anterior fascia, closed at surgery, remains intact. Therefore, the sudden occurrence or persistent presence of pain at a trocar incision site should alert the surgeon to the possible existence of such a hernia. Local wound exploration, even with the opening of an intact anterior fascia, should be undertaken if there is reason for concern.

When complications do occur, the laparoscopic surgeon must follow time-honored surgical principles to minimize the morbidity rates associated with them. Given the high morbidity and mortality rates associated with major vascular injuries and with occult visceral injuries, a high index of suspicion must be constantly maintained. When these injuries are recognized, immediate repair should be undertaken, and the wisdom of continuing with the planned procedure should be evaluated, whether or not the procedure is performed laparoscopically or via a more traditional open approach. Depending on the surgeon's experience and the severity of the injury, conversion to an open approach should be considered for managing a situation that cannot be easily handled laparoscopically. However, the mere existence of a complication or a difficult scenario does not necessarily mandate conversion to an open procedure. As long as the operative dissection is proceeding in a positive fashion, the laparoscopic procedure should be continued. Patients should routinely be made aware of the potential for complications and the need for conversion to an open approach.

ALTERED VISUALIZATION, UNIQUE INSTRUMENTATION, AND THE ROLE OF THE LEARNING CURVE

Several authors cite image reversal and the two-dimensional nature of laparoscopic surgery as influential sources of complications (42–44). Unfortunately, it has not been possible to directly link actual operative complications to the visual alterations experienced during laparoscopic surgery. Nonetheless, the initial, inherent limitations of two-dimensional surgery are well known to most surgeons. This limitation has led several device manufacturers to develop innovative three-dimensional alternatives to the standard two-dimensional laparoscopic image. Interestingly, comparisons between standard two-dimensional laparoscopy and these innovative three-dimensional optical systems have not demonstrated any measurable performance difference among surgeons using the two different systems (42,45). This unexpected finding most likely stems from the fact that such early studies were conducted with very rudimentary three-dimensional systems.

Evidence for the existence of a learning curve stems from several sources. Retrospective studies have demonstrated a clearly identifiable increase in the rate of complications early in a surgeon's experience. For example, more than 80% of bile duct injuries occur during a surgeon's first 50 laparoscopic cholecystectomies (34). In addition to an increased complication rate, studies have also demonstrated that operative times and conversion rates are increased during a surgeon's first 20 to 50 laparoscopic cases. This observation holds true across many types of general surgical procedures, including antireflux surgery (46–48), inguinal herniorrhaphy (49), and colorectal operations (50). Common recommendations for minimizing complications during the learning curve include intensive educational programs that offer didactic instruction, skills training, and laboratory practice. Additional hands-on experience and assistance by surgeons with additional clinical expertise is desirable but not mandatory.

COMMON LAPAROSCOPIC OPERATIONS
Cholecystectomy

After its introduction in the late 1980s, laparoscopic cholecystectomy quickly became the treatment of choice throughout the world for benign gall bladder disease. Several large series involving 12,000 to 115,000 patients have demonstrated that the overall complication rate associated with laparoscopic cholecystectomy is lower than that associated with the open procedure, with the very important exception of bile duct injury. The overall morbidity rates associated with laparoscopic cholecystectomy range from 2.0% to 6.9%, whereas those associated with open cholecystectomy range from approximately 8% to 10.5% (51,52).

Bile Duct Injury

The incidence of serious ductal injuries, including severe bile leaks, in association with laparoscopic cholecystectomy ranges from 0% to 2% (33,53–55). One meta-analysis of more than 40 published series found that the mean incidence of major bile duct injury was 0.5%, two to four times the rate cited for open cholecystectomy (0.1–0.25%) (53). However, the validity of this assessment may be flawed from several vantage points. The actual difference between the risk of bile duct injury for open cholecystectomy and that of laparoscopic cholecystectomy may still be unknown. First, the higher rates of injury found by early studies of laparoscopic cholecystectomy may simply be a reflection of the learning curve for this procedure. Second, many of the large series of open cholecystectomy are retrospective reviews of a solo surgeon's or a single center's experience. Many

of these reports were published in a time when large databases or patient registries and sophisticated data collection systems were not available. The true rate of bile duct injury during open cholecystectomy may therefore have been underestimated.

Careful identification of the important anatomic landmarks is the key to avoiding bile duct injury, regardless of the operative approach. Obviously, meticulous dissection is necessary if this goal is to be accomplished. However, a clear delineation of the individual steps or techniques necessary for performing such a dissection is a much more difficult task. Although individual authors may claim that one discreet surgical technique, such as dissection of the junction of the cystic duct and the common bile duct, can avoid bile duct injury, this assertion has never been proved scientifically. In fact, routine dissection of this junction could put the patient at undue risk and could lead to iatrogenic injury in this anatomic area. Other reports have emphasized additional techniques that may be crucial for completing a safe dissection of the gallbladder, such as dissection of the junction of the cystic duct and the gallbladder, creation of a large window of dissection within Calot's triangle, lateral retraction of the gallbladder neck, and the use of intraoperative cholangiography. Any one or all of these techniques may be used and should be used when they are indicated by the clinical situation. However, it would be unreasonable to claim that all of these techniques must be used in all cases. Therefore, the surgeon's goal should be to do what is necessary in each case to identify the patient's biliary anatomy and to perform a meticulous dissection of Calot's triangle.

Aside from using specific dissection techniques, some surgeons have advocated the use of routine intraoperative cholangiography as a method of avoiding bile duct injuries. The conclusions of reported studies are divided on whether routine cholangiography during laparoscopic cholecystectomy affects the rate of bile duct injury (56–59). Logic would suggest that routine cholangiography does not necessarily decrease the actual incidence of bile duct injury because most cholangiograms are performed via a transcystic approach with clipping of the duct. Therefore, if the surgeon has already erred by identifying the common bile duct as the cystic duct, the common bile duct will be injured by the placement of the cholangiogram catheter itself. The liberal use of cholangiography, however, will identify most bile duct injuries intraoperatively, at a point at which they can be repaired much more easily and with better long-term results than injuries discovered postoperatively (53,54). Bile duct reconstruction and the management of severe bile leaks are discussed in Chapter 8.

Miscellaneous Complications of Laparoscopic Cholecystectomy

The spillage of bile or stones during laparoscopic cholecystectomy has always been of concern to surgeons.

The primary problem is the potential for the development of an intraperitoneal abscess because of the spillage of infected material. Fortunately, in the vast majority of cases, spillage of biliary material does not lead to an increase in morbidity rates (60,61). Memon et al. (62) reported that dropped stones, bile spillage, or both occur with 40% of laparoscopic cholecystectomies but that only 5% of these events are related to any complications as demonstrated by long-term follow-up. All of the complications that did occur were successfully treated by either antibiotics alone or percutaneous drainage (one patient, 0.6% of all patients). Dropped stones can be easily and safely retrieved. The peritoneal cavity should be copiously irrigated so that the possibility of abscess formation can be minimized. However, a lengthy and unrewarding search for lost stones should be avoided because it can increase the risk of visceral and vascular injuries (60,61,63).

A few potential vascular and visceral injuries are unique to laparoscopic cholecystectomy (61). Vascular injuries can often be related to the anomalous nature of the blood supply to the liver and gallbladder. An aberrant right hepatic artery arising from the superior mesenteric artery and passing through or near Calot's triangle is one recognized variation that may predispose patients to injury. Multiple cystic arteries or accessory hepatic arteries passing near the operative field of dissection are also prone to injury during laparoscopic cholecystectomy. Bleeding from the parenchyma of the liver can also be troublesome. Finally, the proximity of the duodenum and the hepatic flexure of the colon to the operative field raise the potential for injury to these organs.

Fundoplication

The complication rate associated with laparoscopic fundoplication (14%) is often reported to be lower than that associated with open fundoplication (25%) (64–67). Impaired visualization of the most superior aspect of the abdomen may account for a portion of the higher morbidity rate associated with open fundoplication. It is possible that additional factors such as decreased immobilization and shorter hospital stays may also decrease the morbidity rate associated with minimally invasive techniques. The recently published series of laparoscopic fundoplication have involved follow-up periods of five years or more, and it is unlikely that serious complications will occur after this time. However, the length of postoperative follow-up in most laparoscopic series is still somewhat limited as compared to that of open series (64).

The most common complication after fundoplication is wrap failure, which occurs after approximately 15% to 20% of open procedures and 5% to 10% of laparoscopic procedures (64–67). Different patterns of failure emerge when open and minimally invasive fundoplication are compared (64). Most laparoscopic failures (84%) are caused by transdiaphragmatic

herniation of the wrap, whereas failures after open fundoplication are evenly distributed between transdiaphragmatic migration, slipped or misplaced fundoplication, and twisted wraps. Overly tight wraps that require reoperation occur with approximately 4% of laparoscopic fundoplications and 10% of open fundoplications (64,68). However, the complication of postoperative paraesophageal hernia appears to be more common after laparoscopic fundoplication (5–6% of all laparoscopic procedures) than after open fundoplication (this complication almost never occurs in such cases) (67,69). In most reported cases of paraesophageal hernia, posterior hiatal narrowing had not been performed during the initial operation, and this finding may account for the higher incidence of this complication in association with the laparoscopic procedure (67).

Complications other than wrap failure are uncommon in association with laparoscopic fundoplication. Most conversions to the open technique (approximately 5% of cases) result from technical difficulties, including adhesions and problems associated with obesity, rather than from intraoperative complications (70,71). The mortality rate was zero and the overall morbidity rate was 7% in one series of more than 600 patients who underwent a variety of different types of laparoscopic fundoplication (70). Infections and pulmonary complications are virtually eliminated during laparoscopic fundoplication (no higher than 1%) but do occur during open fundoplication (1–5% of cases) (67). Serious complications, including gastric, bowel, or esophageal perforation, occurred in association with 0.66% of laparoscopic cases in another large series (71).

Two portions of the fundoplication procedure may pose a greater risk of injury to the esophagus during laparoscopic fundoplication: passage of the dilator and creation of a window posterior to the esophagus. The inability of the surgeon to palpate the bougie or the posterior esophagus during these portions of the minimally invasive procedure could lead to a higher risk of injury.

Herniorrhaphy

The laparoscopic approach has not been widely adopted for the repair of unilateral, primary groin hernias, and its indications in such cases are controversial. It is important, however, for surgeons to be aware of the potential complications of laparoscopic herniorrhaphy because recurrent or bilateral inguinal hernias are often repaired laparoscopically.

Two main laparoscopic herniorrhaphy approaches are currently in use. Although laparoscopic inguinal herniorrhaphy was initially limited to the transabdominal properitoneal approach (TAPP), the advent of balloon dissectors has enabled the development of the totally extraperitoneal repair (TEP). Favorable results have been reported with both types of repairs, with comparable rates of recurrent hernia (72). A large series comparing the two approaches found that intraperitoneal complications (trocar hernias, small-bowel obstructions, and bowel injuries resulting from dissection or trocar placement) occurred at a low rate in the TAPP group (1.5%) but were completely eliminated in the TEP group.

Large series have compared suture and mesh techniques for repairing open inguinal herniorrhaphy. Several studies, including a large meta-analysis involving more than 2400 patients, have found that both types of laparoscopic repair are associated with less postoperative pain and more rapid recovery rates than is the open Shouldice technique (73,74). Recurrence rates are generally better for laparoscopic repair than for nonmesh open repair techniques. A recent randomized controlled trial reported a significantly lower rate of recurrence at a five-years follow-up for TAPP repair (3%) than for Shouldice repair (8%) (74). Equivalent rates of recurrence (2–3%) and severity of postoperative pain (2–3%) are usually reported for laparoscopic and tension-free repairs (73,75). Advances in technique and shortening of the learning curve may be reducing the recurrence rate associated with laparoscopic inguinal herniorrhaphy. A recent multicenter series including more than 10,000 laparoscopic repairs (TAPP and TEP) reported a 0.4% recurrence rate with three years of follow-up (76). Technical errors involving inadequate fixation or the use of a mesh that was too small accounted for most of the recurrences in this study.

Morbidity rates associated with laparoscopic and open approaches are generally equivalent and vary widely depending on which complications are included in the study. Common complications of laparoscopic hernia repair include hematomas, seromas, and hydroceles (8–10%), urinary retention (1–2%), cutaneous nerve injuries (2%), and persistent pain (2–3%) (74,77,78).

Although serious complications are very uncommon during laparoscopic herniorrhaphy, surgeons who choose a laparoscopic approach must keep in mind the special risk to the iliac vessels that is associated with this operation. They should be wary of the so-called "Triangle of Doom" that is bounded by the iliac vessels laterally and the ductus deferens medially (79). Reports of injuries to these structures during laparoscopic herniorrhaphy are rare; however, serious complications associated with this procedure are most likely to occur in this anatomic area.

Appendectomy

The first laparoscopic appendectomy was performed in 1983, nearly five years before the first laparoscopic cholecystectomy. However, laparoscopic appendectomy was not widely used before the widespread acceptance of laparoscopic cholecystectomy (80). The minimal morbidity rates and short hospital stay associated with open appendectomy may account for part of the sluggish enthusiasm for the laparoscopic approach. Additionally, during the past seven years, at least 20 randomized clinical trials comparing laparoscopic to open appendectomy over many variables have yielded equivocal results. No consistent differences have emerged in complication rates (about 15–25%), including superficial wound infections and intra-abdominal infections (81–85). Cost differences have been found between the two approaches, but the results have differed as to which approach is less expensive. This lack of convincing data makes either choice of approach acceptable. Theoretically, the smaller wounds associated with laparoscopy may offer an improved cosmetic outcome. In addition, the ability to view more of the abdomen and pelvis with the camera may be an advantage when the diagnosis is uncertain, particularly for women of childbearing age (80). Regardless of the approach to the abdomen, however, it is important for the surgeon to follow established general surgical principles for the diagnosis and treatment of appendicitis.

Ventral Hernia Repair

Recent prospective and retrospective comparisons of open and laparoscopic techniques for ventral hernia repair have found that the laparoscopic approach has several advantages. Minimally invasive ventral hernia repair is associated with significantly fewer wound complications (3–10%) than are open techniques (12–45%) (86–90). In addition, the reported 10% to 52% recurrence rate associated with open ventral hernia repair is reduced to 3% to 10% when the minimally invasive procedure is used (87–89,91,92). The association of laparoscopic ventral hernia repair with decreased tissue trauma and minimized exposure of the prosthetic material to the environment may account for the decreased infection and recurrence rates. The decrease in recurrence rates may be attributable to the technical advantages of the laparoscopic approach. These include wider coverage with the mesh and the ability to identify all defects and weak areas in the fascia. It is possible, however, that shorter follow-up times (averaging 2–3 years) account for a portion of the lower recurrence rate reported in the laparoscopic series.

Other common complications of ventral hernia repair, including seroma and hematoma, are reduced from 20% or 30% to less than 2% in series of laparoscopic ventral hernia repair (87–89). Hospital stay is significantly reduced when the laparoscopic approach is used, from an average of more than one week to approximately two days (86–88). Of course, any of the general complications of laparoscopy, including needle- and trocar-related visceral and vascular injury, can occur with minimally invasive ventral hernia repair. However, most series suggest equivalent or decreased rates of enterotomy (2–4%) for laparoscopic ventral hernia repair. It is clear that ventral hernias can be performed safely, with decreased morbidity rates, when a laparoscopic approach is used.

Surgery for Morbid Obesity

Two main approaches to laparoscopic surgery for morbid obesity are currently in use: laparoscopic Roux-en-y gastric bypass and laparoscopic placement of an adjustable gastric band (LAPBAND). The LAPBAND was approved for use in the United States in 1999, and initial results from Australia and Europe are encouraging. However, laparoscopic Roux-en-y gastric bypass has been more thoroughly researched; studies have compared the outcomes associated with this procedure to those associated with traditional open gastric bypass. When the complication rates associated with the two techniques are compared, it must be remembered that laparoscopic gastric bypass is a relatively new and complex operation and that many surgeons who perform it may still be on a learning curve. One series reported a very high rate (nearly 25%) of conversion to open surgery (93) and operative times approximately 30 to 40 minutes longer in association with laparoscopic gastric bypass (93,94), findings that may indicate early discomfort with the minimally invasive approach.

Overall complication rates are similar for laparoscopic (26%) and open gastric bypass procedures (23%) (94). Both operations are associated with low rates of anastomotic leak (2–3%), although a significantly higher rate of anastomotic stricture has been reported for the laparoscopic approach (5–25%) than for the open procedure (0–15%) (94,95). Series large enough to evaluate the relative risk of rare but catastrophic events such as pulmonary embolism do not exist. Surgeons performing either open or laparoscopic surgery for morbid obesity must have a high index of suspicion for pulmonary embolism because patients undergoing this procedure comprise a very high-risk population.

In several areas, laparoscopic gastric bypass has advantages over the open procedure. A randomized prospective trial found that patients undergoing minimally invasive gastric bypass procedures experienced significantly shorter hospital stays than those undergoing open procedures; they also experienced shorter times for return to activities of daily living (8 days as compared to 17 days) and to work (32 days as compared to 46 days) (94). In addition, patients undergoing laparoscopic gastric bypass experience less intraoperative bleeding and postoperative pain (93,94) and smaller decreases in postoperative pulmonary function (96) than do patients undergoing open procedures. Importantly, weight loss did not differ between the patients undergoing laparoscopic and those undergoing open surgery in any of the series.

Splenectomy

The laparoscopic approach is widely used for splenic surgery and is considered by many to be the gold standard for elective splenectomy (97–99). Patients undergoing elective laparoscopic splenectomy experience shorter hospital stays (averaging 2–5 days as compared to 7–10 days) and less blood loss (approximately 200 mL as compared to 350–500 mL) than those undergoing open splenectomy (97–100). Complication rates are also lower for patients undergoing laparoscopic splenectomy (6–7%) than for those undergoing open splenectomy (approximately 20%), when those patients are matched for demographic characteristics and underlying disease (99,100). Splenosis associated with missed accessory splenic material can result in failure to accomplish the goal of the operation: the eradication of splenic function. However, with a meticulous technique and an exhaustive search for accessory or dropped splenic material, the incidence of this complication is equivalent for laparoscopic and open splenectomy (100).

Adrenalectomy

Open surgery for benign adrenal disease has traditionally been associated with fairly high morbidity rates (101), but recent reports have found that laparoscopic adrenalectomy is a safer, equally effective option (101,102). Some authors have called this procedure the emerging gold standard of treatment for benign adrenal disease (102,103). Several series have reported that complication rates are lower for laparoscopic adrenalectomy (1–10%) than for open adrenalectomy (10–50%), with mortality rates generally less than 1% (102–104). Although the narrow working space and the paucity of anatomic landmarks might be expected to complicate the retroperitoneal minimally invasive approach to the adrenal gland, studies have found no difference in the rate of complications between retroperitoneal and anterior laparoscopic adrenalectomy (35,104). The importance of radical, wide resection for adrenal malignancies indicates an open approach when cancer is suspected (generally in tumors larger than 6 cm in diameter) (102–104).

Living-Related Donor Nephrectomy

Limited numbers of living-related donor nephrectomy procedures have been performed, and only a subset of these have been performed laparoscopically. Several small series have found that the laparoscopic approach is associated with decreased postoperative pain, shortened hospital stays (2–4 days as compared to 6–7 days for open nephrectomy), and improved cosmesis (105–107). All of the series have reported low complication rates (2–5%) and statistically equivalent post-transplant kidney function (105–108). These early series indicate that laparoscopic living-related donor nephrectomy is a safe alternative to the open approach and has some clear advantages.

CONCLUSIONS

Minimally invasive surgical techniques are increasingly being employed in general surgery; therefore, understanding the causes and incidence of complications associated with laparoscopic surgery is of prime importance for practicing surgeons. Surgeons must remember two important points when they are learning or undertaking a laparoscopic procedure. First, many complications that occur in open versions of an operation can also occur in the laparoscopic version. Time-honored general surgical principles of preventing and managing these complications must be followed no matter which technique is used for abdominal access. Second, other complications are unique to minimally invasive surgical approaches. These complications are best avoided by perfecting and using proper laparoscopic technique and by understanding the unique pitfalls of each laparoscopic operation. Focusing on both of these points can allow surgical procedures to be both minimally invasive and safe.

REFERENCES

1. Makinen MT, Yli-Hankala A. The effect of laparoscopic cholecystectomy on respiratory compliance as determined by continuous spirometry. J Clin Anesth 1996; 8(2):119–122.
2. Pelosi P, Foti G, Cereda M, Vicardi P, Gattinoni L. Effects of carbon dioxide insufflation for laparoscopic cholecystectomy on the respiratory system. Anaesthesia 1996; 51(8):744–749.
3. Rauh R, Hemmerling TM, Rist M, Jacobi KE. Influence of pneumoperitoneum and patient positioning on respiratory system compliance. J Clin Anesth 2001; 13(5):361–365.
4. Volpino P, Cangemi V, D'Andrea N, Cangemi B, Piat G. Hemodynamic and pulmonary changes during and after laparoscopic cholecystectomy. A comparison with traditional surgery. Surg Endosc 1998; 12(2): 119–123.
5. Galizia G, Prizio G, Lieto E, et al. Hemodynamic and pulmonary changes during open, carbon dioxide pneumoperitoneum and abdominal wall-lifting cholecystectomy. A prospective, randomized study. Surg Endosc 2001; 15(5):477–483.
6. Bannenberg JJ, Rademaker BM, Froeling FM, Meijer DW. Hemodynamics during laparoscopic extra- and intraperitoneal insufflation. An experimental study. Surg Endosc 1997; 11(9):911–914.
7. Horvath KD, Whelan RL, Lier B, et al. The effects of elevated intraabdominal pressure, hypercarbia, and positioning on the hemodynamic responses to laparoscopic colectomy in pigs. Surg Endosc 1998; 12(2): 107–114.
8. D'Ugo D, Persiani R, Pennestri F, et al. Transesophageal echocardiographic assessment of hemodynamic function during laparoscopic cholecystectomy in healthy patients. Surg Endosc 2000; 14(2):120–122.
9. Brampton WJ, Watson RJ. Arterial to end-tidal carbon dioxide tension difference during laparoscopy. Magnitude and effect of anaesthetic technique. Anaesthesia 1990; 45(3):210–214.
10. Ortega AE, Richman MF, Hernandez M, et al. Inferior vena caval blood flow and cardiac hemodynamics during carbon dioxide pneumoperitoneum. Surg Endosc 1996; 10(9):920–924.
11. Westerband A, Van De Water J, Amzallag M, et al. Cardiovascular changes during laparoscopic cholecystectomy. Surg Gynecol Obstet 1992; 175(6):535–538.
12. McLaughlin JG, Scheeres DE, Dean RJ, Bonnell BW. The adverse hemodynamic effects of laparoscopic cholecystectomy. Surg Endosc 1995; 9(2):121–124.
13. Dorsay DA, Greene FL, Baysinger CL. Hemodynamic changes during laparoscopic cholecystectomy monitored with transesophageal echocardiography. Surg Endosc 1995; 9(2):128–134.
14. Nguyen NT, Ho HS, Fleming NW, et al. Cardiac function during laparoscopic vs open gastric bypass. Surg Endosc 2002; 16(1):78–83.
15. Zuckerman RS, Heneghan S. The duration of hemodynamic depression during laparoscopic cholecystectomy. Surg Endosc 2002; 16(8):1233–1236.
16. Zuckerman R, Gold M, Jenkins P, Rauscher LA, Jones M, Heneghan S. The effects of pneumoperitoneum and patient position on hemodynamics during laparoscopic cholecystectomy. Surg Endosc 2001; 15(6):562–565.
17. O'Leary E, Hubbard K, Tormey W, Cunningham AJ. Laparoscopic cholecystectomy: haemodynamic and neuroendocrine responses after pneumoperitoneum and changes in position. Br J Anaesth 1996; 76(5): 640–644.
18. Altintas F, Tunali Y, Bozkurt P, et al. An experimental study on the relationship of intra-abdominal pressure and renal ischemia. Middle East J Anesthesiol 2001; 16(1):55–66.
19. Kubota K, Kajiura N, Teruya M, et al. Alterations in respiratory function and hemodynamics during laparoscopic cholecystectomy under pneumoperitoneum. Surg Endosc 1993; 7(6):500–504.
20. Myre K, Buanes T, Smith G, Stokland O. Simultaneous hemodynamic and echocardiographic changes during abdominal gas insufflation. Surg Laparosc Endosc 1997; 7(5):415–419.
21. Myles PS. Bradyarrhythmias and laparoscopy: a prospective study of heart rate changes with laparoscopy. Aust NZ J Obstet Gynaecol 1991; 31(2):171–173.
22. Reed DN Jr., Nourse P. Untoward cardiac changes during CO_2 insufflation in laparoscopic cholecystectomies in low-risk patients. J Laparoendosc Adv Surg Tech A 1998; 8(2):109–114.
23. Reed DN Jr., Duff JL. Persistent occurrence of bradycardia during laparoscopic cholecystectomies in low-risk patients. Dig Surg 2000; 17(5):513–517.
24. Hashizume M, Sugimachi K. Needle and trocar injury during laparoscopic surgery in Japan. Surg Endosc 1997; 11(12):1198–1201.
25. Champault G, Cazacu F, Taffinder N. Serious trocar accidents in laparoscopic surgery: a French survey of 103,852 operations. Surg Laparosc Endosc 1996; 6(5):367–370.
26. Chandler JG, Corson SL, Way LW. Three spectra of laparoscopic entry access injuries. J Am Coll Surg 2001; 192(4):478–491.
27. Schafer M, Lauper M, Krahenbuhl L. Trocar and Veress needle injuries during laparoscopy. Surg Endosc 2001; 15(3):275–279.
28. Bhoyrul S, Vierra MA, Nezhat CR, Krummel TM, Way LW. Trocar injuries in laparoscopic surgery. J Am Coll Surg 2001; 192(6):677–683.

29. Bishoff JT, Allaf ME, Kirkels W, Moore RG, Kavoussi LR, Schroder F. Laparoscopic bowel injury: incidence and clinical presentation. J Urol 1999; 161(3):887–890.

30. Mayol J, Garcia-Aguilar J, Ortiz-Oshiro E, De-Diego Carmona JA, Fernancez-Represa JA. Risks of the minimal access approach for laparoscopic surgery: multivariate analysis of morbidity related to umbilical trocar insertion. World J Surg 1997; 21(5):529–533.

31. Schafer M, Lauper M, Krahenbuhl L. A nation's experience of bleeding complications during laparoscopy. Am J Surg 2000; 180(1):73–77.

32. McGinnis DE, Strup SE, Gomella LG. Management of hemorrhage during laparoscopy. J Endourol 2000; 14(10):915–920.

33. Deziel DJ, Millikan KW, Economou SG, Doolas A, Ko STG, Airan MC. Complications of laparoscopic cholecystectomy: a national survey of 4,292 hospitals and an analysis of 77,604 cases. Am J Surg 1993; 165(1):9–14.

34. Bailey RW, Flowers JL, eds. Complications of Laparoscopic Surgery. St. Louis: Quality Medical Publishing, Inc., 1995:416.

35. Bonjer HJ, Hazebroek EJ, Kazemier G, Guffrida MC, Meijer WS, Lange JF. Open versus closed establishment of pneumoperitoneum in laparoscopic surgery. Br J Surg 1997; 84(5):599–602.

36. Yau P, Watson DI, Lafullarde T, Jamieson GG. Experimental study of effect of embolism of different laparoscopy insufflation gases. J Laparoendosc Adv Surg Tech A 2000; 10(4):211–216.

37. Cottin V, Delafosse B, Viale JP. Gas embolism during laparoscopy: a report of seven cases in patients with previous abdominal surgical history. Surg Endosc 1996; 10(2):166–169.

38. Zaraca F, Catarci M, Gossetti F, Mulieri G, Carboni M. Routine use of open laparoscopy: 1,006 consecutive cases. J Laparoendosc Adv Surg Tech A 1999; 9(1):75–80.

39. Melzer A, Riek S, Roth K, Buess G. Endoscopically controlled trocar and cannula insertion. Endosc Surg Allied Technol 1995; 3(1):63–68.

40. Leibl BJ, Schmedt CG, Schwarz J, Kraft K, Bittner R. Laparoscopic surgery complications associated with trocar tip design: review of literature and own results. J Laparoendosc Adv Surg Tech A 1999; 9(2):135–140.

41. Nezhat C, Nezhat F, Seidman DS, Nezhat C. Incisional hernias after operative laparoscopy. J Laparoendosc Adv Surg Tech A 1997; 7(2):111–115.

42. Hanna GB, Shimi SM, Cuschieri A. Randomised study of influence of two-dimensional versus three-dimensional imaging on performance of laparoscopic cholecystectomy. Lancet 1998; 351(9098):248–251.

43. Hofmeister J, Frank TG, Cuschieri A, Wade NJ. Perceptual aspects of two-dimensional and stereoscopic display techniques in endoscopic surgery: review and current problems. Semin Laparosc Surg 2001; 8(1):12–24.

44. Medina M. Image rotation and reversal—major obstacles in learning intracorporeal suturing and knot-tying. JSLS 1997; 1(4):331–336.

45. Chan AC, Chung SC, Yim AP, Lau JY, Ng EK, Li AMK. Comparison of two-dimensional vs three-dimensional camera systems in laparoscopic surgery. Surg Endosc 1997; 11(5):438–440.

46. Allal H, Captier G, Lopez M, Forgues D, Galifer RB. Evaluation of 142 consecutive laparoscopic fundoplications in children: effects of the learning curve and technical choice. J Pediatr Surg 2001; 36(6):921–926.

47. Soot SJ, Eshraghi N, Farahmand M, Sheppard BD, Deveney CW. Transition from open to laparoscopic fundoplication: the learning curve. Arch Surg 1999; 134(3):278–282.

48. Watson DI, Baigrie RJ, Jamieson GG. A learning curve for laparoscopic fundoplication. Definable, avoidable, or a waste of time? Ann Surg 1996; 224(2):198–203.

49. Edwards CC II, Bailey RW. Laparoscopic hernia repair: the learning curve. Surg Laparosc Endosc Percutan Tech 2000; 10(3):149–153.

50. Agachan F, Joo JS, Weiss EG, Wexner SD. Intraoperative laparoscopic complications. Are we getting better? Dis Colon Rectum 1996; 39(10 suppl):S14–S19.

51. Smith JF, Boysen D, Tschirhart J, Williams T, Vasilenko P. Comparison of laparoscopic cholecystectomy versus elective open cholecystectomy. J Laparoendosc Surg 1992; 2(6):311–317.

52. Moreaux J. Prospective study of open cholecystectomy for calculous biliary disease. Br J Surg 1994; 81(1):116–119.

53. MacFadyen BV Jr., Vecchio R, Ricardo AE, Mathis CR. Bile duct injury after laparoscopic cholecystectomy. The United States experience. Surg Endosc 1998; 12(4):315–321.

54. Krahenbuhl L, Sclabas G, Wente MN, Schafer M, Schlumpf R, Buchler MW. Incidence, risk factors, and prevention of biliary tract injuries during laparoscopic cholecystectomy in Switzerland. World J Surg 2001; 25(10):1325–1330.

55. Fried GM, Barkun JS, Sigman HH, et al. Factors determining conversion to laparotomy in patients undergoing laparoscopic cholecystectomy. Am J Surg 1994; 167(1):35–41.

56. Flowers JL, Zucker KA, Graham SM, Scovill WA, Imbembo AL, Bailey RW. Laparoscopic cholangiography. Results and indications. Ann Surg 1992; 215(3):209–216.

57. Clair DG, Brooks DC. Laparoscopic cholangiography. The case for a selective approach. Surg Clin North Am 1994; 74(4):961–966.

58. Clair DG, Carr-Locke DL, Becker JM, Brooks DC. Routine cholangiography is not warranted during laparoscopic cholecystectomy. Arch Surg 1993; 128(5): 551–555.

59. Woods MS, Traverso LW, Kozarek RA, et al. Biliary tract complications of laparoscopic cholecystectomy are detected more frequently with routine intraoperative cholangiography. Surg Endosc 1995; 9(10): 1076–1080.

60. Schafer M, Suter C, Klaiber C, Wehrli H, Frei E, Krahenbuhl L. Spilled gallstones after laparoscopic cholecystectomy. A relevant problem? A retrospective analysis of 10,174 laparoscopic cholecystectomies. Surg Endosc 1998; 12(4):305–309.

61. Gadacz TR. Update on laparoscopic cholecystectomy, including a clinical pathway. Surg Clin North Am 2000; 80(4):1127–1149.

62. Memon MA, Deeik RK, Maffi TR, Fitzgibbons RJ Jr. The outcome of unretrieved gallstones in the peritoneal cavity during laparoscopic cholecystectomy. A prospective analysis. Surg Endosc 1999; 13(9): 848–857.

63. Memon MA, Fitzgibbons RJ Jr. Assessing risks, costs, and benefits of laparoscopic hernia repair. Annu Rev Med 1998; 49:95–109.
64. Hunter JG, Smith CD, Branum GD, et al. Laparoscopic fundoplication failures: patterns of failure and response to fundoplication revision. Ann Surg 1999; 230(4):595–606.
65. Hinder RA, Filipi CJ, Wetscher G, Neary P, DeMeester TR, Perdikis G. Laparoscopic Nissen fundoplication is an effective treatment for gastroesophageal reflux disease. Ann Surg 1994; 220(4):472–483.
66. Shirazi SS, Schulze K, Soper RT. Long-term follow-up for treatment of complicated chronic reflux esophagitis. Arch Surg 1987; 122(5):548–552.
67. Viljakka MT, Luostarinen ME, Isolauri JO. Complications of open and laparoscopic antireflux surgery: 32-year audit at a teaching hospital. J Am Coll Surg 1997; 185(5):446–450.
68. Lafullarde T, Watson DI, Jamieson GG, Meyers JC, Game PA, Devitt PG. Laparoscopic Nissen fundoplication: five-year results and beyond. Arch Surg 2001; 136(2):180–184.
69. Watson DI, Jamieson GG, Devitt PG, et al. Changing strategies in the performance of laparoscopic Nissen fundoplication as a result of experience with 230 operations. Surg Endosc 1995; 9(9):961–966.
70. Zaninotto G, Molena D, Ancona E. A prospective multicenter study on laparoscopic treatment of gastroesophageal reflux disease in Italy: type of surgery, conversions, complications, and early results. Study Group for the Laparoscopic Treatment of Gastroesophageal Reflux Disease of the Italian Society of Endoscopic Surgery (SICE). Surg Endosc 2000; 14(3):282–288.
71. Collet D, Cadiere GB. Conversions and complications of laparoscopic treatment of gastroesophageal reflux disease. Formation for the Development of Laparoscopic Surgery for Gastroesophageal Reflux Disease Group. Am J Surg 1995; 169(6):622–626.
72. Felix EL, Michas CA, Gonzalez MH Jr. Laparoscopic hernioplasty. TAPP vs TEP. Surg Endosc 1995; 9(9):984–989.
73. Chung RS, Rowland DY. Meta-analyses of randomized controlled trials of laparoscopic vs conventional inguinal hernia repairs. Surg Endosc 1999; 13(7):689–694.
74. Tschudi JF, Wagner M, Klaiber C, et al. Randomized controlled trial of laparoscopic transabdominal preperitoneal hernioplasty vs Shouldice repair. Surg Endosc 2001; 15(11):1263–1266.
75. Khoury N. A randomized prospective controlled trial of laparoscopic extraperitoneal hernia repair and mesh-plug hernioplasty: a study of 315 cases. J Laparoendosc Adv Surg Tech A 1998; 8(6):367–372.
76. Felix E, Scott S, Crafton B, et al. Causes of recurrence after laparoscopic hernioplasty. A multicenter study. Surg Endosc 1998; 12(3):226–231.
77. Rosenberger RJ, Loeweneck H, Meyer G. The cutaneous nerves encountered during laparoscopic repair of inguinal hernia: new anatomical findings for the surgeon. Surg Endosc 2000; 14(8):731–735.
78. Moreno-Egea A, Aguayo JL, Canteras M. Intraoperative and postoperative complications of totally extraperitoneal laparoscopic inguinal hernioplasty.

Surg Laparosc Endosc Percutan Tech 2000; 10(1):30–33.
79. O'Malley KJ, Monkhouse WS, Qureshi MA, Bouchier-Hayes DJ. Anatomy of the peritoneal aspect of the deep inguinal ring: implications for laparoscopic inguinal herniorrhaphy. Clin Anat 1997; 10(5):313–317.
80. Bailey RW. Laparoscopic appendectomy. In: Cameron JL, ed. Current Surgical Therapy. St. Louis: Mosby Year Book, 1995:1039–1052.
81. Huang MT, Wei PL, Wu CC, Lai IR, Chen RJ, Lee WJ. Needlescopic, laparoscopic, and open appendectomy: a comparative study. Surg Laparosc Endosc Percutan Tech 2001; 11(5):306–312.
82. Hellberg A, Rudberg C, Kullman E, et al. Prospective randomized multicentre study of laparoscopic versus open appendicectomy. Br J Surg 1999; 86(1):48–53.
83. Lavonius MI, Liesjarvi S, Ovaska J, Pajulo O, Ristkari S, Alanen M. Laparoscopic versus open appendectomy in children: a prospective randomised study. Eur J Pediatr Surg 2001; 11(4):235–238.
84. Long KH, Bannon MP, Zietlow SP, et al. A prospective randomized comparison of laparoscopic appendectomy with open appendectomy: Clinical and economic analyses. Surgery 2001; 129(4):390–400.
85. Ozmen MM, Zulfikaroglu B, Tanik A, Kale IT. Laparoscopic versus open appendectomy: prospective randomized trial. Surg Laparosc Endosc Percutan Tech 1999; 9(3):187–189.
86. Carbajo MA, del Olmo JC, Blanco JI, et al. Laparoscopic treatment of ventral abdominal wall hernias: preliminary results in 100 patients. JSLS 2000; 4(2):141–145.
87. Carbajo MA, Martin del Olmo JC, Blanco JI, et al. Laparoscopic treatment vs open surgery in the solution of major incisional and abdominal wall hernias with mesh. Surg Endosc 1999; 13(3):250–252.
88. Heniford BT, Park A, Ramshaw BJ, Voeller G. Laparoscopic ventral and incisional hernia repair in 407 patients. J Am Coll Surg 2000; 190(6):645–650.
89. Toy FK, Bailey RW, Carey S, et al. Prospective, multicenter study of laparoscopic ventral hernioplasty. Preliminary results. Surg Endosc 1998; 12(7):955–959.
90. Robbins SB, Pofahl WE, Gonzalez RP. Laparoscopic ventral hernia repair reduces wound complications. Am Surg 2001; 67(9):896–900.
91. LeBlanc KA, Booth WV, Whitaker JM, Bellanger DE. Laparoscopic incisional and ventral herniorrhaphy: our initial 100 patients. Hernia 2001; 5(1):41–45.
92. Larson GM. Ventral hernia repair by the laparoscopic approach. Surg Clin North Am 2000; 80(4):1329–1340.
93. Westling A, Gustavsson S. Laparoscopic vs open Roux-en-Y gastric bypass: a prospective, randomized trial. Obes Surg 2001; 11(3):284–292.
94. Nguyen NT, Goldman C, Rosenquist CJ, et al. Laparoscopic versus open gastric bypass: a randomized study of outcomes, quality of life, and costs. Ann Surg 2001; 234(3):279–291.
95. Matthews BD, Sing RF, DeLegge MH, Ponsky JL, Heniford BT. Initial results with a stapled gastrojejunostomy for the laparoscopic isolated roux-en-Y gastric bypass. Am J Surg 2000; 179(6):476–481.
96. Nguyen NT, Lee SL, Anderson JT, Palmer LS, Canet F, Wolfe BM. Evaluation of intra-abdominal pressure

after laparoscopic and open gastric bypass. Obes Surg 2001; 11(1):40–45.

97. Park A, Marcaccio M, Sternbach M, Witzke D, Fitzgerald P. Laparoscopic vs open splenectomy. Arch Surg 1999; 134(11):1263–1269.

98. Park AE, Birgisson G, Mastrangelo MJ, Marcaccio MJ, Witzke DB. Laparoscopic splenectomy: outcomes and lessons learned from over 200 cases. Surgery 2000; 128(4):660–667.

99. Donini A, Baccarani U, Terrosu G, et al. Laparoscopic vs open splenectomy in the management of hematologic diseases. Surg Endosc 1999; 13(12):1220–1225.

100. Katkhouda N, Hurwitz MB, Rivera RT, et al. Laparoscopic splenectomy: outcome and efficacy in 103 consecutive patients. Ann Surg 1998; 228(4):568–578.

101. Lo CY, Chan WF. From open to laparoscopic adrenalectomy: a review of 16-year experience. Chin Med J (Engl) 1999; 112(12):1080–1084.

102. Guazzoni G, Cestari A, Montorsi F, et al. Current role of laparoscopic adrenalectomy. Eur Urol 2001; 40(1):8–16.

103. Bonjer HJ, Sorm V, Berends FJ, et al. Endoscopic retroperitoneal adrenalectomy: lessons learned from 111 consecutive cases. Ann Surg 2000; 232(6):796–803.

104. Chee C, Ravinthiran T, Cheng C. Laparoscopic adrenalectomy: experience with transabdominal and retroperitoneal approaches. Urology 1998; 51(1):29–32.

105. Waller JR, Veitch PS, Nicholson ML. Laparoscopic live donor nephrectomy: a comparison with the open operation. Transplant Proc 2001; 33(7–8): 3787–3788.

106. Ruiz-Deya G, Cheng S, Palmer E, Thomas R, Slakey D. Open donor, laparoscopic donor and hand assisted laparoscopic donor nephrectomy: a comparison of outcomes. J Urol 2001; 166(4):1270–1274.

107. Hoznek A, Olsson LE, Salomon L, et al. Retroperitoneal laparoscopic living-donor nephrectomy. Preliminary results. Eur Urol 2001; 40(6):614–618.

108. Hensman C, Lionel G, Hewett P, Rao MM. Laparoscopic live donor nephrectomy: the preliminary experience. Aust NZ J Surg 1999; 69(5):365–368.

15

Complications of Liver Transplantation

Gennaro Selvaggi, Andreas G. Tzakis, and David M. Levi
*Department of Surgery, University of Miami, Miami,
Florida, U.S.A.*

Liver transplantation is the most effective form of treatment for end-stage liver disease. With improvements in surgical techniques and more sophisticated immunosuppressive regimens, the patient and graft survival rates after liver transplantation have steadily improved. Many factors are involved in the early outcome of liver transplantation, including preoperative assessment and the clinical status of the recipient, donor-related factors that affect graft quality, and aspects of the surgical technique.

As is true of any complex surgical procedure, liver transplantation may be associated with intraoperative and postoperative complications. Liver transplantation involves resection of a major organ and requires vascular, biliary, and often gastrointestinal anastomoses. Multiple organ systems are often compromised at the time of transplantation, and complications such as hepatorenal syndrome, pulmonary hypertension, and coagulopathic diathesis may occur. Recovery after such complications can pose serious problems. In addition, the immunological barriers to graft tolerance still mandate the use of immunosuppressive regimens. If these regimens are insufficient, organ rejection may occur; if they are excessive, recipients are exposed to an increased risk of infection.

The development of complications has a great impact on morbidity and mortality rates and directly affects resource utilization and costs (1). Clavien et al. (2) classified the negative outcomes associated with solid-organ transplantation on the basis of the severity of their impact on patients' health. Angus et al. (3) applied the Acute Physiology and Chronic Health Evaluation-2 scoring system to cohorts of liver transplant recipients and demonstrated that such a model, with some modifications, can be used to predict outcome, both in the hospital and one year after transplantation.

In this chapter, we have classified the complications related to liver transplantation as early or late because time after surgery is often crucial to an interpretation of the patient's signs and symptoms when a complication occurs. During the early postoperative period, which can be grossly defined as the first three months after transplantation, most complications are technical in nature and are related to the recipient's preoperative organ dysfunction or to early

rejection or infection phenomena. After the first three months, complications usually develop over longer periods of time and are primarily related to those alterations in the recipient's immunological status that are necessary for maintaining graft function and preventing or minimizing the likelihood of infection episodes, rejection, or the development of recurrent or malignant disease.

As is true for all postoperative management, the best outcomes after liver transplantation can be achieved by minimizing the risk of complications. This goal can be achieved by constant vigilance and the implementation of aggressive diagnostic and therapeutic measures if complications occur despite all efforts to prevent them.

EARLY COMPLICATIONS
Extrahepatic Complications
Respiratory Complications

Pulmonary complications are common during the early postoperative course and range from atelectasis and pleural effusion to infiltrates as a marker of infection. If the right phrenic nerve is injured during the transplantation procedure, right hemidiaphragmatic paralysis may result (4). Recipients of liver transplants rarely experience pulmonary embolism during the immediate postoperative course. Pulmonary edema often results from renal dysfunction and is usually managed by restricting fluids and administering diuretics; if renal impairment is severe, hemodialysis may be necessary. Bacterial pneumonia occurs almost exclusively during the first 30 days after transplantation, although *Pseudomonas* pneumonia can occur at any time.

If adult respiratory distress syndrome (ARDS) occurs after liver transplantation, it is usually triggered by sepsis. It occurs among 5% to 17% of patients and is associated with intra-abdominal infections, acute cellular rejection (ACR), pancreatitis, and hepatic artery thrombosis (HAT) with resulting hepatic necrosis (5,6). ARDS must be diagnosed by the use of bronchoalveolar lavage and quantitative cultures to exclude infectious agents. Administering the anti-CD3 monoclonal antibody OKT3 (muromonab-CD3) can induce a "cytokine storm" and can induce ARDS during the treatment of rejection episodes.

Pulmonary hypertension occurs among 2% to 4% of patients with end-stage liver disease and is a significant risk factor for morbidity and mortality after transplantation (7,8). Reperfusion of the liver during transplantation can cause acute right heart failure among patients with relative right-sided decompensation. Patients often require right-heart catheterization before transplantation, and documented severe pulmonary hypertension (mean pulmonary pressure higher than 45 mmHg) is a contraindication for transplantation. Medical therapy is based on the use of vasodilators but is generally ineffective. Agents that have been used with some success are inhalation therapy with nitrous oxide and the intravenous administration of prostacycline (9,10).

Hepatopulmonary syndrome is a rare form of pulmonary insufficiency that usually manifests itself as hypoxemia. This syndrome, which occurs among 1% to 2% of patients with cirrhosis, is characterized by arterial hypoxemia, pulmonary vasodilatation, and the absence of intrinsic cardiopulmonary disease. It is thought to be caused by a ventilation–perfusion mismatch resulting from the opening of multiple arteriovenous shunts in the lung (11). The syndrome usually resolves after hepatic transplantation, but it often requires prolonged therapy with supplemental oxygen.

Renal Complications

Renal insufficiency, whether mild, as caused by renal hypoperfusion, or severe, as associated with hepatorenal syndrome, occurs very commonly after hepatic transplantation. Hepatorenal syndrome is characterized by decreased urinary output, low urinary sodium concentrations, and high blood urea nitrogen concentrations during end-stage liver disease; the syndrome is caused by decreased perfusion to the renal cortex (12). After transplantation, hepatorenal syndrome resolves immediately, but as many as 90% of liver transplant recipients experience an increase in the serum concentration of creatinine. This increase is usually a temporary phenomenon related to intraoperative renal hypoperfusion, allograft dysfunction, and the toxic effects of immunosuppressive regimens (i.e., cyclosporine or tacrolimus). It is important to point out that blood urea nitrogen and creatinine concentrations may appear falsely normal among patients with hepatic failure because of muscle wasting and depletion of total body protein content. Among these patients, oliguria is the best indicator of renal function impairment. Hypovolemic prerenal failure quickly responds to the administration of fluids and colloids. Immunosuppressive medications cause tubular vasoconstriction; their nephrotoxic effects can be reversed by monitoring their plasma concentrations and appropriately lowering their dosages (13). As many as 10% of liver transplant recipients will require hemodialysis, although this procedure is often needed only temporarily until the patient's renal function recovers. For critically ill patients, continuous venous–venous hemodialysis may be preferable to regular hemodialysis.

Hematologic Complications

Coagulopathy is the most common hematologic disorder that occurs after liver transplantation. This condition is caused by deficiencies in vitamin K–dependent coagulation factors, fibrinogen, and prothrombin proteins C and S, all of which are synthesized by the liver. Indeed, one of the most important factors indicating the function of the newly implanted graft is the rapidity with which coagulopathy resolves. Such resolution is indicated by a constant decrease in prothrombin time and partial thromboplastin time, and an increase in the production of fibrinogen. At times, fibrinogen production may be normal, although the recovery of the coagulation indicators is delayed. This condition is often due to a relative lack of vitamin K in the recipient and the graft; it can be corrected by a short course of vitamin K administration. In addition, thrombocytopenia is very common before transplantation primarily because of hypersplenism. After liver transplantation, the platelet counts usually fall to a nadir at approximately postoperative day 4 or 5, but subsequently recover to pretransplantation levels within a week (14). Platelet counts below $100 \times 10^3/\mu L$ have been associated with intracerebral bleeding, such as subdural or epidural hematoma, and must be corrected by the infusion of platelets.

Endocrine and Metabolic Complications

During the immediate postoperative course, hyperglycemia or worsening of diabetes is commonly caused by the high doses of steroids given during the induction phase of immunosuppressive therapy.

Neurologic Complications

Immediately after transplantation, alteration in the mental status of the patient can be due to the resolution of preoperative encephalopathy (which can be monitored by the decline in the ammonia level), but it can also be a consequence of immunosuppressive therapy or of intensive care unit (ICU) sleep deprivation with disorientation and psychosis (15). These metabolic causes of mental status alteration resolve as hepatic function improves, the intensity of the immunosuppressive regimen is reduced, and the patient is transferred out of the ICU. Seizures can occur during the early postoperative period and are usually associated with electrolyte abnormalities (hypomagnesemia, hypokalemia, etc.) or the toxic effects of the immunosuppressive medications administered (e.g., tacrolimus or cyclosporine toxicity) (15). It is important to point out that many of the antiepileptic medications interfere with the metabolism of tacrolimus, rapamycin, and cyclosporine by inducing the formation of cytochrome p54 and lowering the plasma concentrations of such immunosuppressive agents. Phenytoin, valproic acid, phenobarbital, and carbamazepine can negatively affect these plasma concentrations; gabapentin (Neurontin®, Pfizer, New York, New York, U.S.), on the other hand, is metabolized by the kidney and can be safely administered.

Cerebral edema is a common feature of fulminant hepatic failure. It can persist and complicate the postoperative course after liver transplantation. In addition, cerebral edema can be caused by massive fluid shifts after transplantation, especially when hyponatremia is present. In the most severe cases, computed tomography (CT) scans and measurements of intracranial pressure (ICP) can help with the diagnosis and medical management of severe brain edema. The goal is to maintain ICP below 20 mmHg and cerebral perfusion pressure above 50 mmHg. As the graft recovers and its function improves, cerebral edema usually subsides. Another complication associated with altered electrolyte balance is central pontine myelinolysis, which complicates the course of patients with severe sodium disturbances, especially after sudden correction of hypernatremia. The severity of the syndrome ranges from cerebral death to prolonged mild neurologic dysfunction.

Gastrointestinal Complications

When biliary reconstruction is performed with a Roux-en-Y hepaticojejunostomy, patients are at risk of intestinal leaks from the stumps of the transected bowel or from the biliary anastomosis itself. In addition, bowel perforation can complicate the postoperative course, especially if serosal tears have been caused during the hepatectomy. The main complication of intestinal leaks is sepsis. Exploratory laparotomy for repair is mandatory and must be associated with the administration of broad-spectrum antibiotics and antifungal therapy.

Intra-abdominal bleeding complicates the course of 7% to 15% of liver transplant recipients, and approximately half of these patients will require exploratory surgery (16). Intra-abdominal bleeding can arise from the vascular anastomoses, from the suture lines of the intestinal anastomosis for the Roux-en-Y procedure, from the mesentery, or from the exposed surfaces of the retroperitoneum in the subdiaphragmatic space. In addition, recurrent variceal bleeding, gastritis, and ulcerative disease of the stomach and duodenum can cause gastrointestinal bleeding, especially with the added risk factors of coagulopathy, thrombocytopenia, and the administration of high doses of steroids.

Ascites

Ascites is an almost universal feature of end-stage liver disease. It can continue to affect patients after hepatic transplantation primarily because of low plasma albumin concentrations, the exposed raw peritoneal areas of surgical dissection, resolving portal hypertension, or the presence of partial portal system thrombosis. Management usually involves placing drains postoperatively, administering albumin, and correcting malnutrition.

Infections

After liver transplantation, patients are at a high risk of infection because of the immunosuppressive regimens required for avoiding rejection. The mortality rate associated with infections can be as high as 10% (17). The most common infections are bacterial; fungal and viral infections occur less frequently. Depending on the amount of time that has elapsed since transplantation, a pattern of types of infections and causative agents can be observed (18).

During the first month after transplantation, most infections are caused by bacteria. The most common are infections at the sites of intravenous catheters, pneumonia, intra-abdominal (biliary or gastrointestinal) infections, urinary infections, and wound infections. Bacteremia usually occurs among patients with comorbid conditions, such as advanced age, diabetes, or poor nutritional state. Catheter-related sepsis is usually caused by *Staphylococcus* or *Streptococcus* strains. Pulmonary infections are often related to prolonged intubation and are most often caused by gram-negative species.

Infection of the biliary system is usually related to biliary complications or to HAT or hepatic artery stenosis (HAS); these infections are usually associated with mixed, multiple gram-positive, gram-negative, and fungal pathogens. The emergence of vancomycin-resistant *Enterococcus faecium* (VRE) species has resulted from the widespread use of vancomycin to treat severe gram-positive infections. Unfortunately, VRE can colonize as many as 55% of liver transplant recipients postoperatively and is responsible for clinically significant episodes of infection among approximately 10% of patients (19). VRE is usually acquired in the hospital environment via the gastrointestinal route and is normally detectable by rectal swabs with selective cultures. Infection with VRE is more common among patients with biliary complications or after multiple exploratory laparotomy procedures. VRE infections are treated with quinopristine–dalfopristine (Synercid®, Rhone-Poulenc Rorer, Collegeville, Pennsylvania, U.S.) or, more recently, with linezolid (Zyvox®, Pharmacia & Upjohn Company, Kalamazoo, Michigan, U.S.).

The highest incidence of fungal infections occurs during the first two months after transplantation. The spectrum of clinical disease ranges from oral candidiasis to fulminant and often lethal fungemia. The most common form of fungal infection is oral and esophageal candidiasis, which is characterized by oral thrush, dysphagia, and odynophagia. Colonization of the urinary tract by *Candida* species or *Torulopsis glabrata* is also common; the symptoms of such infections are urinary frequency, dysuria, and hematuria. Diffuse fungal infection spreads from a port of entry such as mucosal or skin surfaces, indwelling catheters, or the urinary tract. It usually occurs among highly immunocompromised patients, is associated with a high mortality rate, and can be diagnosed by the presence of disseminated fungal invasion in the retina (chorioretinitis), in blood cultures, or in tissue samples. The number of sites from which a culture positive for fungus is obtained correlates positively with the percentage of increase in the likelihood of disseminated infection (20). Prophylaxis with antifungal agents, such as the administration of oral mycostatin that can be swished and swallowed, is effective in preventing oral candidiasis. Disseminated fungal infections, on the other hand, cannot be prevented by the systematic prophylactic administration of antifungal agents. In addition, fluconazole, the most commonly used agent for fungal prophylaxis, interferes with the metabolism of tacrolimus and cyclosporine by increasing their plasma concentrations. Treatment of fungal infections must be aggressive and prolonged. Amphotericin B and, more recently, liposome-based preparations of Amphotericin B (e.g., Abelcet®, Enzon Pharmaceuticals, Piscataway, New Jersey, U.S.A. and Ambisome®, Astellas Pharma US, Deerfield, Illinois, U.S.A.) are the mainstays of treatment. Amphotericin is effective in treating *Candida* species and *T. glabrata*; *Aspergillus* species resistant to amphotericin may be responsive to prolonged therapy with itraconazole. It is important to point out that part of the treatment strategy for fungal infections is reducing the dosage of immunosuppressive agents.

The infections that occur more than one month after transplantation are usually viral; the highest incidence of such infections occurs during the second or third month after surgery. The viruses that most commonly cause disease during this period are cytomegalovirus (CMV) and Epstein–Barr virus (EBV). For many years, infection with CMV was the most common viral infection that occurred after liver transplantation; today, the incidence of CMV infection has been reduced by the systematic administration of prophylactic therapy with hyperimmune globulin (Cytogam®, Massachusetts, Biologic Laboratories, Massachusetts, U.S.) and antiviral agents (ganciclovir or its equivalent) (21,22). CMV is an endemic DNA virus that belongs to the family of the Herpesviridae. As many as 70% of adults exhibit positive results on immunoglobulin G serologic testing for this virus. The immunosuppression regimens required for organ recipients can favor the reactivation of an existing virus or can allow primary infection, especially during periods of intense suppression, as is the case during treatment with OKT3. The serological status of the donor and of the recipient is important in the development of clinically evident viral disease: patients are at highest risk if they are seronegative but receive a seropositive organ.

The spectrum of disease varies. The first symptoms of CMV syndrome are flu-like symptoms,

malaise, low-grade fever, and arthralgia; the diagnosis is made by polymerase chain reaction (PCR) detection of CMV in blood or by positive results from blood cultures. CMV hepatitis may simulate the symptoms of rejection, such as an increase in the activity of liver enzymes. This condition can be confirmed by biopsy. Treatment consists of reducing the dosages of immunosuppressive agents and initiating antiviral therapy. The symptoms of extrahepatic CMV infection are nausea, vomiting, diarrhea caused by visceral involvement of the gastrointestinal tract, pneumonitis, bone marrow invasion, and chorioretinitis. Prophylaxis varies according to the serologic status of the donor and the recipient: when a seronegative patient is receiving a seronegative organ, attention must be given to transfusing only CMV-negative blood and blood products; no other therapy is needed. When the serologic status of the donor differs from that of the recipient, prophylaxis with ganciclovir is continued for as long as three months postoperatively, in conjunction with the administration of Cytogam.

During the early postoperative period, Epstein–Barr viral infection may manifest itself as mononucleosis syndrome, with flu-like symptoms, or as EBV hepatitis, which causes nonspecific elevations in liver enzyme activity (23). EBV-related illness can be reactivated in a seropositive patient, or it may occur as a new infection related to the transplantation of a seropositive hepatic graft into a seronegative recipient. The risk of clinically significant disease is related to the degree of immunosuppression and to the combination of seropositive donor and seronegative recipient. Diagnosis involves using PCR to detect EBV in the blood. Therapy requires reducing the dosage of immunosuppressive agents and administering antiviral agents such as acyclovir and ganciclovir. The most important complication associated with EBV infection, however, is post-transplant lymphoproliferative disease (PTLD), which develops in the long term and will be discussed further (see "Extrahepatic Complications").

Graft-Related Complications
Primary Nonfunction

Primary nonfunction of the hepatic graft is defined as early (occurring less than 90 days postoperatively) graft failure unrelated to surgical technical factors or rejection (24). It is the most common cause of graft loss in the early postoperative period and has an overall incidence of 7% to 8.5%. This complication is characterized by a lack of bile production, marked coagulopathy, encephalopathy, ascites, marked elevations in liver enzyme activity, and progressive renal and multiorgan system failure. The main cause of primary nonfunction is ischemia-reperfusion injury with massive necrosis of hepatocytes. It is associated with donor-related factors, such as age, degree of steatosis in the graft (macrosteatosis greater than 30%), and severe electrolyte imbalances (hypernatremia), and with technical factors such as a prolonged period of cold ischemia (more than 18 hours). The diagnosis is confirmed by using Doppler ultrasonography to exclude technical complications, such as HAT, or by liver biopsy; both of these tests will demonstrate massive hepatic necrosis. The only successful treatment for primary nonfunction is early retransplantation.

Vascular Complications

Arterial

HAT and HAS are the most common technical complications related to the arterial reconstruction that is involved in liver transplantation. The most common early occurrence is thrombosis.

HAT is the second most common cause of early graft failure after primary nonfunction (25); in fact, HAT in itself is sufficient to justify listing the patient as Status I for retransplantation. This complication occurs after 2% to 10% of all liver transplant procedures and constitutes 60% of all vascular complications related to hepatic transplantation (26,27). The hepatic artery serves as the main blood supply to the biliary tree, and any insult to this artery may lead to biliary complications and sepsis. Risk factors for the development of arterial thrombosis include pediatric age, poor perfusion (as in cases of prolonged hypotension or dehydration), arterial intimal dissection from clamp injury, anastomotic stenosis, arterial reconstruction or kinking (especially when replaced hepatic vessels are present), and, more rarely, recipient factors such as ABO incompatibility, polycythemia, hypercoagulable state, or thrombocytosis.

Early thrombosis within the first week after transplantation can cause an increase in hepatic enzyme activity and progressive hepatic failure. More often, however, the clinical presentation is delayed and first appears two weeks to two months after transplantation. Delayed thrombosis may lead to biliary complications such as delayed bile leak or relapsing biliary sepsis (28). In such cases, intrahepatic necrosis and infected bilomas cause recurrent fevers with bacteremia. In rare instances, HAT may cause no symptoms and may be discovered only incidentally at a later time. In such cases, the arterial revascularization of the hepatic graft has been replaced by collateral vessels. Early HAT is initially diagnosed by Doppler ultrasonography; the diagnosis is confirmed by angiography, CT angiography, or magnetic resonance angiography, which will show thrombosis of the artery.

Early diagnosis of HAT and emergent surgical exploration with arterial thrombectomy and alternative revascularization of the graft can successfully avoid the loss of the organ. At our institution, we have implemented an aggressive policy of graft surveillance for patients at high risk of HAT (pediatric patients and those who have undergone a technically difficult reconstruction). This policy mandates daily Doppler ultrasonography for the first postoperative week and immediate examinations in the following

days if patients experience any alteration in liver enzyme activity or episodes of fever. By using this protocol, we have been able to diagnose early HAT and improve the organ salvage rate (29).

Delayed HAT is usually diagnosed too late for immediate thrombectomy because, in such cases, the patient has already been discharged from the hospital, but returns with a chief complaint of recurrent episodes of fever. In such cases, the hepatic graft has already developed necrosis and bilomas. Therapy involves broad-spectrum antibiotics, fluid resuscitation, drainage of any fluid collection by percutaneous drainage or endoscopic retrograde cholangiopancreatography (ERCP), and the placement of external–internal biliary drains in cases of bile leaks. Rarely, angiographic intervention with thrombolysis of the affected artery has been successful in reopening the thrombosed vessel. The mortality rate associated with HAT is as high as 20%. Emergent intervention with thrombectomy and revascularization can salvage as many as 82% of grafts, but only when HAT is detected early and patients are relatively asymptomatic. Most patients will require urgent retransplantation (30).

HAS is less common than HAT (occurring in fewer than 5% of cases), usually presents later in the post-transplantation course, and is usually related to technical issues at the site of anastomosis. HAS can be diagnosed by Doppler ultrasound, which will show increased blood flow systolic velocities at the site of stenosis, with decreases in resistive indices (less than 0.5) distal to the stenotic segment (31). Angiography confirms the site and severity of stenosis. If discovered early postoperatively, HAS can be corrected by surgical revision of the anastomosis. Delayed HAS can be managed by interventional radiology with balloon angioplasty or stent placement, even though complications such as rupture, intimal dissection, and pseudoaneurysm are possible (32).

Portal Vein

Thrombosis of the portal vein after hepatic transplantation is rare, occuring in only 1% to 3% of all cases (33). This complication manifests itself within one month after transplantation, with symptoms of hepatic failure, elevation of liver enzyme activity, complications of portal hypertension such as variceal bleeding, or persistent refractory ascites. Portal vein thrombosis is usually caused by technical problems, such as previous episodes of portal vein thrombosis or kinking of the anastomosis. Thrombosis can also be caused by poor inflow to the portal vein; it is usually related to the previously existing shunting circuits, such as the coronary vein or a splenorenal bypass, which cause a steal phenomenon. Other risk factors are hypercoagulable state and Budd–Chiari syndrome. Portal vein thrombosis is diagnosed by Doppler ultrasonography, which will show thrombosis of the vein. Therapy consists of emergent reexploration and thrombectomy with possible revision of the anastomosis when the complication is discovered early, or angioplasty when it is discovered late.

Hepatic Veins, Inferior Vena Cava

Obstruction at the outflow of the hepatic graft can occur either at the level of the hepatic veins or at the level of the inferior vena caval (IVC) anastomosis. This complication is rare, occurring in approximately 1% of all cases. During liver transplantation, the venous outflow from the liver can be generally managed in two ways. The first technique, termed *conventional*, involves resecting the liver with the retrohepatic vena cava and implanting the graft with two anastomoses: an infrahepatic IVC and a suprahepatic IVC. The second technique, termed *piggyback*, involves maintaining the retrohepatic vena cava, resecting the liver, and implanting the graft at the level of the hepatic veins, with performance of only one anastomosis. When the conventional technique is used, obstruction can occur at the infrahepatic or the suprahepatic anastomosis. Stenosis at the infrahepatic level does not cause hepatic failure, but does decrease venous drainage from the lower part of the body, mainly the bilateral lower extremities; this condition results in edema of the lower half of the body. Rarely, renal vein thrombosis can complicate infrahepatic stenosis. If stenosis occurs at the suprahepatic caval anastomosis, drainage of the splanchnic district is also impaired for the lower part of the body. In addition to edema of the bilateral lower extremities, patients will experience hepatic dysfunction with a clinical picture similar to that of Budd–Chiari syndrome. When the piggyback technique is used, stenosis at the anastomosis of the hepatic veins will not compromise blood return from the lower half of the body, but will manifest itself as Budd–Chiari syndrome (34). Early in the postoperative course, patients will develop hepatic failure, coagulopathy, jaundice, ascites, portal hypertension, and recurrent variceal bleeding. In the latter stages, the most common symptoms are ascites and hepatomegaly. Risk factors include technical difficulty in constructing the anastomosis, preexisting Budd–Chiari syndrome or hepatocellular carcinoma (HCC), and hypercoagulable state. The diagnosis is indicated by Doppler ultrasonography and confirmed by angiography. Surgical revision of the anastomosis can correct technical problems in the early postoperative period, and chronic outflow obstruction can be managed with diuretics, endovascular or portosystemic shunts, or angioplasty (35).

Biliary Complications

Biliary reconstruction has been defined the Achilles' heel of liver transplantation (36). Because biliary complications are usually diagnosed late and tend to lead to cholangitis infections, the mortality rate associated with these complications is high. Biliary complications are common, occurring among 10% to 20%

of all transplant recipients. These complications usually occur during the early postoperative period (80% occur within the first six months) and can be broadly classified as biliary leaks and biliary strictures (37,38). Biliary leaks usually occur early, whereas strictures tend to occur more than three months after transplantation.

Biliary leaks usually occur at the site of anastomosis. They are caused by technical disruption of the anastomosis or by ischemic necrosis, as in the case of HAT. If a T-tube was placed and then removed, a biliary leak can occur if a fibrous tract did not develop around the T-tube before removal. Rarely, an aberrant duct that went unrecognized during the procedure may cause a postoperative leak. Recognizing the importance of good arterial supply at the cut end of the anastomosed bile duct is essential if ischemia at the anastomotic site is to be avoided. Patients experience pain in the right upper quadrant, fever, and bilious drainage from the peritoneal cavity. The diagnosis is made by the results of laboratory tests, which will indicate hyperbilirubinemia without an increase in liver enzyme activity; by ultrasonography, which will show extrahepatic fluid collections; by biliary scintigraphy with a radiotracer, which will demonstrate the leak; and by percutaneous cholangiography or ERCP, which will show the leak. Doppler ultrasonography should always be used to rule out HAT. Treatment of biliary leaks varies according to their cause. Leaks caused by early removal of a T-tube are managed by nasobiliary drainage or endoscopic stenting. Leaks caused by technical failure or ischemic disruption of the anastomosis will require surgical management. Often, a duct-to-duct anastomosis must be converted to a Roux-en-Y hepaticojejunostomy. Intrahepatic or extrahepatic bilomas can be drained by radiological procedures.

Biliary strictures are usually due to technical problems with the anastomosis or due to chronic ischemic damage to the bile duct. The most important risk factor for stricture is ischemia of the arterial supply to the biliary system, whether due to arterial thrombosis, stenosis, or prolonged periods of hypotension (39). Strictures usually occur more than one month after transplantation. They may cause symptoms of jaundice, cholangitis, and recurrent fevers, or they may cause simple elevations in the bilirubin concentration or in the activity of liver enzymes, particularly alkaline phosphatase and gamma-glutamyl transpeptidase. Strictures caused by ischemic damage to the biliary tree are diffuse and multiple, and the biliary ducts are often filled with biliary sludge. Rarely, recurrent sclerosing cholangitis can cause a similar pattern of biliary strictures; however, recurrent disease in this case appears more than three months after transplantation. The diagnosis is best made by percutaneous transhepatic cholangiography or ERCP, which will show the strictures. In such cases, any manipulation of the biliary tree must be accompanied by the administration of broad-spectrum antibiotics, so that cholangitis and sepsis can be avoided. Balloon dilatation, stenting, and tube drainage are the mainstays of initial therapy. If the stricture is limited to the anastomotic area or the duct and the original anastomosis of the biliary tract was duct-to-duct, surgical revision with conversion to biliary enterostomy can resolve the stricture. Chronic strictures that do not respond to repeated dilatation or stenting will eventually lead to hepatic failure and the need for retransplantation.

Rejection

Hyperacute rejection due to preformed circulating antibodies against epitopes of the donor graft is not encountered in clinical liver transplantation, but it is a potential complication of xenogeneic transplantation (40). It may occasionally occur if liver transplantation is performed across ABO incompatibility barriers, but even so, multiple cases have been described in which transplantation of an ABO-incompatible graft was successful. The most common form of rejection in the immediate postoperative course is ACR.

The mechanism of rejection is based on the allorecognition of specific antigens on the surface of endothelial and parenchymal cells by the circulating T-lymphocyte pool. Engagement and recognition can follow one of two pathways: direct or indirect presentation (41). Direct presentation of the antigen is related to donor-derived antigen-presenting cells (APCs) in the graft; these cells carry their own antigenic epitopes within the human leukocyte antigen (HLA) class II molecules on the cell surface. The recipient's T-lymphocytes recognize these epitopes and activate the cascade of allogeneic response. Indirect presentation is related to recipient-derived APCs, which process antigens from the donor and expose them in the class II molecule groove for recognition by the recipient's own T-lymphocytes. The final effect is selective activation of the lymphocyte population that is responsive to such antigens; this effect is mediated mainly by interleukin-2 and rapid proliferation of clones of T-cells that infiltrate and destroy the graft.

ACR may occur at any time after transplantation of a hepatic graft, but it is most common within the first six weeks after transplantation. As many as 50% of recipients will experience at least one episode of increased liver enzyme activity and pathological evidence of cellular infiltrates (42). Mild episodes of ACR are asymptomatic and are detected only by the elevation in liver enzyme activity; more aggressive episodes lead to hyperbilirubinemia and clinically evident jaundice. Risk factors for ACR are a low level of immunosuppression, younger age of the recipient, and severe HLA-DR mismatch. Conversely, rejection is less common among debilitated patients (such as those who are elderly or malnourished) who have comorbid conditions such as renal failure or episodes of sepsis.

The diagnosis of ACR is confirmed by liver biopsy. Microscopic examination of the biopsy specimen shows mixed periportal infiltrate with a predominantly lymphocytic and eosinophilic population. Important distinguishing features are ductal inflammation (ductulitis), endothelitis (swollen endothelial cells with cellular infiltrates), and, in some instances, centrilobular vein infiltration (central venulitis) (43).

Therapy consists of a drastic increase in the dosage of immunosuppressive agents. Most cases of ACR are managed by administering a pulse of steroids followed by a tapering cyclic schedule and by maintaining a consistently high plasma concentration of tacrolimus, cyclosporine, or rapamycin. If these measures are not successful, or in cases of moderate or severe rejection, antilymphocyte preparations based on antibodies can be used. Among these are antilymphocyte globulin or antithymocyte globulin, which are polyclonal antibody preparations, and OKT3 (muromonab), which is a monoclonal antibody; all are directed against lymphocytes. The use of antilymphocyte antibodies places patients in a strongly immunosuppressed condition and exposes them to the risk of superimposed infections. In addition, OKT3 infusion can evoke a cytokine release syndrome, which, in the most serious cases, causes fever, joint pain, and pulmonary edema.

Only one-third of all cases of rejection requires antilymphocyte therapy; most episodes can be treated with steroid pulses and an increase in the patient's immunosuppressive regimen. Immunologic graft loss because of acute rejection is much more rare after liver transplantation than after the transplantation of other solid organs, such as the kidney or the heart.

LATE COMPLICATIONS

The recent improvement in the survival rate of liver transplant recipients has been remarkable. This improvement is demonstrated by an ever-growing number of patients who survive the first years after transplantation and whose potential complications are related to the long-term use of immunosuppressive agents. In addition to the direct side effects of immunosuppression, patients treated with such regimens are also at risk of malignancies, both in solid organs and in the lymphopoietic system. The original disease that caused liver failure, whether infectious or primary, can recur among patients after transplantation and can pose serious clinical problem.

Extrahepatic Complications
Malignancies

The use of medications to suppress the immune system and avoid rejection exposes patients to the development of malignant disease. The incidence of this complication ranges from 4% to 16% among patients treated with immunosuppressive agents, and most of these malignant diseases are related to viral infection (44). A broad classification of post-transplantation malignancies divides them into solid-organ malignancies and PTLD; among liver transplant recipients, PTLD is more common. The temporal pattern of development of malignancies is shorter for recipients of liver transplants than for recipients of other solid organs (e.g., kidney); the mean time to occurrence is 27 months. Alcoholic patients are at a higher risk of malignant disease.

Most cases of PTLD occur within the first year or two after transplantation. PTLD is linked to EBV infection and the ability of this virus to mutate the proliferation patterns of the lymphoid cell populations it infects (45). Immunosuppression favors the development of EBV infection because T-cells are normally responsible for clearing EBV infection. A decrease in the dosage, or the total withdrawal of the immunosuppressive agents, often leads to complete resolution of PTLD. The most common type of PTLD is B-cell lymphoma, but the spectrum of severity of the disease varies greatly, both in terms of the aggressiveness of the tumor cell lines and in terms of the systemic localization of the tumor cells. The mildest forms of PTLD generally express polyclonal cell lines and are located in the primary lymphoid organs (e.g., tonsils, Peyer's patches of the intestine, spleen, mediastinal lymph nodes, and retroperitoneal lymph nodes). More aggressive forms of lymphoma are diffuse and tend to invade the bone marrow compartment, with monoclonal cell lines that can be detected by gene rearrangement studies. Almost invariably, the malignant cells are infected by EBV; this infection can be diagnosed by PCR or immunohistochemical analysis of tissue samples. Therapy for PTLD involves reducing the dosage or stopping the administration of immunosuppressive agents. If this approach fails, the second line of therapy is the use of interferon-alpha, anti–B-cell monoclonal antibodies, and, in the most severe cases, chemotherapy (46). The survival rate for patients with PTLD has greatly improved over the past 10 years because of our better understanding of the causes of the disease and the recent availability of anti–B-cell monoclonal antibodies.

The most common sites of non-PTLD malignancies are the skin (Kaposi's sarcoma, squamous cell carcinoma, and oropharyngeal carcinoma), the gastrointestinal tract (stomach or colon cancer), and the genitourinary tract (renal, bladder, or cervical cancer) (44). Skin cancers are the most common nonlymphoid malignancies among transplant recipients. Multiple factors have been implicated, including age, sun exposure, race, and viral infection. Specifically, human papillomavirus infection has been linked to cervical cancers and squamous cell carcinoma (47). Kaposi's sarcoma is very often associated with human herpesvirus 8 infection (48). Patients with preexisting inflammatory bowel disease (IBD) are at higher risk of intestinal cancer; for instance, one study found that the incidence of colon cancer among liver transplant recipients was 8% if patients had IBD, but only 0.1% if they did not (49). Interestingly, the rate of incidence of breast cancer among organ transplant recipients is lower than that in the normal population.

The development of malignancies affects patients' survival rates; one study found that the 10-year survival rate for patients with post-transplant malignancies is only 27% (50). The worst survival rates are for patients with metastatic disease, especially if it comes from an unknown primary tumor, Kaposi's sarcoma, or a brain tumor. A high index of suspicion, routine screening tests, and cessation of risk behaviors are essential for the prevention and early detection of all post-transplant malignancies.

Renal Complications

The use of tacrolimus and cyclosporine as primary immunosuppressive agents invariably leads to some degree of renal toxicity (13,51).

The mechanism through which these drugs impair glomerular filtration is tubular vasoconstriction. Renal disease may be exacerbated by the concomitant use of other nephrotoxic medications, especially nonsteroidal anti-inflammatory drugs (NSAIDs), or by dehydration. It is imperative that creatinine and blood urea nitrogen concentrations be monitored in the long-term follow-up of liver transplant recipients. Creatinine concentrations one and three months after transplantation are important predictors of long-term renal outcome (52). In addition, dosages of immunosuppressive drugs must be carefully monitored if toxicity is to be avoided. The new immunosuppressive agent sirolimus (rapamycin) causes virtually no renal toxicity and has been used as primary therapy for some patients; its long-term efficacy, however, has not yet been demonstrated in large clinical trials. Sirolimus can be considered an alternative therapy for patients who have experienced severe nephrotoxic side effects with tacrolimus or cyclosporine.

Cardiovascular Complications

Cardiovascular complications are now emerging as an important factor in long-term morbidity. Such complications are the third most common cause of death occurring more than one year after transplantation. The most common complication after transplantation is hypertension, a well-known problem for patients treated with cyclosporine or tacrolimus. Renal vascular constriction, which is believed to be the common pathogenetic factor, may be mediated by the direct effect of immunosuppressive agents. Therapy must be aggressive and involves the use of vasodilators such as calcium channel blockers, together with lifestyle modifications such as weight loss, a low-salt diet, and exercise.

Endocrine and Metabolic Complications

Strictly related to the development of cardiovascular complications is the spectrum of dysmetabolic alterations in the long term after transplantation.

Hyperlipidemia occurs among as many as 30% of liver transplant recipients. It contributes to accelerated allograft vasculopathy and the development of atherosclerosis (53). Obesity and the use of steroids or cyclosporine contribute to lipemia. The effect of tacrolimus on the development of hyperlipidemia seems to be less pronounced than that of cyclosporine. Triglyceride and cholesterol levels should be monitored at least monthly after transplantation. For patients with significant hyperlipidemia, diet modification and weight loss, together with tapering of the steroid dosage, can reduce cholesterol levels after transplantation.

As many as 64% of patients may become obese after liver transplantation. This condition is related primarily to the patient's improved metabolism and the return of a normal appetite. In addition, the use of steroids improves caloric intake and fuel utilization. The mainstay of therapy is reduced caloric intake, weight control, and exercise programs.

Hyperglycemia is common during the early postoperative period and is primarily related to high-dose steroid regimens. Home monitoring of blood glucose concentrations is often required during the immediate period after discharge from the hospital. However, as many as 17% of patients experience insulin-requiring glucose intolerance more than three months after surgery.

Osteoporosis and bone disease are among the most debilitating complications that occur after liver transplantation (54). During the preoperative period, many patients have already experienced reductions in bone density, especially those with primary biliary cirrhosis (PBC) and chronic cholestatic syndromes because of the decreased absorption of fat-soluble vitamin D, and general malnourishment. After transplantation, the long periods of relative immobility can worsen bone loss, which is also made more acute by the use of corticosteroid agents. Because of this severe osteoporosis, patients can easily experience pathologic fractures, mostly in the spinal column. These fractures can be severely disabling and can cause constant pain and, in some cases, neurological damage or even spinal lesions. There is no specific therapy for osteoporosis in such cases. Diet supplementation with calcium and vitamin D offers only modest benefits. Corticosteroid dosages should be decreased as much as possible or completely stopped. Postmenopausal women should receive hormone replacement therapy. NSAIDs should be avoided for pain control because of their nephrotoxic effects.

Neurologic Complications

Most long-term neurologic complications are related to the use of immunosuppressive therapy (15). The incidence of such complications is high, ranging from 8% to 47% of liver transplant recipients. The most common complaint is headache. Reducing the dosage of immunosuppressive agents or changing the primary immunosuppressive medications can sometimes alleviate this symptom; however, organic causes must always be excluded by a thorough neurological examination and a CT scan of the brain. Tremor is also common and is generally related to the use of cyclosporine and tacrolimus. Tremor may be a sign of the toxic effects of high dosages of these drugs; therefore, constant monitoring of the trough levels of tacrolimus and cyclosporine is mandatory for all patients who experience tremors.

Graft-Related Complications
Rejection

Most episodes of acute rejection occur among liver transplant recipients within the first three postoperative months. However, episodes of ACR can occur at any time after transplantation and pose substantial problems for long-term survival of the graft (55). Most episodes of ACR during the late postoperative period are due to decreases in the plasma concentrations of immunosuppressive agents. These decreases can be caused by multiple mechanisms. For example, patients may wean themselves from their medications or stop taking them altogether. Alternatively, if patients take medications that interfere with the metabolism of immunosuppressive agents, the plasma concentrations will also decrease. Transplant physicians themselves may decrease the dosage of immunosuppressive agents because of side effects or in an attempt to withdraw these agents from long-term patients with previously excellent graft function.

ACR may be asymptomatic and the only abnormal finding may be an increase in serum enzyme activity. If symptoms are present, they usually consist of headaches, general malaise, and tenderness in the right upper quadrant. Physical examination will indicate an enlarged liver with dull borders and occasional tenderness. ACR is confirmed by liver biopsy. The diagnosis is also made by carefully reviewing the patient's history and by monitoring serum transaminase activity and the plasma levels of immunosuppressive agents. Treatment consists of resuming the administration of steroids, if they had been previously discontinued, or increasing their dosage. The dosages of tacrolimus or cyclosporine are usually adjusted until therapeutic levels have been attained. Repeated or steroid-resistant episodes of late rejection pose a substantial risk for loss of the graft and must be aggressively treated, if necessary, with the use of monoclonal antilymphocytic antibodies. Late episodes of ACR are often triggered by concomitant viral infections, perhaps because an episode of infection boosts immunity and disturbs the equilibrium between the graft and the host, thereby making the graft susceptible to rejection. In such cases, if rejection is associated with viral infections, appropriate antiviral therapy must be instituted when the dosage of immunosuppressive agents is increased.

Chronic rejection is also described as ductopenic (56). This complication, which usually occurs from six weeks to six months or more after transplantation, is insidious in its clinical course and is characterized by the development of cholestasis. It occurs in approximately 8% of all cases. Patients usually exhibit no symptoms until jaundice becomes clinically evident. Alkaline phosphatase activity usually increases in proportion to the increase in transaminase activity. The diagnosis of chronic rejection is confirmed by liver biopsy. The main damage to hepatic tissue occurs at the level of the biliary ducts, which progressively decrease in number (therefore the definition *ductopenic*). Chronic vascular changes also occur. The microscopic features of chronic rejection are a cellular infiltrate in the periportal spaces and infiltration, predominantly of macrophages and lymphocytes, around the bile ducts. Bile duct loss occurs in the interlobular areas of the hepatic parenchyma; ductopenia in more than 50% of the visualized portal tracts confirms the diagnosis. Arterial vasculopathy is obliterative at the level of large- and middle-sized arteries; foam cells of macrophage origin are laden with lipids and obliterate the vascular lumen, thereby causing a decrease in blood flow to the liver and specifically to the biliary tree. The standard therapy of increasing the dosages of immunosuppressive agents is not successful in managing chronic rejection, and most patients will require retransplantation. Unfortunately, retransplantation for chronic rejection predisposes patients to a much higher risk of recurrent ductopenic rejection.

Graft Vs. Host Disease

Graft versus host disease (GVHD) is a rare but potentially lethal complication of solid-organ transplantation; it carries substantial risks of morbidity and mortality (57). GVHD is characterized by the presence of immunologically competent cells within the transplanted graft; these cells recognize foreign antigens on recipient tissues and mount a cytotoxic response to such tissues during a period when the recipient's immune system is incompetent and cannot respond to and destroy such cells. Recipients of solid-organ transplants are at risk of GVHD from the graft itself or, more rarely, from the transfusion of cellular blood components. The clinical presentation of GVHD can be limited to a humoral reaction with hemolysis, but the most common and dangerous presentation is T-lymphocyte–mediated destruction of disparate host tissues. When GVHD becomes disseminated, the survival rate is poor: for liver transplant recipients, the mortality rate associated with GVHD can be as high as 50%. Liver transplant recipients are at a higher risk of GVHD than are recipients of other organs, such as the kidney or the heart. This increased risk is believed to be related to the high·number of passenger leukocytes that reside within the large organ.

The diagnosis of GVHD is based on clinical manifestations, histologic findings, and the presence of HLAs from donor leukocytes in the recipient's blood and in the affected organs and tissues. GVHD can occur as early as one week after transplantation, but more commonly occurs a few weeks to a few months after the procedure. After liver transplantation, GVHD most commonly targets the skin and the gastrointestinal tract. Skin manifestations include a macular rash on the trunk and extremities; this rash can progress to frank skin necrosis and sloughing. Gastrointestinal manifestations include nausea, vomiting, and diarrhea. Liver failure, a classic feature of GVHD associated with the transplantation of other organs, is characteristically not seen among liver recipients because the activated T-cells do not see the hepatic graft as foreign. Pancytopenia is also common when the bone marrow compartment is affected; this condition complicates the clinical picture because it exposes the recipient to sepsis. In fact, death usually occurs because of secondary infectious complications. The treatment of GVHD involves increasing the dosages of immunosuppressive agents, using T-cell depleting protocols, and, rarely, using radiation therapy or phototherapy.

Biliary Strictures

Among patients who have not experienced early episodes of rejection, the most common cause of late (more than three months after transplantation) elevation in liver enzyme activity is biliary complications, usually strictures (58). Strictures can result from surgical technique, but are more commonly ischemic and are related to a decrease in arterial inflow to the biliary tree. HAT may cause only biliary symptoms because the hepatic parenchyma has a double vascular supply (portal and arterial). Subsequently, multiple strictures may occur in the large biliary ducts and in the peripheral smaller ductal system. Cold ischemic time of more than 12 hours is an important risk factor for ischemic biliary strictures.

Patients will experience cholestasis, jaundice, pruritus, general malaise, and anorexia. Infectious complications such as ascending cholangitis can pose a serious problem, especially if they are not recognized early enough. Ultrasonography of the liver can demonstrate biliary dilatation and, with Doppler studies, can evaluate the patency of the hepatic artery. Visualization of the biliary tree is possible with ERCP, magnetic resonance cholangiography, or transhepatic cholangiography. Treatment involves dilatation and drainage of the biliary tree by percutaneous or endoscopic means. Occasionally, surgical reconstruction or conversion from a duct-to-duct to a duct-to-jejunum anastomosis can improve localized strictures at the hilum. Retransplantation may be required for those patients who experience cholestatic liver failure as the result of multiple diffuse biliary strictures.

Recurrent Disease

Depending on the cause of the failure, recurrent disease can be classified as follows: recurrence of malignant tumors, recurrence of viral hepatitis B or C infection, or recurrence of the original hepatopathy [e.g., PBC, sclerosing cholangitis, autoimmune hepatitis (AIH), and hemochromatosis].

Recurrent malignant disease is a potential complication of liver transplantation for HCC or biliary malignancy (59). More rarely, patients may have received liver grafts when the original organ was seeded with metastases from other extrahepatic tumors (e.g., neuroendocrine tumors). Recurrent HCC is usually a result of metastases that can reoccur either in the new graft or elsewhere in the body. Risk factors for the recurrence of HCC are size of the original tumor, vascular invasion, and presence of multiple tumors. Screening tests include periodic CT scans, magnetic resonance imaging studies, ultrasonography of the liver, and monitoring of alpha-fetoprotein concentrations, which can confirm the recurrence of the disease. Hepatitis B virus (HBV) is found not only in the liver of infected patients, but also in many other tissues, including spleen, pancreas, and peripheral leukocytes; therefore, recurrent infection of the transplanted hepatic graft is very common. The primary determinant of disease recurrence in the transplanted liver is the presence of antibody to the hepatitis B surface antigen (HbsAg) or viral DNA (HBV-DNA) in the circulation. These factors are associated with histological evidence of liver damage (60). Another risk factor for hepatitis B is the transplantation of a liver from a donor who is positive for antibody to the hepatitis B core antigen (HbcAg) because reactivation of the virus is common in the immunosuppressed environment.

Recurrent hepatitis may occur as early as three weeks after transplantation; it develops into active chronic hepatitis within a few months after the procedure. The disease may progress to cirrhosis, but such progression is usually slow, although some cases rapidly progress to fibrosing cholestatic hepatitis. In such cases, both HbsAg and HbcAg are detected by immunohistochemical staining. The results of retransplantation for patients with recurrent hepatitis B are poor, primarily because of the rapid redevelopment of the recurrent disease. The prevention of HBV recurrent disease is now a mainstay of therapy after transplantation: the infusion of high doses of hyperimmune human hepatitis B immunoglobulin and treatment with the nucleoside-analog lamivudine (Epivir®) have drastically decreased the rate of recurrence from 75% to 20% and have improved graft and patient survival rates (61).

Hepatitis C–related end-stage liver disease occurs among approximately 40% of all liver transplant recipients. For patients with hepatitis C virus (HCV) infection, liver transplantation is almost universally followed by reinfection of the graft and hepatitis in the new organ (62). The course of development of hepatitis can vary from very aggressive early recurrence to a more chronic indolent course. Patients will usually have no symptoms; the only evidence will be an increase in the activity of liver transaminases. The diagnosis is made by the results of liver biopsy. Histologic changes in the biopsy specimens will show periportal infiltrates with lymphocytic predominance and characteristic lobular infiltrates beyond the limiting plane of the portal triad. HCV-RNA detection by PCR is helpful in making the diagnosis. However, the results of this test indicate only that the virus is present in the circulation after transplantation; they do not indicate the degree of damage to the graft. The incidence of recurrence of HCV infection is higher among patients who have experienced episodes of rejection or prolonged exposure to high doses of steroids (63). This increased incidence is believed to be related to the effect of strong immunosuppression that may allow HCV to reinfect the graft and cause earlier and more severe hepatitis recurrence.

Therapy for HCV recurrence relies on two principles: decreasing the dosage of immunosuppressive agents and administering antiviral medications such as interferon and ribavirin (64). Antiviral treatment may cause serious side effects, such as neutropenia, hemolytic anemia, and thrombocytopenia. Interferon alpha has been recently reformulated in a pegylated form for prolonged absorption; this formulation is administered weekly rather than three times per week and may have fewer side effects.

PBC is an autoimmune disease characterized by antimitochondrial antibodies. The disease leads to intrahepatic destruction of the biliary system and eventually to end-stage liver disease. After liver transplantation, PBC may recur; recurrence rates range from 8% to 30% (65). Several studies have shown that the incidence of recurrence is higher among patients treated with tacrolimus than among those treated with cyclosporine. Clinical symptoms of PBC are jaundice, pruritus, and elevations in alkaline phosphatase activity and bilirubin concentration. Liver biopsy is performed to rule out chronic ductopenic rejection, viral hepatitis, and biliary obstruction. Typical features of PBC are granulomatous destruction of interlobular and septal bile ducts, fibrosis, and ductopenia. Patient and organ survival rates are usually good even when PBC recurs; however, long-term follow-up studies are still needed so that the impact of recurrent disease on liver transplant recipients can be fully evaluated.

Primary sclerosing cholangitis (PSC) is an immunologically mediated cholestatic disease that leads to inflammation and fibrosis of the intrahepatic and extrahepatic biliary trees. Typical features of PSC are perinuclear antineutrophil cytoplasmic antibodies and irregular ductal strictures with beading and pruning of the intrahepatic biliary system. The disease eventually leads to hepatic insufficiency and may recur after transplantation (65). The most important consideration in the diagnosis of recurrent PSC is excluding other conditions that may cause biliary strictures, such as biliary complications, ischemic stricture, and chronic rejection. The incidence of recurrent PSC varies from 12% to 41% among recipients of liver transplants. Patients usually have no symptoms other than a slow increase in the bilirubin concentration and in the alkaline phosphatase activity; frank jaundice and pruritus follow. Diagnosis is made by liver biopsy and by cholangiography, which show multiple intrahepatic and extrahepatic strictures, mural irregularities, and diverticulum-like outpouchings.

AIH is an autoimmune destructive disease of the liver parenchyma. It probably results from altered immune presentation of HLAs on the surface of hepatocytes; this altered presentation induces a cytotoxic T-cell response. AIH is associated with hyperglobulinemia and the presence of positive autoantibodies such as antinuclear antibody, smooth muscle antibody, and liver–kidney microsomes. The incidence of AIH shows a bimodal distribution: the rates are highest among juveniles and the elderly . The disease leads to end-stage liver disease, for which transplantation is necessary. The recurrence of AIH is based on clinical, histological, and serological criteria. For 20% to 83% of patients, recurrent AIH is detected by liver biopsy (65), which shows periportal infiltrates and piecemeal necrosis. Haplotype HLA-DR3 is more frequently associated with recurrence. Patients will often have no symptoms or signs other than an increase in transaminase activity. Viral hepatitis, drug toxicity, and rejection must be included in the differential diagnosis. Aggressive forms of recurrent AIH, especially among pediatric patients, can rapidly destroy the graft and mandate retransplantation. Increasing the immunosuppressive regimen is important for slowing down the progression of recurrent AIH and for carefully weaning patients off the immunosuppressive agents initially used after transplantation. Fortunately, disease recurrence does not seem to affect survival rates.

CONCLUSION

Tremendous progress has been made in the field of hepatic transplantation over the past three decades because of innovations in surgical technique, improvements in immunosuppressive therapy, and a better understanding of the pathologic mechanisms that lead to liver failure. The many complications that may affect recipients of a liver transplant can stem from multiple sources: technical issues related to the procurement of the organ and its implantation in the recipient; immunosuppressive regimens that avoid rejection but limit the response to infectious diseases; and recurrent viral or immune-mediated disease. All physicians treating transplant recipients must maintain careful observation, close and long-term follow-up, and a high index of suspicion. Further advances in the field of immunology and tolerance induction will one day eliminate the need for immunosuppressive agents and will therefore drastically decrease the complexity of the management of such issues. Until then, we will continue facing daily challenges in providing the best care and the longest survival times for our patients.

REFERENCES

1. Brown RS Jr, Ascher NL, Lake JR, et al. The impact of surgical complications after liver transplantation on resource utilization. Arch Surg 1997; 132:1098–1103.
2. Clavien PA, Camargo CA Jr, Croxford R, Langer B, Levy GA, Grieg PD. Definition and classification of negative outcomes in solid organ transplantation. Application in liver transplantation. Ann Surg 1994; 220:109–120.
3. Angus DC, Clermont G, Kramer DJ, Linda-Zwirble WT, Pinsky MR. Short-term and long-term outcome prediction with the Acute Physiology and Chronic Health Evaluation II system after orthotopic liver transplantation. Crit Care Med 2000; 28:150–156.
4. McAlister VC, Grant DR, Roy A, et al. Right phrenic nerve injury in orthotopic liver transplantation. Transplantation 1993; 55:826–830.
5. Afessa B, Gay PC, Plevak DJ, Swensen SJ, Patel HG, Krowka MJ. Pulmonary complications of orthotopic liver transplantation. Mayo Clin Proc 1993; 68:427–434.
6. Plevak DJ. Forum on critical care issues in liver transplantation: fluids, electrolytes, and renal disease in the perioperative liver transplant recipient. Liver Transpl 1996; 21:69–86.
7. Kuo PC, Plotkin JS, Gaine S, et al. Portopulmonary hypertension and the liver transplant candidate. Transplantation 1999; 67:1087–1093.
8. Castro M, Krowka MJ, Schroeder DR, et al. Frequency and clinical implications of increased pulmonary artery pressures in liver transplant patients. Mayo Clin Proc 1996; 71:543–551.
9. Fishman AP. Pulmonary hypertension-beyond vasodilator therapy. N Engl J Med 1998; 338:321–322.
10. Kuo PC, Johnson LB, Plotkin JS, Howell CD, Bartlett ST, Rubin LJ. Continuous infusion of epoprostenol for the treatment of portopulmonary hypertension. Transplantation 1997; 63:604–606.
11. Krowka MJ, Cortese DA. Hepatopulmonary syndrome. Current concepts in diagnostic and therapeutic considerations. Chest 1994; 105:1528–1537.
12. Gonwa TA, Morris CA, Goldstein RM, Husberg BS, Klintmalm GB. Long-term survival and renal function following liver transplantation in patients with and without hepatorenal syndrome—experience in 300 patients. Transplantation 1991; 51:428–430.
13. McCauley J. The nephrotoxicity of FK506 as compared with cyclosporine. Curr Opin Nephrol Hypertens 1993; 2:662–669.
14. Chatzipetrou MA, Tsaroucha AK, Weppler D, et al. Thrombocytopenia after liver transplantation. Transplantation 1999; 67(5):702–706.
15. Wszolek ZK, Fulgham JR. Neurologic complications of liver transplantation. In: Maddrey WC, Sorrell MF, Schiff ER, eds. Transplantation of the Liver. Philadelphia: Lippincott Williams and Wilkins, 2001:297–317.
16. Ozaki CF, Katz SM, Monsour HP Jr, Dyer CH, Wood RP. Surgical complications of liver transplantation. Surg Clin North Am 1994; 74:1155–1167.

17. Winston DJ, Emmanouilides C, Busuttil RW. Infections in liver transplant recipients. Clin Infect Dis 1995; 21:1077–1091.

18. Fishman JA, Rubin RH. Infection in organ-transplant recipients. N Engl J Med 1998; 338:1741–1751.

19. Bakir M, Bova JL, Newell KA, Millis JM, Buell JF, Arnow PM. Epidemiology and clinical consequences of vancomycin-resistant enterococci in liver transplant patients. Transplantation 2001; 72(6):1032–1037.

20. Patterson TF. Approaches to fungal diagnosis in transplantation. Transpl Infect Dis 1999; 1:262–272.

21. Rubin RH. Importance of CMV in the transplant population. Transpl Infect Dis 1999; 1(suppl 1):3–7.

22. Gane E, Saliba F, Valdecasas GJ, et al. Randomised trial of efficacy and safety of oral ganciclovir in the prevention of cytomegalovirus disease in liver-transplant recipients. The Oral Ganciclovir International Transplantation Study Group. Lancet 1997; 350:1729–1733.

23. Straus SE, Cohen JI, Tosato G, Mejer J. NIH conference. Epstein-Barr virus infections: biology, pathogenesis, and management. Ann Intern Med 1993; 118:45–58.

24. Bzeizi KI, Jalan R, Plevris JN, Hayes PC. Primary graft dysfunction after liver transplantation: from pathogenesis to prevention. Liver Transpl Surg 1997; 3:137–148.

25. Quiroga J, Colina I, Demetris AJ, Starzl TE, Van Thiel DH. Cause and timing of first allograft failure in orthotopic liver transplantation: a study of 177 consecutive patients. Hepatology 1991; 14:1054–1062.

26. Langnas AN, Marujo W, Stratta RJ, Wood RP, Shaw BW Jr. Vascular complications after liver transplantation. Am J Surg 1991; 161:76–83.

27. Marujo WC, Langnas AN, Wood RP, Stratta RJ, Li S, Shaw BW Jr. Vascular complications following orthotopic liver transplantation: outcome and the role of urgent revascularization. Transplant Proc 1991; 23:1484–1486.

28. Tzakis AG. The dearterialized liver graft. Semin Liver Dis 1985; 5:375–376.

29. Nishida S, Kato T, Levi D, et al. Effect of protocol Doppler ultrasonography and urgent revascularization on early hepatic artery thrombosis after pediatric liver transplantation. Arch Surg 2002; 137(11):1279–1283.

30. Sheiner PA, Varma CV, Guarrera JV, et al. Selective revascularization of hepatic artery thromboses after liver transplantation improves patient and graft survival. Transplantation 1997; 64:1295–1299.

31. Dodd GD III, Memel DS, Zajko AB, Baron RL, Santaguida LA. Hepatic artery stenosis and thrombosis in transplant recipients: Doppler diagnosis with resistive index and systolic acceleration time. Radiology 1994; 192:657–661.

32. Orons PD, Zajko AB, Bron KM, Trecha GT, Selby RR, Fung JJ. Hepatic artery angioplasty after liver transplantation: experience in 21 allografts. J Vasc Interv Radiol 1995; 6:523–529.

33. Lerut J, Tzakis AG, Bron K, et al. Complications of venous reconstruction in human orthotopic liver transplantation. Ann Surg 1987; 205:404–414.

34. Navarro F, Le Moine MC, Fabre JM, et al. Specific vascular complications of orthotopic liver transplantation with preservation of the retrohepatic cava: review of 1361 cases. Transplantation 1999; 68:646–650.

35. Orons PD, Hari Ak, Zajko AB, Marsh JW. Thrombolysis and endovascular stent placement for inferior vena cava thrombosis in a liver transplant recipient. Transplantation 1997; 64:1357–1361.

36. Calne RY. A new technique for biliary drainage in orthotopic liver transplantation utilising the gall bladder as a pedicle graft conduit between the donor and recipient common bile ducts. Ann Surg 1976; 184:605–609.

37. O'Connor TP, Lewis WD, Jenkins RL. Biliary tract complications after liver transplantation. Arch Surg 1995; 130:312–317.

38. Greif F, Bronsther OL, Van Thiel DH, et al. The incidence, timing, and management of biliary tract complications after orthotopic liver transplantation. Ann Surg 1994; 219:40–45.

39. Fisher A, Miller CH. Ischemic-type biliary strictures in liver allografts: the Achilles heel revisited? Hepatology 1995; 21:589–591.

40. Ascher NL. Progress in transgenic pigs for xenotransplantation. Liver Transpl Surg 1998; 4:180–181.

41. Sayegh MH, Watschinger B, Carpenter CB. Mechanisms of T cell recognition of alloantigen. The role of peptides. Transplantation 1994; 57:1295–1302.

42. Wiesner RH, Demetris AJ, Belle SH, et al. Acute hepatic allograft rejection: incidence, risk factors, and impact on outcome. Hepatology 1998; 28:638–645.

43. Banff schema for grading liver allograft rejection: an international consensus document. Hepatology 1997; 25:658–663.

44. Fung JJ, Jain A, Kwak EJ, Kusne S, Dvorchik I, Eghtesad B. De novo malignancies after liver transplantation: a major cause of late death. Liver Transpl 2001; 7:S109–S118.

45. Tanner JE, Alfieri C. The Epstein-Barr virus and post-transplant lymphoproliferative disease: interplay of immunosuppression, EBV, and the immune system in disease pathogenesis. Transpl Infect Dis 2001; 3:60–69.

46. Green M. Management of Epstein-Barr virus-induced post-transplant lymphoproliferative disease in recipients of solid organ transplantation. Am J Transpl 2001; 1:103–108.

47. McGregor JM, Proby CM. The role of papillomaviruses in human non-melanoma skin cancer. Cancer Surv 1996; 26:219–236.

48. Sheldon J, Henry S, Mourad M, et al. Human herpes virus 8 infection in kidney transplant patients in Belgium. Nephrol Dial Transplant 2000; 15:1443–1445.

49. Fabia R, Levy MF, Testa G, et al. Colon carcinoma in patients undergoing liver transplantation. Am J Surg 1998; 176:265–269.

50. Sheil AG. Malignancy following liver transplantation: a report from the Australian Combined Liver Transplant Registry. Transplant Proc 1995; 27:1247.

51. Wheatley HC, Datzman M, Williams JW, Miles DE, Hatch FE. Long-term effects of cyclosporine on renal function in liver transplant recipients. Transplantation 1987; 43:641–647.

52. Fisher NC, Nightingale PG, Gunson BK, Lipkin GW, Neuberger JM. Chronic renal failure following liver transplantation: a retrospective analysis. Transplantation 1998; 66:59–66.

53. Pirsch JD, D'Alessandro AM, Sollinger HW, et al. Hyperlipidemia and transplantation: etiologic factors and therapy. J Am Soc Nephrol 1992; 2:S238–S242.

54. McDonald JA, Dunstan CR, Dilworth P, et al. Bone loss after liver transplantation. Hepatology 1991; 14:613–619.

55. Mor E, Gonwa TA, Husberg BS, Goldstein RM, Klintmalm GB. Late-onset acute rejection in orthotopic

liver transplantation-associated risk factors and outcome. Transplantation 1991; 54:821–824.

56. Wiesner RW, Batts KP, Krom RA. Evolving concepts in the diagnosis, pathogenesis, and treatment of chronic hepatic allograft rejection. Liver Transpl Surg 1999; 5:388–400.

57. Ferrara JL, Deeg HJ. Graft-versus-host disease. N Engl J Med 1991; 324:667–674.

58. Colonna JO II, Shaked A, Gomes AS, et al. Biliary strictures complicating liver transplantation. Incidence, pathogenesis, management, and outcome. Ann Surg 1992; 216:344–352.

59. Wall WJ. Liver transplantation for hepatic and biliary malignancy. Semin Liver Dis 2000; 20:425–436.

60. Villamil FG. Hepatitis B: progress in the last 15 years. Liver Transpl 2002; 8:S59–S66.

61. Lok AS. Prevention of recurrent hepatitis B post-liver transplantation. Liver Transpl 2002; 8:S67–S73.

62. McCaughan GW, Zekry A. Pathogenesis of hepatitis C virus recurrence in the liver allograft. Liver Transpl 2002; 8:S7–S13.

63. Everson GT. Impact of immunosuppressive therapy on recurrence of hepatitis C. Liver Transpl 2002; 8:S19–S27.

64. Gane E. Treatment of recurrent hepatitis C. Liver Transpl 2002; 8:S28–S37.

65. Faust TW. Recurrent primary biliary cirrhosis, primary sclerosing cholangitis, and autoimmune hepatitis after transplantation. Liver Transpl 2001; 7:S99–S108.

16

Complications of Breast Surgery

Qammar Rashid
Department of Surgery, Howard University, Washington, D.C., U.S.A.

Scott McDonald and Frederick L. Moffat
*DeWitt Daughtry Family Department of Surgery, University of Miami School of Medicine,
Miami, Florida, U.S.A.*

The incidence of complications associated with surgery of the breast is low. The superficial location of the breast and its rich blood supply contribute to the paucity of morbidity when surgical management is required.

COMPLICATIONS OF BREAST BIOPSY

Numerous methods exist for procuring diagnostic tissue from breast lesions. For lesions that are nonpalpable but appear on radiographs, the options include ultrasound (US)-guided fine-needle aspiration cytology (FNAC), core needle biopsy (CNB) with US or stereotactic guidance, vacuum-assisted stereotactic (mammotome) CNB, and excisional biopsy with US-guided or mammographically assisted needle localization. FNAC, CNB, incisional biopsy, and excisional biopsy are used for palpable lesions.

Hematoma is usually evident early, but can develop as late as two weeks after surgery. The reported incidence is 1% to 3% (1). Unless hematoma occurs immediately after surgery, management is expectant. Occasionally, resolving hematomas will drain spontaneously through the wound two to three weeks after surgery, and this drainage may cause the patient some anxiety. Educating the patient preoperatively or at the first postoperative visit can allay anxiety and panic in the unlikely event that such drainage occurs. Wound infections are rare; their incidence ranges from 1% to 2%. Infections are managed by drainage; antibiotics are used in a supportive or an adjuvant role.

The diagnostic error (false-negative) rate associated with radiographically guided biopsy is low, ranging from 0.5% to 2%. Immediate imaging of the procured tissue while the procedure is in progress is imperative. If, for example, during a needle localization biopsy the specimen mammogram or the US-guided radiograph demonstrates that the targeted lesion is not within the excised tissue, the surgeon can immediately retrieve more tissue. However, even when the specimen radiograph confirms the presence of a lesion, follow-up mammography, ultrasonography, or both must be performed four months later to confirm that the lesion was completely removed.

COMPLICATIONS OF BREAST CONSERVATION THERAPY FOR BREAST CANCER

Breast conservation therapy for patients with breast cancer combines breast-conserving surgery (resection of the primary tumor with a margin of normal breast tissue) and postoperative adjuvant breast radiotherapy. Both components contribute to morbidity rates; complications attributed to each component separately and to both in combination will be discussed in this chapter.

Wound Complications

Lymphedema and cellulitis of the breast after breast conservation therapy (2–4) should not be confused with the prototypical postsurgical wound infection (characterized by substantial wound site warmth, tenderness, redness, and seropurulent drainage that occurs within the first postoperative week). The lymphatic channels of the breast are compromised by axillary dissection and breast irradiation. The resulting lymphedema is often early and temporary because collateral lymphatic drainage develops through the dermal and subcutaneous lymph vessels of the breast, chest, and shoulder and through higher-level axillary nodes, interpectoral nodes, and internal mammary nodes.

Lymphangitis is a serious consequence of the upper-extremity lymphedema that may occur after axillary lymph node dissection (2–5). Lymphangitis occurs less frequently than in the past because contemporary lymphadenectomy is less invasive than radical mastectomy. Lymphatic obstruction, which results from axillary dissection, may be exacerbated by resection of additional tissue in the lymphatic pathway, by radiation therapy, and by previous or subsequent infection (3,6,7). Clinically significant lymphedema in the upper extremity occurs in 5% to 8% of patients after axillary dissection, whereas debilitating lymphedema rarely occurs (3,4).

Staren et al. (4) reported a 5% incidence of chronic cellulitis or lymphangitis among 184 breast cancer patients treated with conservation therapy (lumpectomy, axillary dissection, and irradiation). Age, volume of breast tissue excised, number of lymph nodes excised, tumor location, stage of disease, and adjunctive therapy were significant risk factors for such complications. For half of the patients in this study, cellulitis persisted for more than a year. It must always be remembered that cellulitis or lymphangitis can represent an aggressive, inflammatory recurrence of breast cancer.

Cellulitis or lymphangitis is not always bacteriological. It may also be caused by an inflammatory reaction to stagnant lymphatic drainage and protein exudates. In such cases, the problem responds to expectant management or anti-inflammatory agents.

Cosmesis

If breast conservation is to be an acceptable alternative to mastectomy, it must routinely achieve a very high cosmetic or aesthetic standard. Surgical factors that contribute to a poor or only fair cosmetic outcome are excessive resection, the use of drains to evacuate fluid from the lumpectomy defect, multiple reexcisions, and excessive undermining of surrounding skin (8). The placement and orientation of the incision are important for cosmesis and optimal local control: transverse or curvilinear incisions are optimal for lumpectomy in the upper hemisphere of the breast; inferior radial incisions also are acceptable.

Radiotherapy factors are important for cosmetic outcome. Whole-breast doses in excess of 50 Gy, the use of tumor bed boosts, the use of multiple radiation fields, and irradiation of the regional lymph vessels are significant risk factors for an adverse cosmetic outcome. The adverse effects of radiotherapy on cosmesis are time dependent, evolving over a period of years (9–11).

Ipsilateral Recurrence of a Breast Tumor

Of the many factors that influence the incidence of ipsilateral recurrence of a breast tumor, only margin status, tumor size, and multicentricity relate directly to the surgical procedure. Excision of all gross disease is essential for control of tumor in the breast. Recurrence is four to five times more likely when gross tumor involves one or more surgical margins, even when the breast is adequately irradiated (12). Tumor

resection with histologically demonstrated tumor-free margins provides optimal disease control (13). Most surgeons and oncologists consider such clear margins the standard of care for breast-conserving surgery in the management of early breast cancer.

There is little agreement among surgeons and pathologists, however, about the optimal method of assessing surgical margins during breast-conserving procedures. The method used in the trials supported by the National Surgical Adjuvant Breast and Bowel Project (NSABP) provides a useful reference point because it has been validated in multiple clinical studies (14). Using intraoperative frozen sections or touch preparations to verify that the margins are clear minimizes the need for repeat lumpectomy or completion mastectomy.

Tumor size and the presence of multicentricity are important factors in determining whether breast-conserving procedures are appropriate. Recurrence is more likely with increased tumor size and with multifocality or multicentricity (15). Tumors larger than 4 cm in diameter are generally not amenable to breast conservation unless the breast is large. One of the most subtle surgical judgments related to management recommendations is the size of the tumor relative to the size of the breast. Histologically demonstrated clearance of tumor must be achieved, and a cosmetically acceptable result should be realized. If the results of the tumor resection are suboptimal, mastectomy with reconstruction is preferable for both tumor control and aesthetics. Excellent results can be achieved with current methods of breast reconstruction (see below).

Late Carcinogenesis

Earlier studies showed that patients who undergo breast or chest wall radiotherapy (XRT) for cancer of the breast have a slightly elevated risk of second neoplasms; this increased risk becomes evident many years after treatment. Therefore, it has been assumed that patients most at risk of late carcinogenesis are those treated for breast cancer at a young age and those with a good prognosis (those who are likely to be long-term survivors). However because the patients included in the studies which led to these assumptions were treated with radiotherapy techniques that are now antiquated, the risk of second neoplasms may have been overstated. The many recent technological improvements in the types of ionizing radiation used and in the methods of delivering such radiation may reduce the risk of late carcinogenesis for patients with breast cancer, who are currently undergoing breast conservation treatment with XRT.

The NSABP trials (16) and a large case–control study of 82,700 patients treated between 1973 and 1985 (17) reported a late increase in the incidence of leukemia among patients with breast cancer who were treated with XRT. The estimated radiation dose to the bone marrow in the 1985 study was 7.5 Gy.

Current methods of irradiating the breast after lumpectomy unavoidably expose the opposite breast to a low dose of ionizing radiation, approximately 0.5 Gy (18). Three large population-based studies (19–21) demonstrated that adjuvant XRT to the breast or chest wall modestly increases the relative risk of contralateral breast cancer. This finding suggests that the magnitude of the carcinogenic effect is very low. A case–control study reported a small but significant increase in the risk of contralateral breast cancer only for patients 45 years of age or younger at the time of XRT (22).

A study of SEER data obtained from 1983 through 1986 showed that patients with breast cancer treated with XRT to the conserved breast or the chest wall were at increased risk of squamous cell carcinoma, small cell carcinoma, and adenocarcinoma of the ipsilateral lung (23). The latency period was 10 years. Radiation dosimetry suggests that whole-breast megavoltage teletherapy at a dose of 6 MeV exposes the ipsilateral breast to 21% of the entire dose and the lungs to 1.2% of the entire dose. A retrospective, population-based cohort study of more than 220,000 patients with breast cancer demonstrated that, after 10 years of follow-up, the relative risk of squamous cell carcinoma of the esophagus for women undergoing XRT was 5.42 [95% confidence interval (CI), 2.33–10.68], whereas that for esophageal adenocarcinoma was 4.22 (95% CI, 0.47–15.25) (24). Soft-tissue sarcomas (angiosarcoma, lymphangiosarcoma, and Stewart–Treves syndrome) may arise in irradiated tissues many years after XRT for breast cancer. Although the incidence of these sarcomas is low and the latency period is long, these are virulent neoplasms (25).

Cardiac Morbidity and Mortality

Excessive rates of late cardiac morbidity and mortality among breast cancer patients treated with XRT have been documented in several long-term studies (26,27). The rate of coronary atherosclerosis is accelerated in these patients; ischemic events predominate over cardiomyopathy or conduction abnormalities. The advent of megavoltage therapy, the avoidance of high-risk radiation fields such as the anterior "hockey stick" portal for irradiation of ipsilateral internal mammary and supraclavicular lymph vessels, and reduced radiation scatter to the heart with newer tangential techniques have decreased the incidence of postirradiation atherosclerosis.

Compromised Surveillance of the Treated Breast

The combined effects of surgery and irradiation can make posttreatment surveillance of the conserved breast a challenge. Early effects such as dermal and parenchymal edema and late effects such as fibrosis and fat necrosis in the treated breast can confound clinical and mammographic surveillance for recurrent disease or new primary tumors (28). Increased cicatricial reaction and fat necrosis may lead to clinical or mammographic changes that cannot simply be observed, given the patient's history of ipsilateral breast cancer. Consequently, in such cases the surgeon must more frequently resort to CNB or open biopsy.

COMPLICATIONS OF BREAST BIOPSY AFTER BREAST-CONSERVING THERAPY

Biopsy of the treated breast is associated with an increased risk of wound complications and is detrimental to cosmesis. The exaggerated postoperative fibrotic response hinders subsequent surveillance of the breast. Pezner et al. (29) reported that wound infections occurred after 8 of 27 open biopsies performed on patients who had undergone breast-conserving therapy. Three infections resolved within four weeks; four required three to seven months for complete resolution; and one failed to resolve. On rare occasions, intractable wound complications, biopsy-induced cosmetic deterioration, or the inability to evaluate the breast for disease can necessitate total mastectomy in the absence of recurrent cancer.

COMPLICATIONS OF SALVAGE SURGERY FOR LOCAL RECURRENCE

Reported complication rates associated with salvage surgery for recurrence after breast conservation range from 7% to 26% (30,31). Wound infection, delayed healing, and flap necrosis are the most commonly reported complications.

COMPLICATIONS ASSOCIATED WITH BREAST RECONSTRUCTION

Postmastectomy breast reconstruction is well accepted as an important part of overall therapy for breast cancer. New information about breast cancer treatment appears frequently, and numerous techniques are available for reconstruction. The surgical oncologist, medical oncologist, and reconstructive surgeon must therefore work together to provide a safe and effective treatment plan that eliminates the cancer and restores the patient's appearance. One of the first decisions is whether breast reconstruction should be performed immediately after mastectomy or be delayed. Both methods are effective, but most reconstructive surgeons believe that immediate reconstruction, especially with the skin-sparing mastectomy technique, provides psychological benefits and better overall results (32–35).

The overall benefit should, however, be placed into the context of new information about adjuvant therapy such as postoperative chemotherapy and irradiation and the effects of immediate reconstruction on the treatment plan. Consequently, the risks and benefits of each type of reconstruction must be carefully discussed with the patient to allow for a completely informed decision about reconstruction. Whether immediate or delayed reconstruction is chosen, it should be initiated only after the patient has recovered from any adjuvant therapy that may have been administered. An adequate recovery period should be allowed after reconstructive surgery so that healing can occur before other potentially complicating therapy such as chemotherapy or irradiation is administered.

Breast reconstruction can be viewed as providing a replacement for the skin and tissue volume that were removed during the mastectomy. Two approaches are used to achieve this result. One approach, tissue expansion and implant placement, expands the adjacent skin and muscle to cover a silicone prosthesis filled with saline solution or silicone gel, which is used to replace lost breast volume. The second technique replaces the lost skin and volume with an autologous tissue flap composed of skin, subcutaneous fat, and, at times, muscle. Some hybrid techniques use the implant to provide missing volume and a flap of tissue to replace the skin deficit. Because a diagnosis of breast cancer is stressful and the treatment decisions are complicated, it is most important that patients have a clear understanding of the options for reconstruction and the necessary risks of reconstruction. Once this understanding has been obtained, most complications associated with breast reconstruction can be treated effectively.

Implant Reconstruction

Implant reconstruction in the form of tissue expansion followed by placement of a permanent implant is an accepted practice. Because the operative time and hospitalization period associated with this procedure are short, implant reconstruction is popular among surgeons and patients. This technique involves placing an underfilled tissue expander into a surgically created pocket behind the lower portion of the pectoralis muscle at the base of the inframammary fold. This procedure can be performed as an immediate reconstruction after a mastectomy or as a delayed or secondary reconstructive procedure. In either case, after the wound has adequately healed, an injection port connected to the implant is accessed with a needle, and normal saline solution is injected at intervals to expand the skin and muscle and thus to create a pocket large enough for the implant. Once the tissue has been expanded, a second surgical procedure is performed to exchange the expander for a permanently placed implant that gives the patient a new breast with volume and adequate soft-tissue coverage. This operation can be followed by nipple reconstruction and, if needed, a symmetry procedure for the opposite breast.

Implant reconstruction is best suited for patients who do not smoke and who have smaller, less ptotic breasts because creating ptosis with implants is difficult (36,37). Although implant reconstruction requires relatively short procedures that are not systemically stressful, the multiple stages and demanding office visits for expansion are undesirable. Most important, the number of potential complications and the frequency with which they occur make tissue expansion and implant reconstruction less attractive than other procedures (38,39). The incidence of capsule contracture associated with tissue expansion and implant reconstruction has been reported to be as high as 50%, particularly with silicone implants (40). Radiation therapy before or after reconstruction further complicates implant reconstruction (41). Radiation therapy after such reconstruction is associated with high infection rates, and many patients who experience this complication will require further flap procedures to cover or replace the implant.

Many other potential complications are associated with implant reconstruction. The Saline Prospective Study (42), conducted over a three-year period and published by implant manufacturer Mentor Corporation, determined the cumulative individual risk rates for the following complications: capsule contracture, 30%; infection, 9%; rupture or deflation, 9%; asymmetry, 28%; wrinkling of the implant, 20%; extrusion, 2%; seroma, 6%; hematoma, 1%; and breast pain or inflammation, 17%. The reported reoperation rate for patients who underwent reconstruction was 40% (42).

Capsule contracture can be very difficult to correct. In such cases, the implants will become firm or even hard and can even be displaced. Capsule contracture can have many causes, but contributing factors may be low-grade infections, undrained hematomas, silicone gel leakage, and foreign-body reactions (43,44). The rates of contracture appear to be lower when implants are placed below the muscle. Saline-filled implants, antibiotic irrigation, and intraluminal administration of steroids may decrease the rate of these complications. Treatment includes removal of the implant and, if possible, total capsulectomy with removal of any leaking gel. A new implant is placed under the muscles.

Infections can be managed with intravenous antibiotics. If improvement is not forthcoming, the implant should be removed. Rupture of a saline implant is easily detected because of the loss of breast volume, but rupture of a silicone gel implant can be more difficult to diagnose because the gel frequently remains in the capsule. Breast US can be helpful, but magnetic resonance imaging performed with a machine equipped with a breast coil is associated with higher sensitivity and specificity (45). Treatment includes removing the implant and any remaining gel and, if possible, a total capsulectomy to remove the excess silicone gel.

Postoperative hematomas usually occur early but may occur as late as 7 to 14 days after surgery (46). The cause is either bleeding from a previously controlled vessel or diffuse oozing. Careful intraoperative hemostasis is the key to prevention. Seromas result from pocket dissection and are generally detectable as a soft, nontender swelling that results in asymmetry. Many seromas will resolve spontaneously within a week or two. Placing a drain can help, but prolonged use of drains can lead to infection. Textured implants have been implicated in the production of serous fluid (47,48).

Implant palpability and rippling can be caused by numerous factors, including underfilling of noncohesive saline implants, surface morphology, thickness of the overlying tissue, and the location of the implant relative to the pectoralis muscle (49). Texturing increases the palpability of implants because textured implants are comparably thick and immobile (50).

One important point that cannot be overlooked is the relationship between breast implants, particularly those used in augmentation mammoplasty, and breast cancer. Even after the moratorium on the use of silicone breast implants, breast augmentation is still a popular procedure. Because reports indicate that one in eight women will experience breast cancer over her lifetime, the effect of breast implants on cancer is very important. If patients are to make an informed decision, they must receive information about the breast implant, mammography, and surveillance.

Breast implants obscure some portion of the breast during mammography. One report demonstrated that as much as 44% of the breast can be obstructed by subglandular silicone gel breast implants and as much as 25% can be obstructed by submuscular implants (51). Capsule contracture also limits the amount of breast tissue that can be seen on mammograms (52). Long-term studies have shown that delayed detection of breast cancer does not appear to be a serious problem for patients with breast implants, nor is their prognosis poorer than that of patients without implants (53). Diagnostic procedures such as needle biopsies and lymphatic mapping may not be recommended for patients with breast implants; open procedures should be used instead. For patients with breast cancer, implants may make lumpectomy impossible and may necessitate mastectomy (54).

Autologous Reconstruction

It is evident that autologous reconstruction provides a more natural and aesthetically pleasing breast than does implant reconstruction (55). The unique aspect of autologous reconstruction is that the entire reconstruction is achieved with the patient's own tissue. Reconstruction without a prosthetic also provides a psychological benefit. Several donor sites can be used for autologous reconstruction, and some of these sites can provide the important vascular supply to the tissue in several ways. Each site is associated with particular types of morbidity and with potential benefits to the patient, but not all options will be possible for all patients. The surgeon and the patient should carefully consider the options and develop a plan that is acceptable to both.

The technique most commonly used for autologous breast reconstruction is the transverse rectus abdominis myocutaneous (TRAM) flap. This ideal flap uses the skin, fat, and muscle of the lower abdomen to replace the breast defect. The TRAM flap can be transferred as a pedicled flap based on the deep superior epigastric artery and the rectus abdominis muscle. Others have used the same abdominal tissue with a segment of the rectus muscle and transferred it as a microvascular free flap based on the deep inferior epigastric artery. Both the free flap and the pedicled flap provide a large amount of viable tissue and allow the reconstruction to be tailored to the desired shape and size. Because it is a complicated procedure, TRAM flap reconstruction requires a lengthy operation and an extended hospitalization. A relatively long recuperation period with limited activity is required for limiting some of the morbidity associated with the procedure, such as incisional hernias or lower abdominal bulges. However, the aesthetic result is better than that achieved with other reconstructive procedures. An outcome study at the University of Michigan found that breast reconstruction with the TRAM flap was generally and aesthetically more satisfying than reconstruction with tissue expansion and implants (56).

Several potential complications are associated with the use of the TRAM flap, including partial or total flap loss, improper wound healing at the donor or recipient site, palpable fat necrosis of the flap, and abdominal bulging, hernia, or weakness. Deep venous thrombosis and pulmonary embolus are extreme complications. Patient choice is crucial if these complications are to be kept at an acceptable level. Hartrampf (57) closely examined the risk factors associated with the poor outcome after TRAM flap reconstructions and created a scoring system to assist surgeons in determining which patients are candidates for such reconstruction. The most important risk factors were obesity, smoking, autoimmune diseases such as scleroderma, diabetes (especially insulin-dependent diabetes), psychosocial problems, abdominal scars that could affect the perfusion of the abdominal flap, and, of course, a serious systemic disease such as chronic lung or heart disease.

Probably the most serious complication of TRAM flap reconstruction is flap necrosis. The incidence of necrosis ranges from 2% to 5% (58–61). Small amounts of fat necrosis are not a problem. Occasionally, contour deformity may require repeated excision of excess tissue. Mammography is made difficult by the associated calcification, but this scarring can be differentiated from carcinoma. Several procedures have been devised to improve the vascular perfusion to the flap tissue.

A delayed TRAM flap procedure performed approximately two weeks before transfer may improve the vascular perfusion of pedicled TRAM flaps and may reduce the incidence of partial or full necrosis of the flap (62). Some surgeons choose to use the free-vascularized TRAM flap for breast reconstruction because of its more direct blood supply, and because clinical evidence shows that the free flap is less subject to fat necrosis than the pedicled TRAM flap (63). Small areas of flap necrosis can be managed by simple observation and local care, and revisions can be performed at a later stage of reconstruction. Large necrotic areas on mastectomy skin flaps or on the TRAM flap should be excised and closed in the earlier stages of reconstruction, so that the optimal final result can be achieved (64).

Bulging and hernia formation are common problems associated with the use of either free or pedicled TRAM flaps for breast reconstruction. Reinforcing the rectus fascia closure with mesh is most helpful in reducing the incidence of this problem (65,66).

More recently, a modification of the TRAM flap, the deep inferior epigastric artery perforator (DIEP) flap, has been shown to be an improvement over the free or pedicled TRAM flap. The DIEP flap uses the same abdominal tissue for reconstruction as the TRAM flap; however, the rectus muscle and the abdominal fascia are completely spared. Although this flap requires a complicated dissection of the perforators passing from the deep inferior epigastric artery and vein through the rectus abdominis muscle to the abdominal fat and also requires a microvascular anastomosis, the reported results have been excellent. Most postoperative abdominal bulges and hernias are eliminated. Muscle strength and function are outstanding. Postoperative pain is reduced and hospitalization may be shorter (67–72). Although the vascular supply to this flap is more compromised than that to the free TRAM flap, careful patient choice will keep flap necrosis rates similar to those associated with the free TRAM flap (72). Some patients, particularly those who are very thin or who have abdominal scars, will not be the candidates for breast reconstruction with abdominal flaps. Alternative autologous flaps, such as the latissimus dorsi flap, the gluteus myocutaneous flap, and the thigh and hip flaps, can be used but donor-site morbidity can be substantial (73). Hybrid flaps such as the TRAM flap or the latissimus dorsi myocutaneous flap with permanent implants are alternatives for reconstruction. Covering a permanent implant with autologous tissue allows the skin defect to be replaced by the flap and the volume to be replaced by an implant. The results obtained by using hybrid flaps can be excellent; however, these

procedures are associated with some of the same long-term problems as are implants, such as infection, rupture, and capsule contracture. The latissimus dorsi myocutaneous flap with implant is the most popular of these hybrid flaps. This flap is quite robust and provides good coverage of the implant. The most common complication associated with this flap is seroma formation at the donor site. This complication can be easily managed by repeated aspiration. The postoperative function of the shoulder muscle is good, with only minimal limitations (74–76).

The gluteus myocutaneous flap and its modification and the superior gluteal artery perforator (S-GAP) flap (a perforator flap based on the superior gluteal artery) are alternatives for autologous reconstruction. These flaps can provide a good volume of adipose tissue, even in thin patients, and can also provide sensory innervation. Donor-site morbidity is minimal and the scar can be well hidden. One criticism of breast reconstruction with the gluteus myocutaneous free flap is that the dissection is difficult and the vascular pedicle is very short. When the perforator to the superior gluteal artery (the S-GAP flap) is used, the pedicle is much longer and the microvascular anastomosis can be performed to the internal mammary artery or the thoracodorsal artery (77). The main complications associated with the S-GAP flap, such as flap loss and necrosis, appear to be similar to those associated with other microvascular breast reconstruction techniques.

CONCLUSION

A critical examination of the findings obtained from the history and physical examination of the patient contemplating breast surgery and a comprehensive discussion of the risks and benefits of possible options are mandatory for maintaining low morbidity rates and high patient satisfaction rates. Patient selection plays a key role in minimizing the complications associated with breast reconstruction. Over the years, several important risk factors for these complications have emerged, including smoking, obesity, and a history of irradiation. In the future, we should be able to identify the causes of breast cancer and limit the need for many reconstructive procedures.

REFERENCES

1. Say CC, Donegan W. A biostatistical evaluation of the complications from mastectomy. Surg Gynecol Obstet 1974; 138:370–376.
2. Aitken DR, Minton JP. Complications associated with mastectomy. Surg Clin North Am 1983; 63:1331–1352.
3. Simon MS, Cody RL. Cellulitis after axillary lymph node dissection for carcinoma of the breast. Am J Med 1992; 93:543–548.

4. Staren ED, Klepac S, Smith AP, et al. The dilemma of delayed cellulitis after breast conservation therapy. Arch Surg 1996; 131:651–654.

5. Gallagher PG, Algird JR. Post radical mastectomy edema of the arm: the role of phlebitis. Angiology 1966; 17:377–388.

6. Veronesi U, Saccozzi R, Del Vecchio M, et al. Comparing radical mastectomy with quadrantectomy, axillary dissection, and radiotherapy in patients with small cancers of the breast. N Engl J Med 1981; 305:6–11.

7. Babb RR, Spittell JA Jr, Martin WJ, Schirger A. Prophylaxis of recurrent lymphangitis complicating lymphedema. JAMA 1966; 195:871–873.

8. Winchester PD, Cox JD. Standards for breast-conservation treatment. CA Cancer J Clin 1992; 42:134–162.

9. Olivotto IA, Rose MA, Osteen RT, et al. Late cosmetic outcome after conservative surgery and radiotherapy: analysis of causes of cosmetic failure. Int J Radiat Oncol Biol Phys 1989; 17:747–753.

10. Van Limbergen E, Rijnders A, van der Schueren E, Lerut T, Christiaens R. Cosmetic evaluation of breast conserving treatment for mammary cancer. 2. A quantitative analysis of the influence of radiation dose, fractionation schedules, and surgical treatment techniques on cosmetic results. Radiother Oncol 1989; 16: 253–267.

11. Wazer DE, DiPetrillo T, Schmidt-Ullrich R, et al. Factors influencing cosmetic outcome and complication risk after conservative surgery and radiotherapy for early-stage breast carcinoma. J Clin Oncol 1992; 10: 356–363.

12. Recht A, Silver B, Schnitt S, Connolly J, Hellman S, Harris JR. Breast relapse following primary radiation therapy for early breast cancer. I. Classification, frequency and salvage. Int J Radiat Oncol Biol Phys 1985; 11:1271–1276.

13. Veronesi U, Volterrani F, Luini A, et al. Quadrantectomy versus lumpectomy for small size breast cancer. Eur J Cancer 1990; 26:671–673.

14. Fisher B, Wolmark N, Fisher ER, Deutsch M. Lumpectomy and axillary dissection for breast cancer: surgical, pathological, and radiation considerations. World J Surg 1985; 9:692–698.

15. Fisher ER, Anderson S, Redmond C, Fisher B. Ipsilateral breast tumor recurrence and survival following lumpectomy and irradiation: pathological findings from NSABP protocol B-06. Semin Surg Oncol 1992; 8: 161–166.

16. Fisher B, Rockette H, Fisher ER, Wickerham DL, Redmond C, Brown A. Leukemia in breast cancer patients following adjuvant chemotherapy or postoperative radiation: the NSABP experience. J Clin Oncol 1985; 3:1640–1658.

17. Curtis RE, Boice JD Jr, Stovall M, et al. Risk of leukemia after chemotherapy and radiation treatment for breast cancer. N Engl J Med 1992; 326:1745–1751.

18. Fraass BA, Roberson PL, Lichter AS. Dose to the contralateral breast due to primary breast irradiation. Int J Radiat Oncol Biol Phys 1985; 11:485–497.

19. Storm HH, Jensen OM. Risk of contralateral breast cancer in Denmark 1943–80. Br J Cancer 1986; 54:483–492.

20. Hankey BF, Curtis RE, Naughton MD, Boice JD Jr, Flannery JT. A retrospective cohort analysis of second breast cancer risk for primary breast cancer patients with an assessment of the effect of radiation therapy. J Natl Cancer Inst 1983; 70:797–804.

21. Harvey EB, Brinton LA. Second cancer following cancer of the breast in Connecticut, 1935–82. J Natl Cancer Inst Monogr 1985; 68:99–112.

22. Boice JD Jr, Harvey EB, Blettner M, Stovall M, Flannery JT. Cancer in the contralateral breast after radiotherapy for breast cancer. N Engl J Med 1992; 326:781–785.

23. Neugut AI, Robinson E, Lee WC, Murray T, Karwoski K, Kutcher GJ. Lung cancer after radiation therapy for breast cancer. Cancer 1993; 71:3054–3057.

24. Inskip PD, Stovall M, Flannery JT. Lung cancer risk and radiation dose among women treated for breast cancer. J Natl Cancer Inst 1994; 86:983–988.

25. Brady MS, Garfein CF, Petrek JA, Brennan MF. Posttreatment sarcoma in breast cancer patients. Ann Surg Oncol 1994; 1:66–72.

26. Cuzick J, Stewart H, Peto R, et al. Overview of randomized trials of postoperative adjuvant radiotherapy in breast cancer. Cancer Treat Rep 1987; 71:15–29.

27. Ebbs SR, Yarnold JR. Patient and anatomical selectivity in postoperative radiotherapy for early breast cancer: a British perspective. Semin Surg Oncol 1992; 8: 167–171.

28. Dershaw DD, McCormick B, Cox L, Osborne MP. Differentiation of benign and malignant local tumor recurrence after lumpectomy. Am J Roentgenol 1990; 155:35–38.

29. Pezner RD, Lorant JA, Terz J, Ben-Ezra J, Odom-Maryon T, Luk KH. Wound-healing complications following biopsy of the irradiated breast. Arch Surg 1992; 127:321–324.

30. Osborne MP, Borgen PI, Wong GY, Rosen PP, McCormick B. Salvage mastectomy for local and regional recurrence after breast-conserving operation and radiation therapy. Surg Gynecol Obstet 1992; 174: 189–194.

31. Stotter A, Kroll S, McNeese M, Holmes F, Oswald MJ, Romsdahl M. Salvage treatment for locoregional recurrence following breast conservation therapy for early breast cancer. Eur J Surg Oncol 1991; 17:231–236.

32. Hidalgo DA, Borgen PJ, Petrek JA, Heerdt AH, Cody HS, Disa JJ. Immediate reconstruction after complete skin-sparing mastectomy with autologous tissue. J Am Coll Surg 1998; 187(1):17–21.

33. Carlson GW, Bostwick J III, Styblo TM, et al. Skin-sparing mastectomy. Oncologic and reconstructive considerations Ann Surg 1997; 225(5):570–578.

34. Wellisch DK, Schain WS, Noone RB, Little JW III. Psychosocial correlates of immediate versus delayed reconstruction of the breast. Plast Reconstr Surg 1985; 76(5):713–718.

35. Schain WS, Wellisch DK, Pasnau RO, Landsverk J. The sooner the better: a study of psychological factors in women undergoing immediate versus delayed breast reconstruction. Am J Psychiatry 1985; 142(1): 40–46.

36. Fan J, Raposio E, Wang J, Nordstrom RE. Development of the inframammary fold and ptosis in breast reconstruction with textured tissue expanders. Aesthetic Plast Surg 2002; 26(3):219–222.

37. Slavin SA, Colen SR. Discussion: analysis of risks and aesthetics in a consecutive series of tissue expansion breast reconstructions. Plast Reconstruct Surg 1992; 89:844.

38. Carlson GW, Losken A, Moore B, Thornton J, Elliott M, Bolitho G, Denson DD. Results of immediate breast reconstruction after skin-sparing mastectomy. Ann Plast Surg 2001; 46(3):222–228.

39. Collis N, Sharpe DT. Breast reconstruction by tissue expansion. A retrospective technical review of 197 two-stage delayed reconstructions following mastectomy for malignant breast disease in 189 patients. Br J Plast Surg 2000; 53(1):37–41.

40. Gylbert L, Asplund O, Jurell G. Capsular contracture after breast reconstruction with silicone-gel and saline-filled implants: a 6-year follow-up. Plast Reconstr Surg 1990; 85:373–377.

41. Spear SL, Onyewu C. Staged breast reconstruction with saline-filled implants in the irradiated breast: recent trends and therapeutic implications. Plast Reconstr Surg 2000; 105(3):930–942.

42. Mentor Corp. Saline Prospective Study (SPS). Saline filled breast implant surgery: making an informed decision, 2000:13.

43. Burkhardt BR. Capsular contracture: hard breasts, soft data. Clin Plast Surg 1988; 15:521–532.

44. Burkhardt BR, Dempsey PD, Schnur PL, Tofield JJ. Capsular contracture: a prospective study of the effects of local antibacterial agents. Plast Reconstr Surg 1986; 77:919–932.

45. Cronin TD, Greenberg RL. Our experiences with the silastic gel breast prosthesis. Plast Reconstr Surg 1970; 46:1–7.

46. Courtiss EH, Goldwyn RM, Anastasi GW. The fate of breast implants with infections around them. Plast Reconstr Surg 1979; 63:812–816.

47. Hester TR, Tebbetts JB, Maxwell GP. The polyurethane-covered mammary prosthesis: facts and fiction (II): a look back and a "peek" ahead. Clin Plast Surg 2001; 28:579–586.

48. Barone FE, Perry L, Keller T, Maxwell GP. The biochemical and histopathologic effects of surface texturing with silicone and polyurethane in tissue implantation and expansion. Plast Reconstr Surg 1992; 90:77–86.

49. Biggs TM, Yarish RS. Augmentation mammoplasty: retropectoral versus retromammary implantation. Clin Plast Surg 1988; 15:549–555.

50. Hester TR Jr, Nahai F, Bostwick J, Cukic J. A 5-year experience with polyurethane-covered mammary prostheses for treatment of capsular contracture, primary augmentation mammoplasty, and breast reconstruction. Clin Plast Surg 1988; 15:569–585.

51. Silverstein MJ, Handel N, Gamagami P. The effect of silicone-gel-filled implants on mammography. Cancer 1991; 68(suppl 5):1159–1163.

52. Deapen D, Hamilton A, Beernstein L, Brody GS. Breast cancer stage at diagnosis and survival among patients with prior breast implants. Plast Reconstr Surg 2000; 105:535–540.

53. Birdsell DC, Jenkins H, Berkel H. Breast cancer diagnosis and survival in women with and without breast implants. Plast Reconstr Surg 1993; 92:795–800.

54. Shons AR. Breast cancer and augmentation mammaplasty: the preoperative consultation. Plast Reconstr Surg 2002; 109:383–385.

55. Kroll SS. Why autologous tissue? Clin Plast Surg 1998; 25(2):135–143.

56. Alderman AK, Wilkins EG, Lowery JC, Kim M, Davis JA. Determinants of patient satisfaction in post-mastectomy breast reconstruction. Plast Reconstr Surg 2000; 106(4):769–776.

57. Hartrampf CR Jr. The transverse abdominal island flap for breast reconstruction. A 7-year experience. Clin Plast Surg 1988; 15:703–716.

58. Bunkis J, Walton RL, Mathes SJ, Krizek TJ, Vasconez LO. Experience with the transverse lower rectus abdominis operation for breast reconstruction. Plast Reconstr Surg 1983; 72:819–829.

59. Trabulsy PP, Anthony JP, Mathes SJ. Changing trends in postmastectomy breast reconstruction: a 13-year experience. Plast Reconstr Surg 1994; 93:1418–1427.

60. Erdmann D, Sundin BM, Moquin KJ, Young H, Georgiade GS. Delay in unipedicled TRAM flap reconstruction of the breast: a review of 76 consecutive cases. Plast Reconstr Surg 2002; 110:762–767.

61. Kroll SS, Gherardini G, Martin JE, et al. Fat necrosis in free and pedicled TRAM flaps. Plast Reconstr Surg 1998; 102(5):1502–1507.

62. Kroll SS. The early management of flap necrosis in breast reconstruction. Plast Reconstr Surg 1991; 87(5):893–901.

63. Kroll SS, Schusterman MA, Reece GP, Miller MJ, Robb G, Evans G. Abdominal wall strength, bulging, and hernia after TRAM flap breast reconstruction. Plast Reconstr Surg 1995; 96(3):616–619.

64. Kroll SS, Marchi M. Comparison of strategies for preventing abdominal-wall weakness after TRAM flap breast reconstruction. Plast Reconstr Surg 1992; 89(6):1045–1053.

65. Blondeel PN. One hundred free DIEP flap breast reconstructions: a personal experience. Br J Plast Surg 1999; 52(2):104–111.

66. Blondeel N, Vanderstraeten GG, Monstrey SJ, et al. The donor site morbidity of free DIEP flaps and free TRAM flaps for breast reconstruction. Br J Plast Surg 1997; 50(5):322–330.

67. Nahabedian MY, Momen B, Galdino G, Manson PN. Breast reconstruction with the free TRAM or DIEP flap: patient selection, choice of flap, and outcome. Plast Reconstr Surg 2002; 110(2):466–477.

68. Futter CM, Webster MH, Hagen S, Mitchell SL. A retrospective comparison of abdominal muscle strength following breast reconstruction with a free TRAM or DIEP flap. Br J Plast Surg 2000; 53(7):578–583.

69. Kroll SS. Fat necrosis in free transverse rectus abdominis myocutaneous and deep inferior epigastric perforator flaps. Plast Reconstr Surg 2000; 106(3): 576–583.

70. de la Torre JI, Fix RJ, Gardner PM, Vasconez LO. Reconstruction with the latissimus dorsi flap after skin-sparing mastectomy. Ann Plast Surg 2001; 46: 229–233.

71. Menke H, Erkens M, Olbrisch RR. Evolving concepts in breast reconstruction with latissimus dorsi flaps: results and follow-up of 121 consecutive patients. Ann Plast Surg 2001; 47:107–114.

72. Clough KB, Louis-Sylvestre C, Fitoussi A, Couturaud B, Nos C. Donor site sequelae after autologous breast reconstruction with an extended latissimus dorsi flap. Plast Reconstr Surg 2002; 109:1904–1911.

73. Allen RJ, Tucker C Jr. Superior gluteal artery perforator free flap for breast reconstruction. Plast Reconstr Surg 1995; 95(7):1207–1212.

74. Dowden RV. Selection criteria for successful immediate breast reconstruction. Plast Reconstr Surg 1991; 88(4):628–634.

75. Padubidri AN, Yetman R, Browne E, et al. Complications of postmastectomy breast reconstructions in smokers, ex-smokers, and nonsmokers. Plast Reconstr Surg 2001; 107(2):342–351.

76. Chang DW, Reece GP, Wang B, et al. Effect of smoking on complications in patients undergoing free TRAM flap breast reconstruction. Plast Reconstr Surg 2000; 105(7):2374–2380.

77. Paige KT, Bostwick J 3rd, Bried JT, Jones G. A comparison of morbidity from bilateral, unipedicled and unilateral, unipedicled TRAM flap breast reconstructions. Plast Reconstr Surg 1998; 101(7):1819–1827.

17

Complications of Thyroidectomy and Parathyroidectomy

George L. Irvin III and Denise M. Carneiro-Pla
*DeWitt Daughtry Family Department of Surgery, Miller School of Medicine,
University of Miami, Miami, Florida, U.S.A.*

Complications associated with surgical procedures involving the thyroid and parathyroid glands are uncommon, but can cause substantial morbidity when they do occur. This chapter will discuss the specific problems that may occur during operations on these important endocrine glands and some methods that can reduce the risk of postoperative hematoma, laryngeal nerve palsy, hypocalcemia, seroma, wound infection, and failure of parathyroidectomy.

POSTOPERATIVE CERVICAL HEMATOMA

Bleeding within the closed deep cervical fascia can be life threatening after thyroid resection. This complication is unusual after parathyroidectomy, occurring in only 0.1% to 1.3% of cases, unless extensive exploration has been done. On the other hand, the thyroid gland is very vascular, and if any cut surface of this gland remains, as is common after lobectomy or partial thyroidectomy, progressive bleeding may occur. Hematoma formation resulting from either venous bleeding or an acute hemorrhage of a major artery can cause airway obstruction that must be recognized early and treated with the utmost urgency. Should obstructive respiratory distress with cyanosis, agitation, stridor, or an expanding neck mass occur, the wound and the deep cervical fascia must be opened immediately at the bedside to relieve pressure on the trachea. This procedure, rather than an attempt to reinsert a tube into the trachea of a patient who is awake or hypoxic, is the best way to obtain airway patency. Once the airway is clear, the patient should be sedated and returned to the operating room for safe evacuation of the remaining hematoma, hemostasis, and wound closure. Although this type of hemorrhage and airway obstruction is unusual, it is life-threatening and calls for emergent therapeutic intervention. In contrast, cervical hematoma without airway compromise can be managed in a less urgent manner with reexploration in the operating room (1,2). This procedure requires careful monitoring of the airway while the patient is being transported to the operating room, and the surgeon should be prepared to open the wound immediately if progressive respiratory distress occurs.

Several factors may help prevent postoperative cervical hematoma. Because many surgical patients may be receiving anticoagulation therapy, a good history should be elicited, and these drugs should be withheld for an appropriate interval preoperatively, depending on the particular anticoagulant used. Meticulous attention to hemostasis is useful and should include double ligation of a divided superior thyroid artery and suture ligation of the cut edge of any incised thyroid tissue with careful cauterization of its surface. A tubular, closed suction drain can be used for patients who have undergone extensive dissection, or who are experiencing continued loss of venous blood, but this drain may not prevent the formation of a hematoma that may lead to a compromised airway. A small incisional dressing, instead of bulky gauze, will allow good monitoring of the neck and because most hematomas occur in the immediate postoperative period or within 24 hours after surgery, an overnight hospital stay for observation seems prudent. Routinely elevating the head to an angle of 20° decreases venous pressure in the neck area. Good anesthesia with spontaneous respirations and deep extubation at the end of the procedure will prevent coughing or retching on the endotracheal tube and will decrease the incidence of hematoma.

LARYNGEAL NERVE INJURY

Injury to the superior or recurrent laryngeal nerves during surgical procedures involving the thyroid gland or the parathyroid gland is a very serious complication with a reported incidence of 1.4% to 5.8% (3,4). Stretching, clamping, pinching, or cutting the nerve or using electrocautery near the nerve can cause palsy that may result in voice change, aspiration, and partial airway obstruction due to paralysis of a vocal cord. If both recurrent nerves are damaged, the paralyzed vocal cords may remain permanently in adduction, causing complete airway obstruction and necessitating reintubation and, possibly, tracheostomy.

The best way to prevent this serious complication is to develop a good understanding of the normal anatomic position of these nerves, including variations that are either natural or caused by a slowly growing goiter. In approximately 20% of cases, the external branch of the superior laryngeal nerve extends inferiorly with the superior thyroid artery to a position at which damage is likely to occur when the blood supply to the superior pole of the thyroid is ligated. During resection of a large goiter, meticulous dissection as close as possible to the capsule of the thyroid, followed by clamping and ligation of individual vessels, will help prevent injury to this nerve, which is often not visualized. The right recurrent laryngeal nerve arises from the vagus in the inferior portion of the neck, passes around the innominate artery, and ascends obliquely in the tracheoesophageal groove until it penetrates the larynx at the level of the inferior horn of the thyroid cartilage lateral to Berry's ligament. In 1% of patients, this nerve is nonrecurrent, traversing directly from the vagus (5). The left recurrent laryngeal nerve arises from the vagus, passes behind the aorta at the level of the ligamentum arteriosum, and then ascends, assuming the same trajectory as the right nerve.

The first step in preventing nerve injury is proper identification of the nerve, using blunt dissection without cautery for hemostasis. The gland is lifted from its bed, while all branches of the nerve along its course to the entrance into the larynx are preserved. The recurrent nerve can be identified in several ways depending on the pathological anatomy. One way is to find the inferior thyroid artery and to follow its medial course to the thyroid gland. The disadvantage of finding the nerve in relation to the inferior thyroid artery is that the anatomy can vary; the nerve can be located medial to, lateral to, or between the branches of this vessel, and it often branches before it reaches this area. Another way of identifying the recurrent nerve is to mobilize the inferior pole of the thyroid to find the nerve in the tracheoesophageal groove. This dissection is also useful, but it is somewhat limited in the presence of a large goiter with substernal extension. Recently, some surgeons have advocated nerve stimulation as helpful, but this technique has yet to gain wide acceptance (6). When the nerve has been found, dissection of the gland is continued, but always with good visualization of the nerve in an attempt to avoid trauma to this delicate structure. It is imperative that patients be informed preoperatively about the risk of damage to the laryngeal nerves and about the consequences of such injury. The informed consent process should include a discussion of the risk of this specific complication and of hypocalcemia (see the following section), and such a discussion should be carefully documented in the patient's chart.

HYPOCALCEMIA

Postoperative hypocalcemia can be a serious complication after total thyroidectomy, excessive parathyroidectomy, or parathyroidectomy in a patient with advanced hyperparathyroidism and osteoporosis. Although this complication cannot always be predicted, it must be anticipated and treated as soon as symptoms appear, usually 6 to 16 hours after surgery. Symptoms will include numbness or tingling in the fingers or toes, or paresthesia around the lips. Chvostek's and Trousseau's signs may be useful in making the diagnosis, but symptoms are more important. Treatment should be started early. A precipitous fall in serum calcium concentrations 12 to 16 hours after surgery, or a total serum calcium concentration of less than 8 mg/dL on the morning after surgery, is an indication that calcium supplementation should be instituted. Permanent hypocalcemia occurs in 3.4% to 8.6% of patients after total thyroidectomy (7,8). This complication has been reported to occur in 1% to 30% of patients after parathyroidectomy, depending on the extent of the resection (9–11). Orally administered calcium preparations of 500 mg given two or three times per day may be sufficient to prevent symptoms in patients undergoing parathyroid or thyroid resections, until the portion of the gland that remains responds to the hypocalcemia and regains function. More severe hypocalcemia resulting in frank tetany may occur either temporarily or permanently. In these cases, vitamin D supplementation or intravenously administrated calcium gluconate may be needed.

The best course of action is prevention of postoperative hypocalcemia. Parathyroid glands of normal size should always be preserved. Performing a biopsy of these glands increases the incidence of postoperative hypocalcemia; therefore, biopsy should be performed only when absolutely necessary, for example, to differentiate a normal parathyroid from a metastatic lymph node in a patient with thyroid cancer (11). During parathyroidectomy, the surgeon should never excise any gland of normal size in an attempt to return the patient to normocalcemia. During unilateral thyroidectomy, normal parathyroid glands should not be resected on the basis of an assumption that contralateral thyroid lobectomy will not be necessary in the future.

Preservation of normal parathyroid gland function is helped by a sound knowledge of topographic anatomy. The superior gland is usually found lateral to the recurrent nerve at the level of the suspensory ligament of the thyroid, and the inferior gland is anterior to the recurrent laryngeal nerve and caudal to the location at which this structure crosses the inferior thyroid artery. The position of the inferior glands can vary. Injury to the parathyroid glands can best be avoided by blunt dissection with good visualization and meticulous hemostasis without cautery. During thyroidectomy, most surgeons try to ligate the branches of the inferior thyroid artery directly on the side of the thyroid lobe because the nutrient branch to the parathyroid can often be seen and preserved. If a parathyroid gland is devascularized and appears compromised, excision and autotransplantation of small pieces of the gland into a muscle are recommended (12).

SEROMA AND WOUND INFECTION

Seroma is a common complication after resection of the thyroid or parathyroid gland, but it rarely requires surgical intervention. Fluid usually collects between the skin flaps and the deep cervical fascia. When the collection is large and cosmetically unsightly, aspiration is indicated. Small collections resolve spontaneously within a few weeks and should not be aspirated so that the risk of bacterial contamination can be avoided. Wound infection is unusual in association with these cervical procedures because of the excellent blood supply in this area. Prophylactic antibiotics are not indicated for these clean, uncontaminated endocrine procedures.

FAILURE OF PARATHYROIDECTOMY

Parathyroidectomy is performed to eliminate the excess secretion of parathyroid hormone. Every disease involving the parathyroid glands requires a different type of resection with extirpation of one or more parathyroid glands in an attempt to correct this imbalance. The extent of the resection will determine not only the operative success, but also the incidence of complications. The ideal way to treat parathyroid disease is to excise only abnormal parathyroid glands and to preserve normally functioning glands.

In most large centers, the operative failure rate is reported to range from 1% to 10% for patients with sporadic primary hyperparathyroidism (SPHPT) (13–15). In institutions where parathyroid disease is treated less frequently, the failure rate is reported to be as high as 30% (16). Operative failure is defined as persistent hypercalcemia with high levels of intact parathyroid hormone (iPTH) within six months after parathyroidectomy, or persistent postoperative hypocalcemia from hypoparathyroidism. These complications are caused by either an insufficient or an overzealous parathyroid resection. An insufficient excision can be due to unrecognized multiglandular disease (MGD) or the inability to find and resect a single abnormal gland. On the other hand, postoperative hypoparathyroidism is due to not having enough normal parathyroid tissue left in situ to support eucalcemia. The reported incidence of hypoparathyroidism, after 3.5 glands have been resected to treat parathyroid hyperplasia, ranges from 12% to 24% (9,10). Furthermore, total parathyroidectomy with autotransplantation results in low normal serum calcium levels in 4% to 30% of cases, depending on the cause of the parathyroid disease (10,17). Because of these complications, resection of 3.5 glands should be reserved for patients with four markedly enlarged glands and should not be used to treat patients with "slightly large" parathyroid glands, or those with hyperplasia diagnosed by frozen section histopathologic analysis alone. The limitations of histopathologic analysis in determining single gland or MGD are well known; thus, the results of such analyses should not be used to determine the

extent of parathyroid resection (14,18,19). For patients with single or double adenoma, biopsy of normal glands substantially increases the incidence of postoperative hypocalcemia (11). Because of this risk and the limited benefit of frozen section histopathologic analysis, many surgeons perform bilateral neck exploration to allow visualization of all four glands and perform parathyroidectomy on the basis of gland size alone. However, judging gland abnormality exclusively on the basis of gross appearance may lead to unnecessary parathyroid resection because the size of the gland is not always correlated with its function (20–22).

Two surgical adjuncts are available to help prevent these complications: (i) the quick intraoperative parathyroid hormone assay and (ii) the use of preoperative localization studies. The intraoperative measurement of parathyroid hormone levels predicts the postoperative outcome and assures the surgeon that all hypersecreting tissue has been excised. At the same time, its results show that the remaining glands are not hypersecreting and therefore neither visualization nor biopsy is necessary (23–26). Furthermore, the results of this assay will indicate the presence of additional hypersecreting parathyroid glands after excision of a suspected adenoma and will guide the surgeon to perform further exploration.

Currently, the most sensitive preoperative localization study is the Tc-99m-sestamibi nuclear scan with tomographic imaging. This study is used to locate hyperfunctioning parathyroid glands, including those in an ectopic position, such as in the mediastinum. The benefit of using preoperative localization studies and intraoperative iPTH assays is that patients with SPHPT can be safely treated with unilateral neck exploration that leaves the normally secreting parathyroid glands in situ. This approach, which is associated with an intraoperative localization success rate of 98%, should also decrease the risk of hypocalcemia (23–25).

Finally, a sure diagnosis and clear surgical indications are of utmost importance in obtaining a successful outcome after parathyroidectomy. Primary hyperparathyroidism is diagnosed when patients exhibit persistent hypercalcemia, elevated intact parathyroid hormone levels, normal renal function, and normal or elevated 24-hour urinary calcium levels. The guidelines for operative management of primary hyperparathyroidism have changed as the surgical approaches to this disease have evolved. With a sure diagnosis and strict surgical indications for parathyroidectomy, the operative results will be satisfactory, with a low incidence of complications (27).

REFERENCES

1. Bergamaschi R, Becouarn G, Ronceray J, Arnaud JP. Morbidity of thyroid surgery. Am J Surg 1998; 176:71–75.
2. Shaha AR, Jaffe BM. Practical management of post-thyroidectomy hematoma. J Surg Oncol 1994; 57:235–238.

3. Lo CY, Kwok KF, Yuen PW. Prospective evaluation of recurrent laryngeal nerve paralysis during thyroidectomy. Arch Surg 2000; 135:204–207.

4. Martensson H, Terins J. Recurrent laryngeal nerve palsy in thyroid gland surgery related to operations and nerves at risk. Arch Surg 1985; 120:475–477.

5. Songun I, Kievit J, van de Velde C. Complications of thyroid surgery. In: Clark OH, Duh QY, McGrew L, eds. Textbook of Endocrine Surgery. Philadelphia: W.B. Saunders, 1997:167–173.

6. Djohan RS, Rodriguez HE, Connolly MM, Childers SJ, Braverman B, Podbielski FJ. Intraoperative monitoring of recurrent laryngeal nerve function. Am Surg 2000; 66:595–597.

7. Pederson WC, Johnson CL, Gaskill HV III, Aust JB, Cruz AB Jr. Operative management of thyroid disease. Technical considerations in a residency training program. Am J Surg 1984; 148:350–352.

8. Glinoer D, Andry G, Chantrain G, Samil N. Clinical aspects of early and late hypocalcemia after thyroid surgery. Eur J Surg Oncol 2000; 26:571–577.

9. Burgess JR, David R, Parameswaran V, Greenaway TM, Shepherd JJ. The outcome of subtotal parathyroidectomy for treatment of hyperparathyroidism in multiple endocrine neoplasia type 1. Arch Surg 1998; 133:126–129.

10. Hellman P, Skogseid B, Juhlin C, Akerstrom G, Rastad J. Findings and long-term results of parathyroid surgery in multiple endocrine neoplasia type 1. World J Surg 1992; 16:718–723.

11. Tibblin S, Bizard JP, Bondeson AG, et al. Primary hyperparathyroidism due to solitary adenoma. A comparative multicenter study of early and long-term results of different surgical regimens. Eur J Surg 1991; 157:511–515.

12. Lo CY, Lam KY. Postoperative hypocalcemia in patients who did or did not undergo parathyroid autotransplantation during thyroidectomy: a comparative study. Surgery 1998; 124:1081–1087.

13. Low RA, Katz AD. Parathyroidectomy via bilateral cervical exploration: a retrospective review of 866 cases. Head Neck 1998; 20:583–587.

14. Kaplan EL, Yashiro T, Salti G. Primary hyperparathyroidism in the 1990s. Choice of surgical procedure for this disease. Ann Surg 1992; 215:300–317.

15. van Heerden JA, Grant CS. Surgical treatment of primary hyperparathyroidism: an institutional perspective. World J Surg 1991; 15:688–692.

16. Malmaeus J, Granberg PO, Halvorsen J, Akerstrom G, Johansson H. Parathyroid surgery in Scandinavia. Acta Chir Scand 1988; 154:409–413.

17. Monchik JM, Bendinelli C, Passero MA Jr., Roggin KK. Subcutaneous forearm transplantation of autologous parathyroid tissue in patients with renal hyperparathyroidism. Surgery 1999; 126:1152–1159.

18. Tezelman S, Shen W, Shaver JK, et al. Double parathyroid adenomas. Clinical and biochemical characteristics before and after parathyroidectomy. Ann Surg 1993; 218:300–309.

19. Ghandur-Mnaymneh L, Kimura N. The parathyroid adenoma. A histopathologic definition with a study of 172 cases of primary hyperparathyroidism. Am J Pathol 1984; 115:70–83.

20. Lietchty RD, Teter A, Suba EJ. The tiny parathyroid adenoma. Surgery 1986; 100:1048–1052.

21. Berger AC, Libutti SK, Bartlett DL, et al. Heterogeneous gland size in sporadic multiple gland parathyroid hyperplasia. J Am Coll Surg 1999; 188:382–389.

22. Carneiro DM, Irvin GL III. Late parathyroid function after successful parathyroidectomy guided by intraoperative hormone assay (QPTH) compared with the standard bilateral neck exploration. Surgery 2000; 128:925–936.

23. Sokoll LJ, Drew H, Udelsman R. Intraoperative parathyroid hormone analysis: a study of 200 consecutive cases. Clin Chem 2000; 46:1662–1668.

24. Garner SC, Leight GS Jr. Initial experience with intraoperative PTH determinations in the surgical management of 130 consecutive cases of primary hyperparathyroidism. Surgery 1999; 126:1132–1138.

25. Irvin GL, Carneiro DM. Rapid parathyroid hormone assay guided exploration. In: van Heerden J, Farley DR, eds. Operative Techniques in General Surgery. Philadelphia: W.B. Saunders Company, 1999; 1:18–27.

26. Molinari AS, Irvin GL III, Deriso GT, Bott L. Incidence of multiglandular disease in primary hyperparathyroidism determined by parathyroid hormone secretion. Surgery 1996; 120:934–937.

27. Irvin GL III, Carneiro DM. Management changes in primary hyperparathyroidism. JAMA 2000; 284:934–936.

18

Complications of Adrenal Gland Surgery

James C. Doherty
*Division of Trauma Surgery, Advocate Christ Medical Center, Oak Lawn, and, Department of
Surgery, University of Illinois College of Medicine at Chicago, Chicago, Illinois, U.S.A.*

Hussein Mazloum
*Department of Surgery, McLaren Regional Medical Center and the College of Human
Medicine–Michigan State University, Flint, Michigan, U.S.A.*

Danny Sleeman
*DeWitt Daughtry Family Department of Surgery, Miller School of Medicine, University of
Miami, Miami, Florida, U.S.A.*

*The adrenal glands are paired structures located at the
superior pole of each kidney. Each adrenal gland is composed
of an inner neuroectoderm-derived medulla surrounded by an
outer mesoderm-derived cortex. The cortex is further subdivided into three functionally distinct layers responsible for
the synthesis and release of mineralocorticoids, glucocorticoids, and sex steroid hormone precursors, respectively. The
adrenal medulla is responsible for the production and release
of the catecholamines, epinephrine, and norepinephrine. The
unique anatomic and physiologic features of the adrenal
gland create an interesting set of preoperative, intraoperative,
and postoperative issues that must be addressed if adrenalectomy is to be safely performed.*

INDICATIONS FOR ADRENALECTOMY

When the potential risks of adrenalectomy are
assessed, the first consideration is the specific disease
process requiring surgical intervention. Among the
common adrenal diseases amenable to surgical therapy are a variety of functional and neoplastic disorders. These include nonfunctional adrenocortical
adenoma, functional adrenocortical adenoma, pheochromocytoma, adrenocortical adenocarcinoma, and
adrenal metastases.

Adrenocortical Adenoma

Adrenocortical adenomas are commonly classified as
functional or nonfunctional. Cortical adenomas, especially those of the nonfunctional type, are often called
"adrenal incidentalomas" because they are frequently
detected by abdominal imaging studies performed for
the purpose of diagnosing other conditions.

Nonfunctional Adrenocortical Adenomas

Nonfunctional adrenocortical adenomas are commonly
resected when they are nonfunctional incidentalomas
of a size sufficient to provoke concerns about the potential for malignancy. Although specific size criteria are debatable, it is generally accepted that any
nonfunctional adrenal mass more than 5 cm in diameter, or with an appearance that is atypical for an
adenoma, should be resected. Smaller nonfunctional
lesions should be followed up with serial imaging studies so that the risk of malignancy can be reevaluated.

Functional Adrenocortical Adenomas
Aldosteronoma

Aldosteronomas are aldosterone-secreting adenomas.
The clinical syndrome associated with this lesion is primary hyperaldosteronism; 62% of patients with this
syndrome have a unilateral functional adenoma that
is amenable to surgical therapy (1). The clinical features
of primary hyperaldosteronism are nonspecific and
include hypertension, hypokalemia, polyuria, weakness, and muscle cramping. Some patients exhibit minimal symptoms or have no symptoms at all. Almost all
patients exhibit suppressed plasma renin activity.

Cortisol-Producing Adenomas

Cortisol-producing adenomas are often associated
with Cushing's syndrome, a clinical syndrome that
includes hypertension, truncal obesity, muscle wasting, diabetes mellitus, and, occasionally, psychological
disturbance. Cortisol-producing adenomas can also
be present without overt signs of hypercortisolism.
Key to the workup of the patient with signs and
symptoms of excess cortisol production is the

determination whether the hypercortisolism is primary (Cushing's syndrome) or secondary to an adrenocorticotrophic hormone (ACTH)–producing pituitary tumor (Cushing's disease). Although 24-hour urinary cortisol excretion studies can suggest a high cortisol state, a dexamethasone suppression test is necessary to confirm the cause of the hypercortisolism. Low plasma ACTH activity in association with a plasma cortisol level that cannot be suppressed by the administration of dexamethasone is consistent with the diagnosis of primary hypercortisolism.

Although Cushing's disease is usually managed with transsphenoidal hypophysectomy, total bilateral adrenalectomy can be indicated under some circumstances. Among these are persistent or severe diseases after hypophysectomy, or contraindications to hypophysectomy, such as the desire to preserve fertility. When performed for this indication, total bilateral adrenalectomy has a cure rate approaching 100% (2).

Pheochromocytoma

Pheochromocytoma is a tumor of the adrenal medulla and of other sympathetic ganglion cells of the peripheral nervous system. Approximately 10% of these tumors are malignant, 10% are bilateral, 10% are familial, and 10% are extra-adrenal. The symptoms caused by these tumors fall into three general groups. One-third of patients with these tumors experience an episode of palpitations, diaphoresis, headache, and a "feeling of impending doom." An additional one-third of patients exhibit normotension with transient symptomatic episodes in conjunction with episodic hypertension. The remaining one-third of these patients exhibit asymptomatic chronic hypertension, which is often misdiagnosed as essential hypertension. Diagnostic testing includes determination of plasma and urinary catecholamine levels, as well as urinary levels of catecholamine degradation products (metanephrines and vanillylmandelic acid). The location of the tumors is determined by computed tomography (CT) or magnetic resonance imaging (MRI) scans of the abdomen, or by 131-iodine metaiodobenzylguanidine (^{131}I-MIBG) scanning when necessary.

Adrenocortical Adenocarcinoma

Adrenocortical adenocarcinoma is a rare tumor often first detected as a large, advanced-stage lesion. Imaging methods such as CT and MRI scans can be very useful in determining the extent of disease preoperatively. Half of these tumors are functional, with clinical evidence of cortisol or androgen excess. Complete surgical resection of adrenocortical adenocarcinoma is the only potentially curative therapy and can substantially palliate the signs and symptoms associated with functional tumors. Initial complete resection is possible in approximately 75% of cases, but recurrent disease develops after 85% of these procedures, with a mean disease-free interval of 2.5 years (3). Reoperation provides a substantially better survival rate than drug therapy.

Adrenal Metastases

Lung, breast, and renal cell carcinomas often metastasize to the adrenal glands. Like nonfunctional adrenocortical adenomas, these tumors sometimes are resected as large incidentalomas that have been diagnosed radiographically. On the other hand, the adrenal mass known to be a metastatic lesion may also be resected for cure under certain circumstances, namely favorable histologic type and the absence of extra-adrenal malignant disease. In clinical practice, these circumstances rarely occur and are an extremely rare indication for adrenalectomy.

ENDOCRINE AND METABOLIC COMPLICATIONS OF ADRENALECTOMY

As can be inferred from the preceding section, adrenalectomy is performed for a variety of indications. Furthermore, the hormonal milieu in which the procedure is performed varies considerably, depending on the underlying adrenal disease process. A number of potential perioperative complications of adrenalectomy arise directly from these endocrinologic factors.

Complications of Adrenalectomy for Hypercortisolism

Patients with hypercortisolism may experience poorly controlled diabetes mellitus before surgery. Glucose levels must be carefully monitored and aggressively treated during the perioperative period so that patients can avoid the complications of hypoglycemia, diabetic ketoacidosis, and poor wound healing. As is true for any elective surgical procedure, adrenalectomy should be delayed until altered potassium metabolism and hypertension have been corrected, so that the complications of anesthesia can be minimized. In severe cases, therapy with the adrenolytic agent mitotane or with steroidogenesis inhibitors such as metyrapone, aminoglutethimide, or ketoconazole may be necessary to control the metabolic derangements of hypercortisolism preoperatively (4).

The obesity associated with Cushing's syndrome and Cushing's disease exposes the patient to substantial risk of a variety of complications, including poor wound healing, wound infection, and respiratory complications. Central obesity may complicate mechanical ventilation, and all patients should be aggressively treated postoperatively so that hypoxemia can be limited or reversed. This treatment usually involves early ambulation and incentive spirometry, measures designed to recover functional residual capacity and reverse alveolar collapse. Patients with hypercortisolism often have thin, easily bruised skin and are susceptible to skin breakdown. Care must be taken to pad all pressure points during the surgical procedure and to aggressively monitor skin integrity postoperatively. Thin skin and vascular fragility may also complicate the establishment of durable intravenous access. In the operating room, patients should be positioned with great care so that pathologic fractures can be prevented because osteopenia is common. Fasciculations related to depolarizing paralytic agents should be minimized for the same reason.

Patients undergoing adrenalectomy for hypercortisolism are at high risk of postoperative adrenal insufficiency. Although the cause of adrenal insufficiency after bilateral adrenalectomy is obvious, the cause is more complicated after unilateral adrenalectomy. A chronic state of cortisol excess induces functional suppression and atrophy of the contralateral gland and chronic suppression of the entire pituitary–adrenal axis. The abrupt withdrawal of cortisol that accompanies adrenalectomy among these patients can cause acute adrenal insufficiency. So that this potentially life-threatening complication can be prevented, all patients undergoing unilateral adrenalectomy for hypercortisolism, or bilateral adrenalectomy, should be given supplemental steroids perioperatively.

No clear recommendations for perioperative glucocorticoid dosing exist for adrenalectomy per se, but in general, one should assume complete adrenal insufficiency postoperatively and a low to moderate degree of surgical stress. When the most recent recommendations for perioperative corticosteroid management are followed, the glucocorticoid target would probably be 50 to 60 mg of hydrocortisone per day on the day of surgery and for the first 24 hours of the postoperative period (5). This dose can be rapidly tapered to a maintenance dosage of approximately 25 mg of hydrocortisone equivalent (usually oral prednisone) daily, given in two divided doses. The daily dose may be decreased to 20 or even 15 mg as tolerated, with adjustment based on the presence of any symptoms of adrenal insufficiency. Function of the pituitary–adrenal axis can be monitored postoperatively by using periodic ACTH stimulation tests. The usual timeframe for normalization of adrenal function is 12 to 24 months. Adrenal autotransplantation has been attempted for the purpose of avoiding the necessity for long-term adrenal replacement therapy after bilateral adrenalectomy, but only 21% of the patients who underwent this procedure were successfully weaned from steroid therapy. Thus, the procedure is generally not recommended (6).

All patients subjected to adrenal replacement therapy should be carefully monitored for clinical signs and symptoms of steroid imbalance. One such sign is the previously mentioned syndrome of adrenal insufficiency, also known as Addison's disease. Chronic adrenal insufficiency after adrenalectomy is characterized by hypotension, hyponatremia, hypoglycemia, fever, and a variety of constitutional symptoms, including weakness, fatigue, weight loss, and anorexia. This weakness may contribute to difficulty in weaning patients with respiratory insufficiency from mechanical ventilation. When the condition of patients with chronic adrenal insufficiency has stabilized, steroid replacement therapy can be started at physiologic doses. For severe acute adrenal insufficiency (Addisonian crisis), hydrocortisone should be given as an initial intravenously administered bolus of 100 mg followed by intravenous administration of 100 to 200 mg over the next 24 hours. Important adjunctive therapy includes aggressive volume expansion with isotonic fluids and treatment of hypoglycemia. Once the patient's condition has stabilized, hydrocortisone dosages can be tapered and maintenance therapy can be instituted.

If a patient receiving chronic steroid replacement therapy requires surgical intervention, careful perioperative glucocorticoid management is essential to the prevention of postoperative adrenal insufficiency. Although "stress dose" perioperative steroid dosing has enjoyed widespread use since the 1950s, this approach has been challenged during the last decade as anecdotal and without scientific justification. Currently, it is recommended that adjustment in perioperative steroid dosing should be based on consideration of the maintenance steroid dose, the duration of steroid therapy, and the extent of the anticipated surgery (5). High doses of corticosteroid, as were commonly given in the past, are rarely necessary.

Recurrent hypercortisolism after adrenalectomy usually indicates residual abnormally functioning adrenal tissue. For nonmalignant adenomas, this condition indicates incomplete resection or failure to diagnose bilateral disease. In the case of adrenalectomy for adrenocortical adenocarcinoma, postoperative hypercortisolism mandates a workup for recurrent tumor or metastatic disease.

A unique complication of bilateral adrenalectomy performed for Cushing's disease is the development of a symptomatic ACTH-secreting pituitary tumor. These tumors are often rapidly growing and can exhibit characteristics of a malignancy. The associated clinical syndrome, known as Nelson's syndrome, is characterized by hyperpigmentation, headache, and visual changes. In one study, this complication occurred in 9% of cases at a median of 9.5 years after the original operation (7). Treatment options include hypophysectomy and irradiation.

Complications of Adrenalectomy for Hyperaldosteronism

Like patients with hypercortisolism, patients with hyperaldosteronism are often first seen with poorly controlled hypertension and metabolic derangements. If inadequately addressed preoperatively, these abnormalities can substantially increase the patient's anesthetic risk. The hypertension associated with primary hyperaldosteronism is salt- and water-dependent and responds well to salt and water depletion. For this reason, several authors recommend two to four weeks of pharmacologic therapy before adrenalectomy for hyperaldosteronism. Combination diuretic therapy with either hydrochlorothiazide or furosemide and either spironolactone or amiloride has been suggested as an appropriate medical approach to primary hyperaldosteronism (8).

Although the hypokalemia associated with hyperaldosteronism is almost always cured by adrenalectomy, the hypertension associated with primary hyperaldosteronism often does respond to surgical therapy. In fact, only 60% to 80% of patients with unilateral benign disease are cured by unilateral adrenalectomy (9,10). The cure rate appears to be higher among patients less than 44 years of age, those whose hypertension responds to spironolactone administration preoperatively, those with hypertension of less than five years' duration before resection, and those whose resected adrenal gland does not demonstrate multinodular disease (11).

Although uncommon in clinical practice, mineralocorticoid deficiency can occasionally occur after adrenalectomy for hyperaldosteronism. This condition is characterized by salt wasting, hyponatremia, and hyperkalemia. Symptoms are usually easily controlled with saline administration and mineralocorticoid replacement with fludrocortisone, and such therapy rarely is required for more than three months postoperatively.

Complications of Adrenalectomy for Pheochromocytoma

The functional nature of pheochromocytoma presents a unique challenge to the surgical team in all phases of perioperative care. Hypertensive crisis, atrial and ventricular arrhythmia, myocardial infarction, cerebrovascular accident, acute congestive heart failure, and pulmonary edema are some of the serious and potentially life-threatening cardiovascular complications associated with resection of these catecholamine-producing tumors. To minimize the risk of these complications, all patients are treated with a combination of antiadrenergic and vasodilatory agents during the perioperative period. Treatment begins with alpha-adrenergic blockade with 30 to 60 mg of phenoxybenzamine daily for at least one week preoperatively. The alpha-blockade is initiated at a low dosage and is increased as needed to control blood pressure. Symptoms such as dizziness and abdominal cramps often accompany the establishment of adequate alpha-blockade. Other antihypertensive agents, including calcium channel blockers and angiotensin-converting enzyme inhibitors, may be added. When hypertension is difficult to control, metyrosine, a tyrosine hydroxylase inhibitor, may also be added. Beta-adrenergic blockade with drugs such as propanolol or atenolol is often necessary for treating tachycardia, but beta-blockers should only be given after initiation of alpha blockade. In the absence of adequate alpha blockade, beta-blockers can induce unopposed vasoconstriction, which can precipitate an acute hypertensive crisis. Another potential drawback of preoperative beta-blockade is that it may cause the body to lose the ability to compensate for episodes of hypotension by developing tachycardia; this loss may complicate blood pressure management. In addition to pharmacologic therapy, all patients are treated with aggressive volume loading before surgery so that intravascular volume status can be optimized.

Even with effective preoperative pharmacotherapy, substantial hemodynamic changes can occur intraoperatively. So that the risk of adverse cardiovascular events related to systemic catecholamine release from the tumor can be minimized, tumor manipulation should be minimized, and the tumor's venous drainage should be controlled and ligated expeditiously. So that changes in hemodynamics can be detected, all patients should undergo invasive arterial blood pressure monitoring, and central venous access should be strongly considered. Acute hypertension during adrenalectomy for pheochromocytoma is best managed with intravenous infusion of sodium nitroprusside. Tachycardia can be effectively managed with intravenously administered beta-blocking agents such as labetalol or esmolol. Again, aggressive fluid resuscitation should be standard for all patients.

Postoperatively, a stay on the intensive care unit may be necessary to ensure adequate hemodynamic monitoring and access to the nursing care and pharmacologic therapy needed for the management of any hemodynamic instability. Loss of adrenergic stimulation can cause hypotension, which can be exacerbated by preoperative beta-blockade. The hypotension can last for several days and is treated with aggressive intravascular volume expansion. In some cases, an alpha-adrenergic agonist may be necessary so that normal blood pressure can be maintained. Patients are slowly weaned from beta-blockade over the first postoperative week so that reflex tachycardia can be avoided.

A relatively uncommon postoperative complication of adrenalectomy for pheochromocytoma is acute hypoglycemia, which occurs in approximately 13% of cases (12). One mechanism proposed as an explanation for this phenomenon is a catecholamine-mediated suppression of endogenous insulin secretion. According to this theory, upon removal of the tumor, excessive rebound secretion of insulin can occur and can result in acute hypoglycemia that often requires an infusion of dextrose. An alternative theory attributes postoperative hypoglycemia to a combination of chronically depleted glycogen stores, chronically reduced sensitivity to catecholamine, and high circulating insulin levels. Regardless of the cause of acute hypoglycemia, blood glucose levels should be closely monitored postoperatively and treatment should be initiated when necessary.

All patients who undergo resection of pheochromocytoma should be carefully monitored for hypertension. Persistent or recurrent hypertension after adrenalectomy raises suspicion of recurrent or residual functional disease. Recurrence rates of malignant disease after adrenalectomy for pheochromocytoma (malignant and benign) have been reported to be as high as 23% (13). Clinical investigation, including biochemical studies and ^{131}I-MIBG scanning, should be performed so that the diagnosis can be confirmed and the disease localized.

Pheochromocytoma is rare among pregnant women, but many of the symptoms of pheochromocytoma (e.g., hypertension, diaphoresis, and nausea) are also seen in association with preeclampsia. Misdiagnosis of the condition can have fatal consequences. The risk of hypertensive crisis makes labor and delivery extremely dangerous for pregnant patients with pheochromocytoma. Maternal mortality rates as high as 40% to 58% and fetal mortality rates of 10% to 56% have been reported (14). During the first trimester, women who do not desire to terminate the pregnancy can be treated medically and resection can be delayed until the second trimester. During the third trimester, medical management should be used and elective Cesarean section should be performed at term. Adrenalectomy can be performed immediately after Cesarean section or at a later date.

TECHNICAL COMPLICATIONS OF ADRENALECTOMY

Unlike the endocrine complications of adrenalectomy, the technical complications are less dependent on the underlying disease than they are on anatomical factors such as size and location. The exception to this rule is adrenocortical carcinoma because the malignant nature of the disease can substantially affect both the extent of resection and the operative approach, factors known to contribute to perioperative complications. Preoperative imaging studies (CT and MRI scans) are extremely important sources of anatomical information about patients undergoing elective adrenalectomy. These studies provide crucial information about tumor size, location, and extent of local invasion, information that strongly influences the choice of operative approach. Ideally, the chosen approach to adrenalectomy should be the one that allows the most effective treatment of the adrenal pathologic state (neoplasm or endocrinopathy), but subjects the patient to the fewest potential complications. A variety of operative approaches are available to the surgeon. Those approaches and the relative advantages and disadvantages of each are listed below.

Transabdominal or Anterior Approach

The earliest approach developed for adrenalectomy, the transabdominal or anterior approach, allows the surgeon to perform a thorough exploration of the entire peritoneal cavity via either a midline or a subcostal incision. Because of the optimal exposure that it affords, this approach is preferred when bilateral or extra-adrenal disease is suspected. Furthermore, in cases of bulky or invasive adrenocortical carcinomas, this method provides excellent exposure of the surrounding organs, thus allowing the surgeon to perform en bloc resection if necessary.

Because of the different anatomic relationships of the right and left adrenal glands, the technique of adrenalectomy and the structures that can be injured differ, depending on which gland is being addressed surgically (15). The right gland sits atop the right kidney posterior to the inferior vena cava (IVC), with its anterior aspect in close proximity to the lateral border of the IVC. The right gland lies anterior to the diaphragm and posterior and inferior to the right lobe of the liver. The right adrenal vein is short and empties directly into the posterior aspect of the IVC. The vein must be dissected with great care so that caval injury and associated massive blood loss can be avoided. The potential for injury to the IVC can be reduced by dissecting the IVC away from the adrenal gland rather than by inferolateral retraction of the adrenal to expose the IVC. Exposure of the right adrenal gland requires mobilization of the hepatic flexure of the colon, retraction of the right lobe of the liver, and mobilization of the duodenum via a Kocher maneuver. When wider exposure of the right adrenal gland is necessary, complete mobilization of the right hepatic lobe may be necessary. This technique requires division of the falciform and right triangular ligaments, and dissection of the bare area of the liver from the diaphragm, thus allowing medial retraction of the entire right lobe (16). This technique may obviate the need for the more morbid thoracoabdominal approach traditionally necessary for large en bloc resections.

The left adrenal gland sits atop the left kidney posterior to the stomach and pancreas and lateral to the aorta and the left crus of the diaphragm. The left adrenal vein is long and drains into the inferior phrenic vein, which courses downward and empties into the left renal vein. Care must be taken to avoid injury to the renal vessels when vascular control of the left adrenal vein is obtained. Exposure of the left adrenal gland requires entry into the lesser sac by division of the gastrocolic omentum, mobilization and cephalad retraction of the pancreatic body, and, occasionally, mobilization and medial rotation of the spleen and distal pancreas.

As one might expect, injuries to each of the structures mobilized in the exposure of the right and left adrenal glands have been reported. In addition to the IVC, the structures that may be injured are the liver, the pancreas, the spleen, and the duodenum, as well as the renal artery, the ureter, the diaphragm, and the pneumothorax. The anterior approach also carries the added operative morbidity associated with violation of the peritoneal cavity and extensive manipulation of the bowel. These complications include ileus, small bowel obstruction, wound infection, and incisional hernia. As is true of any surgical procedure involving the upper abdomen and specifically the subphrenic area, the transabdominal approach is also associated with respiratory complications, including pneumonia and atelectasis. In general, the mortality rate is low (<1%), and the incidence rates of these complications are similarly low (<5%).

Thoracoabdominal Approach

The thoracoabdominal approach provides the best exposure of the adrenal gland. Because it requires entry into both the peritoneal cavity and the pleural cavity, this approach generally is reserved for technically challenging recurrent tumors, very large tumors (10–15 cm), and bulky tumors requiring en bloc resection of the adrenal glands and adjacent organs. The obvious disadvantage of this approach is the extensive operative trauma that it involves. The patient is exposed not only to the morbidity associated with the transabdominal approach, but also to that associated with thoracic exploration. Moreover, the positioning required for this approach greatly limits access to the contralateral adrenal gland and may preclude exploration for bilateral disease.

Posterior Approach

The posterior approach, developed as an alternative to the anterior approach, avoids the morbidity associated with entering the peritoneal cavity. It has been associated with better pain control, fewer wound complications, shorter recovery time, and a reduction in respiratory complications (17). Furthermore, when the posterior approach is used rather than the anterior approach, intraoperative factors such as operative time, intraoperative blood loss, and pancreatic and splenic injury rates are reduced. The disadvantages of the posterior approach are that it does not allow exploration of the abdomen for bilateral or extra-adrenal disease and that it may be inadequate for removal of large tumors. Inadvertent peritoneotomy or pleurotomy can occur when this approach is used, but these injuries are easily repaired primarily at the time of operation. Airtight closure of a pleurotomy can be accomplished with aspiration of air from the pleural cavity under conditions of positive-pressure lung expansion. Tube thoracostomy is rarely necessary. Control of the adrenal vein can be difficult when the posterior approach is used, especially when the procedure is performed on the right adrenal gland. If substantial hemorrhage occurs, packing and emergent repositioning for laparotomy may be necessary. In general, the posterior approach is best for small, unilateral benign tumors.

Lateral Approach

Like the posterior approach, the lateral approach has the advantage of avoiding entry into the peritoneal cavity. However, the exposure it provides is superior to that provided by the posterior approach, especially for obese patients. The lateral approach also allows easier vascular control and removal of larger tumors. Like the posterior approach, the lateral approach does not provide adequate exposure for the assessment of bilateral and extra-adrenal tissue. Postoperative pain can be a significant issue, and recovery time is longer than that associated with the posterior approach. Frequently, resection of the 12th rib is necessary, and postoperative pain can be avoided by sparing the 12th intercostal nerve.

Laparoscopic Adrenalectomy

In recent years, technologic innovations and the expansion of laparoscopic knowledge and experience have broadened the indications for laparoscopic adrenalectomy to include a variety of adrenal lesions. Currently, laparoscopic adrenalectomy is the procedure of choice for resecting most functional adrenal tumors. Laparoscopic adrenalectomy has been associated with less postoperative pain, shorter hospital stay, less blood loss, fewer wound complications and incisional hernias, and faster recovery time than the various open approaches (18–22). The upper size limit of tumors that can be resected laparoscopically depends upon the surgical technique employed, the tumor type, and the relative experience of the surgeon. The laparoscopic approach generally is not recommended for lesions known to be malignant or for lesions more than 8 to 10 cm in diameter because such tumors can be technically difficult to remove and may require en bloc resection. Although previously viewed as controversial, laparoscopic adrenalectomy for pheochromocytoma now appears quite safe and has become a common surgical approach. Furthermore, intraoperative increases in catecholamine levels have been shown to be lower with the laparoscopic approach, a finding suggesting that this approach may be safer than open approaches (23).

Transperitoneal Laparoscopic Adrenalectomy

Like the open lateral approach, the transperitoneal laparoscopic approach is performed with the patient in the lateral decubitus position. However, unlike the open lateral approach, this approach involves entry into the peritoneal cavity and exposure of the left or right adrenal gland. When the procedure is performed on the right adrenal gland, the triangular ligament is dissected, thus mobilizing the right liver for medial retraction and exposure of the adrenal gland. When the procedure is performed on the left adrenal gland, the splenorenal attachment is dissected laterally and the spleen and pancreas are retracted medially to expose the adrenal gland. When left and right adrenalectomy is performed, vascular control is obtained with laparoscopic clips, and an endobag is employed so that the gland can be removed without tumor spillage. The organs that can be injured with this approach are essentially the same as those mentioned previously with respect to the open anterior approach. Complications are relatively minor, with complication rates ranging from 2% to 12%. Conversion from laparoscopic surgery to open laparotomy has been reported to occur in 0% to 14% of cases; hemorrhage is the most common indication (18–22). Operative mortality rates are less than 1%. In several cases, tumor recurrence has occurred after this technique was used for resection of malignant adrenal tumors. As a result, the transperitoneal laparoscopic approach is contraindicated when malignant disease is known to be present or is suspected.

One complication specific to the laparoscopic approach is the occasional difficulty experienced in finding small lesions on the left side. Small adrenal tumors may be indistinguishable from surrounding structures such as pancreas, Gerota's fascia, and retroperitoneal fat. When the laparoscopic approach is used, the ability to perform manual palpation is lost, and small adrenal tumors can be difficult to identify with laparoscopic visualization alone. In such circumstances, laparoscopic ultrasound can be a valuable tool for intraoperative localization.

Posterior Laparoscopic Adrenalectomy

Like the open posterior approach, the posterior laparoscopic approach is performed with the patient in the prone position, and the dissection is carried out entirely in the retroperitoneum. So that exposure can be facilitated, the retroperitoneal space is expanded with a balloon dissector and laparoscopic ultrasonography is used to assist in localization. The overall complication rate for this approach is 10% to 11% (24,25). Intraoperative complication rates are negligible. One unique postoperative complication that has been reported is self-limiting unilateral nerve root pain related to trocar placement (24). The incidence of peritoneal tears, as high as 33% in one study, appears to correlate with the experience level of the surgeon (25). These injuries are easily repaired via the laparoscope and rarely require conversion to open surgery. Conversion to open laparotomy is a relatively uncommon event (4.5%) (25).

CONCLUSION

Adrenalectomy offers the surgeon a unique combination of technical and physiologic challenges. Knowledge and consideration of these issues are essential to the avoidance of complications during the preoperative, intraoperative, and postoperative treatment of patients who undergo this procedure. When the surgeon is experienced and knowledgeable, adrenalectomy can be safe and effective for most patients.

REFERENCES

1. Doppman JL, Gill JR Jr, Miller DL, et al. Distinction between hyperaldosteronism due to bilateral hyperplasia and unilateral aldosteronoma: reliability of CT. Radiology 1992; 184:677–682.
2. Welbourn RB. Survival and causes of death after adrenalectomy for Cushing's disease. Surgery 1985; 97(1):16–20.
3. Pommier RF, Brennan MF. An eleven-year experience with adrenocortical carcinoma. Surgery 1992; 112(6): 963–971.
4. Sonino N, Boscaro M. Medical therapy for Cushing's disease. Endocrinol Metab Clin North Am 1999; 28(1): 211–222.
5. Salem M, Tanish RE Jr, Bromberg J, Loriaux DL, Chernow B. Perioperative glucocorticoid coverage. A reassessment 42 years after emergence of a problem. Ann Surg 1994; 219(4):416–425.
6. Demeter JG, De Jong SA, Brooks MH, Lawrence AM, Paloyan E. Long-term results of adrenal autotransplantation in Cushing's disease. Surgery 1990; 108:1117–1123.
7. Grabner P, Hauer-Jensen M, Jervell J, Flatmark A. Long-term results of treatment of Cushing's disease by adrenalectomy. Eur J Surg 1991; 157:461–464.
8. Bravo EL. Primary aldosteronism. Issues in diagnosis and management. Endocrinol Metab Clin North Am 1994; 23(2):271–283.
9. Lim RC, Nakayama DK, Biglieri EG, Schambelan M, Hunt TK. Primary aldosteronism: changing concepts in diagnosis and management. Am J Surg 1986; 152:116–121.
10. Favia G, Lumachi F, Scarpa V, D'Amico DF. Adrenalectomy in primary aldosteronism: a long-term follow-up study in 52 patients. World J Surg 1992; 16(4):680–684.
11. Celen O, O'Brien MJ, Melby JC, Beazley RM. Factors influencing outcome of surgery for primary aldosteronism. Arch Surg 1996; 131:646–650.
12. Akiba M, Kodama T, Ito Y, Obara T, Fujimoto Y. Hypoglycemia induced by excessive rebound secretion of insulin after removal of pheochromocytoma. World J Surg 1990; 14(3):317–324.
13. Scott HW Jr, Halter SA. Oncologic aspects of pheochromocytoma: the importance of follow-up. Surgery 1984; 96(1):1061–1066.
14. Ellison GT, Mansberger JA, Mansberger AR Jr. Malignant recurrent pheochromocytoma during pregnancy: case report and review of the literature. Surgery 1988; 103(4):484–489.
15. Avisse C, Marcus C, Patey M, Ladam-Marcus V, Delattre JF, Flament JB. Surgical anatomy and embryology of the adrenal glands. Surg Clin North Am 2000; 80(1):403–415.
16. Prinz RA. Mobilization of the right lobe of the liver for right adrenalectomy. Am J Surg 1990; 159:336–338.
17. Russell CF, Hamberger B, van Heerden JA, Edis AJ, Ilstrup DM. Adrenalectomy: anterior or posterior approach. Am J Surg 1982; 144:322–324.
18. Gagner M, Pomp A, Heniford BT, Pharand D, Lacroix A. Laparoscopic adrenalectomy: lessons learned from 100 consecutive procedures. Ann Surg 1997; 226:238–247.
19. Rutherford JC, Stowasser M, Tunny TJ, Klemm SA, Gordon RD. Laparoscopic adrenalectomy. World J Surg 1996; 20:758–761.
20. Thompson GB, Grant CS, van Heerden JA, et al. Laparoscopic versus open posterior adrenalectomy: a case-control study of 100 patients. Surgery 1997; 122:1132–1136.
21. Walz MK, Peitgen K, Hoermann R, Giebler RM, Mann K, Eigler FW. Posterior retroperitoneoscopy as a new minimally invasive approach for adrenalectomy: results of 30 adrenalectomies in 27 patients. World J Surg 1996; 20:769–774.
22. Brunt LM, Doherty GM, Norton JA, Soper NJ, Quasebarth MA, Moley FJ. Laparoscopic adrenalectomy compared to open adrenalectomy for benign adrenal neoplasms. J Am Coll Surg 1996; 183:1–10.
23. Fernandez-Cruz L, Taura P, Saenz A, Benarroch G, Sabater L. Laparoscopic approach to pheochromocytoma: hemodynamic changes and catecholamine secretion. World J Surg 1996; 20(7):762–768.
24. Siperstein AE, Berber E, Engle KL, Duh QY, Clark OH. Laparoscopic posterior adrenalectomy: technical considerations. Arch Surg 2000; 135:967–971.
25. Bonjer HJ, Sorm V, Berends FJ, et al. Endoscopic retroperitoneal adrenalectomy: lessons learned from 111 consecutive cases. Ann Surg 2000; 232(6):796–803.

19

Complications Associated with Surgery for Enteropancreatic Neuroendocrine Tumors

Kenji Inaba and Stephen Brower

Department of Surgery, University of Miami Miller School of Medicine, Miami, Florida, U.S.A.

The islet cells of the pancreas, like all other neuroendocrine cells, are designed to produce peptide hormones for systemic release (1,2). Islet cell tumors may be benign or malignant, similar in this manner to tumors derived from other amine precursor uptake decarboxylase cells, such as the thyroid C cells and adrenal medullary cells. Islet cell tumors produce and release hormones in an unregulated manner, causing unique hormone syndromes. Insulinoma is the most common islet cell tumor, followed by gastrinomas, but all islet cell tumors are rare. Functional islet cell tumors of other types occur much less commonly, and individual series are few and limited. Most islet cell tumors produce one or more peptide hormones, although nonfunctional islet cell tumors have been described. This aids diagnosis and provides tumor markers for follow-up surveillance.

The postoperative outcomes for islet cell tumors are reported in large series of patients from centers with special expertise in this type of surgery (3–6). An understanding of the technical aspects of enteroduodenal–pancreatic surgery for neuroendocrine tumors of the pancreas and of the complications associated with this surgery would not have been possible without the contributions of these centers.

The approach to the diagnosis and treatment of islet cell tumors of the pancreas is different from that of the more common, but also more pernicious, pancreatic adenocarcinomas. Islet cell tumors are associated with unique hormone syndromes and with multiple endocrine neoplasia, are found in unique and multicentric locations, are usually benign, and generally have a good overall prognosis, even if malignant. Therefore, the treatment of these tumors requires special diagnostic methods and specific technical skills. Minimally invasive surgery may be appropriate for the surgical treatment of these tumors and may help in reducing complications.

This chapter will concentrate on the surgical procedures used to treat insulinoma, gastrinoma, and the associated complications, and on nonfunctioning islet tumors. The primary cause of complications associated with the treatment of these rare tumors is incorrect diagnosis, resulting in incorrect treatment.

INSULINOMA

Detecting the aggregate signs and symptoms of insulinoma-caused hypoglycemia is the most important step in establishing the diagnosis and directing treatment. Patients with insulinoma exhibit one of two primary groups of symptoms: neurologic symptoms and the autonomic nervous system response. The most common cause of symptoms is neuroglycopenia; the second is the catecholamine response. The neurologic symptoms are generalized but may, on occasion, be focal (such as seizure) or may simulate a cerebrovascular accident. The release of catecholamines produces symptoms of tremor, sweating, warmth, anxiety, and palpitations. These symptoms are commonly experienced in the morning before breakfast, but can also be provoked by exercise.

A delay in diagnosis is the first potential complication of insulinoma. Whipple's triad of hypoglycemia, a plasma glucose concentration of less than 50 mg/dL, and relief of symptoms with administration of glucose is fundamental for a correct diagnosis. Insulinoma must be included in the differential diagnosis when patients exhibit these symptoms. Various studies have suggested that diagnosis may be delayed for a period ranging from 15 months to 3 years. In one series, the mean time to diagnosis was four years; one unfortunate patient suffered for 52 years before curative resection (7,8).

Before a planned surgical resection is performed, the diagnosis must be confirmed by the following criteria: (i) serum glucose concentration below 40 mg/dL, (ii) elevated insulin levels of 6 μU/mL, (iii) elevated C-peptide levels, and (iv) an absence of sulfonylurea in the plasma. Because there are many other causes of hypoglycemia, the diagnosis of insulinoma must be thorough. Confusing another cause of hypoglycemia with an insulinoma leads to the largest cause of complications in islet cell surgery.

Complications Associated with Localization

Localization of insulinoma has attracted as much attention as any other aspect of surgery for these tumors. The complication of a missed localization of insulinoma leads to a surgical misadventure that in all probability will involve a second and more complicated procedure. Because most insulinomas are located in the pancreas, imaging of the pancreas is helpful. Some surgeons advocate avoiding all preoperative imaging and note that a high percentage of insulinomas can be identified intraoperatively by an experienced endocrine surgeon. However, the rate of incorrect localization of insulinoma is as high as 27% in several series (9).

Many preoperative localization methods can be used but carry a wide range of accuracy. These methods include transabdominal ultrasonography, spiral computed tomography (CT) scan, portal venous sampling, angiography, and magnetic resonance imaging (MRI). Intraoperative localization techniques include laparoscopy, laparoscopic ultrasonography, intraoperative open ultrasonography, and palpation. These tests should be tailored to the specific clinical case, the experience of the surgeon, the experience of the radiologist, and the cost and availability of the procedure. The most effective method is based on the specific success at a particular institution. The Mayo Clinic has achieved a positive predictive value of 89% and a cure rate of 97.2% when patients with insulinoma undergo preoperative ultrasonography (10).

Surgical Considerations and Complications

The standard approach to insulinoma during open resection involves generous exposure of the entire gland before removal of the actual tumor. The pancreatic head is mobilized via the Kocher maneuver, and the duodenum is dissected to the mesenteric vessels to expose the uncinate process. The body and tail are mobilized by incising the peritoneum along the inferior border of the pancreas and then gently dissecting along the posterior aspect to the hilum of the spleen. The vasa brevia are ligated, the spleen and tail are mobilized, and the entire tail is delivered into the surgical field from the left upper quadrant. Usually the tumors are found underlying the rim of normal pancreas. Although bimanual palpation is often successful in detecting these tumors, intraoperative ultrasonography (IOUS) is useful as well. IOUS identifies the pancreatic duct and other relevant structures, thus avoiding injury to the pancreatic duct or the splenoportal veins. In this way, the surgeon can decide whether resection or enucleation should be performed.

Enucleation of the tumor is the standard method of treatment for most insulinomas. These tumors have a pseudocapsule unless the tumor is malignant. A clear dissection plane can usually be developed between the tumor and the pancreatic parenchyma. After the tumor has been enucleated, the operative bed should not be disturbed or should be injected with fibrin glue so as to avoid damage to the normal surrounding pancreas tissue.

A Whipple operation is rarely used to treat a benign insulinoma located in the head of the pancreas. Extensive surgery may be required in the circumstance of multiple endocrine neoplasia type 1 (MEN-1) syndrome in which hypoglycemia is the prominent symptom and multiple neuroendocrine tumors are present throughout the gland.

Complications of Surgery

The morbidity rate (10% to 15%) and the mortality rate (1% to 2%) associated with a major pancreatic resection have been greatly reduced over the last decade (3,11,12). The complications most difficult to manage after surgery are pancreatic fistulae; these fistulae are suspected in cases of high postoperative drainage of amylase. This complication is managed with nonoperative control of the fistula, replacement of lost fluid and electrolytes, and adequate nutrition, and by focusing attention to potential abscesses or phlegmon of the lesser sac. Tube feeding distant to the ligament of Treitz or total parenteral nutrition (TPN) may be warranted when the fistula exhibits a persistently high output. The use of somatostatin analogs to treat enteric or pancreatic fistulas has been well described. Octreotide, administered intravenously or subcutaneously, has also been used to treat pancreatic fistula. A number of studies have documented success in treating pancreatic fistulae with the high-dose somatostatin. Most pancreatic fistulae close spontaneously without operative intervention.

GASTRINOMA

Zollinger–Ellison syndrome (ZES) is caused by a gastrin-secreting tumor called a gastrinoma (13,14), which causes symptoms of peptic ulcer disease including esophagitis and secretory diarrheas. ZES may occur as a part of the familial syndrome of MEN-1. Primary gastrinomas commonly occur in the duodenum and pancreas, but ectopic locations have been reported. Primary gastrinomas are usually malignant and involve both lymph nodes and liver. When surgical treatment is being considered, such metastatic disease should be taken into account. Most patients die because of metastatic liver disease, as most complications related to gastric acid hypersecretion are well controlled by proton pump inhibitors.

Patients with sporadic gastrinoma who do not have diffuse unresectable metastatic disease should undergo surgery. During surgery, the gastrinomas will be identified in most patients and a "biochemical cure" will occur. Resective surgery is indicated for localized metastatic disease because it prolongs survival and may offer some patients long-term survival.

Surgery for the treatment of patients with MEN-1 is more controversial and complex; some physicians recommend an aggressive approach, but most have not been as successful. It is extremely difficult to render a patient with MEN-1 eugastrinemic. Gastrinomas are the most commonly occurring, functionally active islet cell tumor among patients with MEN-1.

Complications of Missed Gastrinoma

Gastrinomas were once believed to occur within the pancreas and to be equally located within the head, body, and tail, as is true for insulinoma. Furthermore, it was believed that duodenal tumors were less common, with an incidence of perhaps 25%. In recent series, both of these beliefs were found to be completely inaccurate. Most gastrinomas (80%) are found within the gastrinoma triangle, the area around the head of the pancreas and the duodenum (15–17). More importantly, the pancreatic head is not the primary site of most of these tumors; rather, they occur most often within the wall of the duodenum. Other sites of gastrinoma include the pancreas, liver, stomach, jejunum, mesentery, spleen, ovary, and heart. An interesting variation is the so-called lymph node primary gastrinoma. These tumors are uncommon, but some patients have been cured after excision of solitary gastrinomas arising within a lymph node. Careful pathologic studies have shown that the incidence of gastrinomas of the duodenum is similar to that of nodal metastases as pancreatic primary tumors. However, the incidence of liver metastases is higher with pancreatic primary tumors, and this factor adversely affects survival rates.

Imaging Studies and the Complication of Missed Gastrinoma

At the time of diagnosis, 20% to 40% of patients with a gastrinoma will have metastatic liver disease. Therefore, imaging studies must accurately assess the liver. Locating small, multicentric, extraduodenal, and pancreatic primary gastrinomas can be difficult. Despite substantial clinical experience with conventional CT or MRI studies, 50% of primary gastrinomas are not detected by preoperative studies.

The accuracy of conventional ultrasonography, CT, and MRI in detecting primary tumors ranges from 10% to 75%. Small extrapancreatic primary tumors (<1 cm in diameter) are seldom detected by conventional preoperative imaging (2,13,14).

Somatostatin receptor scintigraphy (SRS) is the noninvasive imaging study of choice for localizing primary and metastatic gastrinoma (13,18). SRS detects 80% to 90% of tumors. For diagnosing the ZES syndrome, SRS is more accurate than all of the other imaging studies combined. Positive results from an SRS study have a 100% positive predictive value for locating tumors associated with ZES.

Endoscopic ultrasound (EUS) may be a sensitive method for detecting gastrinomas. In one study, EUS demonstrated a sensitivity of 50% for primary gastrinoma of the duodenum, 75% for primary gastrinoma of the pancreas, and 63% for primary gastrinoma of the lymph nodes (19,20).

Complications Associated with the Surgical Management of Gastrinoma

The goal of surgery is complete resection of tumor for a possible cure of ZES. This goal may be achieved when tumors are localized or metastatic. Patients with sporadic gastrinoma and no contraindications for surgery should undergo localization and possibly curative surgery. Resection of the primary tumor can decrease the incidence of liver metastases. Surgery should be performed unless an unresectable bilobar disease is detected. Surgery leads to a complete remission in approximately 60% of patients with sporadic ZES. The experience of the surgeon is the single most important factor in achieving a good surgical outcome because small tumors may be found even when imaging studies are negative.

ZES is the functional pancreatic syndrome most commonly associated with MEN-1. The role of surgery in the treatment of this condition is controversial. Few of these patients are cured, and when multiple neuroendocrine tumors are located in the pancreas and duodenum, it is difficult to determine which tumor is responsible for the syndrome.

Surgery to correct hyperparathyroidism is the initial procedure of choice for the treatment of MEN-1. This procedure may reduce the fasting serum levels of gastrin and the hypersecretion of acid. Pancreatic islet cell tumors that are larger than 2 cm in diameter are very likely to metastasize to the liver and should be resected. Tumors within the pancreatic head are enucleated, whereas the multiple tumors found within the body and tail of the pancreas are treated by distal pancreatectomy with wide margins. The duodenum is explored so that multiple gastrinomas can be located. Peripancreatic lymphadenectomy is required for pancreatic tumors more than 2 cm in diameter and for all duodenal gastrinomas.

The complications associated with this extensive surgical procedure include pancreatic fistulae from the enucleated tumors and an inadequate margin of resection in the case of distal pancreatectomy. Other potential complications are bleeding from splenic vessels, subphrenic collections, and peripancreatic collections. Most of these are managed nonoperatively with bowel rest, TPN, somatostatin administration, and percutaneous drainage.

COMPLICATIONS OF HEPATIC SURGERY FOR METASTATIC PANCREATIC ENDOCRINE TUMORS

Several recent studies of standard surgical resection for hepatic metastases from neuroendocrine tumors have demonstrated excellent relief of symptoms and long-term remission of symptoms. Most series document 80% to 100% relief of symptoms during a follow-up period of 20 to 50 months (21–23).

In the largest series, the operative mortality rate was approximately 2% and the survival rate approached 75%. Most patients have undergone anatomic lobar resection and large nonanatomic segmental resection performed with various techniques, including inflow occlusion and total vascular isolation. With recent advances in the understanding of hepatic anatomy and more experience with major resections, the morbidity rate is less than 10%; complications include bleeding, bile collection, infection, and, very rarely, hepatic insufficiency.

High-frequency electrical energy is an effective means of heating tissue. Radiofrequency ablation is a relatively new technique for the treatment of metastatic neuroendocrine tumors (24,25). Laparoscopic ultrasound-guided ablation has been used to treat patients with metastatic functioning and nonfunctioning islet cell tumors within the liver. Successful ablation can be documented by follow-up CT scans after the procedure.

Most patients are discharged from the hospital on the first postoperative day. Their level of discomfort is similar to that experienced after laparoscopic cholecystectomy and is managed by orally administered pain medications. No patient has exhibited bleeding, bile leak, or late formation of abscess. After ablation, some patients experience low-grade fevers. The procedure is well tolerated and is useful in the treatment of metastatic neuroendocrine tumors.

REFERENCES

1. Chun J, Doherty GM. Pancreatic endocrine tumors. Curr Opin Oncol 2001; 13(1):S2–S6.
2. Azimuddin K, Chamberlain RS. The surgical management of pancreatic neuroendocrine tumors. Surg Clin North Am 2001; 81(3):S11–S25.
3. Phan GQ, Yeo CJ, Hruban RH, Lillemoe KD, Pitt HA, Cameron JL. Surgical experience with pancreatic and peripancreatic neuroendocrine tumors. J Gastrointest Surg 1998; 2(5):472–482.
4. Sarmiento JM, Que FG, Grant CS, Thompson GB, Farnell MB, Nagorney DM. Concurrent resections of pancreatic islet cell cancers with synchronous hepatic metastases: outcomes of an aggressive approach. Surgery 2002; 132(6):976–982.
5. Soga J, Yakuwa Y, Osaka M. Insulinoma/hypoglycemic syndrome: a statistical evaluation of 1085 reported cases of a Japanese series. J Exp Clin Cancer Res 1998; 17(4):379–388.
6. Lo CY, Lam KY, Kung AW, Lam KS, Tung PH, Fan ST. Pancreatic insulinomas. Arch Surg 1997; 132(8):926–930.
7. Christiansen LA, Nielsen OV, Stadil F, Stage JG. Delay in the diagnosis of insulinomas. Scand J Gastroenterol 1979; 53:43–44.
8. Service FJ, McMahon MM, O'Brien PC, Ballard DJ. Functioning insulinoma-incidence, recurrence and long-term survival of patients: a 60 year study. Mayo Clin Proc 1991; 66(7):711–719.
9. Chatziioannou A, Kehagias D, Mourikis D, et al. Imaging and localization of pancreatic insulinomas. Clin Imaging 2001; 25(4):275–283.
10. Grant CS. Insulinoma. Surg Oncol Clin North Am 1998; 7(4):819–844.
11. Lo CY, van Heerden JA, Thompson GB, Grant CS, Soreide JA, Harmsen WS. Islet cell carcinoma of the pancreas. World J Surg 1996; 20(7):878–883.
12. Halloran CM, Ghaneh P, Bosonnet L, Hartley MN, Sutton R, Neoptolemos JP. Complications of pancreatic cancer resection. Digest Surg 2002; 19:138–146.
13. Norton JA, Jensen RT. Current surgical management of ZES in patients without MEN 1. Surg Oncol 2003; 12(2):145–151.
14. Mansour JC, Chen H. Pancreatic endocrine tumors. J Surg Res 2004; 120:139–161.
15. Howard TJ, Stabile BE, Zinner MJ, Chang S, Bhagavan BS, Passaro E. Anatomic distribution of pancreatic endocrine tumors. Am J Surg 1990; 159(2):258–264.
16. Stabile BE, Morrow DJ, Passaro E. The gastrinoma triangle: operative implications. Am J Surg 1984; 147(1):25–31.
17. Norton JA, Fraker DL, Alexander HR, et al. Surgery to cure the Zollinger-Ellison Syndrome. N Engl J Med 1999; 341:635–644.
18. Proye C, Malvaux P, Pattou F, et al. Noninvasive imaging of insulinomas and gastrinomas with endoscopic ultrasonography and somatostatin receptor scintigraphy. Surgery 1998; 124(6):1134–1143.
19. Anderson MA, Carpenter S, Thompson NW, Nostrant TT, Elta GH, Scheiman JM. Endoscopic ultrasound is highly accurate and directs management in patients with neuroendocrine tumors of the pancreas. Am J Gastroenterol 2000; 95(9):2271–2277.
20. Zimmer T, Scherubl H, Faiss S, Stolzel U, Riecken EO, Wiedenmann B. Endoscopic ultrasonography of neuroendocrine tumours. Digestion 2000; 62(suppl 1):45–50.
21. Chen H, Hardacre JM, Uzar A, Cameron JL, Choti MA. Isolated liver metastases from neuroendocrine tumors: does resection prolong survival? J Am Coll Surg 1998; 187(1):88–92.
22. Chamberlain RS, Canes D, Brown KT, et al. Hepatic neuroendocrine metastases: does intervention alter outcomes? J Am Coll Surg 2000; 190(4):432–445.
23. Norton JA, Warren RS, Kelly MG, Zuraek MB, Jensen RT. Aggressive surgery for metastatic liver neuroendocrine tumors. Surgery 2003; 134(6):1057–1063.
24. Siperstein A, Garland A, Engle K, et al. Local recurrence after laparoscopic radiofrequency thermal ablation of hepatic tumors. Ann Surg Oncol 2000; 7(2):106–113.
25. Siperstein A, Garland A, Engle K, et al. Laparoscopic radiofrequency ablation of primary and metastatic liver tumors. Surg Endosc 2000; 14(4):400–405.

20

Gastrointestinal Carcinoid Tumors

Jana B. A. MacLeod

Division of Trauma and Critical Care, Department of Surgery, Emory University School of Medicine, Atlanta, Georgia, U.S.A.

Erik Barquist

Ryder Trauma Center, Department of Surgery, University of Miami, Miller School of Medicine, Miami, Florida, U.S.A.

Håkin Ahlman

Gothenberg University, Sahlgrenska Universitelsjukhuset, Goteborg, Sweden

This chapter reviews the current strategies for managing carcinoid tumors of the gastrointestinal (GI) tract. The discussion highlights the consequences and complications of these strategies and also presents background information concerning the history and epidemiology of carcinoid tumors. Finally, we detail the progression of management strategies and the complications associated with each tumor, according to site of origin.

HISTORY AND EPIDEMIOLOGY OF CARCINOID TUMORS

Lubarsch (1) first described carcinoid tumors of the GI in 1888. The case involved multiple carcinoid tumors of the ileum, which were at the time considered carcinomas. In 1907, Oberndorfer (2) coined the term "Karzinoid" (carcinoma-like) when he reported that the activity of these tumors was more benign than that of carcinomas. Gosset and Masson (3) reported the endocrine nature of these tumors in 1914, when they demonstrated that the cells contained silver salt–reducing granules arising from the Kulchitsky cells of the crypts of Lieberkuhn. The biology of carcinoid tumors was best described in the classification scheme developed by Williams and Sandler (4) in 1963. This scheme, which is still widely used today, classifies carcinoid tumors according to the tissue of their embryologic origin: (i) foregut carcinoid tumors (those appearing in the respiratory tract, stomach, duodenum, biliary system, and pancreas), (ii) midgut carcinoid tumors (those appearing in the small bowel, appendix, caecum, and proximal colon), and (iii) hindgut carcinoid tumors (those appearing in the distal colon and rectum). A revised classification system developed by Rindi et al. (5) takes into account

tumor location, size, angioinvasion, hormone production, degree of neuroendocrine differentiation, histologic grade, and proliferative index, as well as the tumor's clinical activity (benign, low-grade malignant, or high-grade malignant). The World Health Organization (WHO) has solidified these schemes by describing three main groups of endocrine tumors (6): well-differentiated endocrine tumors (carcinoid tumors), differentiated endocrine carcinoma (malignant carcinoid tumors), and poorly differentiated endocrine carcinoma (PDEC). This new classification scheme combines new advances in tumor biology—a description of the tumor's clinical, pathological, and biological patterns and a determination of the disease prognosis.

Although carcinoid tumors are uncommon, they are not rare; their annual incidence is 1 person per 100,000 population (7). During the past 20 years, the incidence of carcinoid tumors of the gut has increased (8), probably because of better diagnostic methods such as endoscopy, ultrasonography, computerized tomography, and, recently, octreotide scintigraphy, which uses a radiolabeled somatostatin analogue that binds to the somatostatin receptors (SSTRs) expressed by endocrine tumors. This supposition is supported by the relatively high incidence of carcinoid tumors in large autopsy series (9) and is also consistent with the asymptomatic nature of carcinoid tumors, which are most often found incidentally during surgery (3). For example, carcinoid tumors are discovered during approximately 1 of every 300 appendectomies (10).

Carcinoid tumors are the most common endocrine tumors, comprising approximately 50% to 75% of all neuroendocrine tumors of the GI tract (11–13). These tumors, which have amine precursor uptake and decarboxylation properties, arise from the histamine-producing enterochromaffin cells (ECL) of the GI tract. They produce a variety of protein and peptide products, the most characteristic of which are serotonin and tachykinins. Foregut and midgut carcinoid tumors produce the highest serotonin levels of the carcinoid tumors (13,14). Foregut tumors produce 5-hydroxytryptophan (5-HTP), 5-hydroxytryptamine or serotonin (5-HT), histamine, and peptides, with a predominance of 5-HTP; midgut tumors produce 5-HT and tachykinins, with a predominance of 5-HT (15). However because the kidney metabolizes both of these products to form 5-hydroxy-indoleacetic acid (5-HIAA), tumors in either location can cause excessive levels of 5-HIAA. Approximately 85% of carcinoid tumors are found in the GI tract; 10% are found in the lungs, mainly as bronchial carcinoid tumors; and the remainder are found in various other organs such as the larynx, thymus, kidney, ovary, prostate, and skin (16). Tumors of the esophagus (0.04%), biliary tract (0.41%), and pancreas (0.55%) were exceedingly rare (8,17). However, the incidental nature of a large proportion of these tumors renders the reports of epidemiological studies about their distribution inconsistent.

CARCINOID TUMORS OF THE STOMACH

The increased use of upper GI endoscopy has increased the frequency with which carcinoid tumors of the stomach are detected; 30% of carcinoids are now reported to occur in this location (18). This has decreased the complication of delayed diagnosis. Pernicious anemia caused by chronic atrophic gastritis type A (A-CAG) and the Zollinger–Ellison syndrome caused by multiple endocrine neoplasia 1 (ZE-MEN1) are risk factors for gastric carcinoid tumors (19,20). A database recently released by the National Cancer Institute (21) showed that the incidence of gastric carcinoid tumors is increasing (0.3% to 0.54% of all gastric malignancies). As with carcinoid tumors found in other locations within the GI tract, patients are most commonly in the sixth or seventh decade of life (22).

Gastric carcinoid tumors can be classified as one of three types according to distinct clinical settings of origin, prognosis, and treatment approaches (23). The tumors associated with A-CAG are called Type I tumors and those associated with ZE-MEN1 are called Type II tumors. Both of these types tend to occur in corpus or fundus of the stomach. Type III tumors arise sporadically in otherwise normal gastric tissue. Type I tumors comprise 70% to 75% of gastric carcinoid tumors, Type III tumors comprise 13% to 20%, and Type II tumors comprise the remainder.

Type I gastric carcinoid tumors characteristically consist of multiple small lesions that are either benign or, less commonly, are of low malignant potential (24). These tumors are consistently associated with hypergastrinemia. The prognosis for Type I tumors is slightly better than that for Type II tumors (25). Rindi et al., in a series of 102 patients with gastric carcinoid tumors, found that no deaths occurred among the 58 patients with Type I tumors (24). A rather benign course is also shared by patients with Type II carcinoids, which arise in approximately 13% of ZE-MEN1 syndromes (24,26). After Type I and Type II tumors have been resected, the patient should undergo testing for parathyroid pathology (27).

The sporadically occurring Type III gastric carcinoid tumors arise in normal gastric mucosa as solitary large lesions. Their activity is moderately aggressive, with invasive growth and a high incidence of metastasis (23,24). At the time of diagnosis, approximately 50% of these tumors have spread beyond the stomach. Approximately 65% of these already involve the liver (26). Some authors report that as many as 30% of patients have carcinoid syndrome (21,28). Type III carcinoid tumors are usually associated with an atypical syndrome because of overproduction of histamine, which produces symptoms of edema, generalized flushing, hypotension, bronchoconstriction, and diarrhea. The production of histamine can be monitored by testing for increased urine levels of the main metabolite of histamine, *tele*-methylimidazoleacetic acid (ô-MIAA) (25). In a retrospective review of cases, Modlin et al. found that in 7.8% of cases, gastric carcinoid tumors were associated with other malignant neoplasms; five-year survival rates were 64.3% for patients with localized disease, 29.9% for patients with regional metastases, and 10% for patients with distant metastases (21). As is true of carcinoid tumors in other locations, metastasis is associated with tumor size (13). However, Kumashiro et al. (29) reported cases of minute gastric carcinoid tumors that were associated with locoregional spread at the time of diagnosis. Similarly. Rindi et al. (30) studied 205 patients with gastric carcinoid tumors and found minute tumors associated with locoregional spread, but no patients with tumors of this type had died after an average 53 months of follow-up.

Hypergastrinemia-associated tumors and sporadic tumors differ in both clinicopathological activity and treatment approach. When hypergastrinemia-associated tumors are smaller than 1 cm in diameter or when fewer than five lesions are present, initial management consists of endoscopic excision of polypoid lesions (27,31). If neither of these criteria is met or if polypectomy fails, local excision of the lesion located in the corpus or fundus should be combined with antrectomy to minimize the secretion of gastrin. Adding antrectomy eliminates the trophic stimulus of gastrin on tumor growth, and regression of such lesions has been reported after antrectomy alone (19,27,32). Other studies have shown no regression of manifest neoplasms but rather continuous hyperplasia or dysplasia (33–35). Unfortunately, lesions that will regress with antrectomy alone cannot be predicted. These lesions need to be excised. Even if the serum concentration of gastrin returns to normal after antrectomy, there is still a risk of tumor recurrence (7,35). A case report from Liverpool, England, suggested the use of an octreotide suppression test to detect either the suppression of histidine decarboxylase or the expression of chromogranin A as a marker for positive response to antrectomy alone (36). Ahlman et al. have proposed a treatment protocol that involves endoscopic treatment alone for as many as five Type I multicentric carcinoid tumors. Antrectomy is performed upon recurrence. If more than five multicentric carcinoid tumors are present, this protocol recommends antrectomy alone. These authors suggest that patients with Type II multicentric carcinoid tumors related to ZE-MEN1 syndrome should undergo resection of the gastrinoma, endoscopic surveillance for small early carcinoid lesions, and gastrectomy for large carcinoid lesions (35). This avoids the complications associated with total or subtotal gastrectomy.

Sporadic gastric carcinoid tumors require a more aggressive surgical approach; some clinicians recommend complete or partial gastrectomy (37). Aranha and Greenlee (38) also include omentectomy and regional lymph-node dissection as part of the standard surgical management for invasive gastric carcinoid tumors larger than 1 cm in diameter. Because the prognosis for Type III carcinoid tumors is substantially more dismal than that for other gastric carcinoid tumors, radical surgical procedures are warranted (35).

CARCINOID TUMORS OF THE SMALL INTESTINE

Carcinoid tumors comprise a substantial component ($\sim$34%) of tumors of the small intestine. Carcinoid tumors of the small bowel are the most common carcinoid tumors, and the frequency of their occurrence from the jejunum to the ileum is increasing (39). In 1997, Soga reviewed 516 published articles from more than 35 countries, which reported a total of 1102 jejunoileal carcinoid tumors (40). Of these, 8.4% occurred within a Meckel's diverticulum. His analysis of these reports showed that jejunoileal carcinoid tumors occur in a slightly older population and are significantly more aggressive than carcinoid tumors in other locations. The rate of metastasis is high, even when lesions are small and invade only the submucosa. Soga also reported a high incidence of argentaffin cell type and serotonin activity with resultant carcinoid syndrome. Rothmund and Kisker found metastatic lesions in 20% to 30% of patients with small midgut carcinoid tumors of less than 1 cm diameter (41). Tumors larger than 2 cm in diameter were associated with an 85% metastatic rate.

It is not uncommon for carcinoid tumors of the small intestine to be asymptomatic for long periods because of their slow growth (39). Various clinicians have reported that 20% to 40% of these tumors are discovered incidentally during laparotomy (17,42). Symptomatic tumors most commonly cause abdominal pain that is associated with partial or complete small-bowel obstruction (17). This may be due to intussusception, but more commonly, the obstruction is caused by a local desmoplastic reaction in the mesentery. Sjoblom found in his case series of GI

carcinoids that 72% of the small-bowel carcinoids had metastatic disease at the time of presentation (43). Ahlman et al. (44) performed preoperative octreotide scintigraphy on 27 patients; for 19 of those patients, this test detected tumors not revealed by noninvasive radiological methods. These tumor deposits were most commonly found in the liver or the periaortic lymph nodes.

It is unusual for a carcinoid tumor of the small intestine to encase mesenteric vessels. An even more infrequent occurrence is the development of a pseudoaneurysm (45). Wangberg et al. (46) advocate aggressive removal or reduction of regional or retroperitoneal lymph-node metastases along with the primary tumor; they dissect all mesenteric lymph-node metastases so as to obtain a tumor-free mesenteric root. These authors also perform sharp dissection of the high-mesenteric lymph nodes, so that the mesenteric vessels and small intestine can be mobilized for adequate resection and so that future local complications such as bleeding and ischemia are reduced in occurrence. Extensive involvement of mesenteric vessels may require vascular shunt grafts or stents.

In 20% to 30% of cases, the carcinoid tumor is multicentric within the bowel wall (17,47). In such cases, the full length of the bowel should be carefully assessed to ensure that a second nidus of tumor is not overlooked. Another 17% to 35% of patients with intestinal carcinoid tumors have a second malignant tumor (48,49). The most common second tumor is adenocarcinoma of the colon. When the carcinoid tumor has caused mild abdominal symptoms and elective surgery can be performed, preoperative radiologic tests often delineate other tumors. Many centers routinely perform preoperative CT scans and octreotide scintigraphy. However, when the small bowel is completely obstructed and emergency surgery is required, any recurrent or unresolved obstructive symptoms warrant an investigation for synchronous malignancy. Gerstle et al. (48) retrospectively reviewed their 20-year experience with 69 cases of GI carcinoid tumors and found that three patients (4%) had metachronous tumors and 29 patients (42%) had second synchronous tumors, 43% of which were in the GI tract and 22% of which were in the colorectal region. Intraoperative enteroscopy is used to detect obscure GI bleeding and can also be considered an adjunct to intraoperative evaluation of synchronous carcinoid lesions. Zaman et al. (50), using the "push enteroscope" for patients with undiagnosed causes of GI bleeding, found that the scope could reach the ileum in 13 of 14 patients, but serious complications occurred in five patients. These complications included an avulsion of the superior mesenteric vein and three serosal tears. Another technique that is associated with fewer reported complications is the use of a hand-held scintillation detector after a preoperative injection of [111]indium-diethyl-triamine pentacetic acid (DTPA)-D-Phe-1-octreotide. This technique allows intraoperative detection and excision of occult tumors during the same surgical procedure (42,51).

Regional lymph-node involvement is found in 45% of cases when small-bowel carcinoids are less than 1 cm in diameter; the incidence of nodal disease increases with the size of the tumor (26,52,53). Therefore, wide segmental resection with corresponding excision of mesenteric lymph nodes should be performed. Lesions in the terminal ileum should be treated by a right hemicolectomy (54). Basson et al. (39) recommend cholecystectomy at the time of tumor resection because long-term octreotide therapy causes bile sludging and can result in cholecystitis. Wangberg and coworkers also recommend cholecystectomy because any future embolization of the hepatic artery can result in gall bladder necrosis (46). Octreotide therapy and hepatic artery embolization are discussed below. Superficial liver metastases can be removed by wedge resection, but formal liver resection is not commonly performed at the same time as intestinal surgery.

Removing most of the tumor mass is advocated even if the tumor involves blood vessels such as the superior mesenteric vessels. Excising the bulk of the tumor mass probably increases survival rates and diminishes the systemic effects of carcinoid syndrome, but to date, no randomized controlled studies have confirmed this observation (55). In one series of patients who had undergone palliative resection, the five-year survival rate was 60% (17,52). However, the remaining bowel must be carefully assessed for viability, so that the risk of postoperative ischemic changes and even frank necrosis can be minimized. The secretory products of carcinoid tumors, such as serotonin and tachykinins, are believed to cause the marked fibrosis that is often seen in the bowel wall and the mesentery (46). New research indicates that connective tissue growth factor may also be involved in this process. Larsson et al. (56) found that patients with GI carcinoid tumors who survived for five years or longer, even in the face of recurrent disease and treatment, perceived their health-related quality of life as being good.

When carcinoid tumors of the small intestine metastasize to other organs, they most frequently affect the liver. Que et al. (57) from the Mayo Clinic reviewed 50 cases of carcinoid tumors that had been treated by resection of liver metastases. The perioperative mortality rate was 2.7%; the four-year survival rate was 73%. The four-year symptom-free survival rate for patients who had preoperative hormone-related symptoms was 30%. They suggest that palliative resection be considered when 90% of the tumor can be safely resected. The postoperative symptomatic response rate was 90%; the mean duration of response was 19.3 months. McEntee et al. (58) performed cytoreduction in 37 patients with hepatic metastases, 24 of whom had carcinoid tumors. Of these 24 patients, nine had symptoms of endocrinopathy, and palliation was achieved in eight. Five of these same nine patients were disease-free postoperatively and experienced a mean disease-free survival

period of 26 months (range 2 to 82 months). There were four major operative complications. Chen et al. (59) compared the outcome of patients with hepatic carcinoid metastases who did or did not undergo hepatic resection. The five-year actuarial survival rates of patients who underwent resection were 44% higher than those of the patients who did not undergo resection.

Reduction of hepatic tumor burden and palliation of carcinoid symptoms are achieved by cytoreduction using surgical resection or hepatic embolization–induced ischemia (60–64). Que et al. suggest that palliative resection be considered when 90% of the tumor can be safely resected (57). Soreide et al. (60) retrospectively reviewed the cases of 75 patients with liver metastases and found a clear relationship between tumor bulk and length of survival; the median survival period of patients treated with resection or embolization (216 months) was superior to that of patients who were not so treated (48 months) ($p < 0.001$). Resection can relieve endocrine tumor symptoms even in the presence of distant metastases. Some authors advocate hepatic cytoreduction by induction of hepatic ischemia through hepatic artery ligation, temporary occlusion, or embolization because this procedure does not carry the risk of major surgical resection (39). The arterial anatomy, blood flow to the tumor, and patency of the portal vein should be demonstrated by angiography before embolization is performed (65). Contraindications to embolization are tumor burden, comprising more than two-thirds of the liver volume, occlusion of the portal vein, hyperbilirubinemia, and persistently elevated liver enzyme in serum testing. Relative contraindications are contrast allergy, coagulopathy, and poor overall patient health (65). The primary side effects of embolization are transient nausea, emesis, fever, abdominal pain, and transient elevation in liver enzymes as measured in serum tests. Occasional paroxysmal episodes of major fluid shifts and alterations in cardiopulmonary function can be safely controlled by the administration of octreotide. The biggest disadvantage of embolization is that collateralization of the arterial supply of the tumor can cause recurrent symptoms; however, this difficulty can be addressed by repeated embolization. In a Swedish series (66), one-third of patients underwent bilateral embolization of the hepatic artery; levels of tumor markers returned to normal, and the size of the hepatic metastases were markedly reduced. During the five-year follow-up period, fewer than 10% of the patients required repeated embolizations for recurrent carcinoid symptoms. The actuarial survival rate was 70% at five years and nearly 60% at 10 years. However, hepatic embolization is not free of complications. Serious complications among individual patients can include gallbladder gangrene, pancreatitis, liver abscess, vascular damage, and the hepatorenal syndrome. In another Swedish series (67), Wangberg et al. found that, among 48 patients treated with embolization, eight complications occurred. These complications included occlusion of the hepatic artery and formation of a pancreatic pseudocyst, both of which were managed conservatively; one hepatic abscess, which was drained percutaneously; and another hepatic artery aneurysm, which required resection. All of these patients had successful outcomes except for one who underwent two embolization procedures and died of disseminated intravascular coagulopathy. At seven-year follow-up, 13 of the 48 patients had died: six deaths were related to the carcinoid disease. The reported mortality rate associated with hepatic artery embolization at major centers is less than 5% (65,68). Whether survival is improved by cytoreduction is still controversial, but Mitty et al. (69) reported that patients with carcinoid tumors who underwent embolization survived two years longer than did historical control patients. Most clinicians agree that, when possible, a potentially curative unilobar hepatic resection is preferable to embolization (39). When such a procedure is not possible, treatment should involve either hepatic artery embolization or resection, depending on the individual patient.

Liver transplantation has been considered an option for patients with bilobar carcinoid disease, especially if hormonal symptoms and pain cannot be controlled medically. To date, few patients have undergone transplantation for this indication; therefore, little is known about the prognostic factors and long-term survival rates associated with transplantation. Lehnert (70) reviewed the cases of 103 patients who had undergone liver transplantation for extensive metastases of neuroendocrine carcinoma. The overall survival rate was 60% at two years and 47% at five years; the recurrence-free five-year survival rate was only 24%. Extended surgical procedures involving upper abdominal exenteration or pancreatoduodenectomy were associated with a poor prognosis. The author concluded that transplantation with curative intent appears to be worthwhile for patients less than 50 years of age who have only hepatic disease. Another study of nine patients treated with transplantation found that the outcome was similar to that achieved with transplantation for liver cirrhosis. However, the patient selection criteria have been strict; transplantation has been reserved for patients less than 60 years of age with isolated liver disease and locoregional disease that can be resected for cure (71).

Small-bowel carcinoid tumors may secrete a wide variety of bioactive agents in addition to serotonin and tachykinins; these secretions cause a cluster of symptoms that are collectively referred to as the carcinoid syndrome. These characteristic symptoms include diarrhea, flushing, wheezing, disease of the valves in the right side of the heart, and cutaneous telangiectasia. The syndrome commonly occurs with carcinoid tumors that have metastasized to the liver, but is also associated with primary ovarian, retroperitoneal, or bronchial carcinoid tumors. However, one study found that, of the 84% of patients with carcinoid tumors and elevated serum serotonin levels, only 18% exhibited the classic carcinoid syndrome (72). Nevertheless, when a patient exhibits symptoms suggestive of the carcinoid syndrome, the biochemical nature of the tumor should be characterized. Resection will be safer when the bioactivity of the tumor is blocked preoperatively with agents such as octreotide and other antagonists (39) because the induction of general anesthesia or manipulation of the tumor can cause a release of bioactive agents and result in carcinoid crisis, which is manifested by profound hypotension or bronchospasm. Carcinoid crisis has been documented by multiple authors (39,73) to be precipitated by the initiation of chemotherapy, during embolization, and even during fine needle biopsy of a liver metastasis. One theory (73) suggests that the carcinoid crisis is elicited by stress-associated endogenous catecholamines that, in turn, stimulate the secretion of serotonin via adenoreceptors on the surface of tumor cell. The use of octreotide prevents these reactions and antagonizes the effects of such products in established crisis situations. Octreotide is given subcutaneously at doses of 100 to 400 µg before, during, and after embolization, attempted surgical resection, or any other manipulation of carcinoid tumor. The usual dosage is 100 mg subcutaneous (SC) twice daily 14 days before the intervention and 100 mg four times on the day of the intervention. Some surgeons use as little as seven preoperative days of octreotide treatment. The pentagastrin provocation test is used to document adequate protection against provoked release of hormones before a procedure is performed. Octreotide inhibits the release and synthesis of bioactive agents from the carcinoid tumor and induces the production of G-proteins that inhibit the intracellular signaling of amines that can lead to peptide secretion. Octreotide is a synthetic analogue of somatostatin, which overcomes the short half-life of native somatostatin (90 to 120 minutes as compared to 1 to 2 minutes). The administration of octreotide controls diarrhea in 85% of patients and also moderates flushing; bronchospasm is the symptom most resistant to treatment. Cyproheptadine, a serotonin and histamine antagonist with additional anticholinergic and sedative side effects, is administered along with more specific serotonin blockers. In Europe, cyproheptadine is not used to treat patients with refractory carcinoid crisis; octreotide is administered intravenously with cortisone (74).

The overall five-year survival rate is 50% to 60% for patients with small-bowel carcinoid tumors, 75% for patients with disease confined to the bowel, and 35% for patients with liver metastases (55).

CARCINOID TUMORS OF THE DUODENUM

Carcinoid tumors of the duodenum are extremely rare; they are polypoid and are usually detected by endoscopy. One half of these tumors are gastrinomas and one-fifth are somatostatinomas. Because they are small, they can be adequately removed by endoscopy. The depth of invasion is assessed by endoluminal ultrasonography (EUS) (8). A small study from Italy suggests that EUS can accurately define the depth of carcinoid invasion, but the small number of patients included in the study precludes a definitive finding (75). If duodenal carcinoid tumors have not invaded the muscularis, local resection is curative and full-thickness resection is not necessary (28). However, accurate assessment of tumors that are not accessible by endoscopy may be more difficult; neuroendocrine carcinoma or PDEC (according to the WHO classification) must be ruled out before a local procedure is performed. In the rare case of full-thickness involvement or more, as is true for small-bowel carcinoid tumors, palliative resection is associated with increased survival rates and is advocated even if portal structures are involved. The prognosis for carcinoid tumors of the second part of the duodenum is better than that for adenocarcinoma in this location. Pancreaticoduodenal resection is warranted if there is no evidence of metastasis and the patient is medically fit (39).

CARCINOID TUMORS OF THE APPENDIX

Appendiceal carcinoid tumors are the most common tumor found in the appendix; they comprise 77% of all malignant tumors found in this organ (7). These tumors are diagnosed primarily by pathological examination of specimens removed during abdominal surgical procedures such as appendectomy. Connor et al. (76) found that the prevalence of incidental carcinoid tumors in their large series of 7970 appendectomies was only 0.9%. Most of these tumors are smaller than 1.5 cm in diameter and are located in the tip of the appendix. Appendiceal carcinoid tumors rarely cause death (77), but they can invade other tissues, metastasize, and produce hormones (78).

Virtually all appendiceal carcinoids infiltrate the muscularis mucosae or the submucosa, but metastasis is uncommon. Muscular and lymphatic invasion was present in all of the 150 cases reviewed by Moertel et al., but metastases occurred in only 4.7% (79). In another series of 46 appendiceal carcinoids, the rate of metastasis was 8.8% (80). In both of these studies, metastasis was associated with tumors larger than 2 cm in diameter, but other studies have found metastasis in association with tumors as small as 1 cm in diameter (81). The risk of lymph-node metastasis in association with tumors larger than 2 cm in diameter ranges from 20% to 30%. The risk of lymph-node involvement for most tumors less than 2 cm in diameter is approximately 1% (52,82).

No further surgical treatment is required beyond the standard appendectomy, which is used to treat most patients with incidentally found appendiceal carcinoid tumors (83). A complete right hemicolectomy is indicated for patients with tumors larger than 1 cm in diameter, but the number of such cases is small and a full evaluation of the effectiveness of the more radical treatment for larger tumors is difficult (52,84). The surgical group in Goteborg, Sweden, recommends ileocecal resection within three to four months of incidental detection of any tumor that is larger than 1.5 cm in diameter, has a basal location, involves the lymph nodes in the mesentery, or is not limited by serosa. These researchers state that carcinoid syndrome rarely occurs if these rules are followed and that the overall five-year survival rate approaches 99%. They also note that it is important to detect those tumors known as "goblet cell carcinoids," which are not neuroendocrine and have a rapidly malignant course.

CARCINOID TUMORS OF THE COLON AND RECTUM

Carcinoid tumors of the colon are rare, especially occurring with carcinoid syndrome. These tumors occur more commonly in the right colon than in the left colon (7). Lymphatic involvement is predicted by the size of the tumor: a diameter of 1.5 to 2.0 cm is associated with a high prevalence of lymph-node metastasis. Most carcinoid tumors of the colon are large and obstructive; thus, formal surgical resection should include lymphatic drainage with a procedure similar to that used for resection of adenocarcinoma (51,60). The biological activity of carcinoid tumors of the colon is similar to that of adenocarcinoma; the five-year survival rate ranges from 20% to 50%, depending on the stage of the tumor (52,53,82).

Rectal carcinoid tumors are the third most common carcinoid tumor and account for 3% of all rectal tumors (84). These tumors are smaller and less likely to metastasize than are colonic carcinoid tumors. Because rectal carcinoid tumors are easier to access by rectal palpation and proctoscopy than are colonic carcinoid tumors, they are more likely to have an early diagnosis. Their resultant small size allows treatment via an endoscopic approach. The prognosis for rectal carcinoid tumors is associated with tumor size; tumors less than 1 cm in diameter are rarely associated with lymph-node involvement, and 90% of tumors larger than 2 cm in diameter are associated with regional nodal spread (overall five-year survival rate, 70% to 85%) (84). Small tumors can be removed by local excision and fulguration. Larger tumors, up to 2 cm in diameter, are removed by transanal excision. The radical approach of abdominoperineal or low anterior resection is reserved for the largest tumors, averaging 4 cm in diameters which carry a higher risk of metastasis (60,85). Soga (87) reviewed 1271 cases of rectal carcinoid reported in 465 international publications since 1912. This review found that rectal carcinoid tumors occurred predominantly among men and were small (10 mm in diameter or less) at the time of detection. Invasion was predominantly submucosal, with a relatively high incidence of metastases and hematogenous spread. The rate of silver-salt reactivity was low, and the tumors were infrequently associated with carcinoid syndrome. The best histopathological marker for neuroendocrine differentiation is the presence of monoclonal antibodies against synaptic vesicle protein (SV2). No relationship has been observed between SV2 expression in tumors and either hormone production or malignant potential (88).

METASTASIS OF CARCINOID TUMOR TO THE LIVER

The most common cause of carcinoid syndrome is the metastasis of small-bowel carcinoid tumor to the liver (13). When carcinoid tumors from other sites metastasize to the liver, the outcome is uniformly poor (87). The most common causes of death are hormone-related heart disease and malignant progression, which lead to liver failure. Before current treatment options existed, the five-year survival rate of patients with metastatic liver tumor was less than 20% (87).

Some patients with carcinoid tumor liver metastasis have no known primary tumor, even when radiological investigation includes octreotide scanning. Staining for vesicular monoamine transporters (VMAT1 and VMAT2) assists in confirming the origin of the tumor as carcinoid. Serotonin-producing endocrine tumors (ileal and appendiceal carcinoid tumors) predominantly express VMAT1, whereas histamine-producing endocrine tumors (gastric carcinoid tumors) express almost exclusively VMAT2 (89). Only a small number of immunopositive tumor cells are observed in peptide-producing endocrine tumors such as rectal carcinoid tumors. If no primary carcinoid tumor is found after exhaustive preoperative and intraoperative investigation, resecting the hepatic metastases can substantially palliate the associated symptoms (39).

Cryosurgical ablation (CSA) and radiofrequency ablation (RFA) are being used to treat patients with carcinoid tumors (90,91). Most centers use a combination of these techniques. RFA of malignant hepatic neoplasms is believed to be safer than CSA, but most practitioners use it only for tumors less than 3 cm in diameter. CSA is more morbid, but is effective for larger, unresectable malignant hepatic neoplasms. Bilchik et al. (92) analyzed the clinical course of 308 patients with liver tumors that could not be surgically resected for cure but were treated with CSA, RFA (percutaneously, laparoscopically, or by celiotomy), or both. RFA used in combination with CSA reduced the morbidity associated with multiple freezing procedures.

Wood et al. reviewed the complications of RFA (93); 7 of 84 patients (8%) had complications: one skin burn, one postoperative hemorrhage, two simple hepatic abscesses, one hepatic abscess associated with diaphragmatic heat necrosis after sequential percutaneous ablations of a large lesion, one postoperative myocardial infarction, and one case of liver failure. There were three deaths, one of which was directly related to the RFA procedure. Three of the complications, including one RFA-related death, occurred after percutaneous RFA. The authors concluded that percutaneous RFA should be reserved for patients at high risk of complications associated with anesthesia, those with recurrent or progressive lesions, and those with small lesions.

McEntee et al. reviewed the use of hepatic resection over a 20-year time period in patients with metastatic neuroendocrine tumors. Seventeen of these resections were curative. The remainder had good relief of symptoms for a mean of six months (58). Norton et al. published their more recent eight-year series of liver resections for metastatic neuroendocrine tumors. They had no operative deaths and reported an 82% actuarial survival rate with a median 32-month follow-up (94). The principles of anatomical resection, wedge resection, and metastasectomy via RFA may be combined, so that good cytoreduction can be achieved.

Liver transplantation has also been used to treat unresectable disease. A series of 1000 orthotopic liver transplants performed in Pittsburgh from 1981 to 1987 stated that five patients had metastatic neuroendocrine tumors and were suitable candidates for transplantation. The authors who reported this series wrote: "Hepatic transplantation broadens the concept of radical excision of tumor" (97). In 1997, the report of a multicenter French retrospective case series stated that 15 patients with metastatic carcinoid tumors underwent hepatic transplantation with a five-year survival rate of 69% (98).

CONCLUSION

Carcinoid tumors vary in biological activity partly because of their location (or embryologic origin). This variance in clinicopathological activity causes the prognosis and management to vary according to the anatomic location of the tumors. The long-term prognosis associated with incidentally found carcinoid tumors is excellent and morbidity is minimal. Treatment of carcinoid syndrome with octreotide, detection of tumors intraoperatively with the use of labeled octreotide, and refinement of cytoreduction techniques have led to prolonged survival and increased quality of life for patients with advanced disease (99).

REFERENCES

1. Thompson GB, van Heerden JA, Martin JK Jr., Schutt AJ, Ilstrup DM, Carney JA. Carcinoid tumors of the gastrointestinal tract: presentation, management, and prognosis. Surgery 1985; 98(6):1054–1063.
2. Hoberock TR, Knutson CO, Polk HC Jr. Clinical aspects of invasive carcinoid tumors. South Med J 1975; 68(1):33–37.

3. Lauffer JM, Zhang T, Modlin IM. Review article: current status of gastrointestinal carcinoids. Aliment Pharmacol Ther 1999; 13(3):271–287.

4. Williams ED, Sandler M. The classification of carcinoid tumors. Lancet 1963; 2(1):238–239.

5. Rindi G, Capella C, Solcia E. Introduction to a revised clinicopathological classification of neuroendocrine tumors of the gastroenteropancreatic tract. Q J Nucl Med 2000; 44(1):13–21.

6. Solcia E, Kloppel G, Sobin LH. Histological Typing of Endocrine Tumors. World Health Organization International Histological Classification of Tumors. 2nd ed. New York: Springer, 2000.

7. Roeher H, Simon D. Carcinoid tumors. In: Clark OH, Quan-Yang D, McGrew L, eds. Textbook of Endocrine Surgery. Philadelphia: WB Saunders, 1997:643–649.

8. Modlin IM, Sandor A. An analysis of 8305 cases of carcinoid tumors. Cancer 1997; 79:813–829.

9. Berge T, Linell F. Carcinoid tumors. Frequency in a defined population during a 12-year-period. Acta Pathol Microbiol Scand [A] 1976; 84:322–330.

10. Moertel CG, Dockerty MB, Judd ES. Carcinoid tumors of the vermiform appendix. Cancer 1968; 21:270–278.

11. Perry RR, Vinik AI. Endocrine tumors of the gastrointestinal tract. Ann Rev Medicine 1996; 47:57–68.

12. Norton JA. Neuroendocrine tumors of the pancreas and duodenum. Curr Probl Surg 1994; 31:77–156.

13. Onaitis MW, Kirshbom PM, Hayward TZ, et al. Gastrointestinal carcinoids: characterization by site of origin and hormone production. Ann Surg 2000; 232(4):549–556.

14. Janson E, Holmerg L, Stridsberg M, et al. Carcinoid tumors: analysis of prognostic factors and survival in 301 patients from a referral center. Ann Oncol 1997; 8(7):685–690.

15. Kolby L. Histamine Metabolism, Peptide Receptors and Monoamine Transporters in Carcinoid Tumors. Thesis, Gothenburg 1999.

16. Godwin DJ II. Carcinoid tumors. An analysis of 2,837 cases. Cancer 1975; 36(2):560–569.

17. Shebani KO, Souba WW, Finkelstein DM, et al. Prognosis and survival in patients with gastrointestinal tract carcinoid tumors. Ann Surg 1999; 229(6):815–823.

18. Solcia E, Fiocca R, Sessa F. Morphology and natural history of gastric endocrine tumors. In: Hakanson R, Sundler F, eds. The Stomach as an Endocrine Organ. Amsterdam: Elsevier Science, 1991:473–498.

19. Sjoblom SM, Sipponen P, Miettinen M, Karonen SL, Jarvinen HJ. Gastroscopic screening for gastric carcinoids and carcinoma in pernicious anemia. Endoscopy 1988; 20:52–56.

20. Cadiot G, Laurent-Puig P, Thuille B, Lehy T, Mignon M, Olschwang S. Is the multiple endocrine neoplasia type 1 gene a suppressor for fundic argyrophil tumors in the Zollinger-Ellison syndrome? Gastroenterology 1993; 105:579–582.

21. Modlin IM, Sandor A, Tang LH, Kidd M, Zelterman D. A 40-year analysis of 265 gastric carcinoids. Am J Gastroenterol 1997; 92:633–638.

22. Robinson EK, Cusack JC Jr., Tyler DS. Small bowel malignancies and carcinoid tumors. In: Feig BW, Berger DH, Fuhrman GM, eds. The M.D. Anderson Surgical Oncology Handbook. 2nd ed. Philadelphia: Lippincott Williams & Wilkins, 1999:161–177.

23. Rindi G, Luinetti O, Cornaggia M, Capella C, Solcia E. Three subtypes of gastric argyrophil carcinoid and the gastric neuroendocrine carcinoma: a clinicopathologic study. Gastroenterology 1993; 104: 994–1006.

24. Rindi G, Azzoni C, La Rosa S, et al. ECL cell tumor and poorly differentiated endocrine carcinoma of the stomach: prognostic evaluation by pathological analysis. Gastroenterology 1999; 116(3):532–542.

25. Solcia E, Fiocca R, Rindi G, Villani L, Cornaggia M, Capella C. The pathology of the gastrointestinal endocrine system. Endocrinol Metab Clin North Am 1993; 22(4):795–821.

26. Caplin ME, Buscombe JR, Hilson AJ, Jones AL, Watkinson AF, Burroughs AK. Carcinoid tumor. Lancet 1998; 352:799–805.

27. Ahlman H. Surgical treatment of carcinoid tumors of the stomach and small intestine. Ital J Gastroenterol Hepatol 1999; 31(suppl 2):S198–S201.

28. Akerstrom G. Management of carcinoid tumors of the stomach, duodenum, and pancreas. World J Surg 1996; 20:173–182.

29. Kumashiro R, Naitoh H, Teshima K, Sakai T, Inutsuka S. Minute gastric carcinoid tumor with regional lymph node metastasis. Int Surg 1989; 74:198–200.

30. Rindi G, Bordi C, Rappel S, La Rosa S, Solte M, Solcia E. Gastric carcinoids and neuroendocrine carcinomas: pathogenesis, pathology, and behavior. World J Surg 1996; 20(2):168–172.

31. Gilligan CJ, Lawton GP, Tang LH, West AB, Modlin IM. Gastric carcinoid tumors: the biology and therapy of an enigmatic and controversial lesion. Am J Gastroenterol 1995; 90:338–352.

32. Richards AT, Hinder RA, Harrison AC. Gastric carcinoid tumors associated with hypergastrinaemia and pernicious anaemia: regression of tumors by antrectomy. A case report. S Afr Med J 1987; 72:51–53.

33. D'Adda T, Annibale B, Delle Fave G, Bordi C. Oxyntic endocrine cells of hypergastrinemic patients. Differential response to antrectomy or octreotide. Gut 1996; 38(5):668–674.

34. Eckhauser FE, Lloyd RV, Thompson NW, Raper SE, Vinik AI. Antrectomy for multicentric, argyrophil gastric carcinoids: a preliminary report. Surgery 1988; 104(6):1046–1053.

35. Ahlman H, Kolby L, Lundell L, et al. Clinical management of gastric carcinoid tumors. Digestion 1994; 55(suppl 3):77–85.

36. Higham AD, Dimaline R, Varro A, et al. Octreotide suppression test predicts beneficial outcome from antrectomy in a patient with gastric carcinoid tumor. Gastroenterology 1998; 114:817–822.

37. Davies MG, O'Dowd G, McEntee GP, Hennessy TP. Primary gastric carcinoids: a view on management. Br J Surg 1990; 77:1013–1014.

38. Aranha GV, Greenlee HB. Surgical management of carcinoid tumors of the gastrointestinal tract. Am Surg 1980; 46:429–435.

39. Basson MD, Ahlman H, Wangberg B, Modlin IM. Biology and management of the midgut carcinoid. Am J Surg 1993; 165(2):288–297.

40. Soga J. Carcinoids of the small intestine: a statistical evaluation of 1102 cases collected from the literature. J Exp Clin Cancer Res 1997; 16(4):353–363.

41. Rothmund M, Kisker O. Surgical treatment of carcinoid tumors of the small bowel, appendix, colon and rectum. Digestion 1994; S3:86–91.

42. Tomassetti P. Clinical aspects of carcinoid tumors. Ital J Gastroenterol Hepatol 1999; 31(suppl 2):S143–S146.

43. Sjoblom SM. Clinical presentation and prognosis of gastrointestinal carcinoid tumours. Scand J Gastroenterol 1988; 23(7):779–787.

44. Ahlman H, Wangberg B, Tisell LE, et al. Clinical efficacy of octreotide scintigraphy in patients with midgut carcinoid tumors and evaluation of intraoperative scintillation detection. Br J Surg 1994; 81(8):1144–1149.

45. Peck JJ, Shields AB, Boyden AM, Dworkin LA, Nadal JW. Carcinoid tumors of the ileum. Am J Surg 1983; 146(1):124–132.

46. Wangberg B, Westberg G, Tylen U, et al. Survival of patients with disseminated midgut carcinoid tumors after aggressive tumor reduction. World J Surg 1996; 20(7):892–899.

47. Herbsman H, Wetstein L, Rosen Y, et al. Tumors of the small intestine. Curr Probl Surg 1980; 17(3):121–182.

48. Gerstle JT, Kauffman GL Jr., Koltun WA. The incidence, management, and outcome of patients with gastrointestinal carcinoids and second primary malignancies. J Am Coll Surg 1995; 180(4):427–432.

49. Brown NK, Smith MP. Neoplastic diathesis of patients with carcinoid: report of a case with four other neoplasms. Cancer 1973; 32(1):216–222.

50. Zaman A, Sheppard B, Katon RM. Total peroral intraoperative enteroscopy for obscure GI bleeding using a dedicated push enteroscope: diagnostic yield and patient outcome. Gastrointest Endosc 1999; 50(4):506–510.

51. Federspiel BH, Burke AP, Sobin LH, Shekitka KM. Rectal and colonic carcinoids. A clinicopathologic study of 84 cases. Cancer 1990; 65(1):135–140.

52. Stinner B, Kisker O, Ziekle A, Rothmund M. Surgical management for carcinoid tumors of small bowel, appendix, colon, and rectum. World J Surg 1996; 20:183–188.

53. Neary PC, Redmond PH, Houghton T, Watson GR, Bouchier-Hayes D. Carcinoid disease: review of the literature. Dis Colon Rectum 1997; 40:349–362.

54. Tilson MD. Carcinoid syndrome. Surg Clin North Am 1974; 54(2):409–423.

55. Norton JA. Surgical management of carcinoid tumors: role of debulking and surgery for patients with advanced disease. Digestion 1994; 55(suppl 3):98–103.

56. Larsson G, Sjoden PO, Oberg K, von Essen L. Importance-satisfaction discrepancies are associated with health-related quality of life in five-year survivors of endocrine gastrointestinal tumors. Ann Oncol 1999; 10(11):1321–1327.

57. Que FG, Nagorney DM, Batts KP, Linz LJ, Kvols LK. Hepatic resection for metastatic neuroendocrine carcinomas. Am J Surg 1995; 169(1):36–43.

58. McEntee GP, Nagorney DM, Kvols LK, Moertel CG, Grant CS. Cytoreductive hepatic surgery for neuroendocrine tumors. Surgery 1990; 108:1091–1096.

59. Chen H, Hardacre JM, Uzar A, Cameron JL, Choti MA. Isolated liver metastases from neuroendocrine tumors: does resection prolong survival? J Am Coll Surg 1998; 187(1):88–93.

60. Soreide O, Berstad T, Bakka A, et al. Surgical treatment as a principle in patients with advanced abdominal carcinoid tumors. Surgery 1992; 111(1):48–54.

61. Akerstrom G, Makridis C, Johansson H. Abdominal surgery in patients with midgut carcinoid tumors. Acta Oncol 1991; 30(4):547–553.

62. Makridis C, Oberg K, Juhlin C, et al. Surgical treatment of mid-gut carcinoid tumors. World J Surg 1990; 14(3):377–385.

63. Agranovich AL, Anderson GH, Manji M, Acker BD, Macdonald WC, Threlfall WJ. Carcinoid tumor of the gastrointestinal tract: prognostic factors and disease outcome. J Surg Oncol 1991; 47(1):45–52.

64. Marshall JB, Bodnarchuk G. Carcinoid tumors of the gut. Our experience over three decades and review of the literature. J Clin Gastroenterol 1993; 16(2):123–129.

65. Ajani JA, Carrasco CH, Wallace S. Neuroendocrine tumors metastatic to the liver. Vascular occlusion therapy. Ann N Y Acad Sci 1994; 733:479–487.

66. Ahlman H, Westberg G, Wangberg B, et al. Treatment of liver metastases of carcinoid tumors. World J Surg 1996; 20(2):196–202.

67. Wangberg B, Geterud K, Nilsson O, et al. Embolization therapy in the midgut carcinoid syndrome: just tumor ischemia? Acta Oncol 1993; 32(2):251–256.

68. Drougas JF, Anthony LB, Blair TK, et al. Hepatic artery chemoembolization for management of patients with advanced metastatic carcinoid tumors. Am J Surg 1998; 175(5):408–412.

69. Mitty HA, Warner RR, Newman LH, Train JS, Parnes IH. Control of carcinoid syndrome with hepatic artery embolization. Radiology 1985; 155(3):623–626.

70. Lehnert T. Liver transplantation for metastatic neuroendocrine carcinoma: an analysis of 103 patients. Transplantation 1998; 66(10):1307–1312.

71. Westberg G. Midgut Carcinoid Tumors: Biochemical and Therapeutic Aspects Ph.D. thesis, Goteborg University, Sweden, 2001.

72. Bax ND, Woods HF, Batchelor A, Jennings M. Clinical manifestations of carcinoid disease. World J Surg 1996; 20:142–146.

73. Ahlman H, Ahlund L, Dahlstrom A, Martner J, Stenquist O, Tylen U. The use of SMS 201–995 and provocation tests in carcinoid patients in preparation for surgery and hepatic embolisation. Anesth Analg 1988; 67:1142–1148.

74. Westberg G, Ahlman H, Nilsson O, Illerskog A, Wangberg B. Secretory patterns of tryptophan metabolites in midgut carcinoid tumor cells. Neurochem Res 1997; 22(8):977–983.

75. De Angelis C, Carucci P, Repici A, Rizzetto M. Endosonography in decision making and management of gastrointestinal endocrine tumors. Eur J Ultrasound 1999; 10(2–3):139–150.

76. Connor SJ, Hanna GB, Frizelle FA. Appendiceal tumors: retrospective clinicopathologic analysis of appendiceal tumors from 7,970 appendectomies. Dis Colon Rectum 1998; 41(1):75–80.

77. Olsson B, Ljungberg O. Adenocarcinoid of the vermiform appendix. Virchows Arch A Pathol Anat Histol 1980; 386:201–210.

78. Syracuse DC, Perzin KH, Price JB, Wiedel PD, Mesa-Tejada R. Carcinoid tumors of the appendix. Mesoappendiceal extension and nodal metastases. Ann Surg 1979; 190(1):58–63.

79. Moertel CG, Weiland LH, Nagorney DM, Dockerty MB. Carcinoid tumor of the appendix: treatment and prognosis. N Engl J Med 1987; 317(27):1699–1701.

80. Glasser CM, Bhagavan BS. Carcinoid tumors of the appendix. Arch Pathol Lab Med 1980; 104:272–275.

81. Dent TL, Batsakis JG, Lindenauer SM. Carcinoid tumors of the appendix. Surgery 1973; 73:828–832.

82. Memon MA, Nelson H. Gastrointestinal carcinoid tumors: current management strategies. Dis Colon Rectum 1997; 40(9):1101–1118.

83. Moertel CL, Weiland LH, Telander RL. Carcinoid tumor of the appendix in the first two decades of life. J Pediatr Surg 1990; 25(10):1073–1075.

84. Pasieka JL, McKinnon JG, Kinnear S, et al. Carcinoid syndrome symposium on treatment modalities for gastrointestinal carcinoid tumors: symposium summary. Can J Surg 2001; 44(1):25–32.

85. Jetmore AB, Ray JE, Gathright JB Jr., McMullen KM, Hicks TC, Timmcke AE. Rectal carcinoids: the most frequent carcinoid tumor. Dis Colon Rectum 1992; 35(8):717–725.

86. Soga J. Carcinoids of the rectum: an evaluation of 1271 reported cases. Surg Today 1997; 27(2):112–119.

87. Godwin JD II. Carcinoid tumors. An analysis of 2,837 cases. Cancer 1975; 36(2):560–569.

88. Jakobsen AM, Ahlman H, Wangberg B, Kolby L, Bengtsson M, Nilsson O. Expression of synaptic vesicle protein 2 (SV2) in neuroendocrine tumors of the gastrointestinal tract and pancreas. J Pathol 2002; 196(1):44–50.

89. Jakobsen AM, Andersson P, Saglik G, et al. Differential expression of vesicular monoamine transporter (VMAT) 1 and 2 in gastrointestinal endocrine tumors. J Pathol 2001; 195(4):463–472.

90. Bilchik AJ, Sarantou T, Foshag LJ, Giuliano AE, Ramming KP. Cryosurgical palliation of metastatic neuroendocrine tumors resistant to conventional therapy. Surgery 1997; 122(6):1040–1048.

91. Siperstein AE, Rogers SJ, Hansen PD, Gitomirsky A. Laparoscopic thermal ablation of hepatic neuroendocrine tumor metastases. Surgery 1997; 122:1147–1155.

92. Bilchik AJ, Wood TF, Allegra D, et al. Cryosurgical ablation and radiofrequency ablation for unresectable hepatic malignant neoplasms: a proposed algorithm. Arch Surg 2000; 135(6):657–664.

93. Wood TF, Rose DM, Chung M, Allegra DP, Foshag LJ, Bilchik AJ. Radiofrequency ablation of 231 unresectable hepatic tumors: indications, limitations and complications. Ann Surg Oncol 2000; 7(8):593–600.

94. Norton JA, Warren RS, Kelly MG, Zuraek MB, Jensen RT. Aggressive surgery for metastatic liver neuroendocrine tumors. Surgery 2003; 134:1057–1065.

95. Farges O, Belghiti J. Options in the resection of endocrine liver metastases. In: Mignon M, Columbel JF, eds. Recent Advances in the Pathophysiology and Management of Inflammatory Bowel Diseases and Digestive Endocrine Tumors. Paris: Libbey Eurotext, 1999:335–337.

96. Carty SE, Jensen RT, Norton JA. Prospective study of aggressive resection of metastatic pancreatic endocrine tumors. Surgery 1992; 112:1024–1032.

97. Makowka L, Tzakis AG, Mazzaferro V, et al. Transplantation of the liver for metastatic endocrine tumors of the intestine and pancreas. Surg Gynecol Obstet 1989; 168:107–111.

98. Le Treut YP, Delpero JR, Dousset B, et al. Results of liver transplantation in the treatment of metastatic neuroendocrine tumors. A 31-case French multicentric report. Ann Surg 1997; 225(4):335–364.

99. Wangberg B, Forssell-Aronsson E, Tisell LE, Nilsson O, Fjalling M, Ahlman H. Intraoperative detection of somatostatin-receptor-positive neuroendocrine tumors using indium-111-labelled DTPA-D-Phe-1-octreotide. Br J Cancer 1996; 73(6):770–775.

21

Complications of Pulmonary and Chest Wall Resection

Rosemary F. Kelly and Romualdo J. Segurola, Jr.
Cardiovascular and Thoracic Surgery, University of Minnesota, Minneapolis, Minnesota, U.S.A.

"I'm better at staying out of trouble than getting out of it."
(H.B. Ward MD, PhD, personal communication, 1999)

Pulmonary and chest wall resection are frequently necessary for the management of benign or malignant thoracic disease. Bronchogenic carcinoma is currently the most frequently occurring malignancy worldwide. Despite advances in chemotherapy regimens, surgical resection remains the only effective cure. In addition, the definitive treatment of benign lung diseases for which medical management has failed to achieve a cure can require resection of involved segments. Such resection may also remove substantial amounts of pulmonary parenchyma, chest wall, or nonvital mediastinal structures. A thorough assessment of the patient and the disease process is crucial before resection is undertaken. Knowledge of associated operative risk, projected loss of pulmonary function, and anticipated recovery time is necessary for a determination of whether the risk is prohibitive. Preoperative attention to detail can optimize the patient's short-term and long-term recovery. Understanding the extent of resection required for curative treatment and refusing to compromise this goal are also important. Achieving the optimal balance between the risks and benefits of curative resection can be challenging.

The ability to resect lung parenchyma and, perhaps, the chest wall or mediastinal structures has depended on the evolution of surgical, anesthetic, and medical techniques. Avoiding complications is a matter of preparation, experience, and careful patient selection. Foremost is the preoperative assessment of the patient. Predictors of operative outcome are especially crucial for an aging population for whom quality-of-life issues are paramount. This chapter will review the indications for diagnostic methods such as bronchoscopy, mediastinoscopy, thoracentesis, and tube thoracostomy and the complications associated with these procedures. It will then present the complications associated with resection of lung parenchyma and the chest wall, as well as strategies for dealing with these complications.

EVALUATION

The evaluation of a patient for possible lung and chest wall resection involves determining the extent of the disease and the patient's ability to undergo surgical intervention. The information obtained from the clinical history and physical examination directs the workup. Initial tests for determining the cardiopulmonary fitness of the patient include studies of pulmonary function and carbon monoxide diffusion capacity (DLCO), ventilation-perfusion scans, exercise testing, and electrocardiography. The diagnostic studies involved in defining the extent of thoracic disease, whether benign or malignant, include chest radiography and computed tomography (CT) with intravenous contrast. For cases involving malignancy, CT scanning of the head with intravenous contrast, bone scanning, and F-18 fluorodeoxyglucose-positron emission tomography (FDG-PET) scanning are used selectively to determine the presence of metastatic disease. The use of chest CT and FDG-PET scans in deciding which diagnostic and therapeutic options should be pursued continues to evolve. The role of invasive procedures such as bronchoscopy, mediastinoscopy, thoracentesis, and tube thoracostomy continues to change as well.

Noninvasive Studies
Cardiopulmonary Tests

The evaluation of patients for elective lung resection begins with an assessment of the patient's physiologic status. Initial assessment includes clinical history, physical examination, and pulmonary function testing. Any abnormality should prompt further evaluation. Noninvasive studies include maximal oxygen uptake (VO_{2max}), cardiac stress testing, quantitative ventilation-perfusion scanning, the six-minute walk, and stair climbing. Invasive studies are uncommonly used but may include pulmonary artery pressure measurement and pulmonary angiography, particularly if pulmonary hypertension is suspected.

Functional evaluation before pulmonary resection allows the assessment of predicted postoperative function. Pulmonary perfusion scans can assist in predicting postoperative forced expiratory volume in one second (FEV_1), DLCO, and VO_{2max}. VO_{2max} is an excellent parameter of pulmonary and cardiovascular reserves and is an easily standardized exercise test. Incorporating the extent of resection with the physiologic reserve of the patient allows the most accurate assessment of risk. An established preoperative algorithm of risk assessment for patients undergoing pulmonary resection permits safe extension of the inclusion criteria to higher risk patients (1). The use of cardiopulmonary exercise testing can assist in determining which patients will be able to tolerate resection despite borderline pulmonary function. Pate et al. (2) determined that surgical resection is safe for patients with a preoperative FEV_1 greater than 1.6 L (40% of its predicted value), those who were able to climb three or more flights of stairs, those with a predicted postoperative FEV_1 of more than 700 mL, and those with a postoperative maximum oxygen consumption of at least 10 mg/kg.

The algorithm developed by Bolliger and Perruchoud (1) supports this conclusion. It indicates that resections as complex as pneumonectomy can be performed if preoperative FEV_1 and DLCO exceed 80% of predicted values. If these preoperative factors are below 80% of predicted values, the patient should undergo exercise testing to determine VO_{2max}. If VO_{2max} exceeds 75% of the predicted value or exceeds 20 mL/kg/min, the patient should be able to safely undergo pneumonectomy. If VO_{2max} is less than 75% of the predicted value, a split function study is performed. If the predicted postresection FEV_1 or DLCO is less than 40%, the patient is deemed inoperable. If either of these measures is more than 40%, the predicted postresection value, VO_{2max}, is the deciding factor. If this factor exceeds 40% of the predicted value or exceeds 10 mL/kg/min, the patient is deemed operable. Using this algorithm, Bolliger and Perruchoud (1) achieved a postoperative mortality rate of only 1.5% and a morbidity rate of 11%.

Another predictor of outcome for patients undergoing lung resection is change in DLCO during exercise (3). Wang et al. (3) found that if DLCO did not increase by more than 10% during exercise, the risk of complications after lung resection was significantly higher.

Nevertheless, reliance on pulmonary function tests alone may overestimate functional loss after lung resection (1). In fact, if the lung to be resected exhibits severe emphysematous changes, resection may even provide a benefit (4). Patients who have undergone lobectomy or lesser resections exhibit an early functional deficit that is usually followed by nearly complete long-term recovery. The permanent functional loss after lobectomy is small and has only a minimal impact on exercise capacity. In contrast, pneumonectomy results in an early, permanent loss of 30% of exercise capacity and pulmonary function.

The evaluation of the patient with significant cardiac risk factors for noncardiac surgery remains controversial. If the patient has significant risk factors but no symptoms, the indication for cardiac evaluation is limited. Instead, the patient should be treated medically with appropriate therapy such as beta-blockers, smoking cessation, control of lipids and hypertension, and aspirin. If the patient has symptomatic angina pectoris, congestive heart failure, or a history of myocardial infarction, a more thorough workup with exercise or thallium stress testing is indicated (5). The results of these tests will determine whether further invasive testing is indicated.

CT of the Chest

Standard posterior–anterior and lateral chest radiographs are almost always the first study performed in an assessment of thoracic pathology. Although radiography has negligible complications, it also has significant limitations. A CT scan, on the other hand, permits a thorough anatomic evaluation of the lungs, mediastinum, and upper abdomen. CT-scanning protocols for thoracic diseases usually recommend the use of intravenous contrast material with 7- to 10-mm cuts that include contiguous images from the thoracic apex to the abdomen, including the liver and adrenal glands. Preoperative CT scanning is crucial for determining location, extent, and spread of disease. It is an easily reproducible study that is highly reliable. Its greatest limitation is the lack of definitive pathologic diagnosis for local and distant disease.

In cases of bronchogenic carcinoma, the ability of chest CT to determine whether metastatic disease has involved mediastinal lymph nodes is particularly limited (6). This limitation is especially applicable to patients with a central tumor, a mass greater than 4 cm in diameter, elevated carcinoembryonic antigen levels, or enlarged lymph nodes (7). Confirmation of disease by tissue biopsy is required for accurate diagnosis and staging.

CT scanning is therefore a fundamental study that should be performed before any surgical intervention is undertaken for chest disease. Notable possible exceptions are spontaneous pneumothorax, massive hemoptysis, and trauma; for these conditions, chest radiography alone may be adequate. In addition to its value in the initial evaluation, CT scanning is also important in assessing complications. It is far more precise than chest radiography in delineating postoperative problems and can also guide interventions such as thoracentesis and tube thoracostomy.

Complications of chest CT scanning are primarily related to the intravenous contrast agent used (8,9). Allergic response to the contrast material can range from mild rash or nausea to respiratory failure. Nephrotoxicity is also a potential complication that is especially concerning for patients with renal insufficiency.

PET Scanning

FDG-PET is an evolving technique that identifies malignancy by using a D-glucose analog concentrated in metabolically active cells. FDG-PET scanning is highly accurate in identifying and staging lung cancer. In defining nodal metastasis in the chest, FDG-PET scanning is 91% accurate, whereas CT scanning is only 64% accurate (10).

Complications associated with PET scanning are extremely uncommon. Rather, it is the failure to appreciate the limitations of PET imaging, which may result in judgment errors. Nodules smaller than 1 cm in diameter are difficult to detect because of limitations in resolution. Also, the uptake of FDG by myocardium may render delineation of a retrocardiac mass difficult. Furthermore, the uptake of FDG depends on the metabolic activity of cells. False-negative or false-positive results may occur when tumors are growing slowly or when active infectious or inflammatory processes are present. FDG-PET scanning is a relatively new addition to the evaluation of lung cancer and should be used in conjunction with established protocols.

Invasive Procedures

Bronchoscopy

Bronchoscopy is an invaluable tool for diagnostic and therapeutic interventions involving the airways. The techniques of rigid and flexible bronchoscopy are complimentary. Both methods allow for tissue biopsy, clearance of secretions and blood, and visualization of proximal airway obstruction. Each method has distinct strengths and limitations.

Flexible bronchoscopy is simpler to perform and more versatile in its application. It can be performed with patients awake or sedated and with spontaneous or ventilated respirations. Biopsy of masses and lymph nodes can be performed via direct or transbronchial approaches. Flexible bronchoscopy provides access for laser therapy and stent placement. It also helps determine the extent of endobronchial tumors, an important component in planning the appropriate extent of resection. Finally, flexible bronchoscopy allows visual inspection up to the level of the tertiary bronchus, far beyond the limits of rigid bronchoscopy.

Complications that occur frequently during diagnostic flexible bronchoscopy are bronchospasm and respiratory failure that occasionally requires intubation (11). If the patient has postobstruction pneumonia, relief of the obstruction can result in contamination of the unaffected lung. Biopsy can cause bleeding or airway perforation. Although rare, these complications are also associated with laser therapy (12). Laser therapy carries the additional risks of air embolism, airway necrosis with delayed perforation, and airway obstruction due to necrotic tumor debris. Stents are also associated with specific risks such as airway obstruction, stent migration, airway perforation, erosion into the pleural space or into vascular structures, and tumor overgrowth (13,14).

Performing rigid bronchoscopy safely is technically more challenging than performing flexible bronchoscopy safely. However, rigid bronchoscopy is a crucial skill for managing such complications as massive hemoptysis or distal trachea stenosis. It allows for complete airway control and can be used in conjunction with flexible bronchoscopy to access more distal airways. General anesthesia is a prerequisite for performing rigid bronchoscopy.

Complications of rigid bronchoscopy include perforation, bleeding, and injury to the teeth. If biopsies are performed or stents are deployed, the complications associated with those procedures are the same as those associated with flexible bronchoscopy. Because general anesthesia is required for rigid bronchoscopy, loss of airway can be a serious complication during induction. Careful planning is required for treating patients with distal airway compromise.

Mediastinoscopy

Mediastinoscopy is an important procedure in the diagnosis and staging of lung cancer. Even patients with small peripheral primary tumors and negative results on CT scanning have an 11% chance of metastatic involvement of the mediastinal nodes (15). Mediastinoscopy determines which patients have advanced-stage disease before resection; this finding allows the consideration of neoadjuvant therapy as part of the treatment plan (16). Mediastinoscopy also provides access to mediastinal masses for tissue biopsy.

Mediastinoscopy is performed through a small curvilinear incision just above the sternal notch. The dissection is carried down to the pretracheal plane. Accessing the proper plane is important for maintaining orientation and a relatively dry field of dissection. Before the mediastinoscope is inserted, digital exploration allows the identification of the innominate artery and potential palpation of a mass or an enlarged lymph node. Once the scope has been inserted, careful blunt dissection with a rigid suction device allows full exposure of any mass before biopsy. Minor bleeding is controlled by electrocautery or tamponade. The structure on which biopsy is to be performed must be clearly identified and delineated. If there is any uncertainty, needle aspiration can be performed to rule out a vascular structure. A feeling of resistance during the biopsy may indicate tumor invasion into a mediastinal structure. Biopsy of tumor, which has invaded a vascular structure, may result in a dramatic vessel tear.

Although mediastinoscopy is generally a safe procedure, it is associated with several known complications (17). Given the proximity of the mediastinum to such crucial structures as the great vessels, knowledge of the relevant anatomy is vital. Also crucial is an understanding of how a disease process may alter the normal anatomy by fibrosis, invasion, or displacement. Complications of mediastinoscopy include hemorrhage, stroke, nerve injury, pneumothorax, and esophageal perforation. Injury to the pulmonary artery, superior vena cava, azygos vein, aorta, innominate artery, or left atrium can result in massive bleeding.

If the hole is very small, tamponade with the scope may control the injury. However, thoracotomy or sternotomy may be required for access and repair. Temporary control of the injury may be possible with scope or sponge tamponade; this temporary control allows time to reposition the patient if necessary and to prepare for exploration. The risk of stroke is low and is related to compression of diseased innominate or carotid arteries. Palpation of calcified vessels before insertion of the scope can heighten the awareness of this potential problem.

Nerve injury can occur at several points. The left recurrent laryngeal nerve is especially prone to injury when the left tracheobronchial angle is dissected. Also, either phrenic nerve may be injured by lateral dissection. If the pleural space is entered, a pneumothorax may result. If pneumothorax is identified during the procedure and if no lung injury has occurred, the condition can be easily remedied by placing a catheter into the pleural space through the incision and closing the incision around the tube. Suction is applied to the catheter during positive-pressure ventilation and the catheter is then removed. A postprocedure chest radiograph will determine whether a residual pneumothorax is present and whether a chest tube is required. Esophageal injury can occur during dissection or biopsy of subcarinal lymph nodes. If the injury involves only the muscle layer, no intervention is required; a mucosal injury, however, requires primary closure.

The use of neoadjuvant chemotherapy for stage IIIA non–small cell lung cancer may require restaging the mediastinal lymph nodes. Because of mediastinal fibrosis, repeat mediastinoscopy is technically much more difficult to perform than the original mediastinoscopy. However, the repeated procedure is highly accurate in evaluating the response to treatment and determining whether pulmonary resection is appropriate (18). Repeat mediastinoscopy has not been replaced by PET-FDG imaging because false-positive results can be caused by inflammatory changes due to radiation and previous surgery. The risks associated with repeat mediastinoscopy are similar to those associated with the initial procedure.

Most complications associated with mediastinoscopy can be avoided if careful attention is maintained to anatomy, dissection, and visualization. The procedure is an essential component in the diagnosis and staging of thoracic diseases. Although mediastinoscopy is often regarded as a minor procedure, given the severity of its potential complications, it should be undertaken with knowledge and respect.

Thoracentesis

Thoracentesis is generally a straightforward, well-tolerated procedure. The use of a needle or small catheter enables physicians to perform a biopsy of a lung mass or of the pleura, or to aspirate an effusion for therapeutic and diagnostic intervention (19). After patients recover from pulmonary resection, drainage of an effusion is occasionally necessary because fluid may accumulate after chest tube removal during the early or late postoperative course. The effusion may be benign, malignant, infectious, or chylous. The location and size of the effusion dictate the need for radiologic guidance with CT or ultrasonography.

Complications associated with thoracentesis primarily include pneumothorax and bleeding. A pneumothorax will occur if the parenchyma is injured at the time of needle entry or as the lung expands. Treatment will require a chest tube if the patient exhibits symptoms or if the pneumothorax results in separation of more than 2 to 3 cm between the chest wall and the lung. Evacuation of pleural effusion may reveal that the remaining lung did not completely fill the hemithorax after lung resection. In such circumstances, tube thoracostomy is not necessary unless the fluid is infected. Insertion of the needle can cause bleeding from an intercostal artery or vein. Bleeding that results from a vascular injury during thoracentesis may require surgical intervention if a large hemothorax develops. A chest radiograph should be performed after thoracentesis, so that the completeness of drainage can be determined and any complications can be evaluated.

A vagal response may occur during thoracentesis. As fluid is removed, reexpansion of the lung may cause the patient to begin coughing. Stimulation of the pleura can cause a sensation of faintness. If the patient is sitting up when this vagal response occurs, the procedure should be immediately terminated and the patient is placed in a supine position. If patients have a history of such a reaction, pretreatment with atropine and a narcotic may prevent this response during future procedures.

Chest Tube Insertion

The proper placement of a chest tube at the bedside or in the operating room after a thoracotomy is a true skill. A properly placed tube can prevent the complications of effusion, empyema, air leak, and atelectasis. In the operating room, creating a subcutaneous tunnel and placing the tube under direct visualization ensure the most effective function of the tube and the rapid closure of the track once the tube is removed. At the bedside, adequate pain control is essential for proper positioning of the chest tube. The trocar technique of chest tube insertion is recommended only if a large effusion is present. Otherwise, an incision large enough for digital exploration of the chest cavity helps assess the extent of the disease and the proper direction of tube placement. It is also possible to palpate pleural studding by tumor, pleural thickening by fibrothorax, lung expansion, and blood clot. Usually the tube is directed apically for evacuation of air and posteriorly for fluid drainage. Guidance by CT or ultrasonography is particularly helpful. When patients have previously undergone thoracotomy, the chest tube should be inserted at or above the level of the incision because the diaphragm can be quite elevated. Guidance by CT or ultrasonography is often invaluable in this situation.

Complications of chest tube insertion include parenchymal or vascular injury, malpositioning, and erosion into vital structures. As with any such technique, resistance during tube placement should be an important indication of improper placement. The chest tube could lacerate lung parenchyma, airway, or mediastinal structures during placement. Such lacerations may cause bleeding and air leak. These parenchymal injuries are usually self-limited. However, other more serious complications can occur with insertion. Major vessels may be injured and massive hemorrhage may result. Similarly, the main stem bronchus may be injured and a large air leak may result. Repair of these injuries requires emergent thoracotomy. Additionally, the diaphragm may be perforated during chest tube insertion. Such perforation could lead to liver, spleen, or intestinal injury requiring laparotomy. A persistent air leak may indicate that the chest tube is in the parenchyma. This malpositioning is often demonstrated by CT scan of the chest. Removing the tube usually results in healing, but placing a second tube is often required while the injury resolves.

Complications of chest tube placement at the site of insertion include bleeding and wound infection. Substantial bleeding is usually the result of an injury to the intercostal vessels. This type of injury is uncommon if the tube is inserted along the upper border of the rib. However, an injury may be unavoidable for patients with small intercostal spaces and may require thoracotomy for control of bleeding. Minor bleeding at the site of chest tube insertion comes from either the skin or the chest wall muscle. A skin suture will often control the problem. However, careful monitoring of chest tube drainage should follow suture placement because the bleeding at the site of insertion may be due to a deeper, more substantial source. Prolonged chest tube drainage may result in wound problems at the insertion site. Seroma, skin erosion, hematoma, and infection are best managed by tube removal. Open wound care to the site often results in rapid resolution. A separate chest tube may be required for treating the ongoing thoracic concern.

A chest tube should be removed immediately after resolution of air leaks and effusion. Failure to remove a tube increases the risk of tube erosion into vital structures. If an air leak persists for days or if an air leak suddenly develops, the drainage system should be checked from the chest wall to the drainage container for confirmation that there is no break in the system. At the same time, chest radiographs should be performed for confirmation that the most proximal tube hole lies within the thoracic cavity. If a tube has moved out of position or is no longer functional, it should be removed and a new tube should be placed. For percutaneously placed small tubes that have suddenly stopped draining but are in good position, irrigation with a lytic agent frequently clears the tube of

fibrinous material and keeps it functioning without the need for a change of position.

A pneumothorax may result when a chest tube is removed. Placing an occlusive dressing as the tube is removed is usually sufficient for avoiding this problem. For thin patients or for tubes without a subcutaneous track, a U-stitch may be placed around the insertion site and tied as the tube is removed. The dressing is usually left in place for 48 hours, so that the track can close. Almost all chest tube sites are associated with some degree of inflammation and drainage during healing. Abscesses or infection are unusual, but if they do occur, local wound care is usually adequate. Antibiotics are required only if substantial cellulitis is present.

RESPIRATORY PROBLEMS
Acquired Postoperative Pneumonia

Pneumonia refers to an infectious inflammation of the lung that is characterized by an exudative consolidation of the respiratory bronchioles, alveolar ducts, and acini. The term "pneumonia" should not be used synonymously with pneumonitis because pneumonitis is limited to a noninfectious inflammation of the lung parenchyma.

Typically, postoperative pneumonitis is a result of the aspiration of gastric contents. Endotracheal intubation, obesity, gastrointestinal dysfunction, and hiatal hernia are among the most frequently encountered risk factors for aspiration. Although the rate of secondary infection may be as high as 50%, the role of antibiotics in treating pneumonitis is less clear. It is generally recommended that antibiotics be withheld until clinical evidence of infection is present and the results of appropriate cultures have been obtained. For example, even though fever, expectoration, and a new infiltrate as demonstrated by chest radiography are considered signs of pneumonia, 50% to 60% of patients with these signs do not have identifiable signs of lung infection (20,21). The best approach to management is the prevention of aspiration, particularly among high-risk patients.

Nosocomial pneumonia is defined as a pulmonary infection that develops 48 to 72 hours after admission to the hospital. The classic triad of fever, a new pulmonary infiltrate, and shortness of breath are nonspecific symptoms of nosocomial pneumonia. The Centers for Disease Control and Prevention (CDC) has proposed the following criteria for the diagnosis of nosocomial pneumonia in adults: (i) a change in the character of the sputum; (ii) culture of a pathogen from blood, lung biopsy, or distal airway secretions; (iii) isolation of a virus or a viral antigen from respiratory secretions; and (iv) histologic evidence of pneumonia. Although gram stains and cultures of sputum are routinely used in the diagnosis of nosocomial pneumonia, they are not included in the CDC criteria (22). More reliable techniques of obtaining distal airway secretions are protected specimen brushing, bronchoalveolar lavage, and protected bronchoalveolar lavage.

Nosocomial pneumonia is usually caused by bacterial infections. The microbiology of nosocomial pneumonia is different from that of community-acquired pneumonia. Most nosocomial pneumonias are caused by gram-negative enteric bacilli. The oropharynx and stomach of a hospitalized patient are colonized by aerobic gram-negative organisms. Approximately one billion bacteria are found in 1 mL of saliva (23). It is supposed that these microorganisms reach the lower respiratory tract by microaspiration or macroaspiration. Therefore, a miniscule inoculum of saliva will carry a generous bacterial load.

Additional risk factors for the development of nosocomial pneumonia include chronic obstructive pulmonary disease (COPD), malnutrition, obesity, indiscriminate use of antibiotics, and thoracic or upper abdominal surgery (24). Surgery to the thorax and upper abdomen has a direct effect on the mechanical properties of the lungs and the chest wall because patients undergoing such surgery will routinely experience a decrease in functional residual capacity (FRC) and will therefore exhibit progressive atelectasis with an impaired cough. The ability to cough effectively is further compromised by pain or by an increase in intra-abdominal pressure caused by postoperative ileus.

A well thought-out clinical approach is warranted for patients with pneumonitis rather than nosocomial pneumonia. The overall mortality rate associated with pneumonitis is estimated to range from 30% to 55%; the risk increases by approximately 1% per day when mechanical ventilation is added to the treatment regimen (25). The rapidity of the process, the immunocompetence of the host, and the clinical condition of the patient should dictate the decision to initiate antibiotics. The antimicrobial regimen selected should be tailored according to the results of gram staining and final cultures.

Postoperative management of patients with pneumonitis includes important preventative measures. These patients require aggressive bronchopulmonary hygiene, including frequent chest physiotherapy, incentive spirometry, nebulized bronchodilators, and, rarely, bronchoscopic aspiration of secretions. In general, aggressive bronchopulmonary hygiene will not be needed after the first postoperative week, provided that pneumonia has not developed.

Air Leaks

Formation of air leaks after pulmonary resection is an extremely common problem that can result in prolonged hospitalization. Despite the frequency of this condition, there are few objective data about its treatment. Air leaks along the divided parenchyma are very common initially. Even though some air leaks persist for several days, most will seal spontaneously. Haste in deciding in favor of aggressive surgical intervention is not warranted.

The approach to air leaks should be systematic. First, one should ensure that the air is leaking from the lung and not from the chest tube system. Second, if the patient underwent closure of a major bronchus and the leak is quite large (inspiratory or continuous), bronchopleural fistula must be ruled out. Bronchoscopy is essential for making this diagnosis. If a bronchopleural fistula has been ruled out by bronchoscopy, the leak can be called an alveolar–pleural fistula. It can then be classified according to size and its relationship to the respiratory cycle. Air leaks most commonly occur during expiration and rarely require operative intervention.

Air leaks may be divided into four main categories: (i) forced expiratory, present only with a cough; (ii) expiratory, present only with expiration; (iii) inspiratory, present only during inspiration; and (iv) continuous, present throughout the respiratory cycle. In their prospective review, Cerfolio et al. (26) analyzed 101-consecutive pulmonary resections and found that most air leaks after resection are expiratory in nature. A low ratio between FEV_1 and forced vital capacity, increased age, increased residual volume, and increased FRC predicted persistent air leaks. Substantial air leaks often result from poor surgical technique or the presence of underlying lung disease such as emphysema. Because most pulmonary fissures are not complete, lobectomies and segmental resections are often accompanied by an initial air leak that will generally stop within the first three or four postoperative days. Meticulous surgical technique is paramount to preventing air leaks. Placing three rows of staples appears to offer the best pneumostasis.

Lungs with normal parenchyma do not need reinforcement. Surgeons must be careful not to tear the lung by using excessive traction or by placing too thick a portion of the lung within the jaws of the stapler. If severe fibrosis or emphysema is present, the staple line may be reinforced with synthetic or bovine pericardial strips. Before the thoracotomy is closed, the lung should be carefully inspected for air leaks, and any such leaks should be closed. Air leaks from the raw surface of the lungs may be controlled by using the coagulative effects of an yttrium-aluminum-garnet laser (27) or an argon beam coagulator. Additionally, in some instances, fibrin glue may be useful in controlling air leaks (28). A chest tube should be placed into the hemithorax after all pulmonary resections. This tube will evacuate air and fluid and will allow the lung to remain completely expanded. Underwater drainage may be supplemented by suction, so that air and fluid can be more efficiently and continuously evacuated from the pleural space. Virtually all parenchymal air leaks will stop if the pleural space is adequately drained and the lung is fully expanded with apposition to the chest wall.

Inspiratory air leaks are extremely unusual and generally require intervention. Apposition of the parietal and visceral pleura is an important factor in sealing air leaks. At times, persistent air leaks may respond better when the chest tube suction level is decreased to $10\,cmH_2O$. Conversion to water seal drainage should not be performed if a pneumothorax develops when the suction is turned off. A small air space that does not increase over time does not require continuous suction. Similarly, if subcutaneous air develops while water seal drainage is being used, the chest tube should be returned to suction. If the pneumothorax still persists, an increase in the suction level may be required at the expense of possible worsening of the air leak.

If the air leak persists for more than seven days, intervention with a sclerotherapeutic agent should be considered. Talc is a readily available and effective sclerosing agent. Talc slurry consists of 5 g of sterile talc dissolved in warm, normal saline solution. This slurry is injected into the chest tube under sterile conditions, and the tube is clamped. If a large air leak is present, the tube should be clamped briefly and then be returned to suction. Rarely, a second pleurodesis is required for full resolution of the air leak. It is important to use no more than 5 g of talc per pleurodesis because larger doses can cause acute pulmonary edema (29).

Alternatively, the patient may be discharged with a Heimlich valve in place in an attempt to avoid the potential complications of sclerotherapy. This is an important alternative for patients who may require future thoracic procedures or those with benign disease. Patients treated in this manner require careful follow-up because the valve may become obstructed with fibrinous exudate. Unfortunately, the air leak may not resolve for several weeks.

Torsion of Lobe or Segment

Pulmonary torsion is a rare but serious complication; it occurs in approximately 0.2% of patients who undergo thoracic surgery and is associated with a mortality rate of 22% (30,31). After pulmonary tissue has been removed, one of the remaining lobes or segments of the lung may twist on its bronchial pedicle, and such twisting may cause total bronchial obstruction and venous outflow. Bronchial or pulmonary arterial inflow is seldom hampered. Massive enlargement of the lobe will result. Patients often exhibit persistently high fever, hemoptysis, and bronchorrhea. Because patients may have a balanced ventilation-perfusion defect, the results of blood gas analysis may be misleadingly normal.

Pulmonary torsion is most often seen after pulmonary resection (lobectomy or bilobectomy), but can occur after any thoracic procedure. The literature contains reports of 28 well-documented cases (32). Pulmonary torsion may occur after procedures such as esophageal myotomy, fundoplication, and aortic repair. Spontaneous pulmonary torsion may also occur after blunt chest trauma (32). By far the most commonly reported form of pulmonary torsion is that of the right middle lobe after right upper lobectomy;

the left upper lobe is the next most frequently involved. The remaining lobes should be routinely fixed together with a suture.

The diagnosis of pulmonary torsion requires maintaining a high level of suspicion. Radiographic and bronchoscopic findings confirm the diagnosis. The chest radiograph shows an enlarged homogenously consolidated lobe. One radiologic clue to the possibility of torsion is the outline of the blood supply to the affected lung area as demonstrated by a posterolateral chest radiograph: in such cases, the blood vessels travel toward the apex of the lung rather than toward the base. CT scanning vividly demonstrates the failure of the affected lobe to take up intravenous contrast and the absence of air in the alveoli. It is the enlargement of the lobe that distinguishes torsion from atelectasis. Bronchoscopy demonstrates a smooth occlusion of the bronchus in the absence of a mucous plug or mucosal irregularities. Interruption of the pulmonary artery may be demonstrated by arteriography. However because time is of the essence, the surgeon should avoid unnecessary delays in confirming the diagnosis if the patient is deemed to have an operable condition.

When the diagnosis of lobar torsion is made, immediate operation is mandatory. Salvage of the lobe by simple detorsion has been advocated (32). However, assessing the amount of ischemic pulmonary insult is almost impossible. Immediate detorsion for hope of lung salvage may cause severe physiologic deterioration. The outcome is usually grave because preserving the affected lobe exposes the patient to the effects of an ischemia-reperfusion injury. Furthermore, secretions trapped in the periphery may flood the main bronchi. For these reasons, lobectomy is recommended more commonly than detorsion. Double-lumen endotracheal tubes are essential for protecting the other lung. Lobectomy should be performed, and detorsion of the lobe should be avoided until the hilum has been isolated and occluded.

Gangrene of the Lung

Gangrene of the lung occurs as a result of total cessation of the venous return of the lung or one of its lobes, or as a result of complete pulmonary artery occlusion in conjunction with an insufficient bronchial artery system (33). Additionally, pulmonary gangrene may be a rare complication of a severe lung infection with devitalization of lung parenchyma and secondary infection (34). This condition usually produces a clinical picture of sepsis, with rapid rise in temperature, chills, hemoptysis, foul-smelling sputum, and even expectoration of necrotic lung tissue. If untreated, gangrene of the lung may lead to uncontrolled sepsis, multiple organ system failure, and death. Pleural empyema commonly accompanies gangrene of the lung. Clinically, the patient will exhibit foul-smelling sputum and the drainage of purulent material from the chest tube. Physicians should maintain a high index of suspicion for pleural empyema and should not be misled by the differential diagnosis of lobar pneumonia. The chest radiograph will demonstrate an area of homogeneous density with sharp margins, and CT of the chest will establish the diagnosis with certainty.

Resection of the gangrenous tissue is mandatory and lifesaving (35). In the presence of pleural empyema, dissection of the hilar structures can lead to mediastinitis, bronchopleural fistula, or both. In this setting, one may consider a two-stage procedure consisting of immediate fenestration and then delayed resection of the gangrenous lung in a clean field with immediate closure of the pleural window (34). Gangrene of the lung is best avoided by meticulous surgical technique. Clear and respectful understanding of the hilar anatomy with gentle and precise dissection is by far the best way of avoiding this complication.

Mediastinal Shift

After pulmonary resection, the mediastinum shifts to compensate for the loss of volume in the involved hemithorax. This shift is part of the compensatory mechanism for obliterating the space after partial or complete lung removal. Other mechanisms at work during this postoperative readjustment phase include expansion of the remaining lung on the ipsilateral side, elevation of the diaphragm, and narrowing of the intercostal spaces on the ipsilateral side. An excessive postoperative mediastinal shift frequently indicates ipsilateral lobar atelectasis, contralateral pulmonary hyperexpansion, fluid accumulation, or even pneumothorax on the side opposite the surgical procedure. Extreme mediastinal shifts may result in an uncommon but life-threatening complication known as postpneumonectomy syndrome.

Postpneumonectomy syndrome was originally believed to occur exclusively among children because their bronchi are softer and more compressible. Now, however, it is readily identified as a possible complication among adults (36). It is caused by airway obstruction resulting from an extreme mediastinal shift after pneumonectomy; such a shift may lead to bronchomalacia. Although almost exclusively described as occurring after pneumonectomy on the right side of the body, postpneumonectomy syndrome may also occasionally occur on the left side (37). After right pneumonectomy, the mediastinum moves posteriorly and counterclockwise to the left. Realignment of the intrathoracic structures results in tracheal displacement to the right and compression of the left main stem bronchus as it angles beneath the aorta and is flattened against the vertebral column or against the descending aorta (36). Similar anatomic distortion after left pneumonectomy occurs typically in the presence of a right-sided aortic arch, but has also been reported with a normally located left-sided aortic arch (37).

In general, patients with postpneumonectomy syndrome fall into one of two groups. The first has mechanical compression alone, whereas the second also has secondary bronchomalacia of the cartilages. The airway compression clearly results from mediastinal displacement. The mediastinal shift occurs within months to years after the pneumonectomy. Symptoms follow soon thereafter on a progressive and severely disabling course (36). Patients may exhibit an acute onset of dyspnea and airway obstruction or may exhibit a more insidious onset of symptoms such as repeated bouts of pulmonary infections, persistent cough, or stridor. Many patients tolerate the symptoms well until critical airway obstruction develops; at this point, patients exhibit acute respiratory distress.

Conventional chest radiography demonstrates the marked lateral and posterior displacement of the trachea and mediastinum toward the side of the pneumonectomy. The exact site of bronchial compression can be confirmed by CT of the chest. Angiography of the affected vessels is usually not indicated as part of the initial workup, but may be useful if aortic bypass is contemplated. Fluoroscopy is recommended for the preoperative diagnosis of bronchomalacia. Although fluoroscopy is very sensitive, it is not very specific. Bronchomalacia confirmed by fluoroscopy may completely resolve after the bronchial compression has been relieved.

Two strategies can be used for avoiding postpneumonectomy syndrome. First, placing a chest tube into the pneumonectomy space will allow repositioning of the mediastinum and hence will permit equilibration and monitoring of fluid output. The tube is usually removed in 24 hours. Second, air can be withdrawn from the pleural space after closure until negative pressure is obtained. This procedure, which is called "setting the mediastinum," avoids the need for a tube.

If the diagnosis of postpneumonectomy syndrome is established, the goal of therapy is surgical restoration of the mediastinum to its normal anatomic position. Such repositioning allows the compromised airway to return to its normal position and patency. Simple replacement and suture fixation of the mediastinum are unreliable. The empty hemithorax must be filled if recurrence of the disorder is to be prevented. Filling the empty hemithorax with silicone or saline breast implants is acceptable and dependable. In comparison with other, more complex surgical procedures, this operation is fairly simple and often achieves immediate and dramatic improvement (38).

The benefit derived from repositioning the mediastinum relates not only to the relief of mechanical obstruction of the bronchus but also to the correction of overdistention and herniation of the lung. This correction is readily demonstrated by marked improvement in the results of pulmonary function tests. If symptoms suggestive of bronchomalacia persist after repositioning of the mediastinum, the patient may require endobronchial stenting.

Mechanical Airway Obstruction

Acute mechanical airway obstruction after pulmonary resection is most commonly due to retained blood clots or thick secretions that were allowed to accumulate during or after the operative procedure. The use of a double-lumen endotracheal tube (Carlen's tube) tends to protect the uninvolved lung during the procedure and to prevent intraoperative accumulation of secretions during surgery by selectively allowing the aspiration of one lung independent of the other. After the operative procedure, each lung is aspirated and the double-lumen tube is removed, or replaced by a single-lumen tube if intubation is to be continued. Indiscriminate use of double-lumen tubes for prolonged respiratory support is not recommended because the tubes are quite rigid and can perforate the airway (39).

Strict attention to the clearance of postoperative airway secretions will prevent postoperative airway obstruction. Careful fluid management is essential to preventing the formation of inspissated secretions. Frequent postoperative bedside auscultation of the lungs will reveal the early signs of airway obstruction due to secretions; these signs include wheezing, rhonchi, stridor, and decreased to absent breath sounds. Chest radiography will reveal air trapping, atelectasis, or pneumonia. Prompt attention with the liberal use of endotracheal suction and bronchoscopy is the most prudent approach to this problem. The use of noninvasive positive-pressure ventilation (inspiratory positive airway pressure, expiratory positive airway pressure, or bilevel positive airway pressure) for certain patients may be effective in treating and preventing postoperative atelectasis.

BRONCHIAL STUMP PROBLEMS
Bronchopleural Fistula

Bronchopleural fistula can occur after lung resection and is associated with a substantial risk of mortality. Fistulas may occur during the immediate or late postoperative course. The combined incidence of bronchopleural fistula after major lung resection ranges from 1% to 2% (40). A study by Sonobe et al. (40) reviewed the incidence of and risk factors for bronchopleural fistulas to determine the indication for preventative stump coverage. The most significant risk factors for bronchopleural fistula were main stem or intermedius bronchial stump; preoperative chemotherapy, radiotherapy, or both; and previous ipsilateral thoracotomy. There was no significant difference in the occurrence of bronchopleural fistula between manual suturing and the use of a stapling device. The authors concluded that preventative stump coverage with a muscle flap is indicated for high-risk resections. A retrospective review by Deschamps et al. (41) concluded that prophylactic coverage of the bronchial stump with viable tissue is indicated for high-risk patients.

Early bronchopleural fistulas occur within one to seven days after surgery and are due to inadequate initial closure. Excessive dissection of the proximal bronchus must be avoided, so that adequate bronchial blood supply can be preserved. Closure should be performed without tension and in an anteroposterior manner, so that the flexible membranous portion is opposed to the rigid cartilaginous portion. Adequate closure is confirmed by filling the hemithorax with saline and temporarily maintaining the airway pressure at 30 to 35 cmH$_2$O. If no air bubbles are seen, the closure is considered adequate.

Late bronchopleural fistulas are a result of ischemia and necrosis, infection of the bronchial stump, or malignant tumor in the bronchial stump. Ischemia can result from perioperative radiation of the tissues or overzealous bronchial dissection (42). Infection of the bronchial stump can result from excessive stump length, bronchitis, or pneumonia. The patient may be at increased risk of infection if preoperative conditions such as postobstructive pneumonia, atelectasis, or bronchitis exist.

The presentation of early bronchopleural fistulas differs slightly from that of late bronchopleural fistulas. An early bronchopleural fistula may be signaled by a sudden, large air leak from the chest tube, substantial loss of volume if the patient is on a ventilator, or hemoptysis. The diagnosis may be established by chest radiography and bronchoscopy. If necessary, the leak can be demonstrated by placing contrast into airway through the bronchoscope under fluoroscopic guidance. Treatment of a confirmed early leak usually involves immediate thoracotomy for reclosure.

A late bronchopleural fistula presents a greater diagnostic and therapeutic challenge. It can occur days to months postoperatively. Symptoms are often subtle and indolent. A chronic cough, a new cough, persistent low-grade fevers, malaise, or recurrent pneumonias are highly suggestive of a bronchopleural fistula. Chest radiography reveals a new air fluid level. Bronchoscopy can identify the location and delineate the size of fistulas and can also detect possible tumor recurrence. CT of the chest is helpful in assessing intrathoracic disease, including tumor recurrence. Treatment can be very complex and is often dictated by the patient's general condition.

The initial intervention for late bronchopleural fistula is conservative, with broad-spectrum intravenous antibiotics and chest tube thoracostomy (43). Care must be taken to avoid contamination of the unaffected lung. Until the infection has been drained, the patient should be kept in the decubitus position with the involved side down. If a small bronchopleural fistula occurs after lobectomy and if there is no evidence of tumor recurrence or tissue necrosis, the fistula may seal with conservative management alone. The additional option of closure by sclerosing or sealing agents may also be used for small fistulas (<7 mm in diameter) (44,45). Conservative management of bronchopleural fistulas that occur after pneumonectomy or in association with empyemas is rarely successful. The complication of postpneumonectomy empyema is associated with a mortality rate of 5% to 10%. Eighty percent of postpneumonectomy empyemas are associated with a bronchopleural fistula (46) and warrant aggressive intervention (47,48). Once the initial infection has been controlled by drainage and antibiotics, surgical treatment can be undertaken. The patient often needs nutritional support and pulmonary physiotherapy. Thoracotomy is required for addressing a bronchopleural fistula. Debridement of the hemithorax is crucial. If a substantial amount of infectious material is present, open wound care is often required. Once the chest cavity is clear of active infection, the fistula can be closed with a muscle flap over the repair. An alternative approach to treating a bronchopleural fistula that has occurred after pneumonectomy is debridement of necrotic tissue, closure of the bronchial stump, and pleural space irrigation. After the pleural drainage has been cleared of infection, as documented by negative results on gram staining, antibiotic solution is instilled into the chest cavity and the drainage catheters are removed (46). This treatment clears the infection with a single operation, but its use is limited to treating relatively early bronchopleural fistulas (those that occur > 30 days postoperatively). If empyema is present, this method will fail.

If the bronchopleural fistula is smaller than 2 mm in diameter, closure is not necessary if the original repair was reinforced with a muscle flap. However, larger fistulae should be debrided back to healthy tissue and closed. For lobectomies, space drainage with suction for at least 10 to 12 days postoperatively will assist the apposition of the muscle flap. A transsternal approach may be used for closing a right bronchopleural fistula after pneumonectomy (49). Such closure is undertaken when drainage of the pleural space is complete and after the chest cavity is clear of infection. Primary closure of the main stem bronchus may not be possible after a bronchopleural fistula has occurred. In this situation, using a muscle flap to fill the bronchus and securing the flap to the edges of the bronchus circumferentially can result in closure of the fistula.

Excessive Length of the Bronchial Stump

When the airway is divided, the length of the bronchial stump should not exceed 1 cm. This guideline is particularly important for left pneumonectomy. The crucial step is clear identification of the carina. The left main stem is approximately 4 cm in length. If the stump is excessively long, secretions can pool in the airway remnant. This pooling leads to ulceration, bronchopleural fistula, aspiration, and hemoptysis. Pooling of secretions is rarely a problem after upper lobectomy because the airways are short and drain easily given their anatomic position.

Complications resulting from excessively long bronchial stumps often occur late in the postoperative course. The diagnosis is based on clinical suspicion and is confirmed by plain radiography and flexible bronchoscopy. If serious purulent bronchitis, hemoptysis, bronchopleural fistula, or chronic aspiration is present, reamputation of the stump is necessary. Muscle flap coverage should also be considered during preoperative planning.

PLEURAL SPACE PROBLEMS
Persistent Airspace

A persistent airspace after pulmonary resection is rare as long as the remaining lung and surrounding structures are healthy. The compliance of lung tissue allows the remaining lung to fill the space left by resection. The compliance of the diaphragm and the chest wall as well as the slight mediastinal shift further reduces the space. It is often possible to anticipate a postoperative space problem on the basis of preoperative studies and the patient's history. Pulmonary function testing, radiographs, and the patient's history usually reveal pulmonary fibrosis resulting from idiopathic, inflammatory, or infectious processes. The same is true of a fixed mediastinum or diaphragm due to previous operations, infections, or pleural thickening.

If an airspace problem is anticipated, several intraoperative maneuvers may aid in alleviating the space. For upper lobe resections, a pleural tent can be created in the apical space. Lower lobe resection may require pneumoperitoneum for elevating the diaphragm. An effective pneumoperitoneum can be created by placing a needle into the peritoneal cavity and insufflating 1.5 L of air (50). The air is slowly reabsorbed over several days. Repeat insufflation may be necessary until the diaphragm is fixed in an elevated position. Such insufflation can be performed by repeated paracentesis or by leaving a small catheter in the peritoneum for this purpose.

If an air space develops postoperatively, several options for management exist. The first choice is to allow the space to fill with serous fluid. This fluid usually will not result in any complications, particularly when the apical air spaces are small. However, an air space that is associated with a persistent air leak may result in empyema. Treatment is then similar to that for bronchopleural fistula and includes antibiotics, possible thoracoplasty directly over the airspace, and filling the space with a muscle flap. Identifying or closing a TEAR in the parenchyma is difficult. Usually, placing tissue in apposition to the muscle flap results in final closure of these air leaks.

Empyema

Empyema rarely occurs after pulmonary resection. Factors that predispose a patient to thoracic space infection include presence of an air space, trapped lung, persistent air leak, bronchopleural fistula, and gross contamination at the time of resection. Mortality and morbidity rates are significantly higher for patients with preoperative empyema due to a destroyed lung (51).

The management of empyema after pulmonary resection begins with immediate drainage of the pleural space, so that pus can be completely evacuated. Tube thoracostomy or open drainage accomplishes gradual sterilization over a period of two to three weeks when appropriate antibiotic coverage is administered concurrently. As a general principle, apposition of parenchyma and parietal pleura is necessary for obliterating the pleural space and resolving the infection. This option is generally feasible only after lobectomy or lesser resections. The greatest management challenge is empyema after pneumonectomy. Eloesser drainage (52), the technique most effective for debriding the cavity, involves open drainage with rib resection at the most dependent aspect of the space. Definitive wound closure is still possible later, once the cavity has been cleared of infection.

For extremely debilitated patients, a large, dependent chest tube placed with the patient under local anesthesia can effectively control infection. The tube is left in place over the long term and the infection resolves very gradually. This method is effective if the space is limited and is the best option for patients who cannot tolerate a more complicated or prolonged procedure.

Wound closure depends on whether a bronchopleural fistula is present. If it is present, closure of either the pneumonectomy cavity or the lobectomy cavity involves muscle flap transposition for coverage of the bronchopleural fistula and obliteration of the space. If no bronchopleural fistula is present, a Clagett procedure (53) for open drainage of the infection may be effective. After several weeks of dressing changes aimed at sterilizing the cavity, an antibiotic solution is instilled into the cavity and the wound is closed. An alternative to the Clagett procedure is allowing granulation tissue to obliterate the space. This method is effective but requires a small residual space; resolution may take one to eight months (54).

Muscle Flap Transposition

The only effective means of treating an infected pleural space associated with a bronchopleural fistula is closure of the fistula and sterilization of the space. Muscle flap transposition is used for reinforcing a bronchial stump closure with well vascularized tissue or for filling a persistent, possibly infected, air space (55).

The choice of muscle flap depends on the location and size of the space (56). Apical spaces are best treated with transposition of the pectoralis major muscle. The latissimus dorsi muscle or serratus anterior muscle may be used for low posterior spaces. It is also possible to use an intercostal muscle flap (57) or a diaphragm muscle flap (58). The decision often depends on whether a previous thoracotomy resulted in division of either the latissimus dorsi muscle or the serratus anterior muscle. Usually, a plastic surgeon works in conjunction with the thoracic surgeon to mobilize the appropriate muscle flap and ensure an adequate blood supply.

The muscle flap must be adequate to fill the space; otherwise, there is potential for recurrent empyema. If the muscle bulk is not quite large enough, thoracoplasty may be required for obliterating a large cavity (59). For the muscle flap to be accommodated without impinging on the vascular pedicle, a portion of one or two ribs should be resected directly over the space. Thoracoplasty may be performed as an initial procedure with debridement of any gross contamination.

Chylothorax

Chylothorax results from injury to the thoracic duct during thoracotomy for pulmonary resection. It has also been reported after pediatric and adult cardiac procedures, esophageal operations, and neck surgeries. Common areas of injury are the left upper part of the chest near the aortic arch and the right lower chest on mobilization of the esophagus. Chylus drainage has a milky appearance because emulsified fats are present in the intestinal lymph. The diagnosis of chylothorax is suggested by persistent chylous chest tube output during the postoperative period. Alternatively, chylothorax may develop after the initial chest tubes have been removed. An effusion develops on the affected side, and thoracentesis or tube thoracostomy is necessary for diagnosis.

Definitive diagnosis of a chylothorax depends on an analysis of the effusion. The triglyceride level is of particular importance. If it is higher than 110 mg/dL, there is a 99% chance that the fluid is chyle (60). Loss of protein, lymphocytes, and fats can lead to serious complications over time. Before a treatment plan can be instituted, the diagnosis must be established, complete drainage with full lung expansion must be allowed, and the daily output must be measured.

Management of chylothorax due to injury during pulmonary resection can be conservative or surgical, depending on the presentation. Management should initially be conservative. This involves allowing nothing orally, draining the pleural space with complete lung expansion, initiating total parenteral nutrition, and perhaps adding somatostatin (61). If the output is less than 500 cc/day while the patient is on this regimen, the likelihood of resolution without surgery is high. Conservative management should be used for as long as 10 to 14 days. The same regimen is recommended if the daily drainage ranges from 500 to 1000 cc. In such cases, the likelihood of success is slightly less, but the initial management strategy is worth trying. If the initial drainage exceeds 1000 cc/day for the first few days, or if the amount of drainage does not decrease after 7 to 10 days of conservative management, spontaneous closure is unlikely, and surgical intervention is recommended (62).

Surgical intervention for persistent chylothorax depends on the injury. The most direct method is ligation at the point of injury. This point may be identified intraoperatively by milky drainage if the patient is given a high-fat diet (e.g., cream) or by lymphangiography just before surgery. Unfortunately, isolating the exact area of injury can be difficult. For this reason, the most effective treatment is ligation of all structures between the aorta and the azygous vein at the level of the diaphragm. This procedure is associated with a 91% success rate (62). Exposure is through a small right thoracotomy incision at the seventh intercostal space. Alternative approaches include talc pleurodesis or video-assisted thoracoscopic closure with clips if the site of injury can be identified. The success of these approaches has been documented, but they are slightly less reliable than open surgical intervention.

CARDIAC PROBLEMS
Arrhythmias

Arrhythmias are the most frequent complications after thoracic surgery. Most commonly, they are of atrial origin and include flutter, fibrillation, and supraventricular tachycardia (63). As is true of arrhythmias after open-heart surgery, these arrhythmias tend to occur within the first 72 hours after surgery. The frequency of postoperative arrhythmias increases with age, history of heart disease, extensive resections, and increased pulmonary vascular resistance (63). The incidence of arrhythmias after pneumonectomy is as high as 40% (64). The exact cause of these arrhythmias remains unclear. Their presentation ranges from asymptomatic rhythm disturbances to hemodynamic collapse. If the patient exhibits no symptoms, the diagnosis is made by physical examination or by electrocardiographic monitoring. Symptoms of atrial arrhythmias include new onset nausea, lightheadedness, palpitations, angina, hypotension, and, rarely, stroke. Evaluation includes physical examination, 12-lead electrocardiography with rhythm strip, and cardiac enzyme profile.

Treatment of atrial arrhythmias focuses on hemodynamic stability, rate control, and possibly anticoagulation. Hemodynamic collapse rarely occurs with atrial arrhythmia; its occurrence should suggest the possibility of associated myocardial infarction or pulmonary embolism. For patients whose condition is unstable, cardioversion using the synchronous mode is indicated. If the patient's condition is stable, the first consideration is rate control. Because cardioversion will usually occur with or without antiarrhythmic therapy within four weeks after surgery, the use of antiarrhythmic agents is controversial. These agents are clearly associated with side effects that limit their safety and efficacy. In addition, the arrhythmia is rarely completely controlled, and the patient will often experience bursts of fibrillation or

flutter. Thus, unless it is contraindicated, anticoagulation is recommended in conjunction with rate control in the immediate postoperative period.

Attempts at preventing postoperative arrhythmias have met with limited success. The administration of digoxin before pneumonectomy has been recommended for preventing atrial fibrillation (65). However, this treatment is successful only in rate control and does not prevent the occurrence of the arrhythmia (66). Only the use of beta-blockers has been shown to significantly reduce the postoperative incidence of atrial fibrillation (67). This treatment is most effective if started preoperatively and continued during the immediate postoperative period. Despite these considerations, arrhythmias after lung surgery are fairly easily managed and do not appear to be associated with higher mortality rates (68).

Pulmonary Hypertension

Postoperative pulmonary hypertension is a difficult problem that may result from either the patient's underlying pulmonary pathology or the extent of resection. Pulmonary hypertension is either primary, which is of unknown cause, or secondary, which is due to left heart failure or pulmonary failure. Among patients who have undergone lengthy lung resection procedures, it is most often associated with a long history of COPD (69).

The diagnosis of pulmonary hypertension is suggested by right heart strain as demonstrated by electrocardiography. It can be confirmed by echocardiography or, if the results of this study are equivocal, by right heart catheterization. Although pulmonary hypertension will rarely preclude lobectomy or segmentectomy, it can contribute to cardiac failure if pneumonectomy is required. A mean pulmonary artery pressure of 35 mmHg or greater is considered pulmonary hypertension. If the pulmonary artery pressure increases by 5 mmHg or more after balloon occlusion, pneumonectomy is associated with serious risks and may be ill advised.

If pulmonary hypertension develops postoperatively, supportive management is necessary. Such treatment includes the administration of nitroglycerin, milrinone, inhaled or intravenous prostaglandins, or inhaled nitric oxide in the short term. Medical intervention for patients with both pulmonary hypertension and COPD includes oxygen, bronchodilators, and antibiotics. In addition, the patient's fluid intake should be restricted. Once positive-pressure ventilation has been removed, the pulmonary artery pressures should normalize somewhat. Because long-term management of pulmonary hypertension is a difficult problem that can lead to progressive respiratory failure and right heart failure, considering this potential complication preoperatively is crucial. The pulmonary artery pressure must be measured preoperatively and if elevated, reduced by pharmacologic means (e.g., endothelin receptor antagonists).

Pulmonary Embolism

Pulmonary resection with ligation of branches of the pulmonary arteries can result in the formation of a thrombus that can dislodge and occlude distal vessels. In the case of pneumonectomy, especially on the right side, the thrombus may embolize into the contralateral lung. If the thrombus is large, such embolization can be a devastating complication because the clot can obstruct the outflow of the right ventricle. If the pulmonary artery stump is suspected as the source of thrombus formation, a rapid diagnosis is crucial. The diagnosis is confirmed by spiral chest CT using an intravenous contrast agent (70). An invasive but more definitive diagnostic method is right heart catheterization with selective angiography of the pulmonary vessels. In addition, the right heart pressures can be assessed at this time, so that the impact of the embolism on the function of the right heart and on the lung can be determined.

If the pulmonary embolus is large, treatment during the immediate postoperative course involves reoperation to divide the pulmonary artery more proximally and remove intra-arterial thrombus. Accomplishing this procedure safely requires cardiopulmonary bypass. If the complication occurs more than several weeks postoperatively, more conventional therapy with thrombolytic agents and heparinization is required. The use of lytic therapy during the early (two to six weeks) postoperative course is not generally recommended; however, there have been case reports of successful use of such therapy during this period. The benefits of thrombolytic therapy during this time period must be weighed against the risk of bleeding, and the decision should be based on each patient's individual condition (71). The best approach is avoiding arterial endothelial injury during the lung resection. The arterial stump should be kept as short as possible, so that the likelihood of thrombus formation can be minimized.

As is true of all major operations, pulmonary resection is also associated with the risk of pulmonary embolism from peripheral sites, especially for patients with malignancy. The prevention, diagnosis, and treatment of this complication are discussed below.

Systemic Embolism

The source of systemic embolization after pulmonary resection is thrombus formation at the stump of the pulmonary vein, often as a result of tumor invading into the pulmonary vein and subsequently embolizing (72). A diagnosis of stroke, peripheral arterial occlusion, or mesenteric ischemia should prompt evaluation of the heart as a possible embolic source. Transesophageal echocardiography allows the most accurate assessment. Treatment is similar to that of an atherosclerotic embolic event: heparinization with emergent embolectomy. Carefully dissecting around the pulmonary veins and creating short vein stumps will minimize the likelihood of this complication.

Careful dissection is especially crucial if tumor invasion into the left atrium is recognized preoperatively.

Cardiac Herniation

For patients with lung cancer, resection of a portion of the right or left pericardium is occasionally required for control of tumor margins. Although lung cancer that has invaded the pericardium is considered to be at a locally advanced stage, complete resection is associated with improvements in the long-term survival rate. However, removal of the pericardium can result in herniation of the heart into the chest cavity, a dramatic complication that usually occurs during the immediate postoperative period. Herniation results in twisting of the vena cavae or obstruction of ventricular outflow. Either event can lead to sudden cardiovascular collapse.

Cardiac herniation toward the right side results in the sudden onset of tachycardia, severe hypotension, cyanosis of the upper half of the body, and elevation in the jugular venous pressure. Herniation into the left chest causes only hypotension and tachycardia because the venous drainage into the heart is not obstructed. The differential diagnosis includes massive intrathoracic hemorrhage, volume loss due to atelectasis of the remaining lung, tension pneumothorax, acute myocardial infarction, and pulmonary embolism. Rapid diagnosis is crucial. A chest radiograph will demonstrate displacement of heart into the hemithorax. The results of chest radiography and the patient's physical presentation are usually sufficient to indicate the need for emergent thoracotomy.

Prevention is the most important means of reducing the likelihood of complications associated with cardiac herniation. Closing any pericardial defect is a simple addition to the original operation. Such closure should be primary if the defect is small. If the defect is larger, replacement of the pericardium with prosthetic material is more appropriate.

Myocardial Infarction

The cardiovascular assessment of patients undergoing noncardiac surgery has been intensively investigated. Patients undergoing thoracotomy have similar risk compared to those undergoing major abdominal or vascular procedures. The rate of cardiac complications is very low for patients with excellent ability to carry out routine daily activities (73). The rate of myocardial infarction or death due to cardiac causes is low for patients who have successfully undergone coronary artery revascularization and remain free of symptoms thereafter; such patients are no different from patients who do not have coronary disease (74–76).

However, several principles of perioperative management may affect cardiac-associated morbidity and mortality rates. Clinical markers are extremely useful in estimating perioperative and long-term cardiac risk. The risk of myocardial infarction is highest for patients with prior myocardial infarction, angina pectoris, congestive heart failure, or diabetes mellitus (77), especially those who are older or whose condition is unstable. The effect of these risk factors appears to be additive (78). The preoperative evaluation may be the first opportunity for appropriate treatment of these patients from a cardiovascular standpoint. For patients with clear evidence of coronary disease, treatment should include aggressive control of elevated serum concentrations of lipids, control of hypertension, smoking cessation, daily administration of aspirin, and administration of beta-blockers. Perioperative use of beta-blockers reduces the long-term risks of both myocardial infarction and death due to cardiovascular causes (79). In particular, patients taking beta-blockers preoperatively should continue taking the medication postoperatively (80). The indication for using beta-blockers to treat patients with cardiac risk factors but with no evidence of disease is less well defined. Patients with congestive heart failure should take angiotensin-converting enzyme inhibitors, in some cases concomitantly with beta-blockers. Because patients who have suffered a nonfatal cardiac event after noncardiac surgery are at risk of later complications, it is critical to use the perioperative period to maximize long-term cardiac care (81).

Patients who have suffered a perioperative myocardial infarction must be aggressively treated with medical therapy and, possibly, revascularization. Presentation is variable and can range from cardiac instability to arrhythmias, angina, or dyspnea. Evaluation with serial enzyme studies and electrocardiography is essential for diagnosis. For an evolving infarction, standard intensive-care management should be instituted while the patient is being prepared for angiographic evaluation, if indicated. The use of lytic therapy is contraindicated during the immediate postoperative period (61). The indications for angioplasty or coronary artery bypass procedures for these patients are the same as those for patients who have not had surgery.

CHEST WALL PROBLEMS
Wound Infection

Wound infections are extremely rare after thoracotomy; when they do occur, they are usually clinically obvious (82). If there is doubt about the diagnosis, fluid for culture should be obtained from the chest wall, the pleural space, or both. If the fluid is infected, the space must be drained. Risk factors associated with infection include inappropriate surgical technique, formation of hematoma within the wound, or fat necrosis in the subcutaneous space. Pyogenic chest wall infection, which may involve bone and cartilage, is caused by processes in the chest wall itself or by extensions of intrathoracic problems that arise in the pleura or the underlying lung.

Perioperative prophylaxis with antibiotics has been demonstrated to reduce the incidence of wound infection from 18% to as low as 1% to 5% (83). A single dose of an antibiotic with gram-positive and gram-negative coverage is given preoperatively; dosing is continued postoperatively for no longer than 24 hours. The incidence of pneumonia and empyema is unaffected by the use of prophylactic antibiotics (83,84).

Any wound infection must be managed in a fashion that will preserve pleural integrity and lung function. Once the infection has been detected, the wound must be opened widely, debrided, and packed so that healthy granulation tissue can form. All chest wall prostheses must be removed. Small wounds may granulate to closure, but larger ones may require secondary closure in the operating room, perhaps including muscle flap closure with split-thickness skin grafting. An attractive alternative for larger wounds is the use of a vacuum dressing device that will act as a suction apparatus for managing wound secretions and will also promote approximation of the wound edges (85).

Chest wall infection may also involve bone and cartilage. It is caused either by the extension of the intrathoracic problem or by primary chest wall involvement. Characteristic bony changes generally occur after the infection has been well established and the bone has been extensively invaded. There is a one- to two-week lag period between the onset of symptoms and the appearance of radiographic changes. Findings include the loss of deep soft-tissue planes and periosteal elevation of the affected bone. In addition to standard radiography, radionucleotide bone scans, CT, and magnetic resonance imaging are helpful in delineating the extent of the infection. It is important to determine the extent of debridement required to eradicate the infection. Osteomyelitis associated with surgical procedures and trauma will routinely require surgical exploration and debridement of the area.

In contrast, primary osteomyelitis may be treated with an initial prolonged course of antibiotics. Bishara et al. (86) reported a series of 106 patients (mostly children and young adults) with primary rib osteomyelitis. The mean duration of symptoms before diagnosis ranged from 16 to 32 weeks. The infectious cause was bacterial, fungal, or protozoal. Common clinical signs were fever, soft tissue mass, and chest pain. Antimicrobial therapy with or without surgery achieved a favorable outcome for 89% of the patients.

Paradoxical Wall Motion

As the aggressiveness of chest wall resection increases, the incidence of postoperative paradoxical wall motion abnormality also increases. Wide resection of a primary malignant chest wall neoplasm is now recognized as essential for curative treatment. King et al. (87), in their report from the Mayo Clinic, evaluated the extent of chest wall resection and the overall survival rates. They reported that a 2-cm margin was adequate for resecting metastatic chest wall tumors. However, for primary chest wall tumors, a resection margin of 4 cm or more resulted in a five-year cancer-free interval for 56% of patients, whereas a margin of 2 cm was associated with a five-year cancer-free interval for only 29% for patients. Long-term survival of patients with primary malignant neoplasms of the chest wall depends on cell type and extent of the chest wall resection. Recurrent neoplasm is an ominous sign associated with a five-year survival rate of only 17% (87). Therefore, the extent of resection should not be compromised.

Paradoxical chest wall motion always occurs after resection of bony elements of the thorax but is not always physiologically detrimental. Defects with a diameter of up to 5 to 7 cm seldom require stabilization (88). Patients with a fixed mediastinum due to previous pleural pathology on either side will have fewer adverse effects from paradoxical motion than will patients whose mediastinum is not fixed. More important is whether the patient can tolerate chest wall resection without serious respiratory embarrassment. The preoperative assessment is the same as that for patients undergoing pulmonary resection and includes pulmonary function studies, arterial blood gas determination, and exercise testing. As a reasonable guiding principle, any patient who could tolerate pulmonary lobectomy should also be able to tolerate major resection of the chest wall (89). Patients who require chest wall resection and concomitant lung resection require special consideration.

The first step in chest wall reconstruction is preservation of function through stabilization. Chest wall reconstruction is generally viewed as a procedure with two aspects: chest wall stabilization and soft-tissue reconstruction. If chest wall stabilization is necessary, both biologic and synthetic materials have been successfully used to preserve chest wall integrity and respiratory mechanics. The location and size of the anticipated chest wall defect is of utmost importance when reconstruction is considered. Previous chemotherapy, steroid dependence, malnutrition, or local wound conditions such as irradiation, infection, or residual tumor may dramatically alter the reconstructive choice. If feasible, primary closure of soft tissue remains the best option.

If full-thickness reconstruction is required, stabilization of the thorax with soft-tissue coverage must be considered. These goals can be accomplished with plastic meshes, fascia lata, musculocutaneous flaps, or any combination of these (90,91). Stabilization is necessary for providing a firm surface on which the soft-tissue flap can be set. Stabilization is best accomplished with a prosthetic material such as Gore-Tex® (W.L. Gore & Associates, Inc., Newark, Delaware, U.S.A.), which is impermeable to water and air. Placing this material under slight tension will improve the rigidity of the chest wall. Currently, reconstruction with meshes impregnated with methyl methacrylate is not recommended because this procedure fails to offer a dynamic environment and is associated with the development of

metabolic acidosis (92). Omentum or muscle flaps using latissimus dorsi, pectoralis major, rectus abdominus, or serratus anterior muscles can be used to reconstruct soft-tissue defects of the chest wall (88).

Most patients who undergo chest wall resection will be treated during the initial postoperative period with volume-dependent ventilation. During the first 48 hours, stabilization of the affected chest wall is optimized by the tissue edema that is generated in surgically manipulated tissue. This tissue edema will render the flap more rigid and, therefore, will reduce paradoxical motion. The flap becomes less rigid as the edema fluid is mobilized, but usually the patient has been weaned from the ventilator by this time (93). Unfortunately, prolonged respiratory support may be unavoidable for certain patients.

Mediastinal and Subcutaneous Emphysema

Mediastinal emphysema and subcutaneous emphysema occur in a large number of patients after pulmonary resection. Even after the chest tube has been removed, subcutaneous emphysema of the chest and neck is common. This condition is usually of limited significance and resolves without complications. Air that leaks into the pleural space may gain access to the mediastinum because of the pleural interruption at the time of surgery; it may then dissect along the mediastinal structures into the supraclavicular areas of the neck. Subcutaneous emphysema of the chest wall can also occur postoperatively because the air within the pleural space finds its way between the ribs and into the muscle layer of the chest. After pneumonectomy, the pleural space is initially filled with air. As blood and serum replace the air, the air is pushed out of the pleural space into the subcutaneous and mediastinal structures.

Subcutaneous emphysema may indicate a persistent air leak, and a chest tube turned to suction may be required to direct the air into the container and eliminate ongoing tissue dissection by air. Occasionally, subcutaneous emphysema may be a sign of a new bronchopleural fistula, a devastating complication whose early diagnosis requires a high index of suspicion. For this reason, new or worsening subcutaneous emphysema requires a thorough evaluation with chest radiography, CT, and, possibly, bronchoscopy. Early intervention is crucial for successful management.

Pain

Pain after thoracotomy is generally more severe and persistent than pain after other types of surgery. The pain can persist for several months postoperatively, but usually resolves by the second month. This pain is caused by transecting major muscles, removing, cutting, or breaking ribs, and spreading the ribs by retractors. A mechanical rib spreader disrupts and may fracture areas of ligamentous attachment to the vertebral body posteriorly and to the sternal cartilage attachments anteriorly.

The intensity of pain after thoracotomy has a direct impact on respiratory mechanics and the potential development of post-thoracotomy pneumonia. Pain generated during ventilatory effort will result in a compromise of tidal volume. The patient will then maintain an adequate minute volume by increasing the respiratory rate but decreasing tidal volume. This activity will decrease the functional respiratory capacity and will lead to atelectasis and ventilation–perfusion mismatch. This problem is compounded by cough suppression, which in the presence of increased secretions will lead to pneumonia and poor oxygenation.

Early, effective pain control is imperative after thoracotomy. Modifying the operative technique can minimize the surgical insult and reduce the resulting pain. Modifications to the conventional thoracotomy technique include muscle-sparing thoracotomy, linear or small transaxillary thoracotomy, and video-assisted thoracoscopy (94). All of these approaches have lessened the degree of postoperative pain, but the difference is most notable two weeks or more after surgery (95).

Effective medical management of pain is a crucial postoperative consideration. Narcotics have been used traditionally because they may be given either intravenously or through an epidural catheter. Patient-controlled analgesia often uses narcotics. In addition, nonsteroidal medications are recommended unless contraindicated.

Thoracic epidural delivery is considered the method of choice for post-thoracotomy analgesia, but it is not suitable for every patient and is associated with some risks and side effects. Risks include hypotension, urinary retention, epidural hematoma, overdose of medication, and malpositioning of the catheter (96). Extrapleural intercostal analgesia is an effective alternative to thoracic epidural anesthesia. Kaiser et al. (96) prospectively studied pain control, recovery of ventilatory function, and pulmonary complications among patients undergoing lobectomy or bilobectomy. Their results suggested that extrapleural intercostal analgesia may be a valuable alternative to thoracic epidural analgesia when the latter is not possible. Important clinical trials are currently evaluating the use of preemptive analgesia. The hypothesis is that the preoperative administration of pain medication will increase patient comfort, thereby, perhaps reducing analgesic requirements and improving respiratory mechanics (97).

Infrequently, prolonged intractable pain after thoracotomy may be associated with the presence of a traumatic intercostal neuroma. Surgical resection results in complete pain relief. This complication is not always recognized; thus, surgical treatment is not used frequently enough (98).

Diminished Sensation

Diminished sensation along the pathway of the dermatome of the fifth or sixth intercostal nerve is a frequent post-thoracotomy complaint. The loss of sensation results from trauma to the nerve when the ribs are spread by the rib spreader. If the intercostal artery, vein, and nerve are divided, the skin dermatome of those nerves will remain numb. Patients should be warned of the possibility of this complication and should be advised that it is permanent. If the nerves have been compressed but not transected, sensation should slowly return to normal.

Keloids and Hypertrophic Scars

Keloids and hypertrophic scars result from abnormal healing processes that occur after injury due to trauma or surgery. Hypertrophic scars remain within the boundaries of the original wound and almost always regress with time. In contrast, keloids extend beyond the boundaries and usually do not regress. Both types of scars are characterized by an overabundant deposition of collagen; however, keloids exhibit a substantially greater rate of collagen synthesis. Growth factors may be very important in the regulation of these lesions.

At present, the clinical treatment of these lesions is not optimal. After excision, hypertrophic scars tend to regress but keloids usually recur. Many trials have evaluated methods of controlling keloids, but most methods have been unsuccessful. Excision may be used for debulking and pharmacologic agents may be used to control abnormal scarring. Perhaps the most popular and effective treatment is an intralesional injection of triamcinolone. In addition to reducing the size of the lesions, triamcinolone relieves the burning and itching associated with keloids. Alternatively, Lee et al. (99) proposed a new surgical technique called "keloid core excision." They excised the inner fibrous core from the keloid and covered the defect with a keloid rind flap, which is arterialized by the subcapsular vascular plexus. Lee et al. have found that this technique works very well in preventing keloid recurrence; no adjuvant therapy is required after surgery (99).

Tumor Implantation

Tumor implantation is exceedingly uncommon after standard thoracotomy. Although rare, tumor implantation does occur after video-assisted thoracotomy and aspiration needle biopsy of thoracic lesions (100,101). Video-assisted thoracic surgery (VATS), which was initially developed for intrapleural lysis of adhesions hindering lung collapse in the treatment of pulmonary tuberculosis by artificial pneumothorax, is now applied in numerous settings (102). VATS has been used for resection of primary and secondary malignant lesions of the lungs. Endoscopic manipulation and the withdrawal of tumors through a rigid and often sharp interspace may result in microscopic or gross tumor spillage within the trocar track or the pleural cavity. The exact mechanism responsible for the seeding remains controversial (103). Care must obviously be taken not to directly hold the tumor with endoscopic forceps and to remove the lesion via endo-bags or surgical gloves (100).

Chest wall implantation may occur at the level of the previous incision or adjacent to it. Temporal and topographical evidence may be helpful in estab-lishing the likelihood of implantation. Todd et al. (101) reported no tumor implantation after 2114 consecutive percutaneous aspirations. However, fine-needle aspiration biopsy has been associated with tumor implantation (104). The low incidence of this problem makes difficult the prospective or even retro-spective evaluation of any precaution modification. If tumor implantation does occur and there is no evi-dence of other metastatic disease, wide chest wall resection with transposition of a musculocutaneous flap is the treatment of choice.

NERVE INJURY
Intercostal Nerves

The intercostal nerves are the anterior rami of the first 11 thoracic spinal nerves. The anterior ramus of the 12th thoracic nerve lies in the abdomen and runs for-ward in the abdominal wall. The intercostal nerves enter the intercostal grooves between the parietal pleura and the internal intercostal muscle. They then run for-ward and inferiorly to enter the intercostal groove and run under the intercostal vessels. The first six nerves are distributed within the intercostal space. The seventh, eighth, and ninth intercostal nerves leave the intercostal space and enter the anterior abdominal wall. The 10th and 11th nerves pass directly into the abdominal wall because the corresponding ribs are floating ribs. The branches of the intercostal nerves are as follows: collateral branch, lateral cutaneous branch, anterior cutaneous branch, muscular branch, pleural and peritoneal sensory branches, and articular branch.

As discussed previously, thoracotomy incisions are known to cause considerable pain. Because the intercostal region is richly innervated, morbidity associated with this incision can hinder the patient's postoperative course. Intercostal pain can be caused by direct or indirect injury to the nerves, iatrogenic rib fractures, stretching of the costovertebral and cost-osternal joints, and direct contusion to the chest wall. A primary focus of postoperative management is pain relief. Persistent pain leads to atelectasis and hypo-ventilation, which predispose the patient to pneumo-nia. In elderly patients, untreated chest pain may lead to marked hypoventilation, carbon dioxide narcosis, and respiratory arrest, especially when the patients have multiple rib fractures (105).

The goal of analgesia is to substantially reduce chest pain without inducing respiratory depression. Traditionally, patients have been treated with patient-controlled analgesia delivery systems. However, high lumbar or thoracic epidural anesthesia and continuous

intercostal nerve blocks may be more effective. Epidural catheters are associated with several compli-cations such as urinary retention, pruritus, sedation, and nausea (105). They may also rarely be associated with epidural hematomas and infections. Hence, they are contraindicated for patients with sepsis. Delayed respiratory depression associated with cephalad migration may occur; therefore, patients with epidural catheters should be continuously monitored.

Alternatively, at the time of thoracotomy, a mul-tiholed catheter of the type used for epidural anesthe-sia is inserted in the subpleural and paravertebral space. The pleura is closed over the catheter, and the catheter is brought out through the skin. A continuous infusion of 0.5% bupivacaine is used to provide analgesia (106). Although both methods offer a similar degree of pain relief, continuous intercostal blocks are associated with less nausea, vomiting, and urinary retention (107).

Phrenic Nerve

The phrenic nerves arise from the anterior rami of the third, fourth, and fifth cervical nerves. The right phre-nic nerve descends in the thorax along the right side of the right brachiocephalic vein and the superior vena cava. It passes in front of hilar structures and runs along the right side of the pericardium. The left phrenic nerve runs along the left side of the left sub-clavian artery. It crosses the left side of the aortic arch and crosses the left vagus nerve. It then descends in front of the hilum of the left lung and descends along the left side of the pericardium. The phrenic nerve possesses efferent and afferent fibers. The efferent fibers are the sole motor supply to the diaphragm. The afferent fibers carry sensory input from the peri-toneum, covering the central undersurface of the diaphragm, the pleura covering the upper surface of the diaphragm and the pericardium and the medi-astinal parietal pleura.

During thoracotomy, the phrenic nerve should always be identified and preserved. Should the phre-nic nerve be directly involved with a malignancy, it should be resected only if the tumor itself can be com-pletely removed. Injury to the nerve will result in a flail diaphragm on the ipsilateral side of surgical resection. The nonfunctioning diaphragm interferes with a rapid, uncomplicated postoperative recovery. Direct injury to the nerve during thoracic surgery may be due to transection, traction of the nerve, pres-sure from a retractor, or use of cautery near the nerve. Unlike bilateral paralysis of the diaphragm, unilateral paralysis is usually fairly well tolerated. An early reduction of 20% to 30% in vital capacity will resolve within approximately six months. However, for 66% of patients with dyspnea on exertion, the symptoms will remain unchanged or will even progress (107).

Diaphragmatic motion as evaluated fluoro-scopically will confirm the diagnosis. Paradoxical motion of the diaphragm is identified with the aid of a "sniff test." Diaphragmatic plication has been used to improve respiratory function because it increases the total and vital capacity of the lung. Plication should be performed when severe symptoms persist, when the nerve is known to have been transected, or when sufficient time has passed so as to preclude regeneration of the phrenic nerve. An exception to this rule is the presence of serious underlying lung disease; patients with this condition may benefit from early plication (107).

Recurrent Laryngeal Nerve

The recurrent nerves are inconspicuous and fragile. On the right side, the recurrent laryngeal nerve arises from the vagus as the latter crosses the first part of the subclavian artery. The recurrent nerve hooks backward and upward behind the artery and ascends in the groove between the trachea and the esophagus. It passes deep to the lobe of the thyroid gland and comes into close relationship with the inferior thyroid artery. The nerve crosses either in front of, behind, or between the branches of the artery. The nerve supplies all of the muscles of the larynx except the cricothyroid, which is supplied by the external laryngeal branch of the superior laryngeal nerve. The nerve supplies the mucous membrane below the vocal folds and the upper trachea. On the left side, the recurrent laryngeal nerve arises from the vagus as the latter crosses the arch of the aorta in the thorax. It hooks around and beneath the arch behind the ligamentum arteriosum. It then ascends into the neck in a fashion similar to that of the right nerve. A nonrecurrent nerve is a special anatomic situation that may occur on the right side with a retroesophageal right subclavian artery or bilaterally with situs inversus with a right-sided arch.

Most laryngeal nerve trauma is iatrogenic. Surgical damage to the recurrent nerves occurs during 0.5% to 37% of operations on the neck and upper chest. Unusual hoarseness or a change in the pitch or force of the voice should alert the surgeon to the possibility of an injury to the recurrent nerve. Direct or indirect laryngoscopy will confirm the diagnosis. The vocal cords may be paralyzed in either an abducted or an adducted position. The left recurrent nerve is more likely than the right to be injured at the time of thoracotomy. If there are malignant lymph nodes at the level of aortopulmonary window, as the left recurrent nerve passes beneath the aortic arch, the surgeon may be forced to sacrifice the nerve to achieve a proper node dissection of the area.

Management consists of early recognition and early treatment to avoid the risk of aspiration. A bruised but intact recurrent nerve possesses remarkable regenerative potential. Bilateral cord paralyses usually require tracheostomy. No repair of the recurrent nerve can restore function of the cord. The patient's clinical course often dictates the management of the injury.

CONCLUSIONS

Lung surgery and chest wall reconstructions can be done with good results, if well-planned operative approaches are taken. Complete workup prior to surgery will lessen complications that occur after these difficult surgeries.

REFERENCES

1. Bolliger CT, Perruchoud AP. Functional evaluation of the lung resection candidate. Eur Respir J 1998; 11:198–212.
2. Pate P, Tenholder MF, Griffin JP, Eastridge CE, Weiman DS. Preoperative assessment of the high-risk patient for lung resection. Ann Thorac Surg 1996; 61:1494–1500.
3. Wang JS, Abboud RT, Evans KG, Finley RJ, Graham BL. Role of CO diffusing capacity during exercise in the preoperative evaluation for lung resection. Am J Respir Crit Care Med 2000; 162:1435–1444.
4. Carretta A, Zannini P, Puglisi A, et al. Improvement of pulmonary function after lobectomy for non-small cell lung cancer in emphysematous patients. Eur J Cardiothorac Surg 1999; 15:602–607.
5. Gauss A, Rohm HJ, Schauffelen A, et al. Electrocardiographic exercise stress testing for cardiac risk assessment inpatients undergoing noncardiac surgery. Anesthesiology 2001; 94:38–46.
6. Tanaka F, Yanagihara K, Otake Y, et al. Biological features and preoperative evaluation of mediastinal nodal status in non-small cell lung cancer. Ann Thorac Surg 2000; 70:1832–1838.
7. Takamochi K, Nagai K, Yoshida J, et al. The role of computed tomographic scanning in diagnosing mediastinal node involvement in non-small cell lung cancer. J Thorac Cardiovasc Surg 2000; 119:1135–1140.
8. Valentini AL, Tartaglione T, Monti L, Marano P. Iomeprol versus iopamidol in contrast-enhanced computed tomography of thoracic and abdominal organs. Eur J Radiol 1994; 18(suppl 1):S88–S92.
9. Lucas LM, Colley CA, Gordon GH. Case report: multisystem failure following intravenous iopamidol. Clin Radiol 1992; 45:276–277.
10. Graeber GM, Gupta NC, Murray GF. Positron emission tomographic imaging with fluorodeoxyglucose is efficacious in evaluating malignant pulmonary disease. J Thorac Cardiovasc Surg 1999; 117:719–727.
11. Colt HG, Matsuo T. Hospital charges attributable to bronchoscopy-related complications in outpatients. Respiration 2001; 68:67–72.
12. Cavaliere S, Venuta F, Foccoli P, Toninelli C, La Face B. Endoscopic treatment of malignant airway obstructions in 2,008 patients. Chest 1996; 110:1536–1542.
13. Beer M, Wittenberg G, Sandstede J, et al. Treatment of inoperable tracheobronchial obstructive lesions with the Palmaz stent. Cardiovasc Intervent Radiol 1999; 22:109–113.
14. Nashef SA, Dromer C, Velly JF, Labrousse L, Couraud L. Expanding wire stents in benign tracheobronchial disease: indications and complications. Ann Thorac Surg 1992; 54:937–940.

15. Tahara RW, Lackner RP, Graver LM. Is there a role for routine mediastinoscopy in patients with peripheral T$_1$ lung cancers? Am J Surg 2000; 180:488–492.

16. Mentzer SJ, Swanson SJ, DeCamp MM, Bueno R, Sugarbaker DJ. Mediastinoscopy, thoracoscopy, and video-assisted thoracic surgery in the diagnosis and staging of lung cancer. Chest 1997; 112(4 suppl): 239S–241S.

17. Hammoud ZT, Anderson RC, Meyers BF, et al. The current role of mediastinoscopy in the evaluation of thoracic disease. J Thorac Cardiovasc Surg 1999; 118:894–899.

18. Pauwels M, Van Schil P, De Backer W, Van den Brande F, Eyskens E. Repeat mediastinoscopy in the staging of lung cancer. Eur J Cardiothorac Surg 1998; 14:271–273.

19. van Sonnenberg E, Wittich GR, Goodacre BW, Zwischenberger JB. Percutaneous drainage of thoracic collections. J Thorac Imaging 1998; 13:74–82.

20. Griffin JJ, Meduri GU. New approaches in the diagnosis of nosocomial pneumonia. Med Clin North Am 1994; 78:1091–1122.

21. Estes RJ, Meduri GU. The pathogenesis of ventilator-associated pneumonia: I. Mechanisms of bacterial transcolonization and airway inoculation. Intensive Care Med 1995; 21:365–383.

22. Garner JS, Jarvis WR, Emori TG, Horan TC, Hughes JM. CDC definitions for nosocomial infections, 1988. Am J Infect Control 1988; 16:128–140.

23. Higuchi JH, Johanson WG Jr. Colonization and bronchopulmonary infection. Clin Chest Med 1982; 3:133–142.

24. Haley RW, Hooton TM, Culver DH, et al. Nosocomial infections in U.S. hospitals, 1975–1976: estimated frequency by selected characteristics of patients. Am J Med 1981; 70:947–959.

25. Torres A, Aznar R, Gatell JM, et al. Incidence, risk, and prognosis factors of nosocomial pneumonia in mechanically ventilated patients. Am Rev Respir Dis 1990; 142:523–528.

26. Cerfolio RJ, Tummala RP, Holman WL, et al. A prospective algorithm for the management of air leaks after pulmonary resection. Ann Thorac Surg 1998; 66:1726–1731.

27. LoCicero J III, Hartz RS, Frederiksen JW, Michaelis LL. New applications of the laser in pulmonary surgery: hemostasis and sealing of air leaks. Ann Thorac Surg 1985; 40:546–550.

28. Matar AF, Hill JG, Duncan W, Orfanakis N, Law I. Use of biological glue to control pulmonary air leaks. Thorax 1990; 45:670–674.

29. Weissberg D. Talc and adult respiratory distress syndrome. J Thorac Cardiovasc Surg 1984; 87:474–477.

30. Rogiers P, Van Mieghem W, Engelaar D, Demedts M. Late-onset post-pneumonectomy empyema manifesting as tracheal stenosis with respiratory failure. Respir Med 1991; 85:333–335.

31. Wong PS, Goldstraw P. Pulmonary torsion: a questionnaire survey and a survey of the literature. Ann Thorac Surg 1992; 54:286–288.

32. Velmahos GC, Frankhouse J, Ciccolo M. Pulmonary torsion of the right upper lobe after right middle lobectomy for a stab wound to the chest. J Trauma 1998; 44:920–922.

33. Mullin MJ, Zumbro GL Jr, Fishback ME, Nelson TG. Pulmonary lobar gangrene complicating lobectomy. Ann Surg 1972; 175:62–66.

34. Refaely Y, Weissberg D. Gangrene of the lung: treatment in two stages. Ann Thorac Surg 1997; 64:970–974.

35. Krishnadasan B, Sherbin VL, Vallieres E, Karmy-Jones R. Surgical management of lung gangrene. Can Respir J 2000; 7:401–404.

36. Grillo HC, Shepard JA, Mathisen DJ, Kanarek DJ. Postpneumonectomy syndrome: diagnosis, management, and results. Ann Thorac Surg 1992; 54:638–651.

37. Kelly RF, Hunter DW, Maddaus MA. Postpneumonectomy syndrome after left pneumonectomy. Ann Thorac Surg 2001; 71:701–703.

38. Wasserman K, Jamplis RW, Lash H, Brown HV, Cleary MG, Lafair J. Post-pneumonectomy syndrome. Surgical correction using Silastic implants. Chest 1979; 75:78–81.

39. Fitzmaurice BG, Brodsky JB. Airway rupture from double-lumen tubes. J Cardiothorac Vasc Anesth 1999; 13:322–329.

40. Sonobe M, Nakagawa M, Ichinose M, Ikegami N, Nagasawa M, Shindo T. Analysis of risk in bronchopleural fistula after pulmonary resection for primary lung cancer. Eur J Cardiothorac Surg 2000; 18:519–523.

41. Deschamps C, Bernard A, Nichols FC III, et al. Empyema and bronchopleural fistula after pneumonectomy: factors affecting incidence. Ann Thorac Surg 2001; 72:243–248.

42. Bonomi P, Faber LP, Warren W, et al. Postoperative bronchopulmonary complications in stage III lung cancer patients treated with preoperative paclitaxel-containing chemotherapy and concurrent radiation. Semin Oncol 1997; 24(4 suppl 12):S12-123–S12-129.

43. Puskas JD, Mathisen DJ, Grillo HL, Wain JC, Wright CD, Moricure AC. Treatment strategies for bronchopleural fistula. J Thorac Cardiovasc Surg 1995; 109:989–996.

44. O'Neill PJ, Flanagan HL, Mauney MC, Spotnitz WD, Daniel TM. Intrathoracic fibrin sealant application using computed tomography fluoroscopy. Ann Thorac Surg 2000; 70:301–302.

45. Varoli F, Roviaro G, Grignani F, Vergani C, Maciocco M, Rebuffat C. Endoscopic treatment of bronchopleural fistulas. Ann Thorac Surg 1998; 65:807–809.

46. Gharagozloo F, Trachiotis G, Wolfe A, DuBree KJ, Cox JL. Pleural space irrigation and modified Clagett procedure for the treatment of early postpneumonectomy empyema. J Thorac Cardiovasc Surg 1998; 116: 943–948.

47. Hollaus PH, Lax F, el-Nashef BB, Hauck HH, Lucciarini P, Pridun NS. Natural history of bronchopleural after pneumonectomy: a review of 96 cases. Ann Thorac Surg 1997; 63:1391–1397.

48. Sirbu H, Busch T, Aleksic I, Lotfi S, Ruschewski W, Dalichau H. Chest re-exploration for complications after lung surgery. Thorac Cardiovasc Surg 1999; 47:73–76.

49. de la Riviere AB, Defauw JJ, Knaepen PJ, van Swieten HA, Vanderschueren RC, van den Bosch JM. Transsternal closure of bronchopleural fistula after pneumonectomy. Ann Thorac Surg 1997; 46:954–959.

50. Handy JR Jr, Judson MA, Zellner JL. Pneumoperitoneum to treat air leaks and spaces after a lung volume reduction operation. Ann Thorac Surg 1997; 64: 1803–1805.

51. Halezeroglu S, Keles M, Uysal A, et al. Factors affecting postoperative morbidity and mortality in destroyed lung. Ann Thorac Surg 1997; 64:1635–1638.

52. Eloesser L. Of an operation for tuberculous empyema. Ann Thorac Surg 1969; 8:355–357.

53. Clagett OT, Geraci JE. A procedure for the management of postpneumonectomy empyema. J Thorac Cardiovasc Surg 1963; 45:141–145.

54. Weissberg D. Empyema and bronchopleural fistula. Experience with open window thoracostomy. Chest 1982; 82:447–450.

55. Regnard JF, Alifano M, Puyo P, Fares E, Magdeleinat P, Levasseur P. Open window thoracostomy followed by intrathoracic flap transposition in the treatment of empyema complicating pulmonary resection. J Thorac Cardiovasc Surg 2000; 120:270–275.

56. Hochberg J, Ardenghy M, Yuen J, et al. Utilization of muscle flaps in the treatment of bronchopleural fistulas. Ann Plast Surg 1999; 43:484–493.

57. Hollaus PH, Huber M, Lax F, Wurnig PN, Bohm G, Pridun NS. Closure of bronchopleural fistula after pneumonectomy with a pedicled intercostal muscle flap. Eur J Cardiothorac Surg 1999; 16:181–186.

58. Mineo TC, Ambrogi V. The diaphragmatic flap. A multiuse material in thoracic surgery. J Thorac Cardiovasc Surg 1999; 118:1084–1089.

59. Garcia-Yuste M, Ramos G, Duque JL, et al. Open-window thoracostomy and thoracomyoplasty to manage chronic pleural empyema. Ann Thorac Surg 1998; 65:818–822.

60. Staats BA, Ellefson RD, Budahn LL, Dines DE, Prakash UB, Offord K. The lipoprotein profile of chylous and nonchylous pleural effusions. Mayo Clin Proc 1980; 55:700–704.

61. Kelly RF, Shumway SJ. Conservative management of postoperative chylothorax using somatostatin. Ann Thorac Surg 2000; 69:1944–1945.

62. Cerfolio RJ, Allen MS, Deschamps C, Trastek VF, Pairolero PC. Postoperative chylothorax. J Thorac Cardiovasc Surg 1996; 112:1361–1366.

63. von Knorring J, Lepantalo M, Lindgren L, Lindfors O. Cardiac arrhythmias and myocardial ischemia after thoracotomy for lung cancer. Ann Thorac Surg 1992; 53:642–647.

64. Harpole DH, Liptay MJ, DeCamp MM Jr, Mentzer SJ, Swanson SJ, Sugarbaker DJ. Prospective analysis of pneumonectomy: risk factors for major morbidity and cardiac dysrhythmias. Ann Thorac Surg 1996; 61:977–982.

65. Shields TW, Ujiki GT. Digitalization for prevention of arrhythmias following pulmonary surgery. Surg Gynecol Obstet 1968; 126:743–746.

66. Ritchie AJ, Danton M, Gibbons JR. Prophylactic digitalisation in pulmonary surgery. Thorax 1992; 47:41–43.

67. Jakobsen CJ, Bille S, Ahlburg P, Rybro L, Hjortholm K, Andresen EB. Perioperative metoprolol reduces the frequency of atrial fibrillation after thoracotomy for lung resection. J Cardiothorac Vasc Anesth 1997; 11:746–751.

68. Rena O, Papalia E, Oliaro A, et al. Supraventricular arrhythmias after resection of the lung. Eur J Cardiothorac Surg 2001; 20:688–693.

69. Stevens D, Sharma K, Szidon P, Rich S, McLaughlin V, Kesten S. Severe pulmonary hypertension associated with COPD. Ann Transplant 2000; 5:8–12.

70. Sostman HD, Layish DT, Tapson VF, et al. Prospective comparison of helical CT and MR imaging in clinically suspected acute pulmonary embolism. J Magn Reson Imaging 1996; 6:275–281.

71. Nasraway SA, Kabani N, Lawrence KR. Thrombolytic therapy for pulmonary embolism: reversal of shock in the early postoperative period. Pharmacotherapy 1994; 14:616–619.

72. MacMahon H, Forrest JV, Weisz D, Sagel SS. Massive tumor embolism occurring during pneumonectomy. Ann Thorac Surg 1974; 17:395–397.

73. Morrow K, Morris CK, Froelicher VF, et al. Prediction of cardiovascular death in men undergoing noninvasive evaluation for coronary artery disease. Ann Intern Med 1993; 118:689–695.

74. Foster ED, Davis KB, Carpenter JA, Abele S, Fray D. Risk of noncardiac operation in patients with defined coronary disease. The Coronary Artery Surgery Study (CASS) registry experience. Ann Thorac Surg 1986; 41:42–50.

75. Hertzer NR, Beven EG, Young JR, et al. Coronary artery disease in peripheral vascular patients. A classification of 1000 coronary angiograms and results of surgical management. Ann Surg 1984; 199:223–233.

76. Thomas P, Giudicelli R, Guillen JC, Fuentes P. Is lung cancer surgery justified in patients with coronary artery disease? Eur J Cardiothorac Surg 1994; 8:287–292.

77. Eagle KA, Coley CM, Newell JB, et al. Combining clinical and thallium data optimizes preoperative assessment of cardiac risk before major vascular surgery. Ann Intern Med 1989; 110:859–866.

78. L'Italien GJ, Paul SD, Hendel RC, et al. Development and validation of a Bayesian model for perioperative cardiac risk assessment in a cohort of 1081 vascular surgical candidates. J Am Coll Cardiol 1996; 27:779–786.

79. 27th Bethesda Conference. Matching the Intensity of Risk Factor Management with the Hazard for Coronary Disease Events. September 14–15, 1995. J Am Coll Cardiol 1996; 27:957–1047.

80. Mangano DT, Browner WS, Hollenberg M, London MJ, Tubau JF, Tateo IM. Association of perioperative myocardial ischemia with cardiac morbidity and mortality in men undergoing noncardiac surgery. The Study of Perioperative Ischemia Research Group. N Engl J Med 1990; 323:1781–1788.

81. Mangano DT, Layug EL, Wallace A, Tateo I. Effect of atenolol on mortality and cardiovascular morbidity after noncardiac surgery. Multicenter Study of Perioperative Ischemia Research Group. N Engl J Med 1996; 335:1713–1720.

82. Nelson JC, Nelson RM. The incidence of hospital wound infection in thoracotomies. J Thorac Cardiovasc Surg 1967; 54:586–591.

83. Wertzel H, Swoboda L, Joos-Wurtemberger A, Frank U, Hasse J. Perioperative antibiotic prophylaxis in general thoracic surgery. Thorac Cardiovasc Surg 1992; 40:326–329.

84. Tarkka M, Pokela R, Lepojarvi M, Nissinen J, Karkola P. Infection prophylaxis in pulmonary surgery: a randomized prospective study. Ann Thorac Surg 1987; 44:508–513.

85. Sposato G, Molea G, Di Caprio G, Scioli M, La Rusca I, Ziccardi P. Ambulant vacuum-assisted closure of skingraft dressing in the lower limbs using a portable mini-VAC device. Br J Plast Surg 2001; 54:235–237.

86. Bishara J, Gartman-Israel D, Weinberger M, Maimon S, Tamir G, Pitlik S. Osteomyelitis of the ribs in the antibiotic era. Scand J Infect Dis 2000; 32:223–227.

87. King RM, Pairolero PC, Trastek VF, Piehler JM, Payne WS, Bernatz PE. Primary chest wall tumors: factors affecting survival. Ann Thorac Surg 1986; 41:597–601.

88. McCormack PM. Use of prosthetic materials in chest-wall reconstruction. Assets and liabilities. Surg Clin North Am 1989; 69:965–976.

89. Seyfer AE, Graeber GM, Wind GG. Pre-operative care and consideration. In: Seyfer AE, Graeber GM, Wind GG, eds. Atlas of Chest Wall Reconstruction. Rockville, MD: Aspen Publishers, 1986:51–58.

90. Bjork VO. Thoracoplasty, a new osteo plastic technique. J Thorac Surg 1954; 28:194–211.

91. Pairolero PC, Arnold PG. Thoracic wall defects: surgical management of 205 consecutive patients. Mayo Clin Proc 1986; 61:557–563.

92. Pass HI. Primary and metastatic chest wall tumors. In: Roth JA, Weisenburger TH, Ruckdeschel JC, eds. Thoracic Oncology. Philadelphia: WB Saunders, 1989:519–537.

93. Graber GM. Chest wall stabilization. In: Pearson FG, Deslauriers J, Ginsberg RJ, Hiebert CA, McKneally MF, Urshel HC Jr, eds. Thoracic Surgery. New York: Churchill Livingstone, 1995:1272–1277.

94. Hazelrigg SR, Landreneau RJ, Boley TM, et al. The effects of muscle-sparing versus standard posterolateral thoracotomy on pulmonary function, muscle strength, and postoperative pain. J Thorac Cardiovasc Surg 1991; 101:394–401.

95. Nomori H, Horio H, Naruke T, Suemasu K. What is the advantage of a thorascopic lobectomy over a limited thoracotomy procedure for lung cancer surgery? Ann Thorac Surg 2001; 72:879–884.

96. Kaiser AM, Zollinger A, De Lorenzi D, Largiader F, Weder W. Prospective, randomized comparison of extrapleural versus epidural analgesia for postthoracotomy pain. Ann Thorac Surg 1998; 66:367–372.

97. Doyle E, Bowler GM. Pre-emptive effect of multimodal analgesia in thoracic surgery. Br J Anaesthesiol 1998; 80:147–151.

98. Wong L. Intercostal neuromas: a treatable cause of postoperative breast surgery pain. Ann Plast Surg 2001; 46:481–484.

99. Lee Y, Minn KW, Baek RM, Hong JJ. A new surgical treatment of keloid: keloid core excision. Ann Plast Surg 2001; 46:135–140.

100. Fry WA, Siddiqui A, Pensler JM, Mostafavi H. Thoracoscopic implantation of cancer with a fatal outcome. Ann Thorac Surg 1995; 59:42–45.

101. Todd TR, Weisbrod G, Tao LC, et al. Aspiration needle biopsy of thoracic lesions. Ann Thorac Surg 1981; 32:154–161.

102. Walsh GL, Nesbitt JC. Tumor implants after thoracoscopic resection of a metastatic sarcoma. Ann Thorac Surg 1995; 59:215–216.

103. Murthy SM, Goldschmidt RA, Rao LN, Ammirati M, Buchmann T, Scanlon EF. The influence of surgical trauma on experimental metastasis. Cancer 1989; 64:2035–2044.

104. Kara M, Alver G, Sak SD, Kavukcu S. Implantation metastasis caused by fine needle aspiration biopsy following curative resection of stage IB non-small cell lung cancer. Eur J Cardiothorac Surg 2001; 20: 868–870.

105. Wisner DH. A stepwise logistic regression analysis of factors affecting morbidity and mortality after thoracic trauma: effect of epidural analgesia. J Trauma 1990; 30:799–805.

106. Sabanathan S, Smith PJ, Pradhan GN, Hashimi H, Eng JB, Mearns AJ. Continuous intercostal nerve block for pain relief after thoracotomy. Ann Thorac Surg 1988; 46:425–426.

107. Graham DR, Kaplan D, Evans CC, Hind CR, Donnelly RJ. Diaphragmatic plication for unilateral diaphragmatic paralysis: a 10-year experience. Ann Thorac Surg 1990; 49:248–252.

22

Complications of Esophageal Surgery and Trauma

Peter P. Lopez

*Division of Trauma and Surgical Critical Care, DeWitt Daughtry Family Department of
Surgery, University of Miami Miller School of Medicine, Miami, Florida, U.S.A.*

*Optimal management of pathology affecting the esophagus
challenges even the most seasoned surgeon. Although the
esophagus is subject to the same complications that affect
other portions of the gastrointestinal (GI) tract (obstruction,
anastomotic leak, perforation, and stricture), several unique
features contribute to the higher morbidity and mortality
rates associated with esophageal surgery. Structurally, unlike
the remainder of the GI tract, the esophagus lacks a serosal
layer; hence, it is particularly susceptible to leaks. This
anatomic fact also contributes to the association between
esophageal surgery and an increased propensity for
perforation and for earlier and easier spread of malignancies
and infections; furthermore, it compounds the difficulty of
operative procedures on the esophagus. In addition, the
esophagus is surrounded by vital structures and is located
within a body cavity that does not lend itself well to direct
examination; thus, the complications that can result are not
only more devastating but also more difficult to diagnose
early than are those associated with other surgical procedures. Finally, restoration of the normal swallowing
mechanisms is an integral component of esophageal surgery
and must be considered during the planning and execution
of any operative intervention.*

*For the reasons mentioned above, there is no substi-
tute for meticulous technique and careful attention to detail
during esophageal surgery. Failure to take such care
invariably results in complications that can have devastating physiologic consequences (1). This chapter will
present the anatomy and physiology of the esophagus as
they pertain to the development of complications, will
discuss the appropriate preoperative assessment of patients,
and will describe some of the more common complications
of esophageal surgery and trauma.*

ANATOMY AND PHYSIOLOGY OF THE ESOPHAGUS

The esophagus is a muscular tube 25 cm in length that
extends from the cricoid cartilage to the stomach. It
functions as a conduit for food and liquid. As measured
endoscopically, the esophagus extends approximately
40 cm from the incisors to the gastric cardia, although
its length varies with the patient's height. The esophagus makes three minor deviations from the midline as
it descends from the neck, through the posterior mediastinum, and into the abdomen. In the neck, it courses to
the left of the midline; at the level of the seventh thoracic
vertebra, it deviates to the right; and finally, just above
the diaphragm, it again deviates to the left.

The esophagus also narrows in three areas, and
injuries caused by foreign bodies, caustic burns, strictures, iatrogenic perforations, and cancer usually occur
at one of these three sites (Fig. 1). The first of these is
the narrowest portion of the GI tract, at the origin
of the esophagus (15 cm from the incisors) and the
level of the sixth cervical vertebra, just above the thoracic inlet. A second narrowing is located 20 cm from
the incisors at the point at which the left main stem
bronchus and the aortic arch cross, at the level of
the angle of Lewis anteriorly and the fourth thoracic
vertebra posteriorly. The resting tone of the lower
esophageal sphincter creates the third narrowing of
the esophagus 40 cm from the incisors.

The esophagus differs from the rest of the GI tract
in that it has no mesentery or serosa. The esophageal
wall is composed of three layers: the outer external longitudinal muscle layer, the inner circular muscle layer,
and the mucosa. In the upper-third of the esophagus,
the muscle fibers are primarily striated (voluntary),
whereas in the distal-third of the esophagus, the muscle
fibers are primarily smooth (involuntary). In the
middle-third of the esophagus, smooth and striated
muscle fibers are intermingled. Because most esophageal motility disorders are due to an abnormality in
smooth muscle fibers, esophageal myotomy needs to
span only these muscle fibers. The submucosa contains
coarse elastic fibers, an arteriolar plexus, fibrous tissue,
and nerve cell bodies of Meissner's plexus. Together
with the mucosa, this thick submucosal layer is the
strongest portion of the esophageal wall. These layers
must be considered as one layer, and both must be sewn
together if a watertight anastomosis is to be created.
The mucosa makes up the inner layer of the esophageal

Distance from incisors

Narrowings

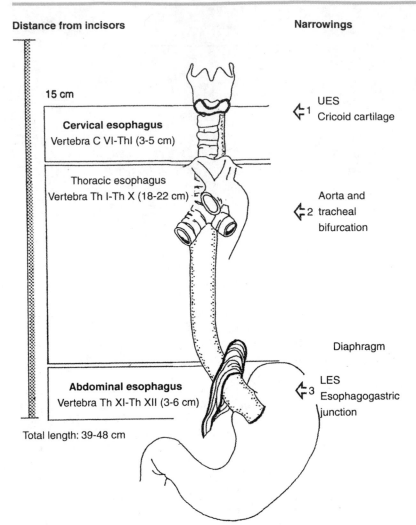

15 cm

Cervical esophagus
Vertebra C VI-ThI (3-5 cm)

Thoracic esophagus
Vertebra Th I-Th X (18-22 cm)

Abdominal esophagus
Vertebra Th XI-Th XII (3-6 cm)

Total length: 39-48 cm

← 1 UES
     Cricoid cartilage

← 2 Aorta and
     tracheal
     bifurcation

Diaphragm

← 3 LES
     Esophagogastric
     junction

Figure 1   Classical division of the esophagus and projection to the cervical (C) and the thoracic vertebrae (Th) as radiologic landmarks. The lengths and narrowings of the esophagus are shown. *Abbreviations*: UES, upper esophageal sphicter; LES, lower esophageal sphicter. *Source*: From Ref. 2.

wall. It is lined with a thick layer of nonkeratinizing, stratified squamous epithelium that is continuous with the mucosa of the oropharynx.

The arterial blood supply of the esophagus is derived from the inferior thyroid artery (neck), the segmental esophageal arteries branching off the aorta (thorax), and the left gastric and splenic artery (abdomen) (Fig. 2) (3). These arteries branch into small vessels some distance from the esophagus before penetrating the esophageal muscle layers. This branching allows blunt mobilization of the esophagus during a transhiatal esophagectomy because these small vessels contract to assist in hemostasis (5). Upon entering the esophagus, these arteries branch at right angles, thereby establishing a longitudinal anastomosing network of vessels. This early branching and collaterization between the cervical, thoracic, and gastric segments desegmentalizes the esophageal blood supply. Thus, the entire esophagus can be mobilized with a blood supply based on the inferior thyroidal artery. Poor technique rather than poor blood supply is the usual reason for anastomotic failure (1). However, the surgeon must exercise caution if the inferior

thyroid arteries have been compromised by prior partial or complete thyroidectomy or by any other previous surgical procedure or radiotherapy.

The venous drainage of the esophagus parallels its arterial supply. The venous system also has an extensive intramural venous plexus in the submucosa, and this plexus may become enlarged in cases of portal venous obstruction; such enlargement can lead to the formation of esophageal varices. Because of its location, the azygos vein may be easily damaged during blunt dissection; if tumor adheres to the vein, blunt dissection can cause massive bleeding. Additionally, esophageal resection through a right thoracotomy may lead to severe hemorrhage if the hemiazygos vein is not ligated (6).

The lymphatic system is made up of capillaries that drain into long and widely anastomosing collecting channels in the submucosa and then out to regional nodes. These nodes may precipitate the intramural spread of cancer, predominately in the submucosa. Because esophageal cancer has been found to spread for approximately 6 to 10 cm both proximally and distally, some surgeons believe that anything less than a

Blood Supply

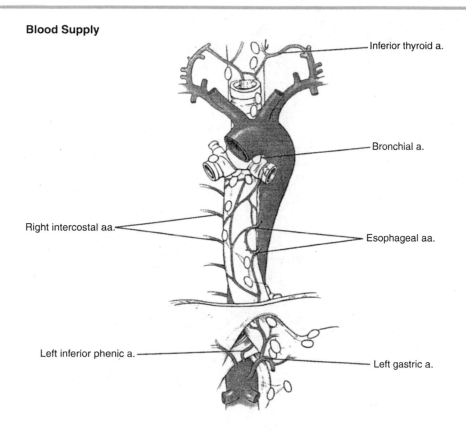

Figure 2 Arterial blood supply of the esophagus. *Source*: From Ref. 4.

subtotal esophagectomy is unwise (4,7). Lymphatic drainage from the upper esophagus flows primarily into the cervical and peritracheal lymph nodes, whereas lymphatic drainage from the lower esophagus flows into the retrocardiac and celiac nodes; however, the lymphatic system of the esophagus is unpredictable and peculiar (Fig. 3) (8).

The esophagus receives both sympathetic and parasympathetic innervation; these types of innervation act antagonistically on the esophagus. The parasympathetic nerve supply arises from the vagus nerve, whose esophageal branches are both motor (to muscles) and seromuscular (to the glands). The recurrent laryngeal nerve, a branch of the vagus nerve, supplies innervation to the upper esophagus. Injury to the recurrent laryngeal nerves during surgery may result in subsequent cervical dysphagia and aspiration (9). Similarly, distal injury to the vagus nerve may produce a lower esophageal motor disorder resembling esophageal spasm or achalasia (10). The sympathetic nerve supply arises from the cervical and thoracic sympathetic chain and the periesophageal, splanchnic, and cardiobronchial nerves from the celiac plexus and ganglia. The sympathetic pathways control contraction of sphincters, relaxation of muscles, and any increase in glandular and peristaltic activity as well as vasoconstriction of vessels to the esophagae.

ASSESSMENT OF OPERATIVE RISK

Careful preoperative assessment of operative risk is essential if the surgeon is to recognize specific clinical variables that may lead to post-operative complications. Often, patients who need esophageal surgery are elderly and malnourished; they may also have other serious medical problems such as coronary artery disease, chronic obstructive pulmonary disease (COPD), and diabetes. Eliciting a thorough history and performing a complete physical examination will often identify which patients are at an increased risk of perioperative and postoperative complications. A history of cardiac dysfunction pulmonary dysfunction, or smoking are all serious risk factors for postoperative adverse events. An objective evaluation of the patient's cardiovascular, pulmonary, renal, hematologic, nutritional, and hepatic status must be completed, so that function can be optimized preoperatively. The incidence of preexisting medical conditions increases with age, and, as the number of medical conditions increases, so do morbidity and mortality rates (11).

Cardiac Risk Factors

For high-risk patients, cardiac complications, including ischemia and infarction along with congestive heart failure (CHF), hypertension, and atrial fibril-

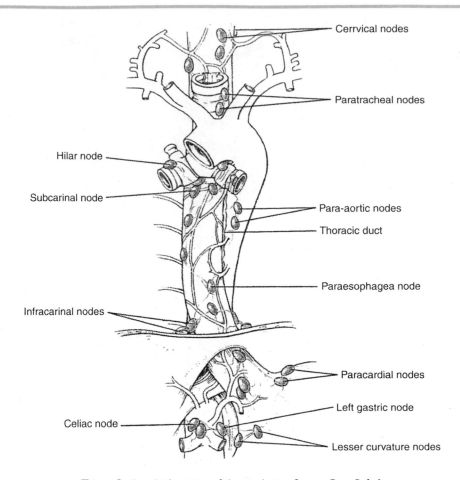

Figure 3 Lymphatic system of the esophagus. *Source*: From Ref. 4.

lation, are the leading causes of death after surgery. Clinical detection and adequate management of these cardiac diseases decrease the risk of postoperative complications. After a thorough history has been elicited and a complete physical examination has been performed, screening for cardiac disease begins with electrocardiography. The clinical risk classification systems proposed by Eagle and coworkers (12) and Lee et al. (13) help to determine the need for further preoperative cardiac tests. In both indexes, for low-risk patients, the risk of a perioperative myocardial event is only 3%. For intermediate-risk patients, the incidence is 15%; this incidence decreases to 3.2% if the results of a thallium stress test are normal, but

increases to 30% if the test results are positive for ischemia. For high-risk patients, the incidence of a perioperative myocardial event may be as high as 50% (Tables 1 and 2). On the basis of available reports, Hanna et al. (14) and Eagle et al. (15) have developed recommendations for the preoperative workup of patients facing major (non-cardiac) surgery (Table 3). All clinically determined intermediate- and high-risk patients undergoing noncardiac surgery should receive beta-blockade preoperatively unless contraindicated (16).

Pulmonary Risk Factors

Postoperative pulmonary complications are an important cause of morbidity, mortality, and increases in the length of stay. Serious pulmonary complications include pneumonia, bronchitis, lobar atelectasis, respiratory failure, and the need for prolonged mechanical ventilation. Postoperative pneumonia reportedly occurs among 5% to 20% of patients and is the most common cause of postsurgical mortality (17). Identifying high-risk patients preoperatively allows the surgeon to develop strategies for preventing postoperative pulmonary complications.

Table 1 Cardiac Risk Factors—Eagle Index

History of myocardial infarction or angina
Q wave on preoperative electrocardiogram
Diabetes requiring drug therapy
Age greater than 70
History of ventricular arrhythmia requiring therapy

Note: The Eagle Index assigns one point for each risk factor. A point total of 0 indicates low risk, a point total of 1 or 2 indicates moderate risk, and a point total of 3 or more indicates high risk.
Source: From Ref. 12.

Table 2 Cardiac Risk Factors—Revised Cardiac Risk Index

High-risk surgery
History of ischemic heart disease as manifested by a history of
   myocardial infarction, positive results from an exercise stress test,
   complaints of current angina, and demonstration of a Q wave by
   preoperative electrocardiography
History of congestive heart failure
History of cerebral vascular disease
Insulin therapy for diabetes
Preoperative serum creatinine concentration >2.0 mg/dL

Note: The Revised Cardiac Risk Index assigns one point for each risk factor.
A point total of 0 indicates Class I risk, a point total of 1 indicates Class II
risk, a point total of 2 indicates Class III risk, and a point total of 3 or more
indicates Class IV risk.
Source: From Ref. 13.

Patient-Related Risk Factors

Risk factors can be either patient related or procedure related (18). Patient-related factors include age, general medical condition, obesity, sleep apnea, pulmonary hypertension, COPD, and smoking. Obese patients exhibit decreases in total lung capacity, functional residual capacity, and vital capacity. Their work at breathing is increased because of increases in elastic load, chest wall resistance, and upper airway resistance. All of these physiologic changes make obese patients more susceptible to hypoxia with a widened alveolar–arterial oxygen gradient and a ventilation-perfusion mismatch.

Patients with chronic lung disease who are wheezing and have productive coughs are also at increased risk of postoperative pulmonary complications. Preoperative pharmacologic treatment of these patients' symptoms is helpful. For men with severe COPD, the preoperative use of oral or inhaled bronchodilators,

Table 3 Recommendations for Cardiac Workup for Patients Undergoing Noncardiac Surgery

Before any elective surgery, patients with an unstable coronary syndrome
   should undergo angiography and appropriate revascularization
Patients with clinical indications for revascularization should undergo these
   procedures before elective noncardiac surgery
Patients with strongly positive results on noninvasive tests such as
   dobutamine stress echocardiography, stress electrocardiography, or
   nuclear perfusion imaging should undergo angiography and appropriate
   revascularization
Patients with symptomatic critical aortic stenosis should undergo aortic
   valve replacement before elective surgery
Noninvasive testing should be limited to patients in the intermediate-risk
   group as stratified by clinical criteria (Eagle Index or Revised Cardiac
   Risk Index). High-risk patients should undergo angiography and
   appropriate revascularization before elective surgery. Low-risk patients
   require no further testing
Patients who have undergone revascularization during the previous five
   years and patients with normal results on noninvasive testing within the
   last two years require no further preoperative testing
All clinically determined intermediate-risk and high-risk patients should
   receive beta-blockade preoperatively unless contraindicated by factors
   such as symptomatic asthma, sinus bradycardia, and second- or third-
   degree heart block (16)

Source: From Refs. 14–16.

corticosteroids, and antibiotics significantly decreases the incidence of postoperative pulmonary complications (19). Kroenke et al. (20) demonstrated that the incidence of pulmonary complications was 20% among patients with severe obstructive pulmonary disease, but the mortality rates for these patients were not higher than those for patients without such disease. This finding implies that patients with severe obstructive pulmonary disease may undergo surgery if necessary. Nevertheless, care must be taken preoperatively to ensure optimization of respiratory function. Regular performance of deep-breathing exercises with an incentive spirometer can decrease the incidence of pulmonary complications from approximately 30% to approximately 10% (21). Instructions about the use of the incentive spirometer are best given preoperatively. Avoiding a supine position helps prevent atelectasis.

Since 1944 (22), smoking has been cited as a risk factor for the development of postoperative pulmonary complications. Patients should be advised to quit smoking at least eight weeks before surgery; however, any period of abstinence before surgery can help decrease postoperative pulmonary complications. Kearney et al. (23) recently showed that an elevation in the arterial partial pressure of carbon dioxide ($PaCO_2$) was not a risk factor for complications among patients undergoing lung resection; therefore, elevations in $PaCO_2$ should not preclude patients from undergoing high-risk surgery. However, the clinician should closely monitor gas exchange during the perioperative period (24).

Nutritional reserve plays a very important role in successful esophageal surgery. A patient with a low serum concentration of albumin (<3.4 g/dL) is at an increased risk of surgical complications involving the cardiovascular, respiratory, and immune systems. Additionally, these patients experience increased rates of anastomotic breakdown, wound dehiscence, and infection. Enteral feeding should be initiated before surgery for patients who have lost more than 10% of their body weight. These feedings can be given by nasogastric tube or through a surgically created gastrostomy or jejunostomy. The use of these tubes is not a contraindication to using the stomach as a conduit. Patients also benefit from these feedings when they are undergoing chemoradiation before surgery. A feeding jejunostomy should be created during the original esophagectomy, not only for immediate postoperative feeding but also as a means of feeding the patient if an anastomotic leak complicates the postoperative course.

Procedure-Related Risk Factors

Procedure-related risk factors include the site and type of surgery and the duration of anesthesia. Thoracic or upper abdominal surgery leads to a reduction in vital capacity and functional residual capacity; these reductions may impair gas exchange, cough, and mucociliary clearance. They are also associated with increased pain, splinting, atelectasis, pneumonia, and, finally, hypoxia. Surgical procedures lasting longer than three hours are associated with a higher risk of postoperative pulmonary complications (25). Neuromuscular blockers, especially the longer-acting blockers, should be avoided for high-risk patients because they are associated with a higher incidence of pulmonary complications than are shorter-acting neuromuscular blockers (26). These risk factors are summarized in Table 4.

Chronic or hospital-acquired renal impairment may deleteriously affect surgical outcomes. Despite its low incidence (1.5 cases per 1000 patients), hospital-acquired renal insufficiency (HARI) leads to increases in complexity of care, length of stay, and mortality rates (27). A two-year review (28) of 2800 patients undergoing cardiac surgery found that 8.6% experienced HARI and 0.7% required dialysis. The mortality rate was 28% for patients who required dialysis, 14% for those who did not require dialysis, and 1% for those without HARI. Few therapeutic interventions exist other than optimizing renal perfusion and limiting nephrotoxin exposure in an attempt to prevent or reverse HARI. Patients with chronic or acute renal failure may benefit from early right-heart catheterization, so that perioperative renal and tissue perfusion can be optimized. Until improved treatment methods are developed, prevention, early detection, and treatment of HARI are essential for decreasing postoperative renal complications.

ESOPHAGEAL PERFORATION
Causes of Perforation

Perforation of the esophagus is a complex and challenging surgical emergency. Most perforations are iatrogenic, occurring during diagnostic and therapeutic endoscopic procedures (Table 5). Successful management depends on four main factors: (i) the age and overall condition of the patient, (ii) the cause and location of the perforation, (iii) the time interval between diagnosis and treatment, and (iv) the presence of any underlying esophageal disease.

Iatrogenic perforations most commonly occur during rigid or flexible esophagoscopy (0.03–0.11%), transesophageal echocardiography (0.01%) (29), pneumatic dilatation (4%), bougienage (0.09%), or sclerotherapy (1%). Perforation is most common at anatomically narrowed areas of the esophagus; the most common site is the cervical esophagus. Spontaneous rupture of the esophagus occurs with a sudden increase in intra-abdominal pressure, usually related to vomiting, weight lifting, excessive coughing, or childbirth. This pressure is transmitted to the lower thoracic esophagus and causes a perforation laterally into the left pleural cavity.

Symptoms of Perforation

The symptoms of esophageal perforation depend on the size and site of the perforation and on the elapsed time since perforation. Patients with cervical perforation usually experience cervical pain lower in the neck; the pain increases with swallowing and neck flexion. Emphysematous crepitus is commonly detected in the neck after cervical perforations; in 60% of such cases, the crepitus is palpable, and in more than 95% of cases, it can be seen on radiographs (30). Thoracic perforations cause pain substernally or in the epigastric area. Mediastinal emphysema and pleural effusions are present in approximately 50% of cases of thoracic perforation. Pleural effusions more commonly occur on the right side after upper perforation and on the left side after middle to distal perforation. Patients with abdominal perforation experience epigastric pain that is often referred to the back or left shoulder; they also experience peritoneal irritation.

Management of Esophageal Perforation

After esophageal perforation, the dissection of oral secretions (bacteria and salivary enzymes) and gastric contents into the fascial planes of the neck and mediastinum initiates a chemical and bacterial inflammatory response. Fever, sepsis, and shock develop with the increasing contamination of the mediastinal, pleural, and abdominal cavities. If this contamination is left untreated, cardiopulmonary collapse and multisystem organ failure occur.

The outcome of treatment of esophageal perforation has traditionally been poor, often because of a

Table 5   Causes of Esophageal Perforation

Iatrogenic
    Endoscopy
    Traumatic endotracheal intubation
    Pneumatic dilation
    Bougienage
    Transesophageal echocardiography
    Mediastinoscopy
    Intraoperative causes (antireflux surgery, paraesophageal hernia repair, vagotomy, etc.)

Not iatrogenic
    Tumors (esophagus, lung, and mediastinum)
    Infection (tuberculosis, AIDS, syphilis, and histoplasmosis)
    Penetrating neck, chest, or abdominal trauma
    Ingestion of caustic agents
    Foreign body
    Barotrauma (postemetic; blunt trauma to neck, chest, or abdomen; seizures)

Table 4   Risk Factors for Postoperative Pulmonary Complications

Patient-related risk factors	Procedure-related risk factors
Chronic lung disease (wheezing, productive cough)	Surgical site (thoracic, upper abdominal surgery)
Smoking: current or within 8 wks	Duration of surgery
General medical condition	Type of anesthesia
Obesity: body mass index >28	Type of neuromuscular blockade
Age >70	

delay in diagnosis brought about by the clinician's failure to consider the diagnosis (31,32). Fifty percent of patients will give a history of recent vomiting or would have undergone esophageal instrumentation or surgery; the presentation will be atypical in the remaining 50% of patients (33). All patients complaining of pain after upper endoscopy or esophageal manipulation should undergo testing to rule out an esophageal perforation. The diagnosis is confirmed with a Gastrografin® (Bracco Diagnostics, Ontario, Canada) or barium swallow. If Gastrografin esophagography shows no leak, a barium study should be performed. These studies are best performed with the patient in the right lateral decubitus position. Esophagoscopy and computed tomography (CT) also aid in making the diagnosis (Table 6).

The optimal management of esophageal perforations is controversial. Any delay in the diagnosis and definitive treatment of esophageal perforation leads to increased complications and poor outcomes (Table 7) (34). The treatment of esophageal perforation should be individualized for each patient and is based on four basic principles: (i) eliminating the source and preventing continued soilage; (ii) performing adequate cervical, mediastinal, and pleural drainage; (iii) providing aggressive resuscitation with fluids, antibiotics, and nutritional support; and (iv) correcting any distal obstructing process, functional or organic. The following factors should be considered when therapy is selected for the individual patient: the clinical toxic effects experienced by the patient, the elapsed time since perforation, the extent of containment of the leak, and any preexisting pathology of the esophagus.

Nonoperative therapy of esophageal perforations has been described (35). Sawyer et al. (36) recommend nonoperative treatment according to strict clinical criteria: (i) a recent perforation (within 24 hours), (ii) no food intake after the perforation occurred, (iii) no high-grade obstruction distal to the perforation, (iv) minor clinical symptoms without sepsis or hemodynamic compromise, (v) containment of the perforation within the mediastinum, and (vi) results of a contrast study showing good and prompt drainage from a small perforation into the esophageal lumen. Strict adherence to these criteria is mandatory if nonoperative management is to have a chance at success.

Most surgeons today recommend immediate surgical treatment of esophageal perforation (37), and multiple surgical options are available (Table 8). All patients with esophageal perforations should undergo a careful examination with a flexible endoscope before

Table 6 Computed Tomography Findings Indicating Esophageal Perforation

Pneumomediastinum
Periesophageal abscess
Mediastinal air fluid level
Pleural effusion
Communication between mediastinum and pleural cavity

Table 7 Esophageal Perforation: Mortality Rates Based on Time Elapsed Before Diagnosis

Report	No. of Patients	<24 hr%	>24 hr%
Goldstein 1982	44	25	44
Larsen 1983	54	14	33
Bladergroen 1985	127	21	33
Nesbitt 1987	51	11	26
Tilanus 1991	59	28	30
Kim-Deobald and Kozarek 1992	13	30	67
White and Morris, 1992	47	10	35
Skinner, 1993	47	9	29
Reeder, 1994	33	5	14
Total	475	19	32

Source: From Ref. 33.

undergoing surgical procedures because visualizing the extent of the esophageal injury and assessing the esophagus for any other pathology are helpful in formulating a surgical plan.

In most cases of acute esophageal perforation, primary closure with buttressing of the suture line is performed along with wide adequate drainage (38–41). Surgeons must maintain an aggressive approach when managing esophageal perforations. Many surgeons are reluctant to be surgically aggressive early on in the management of these injuries; in such cases, the outcome is often poor.

Surgical Management of Cervical Esophageal Perforation

Cervical esophageal perforation is treated with prompt surgical drainage. An incision is made along the lower-third of the medial border of the sternocleidomastoid muscle on the side of the perforation. When the carotid sheath and the internal jugular vein are retracted laterally and the trachea and esophagus are retracted medially, blunt dissection into the retroesophageal space allows adequate drainage of the prevertebral fascia directly posterior to the esophagus. Again, the surgeon must carefully look for and prevent damage to the recurrent laryngeal nerve during dissection. Blunt finger dissection is carried down into the posterior mediastinum.

Once found, the perforation is repaired with a single or double layer of absorbable suture. If the perforation cannot be visualized for repair, closure of the perforation is not required for successful healing as long as there is no distal obstruction and the retroesophageal

Table 8 Surgical Options for the Management of Esophageal Perforations

Primary closure
Primary closure with viable flap buttressing of the suture line
Exclusion and diversion
T-tube drainage
Esophageal resection with primary or delayed reconstruction
Intraluminal stent
Wide drainage only

prevertebral space, along with the superior mediastinum, has been widely dissected, debrided, and drained. The area should be copiously irrigated and a soft drain should be left in place. If the perforation is large, the perforating object has caused significant esophageal wall damage, or there is severe inflammation involving the trachea or the blood vessels, a viable flap of muscle either should be used to close and buttress the repairs or should be interposed between the separate repairs. Oral feeding should be withheld, nasogastric suction applied, and antibiotics given until cervical drainage ceases. Esophagraphy should be performed five to seven days after the repair. At that time, if there is no leak, the patient's diet should be advanced. Once the patient can tolerate a regular diet, the soft cervical drain can be removed.

Surgical Management of Thoracic Esophageal Perforation

For thoracic esophageal perforations, surgical treatment should not be delayed. Intravenous hydration and treatment with antibiotics should be initiated preoperatively. Perforations to the upper- or middle-third of the esophagus are approached through a right posterior lateral thoracotomy between the fourth and fifth intercostal spaces. Lower esophageal perforations are best approached through a left posterior lateral thoracotomy between the sixth and seventh intercostal spaces. Preexisting esophageal disease often must be dealt with at the time of exploration for esophageal perforation. Perforations occurring during pneumatic or hydrostatic dilation for achalasia are managed by primary repair of the perforation and concomitant esophagomyotomy directly opposite the repair (42). Perforations that occur during dilation for benign strictures should be repaired after such dilation has been completed. If the strictures cannot be dilated, an esophagectomy should be performed because healing is unlikely proximal to a stricture or obstruction. Patients with carcinoma who suffer perforation during endoscopy should undergo esophagectomy (43).

Reconstruction may be immediate or delayed, depending on the patient's clinical condition (44). When the patient is a poor candidate for surgery, wide local drainage is performed and a feeding jejunostomy is created. A patient with a malignant esophagorespiratory fistula or a perforated esophageal carcinoma with a mediastinal abscess is a candidate for an endoprosthesis (45) because 80% of these patients die within three months and only 11% survive for six months (46). Palliative bypass procedures are associated with substantial morbidity and mortality rates and usually deprive these patients of the little time they have left with their friends and families.

Posterolateral thoracotomy is performed through the subperiosteally resected fifth rib on the right and the seventh rib on the left. This approach allows construction of a well-vascularized intercostal musculopleural flap that can buttress the repair (Fig. 4).

The chest should be copiously irrigated and debrided of necrotic tissue, and the esophagus should be gently elevated from its bed, so that the opposite mediastinal pleura can be irrigated. If a right or left pleural effusion is found, it must be drained. Next, the perforation should be visualized and the outer muscular coat of the esophagus incised, so that the entire length of the mucosal defect can be seen before it is closed in one or two layers (Fig. 5). Failure to transfix the mucosa with each suture results in an inadequate repair that is at increased risk of an anastomotic leak (49,50).

If the muscular layer cannot be closed primarily, various muscle flaps may be used for closing the defect (51). So that the risk of suture-line disruption or an esophagopleural fistula can be minimized or prevented, the repair should then be buttressed. Flaps that have been used for buttressing repairs have consisted of pleura (52), pedicled intercostal muscle (53), diaphragm (54), pericardium (55), omentum, and gastric fundus (56). However, with minimal inflammatory reaction, the parietal pleura is thin and does not produce a good buttress. Wright et al. (39) used an intercostal muscle buttress over the primary repair and achieved primary healing in 89% of 28 patients with thoracic esophageal perforations.

If a leak develops postoperatively, an esophagram should be performed. If the leak is well drained, the patient exhibits no signs of toxicity, nutritional support is good, and no distal obstruction is present, then the leak should heal with drainage and the patient should take nothing by mouth. If the patient shows signs of sepsis or the leak is not well drained, another exploratory procedure should be performed. The area of the leak should then be widely drained; if this is not possible, the patient should undergo esophagectomy with the creation of a cervical esophagostomy and reconstruction should be performed later.

Esophageal exclusion has been promoted as a good alternative to primary repair and esophagectomy. Urschel et al. (57) modified the technique of total esophageal exclusion in continuity; initially, umbilical tape was tied over a polytetraflouroethylene band at the esophagogastric junction while a tube gastrostomy and a lateral cervical esophagostomy were performed. Many modifications of this technique have been developed. Urschel himself (58) modified the esophagogastric occlusion by using a polypropylene suture snared over a silastic tube and then exteriorizing the snare to obviate the need for a second laparotomy. Ladin et al. (59) reported the primary repair of a postemetic perforation of the thoracic esophagus by stapling the esophagus above and below the repair and performing a gastrostomy and a cervical esophagostomy. Six weeks later, the patient's esophageal lumen was patent without strictures.

Others have reported success with the creation of a T-tube fistula and drainage of the perforation. Abbott et al. (60) constructed a large-bore silastic T-tube, which was placed through a distal esophageal

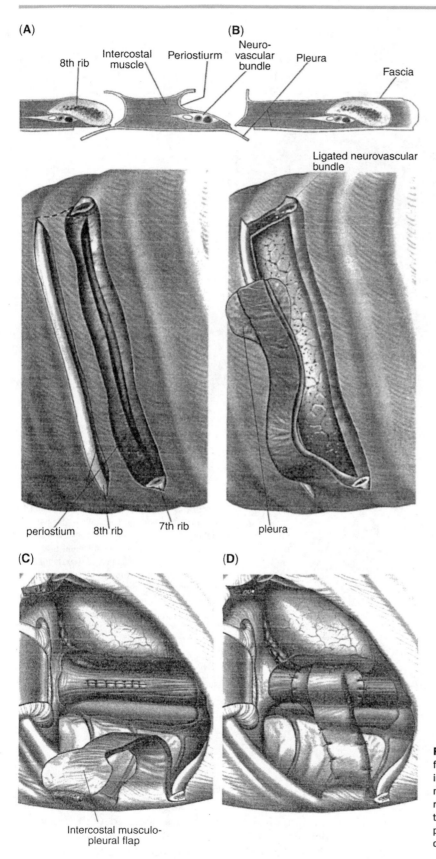

(A)

8th rib Intercostal muscle Periostiurm Neuro-vascular bundle Pleura Fascia

(B)

Ligated neurovascular bundle

periostium 8th rib 7th rib

pleura

(C)

(D)

Intercostal musculo-pleural flap

Figure 4 Construction of intercostal musculopleural flap. (**A**) Periosteum of the rib inferior to thoracotomy incision is incised, and the subjacent pleura is mobilized. (**B**) The neurovascular bundle is divided anteriorly, and the flap is created. (**C**) Two-layer closure of the esophagus is done if possible. (**D**) The musculopleural flap is applied as a buttress or a patch if closure of the perforation is not possible. *Source*: From Ref. 47.

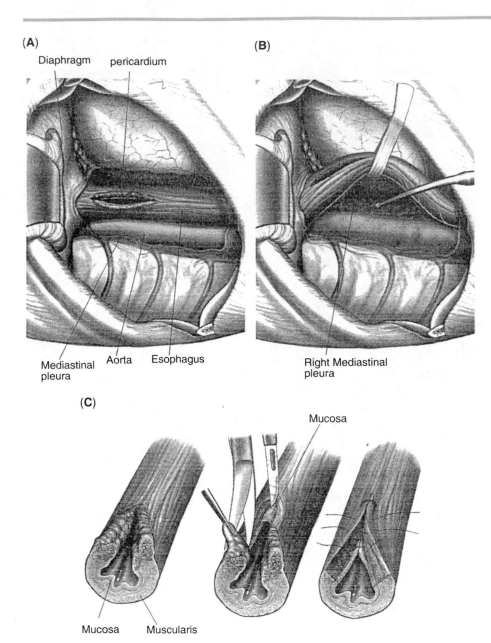

(A)

Diaphragm pericardium

Mediastinal Aorta Esophagus
pleura

(B)

Right Mediastinal
pleura

(C)

Mucosa

Mucosa Muscularis

Figure 5 **(A)** Necrotic mediastinal pleura has been excised and the esophageal tear has been debrided. **(B)** Elevation of the esophagus on a rubber drain allows for debridement of the right mediastinal pleura if indicated. **(C)** Debridement of the esophageal rupture. Muscularis incised superiorly and inferiorly to visualize the extent of mucosal defect prior to two-layer closure of the perforation, if possible. *Source*: From Ref. 48.

perforation. A nasogastric tube was then inserted through the nose, down the esophagus through the T-tube, and into the stomach. The chest cavity was drained with chest tubes. Eventual healing of the perforation requires that perforation be patched by the lung and pleura. Bufkin et al. (61) modified this technique slightly by advocating that the T-tube should be brought out through a lateral incision and sutured to the diaphragm in a position that would avoid aortic erosion.

Surgical Management of Abdominal Esophageal Perforation

The prognosis for patients with abdominal perforation is excellent if the perforation is recognized at the time of injury. Adequate treatment is usually achieved by

primary closure of the perforation and buttressing of the repair with either a partial gastric fundus wrap or an omental wrap. A gastrostomy and a feeding jejunostomy are usually indicated.

Outcome of Surgery for Esophageal Perforation

The overall mortality rate associated with esophageal perforation is 22%, that associated with cervical perforations is 6%, that associated with thoracic perforations is 34%, and that associated with abdominal perforations is 29% (34). All published series demonstrate that early diagnosis and treatment lead to the best outcomes; morbidity and mortality rates increase when diagnosis and treatment occur more than 24 hours after injury. Gouge et al. (62) reviewed the results of a series of 10 primary suture repairs of thoracic perforations; the overall leak rate was 39%, and the overall mortality rate was 25%. In another study (34) involving 99 patients who underwent primary repair with buttressing, the overall leak rate was 13% and mortality rate was 6%.

The overall mortality rate associated with the T-tube technique for draining perforations is 36%, that associated with exclusion and diversion is 35%, and that associated with resection is 26%. The mortality rates associated with T-tube drainage and exclusion may reflect the severity of these patients' illness rather than the severity of the procedure. A surgeon must be ready to use all of the techniques described above and to apply them on an individual basis, so that each patient can be treated appropriately.

ESOPHAGEAL TRAUMA

Today, most injuries to the esophagus are iatrogenic. However, some injuries are caused by blunt or penetrating trauma. Fortunately, esophageal injuries are rare, and most trauma centers see an average of five such cases per year. However, these injuries are associated with high morbidity and mortality rates. Stab wounds and gunshot wounds may injure the esophagus anywhere along its course, but most penetrating injuries occur in the cervical portion of the esophagus.

Blunt Trauma

Blunt esophageal trauma is extremely uncommon (63). It may result from a direct blow to the organ when the neck is hyperextended; such a blow crushes the esophagus against the cervical spine. Blunt trauma may also result from an increased intraluminal pressure against a closed glottis, which causes a burst-type injury. Blunt injuries occur almost exclusively in the neck, but if the intrathoracic portion of the esophagus is injured, the injury usually occurs on the left side just proximal to the esophagogastric junction, where the esophagus is less protected by the pleural lining. This type of injury is thought to be caused by the transmission of increased intra-abdominal pressure to the stomach; the mechanism of injury is similar to that of postemetic esophageal rupture (Boerhaave syndrome). Such injuries are fatal in 30% to 60% of cases (64).

Penetrating Trauma

Penetrating trauma is more common than blunt trauma. Two recent series reported the incidence of esophageal injuries from penetrating wounds to the neck; one study (65) found the incidence to be 7% (7 of 97 patients); the other (66) found it to be 5.5% (39 of 700 patients). Esophageal injuries have been found during 10% to 12% of neck explorations performed because of penetration of the platysma (67,68). Cornwell et al. (69) found only 14 intrathoracic esophageal injuries among 1961 patients (0.7%) with penetrating chest trauma. The rarity of these injuries should not lead to diagnostic complacency in the trauma bay or in the operating suite. Patients with platysmal penetration, posterior chest wounds, transmediastinal penetrating injuries, tracheobronchial injuries, or any wounds whose track may injure the esophagus should undergo testing to rule out esophageal trauma.

Preoperative Assessment of Esophageal Injuries

Clinical signs and symptoms are present among as many as 80% of patients with esophageal injuries. These signs and symptoms include odynophagia, dysphagia, hematemesis, shortness of breath, cervical crepitus, cough, stridor, complaints of neck and chest pain, hoarseness, and bleeding from the oropharynx. Fever, chills, subcutaneous emphysema, abdominal tenderness, and mediastinal crunching upon auscultation of the chest (Hamman's sign) may be present. Clinical findings of pneumothorax, pneumomediastinum, left-sided pleural effusion, a nasogastric tube passing into the pleural space, food particles draining from a chest tube, or bubbles in the chest tube through both inspiration and expiration may suggest esophageal injury (64).

Most reports describing series of traumatic esophageal injuries state that the most common presenting symptom is pain in the neck, chest, or abdomen. Other common signs and symptoms include fever, dyspnea, crepitus, dysphagia, vomiting, and shock (64). The presence of these signs and symptoms depends on the location of the injury, the size of the perforation, the degree of contamination, the length of time since injury, and other associated injuries such as tracheal and vascular injuries (68). Overall, these signs and symptoms are unreliable in predicting esophageal injuries; therefore, the clinician must maintain a high index of suspicion so that the diagnosis can be made.

The results of plain radiography of the neck and chest may be abnormal in as many as 75% of patients with esophageal injuries. More definitive studies are needed if radiographs show hydrothorax, pneumomediastinum, or pneumothorax; air dissecting into the retropharyngeal spaces; or subcutaneous cervical air. If an esophageal injury is suspected or found, the patient should undergo urgent contrast esophagography. Contrast esophagography has been shown to be 89% sensitive and 100% specific for cervical esophageal injuries (70). In their review of esophageal injuries, White and Morris (66) found that contrast esophagography was 100% sensitive and 95% specific. Contrast radiography is usually first performed with Gastrografin®, a water-soluble agent that, unlike barium, does not cause severe mediastinitis but may cause a severe chemical pneumonitis if aspirated. Gastrografin is less radiodense than barium and less likely to demonstrate small leaks or perforations. A barium contrast study is usually performed if the results of the Gastrografin study are negative.

Because the results of esophagraphy may be normal for 15% of patients with esophageal injuries, a high suspicion of injury should prompt the performance of endoscopic esophagoscopy (71). Esophagoscopy, with either a rigid or a flexible scope, has been helpful in identifying esophageal injuries. Rigid esophagoscopy is more sensitive (89%) for cervical esophageal injuries than flexible esophagoscopy (37%) (70). Flexible endoscopy is 100% sensitive and specific for thoracic esophageal injuries (66). Nevertheless, there is a risk (less than 1%) of further esophageal injury or perforation during esophagoscopy (72). When contrast radiography and esophagoscopy are combined, their sensitivity approaches 100% and some clinicians report excellent results with no missed injuries (51).

Management of Esophageal Injuries
Injuries to the Cervical Esophagus

The cervical esophagus is more commonly injured than the thoracic or abdominal esophagus. Some surgeons and institutions consider exploration mandatory for penetrating zone II neck injuries; others recommend a more selective approach. Once a cervical esophageal injury has been diagnosed, the patient is given nothing by mouth, nasogastric suction is begun, and the administration of antibiotics active against oral flora is initiated. Prompt surgical drainage and repair of the esophagus are performed through a collar incision or an incision along the anterior border of the sternocleidomastoid muscle.

Most esophageal injuries are repaired primarily with a single-layer, full-thickness closure with interrupted nonabsorbable 3–0 suture or in two layers with an inner absorbable layer and an outer nonabsorbable layer. Repair by either a single-layer or a two-layer method should ensure complete closure of the mucosa and of all muscular layers, so that delayed leaks can be prevented. Failure of the suture to transfix the mucosa is due to the fatty submucosa, which allows the mucosa to retract under the overlying muscular layers. The mucosa must be identified and deliberately transfixed; each suture must be placed so as to achieve apposition and to avoid anastomotic leaks (1). This principle applies to all repairs performed on all segments of the esophagus.

More complex injuries to the esophagus may require debridement of devascularized segments or resection. Vascularized tissue flaps should be used when defects are large or when the tissues are too friable for primary closure. Flaps are also used when the esophagus is perforated in two places (as is the case with gunshot wounds) or when primary closure of both injuries would result in substantial narrowing of the lumen (71). If the trachea or the carotid arteries are also injured, buttressing the repair with muscle flaps from the sternohyoid, omohyoid, sternothyroid, or sternocleidomastoid muscles is particularly important so that late fistulae can be avoided.

All repairs in the neck should be drained. The drain is placed approximately 2 cm from the esophageal repair and is brought out through a separate wound. Oral intake is started if esophagraphy shows no leak on the fifth postoperative day. The drain is removed after two days of oral intake if no drainage occurs. Most esophageal fistulas that develop after neck trauma drain directly from the esophagus to the skin. Because as many as 50% of all leaks are symptomatic (73), a contrast swallow should be used to confirm the presence of suspected leaks and fistulas. If no distal obstruction is present, most of these fistulas will resolve spontaneously after two to three weeks of adequate drainage, limited oral intake, and antibiotic administration.

Injuries to the Thoracic Esophagus

Thoracic esophageal injuries are less common than cervical esophageal injuries; however, they are more often fatal. These injuries are frequently associated with injuries to the great vessels, trachea, lungs, and diaphragm. During emergent exploration for these other injuries, the surgeon must be careful to rule out esophageal injury. Intraoperative esophagoscopy should be performed when a complete evaluation of the esophagus is impossible. Emergent intraoperative esophagoscopy has been shown to be 100% sensitive and 80% specific for penetrating esophageal injuries (74). During esophagoscopy, insufflation of air is very helpful in identifying the site of injury. Patients who are in stable condition but for whom examination is necessary for ruling out esophageal or other injuries should first undergo contrast-enhanced spiral CT of the chest. This test can rule out associated injuries to lung, great vessels, trachea, and spine and may show the location of esophageal injuries (75).

Surgical treatment involves local debridement, wide drainage, primary repair of the defect, and buttressing of the repair with a viable muscle flap (52). Grillo and Wilkins (52) described the use of pleural flaps for buttressing their repairs.

Wounds to the upper- and middle-thirds of the thoracic esophagus are repaired through a right posterolateral thoracotomy at the fifth intercostal space. After the injury has been identified, the esophageal wall should be circumferentially inspected, so that the presence of an exit wound can be excluded. Primary repair with either a one-layer or a two-layer technique is performed if the injury is repaired within 24 hours (76). After the esophageal wound has been closed, a parietal pleural flap, an intercostal muscle flap, or a pericardial flap should be created to buttress the repair; the pleura, however, may not be sufficiently thickened by inflammation to buttress certain repairs, particularly those between the trachea and the esophagus. Other tissue flaps such as pericardial, intercostal muscle, diaphragm, and rhomboid muscle flaps have been used to buttress these repairs and to close larger defects that cannot be closed primarily. The use of these viable flaps to buttress the repair has been associated with improved anastomotic outcome (77).

The fistulas and leaks that develop after the repair of traumatic esophageal injuries more often than not respond to local drainage and creation of a controlled fistula; usually diversion or resection is unnecessary. If diagnosis has been delayed or if the injury is so severe that primary repair is not feasible because of the degree of contamination and inflammatory reaction, viable alternatives to primary repair are esophageal diversion, exclusion, or resection. Another alternative is dissecting the superior part of the esophagus up to the chest inlet and exteriorizing the esophagus through a new wound, thereby creating an esophagostomy. The distal end is stapled and dissected to the diaphragm and is removed through a separate incision; a gastrostomy is then performed (78). At a later date, reconstruction of the continuity of the GI tract is performed with gastric pull-up or colonic interposition.

Wounds to the lower-third of the thoracic esophagus are repaired through a left posterolateral thoracotomy through the sixth intercostal space. Repair is performed as above except that diaphragm, intercostal muscle, or gastric fundus can be used to buttress the repair. After repair but before closure, the mediastinal pleura must be widely opened, thoroughly irrigated and débrided, and finally drained.

Injuries to the Abdominal Esophagus

Injuries to the abdominal segment of the esophagus are repaired through a laparotomy; the suture line is covered with either omentum or the gastric fundus as in a Thal 180°- or a Toupe 270°-fundoplication. The true Nissan 360°-wrap should probably be avoided because it may cause a functional distal esophageal obstruction. Creating a feeding jejunostomy is sometimes helpful. The rate of esophageal leak or fistula formation has been reported to be 38% (51).

Complications of Surgical Repair of Esophageal Injuries

Esophageal anastomotic leaks are the most common complication after esophageal repair; their incidence is approximately 15% to 25% (79–82). They are frequently the result of technical misadventures such as inadequate debridement of devitalized tissue, devascularization of tissue, closure under tension, inadequate drainage, and the presence or development of infection. Other complications that may occur after repair of esophageal injuries include esophageal stricture, wound infection, mediastinitis, empyema, sepsis, and pneumonia. The incidence of complications after repair increases as the time between injury and repair increases. Shock, spinal cord injuries, the need for emergent tracheostomy, and the presence of other associated injuries also increase the rate of complications.

Outcome of Surgical Management of Esophageal Injuries

Increased morbidity and mortality rates result when diagnosis and treatment of these esophageal injuries are delayed. Both delay in implementing diagnostic investigations aimed at establishing the presence of injuries and difficulty in identifying these injuries when other trauma is present may lead to an increased risk of complications, including death (83). The most important factor contributing to high morbidity and mortality rates is a delay in initiating definitive surgical repair (77,79,84,85). The mortality rate associated with esophageal injuries ranges from 5% to 25% for patients treated definitively within 12 hours after injury, from 10% to 44% for those treated 12 to 24 hours after injury, and from 25% to 66% or more for those treated more than 24 hours after injury (86). The mortality rates associated with injuries to the thoracic esophagus are particularly high because severe suppurative mediastinitis develops within 6 to 12 hours (87).

COMPLICATIONS OF ESOPHAGEAL RESECTION
Pulmonary Complications

Pulmonary complications are the most common cause of morbidity and mortality after esophageal resection (88). Several patient-related and procedure-related factors may predispose the patient to pulmonary complications (Table 4). Postoperative retention of sputum and atelectasis commonly result in hypoxia. The incidence of postoperative atelectasis and respiratory insufficiency is higher after transthoracic incisions, whereas the incidence of pneumonia is similar for the transhiatal approach and the transthoracic approach (89). Risk factors that increase the incidence of respiratory complications include advanced age, COPD, malnutrition, neoadjuvant therapy, loss of more than 1 L of blood during the procedure, and immobility due to pain or malnutrition. Preoperative intervention aimed at optimizing pulmonary hygiene and function can decrease the incidence of pulmonary complications.

Extubation should be performed only after the patient exhibits a good gag reflex and excellent pulmonary mechanics. Postoperative aspiration can occur as the result of retention of secretions in the trachea after mobilization of the esophagus, unrecognized recurrent laryngeal nerve injury with immediate impairment of swallowing, and overdistention of the esophageal conduit by retained secretions. The incidence of pneumonia can be reduced by early ambulation combined with good pain control and aggressive pulmonary toilet, consisting of humidified supplemental oxygen, incentive spirometry, and, at times, chest physiotherapy. If pneumonia develops early, the administration of appropriate antibiotics should be initiated. Early bronchoscopy can improve pulmonary toilet, provide a good specimen for culture, and exclude tracheobronchial injury. If the patient still requires ventilatory support one week after surgery, early tracheostomy should be considered.

A rare but disastrous complication is tracheobronchial fistula. Injury to the trachea or the main stem bronchus can occur during the mobilization of the upper half of the esophagus during both transhiatal and transthoracic esophagectomy. Blunt dissection close to the esophagus and away from the trachea and bronchus avoids this potentially lethal technical error. Intraoperative injury is suggested by a loss in returned tidal volume, inability to ventilate the patient, persistent air bubbles in the mediastinum, and the odor of anesthetic gas. Initial intraoperative management of this complication includes advancing the endotracheal tube past the injury. Once the airway has been secured and the patient's condition is otherwise stable, the planned esophagectomy may proceed; the airway should be repaired via an incision in the right chest, and a buttressed flap should be placed between the repair and the esophageal conduit.

Cardiac Complications

Cardiac complications are infrequent, but may cause serious morbidity or death. Perioperative hypotension is most commonly caused by intravascular volume depletion or excessive vasodilation. Intraoperative hypotension can be caused by blunt dissection around the esophageal hiatus and the posterior mediastinum because such dissection can decrease venous return. However, hypotension may result from myocardial ischemia and is a predictor of postoperative cardiac morbidity. A variety of factors such as anemia, hypotension, tachycardia, hypoxia, and fixed coronary lesions predispose patients to myocardial ischemia. These factors may result in increases in myocardial oxygen demand or decreases in myocardial oxygen supply.

The incidence and severity of perioperative myocardial ischemia appear to be greatest during the first 48 hours after surgery (90). The diagnosis is usually difficult because both perioperative myocardial infarction (MI) and ischemia are usually silent. Symptoms of perioperative MI or ischemia include arrhythmia, hypotension, CHF, impaired mental status, and an increase in the blood sugar level of patients with diabetes. There is now convincing evidence that the use of beta-blockers decreases the incidence of myocardial ischemia and infarction associated with noncardiac surgery (16).

Arrhythmias are common during the perioperative period, but most are clinically benign. The reported incidence of atrial dysrhythmia after esophagectomy ranges from 13% (91) to 60% (92). Important risk factors for dysrhythmia include advanced age and the extent of surgery (93). The administration of beta-blockers has been shown to reduce the incidence of postoperative atrial arrhythmia (94).

Bleeding

Bleeding, both intraoperatively and postoperatively, is not only troublesome but also potentially lethal. The occurrence of hypotension and tachycardia on the first postoperative day is usually related to bleeding due to inadequate hemostasis during surgery. This type of bleeding arises from short gastric arteries that have not been thoroughly ligated. If not recognized intraoperatively, injury to the spleen during gastric mobilization can also lead to postoperative bleeding. The azygous vein is usually ligated during thoracotomy but can be injured by blunt dissection during a transhiatal esophagectomy. Bleeding may also result from injury to the internal mammary artery, from the intercostal arteries, and from the aortic arch. When surgeons are careful to keep dissection planes close to the esophageal wall, bleeding from vessels supplying the esophagus is usually self-limited. When bleeding is severe, the mediastinum should be packed first so that the hemorrhage can be arrested and the patient's condition can stabilize. If possible, the bleeding vessel(s) should be ligated under direct vision. If bleeding is not controlled by packing, a right thoracotomy must be performed so that the source can be identified.

Thoracic Duct Injury

Injury to the thoracic duct may occur anywhere along the esophagus during dissection and mobilization. The reported incidence of injury to the thoracic duct is 1% to 3% (95). Chylothorax is suspected if a large volume of serous drainage from the chest tube persists beyond the fifth postoperative day. The diagnosis may be confirmed by feeding the patient cream, which will turn the chest tube drainage cloudy white. Once the diagnosis has been made, the initial treatment approach is nonoperative. The patient should take nothing by mouth, and total parenteral nutrition should be initiated. Nonoperative treatment, however, is rarely successful. If chest tube output of more than 1 L per day continues for more than five days, if the leak persists for more than two weeks, or if nutritional or metabolic complications occur, exploration is necessary. Routine ligation of the thoracic duct is recommended for preventing chylothorax (96).

Nerve Injury

The incidence of recurrent laryngeal nerve injury after esophageal resection ranges from 2% to 20% (97). Injury to the recurrent laryngeal nerve results in hoarseness and difficulty in swallowing, which predisposes the patient to aspiration. Fortunately, the injury is usually transient and is most likely related to pressure on or stretching of the nerve that is caused by the placement of retractors in the tracheoesophageal groove. Gentle finger retraction during this dissection can decrease the incidence of injury to the recurrent nerve (97). If damage to the left recurrent laryngeal nerve under the arch of the aorta is to be avoided, the esophagus must be very carefully mobilized. Damage to the right recurrent laryngeal nerve may occur during dissection around the subclavian artery at the apex of the right chest cavity. Knowledge of the anatomy and careful dissection near the esophagus can prevent this injury or lessen its associated morbidity rates.

During esophagectomy, the vagus nerves are transected; this procedure results in two problems. The first is pylorospasm and gastric dysmotility, which impair gastric emptying. To avoid this problem, most surgeons today perform a pyloromyotomy or a pyloroplasty during esophageal resection (98). The second problem is the dumping syndrome, which is caused by the vagotomy and can vary in severity. The symptoms of this syndrome are postprandial diarrhea, cramping, nausea, diaphoresis, abdominal pain, and palpitations. These symptoms are usually self-limited and are treated by ensuring that the patient eats frequent small meals, avoids foods with a high carbohydrate content, and drinks liquids with meals. Occasionally, antidiarrheal agents may be necessary.

Anastomotic Leak

Anastomotic leaks are a feared complication of esophageal surgery and lead to increases in morbidity and mortality rates. The reported incidence of leaks after esophageal resection ranges from 2% to 30% (99). Law et al. found that at least 53% of leaks are due to technical errors and are therefore preventable (100). Careful attention to surgical technique is the key to preventing leaks. The anastomosis must be created without any tension, and the remnant of the esophagus and the conduit must have a good blood supply. Again, it is crucial to ensure that each stitch transfixes the mucosal edge, which may retract as far as 1 cm from the cut edge of the esophagus (49). Randomized trials have found that the incidence of leaks is not affected by the type of anastomosis created (stapled or hand sewn, one or two layers, running or interrupted). However, both trials found that the incidence of anastomotic stricture was higher when a stapled anastomosis was created (101,102).

Leaks that occur early, within the first 48 hours, are usually due to necrosis of the conduit. Although rare, this complication can be fatal. Immediate surgical intervention is required so that the conduit can be resected, the mediastinum can be debrided, a cervical esophagostomy can be created, and a feeding jejunostomy can be placed. Preparation of an esophageal conduit that ensures proper length and blood supply will allow the creation of an anastomosis without tension. Careful mobilization of the stomach is essential for preserving the right gastroepiploic artery and, if possible, the right gastric artery. Colon conduits require adequate collateralization through the marginal artery. All conduits must be delivered into the chest or neck in the proper alignment so that twisting or kinking can be avoided.

Although the incidence of cervical leaks is higher than that of thoracic leaks, cervical leaks rarely cause death. In contrast, thoracic leaks often lead to severe mediastinitis and are associated with a mortality rate as high as 50% (88,96). Cervical leaks commonly occur during the fifth to tenth postoperative days; their symptoms are fever, crepitus, increases in wound erythema, and drainage. A barium swallow should be performed to confirm the leak, and a CT scan of the neck and chest should be performed to delineate the degree of contamination. The wound should then be opened and widely drained. Locating and closing the leak should never be attempted. Almost all cervical leaks heal with conservative management; however, anastomotic strictures develop in as many as one-third of cases (88). Thoracic leaks most commonly occur during the first postoperative week. When the first signs of sepsis appear, tests should be performed to rule out a leak. Signs and symptoms include fever, tachycardia, an increasing white blood cell count, an increasing pleural effusion as demonstrated by chest radiographs, and an increasing amount of bile-stained or turbid fluid in the chest tube drainage.

The location and magnitude of a leak are confirmed by radiography with water-soluble contrast material. Treatment of leaks must be patient specific (96). For small, contained leaks with no signs of sepsis, appropriate treatment may be chest tube drainage, CT-guided drainage, or both. Exploration is necessary for large leaks accompanied by sepsis. Direct repair is seldom possible; therefore, the anastomosis must be taken down, the conduit and its return to the abdomen must be debrided, the mediastinum must be widely drained and debrided, and a diverting esophagostomy must be created. Reconstruction may be performed several months later after the patient makes a full recovery. In all cases, the administration of broad-spectrum antibiotics must be initiated; antibiotics active against a specific organism should be used once culture results are available. The patient's nutritional status must be maintained. Asymptomatic leaks that are detected by routine postoperative contrast studies should be treated conservatively by withholding oral feeding until a repeated contrast study shows resolution of the leak (88).

Stricture

Stricture may occur at the anastomotic site regardless of the type of conduit, the type of anastomosis, or the type of surgical approach (81). The reported rate of anastomotic stricture ranges from 2% to 40% (97,102, 103). The incidence of anastomotic stricture is increased if the esophageal pathology is due to the ingestion of lye, the occurrence of a postoperative leak, the creation of a stapled anastomosis (101), or the creation of an anastomosis in an irradiated field (88). Law et al. found that the rate of stricture was 40% after a stapled anastomosis but only 9% after a hand-sewn anastomosis (102). Fortunately, most strictures do not require surgical intervention and may be dilated over a soft, tapered Maloney dilator. Initial dilation should be performed under endoscopic and fluoroscopic guidance so that injury can be prevented and the degree, length, and nature of the stricture can be determined. At this time, a biopsy of all strictures should be performed so that recurrence can be ruled out. Significant symptomatic relief is obtained when the stricture is dilated to 40 to 54 F. Multiple dilations should be performed during the next several weeks so that stricture recurrence can be prevented. The interval between treatments should be gradually extended until a period of six months passes with no recurrence of dysphagia. A few strictures will be chronic and resistant; in these cases, surgical intervention will be required. These resistant strictures can be cured by a variety of stricturoplasty methods using a variety of myocutaneous tissue flaps (104).

Other Complications

Various other complications such as delayed emptying of the conduit, obstruction of the conduit, and herniation of bowel into the chest can be prevented by close attention to operative technique. Delayed emptying of the conduit commonly results from an excess of stomach in the chest when the stomach is used to replace the esophagus. This delayed emptying causes pooling of contents in the posterior costophrenic gutter. Other causes of delayed emptying of the conduit include failure to perform a pyloromyotomy or a pyloroplasty and failure to enlarge the diaphragmatic hiatus. In a randomized study, Fok et al. (98) evaluated the effectiveness of pyloroplasty in preventing delayed emptying of the conduit. No delay in emptying occurred among patients who underwent pyloroplasty but did occur among 13% of patients who did not undergo this procedure. Management of postoperatively identified obstruction at the hiatus usually requires reexploration and enlargement of the hiatus (89). During the laparotomy phase, tacking sutures should be carefully placed from the conduit to the diaphragm so that no space remains through which the bowel can herniate into the chest.

Pneumothorax may occur during transhiatal and transthoracic esophagectomy if the pleural space is inadvertently entered. Careful palpation of the pleura will reveal a tear, and this finding mandates placement of a chest tube, which may be removed according to standard practices. Patients undergoing esophageal surgery have several risk factors that place them at high risk of thromboembolism: they are generally older, may be in a hypercoagulable state because of underlying malignancy, and will require lengthy surgical procedures for disease management. Sequential compression devices should be applied before the induction of anesthesia. The need for additional thromboprophylaxis depends on risk stratification, and additional thromboprophylaxis involves the administration of low-molecular-weight heparins or unfractionated heparin 12 to 24 hours postoperatively. Early ambulation is crucial to preventing this complication and cannot be overemphasized.

CONCLUSION

Although esophageal surgery is fraught with difficulty, a thorough knowledge of the anatomy and an understanding of esophageal function allow such procedures to be performed with an acceptably low morbidity and mortality rate along with a good outcome.

REFERENCES

1. Orringer MB. Complications of esophageal surgery and trauma. In: Greenfield LJ, ed. Complications in Surgery and Trauma. 2d ed. Philadelphia: Lippincott, 1989:302–325.
2. In: Pearson FG, Deslauriers J, Ginsberg RJ, et al. eds. Esophageal Surgery. New York: Churchhill Livingstone, 1995:2.
3. Peters JH, DeMeester TR. Esophagus: anatomy, physiology and gastroesophageal reflux disease. In: Greenfield LG, Mulholland MW, Oldham KT, Zelenock GB, Lillemoe KD, eds. Surgery: Scientific Principles Practice. 3d ed. Philadelphia: Lippincott, Williams and Wilkins, 2001:659–692.
4. Symbas PN, Symbas NP. Esophagus and diaphragm. In: Wood WC, Skandalakis JE, eds. Anatomic Basis of Tumor Surgery. St. Louis: Quality Medical Publishing, 1999:272–303.
5. Liebermann-Meffert DM, Luescher U, Neff U, Ruedi TP, Allgower M. Esophagectomy without thoracotomy; is there a risk of intramediastinal bleeding? A study on blood supply of the esophagus. Ann Surg 1987; 206:184–192.
6. Liebermann-Meffert DM, Duranceau A, Stein HJ. Anatomy and embrology: anatomy of the esophagus. In: Zuidema GD, Yeo CJ, Orringer MB, Heitmiller R, eds. Shackelford's Surgery of the Alimentary Tract. Vol. 1. 5th ed. Philadelphia: Saunders 2002:3–22.
7. Grimes OF, Visalli JA. An embryologic and anatomic approach to the surgical management of gastric cancer. Surg Gynecol Obstet 1956; 103(4):401–408.
8. Skandalakis JE, Ellis H. Embryologic and Anatomic basis of esophageal surgery. Surg Clin North Am 2000; 80:85–155.
9. Henderson RD, Boszko A, VanNostrand AW, Pearson FG. Pharyngoesophageal dysphagia and recurrent laryngeal nerve palsy. J Thorac Cardiovasc Surg 1974; 68:507–512.
10. Guillory JR Jr., Clagett OT. Postvagotomy dysphagia. Surg Clin North Am 1967; 47:833–840.
11. Wilson RF, Tyburski JG. Preoperative risk assessment and perioperative care. In: Corson JD, Williamson RC, eds. Surgery. Philadelphia: Elsevier, 2000:1.1–1.14.
12. Cohen MC, Eagle KA. The role of cardiology consultation. In: Topol EJ, ed. Comprehensive Cardiovascular Medicine. Philadelphia: Lippincott, 1998:1147–1171.
13. Lee TH, Marcantonio ER, Mangione CM, et al. Derivation and prospective valiadation of a simple index for

the prediction of cardiac risk of major noncardiac surgery. Circulation 1999; 100:1043–1049.

14. Hanna MA, Feld M, Sampliner JE. Preoperative cardiac assessment of the candidate for major resective pancreatic surgery. Surg Clin North Am 2001; 81: 575–578.

15. Eagle KA, Berger PB, Calkins H, et al., American College of Cardiology, American Heart Association. ACC/AHA guideline update for perioperative cardiovascular evaluation for non cardiac surgery— executive summary: a report of the American College of Cardiology/American Heart Association Task Force on Practice Guidelines (Committee to Update the 1996 Guidelines on Perioperative Cardiovascular Evaluation for Noncardiac Surgery). J Am Coll Cardiol 2002; 39:542–553.

16. Mangano DT, Layug EL, Wallace A, Tateo I. Effect of atenolol on mortality and cardiovascular morbidity after noncardiac surgery. Multicenter Study of Perioperative Ischemia Research Group. N Engl J Med 1996; 335:1713–1720.

17. Heitmiller RF. Esophageal surgery. In: Gordon TA, Cameron JL, eds. Evidence-Based Surgery. Hamilton, Ontario: BC Decker, 2000:251–262.

18. Smetana GW. Preoperative pulmonary evaluation. N Engl J Med 1999; 340:937–944.

19. Tarhan S, Moffitt EA, Sessler AD, Douglas WW, Taylor WF. Risk of anesthesia and surgery in patients with chronic bronchitis and chronic obstructive pulmonary disease. Surgery 1973; 74:720–726.

20. Kroenke K, Lawrence VA, Theroux JF, Tuley MR, Hilsenbeck S. Postoperative complications after thoracic and major abdominal surgery in patients with and without obstructive lung disease. Chest 1993; 104:1445–1451.

21. Bartlett RH. Respiratory therapy to prevent postoperative pulmonary complications. In: Pierson DJ, ed. Respiratory Intensive Care. Dallas: Daedalus Enterprises, 1986:369–372.

22. Morton HJ. Tobacco smoking and pulmonary complications after surgery. Lancet 1944; 1:368–370.

23. Kearney DJ, Lee TH, Reilly JJ, DeCamp MM, Sugarbaker DJ. Assessment of operative risk in patients undergoing lung resection. Importance of predicted pulmonary function. Chest 1994; 105:753–759.

24. Trayner E Jr., Celli BR, Postoperative pulmonary complications. Med Clin North Am 2001; 85:1129–1139.

25. Celli BR, Rodriguez KS, Snider GL. A controlled trial of intermittent positive pressure breathing, incentive spirometry, and deep breathing exercises in preventing pulmonary complications after abdominal surgery. Am Rev Respir Dis 1984; 130:12–15.

26. Berg H, Roed J, Vilby-Mogensen J, et al. Residual neuromuscular block is a factor for postoperative pulmonary complications. A prospective, randomised, and blinded study of postoperative pulmonary complications after atracurium, vecuronium and pancuronium. Acta Anaesthesiol Scand 1997; 41:1095–1103.

27. Chertow GM, Levy EM, Hammermeister KE, Grover F, Daley J. Independent association between acute renal failure and mortality following cardiac surgery. Am J Med 1998; 104:343–348.

28. Conlon PJ, Stafford-Smith M, White WD, et al. Acute renal failure following cardiac surgery. Nephrol Dial Transplant 1999; 14:1158–1162.

29. Kallmeyer IJ, Collard CD, Fox JA, Body SC, Shernan SK. The safety of intraoperative transesophageal echocardiography: a case series of 7200 cardiac surgical patients. Anesth Analg 2001; 92:1126–1130.

30. Miller DL. Esophageal perforation. In: Bland KI, ed. The Practice of General Surgery. Philadelphia: Elsevier, 2001:326–331.

31. Reeder LB, DeFilippi VJ, Ferguson MK. Current results of therapy for esophageal perforation. Am J Surg 1995; 169:615–617.

32. Ajalat GM, Mulder DG. Esophageal perforations. The need for an individualized approach. Arch Surg 1984; 119:1318–1320.

33. Blom D, Peters JH. Esophageal perforation. In: Cameron JL, ed. Current Surgical Therapy. 7th ed. St. Louis: Mosby, 2001:7–12.

34. Jones WG II, Ginsberg RJ. Esophageal perforation: a continuing challenge. Ann Thorac Surg 1992; 53:534–543.

35. Cameron JL, Kieffer RF, Hendrix TR, Mehigan DG, Baker RR. Selective nonoperative management of contained intrathoracic esophageal disruptions. Ann Thorac Surg 1979; 27:404–408.

36. Sawyer R, Phillips C, Vakil N. Short- and long-term outcome of esophageal perforation. Gastrointest Endosc 1995; 41:130–134.

37. Michel L, Grillo HC, Malt RA. Operative and nonoperative management of esophageal perforation. Ann Surg 1981; 194:57–63.

38. Ohri SK, Liakakos TA, Pathi V, Townsend ER, Fountain SW. Primary repair of iatrogenic thoracic esophageal perforations and Boerhaave's syndrome. Ann Thorac Surg 1993; 55:603–606.

39. Wright CD, Mathisen DJ, Wain JC, Moncure AC, Hilgenberg AD, Grillo HC. Reinforced primary repair of thoracic esophageal perforation. Ann Thorac Surg 1995; 60:245–249.

40. Whyte RI, Iannettoni MD, Orringer MB. Intrathoracic esophageal perforation. The merit of primary repair. J Thorac Cardiovasc Surg 1995; 109:140–146.

41. Wang N, Razzouk AJ, Safavi A, et al. Delayed primary repair of intrathoracic esophageal perforation: is it safe? J Thorac Cardiovasc Surg 1996; 109:114–122.

42. McKinnon WM, Ochsner JL. Immediate closure and Heller procedure after Mosher bach rupture of the esophagus. Am J Surg 1974; 127:115–118.

43. Blalock J. Primary esophagectomy for instrumental perforation of the esophagus. Am J Surg 1957; 94:393–397.

44. Orringer MB, Stirling MC. Esophagectomy for esophageal disruption. Ann Thorac Surg 1990; 49:35–43.

45. Berger RL, Donato AT. Treatment of esophageal disruption by intubation. A new method of management. Ann Thorac Surg 1972; 13:27–35.

46. Hill DC, Murray GF. Malignant tracheoesophageal fistula. In: Grillo HC, Austen WG, Wilkins EW, Mathiesen DJ, Flahakes G, eds. Current Therapy in Cardiothoracic Surgery. St. Louis: Mosby, 1989:56–57.

47. In: Pearson FG, Deslauriers J, Ginsberg RJ, et al., eds. Esophageal Surgery. New York: Churchhill Livingstone, 1995:508–509.

48. In: Pearson FG, Deslauriers J, Ginsberg RJ, et al., eds. Esophageal Surgery. New York: Churchhill Livingstone, 1995:507.

49. Orringer MB. Complications of esophageal surgery. In: Zuidema GD, Yeo CJ, eds. Shackelford's Surgery

of the Alimentary Tract. :Vol. 15th ed. Philadelphia: Elsevier, 2001:444–472.

50. Fell SC. Esophageal perforation. In: Pearson FG, Cooper JD, Hiebert CA, Ginsburg RJ, eds. Esophageal Surgery. 2d ed. Philadelphia: Elsevier, 2002:615–636.

51. Richardson JD, Tobin GR. Closure of esophageal defects with muscle flaps. Arch Surg 1994; 129:541–548.

52. Grillo HC, Wilkins EW Jr. Esophageal repair following late diagnosis of intrathoracic perforation. Ann Thorac Surg 1975; 20:387–399.

53. Dooling JV, Zick HR. Closure of an esophagopleural fistula using onlay intercostal pedicle graft. Ann Thorac Surg 1967; 3:553–557.

54. Jara FM. Diaphragmatic pedicle flap for the treatment of Boerhaave's syndrome. J Thorac Cardiovasc Surg 1979; 78:931–933.

55. Millard AH. "Spontaneous" perforation of the oesophagus treated by utilization of a pericardial flap. Br J Surg 1971; 58:70–72.

56. Thal AP, Hatafuku T. Improved operation for esophageal rupture. JAMA 1964; 188:826–888.

57. Urschel HC Jr., Razzuk MA, Wood RE, Galbraith N, Pockey M, Paulson DL. Improved management of esophageal perforation: exclusion and diversion in continuity. Ann Surg 1974; 179:587–591.

58. Urschel HC. Discussion of: Gouge TH, Depan HJ, Spencer FC. Experience with the Grillo pleural wrap procedure in 18 patients with perforation of the thoracic esophagus. Ann Surg 1989; 209:612–619.

59. Ladin DA, Dunnington GL, Rappaport WD. Stapled esophageal exclusion in acute esophageal rupture: a new technique. Contemp Surg 1989; 35:45–51.

60. Abbott OH, Mansour KA, Logan WD Jr., Hatcher CR Jr., Symbas PN. Atraumatic so-called "spontaneous" rupture of the esophagus. A review of 47 personal cases with comments on a new method of surgical therapy. J Thorac Cardiovasc Surg 1970; 59:67–83.

61. Bufkin BL, Miller JI Jr., Mansour KA. Esophageal perforation: emphasis on management. Ann Thorac Surg 1996; 61:1447–1452.

62. Gouge TH, Depan HJ, Spencer FC. Experience with the Grillo pleural wrap procedure in 18 patients with perforation of the thoracic esophagus. Ann Surg 1989; 209:612–619.

63. Kemmerer WT, Eckert WG, Gathright JB, Reetsma K, Creech O Jr. Patterns of thoracic injuries in fatal traffic accidents. J Trauma 1961; 1:595–599.

64. Riley RD, Miller PR, Meredith JW. Injury to the esophagus, trachea, and bronchus. In: Moore EE, Feliciano DV, Mattox KL, eds. Trauma. 5th ed. New York: McGraw-Hill, 2004:539–552.

65. Demetriades D, Theodorou D, Cornwell E, et al. Transcervical gunshot injuries: mandatory operation is not necessary. J Trauma 1996; 40:758–760.

66. White RK, Morris DM. Diagnosis and management of esophageal perforations. Am Surg 1992; 58:112–119.

67. Sheely CH II, Mattox KL, Beall AC Jr., DeBakey ME. Penetrating wounds of the cervical esophagus. Am J Surg 1975; 130:707–711.

68. Meyer JP, Barrett JA, Schuler JJ, Flanigan DP. Mandatory vs selective exploration for penetrating neck trauma. A prospective assessment. Arch Surg 1987; 122:592–597.

69. Cornwell EE III, Kennedy F, Ayad IA, et al. Transmediastinal gunshot wounds. A reconsideration of the role of aortography. Arch Surg 1996; 131:949–953.

70. Weigelt JA, Thal ER, Snyder WH III, Fry RE, Meier DE, Kilman WJ. Diagnosis of penetrating cervical esophageal injuries. Am J Surg 1987; 154:619–622.

71. Karmey-Jones RC, Wagner JW, Lewis JW Jr. Esophageal injury. In: Trunkey DD, Lewis FR, eds. Current Therapy of Trauma. Philadelphia: Elsevier, 1998:209–216.

72. Nesbitt JC, Sawyers JL. Surgical management of esophageal perforation. Am Surg 1987; 53:183–191.

73. Winter RP, Weigelt JA. Cervical esophageal trauma. Incidence and cause of esophageal fistulas. Arch Surg 1990; 125:849–852.

74. Horowitz B, Krevsky B, Buckman RF Jr., Fisher RS, Dabezies MA. Endoscopic evaluation of penetrating esophageal injuries. Am J Gastroenterol 1993; 88:1249–1253.

75. White CS, Templeton PA, Attar S. Esophageal perforation: CT findings. AJR Am J Roentgenol 1993; 160:767–770.

76. Ivatury RR, Rohman M, Simon RJ. Esophageal injury. In: Maull KI, Wiles CE III, eds. Advances in Trauma and Critical Care. Philadelphia: Elsevier, 1996:245–274.

77. Richardson JD, Martin LF, Borzotta AP, Polk HC Jr. Unifying concepts in treatment of esophageal leaks. Am J Surg 1985; 149:157–162.

78. Symbas PN. Esophageal injuries. In: Symbas PN, ed. Cardiothoracic Trauma. Philadelphia: Saunders, 1989:285–302.

79. Cheadle W, Richardson JD. Options in the management of trauma to the esophagus. Surg Gynecol Obstet 1982; 155:380–384.

80. Iannettoni MD, Vleissis AA, Whyte RI, Orringer MB. Functional outcome after surgical treatment of esophageal perforation. Ann Thorac Surg 1997; 64:1606–1610.

81. Muller JM, Erasmi H, Stelzner M, Zieren U, Pichlmaier H. Surgical therapy of oesophageal carcinoma. Br J Surg 1990; 77:845–857.

82. Katariya K, Harvey JC, Pina E, Beattie EJ. Complications of transhiatal hernia. J Surg Oncol 1994; 57:157–163.

83. Asensio JA, Berne J, Demetriades D, et al. Penetrating esophageal injuries: time interval of safety for preoperative evaluation—how long is safe? J Trauma 1997; 43:319–324.

84. Symbas PN, Tyras DH, Hatcher CR Jr., Perry B. Penetrating wounds of the esophagus. Ann Thorac Surg 1972; 13:552–558.

85. Symbas PN, Hatcher CR Jr., Vlasis SE. Esophageal gunshot injuries. Ann Surg 1980; 191:703–707.

86. Wilson RF, Steiger Z. Esophageal injuries. In: Wilson RF, Walt AJ, eds. Management of Trauma: Pitfalls and Practice. Philadelphia: Lippincott, 1996:388–405.

87. Freidman BC, Pickul DC. Acute mediastinitis. What to do when the case is nonsurgical. Postgrad Med 1990; 87:273–275, 278–280, 285.

88. Yang SC. Complications of esophageal resection. In: Cameron JL, ed. Current Surgical Therapy. 7th ed. St. Louis: Mosby, 2001:66–71.

89. Mathisen DJ. Right thoracoabdominal approaches: Ivor Lewis–Mckeown procedures. In: Pearson FG, Cooper JD, Hiebert CA, Ginsburg RJ, eds. Esophageal Surgery. 2d ed. Philadelphia: Elsevier, 2002:818–828.

90. Mangano DT, Hollenberg M, Fegert G, et al. Perioperative myocardial ischemia in patients undergoing

noncardiac surgery—I: Incidence and severity during the 4 day perioperative period. The Study of Perioperative Ischemia (SPI) Research Group. J Am Coll Cardiol 1991; 17:843–850.

91. Amar D, Burt ME, Bains MS, Leung DH. Symptomatic tachydysrhythmias after esophagectomy: incidence and outcome measures. Ann Thorac Surg 1996; 61:1506–1509.

92. Ritchie AJ, Whiteside M, Tolan M, McGuigan JA. Cardiac dysrhythmia in total thoracic oesophagectomy. A prospective study. Eur J Cardiothorac Surg 1993; 7:420–422.

93. Amar D. Prevention and management of dysrhythmias following thoracic surgery. Chest Surg Clin N Am 1997; 7:817–829.

94. Bayliff CD, Massel DR, Inculet RI, et al. Propanolol for the prevention of postoperative arrhythmias in general thoracic surgery. Ann Thorac Surg 1999; 67:182–186.

95. Cerfolio RJ, Allen MS, Deschamps C, Trastek VF, Pairolero PC. Postoperative chylothorax. J Thorac Cardiovasc Surg 1996; 112:1361–1366.

96. Wong J, Law SYK. Esophagogastrectomy for carcinoma of the esophagus and gastric cardia, and the esophageal anastomosis. In: Baker CC, Fischer JE, eds. Mastery of Surgery. 4th ed. Philadelphia: Lippincott, 2001:813–827.

97. Orringer MB, Marshall B, Iannettoni MD. Transhiatal esophagectomy: clinical experience and refinements. Ann Surg 1999; 230:392–403.

98. Fok M, Cheng SW, Wong J. Pyloroplasty versus no drainage in gastric replacement of the esophagus. Am J Surg 1991; 162:447–452.

99. Urschel JD. Esophagogastrostomy anastomotic leaks complicating esophagectomy: a review. Am J Surg 1995; 169:634–640.

100. Law SY, Fok M, Wong J. Risk analysis in resection of squamous cell carcinoma of the esophagus. World J Surg 1994; 18:339–346.

101. Beitler AL, Urschel JD. Comparison of stapled and hand-sewn esophagogastric anastomoses. Am J Surg 1998; 175:337–340.

102. Law S, Fok M, Chu KM, Wong J. Comparison of hand-sewn and stapled esophagogastric anastomosis after esophageal resection for cancer: a prospective randomized controlled trial. Ann Surg 1997; 226:169–173.

103. Orringer MB, Marshall B, Iannettoni MD. Eliminating the cervical esophagogastric anastomotic leak rate with a side-to-side stapled anastomosis. J Thoac Cardiovasc Surg 2000; 119:277–288.

104. Heitmiller RF, McQuone SJ, Eisele DW. The utility of the pectoralis myocutaneous flap in the management of select cervical esophageal anastomotic complications. J Thorac Cardiovasc Surg 1998; 115:1250–1254.

23

Respiratory Failure After Surgery or Trauma

Fahim A. Habib

Division of Trauma and Surgical Critical Care, DeWitt Daughtry Family Department of Surgery, University of Miami School of Medicine, Miami, Florida, U.S.A.

Respiration is a complex physiologic process that involves coordinated functioning of the different components of the respiratory system. Acute dysfunction of one or more of these components results in an inability to meet the metabolic requirements of the tissues in terms of oxygen delivery or carbon dioxide removal. Such impairment is not infrequent after surgery, trauma, or both and may result from a multitude of causes. Recognition of the more common of these causes will allow the preoperative determination of which patients are at a high risk of respiratory dysfunction and may allow modification of risk factors. Also, a thorough understanding of the principles of mechanical ventilation is crucial to the management of respiratory impairment. Furthermore, an evidence-based approach to the most severe form of respiratory failure, acute respiratory distress syndrome (ARDS), is essential for a potentially successful outcome. Finally, some other causes of respiratory failure in this setting require physicians to maintain a high index of suspicion. Awareness of these conditions may allow earlier recognition and, therefore, earlier treatment.

This chapter emphasizes the definition and scope of problem and provides the basics of mechanical ventilation as it applies to the management of acute respiratory failure, the evidence behind the current strategies used to treat ARDS, and some of the more unusual causes of respiratory failure that are unique to surgical and trauma patients.

RESPIRATORY FAILURE

Definitions

Respiratory failure is defined as the failure of the respiratory system to oxygenate blood or remove carbon dioxide at levels that are commensurate with the metabolic requirements of the tissues. The development of acute severe hypoxemia in the presence of bilateral lung infiltrates and in the absence of evidence of cardiac dysfunction constitutes a severe form of acute respiratory failure. This condition is further characterized on the basis of the ratio of partial pressure of arterial oxygen (PaO_2) to the fraction of inspired oxygen (FiO_2) (the PF ratio). Accordingly, a PF ratio of less than 300 indicates acute lung injury (ALI), whereas a PF ratio of less than 200 indicates ARDS (Box 1) (1).

Classifications

Traditionally, respiratory failure is classified according to the resultant abnormalities in the results of blood gas analysis. It is termed *hypercarbic* if the partial pressure of carbon dioxide in arterial blood ($PaCO_2$) is greater than 45 mmHg, *hypoxemic* if the PaO_2 is less than 55 mmHg at a FiO_2 of greater than or equal to 0.6, or *combined* if a mixed picture exists.

These categories are best understood by dividing the respiratory system into two functionally distinct portions. The *respiratory pump* consists of the central nervous system, the peripheral nervous system, the respiratory muscles, and the chest wall. It functions to deliver air from the atmosphere to the alveoli. Its dysfunction results in hypoventilation characterized predominantly by hypercarbia. Various degrees of associated hypoxemia occur. The alveoli compose the *gas exchange units*. Their dysfunction causes respiratory failure marked by hypoxemia, which results from collapse or flooding of the alveoli. Flooding of the alveoli occurs when the alveoli fill with purulent material, blood, or fluid. The decreased compliance increases the work of breathing and causes dyspnea and tachypnea. Postoperative respiratory failure is often a multifactorial process that results in a combination of hypoxemia and hypercarbia.

Epidemiology

Common respiratory problems that develop after surgery and trauma include atelectasis, bronchospasm, exacerbation of underlying chronic lung disease, pneumonia, pulmonary embolism, ALI, and ARDS. Approximately 5% of patients undergoing surgical intervention will experience one or more of these conditions, and approximately 1% will experience respiratory failure severe enough to necessitate mechanical ventilation for more than 24 hours (2). The occurrence of these problems not only increases the length of stay in the

Definition of ARDS and ALI

Acute onset

PaO_2/FiO_2 ratio less than 300 for ALI and less than 200 for ARDS

Bilateral chest infiltrates as demonstrated by chest radiograph

Pulmonary artery occlusion pressure 18 mmHg or less or the absence of clinical evidence of left atrial hypertension

---

Abbreviations: ALI, acute lung injury; ARDS, acute respiratory distress syndrome; PaO_2, partial pressure of arterial oxygen; FiO_2, fraction of inspired oxygen.

Common Causes of Respiratory Failure

Central nervous system disorders

   Pharmacologic: narcotic overdosage

   Structural: tumors, stroke, vascular abnormalities, and meningoencephalitis

   Metabolic: myxedema, hepatic failure, uremia, obesity-hypoventilation syndrome, and hypercapnia

Peripheral nervous system and chest wall

   Guillain–Barré syndrome, myasthenia gravis, polymyositis, muscular dystrophy, traumatic spinal cord injury, respiratory muscle fatigue, use of paralytic agents, steroid use, aminoglycoside use in myasthenia, severe kyphoscoliosis, flail chest, morbid obesity, massive abdominal distention, and extensive thoracoplasty

Airway

   Acute epiglottitis, aspirated foreign bodies, tracheal tumors, tracheal stenosis, chronic obstructive lung disease, asthma, and cystic fibrosis

Alveolar disease

   Cardiogenic and noncardiogenic pulmonary edema, diffuse pneumonia, pulmonary hemorrhage, aspiration, and near drowning

---

hospital and in the intensive care unit (ICU), but also is responsible for 25% of postoperative deaths (3).

Trauma and burns are an important cause of respiratory failure, especially among patients less than 30 years old (4). During World War I, Pasteur first described the occurrence of respiratory failure after traumatic injuries. This clinical syndrome was given several different names until 1967, when Ashbaugh et al. (5) defined the condition now recognized as ARDS. A less severe form of the disease is called ALI. ARDS occurs among 12% of critically ill trauma patients who are admitted to ICUs and carries a mortality rate of 16%, whereas ALI occurs among 4% of such patients and carries an associated mortality rate of 9% (6). Risk factors that predispose patients to the development of ARDS after trauma include long-bone fractures, pelvic fractures, head injury, direct chest trauma, tissue hypoxia, and massive blood transfusion (7).

Causes

The potential causes of postoperative respiratory failure are many and may involve impaired functioning of any of the components of the respiratory system. These causes include disease processes involving the central nervous system, the peripheral nervous system, the chest wall, the airway, and the alveoli. The more frequently encountered causes are enumerated in Box 2. Most common among these are atelectasis, pneumonia, aspiration of gastric contents, ALI, ARDS, phrenic nerve injury, diaphragmatic dysfunction, pulmonary embolism, and obstructive sleep apnea.

Determination of Risk

Determining the risk factors associated with postoperative respiratory failure is a fundamental step in reducing the morbidity and mortality associated with pulmonary complications. A prudent approach involves not only determining which patients are at high risk, but also determining whether the risk can be reduced or the procedure can be modified. Adopting risk-reduction strategies may improve outcome.

Risk factors may primarily be patient-related, procedure-related, or a combination of the two. Patient-related risk factors include smoking, poor general health status, chronic obstructive pulmonary disease

(COPD), and asthma. The relative risk of complications for smokers is 4.3, whereas that for nonsmokers is 1.4 (8). Smoking cessation for at least eight weeks preoperatively is required if a beneficial effect is to be observed. General health status is best assessed by using indices such as the American Society of Anesthesiologists classification or the Goldman cardiac index (9). The presence of underlying COPD increases the relative risk of pulmonary complications from 2.7 to 4.7 and imposes a 5% risk of respiratory failure (10). Management strategies include preoperative bronchodilators, chest physical therapy, antibiotics, smoking cessation, and corticosteroids. A useful approach is to begin with inhaled ipratropium bromide and beta-adrenergic agents. If this treatment is inadequate, theophylline can be added. If these measures do not control the COPD, a two-week course of antibiotics is employed. Asthma does not increase the risk if there is no wheezing and if the peak flow is more than 80% of predicted values (11). Despite popular beliefs, age and obesity pose no additional risk (12–14).

Procedure-related risk factors include the type of operative procedure performed, the type of anesthesia used, the nature of the neuromuscular agent employed, the duration of surgery, and the adequacy of pain relief. Upper abdominal and thoracic surgical procedures impair respiration by deranging pulmonary mechanics. Therefore, lesser degrees of dysfunction occur with minimally invasive procedures such as laparoscopic operations and video-assisted thoracoscopic surgery (15). The use of general anesthesia is associated with a loss of muscle tone in the diaphragm and intercostal muscles, cephalad movement of the diaphragm, a decrease in transverse thoracic diameter, a drug-induced reduction in the respiratory drive, and an impaired response to CO_2. These effects cause a 20% reduction in functional residual capacity and also result in compressive atelectasis, increased shunt fraction, and impaired hypoxic pulmonary vasoconstriction (16). The use of long-acting neuromuscular blocking agents (e.g., pancuronium) also contributes to impaired muscle function and an increased risk of complications (17). Surgical procedures that last longer than three hours result in greater pulmonary dysfunction (18). Providing inadequate pain relief results in splinting with a reduction in deep breathing and a decrease in coughing. Both of these responses cause atelectasis and retained secretions, which promote respiratory dysfunction.

Preoperative education of patients about techniques for lung expansion, deep-breathing exercises, and the use of incentive spirometry are beneficial. The use of continuous positive airway pressure and nasal bilevel positive airway pressure is more expensive and resource intensive and is also associated with a higher incidence of complications (19). The use of these techniques is best limited to patients who cannot perform deep breathing or intensive spirometry. Options for adequate pain control, such as epidural analgesia and intercostal nerve blocks, can also be planned for patients who are at risk of complications (20).

PRINCIPLES OF MECHANICAL VENTILATION
Overview

The use of mechanical ventilation began during the polio epidemics of the mid-20th century. It initially involved the application of negative pressure with devices such as the iron lung or the lung cuirass. Subsequent development of machines capable of controlling the respiratory rate and inspiratory pressures led to the evolution of positive-pressure ventilation. With further advances, complex measurements of the mechanics of respiration and functional alteration are now possible. Nevertheless, the goal of mechanical ventilation remains the same: to maintain oxygenation and ventilation, thereby allowing time for the underlying disease to heal and for the patient to independently resume these functions. It provides the time required for other measures, normal healing, or both, to bring about healing without causing further damage to the lung.

Methods of Ventilation

The characteristics of the ideal method of mechanical ventilation are enumerated in Box 3 (21). Although no ideal method of ventilation exists, various combinations of these characteristics are present in the more commonly employed methods of ventilation. The key features of these methods are presented in Box 4. Several newer methods of ventilation are under evaluation, including proportional assist ventilation (22), neurally adjusted ventilatory assist (23), fractal ventilation, and biologically variable ventilation (24). Although none of these methods is currently available

Characteristics of the Ideal Method of Ventilation

> Achieves the target for gas exchange
> Unloads the ventilatory muscles
> Does not compromise cardiac function
> Minimizes exposure to high fractions of inspired oxygen
> Does not damage the airways or lung parenchyma
> Is intuitive or easy to apply
> Is comfortable for the patient
> Facilitates weaning
> Requires minimal monitoring
> Is not labor intensive
> Is inexpensive

clinically, the features of those that are closest to clinical utility are presented in Box 5.

Monitoring During Mechanical Ventilation

The goals of monitoring during mechanical ventilation are to minimize ventilator-associated complications, to

Key Features of the More Commonly Employed Methods of Ventilation

> *Assist–Control*: Relates to the control process of the breath. The assist portion is controlled by the patient; the control portion is controlled by the ventilator. The patient's triggering may be based on flow or pressure. Once initiated, the breath may be controlled by flow or pressure
> *Intermittent Mandatory Ventilation/Synchronized Intermittent Mandatory Ventilation*: The ventilator delivers a predetermined number of controlled breaths; the patient breathes spontaneously between mandatory breaths. The controlled breath may be controlled by flow or pressure. The spontaneous breaths may be augmented by pressure support
> *Pressure Support Ventilation*: The breath must be triggered by the patient; after initiation, inhalation is assisted by a predetermined amount of pressure. Inspiration ceases when the flow falls below a certain predetermined rate. Requires an intact respiratory drive; used for weaning
> *Mandatory Minute Ventilation*: In this method, the minimum minute ventilation is set by the clinician. The patient breathes spontaneously with or without pressure support. The difference between the spontaneous and set-minute ventilation is delivered as mandatory breaths with set tidal volume and flow. This method allows patients to take over a greater portion of their breathing efforts
> *Volume-Assured Pressure Ventilation*: Used for patients who are breathing spontaneously. The minimal tidal volume is set. The patient initiates a pressure-supported breath. If the volume falls below the preset minimum, the ventilator completes the breath by delivering additional constant flow at increasing pressures
> *Volume Support*: The patient initiates the breath with clinician-determined pressure support. The machine determines the generated tidal volume and adjusts this pressure support to maintain a minimal target tidal volume
> *Pressure-Regulated Volume Control*: A form of controlled ventilation in which, at a preset rate, the machine regulates the inspiratory pressure to generate a target tidal volume.
> *Airway Pressure Release Ventilation*: Here the upper and lower continuous airway pressure are set as are the pressure release time and the frequency of release.

optimize patient–ventilator interactions, and to determine readiness for discontinuation of ventilator support (25). The factors frequently monitored are presented in Box 6. Respiratory mechanics are measured by using the flow interruption technique, which involves rapid airway occlusion during constant flow inflation (26). The plateau pressure must be routinely monitored and maintained at less than 35 cmH$_2$O. This level minimizes alveolar overdistention, an important cause of lung injury during mechanical ventilation (Fig. 1).

The key components of the pressure–volume curves are the lower and upper inflection points. The lower inflection point reflects the point at which the small airways and the alveoli open. This point is used to determine the optimum positive end–expiratory pressure (PEEP), which is set at 2 cmH$_2$O above this lower inflection point. This setting maximizes oxygenation with minimum lung injury and may result in lower mortality rates (27). The upper inflection point represents encroachment of the total lung capacity. Pressures above this point predispose the patient to lung injury and must be avoided. Measures of resistance, although they have no impact on weaning (28), are useful in the assessment of response to bronchodilator therapy (29). A sawtooth wave pattern on flow–volume curves indicates the need for endotracheal suctioning (30). The work of breathing is the work that the respiratory system must perform to overcome the elastic and functional resistances of the chest and lung wall. By using this measurement, physicians can maintain the necessary degree of ventilatory support for each patient, thereby avoiding unnecessary oxygen consumption.

Noninvasive Positive-Pressure Ventilation

Endotracheal intubation, a key component of positive-pressure mechanical ventilation, is associated with several complications such as upper airway trauma, nosocomial pneumonia, and sinusitis. The use of

Factors Monitored During Mechanical Ventilation

Plateau pressure
Pressure–volume curves
Resistance
Flow–volume curves
Work of breathing
Pressure–time product
PaO$_2$/FiO$_2$ ratio

Abbreviations: PaO$_2$, partial pressure of artevial oxygen; FiO$_2$, fraction of inspired oxygen.

intubation prolongs hospital stay and increases the costs associated with ICU resource utilization. Noninvasive positive-pressure ventilation (NIPPV) combines pressure support and PEEP delivered via a nasal or facial mask. Although initially studied as a means of avoiding intubation during exacerbations of COPD, NIPPV is now increasingly being applied to settings of interest to surgeons (31). These settings include perioperative acute respiratory failure due to obstructive sleep apnea in the morbidly obese, hypoxemic respiratory failure due to pneumonia, ARDS, trauma, and cardiogenic pulmonary edema. NIPPV improves oxygenation, reduces the need for endotracheal intubation, decreases septic complications, reduces the length of ICU stay, and lowers mortality rates (32).

Postoperative indications for NIPPV include a PaCO$_2$ higher than 50 mmHg, a PaO$_2$ lower than 60 mmHg, and respiratory muscle fatigue. Its use may preclude reintubation because of respiratory failure, which may occur in association with 5% to 20% of planned extubations (33) and 40% to 50% of unplanned extubations (34). Its successful application requires the ability to protect the airway, a spontaneously breathing patient, intact dentition, absence of facial trauma, minimal secretions, and the absence of severe acid–base and gas derangement. Contraindications to NIPPV

Newer Methods of Ventilation

Proportional Assist Ventilation: The ventilator instantaneously delivers positive pressure throughout inspiration in proportion to the patient's flow and volume; augmented ventilatory support results from increased support by the ventilator. This method is effective in unloading the ventilatory muscles without imposing a fixed breathing pattern. Enhances patient comfort and patient-ventilator interactions

Neurally Adjusted Ventilatory Assist: Electrical activity of the crural diaphragm is detected by an esophageal array of bipolar electrodes. Requires an intact respiratory drive, an intact phrenic nerve, and neuromuscular junctions that are free of pharmacologic intervention. The amount of support provided is instantaneously adjusted to correspond to the ventilatory demand

Factal Ventilation and Biologically Variable Ventilation: Mimics the spontaneous breath-to-breath variability. Modulates respiratory rate and tidal volume while maintaining a fixed minute ventilation based on a previously generated data file

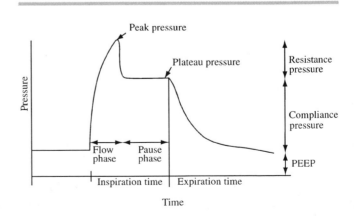

Figure 1 Pressure-time diagram demonstrating the concept of plateau pressure (P_{plat}).

include respiratory arrest, inability to protect the airway, hemodynamic instability, excessive secretions, uncooperative or agitated patients, inability to fit the mask, and upper airway or upper gastrointestinal surgery (31).

NIPPV is administered through an oronasal mask, with a change to a nasal mask if a prolonged duration of support is anticipated. Inspiratory support is begun at 8 to 10 cmH$_2$O and is increased as tolerated. Support is maintained at less than 20 cmH$_2$O so that discomfort due to sinus pain, gastric distention, or both, can be avoided. A trial-and-error method is used to identify the optimal degree of support. Expiratory support begins at 5 cmH$_2$O and is increased as necessary. With increases in expiratory pressure, the inspiratory pressures must be increased so that the pressure support can be kept constant. Supplemental oxygen is provided so that oxygen saturation can be maintained at more than 90%. Humidification improves patient tolerance and the ability to deal with secretions. A nasogastric tube is not routinely used because it breaks the seal. Complications include nasal bridge edema, erythema, and ulceration, as well as nasal congestion, sinus or ear pain, mucosal dryness, eye irritation, and gastric insufflation. Rarely, pneumothorax, hypotension, or aspiration may occur.

Ventilator-Associated Lung Injury

Ventilator-associated lung injury (VALI) is a consequence of mechanical ventilation that is difficult to distinguish clinically from the initial indication for ventilatory support. It worsens the pulmonary status, setting up the inflammatory milieu that may ultimately lead to multisystem organ failure (35).

The mechanisms responsible for VALI are often multifactorial. They include oxygen toxicity, volutrauma, atelectrauma, and barotrauma. All of these mechanisms cause the release of inflammatory mediators, a phenomenon termed *biotrauma*. High levels of FiO$_2$ produce oxygen toxicity in one of two ways: by generating superoxides and free radicals or by predisposing patients to absorption atelectasis (36). The use of large tidal volumes and high distention pressures results in overdistention and is referred to as *volutrauma*. This condition is especially common among patients with ARDS because of the inhomogeneous nature of the disease (Fig. 2), with overdistention of the relatively normal portions of the lung (37). Atelectrauma results from the repeated opening and closing of the alveolar lung units (38). It may be limited by maintaining an adequate level of PEEP (39). Barotrauma is the result of high-pressure ventilation. Its signs include pneumothorax, pneumomediastinum, and subcutaneous emphysema; it also causes alveolar stress injury (5). Limiting the plateau pressure is essential to reducing the incidence of barotrauma.

Preventing VALI involves the adoption of measures termed lung-protective ventilation strategies such

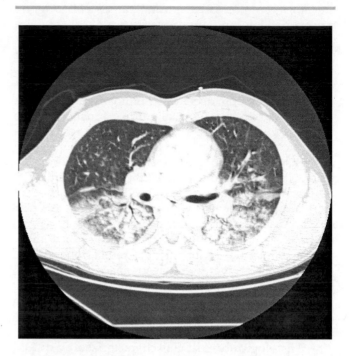

Figure 2 Computed tomogram showing the inhomogeneous nature of the disease process.

as limiting tidal volume, maintaining an adequate PEEP, and using the lowest achievable FiO$_2$ (27). Furthermore, the acceptance of the concept of permissive hypercapnia has allowed limitation of VALI because efforts at maintaining normocapnia may aggravate lung injury (40,41). Here the CO$_2$ is allowed to climb over a period of one to two days. The pH is monitored closely and treated if it falls below 7.2. Such a strategy, in association with aggressive treatment of respiratory acidosis, has resulted in a 9% absolute risk reduction for VALI among patients with ARDS (42). The elevated carbon dioxide levels, however, may increase the release of catecholamines, decrease the seizure threshold, cause cerebral hyperemia, and reduce renal blood flow (43).

ACUTE LUNG INJURY AND ADULT RESPIRATORY DISTRESS SYNDROME

ALI and ARDS are severe forms of respiratory dysfunction that may occur as the result of a multitude of causes. These causes either may involve mechanisms that bring about direct injury to pulmonary tissue or may represent the pulmonary response to a systemic event that sets into motion a cascade of events culminating in an inflammatory event. Common causes of direct injury to pulmonary tissue include aspiration, pneumonia, toxic inhalation, lung contusion, and near drowning. Common causes of indirect injury include severe sepsis, shock, multi-system trauma, burn injury, pancreatitis, cardiopulmonary bypass, and drug overdose. Of these, trauma, aspiration, and sepsis are the most common predisposing causes (44). Among trauma patients, an Injury Severity Scale score of more than 25 and pulmonary contusion are the primary risk factors that predispose patients to the development of ARDS.

Clinically, the condition is characterized by impaired oxygenation, decreased pulmonary compliance, and normal or supranormal cardiac function. These features, which have been incorporated into the definition jointly developed by the American–European Consensus Conference (1), include a PF ratio of less than 300 for ALI and less than 200 for ARDS, bilateral pulmonary infiltrates (Fig. 3), and the absence of evidence of left heart dysfunction, either clinically or on the basis of pulmonary artery catheter (PAC) measurements. Intrapulmonary shunting is a primary mechanism of the observed hypoxemia, whereas the combination of increased dead space fraction and reduced compliance results in an increase in the work of breathing. Together, these factors result in a form of respiratory failure characterized by hypoxemia, hypercarbia, and acidosis.

Histologically, ARDS is characterized by diffuse pulmonary inflammatory infiltrates, interstitial and alveolar edema, loss of type II pneumocytes, depletion of surfactant, deposition of hyaline membranes, and, in long-standing cases, fibrosis (45).

Although ARDS is the most common cause of pulmonary infiltrates associated with hypoxemia in the critically ill patient, it is not the only cause. The differential diagnosis includes acute interstitial pneumonia, acute esosinophillic pneumonia, bronchiolitis obliterans organizing pneumonia, diffuse alveolar hemorrhage, and acute hypersensitivity pneumonitis. These conditions should be suspected in the appropriate clinical setting, especially when acute pulmonary dysfunction with features of ARDS develops in the absence of an identifiable precipitating cause. Diagnosis is made by characteristic findings on bronchoscopy or is based on the appearance of the tissue during open lung biopsy. Treatment depends on the underlying cause and usually involves the administration of steroids.

Because ARDS is associated with high mortality and morbidity rates, the optimal management of the disease remains an elusive goal. However, important advances in our understanding of the pathophysiology of the disease process have led to an evidence-based approach. Key components of a multipronged approach are presented in Box 7.

Identification and Treatment of Underlying Disorders and Infections

Identification and possible control of the inciting event are important first steps in the treatment of ARDS. They remove the source of continued stimulation that generates the inflammatory cascade responsible for perpetuation and potentiation of the lung injury. The early identification of any associated or subsequent infection and its aggressive and appropriate treatment cannot be overemphasized.

Lung-Protective Ventilation Strategies

An important advancement in the management of ARDS has been the recognition of the beneficial effects of lung-protective ventilation strategies. The reduction in mortality rates was demonstrated in two clinical trials (27,43), whereas three other contemporaneous studies failed to demonstrate any benefit (Table 1) (39,46,47). There are several possible explanations for the observed differences in outcome. First, the tidal volumes used in the control arms of the studies that demonstrated a difference were, by current

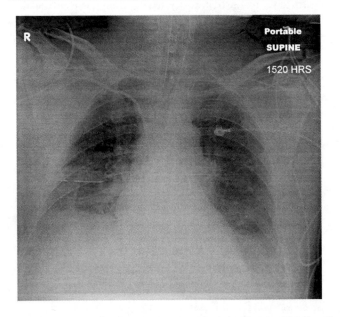

Figure 3 Chest radiograph demonstrating bilateral infiltrates. Acute onset of the process and absence of evidence of left atrial hypertension suggest a diagnosis of acute respiratory distress syndrome.

Approaches to Managing ALI and ARDS

> Identify and treat underlying disorders
> Mechanical ventilation with lung-protective strategies
> Use of alternative methods for patients who are difficult to ventilate
> Hemodynamic management with fluid and pressors
> Pulmonary vasodilators
> Aggressive early identification and appropriate management of infections
> Nutritional support
> Extracorporeal gas exchange
> Prone positioning
> Liquid ventilation
> Anti-inflammatory strategies
> Antioxidant therapy
> Steroids

Abbreviations: ALI, acute lung injury; ARDS, acute respiratory distress syndrome.

standards, excessive. These nonphysiologic tidal volumes may have resulted in excessive mortality in the control arm, thereby giving an impression of benefit from low tidal volumes. Second, in studies showing benefit, additional lung-protective strategies, such as a higher PEEP and lung-recruitment maneuvers, were employed. These strategies may have had an additive effect on limited tidal volumes with resultant benefit. Third, respiratory acidosis was aggressively controlled in the National Institutes of Health (NIH) trial with increases in respiratory rate for a pH lower than 7.30 and bicarbonate infusions for a pH lower than 7.2. Such an approach was not emphasized in the studies that did not show a benefit. Finally, in the NIH trial, the tidal volumes were based on predicted and not actual body weight. Despite these shortcomings, the ARDS Network trial represents the best evidence currently available and should be the benchmark against which future trials are compared. The approach to low tidal volume ventilation as employed in the ARDS Network trial is presented in Box 8 (43). Its implementation led to an absolute mortality reduction of 9% in the largest of these studies (43).

Limitation of airway pressures is another key tenet. The plateau pressure is regularly monitored and maintained at or below 30 cmH$_2$O. Lung-recruitment maneuvers are recommended and should be regularly performed (48). Several techniques of recruitment have been successfully employed, including sustained continuous positive airway pressure for 30 to 40 seconds, traditional sigh breaths, extended sighs, intermittent high levels of PEEP, and brief periods of super PEEP. Higher than normal levels of PEEP are required for maintaining lung volume after a recruitment maneuver. Although these high levels of PEEP produce a short-term improvement in oxygenation, they have not been shown to provide long-term benefits.

Optimal Positive End–Expiratory Pressure for Patients with Adult Respiratory Distress Syndrome

Selection of the optimal level of PEEP is another key component in the management of ARDS. The elastic forces of the lung tissue and the surface tension within the alveoli determine the end-expiratory alveolar volume. Inadequate PEEP and altered surface tension, presumably due to reduced or altered

Clinical approach to Low Tidal Volume Ventilation (42)

1. Calculate the PBW by using the following formula:
   a. Men: PBW (kg) = 50 + 2.3 (height in inches − 60) or 50 + 0.91 (height in cm − 152.4)
   b. Women: PBW (kg) = 45.5 + 2.3 (height in inches − 60) or 45.5 + 0.91 (height in cm − 152.4)
2. Ventilatory mode: synchronized intermittent mandatory ventilation
3. Tidal volume: Begin with 6 mL/kg. Measure the plateau pressure (P_{plat}). If P_{plat} is greater than 30 cmH$_2$O, reduce the tidal volume to 4–5 mL/kg; if the P_{plat} is less than 25 cmH$_2$O and the tidal volume is less than 6 mL/kg, increase the tidal volume by 1 mL/kg
4. Adjust the respiratory rate to maintain minute ventilation that achieves a pH of 7.30–7.45; avoid respiratory rates in excess of 35 breaths/min
5. Use ratios of inspiratory time to expiratory time of 1:3 to 1:1
6. Use the lowest possible FiO$_2$ with adequate PEEP to maintain adequate arterial oxygenation, while maintaining PaO$_2$ at 55–80 mmHg and SaO$_2$ at 88–95%.
7. Correct the acidosis: If pH is less than 7.30, increase the respiratory rate until the pH is more than or equal to 7.30 or the respiratory rate is 35 breaths/min. If the pH remains less than 7.30 despite a respiratory rate of 35 breaths/min, use bicarbonate infusions. If the pH remains below 7.15 after the respiratory rate has been increased to 35 breaths/min and bicarbonate has been administered, increase the tidal volume
8. If the measures listed above fail, consider alternative methods of ventilation

Abbreviations: FiO$_2$, fraction of inspired oxygen; PaO$_2$, partial pressure of arterial oxygen; PBW, predicted body weight; PEEP, positive end-expiratory pressure.
Source: From Ref 42.

production of surfactants (49), allow end-expiratory alveolar collapse. This condition results in shunting and persistent hypoxemia. Furthermore, the alveoli are once again recruited during the inspiratory phase of tidal ventilation. The resultant repetitive derecruitment and recruitment lead to potentiation of the lung injury (50). Using adequate levels of PEEP maintains alveolar volume at the end of expiration, prevents derecruitment, and yields an open lung pattern of ventilation. It additionally attenuates pulmonary edema and maintains an adequate functional residual capacity. At the other end of the spectrum, excessive PEEP is equally detrimental. At high levels of PEEP, cardiac output is diminished as a consequence of decreased venous return due to increased intrathoracic

Table 1 Clinical Studies Using Lung-Protective Ventilation Strategies

Study	Intervention group		Control group		Outcome
	V_T (mL/kg)	PEEP (cmH$_2$O)	V_T (mL/kg)	PEEP (cmH$_2$O)	
ARDS Network (42)	6.2 ± 0.8	9.4 ± 3.6	11.8 ± 0.8	8.6 ± 3.6	Mortality reduction from 40% to 31%
Amato et al. (27)	~6.0	14.7 ± 3.9	~12.0	8.7 ± 0.4	Mortality reduction from 71% to 38%
Stewart et al. (39)	7.0 ± 0.7	8.6 ± 3.0	10.7 ± 1.4	7.2 ± 3.3	No difference
Brochard et al. (46)	7.1 ± 1.3	10.7 ± 2.9	10.3 ± 1.7	10.7 ± 2.3	No difference
Brower et al. (47)	7.3 ± 0.7	8.3 ± 0.5	10.2 ± 0.7	9.5 ± 0.5	No difference

Abbreviations: ARDS, acute respiratory distress syndrome; VT, tidal volume; PEEP, positive end-expiratory pressure.

pressures and impaired distention of the right heart, which limits its filling. Also, the resultant alveolar distention compresses the pulmonary vasculature, thereby increasing the pulmonary vascular afterload. Hence, if maximal benefit is to be obtained, PEEP must be maintained at its lowest effective level.

Several techniques have been used for determining the optimal level of PEEP. It is recognized that the lower inflection point of the pressure–volume curve represents the beginning of recruitment. By using this measure as the reference point, PEEP is maintained at 2 cmH$_2$O above the lower inflection point (Fig. 4) (51). Improved survival is seen when low tidal volumes are combined with a PEEP that has been titrated with this technique (27). Alternatively, PEEP may be titrated above the closing pressure of the deflection limb (52) or may be adjusted by decrements. In this technique, maximal levels of PEEP are applied at the beginning, usually 20 to 25 cmH$_2$O. Then, while the PO$_2$ is monitored, the PEEP is reduced in decrements of 2 cmH$_2$O until the minimum PEEP that results in maximal oxygenation has been determined (53). Yet another technique involves measuring the internal thoracic diameter in centimeters and multiplying this measurement by a factor of 0.8 (54).

High-Frequency Ventilation

Recognition of the beneficial effects of strategies, with an emphasis on strategies that limit VALI (11,27), has generated interest in alternative methods of

ventilation. One such approach is the use of high-frequency ventilation, a technique that employs frequencies of increased Hertz and tidal volumes that are less than the anatomical dead space.

Although several methods of high-frequency ventilation exist [viz., high-frequency oscillatory ventilation (HFOV), high-frequency jet ventilation, and high-frequency positive-pressure ventilation], all employ a similar physiologic principle. In HFOV, oxygenation at a given FiO$_2$ is proportional to the mean airway pressure (P_{aw}) and the resultant lung volume. The P_{aw} is adjusted either by changing the resistance at the end of the bias flow circuit or by changing the rate of bias flow. Ventilation is controlled by changes in the amplitude of the oscillating membrane (ΔP). With this method of ventilation, the tidal volume and frequency are inversely related. Hence, the level of carbon dioxide can be reduced by increasing the ΔP, decreasing the frequency, or both. Because both inspiration and expiration are active events, the incidence of dynamic hyperinflation is reduced.

The efficacy of HFOV is probably the result of several mechanisms, such as bulk convection, penduluft, cardiogenic oscillations, asymmetric velocity profiles, augmented dispersion, and molecular diffusion (55,56). Theoretically, this method of ventilation may have several benefits in preventing VALI. First, the use of small tidal volumes with minimal variation around the mean airway pressure and mean lung volumes allows for more effective oxygenation and reduction of FiO$_2$. Second, HFOV can be adjusted to avoid atelectasis or overdistention. Finally, oxygenation and ventilation are decoupled.

Despite these potential benefits, HFOV is currently used most frequently in the setting of rescue therapy when conventional ventilation fails. Even under such circumstances, its use results in improved oxygenation; however, results are better if HFOV is begun early (57,58). Recognizing the importance of lung recruitment is crucial and is best achieved by setting the mean airway pressure 4 to 8 cmH$_2$O greater than that being used for conventional ventilation. The pressure is then titrated to achieve adequate oxygenation. The patient is weaned from FiO$_2$ before the mean airway pressure is reduced.

Inhaled Nitric Oxide in the Management of Acute Respiratory Distress Syndrome

Nitric oxide (NO) is synthesized by numerous cell types from L-arginine and oxygen by a group of enzymes called nitric oxide synthetases (59). When nitric oxide is administered by the inhaled route (iNO), its high lipid solubility allows rapid diffusion across epithelial cells and access to the pulmonary vasculature. Because NO possesses a high affinity for hemoglobin, a portion of the iNO enters the pulmonary vasculature, where it is rapidly inactivated by binding to the hemoglobin in red cells. The remainder enters the smooth muscle cells of the pulmonary arterioles and causes

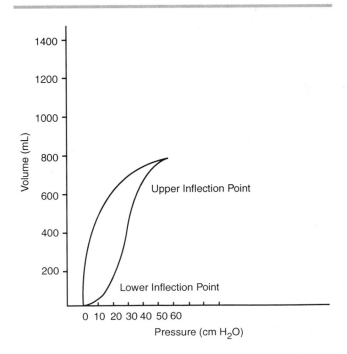

Figure 4 Static pressure–volume curve showing the power and upper inflection points. Pressure just above the lower inflection point prevents derecruitment during expiration.

vasodilatation (60). It modulates pulmonary vascular tone in healthy people (61) and also functions as a pulmonary vasodilator in a variety of conditions that cause pulmonary hypertension (62–64).

When NO is inhaled, its distribution is limited to well-ventilated areas; hence, it does not reverse hypoxic pulmonary vasoconstriction. Furthermore, the resultant distribution of ventilation–perfusion is improved when blood is moved away from poorly ventilated areas to areas with better ventilation (65); this movement improves oxygenation. Additional pulmonary effects include a reduction in the shunt fraction, relaxation of bronchial smooth muscles (66), a decrease in pulmonary capillary permeability because of a reduction in pulmonary venous tone, a decrease in oxidant injury, and a reduction in cytokine levels.

Initial studies (65) found that iNO produces a dose-related pulmonary vasodilatory response, with a decrease in pulmonary artery pressure, without substantial effects on the systemic circulation. They also found greater venous dilation than arterial dilation of the pulmonary system, with resultant reductions in pulmonary capillary pressure. These vascular changes result in acute improvements in oxygenation, a phenomenon associated with rebound on abrupt discontinuation of the drug (67). Several randomized controlled studies (68–70) have observed transient improvements in oxygenation; however, the effects have not been sustained. Furthermore, the improvement in oxygenation has not translated to improvements in mortality rates or in reductions in the number of ventilator-free days. Therefore, iNO improves the physiologic parameters but does not affect outcome.

There are several explanations for the lack of success with iNO. Until now, the dose of iNO has been titrated so that it maximizes oxygenation. At these doses, only small changes in pulmonary artery pressure have been seen. Higher doses that target the pulmonary artery pressure rather than oxygenation may be of benefit. Also, the benefit of improved oxygenation may have been overshadowed by the adverse effects of the toxic levels of oxygen and high levels of airway pressure. Furthermore, the studies were not adequately powered, the patients were a heterogeneous group, and the treatments were not standardized and were employed only for a brief period, which may not have permitted the underlying condition to improve.

Patients most likely to benefit from iNO include those with a high baseline pulmonary vascular tone (71), a high degree of initial venous admixture (72), and increased cardiac output (73). Efforts aimed at improving outcomes have focused on combination therapies involving iNO. Its use in combination with pulmonary vasoconstrictors such as almitrine (74) or norepinephrine (75) increases the PF ratio more than does the use of either agent alone. This outcome is probably the effect of a reduction in the shunt fraction that is the result of generalized pulmonary vasoconstriction

with vasodilatation in the well-ventilated areas. Other combination therapies include the use of phosphodiesterase inhibitors (76), prone positioning, high-frequency ventilation, and partial liquid ventilation.

At the present time, iNO has no proven benefit on outcome. It does, however, produce short-term symptomatic relief. The subgroup of patients who may benefit from such improvement and from the combination of iNO with other treatment strategies needs to be further defined.

Prone-Position Ventilation

Placing patients in the prone position causes gravity-dependent fluid shifts from the dorsal to the ventral aspects of the lungs, thereby increasing the area available for oxygenation (77). Such positioning also restores the functional residual capacity and decreases the vertical transpulmonary pressure gradient, thereby allowing the alveoli to maintain a more uniform size. Such positioning lessens the cyclic opening and closing of unstable alveolar units in the dependent regions and lessens overdistention at end-expiration in nondependent lung regions (78). Additionally, prone positioning alters chest wall compliance (79) and decreases the shunt fraction (80), without any significant change in the hemodynamics. Like iNO, prone positioning improves oxygenation, but no improvement in outcome has been demonstrated.

A response to therapy is defined as an increase in PaO_2 of at least 10 mmHg or an increase in the PF ratio of at least 20. Factors predictive of success include worse oxygenation at baseline (81), shorter duration of ARDS (82), and higher baseline chest wall compliance (80). The use of prone positioning in combination with other therapies, especially iNO, has produced even better response rates (83–85).

Prone-position ventilation may be associated with several complications, including loss of intravenous catheters, skin breakdown, loss or displacement of the endotracheal tube, and transient hemodynamic instability.

Steroids in Acute Respiratory Distress Syndrome

Steroids have been used to treat patients with ARDS in the hope of reducing the systemic response to the inciting event. Neither prophylactic use for high-risk patients nor steroid administration early in the course of the disease process has altered outcome (86,87). Improved survival has, however, been observed with late use of steroid in the fibroproliferative stage of the disease (5,88). The role of steroids remains ill defined, and a NIH-sponsored study is currently under way to address the issue.

Immunomodulation in Adult Respiratory Distress Syndrome

It is now recognized that a local or systemic triggering event brings about a release of mediators [interleukin-8, tumor necrosis factor-α (TNF-α), lipid mediators, platelet-activating factors, etc.] that cause endothelial cell damage. The increased vascular permeability that results causes noncardiogenic pulmonary edema, hypoxemia, and impaired systemic oxygenation. Recognition of the central role played by inflammation has led to attempts at modulating the inflammatory process, and thereby influencing outcome (89). Options include nonsteroidal anti-inflammatory agents, steroids, antioxidants, pentoxyfylline, and ketoconazole.

Ibuprofen has been used as a nonsteroidal anti-inflammatory drug, without benefit (90). Ketoconazole has similarly been used for its anti-inflammatory properties (91). The phosphodiesterase inhibitors pentoxyfylline and lysinophylline also inhibit neutrophil activation, platelet activation, and release of TNF-α. No benefit has been observed with their use (92). One study (93) found that the antioxidants N-acetylcysteine and procysteine reduced the number of days of ALI and lowered the lung injury scores, but had no beneficial effect on mortality. High-dose methylprednisolone is beneficial for certain subgroups of patients, such as those with orthopedic injuries at risk of fat embolism, those with pneumocystis carinii pneumonia (94), and those with ARDS of more than seven days duration (95).

Extracorporeal Life Support

Extracorporeal life support (ECLS) has been an extremely successful treatment for neonates with respiratory distress. Early studies with adult patients (96) failed to demonstrate that ECLS was more beneficial than conventional ventilation. These trials were flawed, however, with mortality rates higher than 90% in the control and treatment arms. This high mortality rate probably occurred because of extremely sick patients who could not be successfully treated. In addition, at that time, there was only limited experience with use of the technique for adult patients, and the standard tidal volumes used were excessive by current standards. Recent trials have been more encouraging (97,98) and have demonstrated higher survival rates than those for historical control subjects.

ECLS is presently indicated for patients who cannot be oxygenated even at a FiO$_2$ of 100%, or for whom peak airway pressures higher than 40 cmH$_2$O are needed for maintaining oxygenation. For patients with adequate cardiac function, venovenous ECLS is sufficient, but for those with cardiac dysfunction, ateriovenous bypass is required.

Other Novel Strategies

New treatment strategies for patients with respiratory distress include the use of surfactant, liquid ventilation, β-adrenergic agents, and dopaminergic agents. Surfactant replacement therapy was recently attempted in a multicenter randomized controlled trial. The trial demonstrated no beneficial effect on lung function, duration of mechanical ventilation, or mortality rates (99–101). Liquid ventilation involves filling the lungs with perfluorocarbon in amounts equal to the functional residual capacity. This treatment has been shown to improve pulmonary hemodynamics and to increase the survival rates of critically ill patients younger than 55 years (102). For trauma patients, although liquid ventilation attenuates the inflammatory response, as demonstrated by a decrease in the level of alveolar proinflammatory cytokines, it has no beneficial effect on outcome (103). Finally, β-adrenergic agents decrease pulmonary vascular permeability (104), whereas dopaminergic agents increase edema clearance.

Fluid Management

Judicious fluid management is an essential component of the management strategy for ARDS. The rationale for using a restrictive fluid strategy is to decrease the pulmonary vascular hydrostatic pressure, thereby limiting transudation across leaky capillaries. At the same time, however, adequate tissue perfusion must be maintained. Using a PAC may be helpful in achieving this fine balance. The pulmonary artery occlusion pressure is maintained at the lowest level that will result in adequate circulation volume and mean arterial pressures, and in cardiac output that meets the oxygen delivery needs of the tissues. For patients without PACs, surrogate markers include central venous pressure, urine output, and acid–base balance. Vasopressors may be used to maintain perfusion if fluid resuscitation is inadequate. There is, however, no role for their use in generating a supranormal patient delivery. Adopting a restrictive fluid strategy with diuresis results in fewer days on mechanical ventilation and improved oxygenation and is associated with better outcomes (105).

Nutritional Support

Adequate nutritional support is essential for meeting the needs of increased metabolic demand and for synthesizing new lean body tissue. Diets low in carbohydrate and high in fat are preferred because diets high in carbohydrate increase the respiratory quotient by producing carbon dioxide, which increases the ventilatory demand. Diets that include eicosapentaenoic acid and gamma-linoleic acid improve outcome (106) because these acids have anti-inflammatory, antioxidant, and vasodilatory properties that improve microvascular permeability and reduce the generation of proinflammatory eicosanoids.

OTHER CAUSES OF RESPIRATORY FAILURE AFTER TRAUMA OR SURGERY
Rib Fractures

Chest wall trauma is most frequently the result of motor vehicle collisions; approximately 10% of patients with chest wall trauma have rib fractures (107). When such fractures are present, the resultant pain limits the ability to breathe deeply or cough, causes retention of sputum and atelectasis, and reduces the functional residual capacity. All of these changes combine to cause reduced lung compliance and to produce ventilation–perfusion mismatch, with resultant hypoxemia. Adequate pain management is, therefore, crucial and may be achieved by one of several methods (108), such as systemic opioids, intercostal nerve blocks, epidural analgesia, intrathecal opioids, intrapleural analgesia, thoracic paravertebral blocks, transcutaneous nerve stimulation, and oral analgesic agents. Each technique has its own unique strengths, weaknesses, and contraindications and must be individualized for each patient. We prefer epidural analgesia when its use is feasible because it has been shown to provide better pain control than intermittent intrapleural injections (109) or patient-controlled analgesia (110).

Pulmonary Contusion

Pulmonary contusion is common after blunt trauma to the chest; its incidence is 17% among patients who suffer multisystem trauma (111). Pulmonary contusion most often follows mechanisms of injury that involve rapid deceleration, such as motor vehicle crashes and falls.

Injury to the lung parenchyma may be direct or indirect. Direct injury is commonly a result of either mechanical tearing of tissue or laceration from overlying injured ribs. Indirect injury results from shearing at the gas–liquid interface, differential rates of movement of the various intrathoracic tissues with varying densities, and the distention of contained air that occurs after a pressure wave passes. These effects result in pulmonary parenchymal injury that is proportional to the severity of the force applied. The resultant injury produces a ventilation–perfusion mismatch, increased intrapulmonary shunting, increased lung water, and reduced compliance. Clinically, these changes manifest themselves as hypoxemia, hypercarbia, and increased work of breathing. Generally, the severity of the injury worsens over the first 24 to 48 hours, reaches a maximum at 72 hours, and then resolves over the ensuing seven days. Long-term consequences may develop as a reaction to blood in the lung tissue, the pulmonary effects of systemic inflammation, or the development of nosocomial pneumonia.

Results of initial chest radiography may be negative; however, infiltrates appear over a period of four to six hours as the process evolves. Chest radiographs, however, underestimate the severity of the disease process. Computed tomography of the chest is much more accurate in delineating the extent of the process (Fig. 5).

Treatment is essentially supportive and includes management of associated injuries, adequate pain control, aggressive pulmonary toilet, and intubation if indicated. In cases of severe unilateral injuries, the patient may be placed in a kinematic bed, with the uninjured lung in the dependent position. This positioning increases blood flow to the lung with better gas exchange capabilities, thereby improving oxygenation. Fluid management remains a challenging issue for this group of patients. Overzealous fluid resuscitation increases the lung water and decreases compliance and gas exchange; therefore, it may be detrimental. The use of hypertonic saline and, more recently, hemoglobin substitutes has been suggested as an alternative to fluid management. Antibiotics are not indicated unless there is evidence of infection. Similarly, prophylactic steroids provide no clear benefit; rather, they increase the risk of infection.

Neuromuscular Acute Respiratory Failure

Neuromuscular acute respiratory failure results from one of two causes: an increase in the load on the respiratory system or a decrease in neuromuscular capacity. An increased load results from greater dynamic resistance, increased dynamic elastance, and increased intrinsic PEEP (auto PEEP). A greater inspiratory effort is required to overcome these increased forces; this increased workload may eventually result in respiratory muscle fatigue and failure.

Decreased neuromuscular capacity may result from neuropathy, myopathy, metabolic abnormalities, decreased oxygen delivery, or medications. Of these, neuropathy and myopathy are being increasingly recognized as consequences of critical illness (112). Diagnosis is often difficult because of the presence of confounding variables.

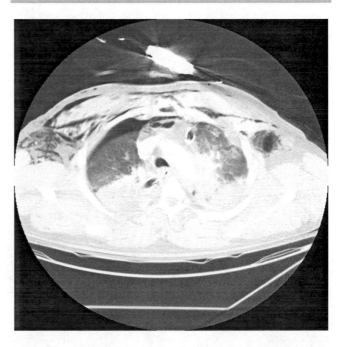

Figure 5 Computed tomogram of a young adult man who suffered substantial blunt trauma to the chest as the result of a motorcycle crash. Bilateral pulmonary contusions are readily evident. A right-sided pneumothorax can also be seen.

Critical illness polyneuropathy is defined as clinically significant muscle weakness that occurs after at least seven days of mechanical ventilation after satisfactory awakening. This condition is characterized by symmetrical distal weakness, with loss of deep tendon reflexes, and absent sensory potential, as demonstrated by nerve conduction studies. Critical illness polyneuropathy is not uncommon; it affects as many as 25% of critically ill patients, and its incidence may be as high 60% in the presence of sepsis and 75% in the presence of septic shock (112). Although this condition will eventually improve for 60% to 90% of patients, it may cause prolonged effects if the initial involvement is severe. Critical illness polyneuropathy may contribute to the occurrence of persistent respiratory failure or to a difficulty in weaning (113). It is believed to be the consequence of axonal degeneration that results from the release of cytokines after trauma or surgery, especially in the face of sepsis.

Critical illness myopathy, which is characterized by generalized muscle weakness, may result from one or more of several causes. The condition includes a form of myopathy that is seen when critically ill patients are treated with glucocorticoids, neuromuscular blocking agents, or both, and especially when these agents are administered for more than two days. Other causes include sepsis-associated myopathy, ventilator-associated respiratory muscle damage, and disuse atrophy.

A combination of critical illness polyneuropathy and critical illness myopathy is called critical illness neuromyopathy. Clinical features include weakness and loss of deep tendon reflexes. The diagnosis can be established by nerve conduction studies. Occasionally, muscle biopsies may be required.

Transfusion-Related Acute Lung Injury

Transfusion-related acute lung injury (TRALI) is a poorly defined, temporary condition that follows allogeneic blood transfusion. Although its true incidence is unknown, it is now being increasingly recognized (114).

TRALI is defined as a new episode of ALI that occurs during or within six hours of a completed transfusion. It is characterized by hypoxemia with a PF ratio of 300 or less or arterial oxygen saturation below 90% on room air. The chest radiograph demonstrates bilateral infiltrates, and there is no evidence of left atrial hypertension. There is no temporal relationship to an alternative risk factor that would explain the development of ARDS. Although the exact pathophysiology remains unknown, the two most favored mechanisms are (i) an antigen–antibody reaction by antibodies contained in the transfused blood against the recipient's white blood cell components and (ii) activation of pulmonary endothelial cells by the transfusion of neutrophils that have been previously primed.

Clinically, the patient exhibits dyspnea, fever, hypotension, tachypnea, tachycardia, and a frothy endotracheal aspirate. Treatment is supportive. Prevention involves limiting the transfusion of blood products, minimizing the inappropriate use of blood products, using blood with a more recent storage date, and using washed cellular products.

Thoracic Compartment Syndrome

The concept of compartment syndrome is well recognized in orthopedic and trauma surgery. Initially described as occurring only in the extremity, the condition is now recognized to affect the abdomen and the thorax as well. It is a clinical syndrome diagnosed by compartment tissue pressures that exceed perfusion pressures; this pressure differential results in decreased capillary perfusion and compromised tissue viability.

Originally described by Riahi (115), thoracic compartment syndrome usually presents with increased airway pressures that occur when the chest is closed after thoracic or cardiac surgery, especially when cases are associated with coagulopathy and uncontrolled bleeding. On occasion, thoracic compartment syndrome may develop more slowly over a period of hours to days; in such cases, it causes reduced cardiac output, hypoperfusion, and worsening acidosis. The diagnosis is usually one of exclusion; hence, physicians must maintain a high index of suspicion.

Therapeutic options include leaving the chest cavity open and packed, or using skin flaps or synthetic materials to provide temporary closure of the chest cavity. Definitive closure can be attempted once the patient's hemodynamic condition stabilizes, and both the coagulopathy and the acidosis have been corrected. The average time to closure is usually two to five days. Diuretics may play an adjunctive role. Mediastinitis is a serious and potentially life-threatening complication.

CONCLUSION

Respiratory failure in not uncommon following surgery or trauma. In this setting, it is often multifactorial due to a combination of patient- and procedure-related factors. Although preoperative risk reduction is ideal, aggressive postopearitve pulmonary care may reduce the impact. In patients requiring mechanical ventilation to support lung function, the data derived from the ARDSNet trial probably represents the current standard of care. The lung protection strategies espoused there should be followed to minimize the occurrence of VALI. A multimodality approach to the most severe form of respiratory failure, ARDS, will most likely lead to a successful outcome. Other unusual causes of respiratory failure in this group of patients must be recognized.

REFERENCES

1. Bernard GR, Artigas A, Brigham KL, et al. The American-European Consensus Conference on ARDS. Definitions, mechanisms, relevant outcomes, and

clinical trial coordination. Am J Respir Crit Care Med 1994; 149(3 Pt 1):818–824.

2. Pedersen T, Eliasen K, Henriksen E. A prospective study of risk factors and cardiopulmonary complications associated with anaesthesia and surgery: risk indicators of cardiopulmonary morbidity. Acta Anaesthesiol Scand 1990; 34:144–155.

3. Lawrence VA, Dhanda R, Hilsenbeck SG, Page CP. Risk of pulmonary complications after elective abdominal surgery. Chest 1996; 110:744–750.

4. Behrendt CE. Acute respiratory failure in the United States: incidence and 31-day survival. Chest 2000; 118: 1100–1105.

5. Ashbaugh DG, Bigelow DB, Petty TL, Levine BE. Acute respiratory distress in adults. Lancet 1967; 2(7511): 319–323.

6. Treggiari MM, Hudson LD, Martin DP, Weiss NS, Caldwell E, Rubenfeld G. Effect of acute lung injury and acute respiratory distress syndrome on outcome in critically ill trauma patients. Crit Care Med 2004; 32: 327–331.

7. White TO, Jenkins PJ, Smith RD, Cartlidge CW, Robinson CM. The epidemiology of posttraumatic adult respiratory distress syndrome. J Bone Joint Surg Am 2004; 86-A:2366–2376.

8. Warner MA, Offord KP, Warner ME, Lennon RL, Conover MA, Jansson-Schumacher U. Role of preoperative cessation of smoking and other factors in postoperative pulmonary complications: a blinded prospective study of coronary artery bypass patients. Mayo Clin Proc 1989; 64:609–616.

9. Goldman L, Caldera DL, Nussbaum SR, et al. Multifactorial index of cardiac risk in noncardiac surgical procedures. N Engl J Med 1977; 297:845–850.

10. Stein M, Cassara EL. Preoperative pulmonary evaluation and therapy for surgery patients. JAMA 1970; 211: 787–790.

11. Expert panel report to provide clinical guidelines for diagnosis and treatment of asthma. J Sch Health 1991; 61:249–250.

12. Wong DH, Weber EC, Schell MJ, Wong AB, Anderson CT, Barker SJ. Factors associated with postoperative pulmonary complications in patients with severe chronic obstructive pulmonary disease. Anesth Analg 1995; 80(2):276–284.

13. Pasulka PS, Bistrian BR, Benotti PN, Blackburn GL. The risks of surgery in obese patients. Ann Intern Med 1986; 104:540–546.

14. Phillips EH, Carroll BJ, Fallas MJ, Pearlstein AR. Comparison of laparoscopic cholecystectomy in obese and non-obese patients. Am Surg 1994; 60:316–321.

15. Rovina N, Bouros D, Tzanakis N, et al. Effects of laparoscopic cholecystectomy on global respiratory muscle strength. Am J Respir Crit Care Med 1996; 153:458–461.

16. Sykes LA, Bowe EA. Cardiorespiratory effects of anesthesia. Clin Chest Med 1993; 14:211–226.

17. Berg H. Is residual neuromuscular block following pancuronium a risk factor for postoperative pulmonary complications? Acta Anaesthesiol Scand Suppl 1997; 110:156–158.

18. Brooks-Brunn JA. Risk factors associated with postoperative pulmonary complications following total abdominal hysterectomy. Clin Nurs Res 2000; 9:27–46.

19. Celli BR, Rodriguez KS, Snider GL. A controlled trial of intermittent positive pressure breathing, incentive spirometry, and deep breathing exercises in preventing pulmonary complications after abdominal surgery. Am Rev Respir Dis 1984; 130:12–15.

20. Cuschieri RJ, Morran CG, Howie JC, McArdle CS. Postoperative pain and pulmonary complications: comparison of three analgesic regimens. Br J Surg 1985; 72:495–498.

21. Pierson DJ. Current limitations of mechanical ventilation: what improvements should the clinician expect? Respir Care 1995; 40:933–941.

22. Navalesi P, Hernandez P, Wongsa A, Laporta D, Goldberg P, Gottfried SB. Proportional assist ventilation in acute respiratory failure: effects on breathing pattern and inspiratory effort. Am J Respir Crit Care Med 1996; 154:1330–1338.

23. Beck J, Gottfried SB, Navalesi P, et al. Electrical activity of the diaphragm during pressure support ventilation in acute respiratory failure. Am J Respir Crit Care Med 2001; 164:419–424.

24. Lefevre GR, Kowalski SE, Girling LG, Thiessen DB, Mutch WA. Improved arterial oxygenation after oleic acid lung injury in the pig using a computer-controlled mechanical ventilator. Am J Respir Crit Care Med 1996; 154:1567–1572.

25. Tobin MJ, Jubran A, Hines E Jr. Pathophysiology of failure to wean from mechanical ventilation. Schweiz Med Wochenschr 1994; 124:2139–2145.

26. Polese G, Rossi A, Appendini L, Brandi G, Bates JH, Brandolese R. Partitioning of respiratory mechanics in mechanically ventilated patients. J Appl Physiol 1991; 71:2425–2433.

27. Amato MB, Barbas CS, Medeiros DM, et al. Beneficial effects of the "open lung approach" with low distending pressures in acute respiratory distress syndrome. A prospective randomized study on mechanical ventilation. Am J Respir Crit Care Med 1995; 152(6 Pt 1): 1835–1846.

28. Jubran A, Tobin MJ. Passive mechanics of lung and chest wall in patients who failed or succeeded in trials of weaning. Am J Respir Crit Care Med 1997; 155:916–921.

29. Tantucci C, Corbeil C, Chasse M, Braidy J, Matar N, Milic-Emili J. Flow resistance in patients with chronic obstructive pulmonary disease in acute respiratory failure. Effects of flow and volume. Am Rev Respir Dis 1991; 144:384–389.

30. Jubran A, Tobin MJ. Use of flow-volume curves in detecting secretions in ventilator-dependent patients. Am J Respir Crit Care Med 1994; 150:766–769.

31. Liesching T, Kwok H, Hill NS. Acute applications of noninvasive positive pressure ventilation. Chest 2003; 124:699–713.

32. Antonelli M, Conti G, Rocco M, et al. A comparison of noninvasive positive-pressure ventilation and conventional mechanical ventilation in patients with acute respiratory failure. N Engl J Med 1998; 339: 429–435.

33. Epstein SK, Ciubotaru RL, Wong JB. Effect of failed extubation on the outcome of mechanical ventilation. Chest 1997; 112:186–192.

34. Chevron V, Menard JF, Richard JC, Girault C, Leroy J, Bonmarchand G. Unplanned extubation: risk factors of development and predictive criteria for reintubation. Crit Care Med 1998; 26:1049–1053.

35. Ranieri VM, Suter PM, Tortorella C, et al. Effect of mechanical ventilation on inflammatory mediators in

patients with acute respiratory distress syndrome: a randomized controlled trial. JAMA 1999; 282:54–61.

36. Bryan CL, Jenkinson SG. Oxygen toxicity. Clin Chest Med 1988; 9:141–152.

37. Roupie E, Dambrosio M, Servillo G, et al. Titration of tidal volume and induced hypercapnia in acute respiratory distress syndrome. Am J Respir Crit Care Med 1995; 152:121–128.

38. Singh JM, Stewart TE. High-frequency mechanical ventilation principles and practices in the era of lung-protective ventilation strategies. Respir Care Clin N Am 2002; 8:247–260.

39. Stewart TE, Meade MO, Cook DJ, et al. Evaluation of a ventilation strategy to prevent barotrauma in patients at high risk for acute respiratory distress syndrome. Pressure- and Volume-Limited Ventilation Strategy Group. N Engl J Med 1998; 338:355–361.

40. Artigas A, Bernard GR, Carlet J, et al. The American-European Consensus Conference on ARDS, Part 2: ventilatory, pharmacologic, supportive therapy, study design strategies, and issues related to recovery and remodeling. Acute respiratory distress syndrome. Am J Respir Crit Care Med 1998; 157(4 Pt 1):1332–1347.

41. Slutsky AS. Mechanical ventilation. American College of Chest Physicians' Consensus Conference. Chest 1993; 104:1833–1859.

42. Ventilation with lower tidal volumes as compared with traditional tidal volumes for acute lung injury and the acute respiratory distress syndrome. The Acute Respiratory Distress Syndrome Network. N Engl J Med 2000; 342:1301–1308.

43. Feihl F, Perret C. Permissive hypercapnia. How permissive should we be? Am J Respir Crit Care Med 1994; 150(6 Pt 1):1722–1737.

44. Sloane PJ, Gee MH, Gottlieb JE, et al. A multicenter registry of patients with acute respiratory distress syndrome. Physiology and outcome. Am Rev Respir Dis 1992; 146:419–426.

45. Hasleton PS. Adult respiratory distress syndrome—a review. Histopathology 1983; 7:307–332.

46. Brochard L, Roudot-Thoraval F, Roupie E, et al. Tidal volume reduction for prevention of ventilator-induced lung injury in acute respiratory distress syndrome. The Multicenter Trial Group on Tidal Volume Reduction in ARDS. Am J Respir Crit Care Med 1998; 158:1831–1838.

47. Brower RG, Shanholtz CB, Fessler HE, et al. Prospective, randomized, controlled clinical trial comparing traditional versus reduced tidal volume ventilation in acute respiratory distress syndrome patients. Crit Care Med 1999; 27:1492–1498.

48. Valente Barbas CS. Lung recruitment maneuvers in acute respiratory distress syndrome and facilitating resolution. Crit Care Med 2003; 31(suppl 4):S265–S271.

49. Bachofen H, Schurch S, Urbinelli M, Weibel ER. Relations among alveolar surface tension, surface area, volume, and recoil pressure. J Appl Physiol 1987; 62: 1878–1887.

50. Dreyfuss D, Saumon G. Role of tidal volume, FRC, and end-inspiratory volume in the development of pulmonary edema following mechanical ventilation. Am Rev Respir Dis 1993; 148:1194–1203.

51. Ranieri VM, Giuliani R, Cinnella G, et al. Physiologic effects of positive end-expiratory pressure in patients with chronic obstructive pulmonary disease during acute ventilatory failure and controlled mechanical ventilation. Am Rev Respir Dis 1993; 147:5–13.

52. Rimensberger PC, Cox PN, Frndova H, Bryan AC. The open lung during small tidal volume ventilation: concepts of recruitment and "optimal" positive end-expiratory pressure. Crit Care Med 1999; 27:1946–1952.

53. Lichtwarck-Aschoff M, Kessler V, Sjostrand UH, et al. Static versus dynamic respiratory mechanics for setting the ventilator. Br J Anaesth 2000; 85:577–586.

54. Gattinoni L, D'Andrea L, Pelosi P, Vitale G, Pesenti A, Fumagalli R. Regional effects and mechanism of positive end-expiratory pressure in early adult respiratory distress syndrome. JAMA 1993; 269:2122–2127.

55. Chang HK. Mechanisms of gas transport during ventilation by high-frequency oscillation. J Appl Physiol 1984; 56:553–563.

56. Drazen JM, Kamm RD, Slutsky AS. High-frequency ventilation. Physiol Rev 1984; 64:505–543.

57. Mehta S, Granton J, MacDonald RJ, et al. High-frequency oscillatory ventilation in adults: the Toronto experience. Chest 2004; 126:518–527.

58. Ferguson ND, Chiche JD, Kacmarek RM, et al. Combining high-frequency oscillatory ventilation and recruitment maneuvers in adults with early acute respiratory distress syndrome: the Treatment with Oscillation and an Open Lung Strategy (TOOLS) trial pilot study. Crit Care Med 2005; 33:479–486.

59. Palmer RM, Rees DD, Ashton DS, Moncada S. L-arginine is the physiological precursor for the formation of nitric oxide in endothelium-dependent relaxation. Biochem Biophys Res Commun 1988; 153: 1251–1256.

60. Pepke-Zaba J, Higenbottam TW, Dinh-Xuan AT, Stone D, Wallwork J. Inhaled nitric oxide as a cause of selective pulmonary vasodilatation in pulmonary hypertension. Lancet 1991; 338(8776):1173–1174.

61. Stamler JS, Loh E, Roddy MA, Currie KE, Creager MA. Nitric oxide regulates basal systemic and pulmonary vascular resistance in healthy humans. Circulation 1994; 89:2035–2040.

62. Rossaint R, Pison U, Gerlach H, Falke KJ. Inhaled nitric oxide: its effects on pulmonary circulation and airway smooth muscle cells. Eur Heart J 1993; 14(suppl I):133–140.

63. Gardeback M, Larsen FF, Radegran K. Nitric oxide improves hypoxaemia following reperfusion oedema after pulmonary thromboendarterectomy. Br J Anaesth 1995; 75:798–800.

64. Capellier G, Jacques T, Balvay P, Blasco G, Belle E, Barale F. Inhaled nitric oxide in patients with pulmonary embolism. Intensive Care Med 1997; 23:1089–1092.

65. Rossaint R, Falke KJ, Lopez F, Slama K, Pison U, Zapol WM. Inhaled nitric oxide for the adult respiratory distress syndrome. N Engl J Med 1993; 328: 399–405.

66. Hogman M, Frostell CG, Hedenstrom H, Hedenstierna G. Inhalation of nitric oxide modulates adult human bronchial tone. Am Rev Respir Dis 1993; 148(6 Pt 1): 1474–1478.

67. Bigatello LM, Hurford WE, Kacmarek RM, Roberts JD Jr, Zapol WM. Prolonged inhalation of low concentrations of nitric oxide in patients with severe adult respiratory distress syndrome. Effects on pulmonary

hemodynamics and oxygenation. Anesthesiology 1994; 80:761–770.

68. Michael JR, Barton RG, Saffle JR, et al. Inhaled nitric oxide versus conventional therapy: effect on oxygenation in ARDS. Am J Respir Crit Care Med 1998; 157(5 Pt 1):1372–1380.

69. Troncy E, Collet JP, Shapiro S, et al. Inhaled nitric oxide in acute respiratory distress syndrome: a pilot randomized controlled study. Am J Respir Crit Care Med 1998; 157(5 Pt 1):1483–1488.

70. Lundin S, Mang H, Smithies M, Stenqvist O, Frostell C. Inhalation of nitric oxide in acute lung injury: results of a European multicentre study. The European Study Group of Inhaled Nitric Oxide. Intensive Care Med 1999; 25:911–919.

71. Puybasset L, Rouby JJ, Mourgeon E, et al. Factors influencing cardiopulmonary effects of inhaled nitric oxide in acute respiratory failure. Am J Respir Crit Care Med 1995; 152:318–328.

72. Rossaint R, Hahn SM, Pappert D, Falke KJ, Radermacher P. Influence of mixed venous PO_2 and inspired O_2 fraction on intrapulmonary shunt in patients with severe ARDS. J Appl Physiol 1995; 78: 1531–1536.

73. Benzing A, Geiger K. Inhaled nitric oxide lowers pulmonary capillary pressure and changes longitudinal distribution of pulmonary vascular resistance in patients with acute lung injury. Acta Anaesthesiol Scand 1994; 38:640–645.

74. Payen DM, Gatecel C, Plaisance P. Almitrine effect on nitric oxide inhalation in adult respiratory distress syndrome. Lancet 1993; 341(8861):1664.

75. Papazian L, Bregeon F, Gaillat F, et al. Does norepinephrine modify the effects of inhaled nitric oxide in septic patients with acute respiratory distress syndrome? Anesthesiology 1998; 89:1089–1098.

76. Ziegler JW, Ivy DD, Wiggins JW, Kinsella JP, Clarke WR, Abman SH. Effects of dipyridamole and inhaled nitric oxide in pediatric patients with pulmonary hypertension. Am J Respir Crit Care Med 1998; 158(5 Pt 1): 1388–1395.

77. Gattinoni L, Pelosi P, Vitale G, Pesenti A, D'Andrea L, Mascheroni D. Body position changes redistribute lung computed-tomographic density in patients with acute respiratory failure. Anesthesiology 1991; 74: 15–23.

78. Piedalue F, Albert RK. Prone positioning in acute respiratory distress syndrome. Respir Care Clin N Am 2003; 9:495–509.

79. Pelosi P, Tubiolo D, Mascheroni D, et al. Effects of the prone position on respiratory mechanics and gas exchange during acute lung injury. Am J Respir Crit Care Med 1998; 157:387–393.

80. Pappert D, Rossaint R, Slama K, Gruning T, Falke KJ. Influence of positioning on ventilation-perfusion relationships in severe adult respiratory distress syndrome. Chest 1994; 106:1511–1516.

81. Vollman KM, Bander JJ. Improved oxygenation utilizing a prone positioner in patients with acute respiratory distress syndrome. Intensive Care Med 1996; 22: 1105–1111.

82. Blanch L, Mancebo J, Perez M, et al. Short-term effects of prone position in critically ill patients with acute respiratory distress syndrome. Intensive Care Med 1997; 23:1033–1039.

83. Guerin C, Badet M, Rosselli S, et al. Effects of prone position on alveolar recruitment and oxygenation in acute lung injury. Intensive Care Med 1999; 25:1222–1230.

84. Johannigman JA, Davis K Jr, Miller SL, et al. Prone positioning and inhaled nitric oxide: synergistic therapies for acute respiratory distress syndrome. J Trauma 2001; 50:589–596.

85. Papazian L, Bregeon F, Gaillat F, et al. Respective and combined effects of prone position and inhaled nitric oxide in patients with acute respiratory distress syndrome. Am J Respir Crit Care Med 1998; 157:580–585.

86. Weigelt JA, Norcross JF, Borman KR, Snyder WH III. Early steroid therapy for respiratory failure. Arch Surg 1985; 120:536–540.

87. Bernard GR, Luce JM, Sprung CL, et al. High-dose corticosteroids in patients with the adult respiratory distress syndrome. N Engl J Med 1987; 317:1565–1570.

88. Hooper RG, Kearl RA. Established ARDS treated with a sustained course of adrenocortical steroids. Chest 1990; 97:138–143.

89. Matthay MA, Zimmerman GA, Esmon C, et al. Future research directions in acute lung injury: summary of a National Heart, Lung, and Blood Institute working group. Am J Respir Crit Care Med 2003; 167: 1027–1035.

90. Bernard GR, Wheeler AP, Russell JA, et al. The effects of ibuprofen on the physiology and survival of patients with sepsis. The Ibuprofen in Sepsis Study Group. N Engl J Med 1997; 336:912–918.

91. The ARDS Network. Ketoconazole for early treatment of acute lung injury and acute respiratory distress syndrome: a randomized controlled trial. JAMA 2000; 283:1995–2002.

92. Anonymous. Randomized, placebo-controlled trial of lisofylline for early treatment of acute lung injury and acute respiratory distress syndrome. Crit Care Med 2002; 30:1–6.

93. Bernard GR, Wheeler AP, Arons MM, et al. A trial of antioxidants N-acetylcysteine and procysteine in ARDS. The Antioxidant in ARDS Study Group. Chest 1997; 112:164–172.

94. Luce JM. Corticosteroids in ARDS. An evidence-based review. Crit Care Clin 2002; 18:79–89,vii.

95. Meduri GU, Headley AS, Golden E, et al. Effect of prolonged methylprednisolone therapy in unresolving acute respiratory distress syndrome: a randomized controlled trial. JAMA 1998; 280:159–165.

96. Zapol WM, Snider MT, Hill JD, et al. Extracorporeal membrane oxygenation in severe acute respiratory failure. A randomized prospective study. JAMA 1979; 242:2193–2196.

97. Anderson H III, Steimle C, Shapiro M, et al. Extracorporeal life support for adult cardiorespiratory failure. Surgery 1993; 114:161–173.

98. Kolla S, Awad SS, Rich PB, Schreiner RJ, Hirschl RB, Bartlett RH. Extracorporeal life support for 100 adult patients with severe respiratory failure. Ann Surg 1997; 226:544–566.

99. Anzueto A, Baughman RP, Guntupalli KK, et al. Aerosolized surfactant in adults with sepsis-induced acute respiratory distress syndrome. Exosurf Acute Respiratory Distress Syndrome Sepsis Study Group. N Engl J Med 1996; 334:1417–1421.

100. Spragg RG, Gilliard N, Richman P, et al. Acute effects of a single dose of porcine surfactant on patients with

the adult respiratory distress syndrome. Chest 1994; 105:195–202.

101. Walmrath D, Gunther A, Ghofrani HA, et al. Broncho-scopic surfactant administration in patients with severe adult respiratory distress syndrome and sepsis. Am J Respir Crit Care Med 1996; 154:57–62.

102. Bartlett RH. Extracorporeal Life Support Registry Report 1995. ASAIO J 1997; 43:104–107.

103. Croce MA, Fabian TC, Patton JH Jr, Melton SM, Moore M, Trenthem LL. Partial liquid ventilation decreases the inflammatory response in the alveolar environment of trauma patients. J Trauma 1998; 45:273–282.

104. Basran GS, Hardy JG, Woo SP, Ramasubramanian R, Byrne AJ. Beta-2-adrenoceptor agonists as inhibitors of lung vascular permeability to radiolabelled transferrin in the adult respiratory distress syndrome in man. Eur J Nucl Med 1986; 12:381–384.

105. Martin GS, Mangialardi RJ, Wheeler AP, Dupont WD, Morris JA, Bernard GR. Albumin and furosemide therapy in hypoproteinemic patients with acute lung injury. Crit Care Med 2002; 30:2175–2182.

106. Pacht ER, DeMichele SJ, Nelson JL, Hart J, Wennberg AK, Gadek JE. Enteral nutrition with eicosapentaenoic acid, gamma-linolenic acid, and antioxidants reduces alveolar inflammatory mediators and protein influx in patients with acute respiratory distress syndrome. Crit Care Med 2003; 31:491–500.

107. Mayberry JC, Trunkey DD. The fractured rib in chest wall trauma. Chest Surg Clin N Am 1997; 7:239–261.

108. Karmakar MK, Ho AM. Acute pain management of patients with multiple fractured ribs. J Trauma 2003; 54:615–625.

109. Luchette FA, Radafshar SM, Kaiser R, Flynn W, Hassett JM. Prospective evaluation of epidural versus intrapleural catheters for analgesia in chest wall trauma. J Trauma 1994; 36:865–870.

110. Moon MR, Luchette FA, Gibson SW, et al. Prospective, randomized comparison of epidural versus parenteral opioid analgesia in thoracic trauma. Ann Surg 1999; 229:684–692.

111. Cohn SM. Pulmonary contusion: review of the clinical entity. J Trauma 1997; 42:973–979.

112. Latronico N, Peli E, Botteri M. Critical illness myopathy and neuropathy. Curr Opin Crit Care 2005; 11:126–132.

113. Garnacho-Montero J, Amaya-Villar R, Garcia-Garmendia JL, Madrazo-Osuna J, Ortiz-Leyba C. Effect of critical illness polyneuropathy on the withdrawal from mechanical ventilation and the length of stay in septic patients. Crit Care Med 2005; 33:349–354.

114. Kleinman S, Caulfield T, Chan P, et al. Toward an understanding of transfusion-related acute lung injury: statement of a consensus panel. Transfusion 2004; 44: 1774–1789.

115. Riahi M, Tomatis LA, Schlosser RJ, Bertolozzi E, Johnston DW. Cardiac compression due to closure of the median sternotomy in open heart surgery. Chest 1975; 67:113–114.

24

Complications of Lung Transplantation

Xiao-Shi Qi
*Division of Cardiothoracic Surgery, DeWitt Daughtry Family Department of Surgery,
University of Miami Miller School of Medicine, Jackson Memorial Hospital,
Miami, Florida, U.S.A.*

Debra Fertel
*Division of Pulmonary and Critical Care Medicine, Department of Medicine,
University of Miami Miller School of Medicine, Miami, Florida, U.S.A.*

*Lung transplantation has evolved into an accepted
therapeutic option for many patients with end-stage lung
disease. Advances in immunosuppression, surgical
techniques, and postoperative management have
contributed to improved outcomes. Nevertheless, lung
transplantation is still associated with several potential
complications that may limit long-term graft function and,
ultimately, patient survival. Prevention of complications
requires attention to proper selection of donor and recipient.
However, despite all due diligence, patients receiving
lung transplants are prone to several complications. This
chapter will review the complications that are currently
associated with lung transplantation.*

HISTORICAL PERSPECTIVE

Hardy et al. (1), at the University of Mississippi,
performed the first human lung transplantation in
1963. The recipient had a central squamous carcinoma and an inadequate pulmonary reserve that
precluded pneumonectomy. The transplanted organ
was a lung allograft harvested postmortem from a
donor who had died of cardiac arrest. The postoperative immunosuppressive regimen included steroids,
azathioprine, and thymic radiation. The patient died
of renal failure 18 days after the transplant procedure.
No signs of rejection were found during autopsy.

Between 1963 and 1983, approximately 38 single-
lung transplantations (SLTs) were performed worldwide; only 12 recipients survived for more than two
weeks. Seven of these 12 patients eventually died of
complications related to bronchial anastomotic leaks.
The patient who survived longest had silicosis and
lived for 10 months, all but two weeks of that time in
the hospital (2,3). These reports show that bronchial
complications related to anastomotic healing were a
crucial limiting factor in the early days of lung

transplantation. Systemic arterial reanastomosis,
which was routine with solid organ transplantation,
was not routinely performed for lung transplantation. Thus, blood supply to the donor bronchus relied
entirely on collateral vessels from the pulmonary
arterial system.

In 1981, Shumway and coworkers reported their
series of three patients who underwent successful
heart–lung transplant for pulmonary vascular disease
(4). In 1983, the Toronto Lung Transplant Group (5)
performed their first successful single-lung transplant
on a patient with pulmonary fibrosis. Their surgical
technique included reinforcing the bronchial anastomosis with an omental graft so as to increase blood
flow via omental collateral vessels. They also emphasized the importance of early patient rehabilitation
and of minimizing early administration of corticosteroids. The patient lived for six years before dying of
renal failure.

In 1986, the Toronto Lung Transplant Group (6)
and later Yacoub and coworkers (7) independently
began performing en bloc double-lung transplantation. However, more than half of the patients died of
complications related to dehiscence of the tracheal
anastomosis (6). Yacoub and coworkers (7) were able
to achieve success by directly revascularizing the
bronchial arteries, but the en bloc procedure was
eventually abandoned. In 1989, Cooper and coworkers (8,9) reported the use of the transverse anterior
thoracosternotomy incision (the clamshell incision)
for bilateral sequential SLT. This technique improved
the morbidity and mortality rates associated with lung
transplantation and ultimately obviated the need for
heart–lung transplantation in patients who required
two lungs because of parenchymal lung diseases.
Since 1990, improved results have led to a resurgence
of lung transplantation worldwide. However, continued growth has been limited by the lack of an
adequate supply of cadaveric donors; thus, the annual
rate of lung transplantation has leveled off (10).

RECIPIENT SELECTION

Inherent to any strategy aimed at reducing potential surgical complications is the appropriate selection of candidates for lung transplantation (11). General guidelines are outlined in Table 1. Appropriate candidates must have advanced lung disease for which all therapeutic options have been exhausted. Timing of the referral and listing must take into account a waiting period of one to two years. Choosing poor candidates out of compassion or desperation should be avoided. Candidates should be disabled by their pulmonary disease but should be ambulatory and free of extrapulmonary disease. They should have an estimated life expectancy of less than two years, with acceptable nutritional status and rehabilitation potential; additionally, they should have no other serious medical illnesses. Because the potential for a successful outcome decreases with age, the following age limits have been recommended: 55 years for heart–lung transplantation, 60 years for bilateral lung transplantation (BLT), and 65 years for SLT. Disease-specific guidelines have also been recommended and are outlined in Table 2. Relative and absolute contraindications to lung transplantation are presented in Table 3.

Patients who have undergone previous thoracic surgery or pleurodesis are at higher risk of bleeding, particularly if cardiopulmonary bypass (CPB) is used; however, successful outcomes can be achieved in carefully selected candidates (12,13). Likewise, preoperative corticosteroid therapy, once believed to be the direct cause of bronchial anastomotic complications, no longer precludes a successful outcome if administered at moderate doses (14). Mechanical ventilation, once viewed as a relative contraindication to lung transplantation because of its association with higher postoperative mortality rates, can be beneficial for selected patients and can lead to successful transplantation and long-term survival (15,16).

Finally, allosensitized recipients present a unique problem. Blood transfusion or pregnancy can produce alloantibodies to human leukocyte antigens (HLAs). These antibodies are identified by determining the panel-reactive antibody (PRA) level of the potential recipient's serum; the results of this test are read as either positive or negative for HLA antibodies. A positive result indicates an increased risk of hyperacute rejection if the patient's serum also tests positive for lymphocyte-reactive antibodies. Although a high PRA

Table 1 Indications for Lung Transplantation

End-stage lung disease for which all medical and surgical options have been exhausted
Estimated life expectancy <2 yr
Stable psychosocial profile
Rehabilitation potential
Compliance with medical regimens
Absence of systemic disease
Abstinence from smoking >6 mo

Source: Adapted from Ref. 11.

Table 2 Disease-Specific Guidelines for Lung Transplant Referral

Chronic obstructive pulmonary disease
$FEV_1 < 25\%$ predicted without reversibility
$PaCO_2 \geq 55$ mmHg, elevated pulmonary artery pressures, or both
Progressive deterioration with elevated $PaCO_2$ and chronic hypoxemia
Cystic fibrosis
$FEV_1 \leq 30\%$ predicted
$FEV_1 > 30\%$ predicted but with progressive deterioration (frequent hospitalization, rapid decrease in FEV_1, massive hemoptysis, and weight loss)
Females <18 yr old with rapid deterioration (poorer prognosis)
Idiopathic pulmonary fibrosis
Symptomatic progressive disease unresponsive to medical therapy
Vital capacity <60–70% and diffusing capacity of carbon monoxide <50–60%
Primary pulmonary hypertension
New York Heart Association functional class III or IV
Mean pulmonary artery pressure ≥ 55 mmHg, mean RA pressure >15 mmHg, or cardiac index < 2 L/min/m^3
Severe progressive symptoms despite optimal medical treatment

Abbreviations: FEV_1, forced expiratory volume in one second; $PaCO_2$, partial pressure of carbon dioxide; RA, right atrial.
Source: Adapted from Ref. 11.

level may exclude a patient from consideration for transplantation, treatment with plasmapheresis, cytoxan, and intravenous immune globulin, as is used for recipients of other solid organ transplants, may reduce alloreactivity and allow transplantation (3,17,18).

Size matching is based on measurements taken on a frontal chest radiograph. The vertical measurement is made from the apex to the diaphragm at the mid-clavicular line, and the horizontal measurement is made at the level of the dome of the diaphragm. Substantial undersizing should be avoided; oversizing is tolerated and can be advantageous for recipients of single lungs.

Table 3 Contraindications to Lung Transplantation

Absolute contraindications
Active malignancy
HIV infection
Active smoking; alcohol or drug abuse
Severe dysfunction of other organs (liver, kidney, and heart)
Positive test for hepatitis B antigen
Hepatitis C viral activity with biopsy-proven histologic evidence of liver disease
Relative contraindications
Osteoporosis
Kyphoscoliosis
Corticosteroid use ≥ 20 mg/day
Body weight >130% ideal body weight or <70% of ideal body weight for height and age
Mechanical ventilation
Physiologic age >55 for heart–lung transplantation, >60 for bilateral lung transplantation, and >65 for single-lung transplantation
Coronary artery disease or left ventricular dysfunction
Psychosocial problems
Colonization with resistant bacteria, atypical mycobacteria, or *Aspergillus*

Abbreviation: HIV, human immunodeficiency virus.
Source: Adapted from Ref. 11.

DONOR SELECTION

Despite improvements in the treatment of potential donors, the lungs of brain-dead patients are often damaged, typically by aspiration, excessive administration of fluids, neurogenic edema, and ventilator-associated pneumonia. Fewer than 20% of cadaveric donors contribute to the lung donor pool. What were once standard criteria for potential donor candidates (Table 4) are often relaxed because of the shortage of suitable donor organs. The ideal donor is less than 55 years old with a history of less than 20 pack-years of smoking, a clear chest radiograph, acceptable oxygenation (arterial oxygen pressure >350 mmHg at a fraction of inspired oxygen of 100% and a positive end-expiratory pressure of 5 cmH$_2$O), normal airways as confirmed by bronchoscopy, and no evidence of chest trauma or contusion.

The increased demand for donors has led to the use of marginal donors who were once considered unacceptable. In fact, acceptable outcomes have been achieved by transplantation of lungs with secretions that can be lavaged clear with a bronchoscope, revealing normal underlying mucosa; lungs with marginal oxygenation; and lungs with unilateral infiltrates. However, the use of marginal donors increases the risk of graft dysfunction and postoperative complications. The decision to use any particular donor is often weighed against the risks for the intended recipient. A marginal donor may be acceptable for a recipient whose condition has deteriorated to the point at which mechanical ventilation is required; on the other hand, because of the risk of reperfusion injury, a nearly perfect donor is required for patients who need SLT for pulmonary vascular disease.

Techniques for procuring and preserving donor lungs are continuing to evolve. Most centers use a cold, crystallized solution [Celsior™ (Genzyme Corporation, Cambridge, Massachusetts, U.S.A.) or Perfadex™ (Transplantation Systems, Goteborg, Sweden)] with a single-flush technique, preceded by an injection of prostaglandin E$_1$ into the pulmonary artery or as a systemic infusion titrated to the donor's blood pressure (19). Celsior and Perfadex are extracellular electrolyte solutions containing low concentrations of potassium; the administration of these solutions has been shown to reduce the likelihood and severity of ischemia-reperfusion injury (IRI) and to improve postischemic oxygenation and functional outcome. Prostaglandin E$_1$, a potent pulmonary vasodilator, improves distribution of the flush solution. Instilling the flush under a monitored pressure of 20 to 40 cmHg may avoid perfusion injury (20). Furthermore, inflating the lung with 100% oxygen, using moderate pressures (21), and transporting the lung at 4°C (22) have produced better graft outcomes in experimental models.

INTRAOPERATIVE MANAGEMENT
Surgical Techniques

The technique of performing lung transplantation has evolved substantially over the past two decades. Single and bilateral sequential lung transplantations are the procedures of choice; BLT with tracheal anastomosis has largely been abandoned because of problems related to ischemia at the anastomotic site. The recipient's condition is monitored with a pulmonary artery catheter, a peripheral artery catheter, and an end-tidal CO$_2$ monitor. Anesthesia may be initiated with a single-lumen endotracheal tube, particularly for patients with septic lung diseases who require preoperative (bronchoscopic) clearance of large airway secretions. However, the preferred approach requires changing to a double-lumen endotracheal tube for the operative procedure. Transesophageal echocardiography (TEE) should be performed so that right and left ventricular function can be assessed and the need for CPB can be determined. TEE can also help in assessing the outcome of the anastomosis between the pulmonary vein and the left atrium.

SLT is usually performed through a standard posterolateral thoracotomy incision, although anterior incisions have been used. The lung to be removed is deflated while ventilation to the contralateral lung is continued. BLT is performed through a transverse thoracosternotomy incision; transplantation of the right and left lungs is achieved by sequential single-lung transplant procedures. The lung with the poorer function is removed first. Clamping the pulmonary artery may worsen hypoxemia, hemodynamic instability, and echocardiographic evidence of right ventricular failure; inotropic support, pulmonary vasodilators (nitric oxide or prostaglandin E$_1$), or both may be necessary. CPB may become necessary at this point. Removal of the lung is completed by dividing the pulmonary artery and veins as far distally as possible and resecting the bronchus at the level of the takeoff of the upper lobe. Care must be taken not to injure the phrenic, vagus, and recurrent laryngeal nerves.

Graft implantation is begun with the bronchial anastomosis; next, the pulmonary artery is anastomosed; finally, the pulmonary vein is sutured to the left

Table 4 Criteria for Suitable Lung Donor

Preliminary assessment
  Age <55
  Clear lungs as documented on chest radiograph
  Oxygenation PaO$_2$ > 350 mmHg on FiO$_2$ 100% and PEEP 5 cmH$_2$O
  Adequate size match and ABO compatibility
  Negative history of smoking (≤20 pack years), chest trauma or thoracic
    surgery, aspiration, or sepsis
Final assessment
  Chest radiograph and oxygenation show no deterioration
  Results of bronchoscopy negative for aspiration
  Visual and manual assessment negative for contusions, trauma,
    and adhesions

Abbreviations: PaO$_2$, partial pressure of oxygen; FiO$_2$, fraction of inspired oxygen; PEEP, positive end-expiratory pressure; ABO, blood type A,B,O.
Source: Adapted from Ref. 16.

atrium. The donor bronchus is cut two cartilaginous rings above the takeoff of the upper lobe, and the membranous bronchi are approximated. The cartilaginous bronchi are telescoped, with intussusception of the donor and recipient bronchi. The pulmonary artery is anastomosed; then the left atrial anastomosis is performed with excision of the pulmonary venous stumps.

Before the anastomosis is completed, the clamps are removed from the pulmonary artery and vein, and air is evacuated from these vessels by flush irrigation. The vessels are then perfused with leukocyte-depleted blood. This sequence is repeated if BLT is performed. Hypoxemia or hemodynamic instability necessitates the use of CPB. After the chest has been closed, the double-lumen endotracheal tube is replaced by a large single-lumen endotracheal tube. The bronchial anastomosis is inspected by fiberoptic bronchoscopy and any blood clots or residual secretions are removed.

Application of Extracorporeal Membrane Oxygenation

Extracorporeal membrane oxygenation (ECMO) has been used intraoperatively to support the patient with immediate graft dysfunction that is refractory to medical treatment and standard methods of ventilation. ECMO is a useful bridge treatment for patients with severe IRI; it allows time for recovery and for retransplantation if the graft completely fails. ECMO differs from CPB in its artificial lung and blood reservoirs, mode of ventilator setting, methods of anticoagulation employed, temperature, and duration (23–25).

Circuits are placed either vein to vein (also called venovenous or V-V ECMO), for patients whose hemodynamic condition is stable, or vein to artery (venoarterial or V-A ECMO), for patients whose cardiac function is unstable. Access may be peripheral (via percutaneous catheter) or central (within the thoracic cavity). V-A ECMO requires minimal ventilator support, whereas V-V ECMO requires moderate ventilator settings. Small tidal volumes should be used with both methods so that the likelihood of lung injury can be reduced. The use of ECMO has been associated with an increased risk of renal and neurologic impairment (23). However, when used early to treat reversible lung injury, it can support the patient by providing adequate gas exchange and systemic perfusion (21–25).

COMPLICATIONS RELATED TO IMMEDIATE GRAFT DYSFUNCTION
Hyperacute Rejection

Hyperacute rejection results from preformed antibodies that target major allograft antigens; these antibodies result in rapidly progressive injury and graft failure within minutes to hours after transplantation. Pathologic findings include the presence of fibrin and platelet thrombi in arterioles and capillaries of the allograft, in association with prominent neutrophilia. Immunohistochemical analysis shows the presence of antibodies on the endotracheal surface and within vessel walls (26). This is followed by endothelial damage, leading to edema, hemorrhage, and infarction. Clinically, the graft becomes edematous, cyanotic, and mottled. Preformed antibodies to HLA antigens are almost always found and the outcome is uniformly fatal (26,27,29). Better techniques for detecting antibodies and improvements in crossmatching techniques are needed if this devastating problem is to be eliminated.

Ischemia-Reperfusion Injury

IRI is the most common cause of immediate graft dysfunction after lung transplantation. Although it has not been well defined, IRI, also called the reimplantation response, is a syndrome characterized by edema and infiltrates, worsening gas exchange, and histologic evidence of diffuse alveolar damage (28,30,31). Radiographic studies have demonstrated that as many as 97% of lung allografts exhibit perihilar edema in the immediate postoperative period (30,32). However, severe graft dysfunction has been reported among only 20% to 37% of recipients; the most severe cases produce a pattern similar to that of adult respiratory distress syndrome (30,33–35). Infection, rejection, volume overload, and pulmonary venous obstruction must be excluded. The cause of IRI appears to be increased vascular permeability related to ischemia and preservation, although no direct association with ischemic time, age, sex, or underlying disease has been found (34,35). CPB appears to increase the incidence and severity of IRI (35,36).

Treatment is largely supportive, but nitric oxide has been used (37). Selective lung ventilation has been attempted if lung injury is unilateral. ECMO may be required (38) and has been useful in allowing time for graft recovery. The risk of posttransplantation morbidity is increased for patients with IRI, if mechanical ventilation and intensive care unit stay are prolonged for more than 10 days. Mortality rates as high as 40% have been reported with severe injury (28). The condition of the graft with regard to donor abnormalities (contusion, aspiration, and preservation) may play a role in the severity of IRI. Efforts aimed at improving the outcomes associated with IRI must focus on preventing the release of cytokines, platelet activating factor, and complement; on preventing vascular endothelial injury; and on developing better preservation techniques.

PERIOPERATIVE COMPLICATIONS
Airway Complications

Anastomotic necrosis with dehiscence, once the primary limitation of lung transplantation, is now a rare occurrence; this fact reflects improvements in surgical techniques (40,41). Routine intussusception of the donor and recipient bronchi has helped to substantially reduce this once frequent complication (42,43). When it does occur, partial dehiscence is treated conservatively by placing a chest tube and reducing the steroid dosage; complete dehiscence may require surgical intervention (44). However, if necrosis is extensive and involves the upper lobe bronchus, resection with reanastomosis may not be possible and emergency retransplantation may be the only viable option (44).

Currently, the most common airway complications are bronchomalacia and stenosis at the site of the anastomosis; they occur in approximately 12% to 17% of cases (45–47). These complications can occur weeks to months after transplantation and often produce dyspnea, wheezing, and a decline in lung function with worsening airflow limitation as detected by spirometry. The definitive diagnosis is made with bronchoscopy, which shows luminal narrowing at the site of the anastomosis (34,35,43). Bronchial ischemia is related to resection of the bronchial arteries; reliance on retrograde pulmonary arterial blood to supply the airways has been implicated as a causative factor (35,44). Groups that perform revascularization of the bronchial arteries have reported better healing and a reduction in the rate of late stricture complications (3,40,46,47). However, this procedure adds technical complexity to the operation, and more data are needed if we are to determine how this added procedure might affect overall outcome.

Attempts at identifying other causes of airway complications, such as lung preservation and ischemic times, anastomotic techniques, corticosteroid dosing, and rejection, have led to inconclusive results (43). An association has been noted between *Aspergillus* colonization or infection and airway necrosis (44), whether *Aspergillus* infection results from or causes the necrosis is unclear.

The management of airway complications depends on the degree and location of the problem. A thin, web-like lesion may be amenable to laser therapy or bronchial balloon dilatation. However, most lesions require placement of an airway stent via bronchoscopy (43,44,47,48).

Complications of Native Lung Hyperinflation

Both SLT and BLT have been successfully used to treat patients with emphysema. Although there is no difference in the three-year survival rates associated with SLT and BLT, SLT has been preferred for older, high-risk patients because it is associated with a lower rate of perioperative complications (49). Radiographs of patients who have undergone SLT for emphysema frequently demonstrate mediastinal shift and ipsilateral diaphragmatic flattening, findings suggestive of native lung hyperinflation (NLH) (50–52). Symptomatic NLH has been reported to cause hemodynamic instability and respiratory dysfunction requiring independent lung ventilation (50). However, most studies have shown that NLH is not responsible for severe graft dysfunction or substantial increases in mortality rates (49–52). When it occurs, symptomatic NLH has been successfully treated with lung-volume reduction procedures on the native lung (53).

Renal Complications

Renal dysfunction among recipients of lung transplants has several causes. It may be a consequence of renal hypoperfusion during surgery, resulting from either hemodynamic instability or hypovolemia. Alternatively, it may occur as the result of acute renal tubular necrosis, often caused by immunosuppressive medications such as calcineurin inhibitors (tacrolimus or cyclosporine) and lympholytic agents. Close monitoring of calcineurin inhibitor levels and appropriate dose adjustments are essential. Drug interactions are common and can exert additive nephrotoxic effects.

Renal function declines most rapidly during the first six postoperative months. The clinical picture of chronic nephropathy is characterized by elevations in the serum creatinine concentration, decreases in creatinine clearance, disproportionate azotemia, hyperkalemia, proteinuria, decreases in sodium excretion, hypertension, and fluid retention. Diuresis is attempted first; if it is unsuccessful, hemodialysis is usually required.

Gastrointestinal Complications

Gastrointestinal problems have been reported to occur among as many as 42% of patients undergoing lung and heart–lung transplantation (54,55). Diarrhea, ileus, gastroparesis, ulcers, and ischemic bowel occur during the early posttransplantation period (55,56), whereas problems related to diverticulitis and posttransplantation lymphoproliferative disorders (PTLD) occur among long-term survivors (57). Symptomatic gastroparesis is a serious complication and has been reported to occur in as many as 25% of cases (58). Symptoms include early satiety with nausea, vomiting, and abdominal complaints; these symptoms are associated with prolonged gastric emptying. The pathophysiology of symptomatic gastroparesis is not completely understood, but inadvertent thermal or traumatic injury to the vagus nerve has been implicated (58). Direct toxic effects of immunosuppressive medicines have also been implicated (55,58), although gastroparesis has not been reported to occur among recipients of kidney and liver transplants who receive the same medications (58). Treatment may include the temporary use of jejunal feeding tubes and cholinergic stimulants, but subtotal gastrectomy or gastric bypass may occasionally be required (56).

Posttransplantation diarrhea is common and may be related to infection with agents such as *Clostridium difficile*, to colitis caused by cytomegalovirus (CMV), or to immunosuppressive medications such as mycophenolate mofetil (MMF). Differentiating immunosuppression-related disease from infection-related disease may be difficult. The presence of fever, inflammatory cells in the stool, moderate leukocytosis, and abnormal results on endoscopy, colonoscopy, or computed tomography suggest an infectious process (55). Reduction of the immunosuppressive regimen may be required.

Bone Complications

Osteoporosis can contribute substantially to morbidity after lung transplantation by limiting rehabilitation potential and impairing quality of life. As many as 35% to 40% of transplant recipients with osteoporosis can experience vertebral fractures; avascular necrosis of weight-bearing joints seems to occur less frequently (33). Most fractures are diagnosed by routine radiographs; however, more sophisticated methods are required for assessing bone mass and bone mineral content. The bone density scan has been used most often as a reliable assessment of osteoporosis.

Withdrawing corticosteroids from the treatment regimen of lung transplant recipients substantially slows the progression of osteoporosis. Regular active exercise, appropriate exposure to sunshine, oral calcium supplementation, and the administration of calcitonin, testosterone, estrogen, vitamin D, and biphosphonates have been successful in preventing osteoporosis among recipients of lung transplants.

Rejection
Acute Rejection

Acute rejection has been reported to occur as early as days and as late as years after lung transplantation. However, most episodes of acute rejection occur within the first three months after transplantation; the incidence declines thereafter (59,60). Substantial HLA mismatching, particularly at the HLA-DR and HLA-B foci, may be important risk factors (60,61). The clinical signs are nonspecific and may include fever, dyspnea, and impaired gas exchange. New infiltrates may be observed on radiographs within the first four to six weeks after transplantation; however, after that, changes in the results of chest radiography are uncommon (62). A decline in the forced expiratory volume in one second (FEV_1) is common; a 10% decrease in FEV_1 should signal the need for further diagnostic testing to rule out infection or rejection (63,64). When clinical findings suggest acute rejection, bronchoscopy with transbronchial biopsy is indicated and is the key to diagnosis (65,66).

The histologic classification of rejection was instituted in 1990 and revised in 1995 (29). Acute rejection is based on the intensity of perivascular mononuclear cell infiltrates and the extent of their extension into adjacent alveolar septae. Classification starts with Grade 0, normal pulmonary parenchyma, and Grade 1, minimal acute rejection with no obvious perivascular mononuclear infiltrates around blood vessels at low magnification. The classification extends to Grade 4, severe acute rejection with diffuse perivascular, interstitial, and airspace mononuclear cells, often associated with intra-alveolar macrophages, hyaline membranes, neutrophilic infiltrates, and hemorrhage (29). Infection can coexist with rejection and must be excluded before the immunosuppressive regimen is augmented.

Controversy exists about the need for routine surveillance bronchoscopy for patients with no clinical symptoms, and whose condition is physiologically stable. However, histologic rejection, usually minimal to mild, has been observed in as many as 39% of biopsy specimens (65,66). Discrepancies between clinical impression and histologic diagnosis appear to be greatest during the first six months after transplantation (67).

Standard treatment of acute rejection is 10 to 15 mg/kg of intravenously administered methylprednisolone daily for three successive days, followed by an increase in the maintenance dose of prednisone and subsequent tapering of the dose over one to two weeks. Most patients respond well to this treatment; follow-up biopsy is recommended. Recurrent or persistent acute rejection may be treated by repeated steroid boluses, by changing the immunosuppressive regimen from cyclosporine to tacrolimus, or from azathioprine to MMF, or by both. Antithymocyte globulin (ATG) and OKT3 monoclonal antibody have been used (68,69). Recurrent or refractory rejection is the primary risk factor for the subsequent development of bronchiolitis obliterans (70–75).

Chronic Rejection

Chronic rejection, characterized clinically by progressive allograft dysfunction and histologically by bronchiolitis obliterans, is the key factor limiting the long-term survival of recipients of lung transplants. Bronchiolitis obliterans is unusual during the first six months after transplantation but affects 60% to 70% of patients who survive for five years or longer (73–75). The clinical presentation includes progressive dyspnea and airflow limitation. Histologic studies show dense eosinophilic plaques in the submucosa of small airways; these plaques result in luminal narrowing (63). Chest radiographs may be nondiagnostic, but high-resolution computed tomography may show a reduction in graft volume, bronchiectasis, air space disease, atelectasis, and nodular opacities (76).

The diagnosis of bronchiolitis obliterans is often missed when the results of transbronchial biopsy are reviewed because of the characteristic patchy distribution of the disease and because of sampling error (77). As a result, the clinical criteria of bronchiolitis obliterans syndrome (BOS) have been developed on the basis of spirometric parameters (73). BOS is characterized by a decline in FEV_1 that is present for at least one month and is not caused by infection or acute rejection (73). Multiple treatment methods that augment the immunosuppressive regimen have been attempted (72) and may slow the decline in lung function. However, to date none of these methods have been proved to completely stop the progression of the disease (67,72,73,75).

Complications Related to Infection

Infectious complications are an important cause of morbidity and mortality among recipients of lung transplants (11,61,76). Their incidence appears to be much higher among recipients of lungs than among recipients of other solid organs (63), perhaps because the lung is the only allograft that is exposed to the environment. Associated factors such as lung denervation (which impairs cough reflex), lymphatic disruption, and impaired mucociliary clearance also play a role. Furthermore, infections can be transmitted from the donor or from the native lung or proximal airways of the recipient; they may also develop as a result of the decrease in immune defenses related to immunosuppression.

The lung is placed at an increased risk by airway instrumentation and is constantly at risk of aspiration. Anastomotic narrowing and airway mucosal edema may impair adequate clearance of organisms. Most infections among recipients of lung transplants occur within the lung allograft (35,77), although infections in the native lung have occurred among patients who have undergone SLT (78,79). Bacterial pathogens, frequently gram-negative organisms, predominate during the early posttransplantation period (33,76,77,80). Most centers empirically administer broad-spectrum antibiotics perioperatively and continue such administration until the specific organism involved has been determined by cultures from donor and recipient. Patients with septic lung diseases such as cystic fibrosis will require broad-spectrum antibiotics to cover the pathogens they carried before transplantation. Patients among whom BOS develops later are at an increased risk of colonization and infection with bacterial pathogens, predominantly *Pseudomonas* species (80).

Recipients of lung transplants frequently become colonized with *Candida* and *Aspergillus* species, but it is clinical infection with *Aspergillus*, which is associated with increased morbidity and mortality rates (33,77,80). Aspergillosis is acquired by inhaling spores and therefore occurs far more frequently among recipients of lung transplants (as many as 48%) than among recipients of other organs (81–85). The clinical presentation of Aspergillosis includes colonization, ulcerative tracheobronchitis, pseudomembranous tracheobronchitis, and invasive pneumonia (81–83). Aspergillosis has also been associated with ulcerative lesions that occur primarily at the anastomotic site. Scarring associated with the healing of these lesions results in stricture formation (82,85). Aspergillosis has been strongly associated with endobronchial

abnormalities and narrowing of airway anastomoses (82). Treatment includes the administration of 200 to 400 mg of itraconazole daily, with or without the addition of nebulized amphotericin B (86,87,89). Systemic amphotericin B and its lipid formulations have been the mainstay of therapy, but their use has been limited by toxic effects (84). Caspofungin, a new class of antifungal medications, has good activity against *Aspergillus* and offers an additional treatment option (88,89).

CMV is second to bacterial organisms as a cause of infection among recipients of lung transplants and has been frequently associated with the development of BOS (33,73,90,91). The prevalence of CMV infection in the United States is high; results of serologic testing for CMV indicate that more than half of the adults in the United States have been infected with this virus sometime during their lives. The risk of CMV disease after transplantation depends on the CMV status of the donor and the recipient. The risk is greatest when the recipient is seronegative and the donor is seropositive; CMV disease occurs among as many as 90% of patients in this group. When both the donor and the recipient are seronegative, the incidence of CMV disease is less than 15% (33,90–92). Seropositive recipients can experience reactivation of disease, particularly when their immunosuppressive regimen is augmented. Infection will usually occur between two weeks and three months after transplantation. The most common presentation of CMV disease is pneumonitis; however, gastroenteritis, hepatitis, colitis, and bone marrow depression have also been documented.

The diagnosis of CMV infection requires identification of the virus by culture, shell-vial assay, or polymerase chain reaction amplification of viral DNA from blood, urine, or bronchioalveolar lavage fluid. Definitive diagnosis of the disease requires histologic evidence of the characteristic cells in cytology or biopsy specimens (33). Ganciclovir and its derivative, valganciclovir, are the drugs of choice for the prophylaxis and treatment of CMV disease, but guidelines for their use appear to be center specific. Ongoing studies are needed to determine the best prophylactic and treatment regimens for this disease.

COMPLICATIONS OF IMMUNOSUPPRESSION

Standard immunosuppression for recipients of lung transplants is a triple-drug regimen that includes a calcineurin inhibitor (cyclosporine or tacrolimus), an inhibitor of purine biosynthesis (azathioprine or MMF) and corticosteroids. Acute rejection necessitates therapy with high doses of corticosteroids, whereas refractory acute rejection often requires lympholytic agents [rabbit ATG or horse antilymphocyte globulin (ALG)] or murine monoclonal antibody against the human CD3 T-cell antigen (OKT3). Serious toxic effects are associated with all immunosuppressive agents, and all patients must be diligently monitored for side effects and drug interactions. Both cyclosporine and tacrolimus can cause nephrotoxicity, neurotoxicity (including headache and tremors), and hypertension. Tacrolimus more commonly causes hyperglycemia, whereas cyclosporine more commonly causes hirsutism and gingival hyperplasia. Azathioprine can cause bone marrow depression and toxicity to the pancreas and liver, whereas MMF more commonly causes gastrointestinal side effects, particularly diarrhea. Complications related to steroid use are well known and include Cushing's syndrome, hyperglycemia, hyperlipidemia, osteoporosis, peptic ulcer disease, and cataracts. OKT3 can cause a cytokine-release syndrome with hypotension and pulmonary edema, whereas ATG and ALG can produce a serum sickness reaction. All immunosuppressive agents enhance the risk of opportunistic infections and malignancy such as PTLD (33,93).

LIVING-DONOR LUNG TRANSPLANTATION

The limited number of cadaveric lung donors prompted Starnes et al. to initiate living-donor lung transplantation in 1993 (94). By December 2000, 139 such procedures had been performed (95). Two donors are required, one to provide a right lower lobe and the other to provide a left lower lobe. Donors must be aged between 18 and 55, be in good health, and have undergone no thoracic procedures on the side from which the lung is to be donated. Donors are matched on blood type and should be taller than the recipient. They must pass through rigorous psychosocial screening (96). Although for adults, the outcomes of living-donor lung transplantation are similar to those of cadaveric lung transplantation (97), living-donor lung transplantation has been associated with improved graft function and fewer cases of BOS among children (98). Studies of complication rates have therefore focused on donors. In one group, 61.3% of donors (38 of 62 patients) suffered postoperative complications; the most severe were pleural effusions requiring drainage, bronchial stump fistulas, phrenic nerve injury, atrial flutter necessitating ablation, and bronchial stricture (99). Clearly, more data are needed for evaluating morbidity rates among the donors before living-donor lung transplantation is universally accepted as an alternative to cadaveric lung transplantation.

CONCLUSION

Lung transplantation is continuing to evolve as an acceptable option for patients with end-stage lung disease. The complication of anastomotic dehiscence, once thought to be the limiting factor in lung transplantation, has been overcome and has given way to problems related to IRI, hyperacute and acute rejection, airway dysfunction, infection, and bronchiolitis obliterans. However, continued improvements in immunosuppressive regimens, antibiotic choices, crossmatching, and organ preservation techniques, as well as research focused on vascular endothelial injury and immune tolerance, should help reduce the complications of lung transplantation in the future.

REFERENCES

1. Hardy JD, Webb SR, Dalton ML Jr, Walker GR Jr. Lung homotransplantation in man. JAMA 1963; 186:1065–1074.
2. Veith FJ. Lung transplantation. Surg Clin North Am 1978; 58:357–364.
3. Daly RC, McGregor CG. Surgical issues in lung transplantation: options, donor selection, graft preservation, and airway healing. Mayo Clin Proc 1997; 72:79–84.
4. Reitz BA, Wallwork JL, Hunt SA, et al. Heart-lung transplantation: successful therapy for patients with pulmonary vascular disease. N Engl J Med 1982; 306:557–564.
5. Toronto Lung Transplant Group. Unilateral lung transplantation for pulmonary fibrosis. N Engl J Med 1986; 314:1140–1145.
6. Patterson GA, Todd TR, Cooper JD, Pearson FG, Winton TL, Maurer J. Airway complications after double lung transplantation. Toronto Lung Transplant Group. J Thorac Cardiovasc Surg 1990; 99:14–21.
7. Daly RC, Tadjkarimi S, Khaghani A, Banner NR, Yacoub MH. Successful double-lung transplantation with direct bronchial artery revascularization. Ann Thorac Surg 1993; 56:885–892.
8. Cooper JD, Patterson GA, Grossman R, Maurer JR. Double-lung transplant for advanced chronic obstructive lung disease. Am Rev Respir Dis 1989; 139(2):303–307.
9. Pasque MR, Cooper JD, Kaiser LR, Haydock DA, Triantafillou A, Trulock RJ. Improved technique for bilateral lung transplantation: rationale and initial clinical experience. Ann Thorac Surg 1990; 49:785–791.
10. Hosenpud JD, Bennett LE, Keck BM, Boucek MM, Novick RJ. The Registry of the International Society for Heart and Lung Transplantation: seventeenth official report-2000. J Heart Lung Transplant 2000; 19:909–931.
11. Maurer JR, Frost AE, Estenne M, Higenbottam T, Glanville AR. International guidelines for the selection of lung transplant candidates. The International Society for Heart and Lung Transplantation, the American Thoracic Society, the American Society of Transplant Physicians, the European Respiratory Society. J Heart Lung Transplant 1998; 17:703–709.
12. Detterbeck FC, Egan TM, Mill MR. Lung transplantation after previous thoracic surgical procedures. Ann Thorac Surg 1995; 60:139–143.
13. Dusmet M, Winton TL, Kesten S, Maurer J. Previous intrapleural procedures do not adversely affect lung transplantation. J Heart Lung Transplant 1996; 15:249–254.
14. Schafers HJ, Wagner TO, Demertzis S, et al. Preoperative corticosteroids. A contraindication to lung transplantation? Chest 1992; 102:1522–1525.

15. Baz MA, Palmer SM, Staples ED, Greer DG, Tapson VF, Davis DD. Lung transplantation after long-term mechanical ventilation: results and 1-year follow-up. Chest 2001; 119:224–227.
16. Davis RD Jr., Pasque MK. Pulmonary transplantation. Ann Surg 1995; 221:14–28.
17. Tyan DB, Li VA, Czer L, Trento A, Jordan SC. Intravenous immunoglobulin suppression of HLA alloantibody in highly sensitized transplant candidates and transplantation with a histoincompatible organ. Transplantation 1994; 57:553–562.
18. Halldorsson AO, Kronon MT, Allen BS, Rahman S, Wang T. Lowering reperfusion pressure reduces the injury after pulmonary ischemia. Ann Thorac Surg 2000; 69:198–204.
19. Date H, Matsumura A, Manchester JK, Cooper JM, Lowry OH, Cooper JD. Changes in alveolar oxygen and carbon dioxide concentration and oxygen consumption during lung preservation. The maintenance of aerobic metabolism during lung preservation. J Thorac Cardiovasc Surg 1993; 105:492–501.
20. Wang LS, Nakamoto K, Hsieh CM, Miyoshi S, Cooper JD. Influence of temperature of flushing solution on lung preservation. Ann Thorac Surg 1993; 55:711–715.
21. Meyers BF, Sundt TM III, Henry S, et al. Selective use of extracorporeal membrane oxygenation is warranted after lung transplantation. J Thorac Cardiovasc Surg 2000; 120:20–26.
22. Zenati M, Pham SM, Keenan RJ, Griffith BP. Extracorporeal membrane oxygenation for lung transplant recipients with primary severe donor lung dysfunction. Transplant Int 1996; 9:227–230.
23. Vlasselaers D, Verleden GM, Meyns B, et al. Femoral venoarterial extracorporeal membrane oxygenation for severe reimplantation response after lung transplantation. Chest 2000; 118:559–561.
24. Choi JK, Kearns J, Palevsky HI, et al. Hyperacute rejection of a pulmonary allograft. Immediate clinical and pathologic findings. Am J Respir Crit Care Med 1999; 160:1015–1018.
25. Christie JD, Bavaria JE, Palevsky HI, et al. Primary graft failure following lung transplantation. Chest 1998; 114:51–60.
26. Frost AE, Jammal CT, Cagle PT. Hyperacute rejection following lung transplantation. Chest 1996; 110:559–562.
27. Zander DS, Baz MA, Visner GA, et al. Analysis of early deaths after isolated lung transplantation. Chest 2001; 120:225–232.
28. King RC, Binns OA, Rodriguez F, et al. Reperfusion injury significantly impacts clinical outcome after pulmonary transplantation. Ann Thorac Surg 2000; 69:1681–1685.
29. Yousem SA, Berry GJ, Cagle PT, et al. Revision of the 1990 working formulation for the classification of pulmonary allograft rejection: Lung Rejection Study Group. J Heart Lung Transplant 1996; 15:1–15.
30. Anderson DC, Glazer HS, Semenkovich JW, et al. Lung transplant edema: chest radiography after lung transplantation—the first 10 days. Radiology 1995; 195:275–281.
31. Haydock DA, Trulock EP, Kaiser LR, Knight SR, Pasque MK, Cooper JD. Management of dysfunction in the transplanted lung: experience with 7 clinical cases. Washington University Lung Transplant Group. Ann Thorac Surg 1992; 53:635–641.
32. Paradis IL, Duncan SR, Dauber JH, Yousem S, Hardesty R, Griffity B. Distinguishing between infection, rejection, and the adult respiratory distress syndrome after human lung transplantation. J Heart Lung Transplant 1992; 11:S232–S236.
33. Trulock EP. Lung transplantation. Am J Respir Crit Care Med 1997; 155:789–818.
34. Chapparro C, Chamberlain D, Maurer J, De Hoyos A, Winton T, Kesten S. Acute lung injury in lung allografts. J Heart Lung Transplant 1995; 14:267–273.
35. Khan SU, Salloum J, O'Donovan PB, et al. Acute pulmonary edema after lung transplantation: the pulmonary reimplantation response. Chest 1999; 116:187–194.
36. Aeba R, Griffith BP, Kormos RL, et al. Effect of cardiopulmonary bypass on early graft dysfunction in clinical lung transplantation. Ann Thorac Surg 1994; 57:715–722.
37. Date H, Triantafillou AN, Trulock EP, Pohl MS, Cooper JD, Patterson GA. Inhaled nitric oxide reduces human lung allograft dysfunction. J Thorac Cardiovasc Surg 1996; 111:913–919.
38. Glassman LR, Keenan RJ, Fabrizio MC, et al. Extracorporeal membrane oxygenation as an adjunct treatment for primary graft failure in adult lung transplant recipients. J Thorac Cardiovasc Surg 1995; 110:723–727.
39. Whyte RI, Deeb GM, McCurry KR, Anderson HL III, Bolling SF, Bartlett RH. Extracorporeal life support after heart or lung transplantation. Ann Thorac Surg 1994; 58:754–759.
40. Kshettry VR, Kroshus TJ, Hertz MI, Hunter DW, Shumway SJ, Bolman RM III. Early and late airway complications after lung transplantation: incidence and management. Ann Thorac Surg 1997; 63:1576–1583.
41. Date H, Trulock EP, Arcidi JM, Sundaresan S, Cooper JD, Patterson GA. Impaired airway healing after lung transplantation. An analysis of 348 bronchial anastomoses. J Thorac Cardiovasc Surg 1995; 110:1424–1433.
42. Kirk AJ, Conacher ID, Corris PA, Ashcroft T, Dark JH. Successful surgical management of bronchial dehiscence after single-lung transplantation. Ann Thorac Surg 1990; 49:147–149.
43. Shennib H, Massard G. Airway complications in lung transplantation. Ann Thorac Surg 1994; 57:506–511.
44. Herrera JM, McNeil KD, Higgens RS, et al. Airway complications after lung transplantation: treatment and long-term outcome. Ann Thorac Surg 2001; 71:989–994.
45. Daly RC, McGregor CG. Routine immediate direct bronchial artery revascularization for single-lung transplantation. Ann Thorac Surg 1994; 57:1446–1452.
46. Couraud L, Baudet E, Martigne C, et al. Bronchial revascularization in double-lung transplantation: a series of 8 patients. Bordeaux Lung and Heart-Lung Transplant Group. Ann Thorac Surg 1992; 53:88–94.
47. Norgaard MA, Olsen PS, Svendsen UG, Pettersson G. Revascularization of the bronchial arteries in lung transplantation: an overview. Ann Thorac Surg 1996; 62:1215–1221.
48. Susanto I, Peters JI, Levine SM, Sako EY, Anzueto A, Bryan CL. Use of balloon-expandable metallic stents in the management of bronchial stenosis and bronchomalacia after lung transplantation. Chest 1998; 114:1330–1335.

49. Trulock EP III. Lung transplantation for COPD. Chest 1998; 113:269S–276S.

50. Mal H, Brugiere O, Sleiman C, et al. Morbidity and mortality related to the native lung in single lung transplantation for emphysema. J Heart Lung Transplant 2000; 19:220–223.

51. Weill D, Torres F, Hodges TN, Olmos JJ, Zamora MR. Acute native lung hyperinflation is not associated with poor outcomes after single lung transplant for emphysema. J Heart Lung Transplant 1999; 18:1080–1087.

52. Yonan NA, el-Gamel A, Egan J, Kakadellis J, Rahman A, Deiraniya AK. Single lung transplantation for emphysema: predictors for native lung hyperinflation. J Heart Lung Transplant 1998; 17:192–201.

53. Kroshus TJ, Bolman RM III, Kshettry VR. Unilateral volume reduction after single-lung transplantation for emphysema. Ann Thorac Surg 1996; 62:363–368.

54. Berkowitz N, Schulman LL, McGregor C, Markowitz D. Gastroparesis after lung transplantation. Potential role in postoperative respiratory complications. Chest 1995; 108:1602–1607.

55. Smith PC, Slaughter MS, Petty MG, Shumway SJ, Kshettry VR, Bolman RM III. Abdominal complications after lung transplantation. J Heart Lung Transplant 1995; 14:44–51.

56. Hoekstra HJ, Hawkins K, de Boer WJ, Rottier K, van der Bij W. Gastrointestinal complications in lung transplant survivors that require surgical intervention. Br J Surg 2001; 88:433–438.

57. Arcasoy SM, Kotloff RM. Lung transplantation. N Engl J Med 1999; 340:1081–1091.

58. Akindipe OA, Faul JL, Vierra MA, Triadafilopoulos G, Theodore J. The surgical management of severe gastroparesis in heart/lung transplant recipient. Chest 2000; 117:907–910.

59. Bando K, Paradis IL, Komatsu K, et al. Analysis of time-dependent risks for infection, rejection, and death after pulmonary transplantation. J Thorac Cardiovasc Surg 1995; 109:49–59.

60. Wisser W, Wekerle T, Zlabinger G, et al. Influence of human leukocyte antigen matching on long-term outcome after lung transplantation. J Heart Lung Transplant 1996; 15:1209–1216.

61. Schulman LL, Weinberg AD, McGregor C, Galantowicz ME, Suciu-Foca NM, Itescu S. Mismatches at the HLA-DR and HLA-B loci are risk factors for acute rejection after lung transplantation. Am J Respir Crit Care Med 1998; 157:1833–1837.

62. Millet B, Higenbottam TW, Flower CD, Stewart S, Wallwork J. The radiographic appearances of infection and acute rejection of the lung after heart-lung transplantation. Am Rev Respir Dis 1989; 140:62–67.

63. Otulana BA, Higenbottam T, Ferrari L, Scott J, Igboaka G, Wallwork J. The use of home spirometry in detecting acute lung rejection and infection following heart-lung transplantation. Chest 1990; 97:353–357.

64. Becker FS, Martinez FJ, Brunsting LA, Deeb GM, Flint A, Lynch JP III. Limitations of spirometry in detecting rejection after single-lung transplantation. Am J Respir Crit Care Med 1994; 150:159–166.

65. Guilinger RA, Paradis IL, Dauber JH, et al. The importance of bronchoscopy with transbronchial lung biopsy and bronchoalveolar lavage in the management of lung transplant recipients. Am J Respir Crit Care Med 1995; 152:2037–2043.

66. Sibley RK, Berry GJ, Tazelaar HD, et al. The role of transbronchial lung biopsies in the management of lung transplant recipients. J Heart Lung Transplant 1993; 12:308–324.

67. Fertel DP, Qi XS, Pham SM. Treatment strategies for obliterate bronchiolitis. Curr Opinion in Organ Transplant 2001; 6:231–238.

68. Shennib H, Massard G, Reynaud M, Noirclerc M. Efficacy of OKT3 therapy for acute rejection in isolated lung transplantation. J Heart Lung Transplant 1994; 13:514–519.

69. Shennib H, Mercado M, Nguyen D, et al. Successful treatment of steroid-resistant double-lung allograft rejection with Orthoclone OKT3. Am Rev Respir Dis 1991; 144:224–226.

70. Bando K, Paradis IL, Similo S, et al. Obliterative bronchiolitis after lung and heart-lung transplantation: an analysis of risk factors and management. J Thorac Cardiovasc Surg 1995; 110:4–14.

71. Scott JP, Higenbottam TW, Sharples L, et al. Risk factors for obliterative bronchiolitis in heart-lung transplant recipients. Transplantation 1991; 51:813–817.

72. Reichenspurner H, Girgis RE, Robbins RC, et al. Stanford experience with obliterative bronchiolitis after lung and heart-lung transplantation. Ann Thorac Surg 1996; 62:1467–1473.

73. Heng D, Sharples LD, McNeil K, Stewart S, Wreghitt T, Wallwork J. Bronchiolitis obliterans syndrome: incidence, natural history, prognosis, and risk factors. J Heart Lung Transplant 1998; 17:1255–1263.

74. Girgis RE, Tu I, Berry GJ, et al. Risk factors for the development of obliterative bronchiolitis after lung transplantation. J Heart Lung Transplant 1996; 15:1200–1208.

75. Boehler A, Estenne M. Obliterative bronchiolitis after lung transplantation. Curr Opin Pulm Med 2000; 6:133–139.

76. Soyer P, Devine N, Frachon I, et al. Computed tomography of complications of lung transplantation. Eur Radiol 1997; 7:847–853.

77. Kramer MR, Stoehr C, Whang JL, et al. The diagnosis of obliterative bronchiolitis after heart-lung transplantation: low yield of transbronchial lung biopsy. J Heart Lung Transplant 1993; 12:675–681.

78. Cooper JD, Billingham M, Egan T, et al. A working formulation for the standardization of nomenclature and for clinical staging of chronic dysfunction in lung allografts. International Society for Heart and Lung Transplantation. J Heart Lung Transplant 1993; 12:713–716.

79. Horvath J, Dummer S, Loyd J, Walker B, Merrill WH, Frist WH. Infection in the transplanted and native lung after single lung transplantation. Chest 1993; 104:681–685.

80. Flume PA, Egan TM, Paradowski LJ, Detterbeck FC, Thompson JT, Yankaskas JR. Infectious complications of lung transplantation. Impact of cystic fibrosis. Am J Respir Crit Care Med 1994; 149:1601–1607.

81. Yeldandi V, Laghi F, McCabe MA, et al. Aspergillus and lung transplantation. J Heart Lung Transplant 1995; 14:883–890.

82. Nathan SD, Shorr AF, Schmidt ME, Burton NA. Aspergillus and endobronchial abnormalities in lung transplant recipients. Chest 2000; 118:403–407.

83. Westney GE, Kesten S, De Hoyos A, Chapparro C, Winton T, Maurer JR. Aspergillus infection in single and double lung transplant recipients. Transplantation 1996; 61:915–919.

84. Nunley DR, Ohori P, Grgurich WF, et al. Pulmonary aspergillosis in cystic fibrosis lung transplant recipients. Chest 1998; 114:1321–1329.

85. Kramer MR, Denning DW, Marshall SE, et al. Ulcerative tracheobronchitis after lung transplantation. A new form of invasive aspergillosis. Ann Rev Respir Dis 1991; 144:552–526.

86. Boettcher H, Bewig B, Hirt SW, Moller F, Cremer J. Topical amphotericin B application in severe bronchial aspergillosis after lung transplantation: report of experiences in 3 cases. J Heart Lung Transplant 2000; 19:1224–1227.

87. Monforte V, Roman A, Gavalda J, et al. Nebulized amphotericin B prophylaxis for Aspergillus infection in lung transplantation: study of risk factors. J Heart Lung Transplant 2001; 20:1274–1281.

88. Andriole VT. The 1998 Garrod lecture. Current and future antifungal therapy: new targets for antifungal agents. J Antimicrob Chemother 1999; 44:151–162.

89. Wood DE, Raghu G. Lung transplantation. Part II. Postoperative management and results. West J Med 1997; 166:45–55.

90. Keenan RJ, Lega ME, Dummer JS, et al. Cytomegalovirus serologic status and postoperative infection correlated with risk of developing chronic rejection after pulmonary transplantation. Transplantation 1991; 51:433–438.

91. Duncan SR, Paradis IL, Yousem SA, et al. Sequelae of cytomegalovirus pulmonary infections in lung allograft recipients. Am Rev Respir Dis 1992; 146:1419–1425.

92. Griffith BP, Bando K, Armitage JM, et al. Lung transplantation at the University of Pittsburgh. Clin Transpl 1992; 13:149–159.

93. Hausen B, Morris RE. Review of immunosuppression for lung transplantation. Novel drugs, new uses for conventional immunosuppressants, and alternative strategies. Clin Chest Med 1997; 18:353–366.

94. Starnes VA, Barr ML, Cohen RG. Lobar transplantation. Indications, techniques, and outcome. J Thorac Cardiovasc Surg 1994; 108:403–411.

95. DeMeo DL, Ginns LC. Clinical status of lung transplantation. Transplantation 2001; 72:1713–1724.

96. Barr ML, Baker CJ, Schenkel FA, et al. Living donor lung transplantation: selection, technique, and outcome. Transplant Proc 2001; 33:3527–3532.

97. Starnes VA, Woo MS, MacLaughlin EF, et al. Comparison of outcomes between living donor and cadaveric lung transplantation in children. Ann Thorac Surg 1999; 68:2279–2284.

98. Woo MS, MacLaughlin EF, Horn MV, Szmuszkovicz JR, Barr ML, Starnes VA. Bronchiolitis obliterans is not the primary cause of death in pediatric living donor lobar lung transplant recipients. J Heart Lung Transplant 2001; 20:491–496.

99. Battafarano RJ, Anderson RC, Meyers BF, et al. Perioperative complications after living donor lobectomy. J Thorac Cardiovasc Surg 2000; 120:909–915.

25

Complications After Cardiopulmonary Resuscitation and Cardiac Arrest

Abhijit S. Pathak, Amy J. Goldberg, and Robert F. Buckman, Jr.
*Department of Surgery, Temple University School of Medicine,
Philadelphia, Pennsylvania, U.S.A.*

Cardiopulmonary resuscitation (CPR) is typically performed in one of three locations: the emergency department, the operating room, or the intensive care unit (ICU). The surgeon's initial response to cardiac arrest depends on the presumed cause of the arrest, on whether the arrest was witnessed, and on the patient's clinical status (e.g., whether the arrest occurred intraoperatively while the patient's abdomen or chest was open).

Whenever cardiac arrest occurs, the well-known airway, breathing, circulation (ABC) algorithm must be emphasized. Furthermore, because the surgeon is most likely to encounter cardiac arrest in a hospital environment, it is likely that adequate monitoring will be in place and that support personnel competent to initiate CPR will be available.

Only rarely will surgeons be involved in treating a patient who suffers sudden cardiac death. With a few exceptions, such as trauma, sudden massive pulmonary thromboembolism, or massive myocardial infarction, most episodes of cardiac arrest with which surgeons are involved are associated with serious multiorgan dysfunction.

CAUSES OF AND FACTORS UNDERLYING CARDIAC ARREST

If cardiac arrest is to be successfully managed, certain underlying factors must be recognized and corrected. In general, cardiac compromise or arrest can be broadly categorized as due to nontraumatic or traumatic causes. Nontraumatic arrest can be further categorized as resulting from respiratory factors, cardiac factors, neurologic factors, or metabolic or electrolyte disturbances. Table 1 outlines the causes of nontraumatic arrest, and Table 2 outlines the causes of traumatic arrest.

PATHOPHYSIOLOGY OF CARDIAC ARREST

Understanding the pathophysiology of the precipitating event will help guide and direct the management of cardiac arrest during the resuscitation phase and the postresuscitation period.

Cardiac arrest results in cessation of blood flow; however, the vulnerability of organs to ischemic injury differs. The central nervous system, particularly the brain, is the most susceptible to such injury; the most vulnerable areas of the brain are the cerebral cortex, the hippocampus, and the cerebellum. Irreversible brain damage can be expected after five minutes of normothermic cardiac arrest. If the blood flow to the brain is not restored within ten minutes, restoration of neurologic function rarely occurs. The heart is the second most vulnerable organ to ischemia; the endocardium is more sensitive than the epicardium. The kidneys, gastrointestinal tract, and musculoskeletal system are much more tolerant to the disruption of blood blow and can tolerate long periods of normothermic ischemia (up to one hour) without permanent damage, if adequate reperfusion is reestablished.

Cessation of cardiac function results from one of three causes: ventricular fibrillation (VF) or pulseless ventricular tachycardia (VT); ventricular asystole; or pulseless electrical activity (PEA) (1).

Ventricular Fibrillation or Pulseless Ventricular Tachycardia

VF or pulseless VT usually results from a primary cardiac event such as acute myocardial infarction or ischemia. The presence of antecedent multifocal premature ventricular contractions may serve as a warning sign for these serious conditions. Certain electrolyte disturbances, such as hypokalemia, hypomagnesemia, or hypocalcemia, may complicate or contribute to this scenario (Table 1). In cases of traumatic cardiac arrest, ventricular irritability may suggest air embolism or cardiac compression caused by a tension pneumothorax or pericardial tamponade. Electrocution with alternating current in the range of 100 mA to 1 A can also cause VF (Table 2).

Table 1 Factors Causing or Contributing to Nontraumatic Cardiac Arrest

Respiratory factors	*Neurologic factors*
Airway obstruction	Central depression
CNS injury	Stroke
Foreign body	Anesthesia
Infection	Drugs or toxins
Trauma	
Tumor	*Metabolic or electrolyte factors*
Insufficient ventilation	Acidosis
CNS injury	Alkalosis
Neuromuscular disease	Hypokalemia or hyperkalemia
Drugs	Hypomagnesemia or
Hypoxemia or pulmonary dysfunction	hypermagnesemia
COPD	Hypocalcemia
Asthma	Hypothermia
Pulmonary edema	
Venous thromboembolism	*Drugs or toxins*
Pneumonia	Beta-blockers
	Calcium channel blockers
Cardiovascular factors	Digoxin
Cardiac factors	Antiarrhythmics
Acute coronary occlusion	Tricyclic antidepressants
Coronary artery disease	Carbon monoxide
Drugs	Cyanide
Reduced cardiac output	Cocaine
Cardiomyopathy	
Valvular or structural abnormalities	
Tension pneumothorax	
Pericardial tamponade	
Pulmonary embolism	
Circulatory factors	
Hypovolemia or hemorrhage	
Vasodilatory shock	
Sepsis	
Neurogenic shock	

Abbreviations: CNS, central nervous system; COPD, chronic obstructive pulmonary disease.

Ventricular Asystole

Asystole usually results from cardiac arrest while the heart was in diastole. Asystole may be the final outcome of a process beginning with bradycardia in patients with hypoxemia caused by respiratory failure, by a vasovagal event, or by a metabolic disturbance such

Table 2 Factors Causing or Contributing to Traumatic Cardiac Arrest

Exsanguination
Hypovolemia or hemorrhage
Cardiac injury
Pericardial tamponade
Tension pneumothorax
Air embolism
Airway obstruction
Extrinsic compression
  CNS depression
  Direct injury
  Intraluminal or oropharyngeal bleeding
Hemic drowning
Drowning or near-drowning
Severe brain injury
Spinal cord injury
Electrocution
Hypothermia

Abbreviation: CNS, central nervous system.

as hyperkalemia. Furthermore, asystole may be the result of exsanguination: in this event, the progression from tachycardia to bradycardia and PEA finally degenerates to asystole. Electrocution with alternating current of more than 10 A can also result in ventricular asystole.

Pulseless Electrical Activity

PEA occurs when a heart rhythm is present but cardiac output is absent. Common causes of PEA include severe hypoxia, hypovolemia, hypothermia, acidosis, tension pneumothorax, and pericardial tamponade.

PHYSIOLOGY OF STANDARD CLOSED-CHEST CARDIOPULMONARY RESUSCITATION
Cardiac Pump Model

Kouwenhoven et al. (2) first suggested that CPR works as a cardiac pump by squeezing the heart between the sternum and the spine. Each chest compression results in systole, with the left ventricle compressed and blood propelled forward. Because the cardiac valves operate in only one direction, prograde flow into the arterial circulation is guaranteed. The relaxation phase of CPR, which allows the sternum to return to its normal position, corresponds to diastole, during which intracardiac pressures fall, the atrioventricular valves open, and venous return occurs.

Thoracic Pump Model

Most physiologists favor the thoracic pump model of CPR (3). In this model, forward flow is generated by an arteriovenous pressure gradient that is established by chest compression. External compression of the chest generates an increase in thoracic pressure that is transmitted throughout the thorax, including the heart, the aorta, and the great veins. According to this model, the mitral and tricuspid valves are incompetent and no significant atrioventricular or ventriculo-aortic pressure gradients are present.

Perfusion During Cardiopulmonary Resuscitation

Closed-chest CPR results in only limited perfusion of vital organs. Cardiac output is believed to be no more than 25% of normal and cerebral blood flow is believed to be only about 15% of normal (3,4). Furthermore, coronary blood flow during standard CPR may be as low as 5% of normal (4).

MANAGEMENT OF CARDIAC ARREST

The American Heart Association has established standards for basic life support, advanced cardiac life support, and CPR (5,6). These standards and guidelines are readily available and will not be discussed here.

The management of cardiac arrest begins with the ABC algorithm mentioned above. However, there is one instance in which this orderly rule may be circumvented: when patients who are being monitored experience VF, immediate defibrillation takes precedence over airway management, pharmacotherapy, and CPR because hypoxemia and prolonged fibrillation have not yet developed.

As stated above, closed-chest compressions provide only a fraction of the normal cardiac output, even under optimal conditions. If standard closed-chest CPR fails to provide effective circulation, the surgeon may consider using open-chest cardiac massage. Under certain circumstances, resuscitative thoracotomy and open-chest cardiac massage may be the only means of effective resuscitation after nontraumatic cardiac arrest. Because most physiologists subscribe to the thoracic pump model of CPR, effective circulation may not be provided when the transmission of pressure throughout the thorax is impossible, such as when the abdomen or chest is open. Especially for trauma victims, the situation may be compounded by hypovolemia or an unstable chest wall, which renders conventional CPR ineffective. These conditions are most commonly encountered in the operating room, during laparotomy or thoracotomy, and in the ICU, where patients may have an open abdomen because a laparotomy has been performed to treat injuries. In such circumstances, open cardiac massage via resuscitative thoracotomy or a transdiaphragmatic route (if done during laparotomy) may be the only hope for survival.

Direct cardiac massage through a minimally invasive approach rather than an open thoracotomy has been reported (7,8). This procedure, called minimally invasive directed cardiac massage, involves inserting a heart-contracting padded baseplate, connected to a handle, through a 2- to 3-cm incision in the left parasternal area. The handle remains outside the chest, and the baseplate is positioned directly on the ventricles with the pericardium intact. Manual decompression of the device compresses the heart and causes an artificial systole. In a swine model of cardiac arrest (7), this technique provided coronary and cerebral perfusion similar to that achieved using standard open-chest cardiac massage. A European pilot study (8) using this technique in the prehospital setting demonstrated promising results.

The management scheme described above is appropriate in cases of nontraumatic cardiac arrest. In cases of trauma, resuscitative thoracotomy is vital for patients who are in extremis or whose condition deteriorates so that cardiac arrest appears imminent. For trauma victims, thoracotomy may be necessary to relieve pericardial tamponade, control thoracic bleeding, control air embolism, allow open cardiac massage, provide temporary aortic occlusion so as to maximize cerebral and coronary perfusion, and limit infradiaphragmatic bleeding (9).

TECHNIQUE OF RESUSCITATIVE THORACOTOMY AND OPEN CARDIAC MASSAGE

The technique of resuscitative thoracotomy and open cardiac massage has been reviewed by Buckman

et al. (10). In most instances, the patient is placed supine with the left arm raised above the head. For men, a standard left anterolateral thoracotomy incision is begun just lateral to the left border of the sternum and carried in a straight line laterally to a point just below the nipple (Figs. 1 and 2). For women, the incision is placed in the inframammary crease, and the breast is held under cephalad traction. The chest is entered through the fifth intercostal space. During most emergency thoracotomy procedures, the pericardium is opened with an incision that begins anterior to the phrenic nerve and proceeds longitudinally so as to avoid transecting the nerve. The pericardium must be opened widely so that the heart can be delivered through the incision (Fig. 3). An inadequate pericardiotomy may impede effective cardiac output during open massage or result in cardiac arrest because inflow is occluded.

Manual cardiac massage should be performed with both hands. In this technique, the hands should be slightly cupped and placed on the anterior and posterior surfaces of the heart. The ventricles are cyclically compressed as shown in Figure 4. The fingertips should be flat against the epicardial surface. Most studies have indicated that the optimal rate of manual cardiac massage is approximately 60 beats/min.

Aortic cross clamping is generally performed at the outset of cardiac massage; its purpose is to help maximize cerebral and coronary flow. The first step in clamping the aorta is to locate the descending vessel by anteriorly retracting the left lung with the left hand, a maneuver that is facilitated if the lung is deflated. Direct visualization of the aorta is ideal but can be very difficult to achieve; blind dissection may be necessary. The surgeon should run the fingers over the anterior spine until the space between the spine and

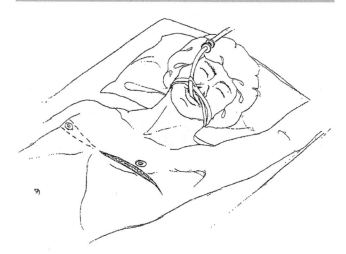

Figure 1 The standard skin- and soft-tissue incision for a left anterolateral resuscitative thoracotomy extends in a straight line from the left border of the sternum to the posterior axillary line. The incision may be extended into the right chest at the same level or one intercostal space higher.

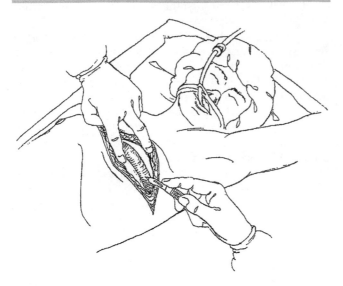

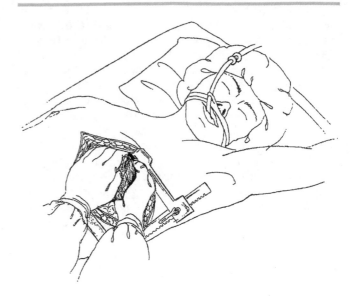

Figure 2 Once the plane of the ribs and intercostal muscles has been reached, the intercostal muscle is thinned with a knife, but the pleura is entered with a finger or blunt-tipped scissors to avoid iatrogenic laceration of the heart or the lungs. The intercostal space is then opened widely with scissors.

Figure 4 Bimanual cardiac massage is performed via a left anterolateral thoracotomy. The fingertips must be kept flat on the cardiac surface to avoid iatrogenic cardiac penetration. Excessive traction on the heart should be avoided because it can result in obstruction of venous inflow.

aorta can be palpated; this space should be entered by blunt dissection with the surgeon's fingers. The pleura is opened just anterior and posterior to the aorta at the site of intended occlusion. The jaws of the clamp are then passed through the created apertures to securely

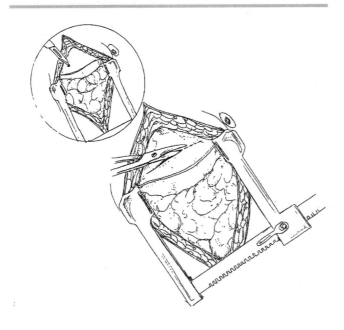

Figure 3 In cases of cardiac tamponade, the pericardium is initially nicked with a knife anterior to the phrenic nerve, as shown in the inset. The pericardium is then widely opened with scissors with care to avoid injury to the heart.

grasp the aorta, as shown in Figure 5. Complete occlusion of the aorta must be ensured.

COMPLICATIONS OF CARDIOPULMONARY RESUSCITATION

Standard Closed-Chest Cardiopulmonary Resuscitation

Most complications after closed-chest CPR are related to thoracic wall damage and include rib or sternal fractures and costochondral separation. These injuries can lead to more severe problems such as pneumothorax, hemothorax, cardiac injury, and even aortic injury.

The thorax is not the only cavity at risk of damage from CPR. Compression of the liver against the xiphoid process can damage that organ (11). In addition, gastric injury, splenic injury (12), or fat embolism may occur. It is important to remember that an endotracheal tube may become dislodged or malpositioned by closed-chest compression. Thus, chest radiographs should be obtained as soon as possible after resuscitation. The true incidence of complications after CPR may not be accurately estimated or known because the primary event that caused the cardiac arrest usually causes death.

Open-Chest Cardiac Massage and Thoracotomy

When an emergency thoracotomy is performed, technical complications can occur. Iatrogenic injuries to the lung, pericardium, heart, phrenic nerves, aorta, esophagus, and chest wall have been described (13).

The standard approach for left anterolateral thoracotomy, as noted above, is through the fifth

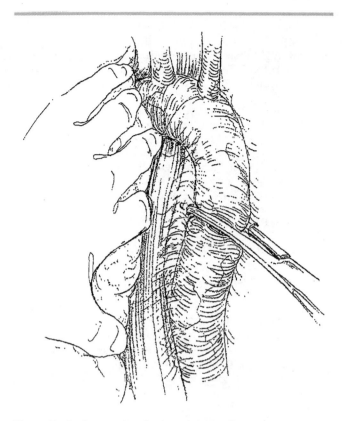

Figure 5 Aortic cross-clamping is carried out after anterior retraction of the left lung and penetration of the mediastinal pleura, so that the jaws of the vascular clamp securely grip the aortic adventitia.

intercostal space below the nipple of male patients and in the inframammary crease of female patients. Exposure can be limited if the skin incision is improperly placed or if the correct intercostal space is not entered. Bleeding from the chest wall, especially from the internal mammary vessels, can be troublesome, and these vessels should be ligated if they are injured. During attempts at occluding the descending thoracic aortic, damage to the aorta, the esophagus, or the intercostal branches of the aorta may occur (13).

Cardiac injuries can occur during an open cardiac massage. Perforation of the right ventricle is a serious complication and is usually caused by incorrectly applied cardiac compression. This lethal complication can be avoided if compression is performed with both hands and with the digits flat rather than curled. The right ventricle is particularly susceptible to injury because it is thinner than the left ventricle and is often distended as a result of fluid resuscitation (1). If perforation occurs, it should be repaired with sutures buttressed with pledgets. As a temporary measure, skin staples can be applied to the perforation until a definitive repair can be performed. Under these circumstances, the right ventricle is usually very friable and repair can be difficult.

Infection and bleeding are the two most serious concerns after emergency thoracotomy. After successful resuscitation, the patient should be taken to the operating room for hemostasis, wound irrigation, and closure.

The most serious complication of either closed-chest or open-chest CPR, of course, is failure to resuscitate. The rates of successful resuscitation vary depending on the cause of cardiac arrest but are, in general, poor. Investigations continue in an attempt to improve the outcome of CPR (14).

MANAGEMENT AFTER SUCCESSFUL CARDIOPULMONARY RESUSCITATION

Once spontaneous circulation has resumed, the underlying cause of arrest should be identified and treated and the adequacy of tissue perfusion should be assured and maintained. Cardiovascular and hemodynamic dysfunctions are common after cardiac arrest; such dysfunctions include hypovolemic shock, cardiogenic shock, and the systemic inflammatory response syndrome (6). Invariably, some form of cardiovascular dysfunction is present, and normal cardiac function may not return for 12 to 24 hours (6). The primary goal of management after CPR is reestablishing global and regional perfusion of tissues. Traditional end points, such as restoration of blood pressure, may not adequately reflect peripheral organ perfusion. Regional tissue malperfusion may exist particularly in the splanchnic bed, and this condition is believed to contribute to the multiple-organ dysfunction syndrome. Physicians should strongly consider the use of invasive hemodynamic monitoring, such as pulmonary artery catheterization, to guide therapy after CPR.

Neurologic impairment is common among survivors of cardiac arrest; approximately 80% of patients remain comatose for various time periods (15). As many as 40% of survivors enter a persistent vegetative state and 79% die within one year (16). This generally poor outcome after cardiac arrest has prompted many physicians to attempt to develop a means of predicting outcome during the early postresuscitative phase. When coma lasts for more than six hours after CPR, the prognosis for full neurologic recovery is poor. The prognosis worsens when the coma persists for more than three days; in such cases, patients rarely survive without severe disability (16).

The Glasgow Coma Scale score is the most common objective method of monitoring the neurologic status and progression of coma. A recent meta-analysis (17) concluded that somatosensory-evoked potentials are useful in predicting the outcome after severe brain injury and are particularly useful in predicting poor outcome: the false-positive rate was less than 0.5%. However, no single variable or technique has been found to be useful in predicting outcome.

CONCLUSION

Despite significant advances in acute care medicine, little advancement has been made in the care of the cardiac arrest patient. Little improvement to complete recovery (hospital discharge to independent living) has occurred. Perhaps a complete reevaluation of CPR, questioning every step that is currently a protocol, needs to be done to alter that uniformly poor outcome.

REFERENCES

1. Greenfield LJ. Complications after cardiopulmonary resuscitation. In: Greenfield LJ, ed. Complications in Surgery and Trauma. 2d ed. Philadelphia: Lippincott, 1984:351–358.
2. Kouwenhoven WB, Jude JR, Knickerbocker CG. Closed-chest cardiac massage. JAMA 1960; 173:1064–1067.
3. Niemann JT. Cardiopulmonary resuscitation. N Engl J Med 1992; 327(15):1075–1080.
4. Ditchey RV, Winkler JV, Rhodes CA. Relative lack of coronary blood flow during closed-chest resuscitation in dogs. Circulation 1982; 66:297–302.
5. Kern KB, Halperin HR, Field J. New guidelines for cardiopulmonary resuscitation and emergency cardiac care: changes in the management of cardiac arrest. JAMA 2001; 285(10):1267–1269.
6. Guidelines 2000 for Cardiopulmonary Resuscitation and Emergency Cardiovascular Care. Part 6: advanced cardiovascular life support: section 8: postresuscitation care. The American Heart Association in collaboration with the International Liaison Committee on Resuscitation. Circulation 2000; 102(suppl 8):I166–I171.
7. Buckman RF Jr, Badellino MM, Mauro LH, et al. Direct cardiac massage without major thoracotomy: feasibility and systemic blood flow. Resuscitation 1995; 29(3):237–248.
8. Rozenberg A, Incagnoli P, Delpech P, et al. Prehospital use of minimally invasive direct cardiac massage (MID-CM): a pilot study. Resuscitation 2001; 50(3):257–262.
9. Biffl WL, Moore EE, Johnson JL. Emergency department thoracotomy. In: Moore EE, Feliciano DV, Mattox KL, eds. Trauma. 5th ed. New York: McGraw-Hill, 2004: 239–253.
10. Buckman RF, Ballard RB, Eynon CA. Resuscitative thoracotomy for trauma: critical techniques. Trauma Q 1995; 12(2):105–132.
11. Adler SN, Klein RA, Pellecchia C, Lyon DT. Massive hepatic hemorrhage associated with cardiopulmonary resuscitation. Arch Intern Med 1983; 143:813–814.
12. Fitchet A, Neal R, Bannister P. Lesson of the week: splenic trauma complicating cardiopulmonary resuscitation. BMJ 2001; 322:480–481.
13. Ivatury R. Cardiac injuries and resuscitative thoracotomy. In: Maull KI, Rodriguez A, Wiles CE, eds. Complications in Trauma and Critical Care. Philadelphia: W.B. Saunders, 1996:279–288.
14. Thel MC, O'Connor CM. Cardiopulmonary resuscitation: historical perspective to recent investigations. Am Heart J 1999; 137(1):39–48.
15. Madl C, Kramer L, Domanovits H, et al. Improved outcome prediction in unconscious cardiac arrest survivors with sensory evoked potentials compared with clinical assessment. Crit Care Med 2000; 28(3):721–726.
16. Edgren E, Hedstrand U, Kelsey S, Sutton-Tyrell K, Safar P. Assessment of neurological prognosis in comatose survivors of cardiac arrest. BRCT I Study Group. Lancet 1994; 343:1055–1059.
17. Carter BG, Butt W. Review of the use of somatosensory evoked potentials in the prediction of outcome after severe brain injury. Crit Care Med 2001; 29(1):178–186.

26

Complications of Vascular Surgery

Frank B. Pomposelli, Jr. and Allen D. Hamdan
*Harvard Medical School and Division of Vascular Surgery, Beth Israel Deaconess
Medical Center, Boston, Massachusetts, U.S.A.*

Malachi G. Sheahan
*Division of Vascular Surgery, Louisiana State University School of Medicine, New Orleans,
Louisiana, U.S.A.*

Guatam V. Shrikhande
*Department of Surgery, Harvard Medical School and Beth Israel Deaconess Medical Center,
Boston, Massachusetts, U.S.A.*

Advancements in surgical techniques, better instruments and graft materials, and substantial improvements in diagnostic imaging have made it possible for vascular surgeons to execute vascular surgical procedures with a high likelihood of success in most circumstances. In addition, a better understanding of how to treat patients before, during, and after vascular surgery has contributed greatly to a reduction in the morbidity and mortality rates associated with these operations. Nonetheless, procedure-related and systemic complications continue to occur and can probably never be totally eliminated because most patients undergoing vascular surgery are elderly and the procedures are complicated by atherosclerosis.

The demands of operating on the circulatory system in these patients are great, and meticulous attention to detail is required so that potential complications, which are often difficult to treat and can have catastrophic consequences, can be avoided or prevented. Indeed, the old adage that it is easier to stay out of trouble than to get out of trouble is particularly relevant to vascular surgery and, in the authors' opinion, describes the best strategy for decreasing the likelihood of operative complications.

Preventing complications depends on the following basic principles:

1. *A careful and comprehensive preoperative evaluation, including assessment of the severity of associated diseases that may adversely affect outcome*
2. *A thorough understanding of the natural history of the disease process so that the surgeon can properly assess the risk of treatment and opt for no treatment when such a decision is appropriate*
3. *High-quality preoperative imaging studies that provide an anatomic picture of the disease process and form the basis of the ultimate surgical treatment plan*
4. *A surgical strategy that appropriately balances the following factors: achieving the treatment goal and providing the least risk to the patient, the best chance of success, and a level of durability that will, ideally, allow the results of the procedure to last for the rest of the patient's life*
5. *An operation performed with a flawless technique so that the need for early reoperation due to technical errors can be minimized because reoperation invariably increases the risk of systemic complications and may adversely affect survival or long-term results*
6. *Excellent and attentive postoperative care under the direction of the vascular surgeon*

When complications do occur, early recognition and prompt treatment are crucial for diminishing their impact and maintaining a good result. This chapter will discuss complications common to all vascular surgical procedures and those specific to the most commonly performed procedures. Emphasis will be given to early recognition and treatment but also to avoidance and prevention.

ASSOCIATED DISEASES AND THEIR IMPLICATIONS FOR COMPLICATIONS OF VASCULAR SURGERY
Coronary Artery Disease

Approximately 80% of patients undergoing vascular surgery have coronary artery disease (CAD) (1), which is the most common cause of both early and late death after such procedures (2–4). Most surgeons believe that there is a direct relationship between the extent of CAD and the likelihood of cardiac complications. When patients have overt symptoms of CAD or have recently suffered a myocardial infarction (MI), the risk of an event during vascular surgery is high enough to warrant a thorough preoperative evaluation, including coronary angiography and angioplasty, or even coronary bypass grafting when indicated (4). Clearly, however, many patients have clinically significant coronary disease without obvious symptoms (5). Determining which of those patients will probably suffer an adverse event related to vascular surgery has become a controversial and widely studied topic that is beyond the scope of this text. Most vascular surgeons augment the medical history and the results of clinical examination and baseline electrocardiography (ECG) with the results of some other noninvasive tests as a means of assessing the degree or severity of coronary disease. Dipyridamole thallium imaging in particular has emerged as the most widely used screening test (6,7). On the basis of a clinical evaluation and the results of noninvasive testing, patients are classified as being at low, intermediate, or high risk of cardiac complications in association with vascular surgery (8,9). Studies have demonstrated an association between a positive risk assessment and the likelihood of a cardiac event (10). No study, however, has conclusively demonstrated that preoperative interventions for treating CAD improve the outcomes associated with peripheral vascular surgery, and this lack of findings raises questions about the cost-effectiveness and the usefulness of such an approach. In spite of this controversy, it is important to recognize that perioperative cardiac complications are common among patients with CAD. All patients should be monitored closely, especially during the first 48 hours after surgery, when most events are likely to occur. Many cardiac complications can be avoided, in the authors' opinion, by judicious fluid management, especially by avoiding hypervolemia and congestive heart failure (CHF). Pulmonary artery catheters may be helpful in fluid management, especially for elderly patients, those with diabetes, and those with left ventricular dysfunction, pulmonary disease, or renal insufficiency.

Pulmonary Disease

Patients undergoing vascular surgery often have chronic obstructive pulmonary disease, and many are current or former smokers. Carefully eliciting a history of chronic cough, sputum production, and shortness of breath upon minimal exertion can usually determine which patients are at high risk of complications. Occasionally, pulmonary function studies and measurements of preoperative arterial blood gases may be needed. Patients with alveolar oxygen pressure below 70, carbon dioxide partial pressure above 45, or forced expiratory volume in one second below 1 L are considered to be at especially high risk (11,12). For such patients, the chance of pulmonary complications may be diminished by methods such as pretreatment with bronchodilators, smoking cessation, or pulmonary physiotherapy (13). The presumed risk of complications can suggest modifications in surgical decisions, including such measures as the preferential use of regional anesthesia, retroperitoneal as

opposed to transabdominal approaches to intra-abdominal operations, the use of extra-anatomic (axillobifemoral) bypass, or angioplasty and stenting rather than open aortofemoral reconstructions. Laparotomy for aortic aneurysm surgery can also be avoided by the use of stent grafts inserted through the femoral artery, if the patient's anatomical structure is suitable.

If unrecognized, respiratory failure can rapidly lead to death (14), but it is usually relatively short-lived and reversible if properly treated. Although pulse oximetry has greatly simplified monitoring for hypoxemia (15), a high index of clinical suspicion is important if physicians are to recognize and treat respiratory failure before a catastrophic complication ensues. Unexplained agitation in the postoperative period should be considered to be caused by hypoxia until proven otherwise. Causes of postoperative pulmonary problems include ventilatory compromise due to abdominal incisions, atelectasis, poor cough and clearance of secretions, respiratory failure due to pneumonia, fluid overload, as well as adult respiratory distress syndrome and pulmonary embolism (PE).

Renal Disease

Patients with preexisting renal insufficiency are most at risk of deterioration of renal function after vascular surgery. Elevated serum creatinine concentrations and hemodialysis have been markers of poorer outcomes and more complications after many vascular surgery procedures. When the patient's renal function is compromised, proper hydration and maintenance of adequate intravascular volume and cardiac output are fundamental if further renal parenchymal injury is to be avoided. In addition, minimizing warm renal ischemic time during surgery and taking particular care with aortic cross-clamping are other important factors in avoiding atheroembolism.

Chemical agents, such as aminoglycoside antibiotics and contrast agents used for angiography, can cause renal injury. The risk of contrast-induced renal injury is higher among patients who are dehydrated and those with diabetes mellitus and multiple myeloma. The risk of renal failure can be reduced by intravenous prehydration with 0.45% normal saline (16). Myoglobinuria can cause renal failure among patients undergoing revascularization after a prolonged period of limb ischemia. Inducing a brisk diuresis with vigorous hydration and intravenous administration of mannitol, administering diuretics, and alkalinizing the urine with intravenous sodium bicarbonate can reduce the risk of renal injury (17).

In patients being treated with hemodialysis, expectations for vascular surgery must be tempered by the poorer outcomes often experienced by this group. Surgical decisions should be individualized and made by balancing a careful evaluation of the patient's life expectancy, functional status, and likely benefit with the expected rate of complications.

Coagulopathy

A history of blood-clotting abnormalities, such as inherited disorders (von Willebrand's disease and hemophilia) or acquired problems (liver disease, vitamin K deficiency, use of anticoagulants or antiplatelet agents, and uremia), should be elicited as part of the initial evaluation of all patients who may require vascular surgery. Technical errors leading to excessive bleeding can result in consumptive coagulopathy and hypothermia, which further aggravate blood-clotting problems (see below). Underlying coagulation abnormalities should be corrected with appropriate clotting factors before surgery when possible. The administration of warfarin should be discontinued 48 to 72 hours before surgery, and the administration of antiplatelet agents should be discontinued one week before the procedure. Intravenous administration of heparin should be discontinued at least four hours before vascular surgery, if possible.

COMPLICATIONS COMMON TO ALL VASCULAR PROCEDURES
Early Graft Thrombosis

Early graft thromboses (those that occur less than 30 days postoperatively) are usually due to errors of commission on the part of the surgeon. Hemodynamic causes of graft failure include inadequate inflow or outflow, or hypoperfusion as a result of shock or cardiac failure. Most inflow or outflow problems are a result of choosing the wrong operation. A comprehensive arteriogram is the cornerstone of most treatment plans in vascular surgery and is essential for choosing the proper locations of inflow and outflow anastomoses. In general, all arteries proximal to the inflow anastomosis should be free of significant stenosis, and the outflow target artery should have unimpeded and continuous flow to the end organ. In some circumstances, inflow can be improved by adjunctive measures such as balloon angioplasty and stenting. If the outflow artery is diseased, collateral vessels must be adequate to support graft flow; if they are not, thrombosis will occur. These surgical decisions are not always straightforward and can require considerable judgment and experience.

Mechanical causes of early graft failure are innumerable, and almost all are avoidable. Poor anastomotic technique can lead to a stenotic anastomosis or intimal flaps. Injudicious clamping can cause traumatic dissection, tears, or crush injuries, particularly in diseased or calcified arteries. Conduits can get twisted when tunneled or can kink if they are too long or improperly placed. Poor hemostasis can lead to graft compression by hematomas. Wound closure sutures can perforate or constrict underlying grafts. Vein grafts are prone to all of these complications and to specific problems related to harvesting and preparation (see below). The potential for mechanical failure is substantial enough that some objective method of assessing the result at the end of the procedure should be used in most circumstances. These methods include hand-held continuous-wave Doppler ultrasonography, angiography (18), angioscopy (19), and intraoperative duplex scanning (20).

When early postoperative thrombosis occurs, immediate reoperation and thrombectomy with some imaging modality should be carried out to identify the underlying problem. Generally, good results can be expected with this approach when a mechanical defect can be identified and corrected. Patients with no identifiable problem should be evaluated for a hypercoagulable state (antithrombin 3 deficiency, factor V Leiden mutation, protein C or S deficiency, anticardiolipin antibodies, etc.) (21). These patients should be given anticoagulant therapy, although the long-term prognosis for graft patency is poor.

Perioperative Hemorrhage

Perioperative hemorrhage can occur as a result of an uncorrected, preexisting coagulopathy (see above), but it is most commonly due to technical error. Important basic measures for preventing this complication include the use of electrocautery for dissection, meticulous hemostasis, and the avoidance of excessive heparin doses (and the reversal of excessive doses with protamine sulfate when they do occur). Dissection of any arterial structure can result in injury and substantial bleeding from adjacent veins. Knowledge of the anatomy, dissection in the plane immediately adjacent to the artery, and avoidance of circumferential dissection when possible can avoid vein injury. Arterial anastomosis should be performed with proper suture bites and graft tension. Proximal graft anastomoses should be tested for leaks before flow is restored. Atraumatic clamps should be used and should be applied carefully so that the risk of injury related to their use can be reduced.

When intraoperative hemorrhage does occur, a careful systematized approach must be undertaken. It is important to notify the anesthesiologist immediately about the problem at hand. Initial application of local pressure or packs will control most of the bleeding. Once the problem has been identified, suture repair, topical hemostatic agents (oxidized cellulose, microfibrillar collagen, and thrombin-soaked gelatin sponges), or both can be used for repair. Venous injuries require particular care. Hastily clamping bleeding veins is inadvisable because this procedure can worsen the injury and exacerbate the problem. Good results can usually be achieved by applying manual pressure with good exposure and suction and using a technique of partial and advancing exposure of the injury with continuous suture repair.

If blood products must be transfused in large amounts, they should be warmed. One or two units of fresh frozen plasma should be given for approximately every four to six units of blood transfused, and a platelet pack should be given after eight units of packed cells have been transfused. Particular care must be taken when lost blood is replaced with blood retrieved from the cell saver because cell-saver blood is completely devoid of clotting factors and its administration can result in severe coagulopathy. Massive hemorrhage may also lead to disseminated intravascular coagulation (22). Good communication and cooperation between the surgeon and the anesthesiologist are crucial to avoiding exsanguination and shock during repair of a vascular injury.

As a general rule, patients who experience postoperative bleeding in the recovery room are best treated by an exploratory procedure. Intra-abdominal bleeding after intracavitary procedures is particularly worrisome because there are no external signs of bleeding. Often, the first indication of postoperative hemorrhage after an abdominal or a thoracic procedure is not hypotension and shock but rather low urine output that is unresponsive to volume replacement.

Wound hematomas can compromise the airway and the function of the graft, can cause compartment syndromes, and can lead to weeks of wound morbidity or infection. If the surgeon is undecided about whether to drain a hematoma, it is generally a good policy to err on the side of a return trip to the operating room.

Myocardial Infarction and Respiratory Failure

Acute respiratory decompensation has already been addressed. As previously outlined, prompt intubation and institution of mechanical ventilatory support is the first treatment. Correction of the underlying problem can then be addressed. It is important to remember that agitation may be the first sign of hypoxia among elderly demented patients who are about to suffer respiratory collapse. It is inappropriate to sedate such patients until their respiratory status has been fully evaluated.

Chest pain, shortness of breath, or both are often the first indications of coronary ischemia and myocardial compromise. The only symptom among patients with diabetes may be nausea or diaphoresis in the absence of chest pain. When coronary ischemia is suspected, ECG should be performed and then followed by electrocardiographic monitoring. Treatment with oxygen, intravenous morphine, and nitrates to control chest pain should be initiated. Tachyarrhythmias should be aggressively treated with beta-blockers, calcium channel blockers, and diuretics as needed. Creatine phosphokinase concentrations, isoenzyme activity, and troponin levels should be determined every eight hours for 24 hours. Patients whose hemodynamic condition is unstable or confusing should be monitored with a pulmonary artery catheter, and those whose condition does not rapidly respond to therapy may require urgent coronary arteriography and surgical intervention.

Acute Renal Failure

The most common cause of oliguria in the early postoperative period is hypovolemia due to third spacing. Low urine output that does not respond as expected to volume replacement can be due to several factors, including continued bleeding, deteriorating myocardial function, mechanical problems with the Foley catheter or urinary system (ureteral injury), or acute renal failure (Table 1). When acute renal failure is suspected, a pulmonary artery catheter should be placed to help optimize fluid status and eliminate potential prerenal causes. Urinalysis should be performed to detect characteristic tubular casts. The administration of all potentially nephrotoxic drugs should be discontinued. In some cases, perfusion scans or even arteriography may be indicated if compromised arterial flow to the kidney is suspected. An increase in the serum creatinine concentration is usually seen within 24 hours after the vascular procedure.

Patients with nonoliguric renal failure should be treated with fluid replacement adequate to maintain urine flow. Anuric patients may benefit from one large dose of a loop diuretic in an attempt to convert the renal failure to a nonoliguric state, for which the prognosis is better (23). Electrolyte levels, especially serum potassium concentration, acid–base balance, and volume status, must be carefully monitored. When hemodialysis is required, a temporary indwelling double-lumen venous access catheter should be placed.

The cause of acute renal failure should be investigated and, when possible, treated, although most causes are diagnosed after the fact and are not correctable. Treatment is therefore directed at support and maintenance of metabolic homeostasis until renal function returns. Conditions such as contrast-induced nephropathy and ischemic injury are reversible, although recovery may not occur for days or weeks. Renal failure caused by renal infarction or atheroembolism often results in an irreversible injury to the renal parenchyma. Protection of renal function is especially crucial when aortic or renal artery reconstruction is performed (24). The mortality rate associated with anuric renal failure remains high, a fact that underscores the importance of avoiding its occurrence in the first place.

Table 1 Classification of Events Causing Renal Dysfunction in Vascular Surgery

Prerenal	Parenchymal	Postrenal
Low cardiac output	Acute tubular necrosis	Foley catheter obstruction
Shock due to any cause	Renal ischemia	Ureteral obstruction
Hypovolemia	Nephrotoxic agents	Clot in pelvis, ureter, and bladder
Third-spacing losses	Aminoglycosides	
Bleeding	Contrast agents	Abdominal compartment syndrome
Dehydration	Others	

Wound Infection

Wound infection after vascular surgery is particularly worrisome when it occurs in wounds containing vascular grafts. The spectrum of wound infection ranges from mild cellulitis to extensive necrosis, with abscess formation and involvement of deep structures, including grafts. Contiguous involvement of a vascular graft by an infection starting in the adjacent soft tissues can result in graft exposure, disruption, and limb loss, even death. Although prosthetic grafts are most at risk, autogenous grafts can also become infected under some circumstances.

The management of graft infections is discussed in more detail in the sections on aortic and lower-extremity bypass. The management of surgical wound infections depends on their severity. Appropriate antibiotics, drainage, and dressing care are the cornerstones of therapy. Complex wounds may require additional measures that may challenge the skills of even the most experienced vascular surgeon, including graft excision, repeated bypass through uninfected tissues, extensive debridement, and closure with myocutaneous flaps or free tissue transfers.

Many wound infections result from poor surgical techniques. Exposure of vascular structures should be accomplished without the creation of large flaps, which may become necrotic and infected. Care should be taken to minimize the disruption of the lymph vessels during vascular exposure and to carefully ligate or cauterize those vessels that are disrupted so that the formation of lymph leaks or lymphocele can be avoided. Meticulous hemostasis is important in avoiding wound hematomas, which are perhaps the most common cause of vascular wound infections. When large hematomas do occur, they should be drained promptly. If a patient has both an infection and ischemia, as is commonly the case with lower-extremity ulcers and gangrene, the infection should be aggressively treated before a vascular graft is implanted.

Late Complications

Arterial constructions may fail as a result of neointimal hyperplasia, an incompletely understood mechanism related to the response of blood vessels to injury. This complication consists of a hypertrophic, subintimal smooth muscle proliferation leading to stenosis at the location of anastomoses, within vein grafts, on arterial surfaces after endarterectomy or angioplasty, and within previously placed stents (25). Neointimal hyperplasia most commonly occurs 6 to 18 months after arterial interventions.

Anastomotic false aneurysms can occur as a result of the failure of sutures or graft materials or as a result of the loss of the structural integrity of the arterial wall at the anastomosis because of degeneration or infection (26). Many false aneurysms occur several years after implantation of a graft. The incidence of anastomotic aneurysms has decreased substantially since the abandonment of silk sutures for vascular anastomosis (27). Avoiding endarterectomy at the site of anastomoses, taking proper suture bites in grafts and in the arterial wall, avoiding excessive tension of grafts, and using polypropylene or polyester sutures are important principles in preventing false aneurysms.

Failure of reconstructions more than 18 months after their placement is usually due to the progression of atherosclerosis. The fact that all vascular surgery for atherosclerosis is palliative for an incurable disease mandates that patients be followed up for life so that disease progression can be detected and treated when necessary and so that the function of previously placed grafts can be preserved. Risk factor reduction, especially smoking cessation, should also be part of the overall treatment strategy recommended by the vascular surgeon to slow the progression of disease.

COMPLICATIONS OF LOWER-EXTREMITY BYPASS FOR CHRONIC ISCHEMIA

During the last two decades, the technical aspects of arterial reconstruction in the lower extremity have changed tremendously. Improvements in suture materials and vein preparation techniques and the routine use of magnification, fine cardiovascular sutures, and specialized instruments have made it possible for vascular surgeons to bypass essentially any artery in the lower extremity, from the common femoral artery to the pedal and plantar arteries in the foot. Arteries as small as 1 mm in diameter can be successfully bypassed with results comparable to those achieved by more proximal arterial reconstructions. The technical challenges of performing distal arterial bypass of small vessels are substantial, and avoiding errors that might lead to graft thrombosis is especially important during these procedures. An incomplete list of the potential pitfalls of arterial reconstructive surgery in the lower extremity is presented below.

Early Graft Thrombosis

Technical errors of vein graft preparation are usually related to improper handling of the greater saphenous vein. When this vein is harvested, the surgeon must be careful not to avulse side branches. Branch avulsion usually requires suture repair, which can be difficult and can lead to areas of stenosis or stricture in the vein graft. During the last 20 years, the in situ saphenous vein bypass technique (28) has become quite popular. Cutting the valves and leaving the vein in its bed creates a tapered venous conduit, which more closely matches the size and configuration of the inflow and outflow artery. The favorable size match makes the use of this vein very appealing, especially for tibial artery reconstructions, in which veins as small as 2.5 mm in diameter work extremely well. Preparing a saphenous vein for use as an in situ conduit is fraught with many technical errors. Most problems occur when the valves are cut. Numerous valvulotomes are now commercially available and can simplify the process. Each of these instruments has advantages and disadvantages, and the use of each is associated with a steep learning curve. As a general principle, any valve-cutting technique should involve careful cutting of the leaflets of the valve without injuring the adjacent wall. Intimal injuries of the adjacent vein wall, transmural perforations, and tears or cuts in the vein that are caused by valvulotomes can lead to areas of thrombosis and stricture formation, which can cause both early and late graft failures. The authors have found that using angioscopy (29) reduces the number of valvulotome injuries related to in situ vein preparation (Fig. 1). The proximal and distal ends of in situ saphenous vein grafts should be harvested adequately so that undue tension can be avoided and so that no kinking or compression occurs when the graft is connected to the artery. An especially acute angle can occur when an in situ saphenous vein graft is tunneled from the subcutaneous bed to the popliteal space. This acute angle can lead to early graft thrombosis or late stenosis at the angulation point. For this reason, when performing femoral-popliteal reconstructions, the authors prefer to remove the vein, cut the valves, and tunnel the graft in an anatomic plane as is traditionally done with reversed vein grafts. The "nonreversed" vein graft lies straight and avoids acute angles but maintains the size-match advantage.

Before using saphenous vein grafts, vascular surgeons commonly distend them gently, usually using a syringe distension technique with a balanced salt solution containing heparin and papaverine. Studies have shown that using excessive pressure to distend saphenous veins can cause extremely high hydrostatic pressures within the vein, and these pressures may damage endothelial cells. Many authors recommend using chilled heparinized blood as a preparation solution and avoiding syringe distension (30).

Anastomoses should be performed with great care. It is not uncommon for either inflow or outflow target arteries in lower-extremity arterial reconstructions to have some degree of atherosclerosis. Arteries may be heavily calcified, especially among patients with diabetes mellitus. Gentle occlusion clamps should be used to control flow before arteriotomies are performed. The authors prefer to use soft-jawed hydrogrip-type clamps for proximal control of larger arteries and silicone plastic vessel loop slings for control of smaller arteries. When performing arteriotomies, surgeons must avoid injuring the posterior wall of the artery when opening it with a knife or Potts scissors. When anastomoses are created, attention must be paid to avoiding intimal flaps and strictures. It is important to evert the ends of the graft and the artery when sutures are placed so that a smooth flow surface can be promoted. Hemostatic control of distal calcified arteries can be quite challenging. As a general rule, heavily calcified arteries should not be clamped because clamping can crush or crack the vessel. Proximal control with tourniquets (31) or intraluminal vascular occluders is effective in these circumstances.

Tunneling of grafts requires meticulous attention. It is important to be sure that grafts passing through the popliteal space rest in the space between the medial and lateral heads of the gastrocnemius muscle. Inadvertently tunneling a graft through the muscle belly of the medial head of the gastrocnemius muscle can lead to graft compression and thrombosis. Similar concerns apply when grafts pass beneath the sartorius muscle in the thigh. In aortofemoral reconstructions, grafts should pass posterior to the ureters to avoid entrapping the ureter between the iliac artery and the graft. Creating aortofemoral graft tunnels can also damage the sigmoid colon, the cecum, and the bladder. When tunnels are created in a subcutaneous plane, they must be of an adequate caliber to allow grafts to pass through them without compression or kinking. Excessive hemorrhage in the tunnel can be avoided by creating the tunnel before heparin is administered. The authors find it useful to perform the proximal anastomosis first and then to pass the fully distended graft through the tunnels under arterial pressure so that potential kinking and twisting can be avoided. This procedure also allows the surgeon to observe blood flow from the distal end of the graft before performing the distal anastomosis. Tunneling devices are commercially available and are often quite helpful, but they are not absolutely necessary if the previously described principles are adhered to before grafts are tunneled.

Judgment errors have already been discussed. The proper selection of inflow and outflow arteries should be made only on the basis of a high-quality, comprehensive arteriogram. The ability to image the

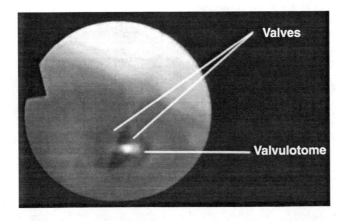

Figure 1 The use of angioscopy reduces the number of valvulotome injuries related to in situ vein preparation.

entire arterial circulation of the lower extremity, from the infrarenal aorta to the toes, has been greatly enhanced in the last 15 years by the routine use of intra-arterial digital subtraction angiography (32). Currently available equipment provides images with resolution quality as good as or superior to that obtained by conventional cut-film techniques. Recently, it has been suggested that magnetic resonance arteriography (MRA) provides images of the distal infrageniculate arterial circulation that are of superior quality to those obtained by other imaging methods (33). Our experience has not supported this concept. We continue to rely mostly on intra-arterial digital subtraction contrast angiography, although we have used MRA imaging selectively in our practice when the use of contrast agents was strongly contraindicated.

When early graft failure does occur, it usually does so within the first 12 to 24 hours after the surgical procedure has been completed. Managing an acutely thrombosed graft requires a systematized approach. As a general rule, all patients should be treated with heparin and immediate reexploration. The authors usually expose the distal anastomosis first. The pattern of thrombosis will often provide some clues about the cause of the problem. If thrombus is present at the terminal end of the vein graft but most of the graft is still pulsating, a technical problem will usually be found at the distal anastomosis. The hood should be opened and the thrombus carefully removed. Any intimal flaps, strictures, or stenoses can then be identified and treated appropriately. If the distal portion of the vein graft is not thrombosed, the wound must be opened completely and the vein graft examined in its entirety.

Thrombosis generally starts at the point of some abnormality in the vein graft, such as a kink, twist, stricture, extrinsic compression point, uncut valve, injury from the valvulotome, etc. If the entire vein graft is clotted, the problem may be either at the anastomosis or in the vein itself. A thrombectomy should be performed, flow reestablished, and an angiogram obtained to disclose the problem. Vein graft thrombectomy should be performed with great care. A thrombectomy catheter can be used, although often the fresh nonadherent thrombus can be milked out from either the proximal or the distal end of the vein graft. This procedure avoids the passage of balloon catheters that will severely damage the endothelium and compromise long-term graft patency.

When a mechanical defect in a graft has been discovered and corrected, the long-term prognosis for graft survival is reasonably good. When graft thrombosis occurs with no identifiable cause but outflow is considered reasonable, a hypercoagulable state must be suspected. Patients with this complication should be treated with anticoagulants and evaluated for thrombophilia (21). In general, even when anticoagulation is administered, the long-term prognosis for graft patency, whether or not mechanical or technical defects have been discovered, is poor (34).

Hemorrhage

Hemorrhage in lower-extremity arterial reconstructions is usually caused by avoidable technical errors. Poor hemostasis or excessive anticoagulation can lead to the formation of wound hematomas, which may not be apparent until several hours after surgery. As previously stated, all large wound hematomas in the lower extremity should be drained in the operating room. Leaving large hematomas in the lower extremity will result in a draining wound, which is susceptible to secondary infection. Wound morbidity related to hematomas can plague the patient and the surgeon for many months and can ruin an otherwise good result. Improper ligation of vein branches on saphenous vein grafts can lead to loss of the ligature and bleeding through a side branch. Side branch bleeding is usually profuse and dramatic and requires immediate surgery. Poorly performed anastomoses can also cause bleeding between suture bites because of tears in the arterial wall or breakage of sutures that have been improperly tied. Polypropylene suture material is particularly susceptible to fracture and breakage when insufficient care is taken in tying sutures or when the suture material is crushed or clamped by metal clamps or forceps.

Cardiac Complications

More than 80% of patients who undergo lower-extremity arterial reconstructive surgery will have CAD, and 20% to 30% of these patients will have severe disease (1). Many patients may have few or no symptoms because of poor physical condition and inactivity or because of diabetes. It is often impractical or impossible to completely evaluate and correct the underlying coronary artery occlusive disease among patients with severe limb-threatening arterial ischemia of the lower extremity. Many patients will therefore undergo lower-extremity surgery with uncorrected coronary occlusive disease and must be monitored closely for signs of coronary ischemia. Continuous ECG monitoring and close nursing supervision are necessary in the early postoperative period, when most cardiac complications occur (24–48 hours after surgery). A common cause of cardiac decompensation in a patient undergoing lower-extremity reconstruction is hypervolemia due to excessive replacement of intravenous fluid. Patients undergoing lower-extremity bypass do not have large third-spacing requirements. On average, approximately 1.5 to 2 L of fluid will be necessary to adequately replace insensible losses during a 3.5- to 4-hour surgical procedure. After surgery, fluid requirements rarely exceed 1 to 2 L/day. Most patients will require monitoring of central venous pressure, and those patients who are known to have compromised myocardial function will require measurement of pulmonary artery pressures. Patients with diabetes may exhibit atypical signs of coronary ischemia. Diaphoresis, nausea, and vomiting in the absence of chest pain may be the first signs of an impending MI.

Surgeons must maintain a high index of suspicion and order ECG promptly when patients exhibit these symptoms. Patients who show signs of fluid overload should undergo aggressive diuresis with a loop diuretic such as furosemide. As a general rule, patients should gain no more than 1 to 2 kg of body weight after lower-extremity arterial reconstruction. After the first 48 hours, it is prudent to use mild diuresis to return patients to their preoperative body weight within four to five days after surgery. When blood products are needed, they should be administered slowly so that sudden fluid overload can be avoided. Fluid overload can also be avoided by administering a dose of a loop diuretic after one or two units of packed red blood cells have been given to patients with compromised ventricular function.

Wound Complications

The skin in areas of proposed surgical incisions should be free of superficial infection. Spreading cellulitis and infection should be adequately controlled before arterial reconstruction is performed. Prophylactic antibiotics with activity against staphylococcal and streptococcal organisms should be administered before surgery. Diabetic patients with multimicrobial foot infections should be treated with broad-spectrum antibiotics. Surgical incisions should be made directly over the femoral artery, the saphenous vein, and other structures; large flaps, which predispose patients to seroma, hematoma, and wound edge necrosis, should be avoided. Lymph nodes and lymph vessels that are encountered in the groin should be reflected medially so that disruption can be avoided; if these structures are disrupted, they should be carefully ligated or electrocauterized so that spillage of lymph, which may be contaminated with bacteria in patients with distal foot wounds, can be avoided. It is not unusual for patients to have some small amount of lymphatic fluid leakage from wounds caused by lower-extremity surgery, particularly groin wounds, for a few days after surgery. Likewise, small contained lymphoceles may be evident, particularly during the first postoperative visit; most will resolve spontaneously. Small lymph leaks can be contained with appropriate dry sterile dressings until they close. If any signs of infection are present, the drainage should be cultured and appropriate antibiotics should be given. Persistent lymph leaks that do not close during the first few weeks after surgery and large lymphoceles are probably best treated by reexploration and ligation, although this procedure can sometimes prove difficult. Large lymphoceles can sometimes be managed with repeated percutaneous aspiration. If lymphoceles and seromas are aspirated, sterile technique should be used so that contamination can be avoided. Infected hematomas and fluid collections require prompt incision and appropriate packing, as well as dressing care so that open wounds can heal by secondary intention.

Limb Swelling

Limb edema of the extremity after arterial reconstruction is very common. Virtually all patients will experience some degree of leg swelling. Edema usually resolves within two to three months, but can persist for many months and may be permanent for some patients. Many factors can cause edema of the lower extremity after arterial reconstruction, including a combination of lymphatic insufficiency, endothelium dysfunction, and increased perfusion pressure (35). Most leg edemas can be treated by encouraging leg elevation and reassuring the patient that the condition is temporary. For persistent edema, a graduated compression stocking can be helpful.

Infection

Graft infection after lower-extremity arterial reconstruction can cause graft thrombosis or catastrophic hemorrhage. Proper sterile technique, adequate treatment of preexisting infection, and avoidance of wound complications are the most important principles of prevention. Wound infections involving underlying saphenous vein grafts can be treated successfully without removing the graft, even when it is exposed. Adequate debridement and drainage of infected tissues, as well as dressing care designed to maintain a moist environment over the graft, will occasionally allow healing by formation of granulation tissue and by secondary intention. Many surgeons will use a muscle flap to cover the exposed portion of the graft (36,37). Infections caused by gram-negative organisms, particularly *Pseudomonas* species (38), can result in necrosis of the vein graft wall, with disruption and hemorrhage. Such grafts must be ligated.

It is occasionally possible to save an exposed prosthetic graft, provided that there is minimal surrounding infection, that most of the graft is incorporated into surrounding tissues, and that the anastomosis is not involved. Most of these grafts, however, will need to be removed (39). All patients with exposed grafts of any type are at risk of bleeding and must be followed up very closely.

Late Graft Failure

The time course of graft failure will usually give some indication of the underlying cause of the failure. When grafts fail within 30 days after surgery, the cause is usually a technical error, inadequate inflow or outflow, or a hypercoagulable state. When grafts fail more than 30 days but less than 18 months after surgery, the cause is usually neointimal hyperplasia. Neointimal hyperplasia often occurs in saphenous vein grafts and in other autogenous vein grafts as a result of intimal injuries at the time of graft preparation, or in arm vein grafts in areas of previous venipuncture. In the authors' experience, the results achieved with arm vein grafts have improved with the use of angioscopy (40) to identify and discard arm veins that are of poor quality because of previous venipuncture. Such veins quickly form strictures because of intimal hyperplasia, and grafts using these veins usually fail.

Intimal hyperplasia in vein grafts is often focal and can cause graft thrombosis before the onset of symptoms or before ankle pressures are reduced. Graft patency has improved with the use of duplex ultrasonography to detect areas of stenosis, which may cause graft failure (41). Findings of reduced blood flow velocity or focal areas of stenosis with blood flow velocities 2.5 to 3.5 times the baseline values should be investigated with arteriography so that the area of stenosis can be identified. Many such areas can be repaired with vein patch angioplasties or interposition grafting. Intimal hyperplasia can sometimes be diffuse in nature, involving long segments or even the entire vein graft. Such vein grafts are unsalvageable and should be replaced. When arterial reconstructions fail more than 18 months after surgery, the cause is usually progression of the disease in either the inflow tract or the outflow tract.

When an arterial reconstruction fails after a period of normal function, the most important factor in determining a course of action is whether ischemic symptoms return. Approximately 10% to 20% of arterial reconstructions will fail late without the return of symptoms. In such cases, patients should be followed up expectantly without another arterial reconstruction. When severe symptoms do occur, a secondary bypass procedure will be necessary and an arteriogram should be obtained. Secondary arterial reconstructions can often be challenging because previously dissected arteries that are now in scar tissue will need to be exposed because usable saphenous vein is absent, and because outflow will have to be extended to more distal and smaller target arteries. The results of secondary arterial reconstructions are generally inferior to those obtained with primary procedures, and this fact underscores the need to do it right the first time.

COMPLICATIONS OF LIMB AMPUTATION

Amputations are an inevitable and important part of the treatment of many patients with vascular diseases. Amputation should be performed with the same care and attention to detail that the surgeon devotes to arterial reconstructions. To do otherwise does the patient a great disservice. Amputations are usually performed when some other procedure, usually a lower-extremity bypass, has led to a complication or has failed, or as treatment for gangrene or infection. An amputation can relieve pain, improve the quality of life, and end a long course of recurrent problems. Amputations should not be assigned to junior staff.

Surgeons should be sensitive to patients' fears about all amputations. A recommendation for amputation should be given to the patient in an unhurried and compassionate manner. No amputation is complete until the patient has been rehabilitated to the fullest extent possible. The surgeon's burden of responsibility does not end until this goal has been achieved.

Lack of Healing

Amputations fail to heal when they are performed in areas of ischemia. Necrosis is usually not evident for several days. A variety of tests have been used to predict the chance of healing, including segmental pressure measurements, pulse volume recordings, xenon flow studies, laser Doppler flow studies, and transcutaneous oxygen measurements (42). No test is completely reliable, and may predict failure at a level where healing can still occur. The authors continue to rely on physical examination and clinical judgment to determine the level of amputation (43). This practice results in the need to revise some failed amputations but avoids amputating a limb too proximally on the basis of erroneous test results (44).

Infection

Patients who undergo amputation often experience active tissue loss and infection. As many as 10% of stumps will become infected, but most infections will respond to antibiotics and will not require operative incision and drainage. When infections are severe, more proximal revisions may be required (45). When patients require below-knee amputation for severe foot sepsis, performing the procedure in two stages can reduce the risk of stump infection. In the first stage, the foot is removed at the ankle (guillotine amputation) so that the infection can be controlled. After the infection has resolved, a formal below-knee amputation is performed.

Venous Thromboembolism

Patients are often bedridden or limited in their physical activity for a period of time before and after amputation. Deep venous thrombosis (DVT) occurs in as many as 12.5% of patients. A high index of suspicion is necessary for diagnosing this complication, and appropriate prophylaxis with subcutaneously administered heparin may prevent its occurrence (46).

Myocardial Infarction and Death

The mortality rate associated with major amputations is 7% to 15%, 5 to 10 times higher than that associated with lower-extremity revascularization (47). Advanced CAD is the most common cause of this complication, although uncontrolled sepsis and PE also contribute to its occurrence.

COMPLICATIONS OF CAROTID ENDARTERECTOMY

Carotid endarterectomy (CEA) is one of the most studied and scrutinized vascular surgery procedures. Although innumerable studies of this procedure have been performed, including several large, randomized prospective trials, controversy still exists about its proper role in the prevention of ischemic stroke, especially in patients without symptoms. All studies emphasize the importance of a low complication rate, especially a low rate of perioperative stroke, if endarterectomy is to be of benefit in preventing ischemic stroke.

Stroke

The intolerance of the brain to even brief periods of loss of blood flow is the fundamental issue that surgeons must keep in mind when performing CEA. A mishap can turn an otherwise enjoyable and usually straightforward technical exercise into a surgical nightmare, the end result of which is a devastating neurologic injury or death. More than any vascular surgery procedure, CEA requires vigilance and a clear understanding of how to stay out of trouble. The most feared complication is stroke, which can occur for a number of reasons.

Diagnostic Arteriography

At one time, all patients scheduled for CEA routinely underwent diagnostic arteriography, and this test is still the gold standard for determining the degree of stenosis in the internal carotid artery. The risk of stroke associated with arteriography itself ranges from 0.5% to 1.5% (48). In recent years, arteriography has been used much more selectively because of the accuracy of duplex ultrasonography (49) and MRA in determining the severity of stenosis. Currently, fewer than 5% of patients at our institution undergo diagnostic arteriography before CEA.

Perioperative Stroke

Intraoperative strokes (Table 2) are caused by technical errors, dislodgement of atheroma during dissection, or clamping ischemia (50). The most common error is poor management of the end point of the endarterectomy in the internal carotid artery. The end point should be visualized and care should be taken to ensure that all loose debris has been removed so that an intimal flap is not created upon restoration of blood flow (51). In the authors' experience, tacking sutures should be rarely necessary if an effort has been made to completely remove the atheroma and to be sure that the end point is well adhered; however, such sutures may occasionally be needed. Arterial closures should be performed with care so that the lumen is not narrowed at the end point because such narrowing may cause thrombosis. Small arteries (less than 4 mm in diameter) are best closed with a patch. Many vascular surgeons, including the authors, now routinely use patch closure. Arterial dissection should be performed gently, especially around the atheroma-filled bulb.

Table 2   Causes of Stroke After Carotid Endarterectomy, from Most Common to Least Common

Technical errors
Plaque embolism
Clamping ischemia
Cerebral hemorrhage

Adhering to the principle that the patient is dissected away from the artery and not the artery away from the patient will minimize the chance of plaque dislodgement. Clamping ischemia is uncommon and can be avoided by proper cerebral monitoring, including regional anesthesia with neurological assessment or general anesthesia with EEG monitoring, measurement of internal carotid backpressure, and other techniques. Patients with clamping ischemia should be treated with insertion of an indwelling shunt. An alternative approach favored by the authors is to use shunts for all patients and to insert the shunts while patients are under general anesthesia.

Perioperative neurologic deficits usually occur within the first 12 to 24 hours after surgery, after an initial period of normalcy (52). A standardized, systematic approach must be carried out when such deficits occur. The patient should be placed under general endotracheal anesthesia, and the wound should be opened and the artery examined by palpation and hand-held Doppler ultrasonography. If there is no pulse, the artery should be opened and cleared of thrombus, and the cause of the problem should be identified and repaired. Patch closure should always be used, and arteriography is usually performed after the procedure. If the artery has a pulse, an angiogram is performed while the patient is on the operating table, and the artery is opened if a defect is identified. In more than 70% of cases, a technical error of some type will be identified. When such treatment is performed promptly and a correctable technical error is identified and corrected, the prognosis is favorable, and many patients recover fully.

Stroke occurs in 1% to 5% of patients (according to single-institution studies), is mainly dependent on the severity of presenting symptoms (symptomatic or asymptomatic disease preoperatively), and may be influenced by the presence of contralateral occlusion of the internal carotid arteries. Nonetheless, most strokes are caused by surgical errors and are therefore preventable. The American Heart Association consensus statement suggests that the perioperative stroke rate associated with CEA should be less than 3% for patients without symptomatic disease and less than 6% for patients with symptomatic disease. Surgeons unable to achieve these outcomes should not perform CEA.

Cerebral Hemorrhage

Cerebral hemorrhage, which is an uncommon cause of stroke and carries a mortality rate of 50%, can occur several days after CEA and is often heralded by a severe headache. The causes of cerebral hemorrhage are unclear, but relief of critical stenosis and postoperative hypertension are common features (53). When patients have suffered ischemic stroke, when computed tomography (CT) scans show large infarcts, and when severe neurologic deficits are present, delaying CEA for four to six weeks is advisable so that conversion of an ischemic infarct into a hemorrhagic infarct can be avoided.

Neck Hematoma

Neck hematomas occur in as many as 5% of patients (54). Most result from technical errors associated with poor hemostasis or arterial closure. Airway compromise and death can occur. Tracheal deviation with large hematomas can make intubation difficult and tracheostomy impossible. Smaller hematomas are painful and unsightly, and they delay recovery. Avoiding severe postoperative hypertension is an important principle in preventing hematoma. As a general rule, the authors evacuate all but the smallest neck hematomas. Patients with rapidly expanding hematomas should be immediately intubated before they are transported to the operating room. Opening the wound and evacuating the clot at the bedside may be necessary to facilitate attempts at intubation.

Nerve Injury

The vagus, hypoglossal, glossopharyngeal, and mandibular branches of the facial nerves and the spinal accessory nerves can be injured during dissection. Injury rates are higher in association with operations for recurrent stenosis (55). Nerve injuries can be prevented by knowing the anatomy, avoiding electrocautery in areas adjacent to nerves, and exposing vein branches circumferentially before ligature. Most injuries resolve, assuming the nerve has not been transected, but they can cause many months of morbidity. Bilateral injury to the vagus nerve can lead to airway compromise.

Myocardial Infarction

A high percentage of patients with carotid disease will also have underlying CAD, but the rate of MI is usually less than 2% (51).

Patch Disruption or Infection

Patch disruption is rare but can occur with vein patch closure and may be more common with saphenous vein harvested from the ankle (as opposed to the groin). Most surgeons now use prosthetic patches, which rarely become infected. We have encountered only four patch infections in our last 1000 consecutive CEAs. Treatment involves removal of the infected synthetic patch and repair with a vein patch (Fig. 2). All patients should receive a dose of antibiotics before undergoing CEA. Meticulous sterile technique and avoidance of hematoma formation are preventative measures.

Restenosis

Restenosis occurs in 10% to 45% of cases, especially among women, in patients with arteries less than 4 mm in diameter, and in smokers. Most cases of restenosis are due to neointimal hyperplasia and occur in the first 6 to 18 months after surgery. Symptomatic restenosis is uncommon and the risk of stroke is low. Most lesions occlude less than 70% of the artery

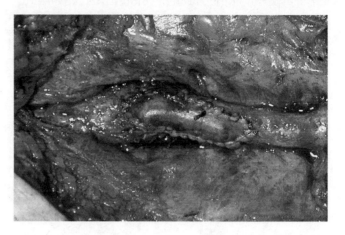

Figure 2 Vein patch repair for carotid endarterectomy.

and some may occasionally regress. Patch closure may decrease the incidence of restenosis, especially in patients with small arteries and among women (56). Restenosis occurring more than two years after endarterectomy is usually due to progression of atherosclerosis. The precise indications for reoperation are unknown, and the complication rates associated with a second procedure are higher than those associated with the original CEA. Most surgeons will operate when patients exhibit symptoms or when critical asymptomatic lesions are at risk of thrombosis (57). Angioplasty with stenting is currently being investigated as a treatment for restenosis after CEA.

Hyperperfusion Syndrome

Hyperperfusion syndrome, which occurs in fewer than 1% of patients, is manifested by cerebral edema, headache, and seizures. It usually occurs 3 to 11 days after CEA. Characteristics that predispose patients to this complication are critical contralateral disease and preoperative and perioperative hypertension. The cause of this syndrome is thought to be loss of autoregulation of cerebral blood flow; this loss leads to cerebral edema. Treatment consists of controlling seizures, which can be difficult, and correcting hypertension. If hyperperfusion syndrome is mistaken for thrombotic infarct and is treated with intravenous administration of heparin, fatal intracerebral hemorrhage can occur.

COMPLICATIONS OF SURGERY TO THE AORTA AND ITS BRANCHES
Open Aortic Aneurysm Repair and Aortofemoral Bypass for Occlusive Disease

Since Dubost performed the first successful abdominal aneurysm resection in 1951, substantial improvements have been made in anesthesia, critical care, and surgical technology. These developments have led to a decline in operative mortality rates, from 14–20% in early reports to 2–5% today (58). Some large series have even found perioperative death rates below 1% (59). Because the natural history of abdominal aneurysms involves progressive dilation, surgical repair is now being advocated for patients with smaller aneurysms and for older, higher-risk patients than patients with those that could have been treated in the past. In this section, we will consider many of the commonly occurring complications associated with abdominal aneurysm surgery in conjunction with the complications associated with aortofemoral bypass because the clinical outcomes of these procedures are similar.

Hemorrhage

The aorta is a large artery surrounded by veins. An old surgical pearl states that the safest place in aneurysm surgery is inside the aneurysm itself. Limiting dissection to the space immediately surrounding the aorta is an important principle in avoiding many problems with bleeding. Intraoperative bleeding usually results from injury to an adjacent venous structure, injury to the aorta itself, or inadequate hemostatic integrity of the anastomosis. Venous injury can be avoided by minimal dissection of the aneurysm and the iliac arteries. Encircling the aorta with tapes is both unnecessary and dangerous. Aortic tissue at the neck of the aneurysm is often thickened due to thrombus or atheroma, or it may be thin walled and friable. The aortas of patients with occlusive disease may be heavily calcified. Aortic clamping should be performed carefully, with appropriately sized, soft-jawed clamps. It is often prudent to lower the systolic blood pressure before the clamp is applied. If suprarenal clamping is necessary, the renal arteries should be clamped first so that emboli from the aorta do not reach the renal arteries. The left renal vein can be ligated to improve exposure as long as ligation is performed to the right of the left adrenal and gonadal veins, which are important collateral vessels. Transecting the aorta is rarely necessary in treating aneurysmal disease. The graft inclusion technique works well in most circumstances and avoids the hazard of injuring posterior structures when the aorta is divided.

If anastomoses are erroneously placed in the proximal aneurysm rather than in its neck, bleeding may occur upon restoration of flow, or anastomotic or juxta-anastomotic aneurysms (60) may develop later. The aorta should be exposed to the level of the left renal vein, which crosses the anterior aorta at the approximate level of the renal arteries. In approximately 10% of cases, the left renal vein crosses the aorta posteriorly; in such cases, the vein may be injured during cross-clamping if its aberrant location is not recognized. The proximal anastomosis should be placed as close to the renal arteries as possible to ensure that all of the aneurysm has been excluded

from blood flow. Injury to adjacent structures and anastomotic bleeding may also be avoided by large suture bites, a running suture using the graft inclusion technique, and grafts of the proper size. Plates of calcium should not be incorporated into suture bites because they will prevent a snug approximation of the graft to the artery. These structures should be carefully removed. Occasionally, sutures may require reinforcement with felt pledgets, either in a running closure or as a series of interrupted sutures when the neck of the aneurysm is very thin and friable.

Different principles apply when aortic occlusive disease is present. Because the aorta is not aneurysmal, the anastomosis can be placed at the most distal disease-free point in the aorta. Both end-to-end and end-to-side anastomoses work well. The authors generally prefer end-to-end grafts unless the patient is a sexually potent man with disease confined principally to the external iliac arteries. In such cases, an end-to-side graft will preserve flow to the pelvis, and this blood flow, it is hoped, will maintain erectile function. Surgical procedures can be challenging when the arteries are heavily calcified. Clamping the aorta can cause cracking of the arterial wall and catastrophic hemorrhage. When aortic calcification is severe, the most prudent option may be to abort the planned aortic procedure and perform an axillary-bifemoral bypass instead.

Renal and visceral artery bypass may be performed in conjunction with aortic surgery or as a separate procedure. Blood flow into renal reconstructions usually comes from the infrarenal aorta, but when the aorta is diseased, extra-anatomic bypass from the hepatic or splenic artery (61) may be used and is less hazardous. Retrograde mesenteric bypasses can be created from the infrarenal aorta or iliac arteries. If these grafts are improperly positioned, they can easily kink or twist when the bowel is returned to its normal position. Antegrade bypasses, created from the supraceliac aorta (62), are not as likely to kink as retrograde grafts but are technically more demanding to create, are prone to the hazards associated with clamping the aorta in the distal thorax (paraplegia and visceral emboli), and are tunneled posterior to the pancreas, a procedure that can cause troublesome bleeding. Proper patient selection and the experience of the surgeon are important factors in avoiding the complications associated with renal and visceral artery bypass.

Hemodynamic instability accompanied by low hemoglobin levels and poor urine output during the postoperative period commonly indicates continued blood loss. Most postsurgical bleedings occur at the sites of anastomoses, through the graft interstices, or in the periaortic retroperitoneal tissues. Reversal of heparin at the conclusion of the procedure can generally limit such bleeding. Postsurgical bleeding may be self-limiting, but unresponsive hypotension combined with signs of hemorrhage mandates surgical intervention. Postoperative bleeding is more likely after intervention for ruptured aneurysms because of the development of coagulopathy as a result of preoperative hypothermia and the transfusion of large volumes of blood. Using intraoperative autotransfusion to treat patients who have suffered an acute ruptured aneurysm reduces the requirement for homologous red blood cell transfusions and is associated with a lower mortality rate for hospitalized patients (63).

Limb Ischemia and Thrombosis of the Graft Limb

Acute lower-limb ischemia immediately after aortic surgery, the so-called "trash foot" syndrome (Fig. 3), is usually due to emboli from either the graft or the native vessels. Distal small-vessel thrombosis is another possible culprit. This phenomenon is best prevented by early mobilization and clamping of the iliac arteries and copious irrigation of the graft and anastomoses with heparin saline solution (64).

Thrombosis of one or both limbs of an aortic graft will usually occur during the first two years after the repair. Early thrombosis (less than 30 days after graft placement) is normally due to a technical error; the most common cause is an intimal flap. Treatment requires thrombectomy and repair of the technical problem. Late thrombosis at the distal anastomosis is probably the result of neointimal hyperplasia or recurrent atherosclerosis. Treatment options include femorofemoral bypass, reconstruction of the distal anastomosis with graft interposition, and patch angioplasty.

Myocardial Infarction

Acute MI is the principal cause of hospital death after elective aortic repair. One large series demonstrated that cardiac problems accounted for 39.8% of all major postoperative complications (58). Risk factors for acute MI include a history of CHF, a prior Q-wave MI, rupture of an abdominal aortic aneurysm,

preoperative hypotension, excessive bleeding, and prolonged cross-clamping time. Many studies have attempted to determine the benefit of extensive preoperative cardiac screening (thallium scanning, echocardiography, and cardiac catheterization), but the most predictive findings are those obtained by a detailed history and a complete physical examination (65,66).

Ischemic Colitis and Gastrointestinal Complications

Clinically evident ischemic colitis complicates 1% to 2% of cases of elective aortic repair and as many as 35% of cases with ruptured aneurysms (67). Patients usually experience bloody diarrhea one to seven days after the surgical procedure. Leukocytosis, abdominal distension, and abdominal pain should also alert the surgeon to the possibility of ischemic colitis. Sigmoidoscopy is the initial diagnostic test of choice, although it will not differentiate mucosal ischemia from full-thickness infarction. Approximately 50% of cases will be self-limiting, although some will progress to stricture formation. If transmural bowel infarction is present, surgical resection with colostomy and creation of a mucous fistula should be expediently performed. Creating two stomas will allow the surgeon to monitor further bowel necrosis, if it occurs. In an attempt to prevent ischemic colitis, many surgeons reimplant the inferior mesenteric artery (IMA) after aneurysm resection if that vessel does not demonstrate brisk back-bleeding. This technique, however, has not been shown to decrease the incidence of postoperative ischemic colitis (68).

Other gastrointestinal complications of abdominal aortic surgery include paralytic ileus, *Clostridium difficile* enterocolitis, mechanical obstruction, and acute cholecystitis.

Acute Renal Failure

Defined as a 20% increase in the blood urea nitrogen or serum creatinine concentration, acute renal failure complicates 3% to 7% of elective infrarenal aortic procedures and approximately 75% of aneurysmal ruptures. The mechanism of injury after rupture is decreased renal perfusion leading to acute tubular necrosis. In elective cases, atheroemboli are most commonly responsible for the renal failure. The hospital mortality rate is substantially increased for patients who require dialysis (69), but 75% of the survivors will regain renal function. Although in the past the preoperative administration of low-dose dopamine was advocated for preventing acute renal failure, this agent is no longer believed to be beneficial. The best preventative measure is careful monitoring of the fluid status in an attempt to maintain ideal renal perfusion.

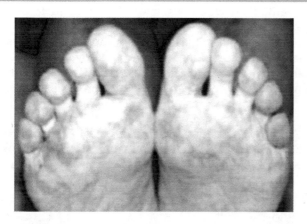

Figure 3 Acute lower extremity ischemia immediately after aortic surgery – "trash foot syndrome".

Impotence

Although commonly overlooked, impotence is one of the most common forms of morbidity associated with aortic surgery. Although nearly half of all men undergoing aortic surgery are impotent to begin with, of the remainder, as many as 75% will experience loss of potency postoperatively (70). Preventing this complication requires avoiding the sympathetic plexus, which travels along the inferior abdominal aorta on the left, in close proximity to the IMA, and using an end-to-side graft configuration when appropriate, as previously described.

Paraplegia

Paraplegia, a rare but devastating complication, occurs in association with fewer than 1% of infrarenal aortic procedures and 5% to 25% of thoracoabdominal aortic aneurysm repairs. The clinical presentation ranges from anterior or posterior arterial ischemic syndromes to a complete transverse myelopathy. Once the symptoms appear, the possibility of improvement is remote. Paraplegia in association with infrarenal aortic procedures is due to pelvic devascularization and can usually be prevented by ensuring the perfusion of at least one hypogastric artery. Paraplegia in association with thoracoabdominal aortic surgery is usually due to spinal cord ischemia. Many factors, both anatomic and physiologic, may cause this complication. The precise method of prevention is unknown, but several methods have been suggested, including reimplantation of intercostal vessels, reduction of cerebrospinal fluid pressure, epidural cooling of the spinal cord, the use of various pharmacologic "neuroprotective" agents, and partial cardiopulmonary bypass (71).

Incisional Hernia

The infrarenal aorta can be approached through either a retroperitoneal or a transperitoneal (midline) incision. The retroperitoneal approach is beneficial when patients are morbidly obese, when they have undergone multiple abdominal surgical procedures, and when exposure to the suprarenal aorta is necessary. The incision required for the retroperitoneal approach carries a 3% to 7% risk of hernia; however, a much more frequent problem is a persistent flank bulge. Occurring in 10% to 30% of patients, this bulge is related to intercostal nerve injury and can be prevented by avoiding extension into the 11th intercostal space (72).

A midline incision is appropriate when access to the right renal artery or the intraperitoneal organs is necessary. This approach is associated with a 5% incidence of hernia, a rate similar to that associated with midline incisions for other surgical procedures.

Graft Infection

The risk of graft infection is permanent and increases with time. The pathogenesis is usually bacterial seeding of the graft through a hematogenous route. Colonic bacterial translocation during surgery may contribute to the condition. The usual treatment involves removing the entire graft and performing an extra-anatomic bypass. One recent study reported a hospital mortality rate of 11%, with 64% primary patency and 100% secondary patency 60 months after placement with an axillofemoral technique (73). When an extra-anatomic bypass is not feasible, reconstruction of the aorta with autogenous superficial femoropopliteal vein (74) or cryopreserved arterial homograft (75) may be possible.

Aortoduodenal Fistula

Often discussed but rarely seen, aortoduodenal fistula is a life-threatening complication of late graft infection (76). Months to years after surgery, patients may experience the so-called "herald" hemorrhage. Surgeons should maintain a high index of suspicion for this complication whenever a patient with a gastrointestinal hemorrhage has a history of aortic surgery. The first step in the diagnosis of this complication is an emergent esophagogastroduodenoscopy, which should demonstrate the fistula if one is present. Equally important, the procedure may reveal other more common causes of gastrointestinal hemorrhage, such as peptic ulcer disease or diffuse hemorrhagic gastritis. Aortoduodenal fistula usually occurs between the proximal suture line and the duodenum. Aorto-sigmoid fistulas have also been described.

Other Complications

Additional types of morbidity that have been associated with aortic surgery include chyloperitoneum, ureteral obstruction, gluteal infarction, and obturator nerve injury.

Complications of Endovascular Aneurysm Repair

The placement of aortic stent grafts to repair or exclude infrarenal aortic aneurysms was first attempted in 1991 but did not become widespread until the Food and Drug Administration approved two devices in October 1999. Stent grafts gave vascular surgeons an alternative to conventional open repair, particularly for treating high-risk or elderly patients who would probably be expected to poorly tolerate laparotomy and aortic clamping. In addition because endovascular aneurysm repair (EAR) is associated with less pain and shorter recovery times than other procedures, it is a beneficial alternative for all patients. Initial results have demonstrated the technical feasibility of EAR, as well as its advantages and shortcomings. As is true for all new surgical procedures, EAR is associated with a number of complications, some specific to the new procedure and some common to both the new and the old procedures.

Patient Selection, Improper Positioning, and Device Failure

The most important determinant of the success of aortic stent grafts is the anatomy of the aneurysm and the iliac arteries. Proper proximal fixation requires a suitable length of infrarenal aorta (at least 1 cm) that is free of thrombus and is not heavily calcified or too severely angulated (77). Aortic necks larger than 26 mm in diameter are too large for adequate sealing of the graft to the aortic wall. Similar criteria are important to assure proper distal fixation; in addition, the iliac arteries must be large enough to allow safe passage of the introducer (see below). During the procedure, proper proximal fixation based on the results of intraoperative arteriography, fluoroscopy, and road-mapping is crucial. If the stent graft is deployed too proximally, one or both renal arteries can be inadvertently covered. If placed too distally, it will not attach and could slip into the aneurysmal sac. Both occurrences require immediate conversion to open repair.

Some devices are fixed to the aortic wall by hooks; others are fixed by the radial force of the stent. Device failure can result from hook fracture or continued expansion of the aortic neck, and such failure is perhaps the greatest concern associated with the concept of stent grafting. Because neither causative factor can be prevented, careful lifelong follow-up is mandatory for patients treated with stent grafts (see below).

Endoleak

The stent graft is deployed from a remote site, usually the femoral artery, and is connected to the aortic wall by a metallic stent connected to a graft proximal to the aneurysm and distal to the iliac arteries. The aneurysm is thus excluded from blood flow; the blood moves through the device into the distal circulation. The blood in the aneurysmal sac clots and the aneurysm eventually shrinks. Persistence of blood flow in the space between the stent graft and the aortic wall is called an endoleak (78).

There are four types of endoleak (79). Type I endoleaks occur when the attachment between the graft and the aorta or iliac arteries is faulty (Fig. 4). The aneurysm is not excluded from blood flow, remains pressurized, and can still rupture. Endoleaks of this type must be corrected when they are discovered. Type II leaks are caused by retrograde bleeding into the aneurysmal sac from branch vessels, usually the inferior mesenteric or lumbar arteries. Many of these endoleaks will clot within days or weeks. Type III leaks are specifically associated with modular stent grafts, which are composed of multiple pieces joined together at the time of implantation. Junction points can separate, thereby allowing blood flow into the aneurysmal sac. These endoleaks must be treated so that further expansion and possible rupture can be avoided. Type IV leaks result from defects or tears in the fabric of the graft, and most are self-limiting.

Type II endoleaks are the most common; they occur in association with 20% to 30% of procedures. Their clinical significance is not fully understood; although they are generally considered benign, they have been associated with a continued increase in

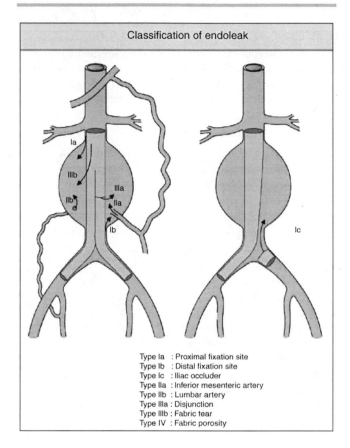

Figure 4 Types of endoleak. Obtained with permission from Comprehensive Vascular and Endovascular Surgery, Elsevier 2004.

the size of the aneurysm and with rupture in some cases (80). These endoleaks should be treated when they are associated with aneurysmal expansion. The treatment of endoleaks is complex and beyond the purview of this chapter. Most can be corrected with additional endovascular techniques, but some may require open surgical repair or replacement of the stent with a conventional aortic graft (80). Lifelong follow-up is necessary for patients who have experienced endoleak complications; the function of the aortic stent graft must be evaluated with CT scans every six to twelve months.

Rupture of an Aneurysm or Vessel

The stent graft is housed in an introducer sheath, which is inserted through a femoral artery cutdown and must traverse the iliac arteries. Such sheaths can be as large as 8 mm in diameter. Exerting undue force during insertion can cause arterial rupture or perforation, which results in substantial and even fatal hemorrhage. Patients with small or diseased iliac arteries are poor candidates for stent graft repair.

Recent reports have described cases of aneurysmal rupture after seemingly successful placement of stent grafts (81). Most of these cases involved either short and angulated proximal aneurysm necks, which were poorly suited to stent graft placement, or a known endoleak, with continued expansion of the aneurysm (82). Some ruptures have occurred in grafts thought to be in proper position and without obvious endoleaks or other defects. These problems underscore the fact that our understanding of the endovascular treatment of aneurysms is still incomplete and that proper patient selection and careful follow-up are crucial.

Graft Limb Thrombosis

Graft limbs may occlude early, usually because of technical errors such as kinking or twisting the limb, or because of attachment site problems such as dissection or stenosis (82). When defects are seen on an angiogram obtained after the procedure has been completed, angioplasty, placement of an additional stent, or both can correct most problems. Late limb thrombosis is usually caused by changes in the shape of the aneurysm as it shrinks. Most aneurysms will shorten and will also decrease in diameter. When this happens, iliac limbs may kink, especially in the externally reinforced type of graft, which is relatively inflexible. The initial sign of this kinking may be severe limb ischemia; in such cases, an urgent femorofemoral bypass procedure is necessary. Patients without critical symptoms can often be treated with thrombolysis and an additional endovascular procedure, such as angioplasty and stenting.

Limb Ischemia Due to Emboli

A thrombus or an atheroma may be dislodged by the wire sheath and by the passage of the device. Clamping the distal femoral arteries and initiating full anticoagulation before passing any devices can reduce the incidence of this problem.

Claudication and Paralysis

Aneurysms of the common iliac artery are present in 50% to 60% of patients with aortic aneurysms. When the common iliac arteries are too large to allow the graft to be sealed properly, terminating the graft in the external iliac artery may be necessary; in such cases, one or two of the internal iliac arteries are covered by the stent graft. The internal iliac artery is often embolized with coils so as to prevent back-bleeding and the resultant large endoleak. It has become apparent that such embolization is not a benign maneuver: 20% to 40% of patients will experience substantial claudication in the buttocks, a condition that usually improves but does not resolve completely (83). Lower-extremity paralysis and ischemic colitis are recognized complications of bilateral internal iliac occlusion.

VENOUS DISEASES
Complications of Varicose Vein Surgery

For decades, the stripping and ligation method has been touted as a safe and effective means of dealing with venous incompetence in the lower extremity. Postoperative hospital stays are usually brief, and many procedures are even performed on an outpatient basis. Although functional improvement occurs in most cases, reports of patient satisfaction are not consistently positive. Most dissatisfaction is related to the procedure's failure to achieve the desired cosmetic result. Minor complications are fairly common and include bruising, pain, and slight numbness. Major complications are rare but include injury to the femoral vein or artery, PE, DVT, compartment syndrome, and lymphatic injury. Lymphedema and groin lymphatic fistula seem to occur most frequently after reexploration of the groin for recurrent varicosities. The incidence of major complications is less than 1% and that of minor complications is 17% (84).

Complications of Sclerotherapy

The use of injectable irritating agents is an increasingly popular method of treating varicose veins and telangiectasia. Some of the more severe complications of this therapy are due to erroneous extravenous infusion of the sclerosing agent. Intradermal injection can result in ulcers or tissue necrosis, which may require wide debridement. Inadvertent intra-arterial injection is often associated with attempted injection of the agent into the lesser saphenous vein. The consequences of erroneous infusion can be severe enough to require limb amputation. Other untoward outcomes, such as allergic reaction, DVT, and PE, are rare (85).

Complications of Vena Cava Filter Placement

Traditionally, vena cava filters were used to treat patients at high risk of PE for whom anticoagulation was either contraindicated or had failed to prevent thrombus formation. Many authors advocate using these filters to treat all patients at high risk of PE (86). In general, filters can be placed expediently in the operating room or even in the intensive care unit (87). Complications that may occur during filter placement include pneumothorax, PE, bleeding at the insertion site, and guidewire mishaps such as entrapment of the wire in the filter device or migration of the filter device (88). Surgeons should also recognize that the incidence of intra-atrial shunts is high among patients with chronic thromboembolic disease and that such shunts can lead to paradoxical cerebral embolism (89). Late complications include filter migration, filter fracture, and vena cava occlusion, which occurs in 6% to 7% of cases reported in most long-term series (88).

COMPLICATIONS OF SURGERY FOR ACUTE ARTERIAL INSUFFICIENCY
Complications of Balloon Embolectomy

For patients with acute lower-extremity ischemia due to embolism, balloon catheter embolectomy is still the treatment of choice. Limb salvage procedures are successful in 75% to 90% of cases. Still, complications are common and sometimes severe. Mortality rates range from 10% to 20%. Local mechanical effects of the balloon on the vessel wall can include injury, perforation, or rupture. Wall injury leading to myointimal hyperplasia may result in stricture or, less commonly, in diffuse arterial narrowing. Preventing arterial injury requires using meticulous surgical technique, checking the balloon for leaks or eccentricity, and using the smallest effective catheter. Other risks associated with balloon embolectomy are groin hematoma at the insertion site and ischemia–reperfusion injury.

Complications of Ischemia and Reperfusion

Haimovici first described the ischemia–reperfusion syndrome in 1960 (90). The pathological insult occurs when an acutely ischemic limb is suddenly reperfused with warm blood. Acute muscle edema leads to elevated compartment pressures, which in turn lead to neuromuscular dysfunction. The syndrome is mediated by the release of potassium, myoglobin, free radicals, cytokines, and tumor necrosis factor-α from the injured muscle. Acute myoglobinuria can result in renal failure. Tumor necrosis factor-α is believed to lead to pulmonary injury and even to death in severe cases. The extent of the initial muscle injury is determined by ischemia time, limb temperature, and muscle location and type.

Many treatment options exist for ischemia–reperfusion syndrome. Fluid support and aggressive monitoring of the patient's electrolyte levels, especially the potassium concentration, are essential. Perioperative administration of hypertonic mannitol may be protective. Controlled limb reperfusion with a mixture of blood and a crystalloid solution and with limb hemodialysis has been advocated to control the metabolic derangements that lead to ischemia–reperfusion syndrome. Prophylactic fasciotomy is indicated when ischemia is prolonged (for more than six hours) (91).

Complications of Fasciotomy

When performed in a timely and expedient manner, a fasciotomy can literally save both life and limb. In light of this fact, complications arising from fasciotomy, although frequent, are relatively minor. Wound pain, altered skin sensation, pruritus, skin discoloration, and substantial scarring are the most commonly reported complaints. Infections are rare but can cause tibial osteomyelitis; excellent wound care is required to avoid this complication. The authors prefer to close all fasciotomies, usually with a split-thickness skin graft, as soon as possible. Patient education and reassurance provide adequate therapy in most cases. Bleeding and nerve injury are less common than infection and should be recognized and treated early.

Complications of Surgery for Hemodialysis

Surgical creation of hemodialysis access is a leading cause of morbidity among patients with end-stage renal disease. Complications associated with these procedures lead to frequent hospital admissions for the patient, large costs to the community, and a great deal of frustration for both the doctor and patient. Therefore, every effort should be made to minimize these untoward outcomes.

Temporary Devices

Providing emergent access for dialysis when patients have not yet undergone placement of permanent access or when the access has not yet matured often requires the insertion of a venous catheter. These catheters must be placed in a large vein, such as the subclavian vein or the femoral vein, so that the high flow rates necessary for hemodialysis can be accommodated. Temporary dialysis catheters are subject to the same complications that plague all central lines, including pneumothorax, hemothorax, hematoma, infection, and thrombosis.

Arteriovenous Fistulas and Grafts

Because it is associated with higher rates of patency and a lower incidence of complications, creating an arteriovenous fistula (AVF) is the procedure of choice for obtaining permanent access for hemodialysis. When creating an AVF is not possible because of anatomic constraints or poor vein quality, an arteriovenous graft (AVG) of polytetrafluoroethylene is the primary alternative. The problems most frequently encountered with each procedure will be discussed below.

Lack of Maturation of Arteriovenous Fistula

Although the long-term patency rate of AVFs is higher than that of AVGs, their initial failure rate is also higher. This lack of development is usually due to small-diameter veins (less than 2 mm). In some series, this complication has been reported to occur in as many as 15% to 25% of cases. Once technical problems have been ruled out as a cause of the fistula's failure, little can be done to salvage the site. The surgeon may then elect to place a fistula at an alternative site, such as the antecubital fossa if the wrist was the primary site, or to construct an AVG. If risk factors for lack of maturation are present (patients with diabetes, women, and older patients), using the upper arm as the initial site may yield improved results.

Ischemic Steal

A complication associated with both AVGs and AVFs is the vascular steal phenomenon, which can lead to hand ischemia (Fig. 5). This complication occurs most commonly when the brachial artery is used. The size of the arterial anastomosis is crucial; the diagnosis is correlated with a wrist–brachial index of less than 0.75, which improves with digital occlusion of the fistula. Treatment options include fistula ligation, arterial banding, and graft lengthening (92).

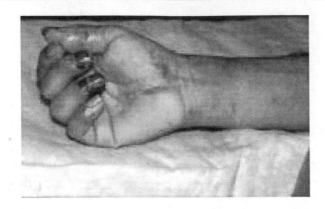

Figure 5 Vascular steal phenomenon leading to hand ischemia.

Early and Late Thrombosis

The leading cause of fistula loss is thrombosis, which can be classified as either early (less than six weeks after placement of the fistula) or late. Early thrombosis is often due to a technical problem, but it can also occur when the diameter of the native vessels is small—especially the vessels on the venous end.

Late thrombosis can be caused by multiple factors, including stenosis (which reduces the flow of blood through the graft), coagulation abnormalities, and cardiac dysfunction. Factors that confer a negative prognosis for graft survival are diabetes, advanced age, female sex, hypoalbuminemia, and hyperfibrinogenemia. The stenosis forms at the venous anastomosis, in the graft itself, or in the central venous system. Approximately 90% of stenoses occur at the venous anastomosis. Thrombectomy, graft revision, or both can often restore function. Thrombolysis with endovascular therapy has been reported to achieve patency rates equivalent to those achieved by thrombectomy or graft revision but at a substantially greater cost and with a high rate of technical failure, which requires surgical intervention (93).

Infection and False Aneurysm

Infection, although rare in association with autogenous fistulas, complicates 3% to 8% of all AVGs. The causative organism is predominantly *Staphylococcus aureus* (94). The ideal treatment is complete removal of the graft; however, when access is limited, some success has been achieved by partial removal of the graft or by incision and drainage with administration of intravenous antibiotics.

The formation of a pseudoaneurysm, which is fairly common in association with AVGs, results from continued puncture of the graft with large-bore needles. When puncture wounds become excessively large or numerous, surgical revision is indicated.

Venous Hypertension

Venous hypertension is a rare complication most often seen when side-to-side Brescia–Cimino fistulas are created. The hypertension results from arterialization of the venous system proximal to the fistula. If the venous valves are incompetent, retrograde flow can develop.

Physical findings include distal edema, venous congestion, and discoloration that can progress to ulceration. The most common cause is subclavian vein thrombosis proximal to a patent AVF, which causes a painful swollen arm. The diagnosis of venous hypertension can be made by duplex ultrasonography, magnetic resonance venography, or contrast venography.

Surgical treatment of venous hypertension caused by a Brescia–Cimino shunt is ligation of the vein distal to the fistula and conversion to a functional venous end-to-side anastomosis. Treatment of other forms of venous hypertension involves control of venous hypertension either by ligation of the fistula or by relief of the subclavian vein stenosis, usually by balloon angioplasty with or without stenting (95).

SUMMARY

The practice of vascular surgery is perhaps one of the more demanding of the medical specialties. Given the significant premorbid conditions of most patients that come to the attention of the vascular surgeon, and the physiological stress of the surgical procedures, complications can be frequent and significant. While not entirely unavoidable, a high degree of expertise and attention to detail can lessen the incidence of these adverse events.

REFERENCES

1. Hertzer NR, Beven EG, Young JR, et al. Coronary artery disease in peripheral vascular patients. A classification of 1000 coronary angiograms and results of surgical management. Ann Surg 1984; 199(2):223–233.
2. L'Italien GJ, Cambria RP, Cutler BS, et al. Comparative early and late cardiac morbidity among patients requiring different vascular surgery procedures. J Vasc Surg 1995; 21(6):935–944.
3. Mangano DT. Perioperative cardiac morbidity. Anesthesiology 1990; 72(1):153–184.
4. Hertzer NR. The natural history of peripheral vascular disease. Implications for its management. Circulation 1991; 83(suppl 2):I12–I19.
5. Cohn PF. Silent myocardial ischemia. Ann Intern Med 1988; 109(4):312–317.
6. Boucher CA, Brewster DC, Darling RC, Okada RD, Strauss HW, Pohost GM. Determination of cardiac risk by dipyridamole-thallium imaging before peripheral vascular surgery. N Engl J Med 1985; 312(7):389–394.
7. Cutler BS, Leppo JA. Dipyridamole thallium 201 scintigraphy to detect coronary artery disease before abdominal aortic surgery. J Vasc Surg 1987; 5(1):91–100.

8. Eagle KA, Coley CM, Newell JB, et al. Combining clinical and thallium data optimizes preoperative assessment of cardiac risk before major vascular surgery. Ann Intern Med 1989; 110(11):859–866.

9. Eagle KA, Singer DE, Brewster DC, Darling RC, Mulley AG, Boucher CA. Dipyridamole-thallium scanning in patients undergoing vascular surgery. Optimizing preoperative evaluation of cardiac risk. JAMA 1987; 257(16):2185–2189.

10. Eagle KA, Boucher CA. Cardiac risk of noncardiac surgery. N Engl J Med 1989; 321(19):1330–1332.

11. Jayr C, Matthay MA, Goldstone J, Gold WM, Wiener-Kronish JP. Preoperative and intraoperative factors associated with prolonged mechanical ventilation. A study in patients following major abdominal vascular surgery. Chest 1993; 103(4):1231–1236.

12. Kispert JF, Kazmers A, Roitman L. Preoperative spirometry predicts perioperative pulmonary complications after major vascular surgery. Am Surg 1992; 58(8): 491–495.

13. Bartlett RH, Gazzaniga AB, Geraghty TR. Respiratory maneuvers to prevent postoperative pulmonary complications. A critical review. JAMA 1973; 224(7): 1017–1021.

14. Shanley CJ, Bartlett RH. The management of acute respiratory failure. Curr Opin Gen Surg 1994:7–16.

15. Barker SJ, Tremper KK. Pulse oximetry: applications and limitations. Int Anesthesiol Clin 1987; 25(3):155–175.

16. Solomon R, Werner C, Mann D, D'Elia J, Silva P. Effects of saline, mannitol, and furosemide to prevent acute decreases in renal function induced by radiocontrast agents. N Engl J Med 1994; 331(21):1416–1420.

17. Eneas JF, Schoenfeld PY, Humphreys MH. The effect of infusion of mannitol-sodium bicarbonate on the clinical course of myoglobinuria. Arch Intern Med 1979; 139(7):801–805.

18. Liebman PR, Menzoian JO, Mannick JA, Lowney BW, LoGerfo FW. Intraoperative arteriography in femoropopliteal and femorotibial bypass grafts. Arch Surg 1981; 116(8):1019–1021.

19. Miller A, Stonebridge PA, Jepsen SJ, et al. Continued experience with intraoperative angioscopy for monitoring infrainguinal bypass grafting. Surgery 1991; 109(3 Pt 1):286–293.

20. Yu A, Gregory D, Morrison L, Morgan S. The role of intra-operative duplex imaging in arterial reconstructions. Am J Surg 1996; 171(5):500–501.

21. Donaldson MC, Belkin M, Whittemore AD, Mannick JA, Longtine JA, Dorfman DM. Impact of activated protein C resistance on general vascular surgical patients. J Vasc Surg 1997; 25(6):1054–1060.

22. Bick RL. Disseminated intravascular coagulation and related syndromes: a clinical review. Semin Thromb Hemost 1988; 14(4):299–338.

23. Anderson RJ, Linas SL, Berns AS, et al. Nonoliguric acute renal failure. N Engl J Med 1977; 296(20):1134–1138.

24. Miller DC, Myers BD. Pathophysiology and prevention of acute renal failure associated with thoracoabdominal or abdominal aortic surgery. J Vasc Surg 1987; 5(3): 518–523.

25. Clowes A. Pathologic intimal hyperplasia as a response to vascular injury and reconstruction. In: Rutherford R, ed. Vascular Surgery. Vol. 1. 5th ed. Philadelphia: W.B. Saunders Company, 2000:408–418.

26. Sedwitz MM, Hye RJ, Stabile BE. The changing epidemiology of pseudoaneurysm. Therapeutic implications. Arch Surg 1988; 123(4):473–476.

27. Moore WS, Hall AD. Late suture failure in the pathogenesis of anastomotic false aneurysms. Ann Surg 1970; 172(6):1064–1068.

28. Corson JD, Leather RP, Naraynsingh V, Shah DM, Young HL, Karmody AM. In situ femoral, popliteal and distal bypass for limb salvage. Br J Surg 1983; 70(12):744–745.

29. Miller A, Stonebridge PA, Tsoukas AI, et al. Angioscopically directed valvulotomy: a new valvulotome and technique. J Vasc Surg 1991; 13(6):813–820.

30. Adcock OT Jr, Adcock GL, Wheeler JR, Gregory RT, Snyder SO Jr, Gayle RG. Optimal techniques for harvesting and preparation of reversed autogenous vein grafts for use as arterial substitutes: a review. Surgery 1984; 96(5):886–894.

31. Bernhard VM, Boren CH, Towne JB. Pneumatic tourniquet as a substitute for vascular clamps in distal bypass surgery. Surgery 1980; 87(6):709–713.

32. Blakeman BM, Littooy FN, Baker WH. Intra-arterial digital subtraction angiography as a method to study peripheral vascular disease. J Vasc Surg 1986; 4(2): 168–173.

33. Hertz SM, Baum RA, Owen RS, Holland GA, Logan DR, Carpenter JP. Comparison of magnetic resonance angiography and contrast arteriography in peripheral arterial stenosis. Am J Surg 1993; 166(2):112–116.

34. Robinson KD, Sato DT, Gregory RT, et al. Long-term outcome after early infrainguinal graft failure. J Vasc Surg 1997; 26(3):425–437.

35. Gloviczki P, Lowell RC. Lymphatic complications of vascular surgery. In: Rutherford R, ed. Vascular Surgery. Vol. 1. 5th ed. Philadelphia: W.B. Saunders Company, 2000:781–789.

36. Meyer JP, Durham JR, Schwarcz TH, Sawchuk AP, Schuler JJ. The use of sartorius muscle rotation-transfer in the management of wound complications after infrainguinal vein bypass: a report of eight cases and description of the technique. J Vasc Surg 1989; 9(5):731–735.

37. Tukiainen E, Biancari F, Lepantalo M. Deep infection of infrapopliteal autogenous vein grafts—immediate use of muscle flaps in leg salvage. J Vasc Surg 1998; 28(4):611–616.

38. Campbell DR, Bartlett FF. Postoperative Pseudomonas urinary tract infections as a source of bacterial contamination of an autogenous vein graft. J Vasc Surg 1987; 5(3):492–494.

39. Cherry KJ Jr, Roland CF, Pairolero PC, et al. Infected femorodistal bypass: is graft removal mandatory? J Vasc Surg 1992; 15(2):295–303.

40. Stonebridge PA, Miller A, Tsoukas A, et al. Angioscopy of arm vein infrainguinal bypass grafts. Ann Vasc Surg 1991; 5(2):170–175.

41. Mills JL, Bandyk DF, Gahtan V, Esses GE. The origin of infrainguinal vein graft stenosis: a prospective study based on duplex surveillance. J Vasc Surg 1995; 21(1):16–22.

42. Keagy BA, Schwartz JA, Kotb M, Burnham SJ, Johnson G Jr. Lower extremity amputation: the control series. J Vasc Surg 1986; 4(4):321–326.

43. Fearon J, Campbell DR, Hoar CS Jr, Gibbons GW, Rowbotham JL, Wheelock FC Jr. Improved results with

diabetic below-knee amputations. Arch Surg 1985; 120(7):777–780.

44. Gibbons GW, Wheelock FC Jr, Hoar CS Jr, Rowbotham JL, Siembieda C. Predicting success of forefoot amputations in diabetics by noninvasive testing. Arch Surg 1979; 114(9):1034–1036.

45. Moller BN, Krebs B. Antibiotic prophylaxis in lower limb amputation. Acta Orthop Scand 1985; 56(4):327–329.

46. Yeager RA, Moneta GL, Edwards JM, Taylor LM Jr, McConnell DB, Porter JM. Deep vein thrombosis associated with lower extremity amputation. J Vasc Surg 1995; 22(5):612–615.

47. Feinglass J, Pearce WH, Martin GJ, et al. Postoperative and late survival outcomes after major amputation: findings from the Department of Veterans Affairs National Surgical Quality Improvement Program. Surgery 2001; 130(1):21–29.

48. Executive Committee for the Asymptomatic Carotid Atherosclerosis Study. Endarterectomy for asymptomatic carotid artery stenosis. JAMA 1995; 273(18): 1421–1428.

49. Muto PM, Welch HJ, Mackey WC, O'Donnell TF. Evaluation of carotid artery stenosis: is duplex ultrasonography sufficient? J Vasc Surg 1996; 24(1):17–22.

50. Riles TS, Imparato AM, Jacobowitz GR, et al. The cause of perioperative stroke after carotid endarterectomy. J Vasc Surg 1994; 19(2):206–214.

51. Hamdan AD, Pomposelli FB Jr, Gibbons GW, Campbell DR, LoGerfo FW. Perioperative strokes after 1001 consecutive carotid endarterectomy procedures without an electroencephalogram: incidence, mechanism, and recovery. Arch Surg 1999; 134(4):412–415.

52. Rockman CB, Jacobowitz GR, Lamparello PJ, et al. Immediate reexploration for the perioperative neurologic event after carotid endarterectomy: is it worthwhile? J Vasc Surg 2000; 32(6):1062–1070.

53. Pomposelli FB, Lamparello PJ, Riles TS, Craighead CC, Giangola G, Imparato AM. Intracranial hemorrhage after carotid endarterectomy. J Vasc Surg 1988; 7(2): 248–255.

54. North American Symptomatic Carotid Endarterectomy Trial Collaborators. Beneficial effect of carotid endarterectomy in symptomatic patients with high-grade carotid stenosis. N Engl J Med 1991; 325(7):445–453.

55. Schauber MD, Fontenelle LJ, Solomon JW, Hanson TL. Cranial/cervical nerve dysfunction after carotid endarterectomy. J Vasc Surg 1997; 25(3):481–487.

56. Das MB, Hertzer NR, Ratliff NB, O'Hara PJ, Beven EG. Recurrent carotid stenosis. A five-year series of 65 reoperations. Ann Surg 1985; 202(1):28–35.

57. O'Donnell TF Jr, Rodriguez AA, Fortunato JE, Welch HJ, Mackey WC. Management of recurrent carotid stenosis: should asymptomatic lesions be treated surgically? J Vasc Surg 1996; 24(2):207–212.

58. Galland RB, Wolfe JH. Mortality after elective abdominal aortic aneurysm repair: not where … but how many and by whom. Ann R Coll Surg Engl 1998; 80(5):339–340.

59. Whittemore AD, Clowes AW, Hechtman HB, Mannick JA. Aortic aneurysm repair. Reduced operative mortality associated with maintenance of optimal cardiac performance. Ann Surg 1980; 192(3):414–421.

60. Hagino RT, Taylor SM, Fujitani RM, Mills JL. Proximal anastomotic failure following infrarenal aortic reconstruction: late development of true aneurysms, pseudoaneurysms, and occlusive disease. Ann Vasc Surg 1993; 7(1):8–13.

61. Moncure AC, Brewster DC, Darling RC, Atnip RG, Newton WD, Abbott WM. Use of the splenic and hepatic arteries for renal revascularization. J Vasc Surg 1986; 3(2):196–203.

62. Farber MA, Carlin RE, Marston WA, Owens LV, Burnham SJ, Keagy BA. Distal thoracic aorta as inflow for the treatment of chronic mesenteric ischemia. J Vasc Surg 2001; 33(2):281–287.

63. Marty-Ane CH, Alric P, Picot MC, Picard E, Colson P, Mary H. Ruptured abdominal aortic aneurysm: influence of intraoperative management on surgical outcome. J Vasc Surg 1995; 22(6):780–786.

64. Kuhan G, Raptis S. 'Trash foot' following operations involving the abdominal aorta. Aust N Z J Surg 1997; 67(1):21–24.

65. D'Angelo AJ, Puppala D, Farber A, Murphy AE, Faust GR, Cohen JR. Is preoperative cardiac evaluation for abdominal aortic aneurysm repair necessary? J Vasc Surg 1997; 25(1):152–156.

66. Klonaris CN, Bastounis EA, Xiromeritis NC, Balas PE. The predictive value of dipyridamole-thallium scintigraphy for cardiac risk assessment before major vascular surgery. Int Angiol 1998; 17(3):171–178.

67. Brewster DC, Franklin DP, Cambria RP, et al. Intestinal ischemia complicating abdominal aortic surgery. Surgery 1991; 109(4):447–454.

68. Killen DA, Reed WA, Gorton ME, et al. Is routine postaneurysmectomy hemodynamic assessment of the inferior mesenteric artery circulation helpful? Ann Vasc Surg 1999; 13(5):533–538.

69. Katz DJ, Stanley JC, Zelenock GB. Operative mortality rates for intact and ruptured abdominal aortic aneurysms in Michigan: an eleven-year statewide experience. J Vasc Surg 1994; 19(5):804–815.

70. Lee ES, Kor DJ, Kuskowski MA, Santilli SM. Incidence of erectile dysfunction after open abdominal aortic aneurysm repair. Ann Vasc Surg 2000; 14(1):13–19.

71. Cambria R. Thoracoabdominal aortic aneurysms. In: Rutherford R, ed. Vascular Surgery. Vol. 2 5th ed.. Philadelphia: W.B. Saunders Company, 2000:1303–1325.

72. Gardner GP, Josephs LG, Rosca M, Rich J, Woodson J, Menzoian JO. The retroperitoneal incision. An evaluation of postoperative flank 'bulge'. Arch Surg 1994; 129(7):753–756.

73. Seeger JM, Pretus HA, Welborn MB, Ozaki CK, Flynn TC, Huber TS. Long-term outcome after treatment of aortic graft infection with staged extra-anatomic bypass grafting and aortic graft removal. J Vasc Surg 2000; 32(3):451–459.

74. Gordon LL, Hagino RT, Jackson MR, Modrall JG, Valentine RJ, Clagett GP. Complex aortofemoral prosthetic infections: the role of autogenous superficial femoropopliteal vein reconstruction. Arch Surg 1999; 134(6):615–620.

75. Locati P, Socrate AM, Costantini E. Surgical repair of infected peripheral graft and abdominal aortic aneurysm using arterial homograft. Ann Vasc Surg 2000; 14(2):176–180.

76. Pegoraro M, Ferrero F, Palladino F, Baracco C, Merlo M, Bretto P. Aorto-enteric fistula as a rare complication of reconstructive surgery of the abdominal aorta. Minerva Cardioangiol 1984; 32(3):113–118.

77. Buth J, Laheij RJ. Early complications and endoleaks after endovascular abdominal aortic aneurysm

repair: report of a multicenter study. J Vasc Surg 2000; 31(1 Pt 1):134–146.

78. Schurink GW, Aarts NJ, van Bockel JH. Endoleak after stent-graft treatment of abdominal aortic aneurysm: a meta-analysis of clinical studies. Br J Surg 1999; 86(5): 581–587.

79. Wain RA, Marin ML, Ohki T, et al. Endoleaks after endovascular graft treatment of aortic aneurysms: classification, risk factors, and outcome. J Vasc Surg 1998; 27(1):69–78.

80. Zarins CK, White RA, Hodgson KJ, Schwarten D, Fogarty TJ. Endoleak as a predictor of outcome after endovascular aneurysm repair: AneuRx multicenter clinical trial. J Vasc Surg 2000; 32(1):90–107.

81. Zarins CK, White RA, Fogarty TJ. Aneurysm rupture after endovascular repair using the AneuRx stent graft. J Vasc Surg 2000; 31(5):960–970.

82. Zarins CK, White RA, Moll FL, et al. The AneuRx stent graft: four-year results and worldwide experience 2000. J Vasc Surg 2001; 33(suppl 2):S135–S145.

83. Lee WA, O'Dorisio J, Wolf YG, Hill BB, Fogarty TJ, Zarins CK. Outcome after unilateral hypogastric artery occlusion during endovascular aneurysm repair. J Vasc Surg 2001; 33(5):921–926.

84. Mildner A, Hilbe G. Complications in surgery of varicose veins. Zentralbl Chir 2001; 126(7):543–545.

85. Goldman M. Complications and adverse sequelae of sclerotherapy. In: Goldman MP, Bergan JJ, eds. Sclerotherapy: Treatment of Varicose and Telangiectatic Leg Veins. 3rd ed. St. Louis: Mosby, 2001:191–240.

86. Proctor MC. Indications for filter placement. Semin Vasc Surg 2000; 13(3):194–198.

87. Ebaugh JL, Chiou AC, Morasch MD, Matsumura JS, Pearce WH. Bedside vena cava filter placement guided with intravascular ultrasound. J Vasc Surg 2001; 34(1): 21–26.

88. Greenfield LJ, Proctor MC. Filter complications and their management. Semin Vasc Surg 2000; 13(3): 213–216.

89. Krieter DH, Rumpf KW, Muller GA, Werner GS. Paradoxical cerebral embolism during fibrinolytic therapy in deep venous thrombosis of the leg and pulmonary embolism. Dtsch Med Wochenschr 1994; 119(22):825.

90. Haimovici H. Arterial embolism with acute massive ischemic myopathy and myoglobinuria: evaluation of a hitherto unreported syndrome with report of two cases. Surgery 1960; 47:739–747.

91. Patman RD, Thompson JE. Fasciotomy in peripheral vascular surgery. Report of 164 patients. Arch Surg 1970; 101(6):663–672.

92. Haimov M, Schanzer H, Skladani M. Pathogenesis and management of upper-extremity ischemia following angioaccess surgery. Blood Purif 1996; 14(5):350–354.

93. Brooks JL, Sigley RD, May KJ Jr, Mack RM. Transluminal angioplasty versus surgical repair for stenosis of hemodialysis grafts. A randomized study. Am J Surg 1987; 153(6):530–531.

94. Mennes PA, Gilula LA, Anderson CB, Etheredge EE, Weerts C, Harter HR. Complications associated with arteriovenous fistulas in patients undergoing chronic hemodialysis. Arch Intern Med 1978; 138(7): 1117–1121.

95. Bhatia DS, Money SR, Ochsner JL, et al. Comparison of surgical bypass and percutaneous balloon dilatation with primary stent placement in the treatment of central venous obstruction in the dialysis patient: one-year follow-up. Ann Vasc Surg 1996; 10(5):452–455.

27

Acute Complications of Cardiovascular Surgery and Trauma

Riyad C. Karmy-Jones
Division of Cardiothoracic Surgery, University of Washington, and Thoracic Surgery, Harborview Medical Center, Seattle, Washington, U.S.A.

Edward M. Boyle
Division of Cardiothoracic Surgery, University of Washington, Seattle, Washington, U.S.A.

John C. Mullen
Department of Cardiac Sciences, University of Alberta, Edmonton, Canada

The spectrum of cardiac surgery has changed substantially in the past decade. The complexity of cases has increased, with increases in the number of repeated procedures and the number of older and sicker patients referred for surgery. At the same time, surgical practice has changed to include minimal access approaches, off-pump cardiopulmonary bypass techniques, bypass modifications to alleviate inflammatory responses, biochemical investigations to ameliorate ischemia–reperfusion injury, and improved artificial valves (such as stentless valves). These changes have substantial implications for the long-term outcome of patients undergoing surgical interventions, and a detailed discussion of these implications is beyond the scope of this chapter. However, the prevention and treatment of acute complications remain important, particularly as the surgical population becomes older and more likely to have comorbid conditions (1). Bojar noted that after coronary bypass procedures, approximately 10% of patients will experience a complication that will require treatment, prolonged hospitalization, or both (Table 1) (1).

The incidence of traumatic cardiovascular injury continues to increase (2,3). Advances in prehospital care mean that more severely injured patients will arrive at the hospital alive, although in extremis, and that more of them will survive. At the same time, newer diagnostic and therapeutic approaches have changed the management of these traumatic injuries, e.g., the use of endovascular stent grafts for the nonoperative treatment of patients with blunt aortic injury (4).

This chapter will focus on the immediate and early postoperative complications that may be encountered and should be anticipated in association with treatment of traumatic cardiovascular injuries. The primary emphasis is on the technical aspects and acute management of cardiovascular diseases.

TECHNICAL COMPLICATIONS RELATED TO CARDIOPULMONARY BYPASS
Iatrogenic Arterial Dissection

Iatrogenic dissection of the ascending aorta occurs in as few as 0.12% of cases in which cardiopulmonary bypass is used (5). Factors predisposing patients to undergo iatrogenic dissection include hypertension and connective tissue disorders, but the primary risk factor is calcification of the aorta (6). Dissection can occur from cannulation, clamping, or cardioplegia, or because of the creation of proximal anastomotic sites (7). In two-thirds of cases, dissection of the ascending aorta occurs acutely, with a rapidly expanding hematoma, bleeding, and, eventually, decreased return from the venous pump, which reflects blood loss (8). In the remaining third of cases, dissection occurs postoperatively.

The overall mortality rate associated with acute dissection of the ascending aorta is nearly 30% (8). When the dissection is discovered intraoperatively, the

Table 1 Complications After Coronary Bypass Procedures

Complications	Average incidence (%)
Arrhythmias	
Atrial	30
Ventricular	5
Infectious complications	
Leg wound	5
Sternal wound	3
Myocardial infarction	5
Respiratory failure	5
Reoperation for bleeding	3
Stroke	2
Gastrointestinal complications	2
Renal failure	2

Source: From Ref. 1.

mortality rate is approximately 20%; if it is recognized postoperatively, the mortality rate increases to 50% (7). Management of this condition requires removal of the cause (if it occurs at the site of arterial cannulation, the cannula must be replaced at another site), deepening hypothermia, and repair. Repair may be simple, using gelatin–resorcin–formalin glue or pledgeted sutures, but aortic tube grafts may also be required (6).

The symptoms of postoperative dissection of the ascending aorta are similar to those of acute aortic dissection, including tamponade (6). The primary methods of preventing this complication are to ensure that the surgical procedure avoids areas of aortic calcification that have been defined by palpation and echocardiography and to carefully control blood pressure during manipulation of the aorta.

Aortic dissection may occur more commonly after cannulation of the femoral artery (9). Manifestations can include high pressures, which reflect obstruction, or acute rupture of the vessel. More common complications after cannulation of the femoral artery, however, are occlusion or emboli, which can cause postoperative limb ischemia. As is true of the ascending aorta, palpation of the femoral artery at the time of surgery may indicate that one site is safer than another. Limited arterial dissections may be medically managed, but extensive dissections require surgical repair.

Rupture of the Coronary Sinus

Rupture of the coronary sinus occurs during retrograde cardioplegia in fewer than 1% of cases. It manifests itself as vigorous retrocardiac bleeding into the pericardial sac (10,11). Management depends upon how large the rupture is, when it occurred, and whether antegrade cardioplegia is possible. If antegrade cardioplegia is possible, reasonable treatment consists of cooling, antegrade cardioplegia, and subsequent cardioplegia through successive vein grafts, followed by repair at the end of the case. If antegrade cardioplegia is not a reliable option (e.g., in the case of reoperation using a patent mammary artery for repair, or because of severe obstructive lesions in the coronary arteries), then one of two treatments may be used: rapid cooling and bypass with the patient under fibrillatory arrest to ensure adequate venting of the heart and with antegrade cardioplegia through successive vein grafts, or immediate repair over the catheter. Although immediate repair may initially seem to be the "best" approach, it must be remembered that the repair will have to withstand the pressures created by delivering cardioplegia and that the catheter tip will most likely be advanced past the tributary that drains a substantial portion of the right ventricle and atrium; thus, less protection will be provided to these areas. If this option is chosen, the first anastomosis should be to the right coronary distribution.

The actual repair can be performed over the catheter, which acts as a stent. Primary repair, vein patch, and, occasionally, Gore-Tex® (W.L. Gore & Associates,

Inc., Newark, Delaware U.S.A.) patch repairs that connect to the right atrium have been used (10,11).

Venous Air Lock

Occasionally, a large amount of air will be entrained into the venous cannula. This complication most commonly occurs during operations on the right side of the heart, such as closure of a patent foramen ovale or tricuspid valve repair, when snares around the cannula loosen. If a substantial air lock occurs, the pump will stop automatically until the reservoir level has been replenished. Management includes the use of "sucker bypass" to refill the reservoir, purging the venous lines with saline solution, and repositioning the cannula and securing its snares.

Systemic Air Embolism

One large study has documented the occurrence of systemic air embolism in 458 of 575,000 cases (12). The impact of this complication is predominantly noted postoperatively; left hemiparesis is observed as a consequence of embolization of the right carotid artery (13). Massive systemic air embolism is associated with an immediate mortality rate of 22% (14). Air embolism has many potential causes (Table 2). The use of membrane oxygenators rather than bubble oxygenators has reduced the risk of air embolism, particularly the risk of a drop in the reservoir level (15). In general, there is no substitute for carefully checking the pump circuits and connections and for having an organized plan for removing air, particularly during open heart procedures. The left atrial appendage should be invaginated, the lungs should be ventilated with restricted venous return, and residual blood should be aspirated. If the left atrium has been opened, a catheter placed across the mitral valve will prevent

Table 2 Sources of Systemic Air Embolism

Bypass machine
  Drop in reservoir level
  Pressurization of cardiotomy
  Reservoir reversal of pump-head rotation
  Disconnection of oxygenator
  Inadequate debubbling of lines
Venting
  Excessive suction on atrial vent lines
  Air entering aorta retrograde via nonoccluded coronary arteries
    when excessive aortic venting is applied
Heart
  Retained air in atrial appendage
  Retained air in trabeculae
  Retained air in pulmonary veins
  Unexpected resumption of cardiac activity when heart is open
  Unexpected patent foramen ovale when the patient is on
    cardiopulmonary bypass but heart is not arrested
Other
  Continued use of intra-aortic balloon pump, which can suck air
    when arch is opened
  Air introduced from venous lines in setting of patent foramen ovale
  Entry via partial occlusion clamp when proximal anastomoses
    are performed

ventricular ejection until deairing is complete. Aortic clamping should be maintained until all air bubbles have been removed.

If air is pumped into the patient, a sequence of events must be undertaken quickly (Fig. 1). Retrograde perfusion at 20°C, with flows of 1 to 2 L/min in the average adult, can prevent injury in 61% of cases (12). Maintaining hypothermia at 20 to 22°C will reduce cerebral metabolic requirements and encourage gas solubility (13). Administering high-dose steroids, mannitol, glycerol, or some combination of the three has been shown to reduce the likelihood of injury (16,17). Increasing cerebral perfusion by augmenting flow (6.0–6.6 L/min) and blood pressure (including administering vasopressor drugs) may help purge the cerebral vasculature. Cerebral perfusion can be further enhanced by temporarily clamping the descending thoracic aorta (13). Thiopental (40 mg/kg) has been used to quiet brain activity until bypass is complete (18). Although the use of thiopental is attractive, it is associated with substantial negative effects, including myocardial depression and a delay in early return of consciousness, which would otherwise be the best indicator of a good prognosis (19). If the necessary equipment is available, hyperbaric oxygenation may be a useful adjunct (20).

Coronary Air Embolism

Air may be introduced into the coronary arteries by any of the mechanisms described above, but it may also be inadvertently injected through the cardioplegia lines. When the source of the air is systemic, the right coronary artery, which is more anterior, is most often involved. Heart block, right ventricular dysfunction, or both will result (13). Prevention includes all of the techniques described above. In addition, removing air from the aortic root by means of a clamp placed across the valve and using a venting needle in the anterior aorta during slow removal of the cross clamp have proved useful (21). If air introduction is recognized, purging the coronary arteries by elevating aortic root pressure or by retrograde flushing will assist in return of function (13).

Protamine Reactions

Adverse reactions to protamine, which is used to reverse the effects of heparin, may be the most common intraoperative complication associated with cardiopulmonary bypass (22,23). Various reactions have been characterized and loosely categorized as "predictable" (nonspecific) hypotension and "idiosyncratic" reactions (24). Nonspecific hypotension appears to be related to direct or histamine-mediated vasodilatation rather than to a direct myocardial depressant effect (25). Slow administration of protamine over a period of 10 to 15 minutes will reduce the incidence and magnitude of the hypotension, but the condition may still occur. Treatment includes temporarily stopping protamine administration and, if the reaction is serious, administering short-acting vasoconstrictor drugs.

Idiosyncratic reactions include an anaphylactic reaction mediated by immunoglobulins and an anaphylactoid reaction not mediated by immunoglobulins. Both reactions result in histamine release, which leads to bronchospasm, edema, and decreased systemic and pulmonary vascular resistance; this sequence, in turn, leads to low systemic and pulmonary pressures. These reactions may be more likely when patients have received neutral protamine Hagedorn insulin or have fish allergies. Initial management includes reinstitution of bypass if the reaction is too severe to allow time for medical intervention to take effect. Medical treatments include volume expansion, administration of epinephrine, steroids, and antihistamines (both H1 and H2 blockers), and administration of aminophylline if bronchospasm is persistent.

Catastrophic pulmonary vasoconstriction differs from protamine reactions in that systemic hypotension is coupled with pulmonary hypertension and acute right heart failure. Heparin–protamine complexes are believed to cause the release of thromboxane by means of the complement cascade (26,27). Treatment includes repeated administration of heparin, reinstitution of bypass, and administration of pulmonary vasodilator drugs (28).

Atrial Cannulation During Left Heart Bypass

The left atrial appendage is often extremely friable and can tear with catastrophic results. In addition, passing a cannula into the left atrium is associated with the risk of posterior atrial rupture. Furthermore, in the setting

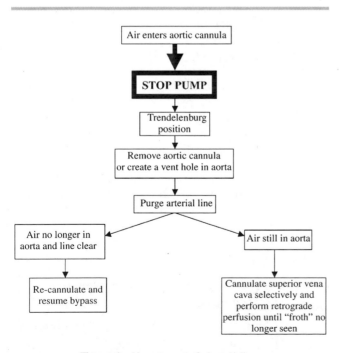

Figure 1 Management of air embolism.

of traumatic injury, hematoma can obscure landmarks and cardiac irritability can increase the risk of malignant arrhythmias (29). Accessing the left atrium extrapericardially through the pulmonary veins is associated with a marked reduction in the incidence of complications. Karmy-Jones et al. (30) noted a 37% incidence of significant complications (including ventricular fibrillation leading to arrest) when the atrial appendage was cannulated for bypass during repair of traumatic aortic rupture, as opposed to 7% when the pulmonary veins were used.

COMPLICATIONS OF REPEAT CARDIAC OPERATION

The cumulative incidence of repeated coronary bypass is approximately 11% by 10 years after the initial bypass procedure. The incidence increases if internal mammary arteries (IMAs) were not used or if incomplete revascularization was performed (31). Indications for repeated operation [as opposed to percutaneous transluminal coronary angioplasty (PTCA)] include (32):

1. Vein graft stenosis of more than 50%, occurring more than five years after initial surgery, particularly if large areas of myocardium [usually the left anterior descending artery (LAD)] are at risk
2. Left main or multiple-vessel disease and decreased left ventricular function, or proximal LAD stenosis in large vessels with no patent grafts
3. Disabling angina

The operative mortality rate associated with second coronary bypass is approximately 3% to 4%, whereas that associated with a third procedure is 7% (33,34). Independent risk factors are the age of the patient being more than 70 years and diminished ventricular function (33,34). However, encouraging results indicate that the five-year survival rate after a third coronary artery bypass operation is 84% and the 10-year survival rate is 66% (35).

Technical issues related to repeated surgery include the risk of catastrophic bleeding when the sternotomy is reopened, potential damage to a patent graft (particularly the IMA), difficulty in achieving adequate myocardial protection, and atheroembolism in patent grafts. Because of these issues, the incidence of perioperative infarction is two to three times greater for repeated procedures than for primary surgery (1).

Most repeated operations will require sternotomy. Occasionally, minimally invasive approaches can be used, for example, if only the LAD needs to be grafted and the IMA was not used originally (32). Preparation includes evaluating potential conduits (right internal mammary and radial arteries, available arm and leg veins, gastroepiploic artery, etc.). When sternotomy is performed during a repeated procedure, the initial concern is avoiding tears of the right ventricle. The density of adhesions between the sternal incision and the surface of the heart (particularly the right ventricle and aorta) may be estimated by viewing the lateral chest radiograph. If little or no retrosternal space is seen, the bypass lines should be brought into the operative field. In some instances, cannulating the femoral or axillary artery may be advisable before the sternotomy is begun. The axillary artery is less atherosclerotic than the femoral artery and provides antegrade rather than retrograde flow; these factors may reduce the risk of embolization (36). Defibrillator paddles should be placed before the procedure is started. The sternal wires are left intact posteriorly, and the approach starts cautiously from the xiphoid level, with elevation provided by pulling up on the costal margin. As the dissection proceeds, an oscillating saw is used to open the sternum carefully by steps. If adhesions are particularly dense, a small right anterolateral thoracotomy may allow the surgeon to place a hand under the sternum (32). Should catastrophic bleeding occur, bypass can be initiated by instituting "sucker" bypass, draining venous blood by pump suckers, and returning flow by the femoral cannula. If the left IMA (LIMA) is patent, exposure may be assisted by entering the left pleural space at the level of the diaphragm and dissecting superiorly. The pericardium can be divided to the left of the LAD, creating a flap of tissue containing the LIMA if it is patent.

Once conduits have been prepared, cannulation of the right atrium can be performed, but care must be taken not to manipulate patent grafts. Retrograde cardioplegia will allow adequate and uniform protection in most cases, with the added advantage of not creating embolization in partially patent grafts. Because of the theoretical disadvantage of decreased right ventricular protection, and because performing distal anastomoses can be difficult when continuous warm cardioplegia is used, many surgeons prefer to use intermittent retrograde and antegrade cardioplegia, although the latter can be used less frequently if it is clear that retrograde cardioplegia results in adequate cooling and arrest (32). In addition, patent IMA grafts must be clamped during arrest to prevent rewarming of the heart. As revascularization proceeds, antegrade cardioplegia can be provided through each of the newly anastomosed vein grafts.

Injury to a patent LIMA occurs in 5% to 8% of cases. In nearly 60% of these cases, the graft can be preserved by using a variety of techniques, ranging from repair to repeated bypass with a vein graft (37). The perioperative infarction rate is increased (40%) with higher overall mortality (8%). The risk can be reduced during the first bypass procedure by positioning the LIMA graft in the left chest away from the sternal table (37).

POSTOPERATIVE MYOCARDIAL INFARCTION AND CORONARY SPASM

The incidence of postoperative myocardial infarction varies depending on the circumstances in which the surgery occurred. The incidence is 2% to 3% among patients with stable angina, 5% to 10% among those with unstable angina, and 30% to 50% among those undergoing emergency bypass after a failed PTCA procedure (1). Others have reported the occurrence of myocardial ischemia within six hours of operation in as many as 40% of cases and of infarction in 5% to 25% of cases (38,39). The diagnosis can be suggested by new-onset low cardiac output, electrocardiography (ECG) changes, creatinine phosphokinase (CPK)-2–myocardial band (MB) activity greater than 50 U/L, or elevated levels of the cardiac isoenzymes troponin T or troponin I. Patients at the highest risk of infarction and death are those whose condition does not respond to preoperative intra-aortic balloon pump (IABP) support (40). For these patients, outcomes are related to timing, with mortality rates as low as 3% if bypass can be instituted within four hours of the acute event (41,42). In addition, coronary atheroembolism, particularly in repeated operations, remains a risk. Finally, the inflammatory cascade initiated by cardiopulmonary bypass may play a role in the occurrence of postoperative myocardial infarction. Aldea (43) noted that the perioperative infarction rate decreased from 3.96% to 0.99% when heparin-bonded circuits were used. For patients with severe ischemia at the start of the operation, an IABP should be used, bypass and hypothermia should be instituted early to decrease metabolic demands, and warm-blood cardioplegia should be delivered to areas of the myocardium as a resuscitative tool (44). Postoperative management should be simplified if complete revascularization was performed because the issues of coronary perfusion pressure are not so prevalent. Management is directed at decreasing workload by using an IABP and, if necessary, by administering pressor drugs with some vasodilating properties.

Coronary artery spasm occurs after myocardial revascularization in only approximately 0.1% of cases (45). This complication is believed to be due to a combination of injury to coronary arteries during operation and production of thromboxane A2 during bypass (46). Coronary artery spasm manifests itself as acute ventricular dysfunction coupled with diffuse ECG changes, often with catastrophic cardiovascular collapse. It usually occurs shortly after bypass has been terminated and carries a high mortality rate (46,47). Initial management requires administration of heparinization, reinstitution of cardiopulmonary bypass, and rapid assessment of graft patency. Injecting nitroglycerin directly into the grafts will quickly reverse the condition, but sublingual or systemic administration of calcium channel blockers (e.g., diltiazem 5–25 mg/hr intravenously) is also effective (48). Administration of intravenous calcium channel blockers should be maintained after the operation to prevent the recurrence of coronary artery spasm, although there are as yet no clear guidelines for safely discontinuing these drugs. Administering calcium channel blockers indefinitely is a reasonable treatment for patients who have experienced coronary artery spasm.

POSTOPERATIVE BLEEDING AND TAMPONADE

Persistent hemorrhage will necessitate a return to the operating room for 2% to 5% of patients (48). Patients at increased risk for this complication are primarily those receiving preoperative antiplatelet or thrombolytic agents and those who have undergone a repeated procedure, but multiple factors can play a role (Table 3). Postoperative bleeding should always be considered surgically related until proven otherwise (49). This bleeding will generally manifest itself as persistent drainage from the mediastinal tubes or as an increase in pleural effusion. Surgical treatment is indicated if bleeding exceeds 400 mL/hr in any hour, if it exceeds 200 mL/hr for two to four hours, or if there is any hemodynamic instability. Nonspecific interventions include avoiding hypertension; some surgeons recommend the use of high levels of positive end-expiratory pressure (PEEP) (up to 20 cmH$_2$O) to "tamponade" bleeding. However, the prophylactic use of PEEP does not appear to reduce the incidence of repeated operation and can potentially complicate the postoperative course by aggravating cardiac dysfunction through physiologic tamponade or by putting pressure on an internal mammary graft (48). Apart from surgical bleeding, multiple coagulation disorders may be quickly assessed by using a thromboelastogram; however, the results of this procedure do not reliably predict the likelihood of bleeding complications preoperatively (50,51).

The most common coagulopathic cause of bleeding is platelet dysfunction (48). Inciting factors include hypothermia, contact with inert surfaces during bypass, and platelet consumption (43). The occurrence of platelet dysfunction can be combated with combinations of rewarming, administering D-amino-D-arginine vasopressin (DDAVP) at a dose of 0.3 mg/kg, and transfusing 6 to 10 platelet packs to maintain a platelet

Table 3 Causes of Postoperative Bleeding

Preoperative factors
  Reoperation
  Preoperative anticoagulation
    Antiplatelet agents
    Thrombolytic agents
Cyanotic heart disease
Liver dysfunction
Coagulation disorders
  Von Willebrand's disease
  Uremia
Intraoperative factors
  Inadequate surgical hemostasis (most common cause)
  Long pump run
  Core cooling to <32°C
  Coagulation impact of bypass
    Platelet dysfunction or depletion
    Residual heparin effect
    Fibrinolysis
    Excessive use of cell-saver blood

count of more than 100,000/mm^3, depending on the circumstances.

Excessive administration of heparin, resulting in prolonged activated clotting time, occurs because of either inadequate reversal or heparin rebound (52). The latter is a consequence of the shorter half-life of protamine, which may mobilize heparin from both intravascular and extravascular spaces after heparin has been initially bonded. For this reason, protamine at doses of 25 to 50 mg should be given slowly to compensate for excessive heparin activity.

Coagulation defects can be documented by an elevated prothrombin time (PT) in conjunction with the international normalized ratio. An elevated PT supports the use of fresh frozen plasma (three to four units), cryoprecipitate, or both. Fibrinolysis can occur; if elevated fibrin split products are documented or if fibrinogen concentrations fall to less than 100 mg/dL (1 g/L), cryoprecipitate can be administered. Each unit of cryoprecipitate should increase fibrinogen concentrations by 10 mg/dL (0.1 g/L). Adults are usually given 10 units (48). Epsilon-aminocaproic acid (EACA), an inhibitor of fibrinolysis, can also be administered at a dose of 10 to 20 g.

Repeated operation is a particular risk factor for bleeding if surgery is performed after thrombolysis has been attempted. In such cases, preoperative administration of aprotinin, a serine protease inhibitor, dramatically reduces blood loss (53). Avoiding reinfusion of shed blood and using heparin-bonded circuits also reduces the risk of postoperative bleeding (43). Prophylactic administration of DDAVP, EACA, or both has also been useful (48).

Cardiac tamponade in the postoperative setting may manifest itself in the classic manner, with elevated right heart pressures, jugular venous distention, and shock. This complication may be recognized, before clinical features are noticeable, by chest radiographs showing a widening cardiac silhouette, by decreased cardiac output with no apparent cause, or by equalization of right-sided filling pressures. It is crucial to recognize that chest tubes may appear to be patent when in fact they are not and that a small, contained clot in the retrocardiac space can result in critical impairment for patients with poor cardiac function. Early echocardiography should be considered, but if there is no obvious explanation for a sudden deterioration in function, there must be a low threshold for reexploration. Tamponade will occur in 50% of patients with arrest or profound hypotension, and an identifiable source is documented in nearly 80% of patients with vigorous bleeding (54). Patients in extremis should undergo immediate reexploration in the intensive care unit, without the delay caused by transport to the operating room. When simple sterile precautions are taken, the risk of infection does not appear to be higher when urgent reexploration is performed in the intensive care unit rather than in the operating suite (54).

POSTOPERATIVE DYSRHYTHMIAS

Dysrhythmias may be the most common complication after cardiac surgery, affecting as many as 25% of patients undergoing myocardial revascularization and 75% of those undergoing valve surgery (55). Supraventricular tachyarrhythmias are most common and appear to have a greater impact on length of stay because they are more persistent (56). Atrial fibrillation or flutter occurs in 40% of cases. Many factors may cause postoperative dysrhythmia, including preexisting dysrhythmias, catecholamine release during operation, atrial enlargement or stretch, areas of patchy ischemia, and electrolyte disturbances (56). Preoperative risk factors include age greater than 70 years, preoperative left ventricular end-diastolic pressure higher than 20 mmHg, a history of atrial dysrhythmia, chronic obstructive pulmonary disease, and acute cessation of the administration of beta-blockers or calcium channel blockers (48). Hypomagnesemia is particularly common after cardiac operations and has been related to loss of urinary function; preoperative use of digoxin, beta-blockers, or diuretics; and diabetes mellitus. Administering magnesium is important for maintaining potassium levels and myocardial cell contractility. In addition, a combination of manipulation of the atrium (although the incidence is substantial even for cases performed off-pump) and inadequate preservation of the atrium and the conduction system appear to be important causes of both supraventricular tachyarrhythmias and bradyarrhythmias (including heart block). The atrium cools more slowly and rewarms more quickly than do the ventricles, in part because of noncoronary collateral flow (44). Blood cardioplegia may be more effective than crystalloid cardioplegia in reducing atrial activity during bypass, thus lowering the incidence of postoperative arrhythmias (57). Topical cooling of the atrium may similarly reduce the incidence. In addition, particularly when bicaval snares are used, surgeons must take care not to manipulate the junction of the superior vena cava with the atrium, the site of the sinoatrial node.

Bradyarrhythmias, notably second- and third-degree heart block, are usually transient and can be managed by pacing with temporary leads placed at the time of surgery. Because arrhythmias are so common, ventricular leads are always placed, and atrial leads are usually placed as well. Placing these leads allows sequential pacing, which is preferred because it maintains more effective cardiac output. The rate can be varied, but the target is generally 80 to 90 beats/min. The atrioventricular (AV) delay should also be individualized, but in general a delay of 150 msec provides the most effective output. A shorter delay may more effectively suppress ventricular arrhythmias. Metabolic or pharmacological causes of bradyarrhythmias should be explored, including hypothermia, elevated calcium or potassium concentrations, or the administration of beta-blockers. In most cases, the bradycardia is of short duration, but in a few cases, it persists for more than six days and a permanent pacemaker may be required.

To some extent, the clinical significance of ventricular tachyarrhythmias has diminished. Magnesium prophylaxis substantially reduces the incidence and severity of these arrhythmias (56). They may be caused by patchy changes in ventricular function as rewarming occurs or by different areas of ischemia, but they are generally self-limiting and do not require treatment. Overaggressive treatment can lead to complications because all antidysrhythmic drugs have proarrhythmic side effects (in as many as 15% of patients) and function to a certain degree as myocardial depressants (56). However, frequent premature ventricular contractions (more than six per minute) multifocal that demonstrate the R-on-T phenomenon, or those associated with hypotension are usually managed with antidysrhythmic drugs. Ventricular tachycardia associated with hypotension and ventricular fibrillation requires cardioversion (at 100–400 J). Stable ventricular tachycardia can be managed in the standard fashion (Fig. 2) (58).

Supraventricular disturbances, including atrial fibrillation, are more difficult to treat. Magnesium prophylaxis does not appear to be useful. Patients in an unstable condition should be treated with synchronized cardioversion (40 J). Once metabolic disturbances (notably hypokalemia) have been corrected, standard pharmacological approaches can be used, first to control the rate and then to attempt cardioversion to a normal rhythm (Table 4, Fig. 3) (58). Persistent atrial fibrillation will necessitate long-term anticoagulation. In some cases, the fibrillation is related to atrial enlargement; in the case of valve surgery, this enlargement may remodel itself in the ensuing months, thus allowing a chance for cardioversion at a later date.

LOW CARDIAC OUTPUT

Myocardial failure after cardiac surgery is generally defined as a cardiac index of less than 2.0 L/min/m². It can be further defined by the presence of low mixed venous saturation (less than 60%), which implies increased oxygen consumption because of inadequate systemic delivery (59). Clearly, some patients can be expected to have chronic poor function [for example, those with extremely low preoperative ejection fraction (EF) who undergo salvage bypass]; in these cases, artificially driving the output may be counterproductive. However, in general, attempts must be made to increase myocardial function to avoid progressive end-organ failure.

Substantial right ventricular failure is less common than left ventricular failure after cardiac surgery because the right ventricle is less sensitive to ischemia for two reasons: the right ventricle has lower energy requirements than the left ventricle and coronary blood flow is well distributed transmurally. However, in the presence of right ventricular infarction, pressure overload (e.g., in the setting of mitral stenosis), or both, inadequate protection or persistent pulmonary hypertension can trigger failure (44). Antegrade cardioplegia appears to cool the right ventricle more reliably than the left ventricle, partly because the noncoronary sinus tributaries that provide right-sided

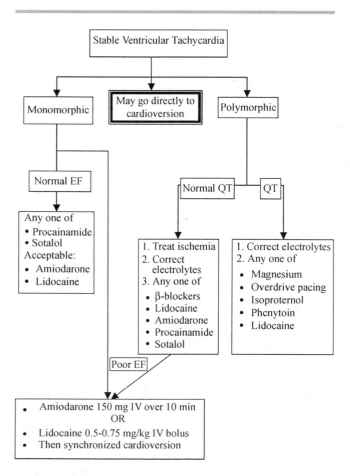

Figure 2 Management of ventricular tachycardia.

Table 4 Atrial Fibrillation and Flutter

	Control rate	Convert rhythm (less than or equal to 48 hrs)	Convert rhythm (more than 48 hrs)
EF≥40%	Use one: Calcium channel blockers Beta-blockers Note: in case of flutter, try overdrive pacing	Consider cardioversion Use: Amiodarone Procainamide Propafenone Flecainamide Ibutilde	Delayed cardioversion after 3 wk anticoagulation or early cardioversion if TEE excludes clot, after 24 hrs of heparin
EF < 40%	Use one: Digoxin Diltiazem Amiodarone	DC cardioversion or amiodarone	As above

Abbreviations: EF, ejection fraction; TEE, transesophageal echocardiography; DC, direct current.

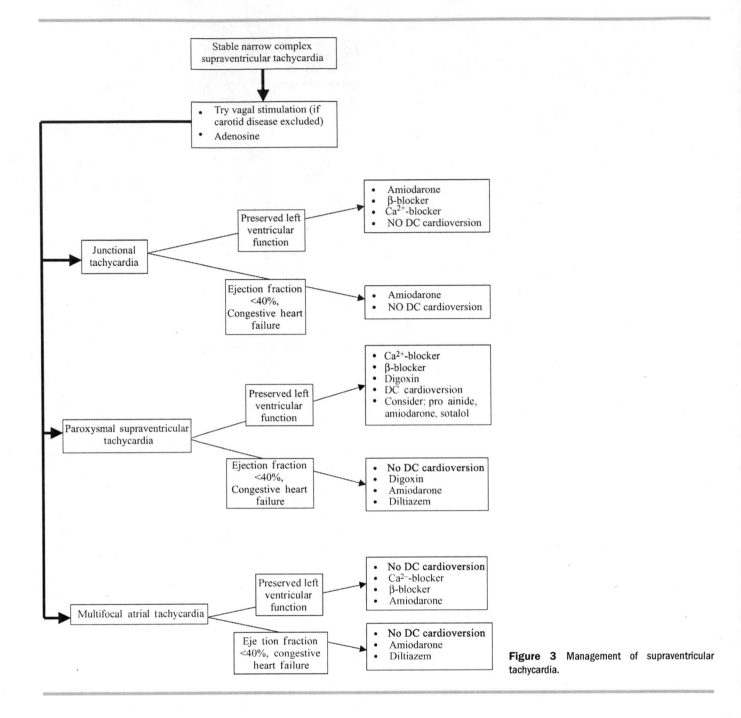

Figure 3 Management of supraventricular tachycardia.

drainage include not only the right atrium but also the anterior right ventricular free wall (44,60). Because of extensive collateral drainage, retrograde cardioplegia still provides excellent protection against right ventricular failure, but in some instances, adding antegrade cardioplegia after grafting the right coronary system may be advisable. Right ventricular failure, when it occurs, can lead to a combination of decreased left ventricular preload and leftward shift of the septum, thus creating a spiral of decompensation. Clinically, right ventricular failure will manifest itself as low cardiac output with elevated right-sided filling pressures that are disproportionately higher than pressures

caused by pulmonary occlusion or that directly measured left atrial pressures.

Left ventricular dysfunction is often characterized by a temporary depression in contractility. Diastolic dysfunction is often the predominant early characteristic of this complication, preceding systolic changes that are more clinically appreciable. Recognizing the significance of diastolic dysfunction enables a better understanding of afterload reduction in conjunction with careful volume management. For example, a "stiff" ventricle often requires higher filling pressures initially, until relaxation recovers. The acute ventricular changes relate primarily to myocardial edema, ischemia–reperfusion injury, or the effect of cooling (61,62). If myocardial protection has been adequate and preoperative function well preserved, the impact is usually transient and minimal intervention is required. Techniques for alleviating the inflammatory impact of bypass, such as the use of heparin-bonded circuits and the avoidance of excessive cell-saver transfusion, may further reduce the impact of bypass (43). Preoperative deterioration is a crucial factor and it is important to distinguish between perioperative "stunning" and "hibernation," particularly when coronary atherosclerosis is present. These conditions represent different parts of the spectrum of myocardial cell dysfunction. Stunning implies an acute but reversible reduction in ventricular function, usually in the setting of myocardial ischemia or after coronary artery bypass grafting. Hibernation reflects a more chronic downregulation in response to more chronic ischemia or stress; this condition may be present in as many as 50% of patients with congestive heart failure (63,64). In both cases, once reperfusion has been achieved, the myocardium should eventually recover; recovery will occur within hours after stunning but may require days after hibernation. Recognizing areas of reversible ischemia (by history of angina or nuclear studies) will support the decision to revascularize a patient with very low EF, in anticipation of eventual rescue of some myocardial function (65). A persistently low cardiac index will ultimately lead to worsening pulmonary function, systemic end-organ failure, and progressive metabolic collapse.

Nonspecific measures are important in avoiding this sequence of deterioration. Although coronary perfusion pressure should not be as crucial after complete revascularization as before the procedure, arterial pressures below a mean of 65 mmHg can lead to inadequate conduit perfusion, particularly through IMA grafts (66). General interventions include reducing metabolic demands by preventing shivering, correcting electrolyte and acid–base disturbances, optimizing oxygenation, and preventing hyperthermia. Chemical paralysis may be needed. Maintaining sinus rhythm can be crucial, with pacing if needed; conversion from atrial fibrillation to sinus rhythm can increase EF by as much as 30% in patients with severely compromised ventricular function (59). The goal should be a rate of 80 to 100 beats/min. A quick assessment must be made to ensure that there are no technical complications, such as graft occlusion leading to acute ischemia or tamponade. Preload, with a target central venous pressure (CVP) of 15 mmHg, is optimized as well, although, as noted previously, patients with a "stiff" ventricle may require levels up to 20 mmHg. A simple technique is to perform a "CVP challenge:" a bolus of fluid (usually 500 cc) is given, and the cardiac output is calculated before the bolus, immediately thereafter, and 10 to 20 minutes later. If the cardiac output improves only transiently, more volume is required. If the CVP increases with no improvement in cardiac output, further volume expansion will not be helpful.

Some form of inotropic support is commonly required. Agents with some vasodilating properties are preferred because they will reduce myocardial oxygen demand (59). Dobutamine has β-adrenergic myocardial effects and is associated with pulmonary and systemic vasodilatation. It is usually administered at a beginning dosage of 3 to 5 μg/kg/min, which is increased to 15 μg/kg/min. Dobutamine leads to greater myocardial perfusion than dopamine (67). Amrinone and other phosphodiesterase inhibitors (such as milrinone) have also proved useful, with improved contractility and decreased afterload. Amrinone is administered as a bolus of 0.75 μg/kg and then at a dosage of 5 to 10 μg/kg/min. Complications include thrombocytopenia, which should be monitored. Newer "inodilators" include dopexamine, a β₂-adrenergic agonist with effects similar to those of dobutamine (68). Dopexamine is administered at doses of 1 to 4 μg/kg/min; complications (tachycardia and hypotension) occur at doses greater than 4 μg/kg/min (68). Isoproterenol, a pure myocardial β₂-adrenergic agonist, is both a potent inotropic agent and a vasodilator. The dosage ranges from 0.01 to 0.2 μg/kg/min. Its efficacy is limited by its chronotropic and arrhythmogenic effects that increase myocardial oxygen consumption, but isoproterenol is particularly useful for the management of right heart failure or pulmonary hypertension. Nitroglycerin tends to lead to greater pulmonary than systemic vasodilation, but is useful for managing hypertension, postoperative ischemia, right ventricular failure, and pulmonary hypertension. Nitroprusside at a dosage of 0.3 to 1.0 μg/kg/min is also effective but may cause reflex tachycardia, which can aggravate myocardial oxygen consumption and cause extreme fluctuations in pressure, increased pulmonary shunt, and, in more chronic settings, cyanide toxicity (69). Some centers routinely determine thiocyanate levels if nitroprusside is used for more than 24 hours (48). Although most inotropic agents used after cardiac surgery ideally have some vasodilating properties, agents that are purer agonists are often required. The most commonly used such agent is dopamine, a direct myocardial β-adrenergic agonist that will increase both inotropy and chronotropy. Traditionally, dopamine is believed to have three dose-related effects. At dosages of 0.5 to 3.0 μg/kg/min, splanchnic (particularly renal) vasodilation occurs. At dosages of 2 to 8 μg/kg/min β-adrenergic stimulation becomes predominant, with increased contractility. At dosages of 8 to 15 μg/kg/min, increasing α-adrenergic stimulation results in systemic vasoconstriction. We have not found these divisions to be uniform; because dosages have different effects in different patients, dosing should be individualized. Epinephrine, which causes both α- and β-stimulation, has been used as a first-line agent by some and as a second-line inotropic agent by others. At dosages of 0.01 to 0.06 μg/kg/min, the β-adrenergic effects predominate, with increases in both inotropy and chronotropy, coupled with some vasodilation. Epinephrine is particularly useful for treating patients with long-standing ventricular dysfunction (66). At higher dosages, systemic vasoconstriction increases. Norepinephrine is characterized by its predominantly vasoconstrictive action. It may be most useful for treating patients with transient systemic vasodilation and hyperdynamic states, such as during rewarming, to avoid the need for excessive fluid administration. Triiodothyronine has also been used preoperatively to increase cardiac output in patients with depressed cardiac function (EF less than 30%); administering this agent decreases the need for postoperative inotropic support (70).

It has been noted that increasing requirements for inotropic support should prompt consideration of mechanical support earlier rather than later. The principal mechanical support is the IABP, which results in increased coronary perfusion, decreased systemic vascular resistance, and, consequently, improved myocardial output and decreased myocardial oxygen demand. IABP use can increase cardiac output by as much as 0.7 to 1.0 L/min. After cardiac surgery, IABP use should be considered, particularly if the cardiac index is less than 2.0 L/min/m^2, with left atrial pressures greater than 20 to 25 mmHg or mean blood pressure less than 60 mmHg (71).

More advanced assist devices are available. The roles of extracorporeal life support and ventricular assist devices are discussed elsewhere in this text, but as many as 50% of patients can be weaned from these devices, and approximately 30% will be discharged from the hospital (71,72).

Finally, newer pharmacological interventions are being studied, notably with respect to the problem of pulmonary hypertension leading to heart failure. Both prostacyclin and nitric oxide appear to have some benefit for selected patients (73).

NEUROLOGICAL COMPLICATIONS

Neurological complications are an important focus of research in attempts to improve survival and quality of life after cardiac procedures. Complications can be grouped into three categories: central nervous system (CNS) insults, spinal cord ischemia, and peripheral nerve injuries. CNS injuries can be further categorized as those occurring during routine bypass and those occurring during operations that require hypothermic circulatory arrest.

Central Nervous System Injury During Cardiopulmonary Bypass

A spectrum of CNS injuries associated with cardiopulmonary bypass has been described; these injuries are related to embolic phenomena and to the inflammatory effect of cardiopulmonary bypass (Table 5) (74).

Table 5 Definition of Neurological Sequelae

Stroke	Focal motor, sensory, or visual alteration lasting longer than 24 hr
Cognitive injury	Alteration in thou!ght, behavior, or consciousness, with or without detectable focal signs
Encephalopathy	Obtundation, drowsiness, lethargy, or delirious state without focal changes

Stroke affects approximately 5% of patients undergoing isolated coronary bypass, 8% of those undergoing isolated valve surgery, and 11% of those undergoing combined procedures (75–77). More than 90% of strokes occur within 24 hours after surgery, and the associated mortality rate is as high as 36% (74,78,79). Cognitive defects, predominantly psychomotor changes, affect as many as 80% of patients after elective cardiac procedures (79). However, the actual incidence of such defects depends on how they are specifically defined and which method is used to detect them. Fortunately, these defects usually resolve with time. One study documented a 52% incidence of stroke-related sequelae in the immediate postoperative period; this incidence decreased to 35% by one year after surgery and to 22% at three years after surgery (80).

Encephalopathy affects as many as 35% of patients but generally resolves relatively quickly; only 10% of patients still exhibit symptoms by the fourth postoperative day (74). Unlike other neurological injuries, encephalopathy is related not to embolic phenomena but instead to advanced age, alcoholism, and the use of sedative hypnotics and other agents (81). Hypoperfusion and vasospasm also play a role. Risk factors include preexisting carotid disease and atheroma of the aorta. Patients at particular risk of encephalopathy are those with preoperative uncontrolled hypertension, diabetes mellitus, chronic renal failure, or extensive peripheral vascular disease (82).

Fewer than 3% of patients undergoing cardiac surgery have a combination of symptomatic carotid disease and coronary artery or aortic valve disease; however, these patients do appear to benefit from combined procedures (83). There are two approaches, depending on institutional experience. The carotid endarterectomy can be performed before the cardiac procedure, with the wound left packed until completion of the operation, or endarterectomy can be performed while the patient is on cardiopulmonary bypass to take advantage of relative cooling (84). Currently, with combined procedures, the risk of serious neurological events has been reported to be as low as 2% and the risk of death 9% (83). The best treatment for patients who have suffered a stroke or who have asymptotic carotid lesions or stable cardiac disease is not clear; staged repair is probably reasonable, especially when the carotid endarterectomy can be performed with the patient under local anesthesia.

The primary source of emboli is the aorta itself, and each manipulation (clamping, partial clamping,

Table 6 Transesophageal Echocardiographic Grading of Aortic Atheroma

Extent of atheroma	Grade
Normal to mild intimal thickening	1
Severe intimal thickening	2
Protrusion <5 mm	3
Protrusion >5 mm	4
Mobile components	5

Source: Modified from Ref. 74.

and unclamping) is associated with the release of echogenically detectable material into the cerebral circulation (82,85–87). This knowledge has led to attempts to avoid manipulation of the aorta in patients at risk of emboli, or at least to identify disease-free areas of the aorta. However, palpation is unreliable in detecting lesions, especially if soft atheroma is present. The best studies for defining the grade of disease are transesophageal echocardiography (TEE), epiaortic imaging, or intravascular ultrasound (Table 6) (82,88). Attempts to reduce aortic manipulation appear to be associated with improved outcomes, particularly for patients with grade 4 or 5 disease; these techniques include completely avoiding aortic clamping (e.g., off-pump bypass, bypass during fibrillatory arrest, circulatory arrest, and use of endoaortic balloon occlusion) and manipulation for bypass (e.g., arterial grafts and vein grafts from great vessels) (74,89). Aortic resection has been proposed for selected patients with extensive disease, but in general the no-touch techniques described above are favored (74). Femoral cannulation should be avoided in patients with evidence of descending aortic disease because lesions can thus be driven into the cerebral circulation. In this regard, subclavian or innominate cannulation has the advantage of moving any potential debris into the distal aorta rather than to a location that could affect the brain (74).

Apart from avoiding emboli, a number of other techniques associated with cardiopulmonary bypass deserve consideration. Avoiding or minimizing cardiotomy suction and using heparin-bonded circuits appear to reduce the number of emboli and the inflammatory changes that promote CNS injury (43). Arterial line filtration, in particular leukocyte filtration, appears to provide some protection as well (90). Other factors that play a crucial role in reducing the incidence of emboli include avoiding extreme variations in glucose or osmolarity, rapid rewarming, careful deairing, using pulsatile flow for extended cases, and using membrane oxygenators rather than other types of oxygenators (90).

Central Nervous Injury During Hypothermic Circulatory Arrest

Complete interruption of blood flow is a crucial adjunct in complex neonatal and adult cardiac and aortic procedures, especially those that involve the aortic arch. In this regard, hypothermic circulatory arrest has proved invaluable. A substantial potential advantage is the elimination of the need to clamp atherosclerotic vessels; this factor may in itself reduce embolic phenomena. Strategies for protecting the CNS include not only understanding the issues discussed in the previous section of this chapter but also minimizing the period of global ischemia to which the CNS is subjected. The primary protective mechanism is hypothermia, which decreases metabolic demand, preserves tissue levels of adenosine triphosphate, maintains cellular pH concentrations, and inhibits the release of neurotransmitters that may cause damaging excitation, including glutamate and aspartate (91,92). Substantial metabolic and electroencephalographic activity is still present at 18°C (93). On the basis of measurement of the cerebral metabolic rate for oxygen, the safe time for hypothermic arrest has been estimated to be 30 minutes at 15°C and 40 minutes at 10°C (94).

In attempts to increase cerebral protection, surgeons have used strategies for maintaining some cerebral flow. Selective antegrade perfusion requires cannulation of two or all three of the great vessels. Problems associated with this approach include the risk of emboli and of "cluttering" the operative field. When performed under moderate hypothermia, selective antegrade perfusion requires the maintenance of distal body perfusion. When arrest is expected to last for more than 40 minutes, an island can be created with the portion of the arch containing the cerebral vessels. Perfusion is achieved at 10°C by means of a graft anastomosed to this island, and a pressure of 50 mmHg is maintained. The graft can then be sewn to the aortic graft to complete reconstruction (95).

Retrograde cerebral perfusion via the superior vena cava appears to maintain cerebral hypothermia and may provide some substrate to the brain during circulatory arrest, despite evidence that more than 95% of the perfusate does not reach brain tissue (92,96). In addition, retrograde cerebral perfusion may dislodge particulate emboli and may reduce the extent of embolic injury when it does occur (95,97). Superior vena cava pressures should be maintained at 15 to 20 mmHg; higher pressures should be avoided because of their association with an increased likelihood of cerebral edema (98). Retrograde cerebral perfusion should be used only with hypothermic circulatory arrest and without attempting to extend the duration of cardiac arrest beyond times that have been demonstrated to be relatively safe (92).

Metabolic management during hypothermic arrest is also important and is somewhat controversial. Two pH management strategies can be used: pH-stat and alpha-stat (Table 7). The addition of hyperoxia before circulatory arrest appears to confer added protection against CNS injury, particularly when used in conjunction with pH-stat management (99). Some surgeons combine these management strategies, either cooling with pH-stat until just before arrest and then

Table 7 Strategies for Managing pH

pH management	Definition	Potential advantages	Potential disadvantages
pH-stat	Adds CO_2 to the system to maintain pH at 7.4, at which the temperature is collected, thus correcting the alkaline shift that occurs with cooling	Increased vasodilation leading to improved cooling and potential oxygen delivery	Abolishes cerebral autoregulation, leading to increased luxury perfusion and risk of emboli
Alpha-stat	Allows normal alkaline shift to occur, keeping the pH at 7.4 when samples are corrected to 37°C	Preserves autoregulation, thus leading to luxury perfusion and associated risk of increased embolic load	Less efficient cerebral cooling and potentially decreased perfusion

switching to alpha-stat principles or using pH-stat for cooling and alpha-stat for rewarming (100). Finally, attempts to inhibit the reperfusion aspect of ischemia–reperfusion injury continue to be studied, including the potential role of calcium channel blockers in attenuating the inflammatory response.

Spinal Cord Injury During Replacement of the Descending Thoracic Aorta

Spinal cord ischemia remains a serious problem in the treatment of patients who require replacement of the descending thoracic aorta. However, continued refinement of techniques has markedly reduced the incidence of postoperative paralysis to as low as 3% to 10% after complex thoracoabdominal aortic replacement (101). Much of the effort in prevention of cord injury has concentrated on shortening ischemic time; but more recently, attention to ameliorating the reperfusion response has increased. Attempts to reduce the impact of ischemia have concentrated on reducing cross-clamp time, maintaining distal perfusion with left heart bypass, and performing early revascularization of key intercostal arteries, notably T7-L1 (101,102). A sequential approach has been advocated as the quickest and most reliable method for reducing cross-clamp time and maintaining important spinal arterial perfusion; in this approach, the proximal anastomosis is performed, reperfusion via the subclavian artery is allowed while the intercostal arteries are being reattached, and distal anastomosis is then performed (often with an open technique) (102–104). Reanastomosing patent intercostal arteries in the T10-L1 distribution is particularly important because ligation of these arteries alone has been documented to result in a paralysis rate as high as 63% (105). These vessels should be located during preoperative angiography and plans should be made to reestablish flow during surgery. During the operation, back-bleeding through these vessels should be controlled until ligation or reimplantation so as to prevent a steal phenomenon. Mechanical circulatory support, usually left heart bypass, is particularly useful if cross-clamp times exceed 40 minutes (106). Topical hypothermia and moderate systemic hypothermia (30°C) ameliorate both ischemic and reperfusion insults to the spinal cord (107). Avoiding preoperative administration of sodium nitroprusside, which may aggravate spinal

cord "steal," has also reduced the incidence of injury (108). Reperfusion injury appears to be reduced by cerebrospinal fluid (CSF) drainage to keep CSF pressures below 10 mmHg during cross-clamping (109). The addition of intrathecal papaverine may further reduce the risk of injury (101). Future advances in reducing the risk of injury may include inhibition of reperfusion injury responses by inhibiting cellular responses such as the production of tissue factor; such responses promote thrombosis and inflammation (110).

Although spinal cord monitoring of evoked potentials may help by identifying key intercostal arteries and warning the operating team of impending ischemia, the practicality and usefulness of this technique have not been uniformly demonstrated. In addition, neuromuscular blockade, anesthetic agents, intrathecal medications, and cooling can inhibit interpretation of both motor and sensory evoked potentials (111).

Once paralysis has occurred, there is little effective treatment. A few reports indicate some success in reversing injury with CSF drainage and intrathecal papaverine, and steroids may help if the injury has an acute inflammatory component (101).

Peripheral Nerve Injuries

Brachial plexus injury occurs after sternotomy in 6% to 15% of cases (112). The precipitating event is compression of the lowest roots of the brachial plexus by the first rib during excessive retraction. The most common symptoms of this injury are paresthesias of the ring and small fingers, with weakness in nearly one-third and pain in 26% of cases (113). Brachial plexus injuries can be prevented by carefully expanding the sternal retractor and by avoiding excessive spreading at the superior aspect of the incision (114). More than 90% of complaints will resolve within three months, and therapy is generally supportive (113).

Phrenic nerve injury can occur during mobilization of the IMA, but more commonly results from "cold" injury. One study noted diaphragmatic elevation in 73% of patients when phrenic nerve protection (with a pad or sponge) was not used but in only 17% of patients when it was used (115). The predominant impact is on postoperative respiratory function; however, prolonged gastric paresis may also occur, although the mechanism causing this complication is unclear. In general, therapy is supportive, but recovery usually takes several months.

Recurrent nerve injury most commonly occurs after operations on the descending aorta. It affects as many as 10% of patients who require clamping of the aorta proximal to the left subclavian artery (116). The best method of preventing recurrent nerve injury is avoiding excessive traction on the vagus nerve proximal to the origin of the recurrent nerve. Approximately half of traction injuries will resolve within six months, but if hoarseness or ineffective cough presents a problem, medialization of the vocal cord with collagen injection may be required.

END-ORGAN COMPLICATIONS OF CARDIOPULMONARY BYPASS

Cardiopulmonary bypass is associated with a number of deleterious effects on the pulmonary, renal, and gastrointestinal systems. These effects are mediated by a combination of inflammatory changes, lack of pulsatile flow, and microemboli (24,43). Although the inflammatory response to cardiopulmonary bypass often remains at subclinical levels, it can lead to substantial organ dysfunction and multiple organ failure. Because of the heterogeneity of individual responses to injury and the various degrees of preoperative acute and chronic organ dysfunction in patients undergoing heart surgery, clinically defining the extent of injury that results from cardiopulmonary bypass can be difficult. Defining the extent of injury is further complicated by the effects of a number of factors, such as the length of the bypass run, the duration of ischemia, the use of deep hypothermic circulatory arrest, and the circuitry of the pump. For most patients, the likelihood of difficulties related to inflammatory responses to cardiopulmonary bypass seems to increase as the perfusion time extends beyond approximately three hours, and it probably increases sharply after four hours. In addition, patients may be in shock at the time of surgery or may experience various degrees of hypoperfusion during and after cardiopulmonary bypass; such problems compound the degree of injury and worsen the patients' tolerance to surgery. Despite the difficulty of delineating exactly what degree of injury results from cardiopulmonary bypass, it is clear to most clinicians that end-organ changes resulting from the consequences of extracorporeal circulation can affect nearly every organ system and can thus contribute to higher morbidity and mortality rates and to longer hospital stays (61). These complications can at times affect the decision to proceed with surgery or the decision about the type of surgery chosen for a given patient. Although in some patients only a single organ system appears to be affected, careful examination will reveal impaired organ function in nearly all of the body's physiologic systems.

Respiratory Complications

Acute postoperative pulmonary dysfunction is one of the most noticeable systemic effects of cardiopulmonary bypass, and a broad spectrum of acute pulmonary complications can occur postoperatively. Acute lung injury after cardiopulmonary bypass is best appreciated by measuring the alveolar–arterial oxygenation gradient, intrapulmonary shunt, degree of pulmonary edema, pulmonary compliance, and pulmonary vascular resistance. After cardiopulmonary bypass, pulmonary hypertension and lung injury are affected by inflammatory changes; these changes are exacerbated by lung ischemia that occurs intraoperatively when the lungs are left without their primary sources of oxygen (117).

Clinically, pulmonary dysfunction manifests itself as increased time to extubation in the early postoperative period. In most cases, mechanical ventilation is required during the early postoperative period, and the likelihood of pulmonary complications such as pneumonia due to impaired pulmonary host defenses is increased. Once pulmonary dysfunction becomes severe enough to require ventilation for more than a few days, the mortality rate increases substantially. Kollef et al. (118) found a mortality rate of nearly 20% among 107 patients ventilated for more than 48 hours after cardiac surgery. When acute respiratory distress syndrome develops after cardiopulmonary bypass, the mortality rate can be as high as 90% (118).

Additional respiratory complications can be linked to technical factors. Direct cold injury to the left phrenic nerve should be minimized by using cardiac "pads" behind the left ventricle so that the nerve can be protected from iced solution. Topical injury to the nerve in this area, or possibly to the left lower lobe bronchus, manifests itself as persistent left lower lobe collapse that must be aggressively treated if pneumonia is to be prevented.

Renal Failure

New renal failure occurs among 1% to 3% of patients who undergo cardiopulmonary bypass (119). Risk factors include decreased preoperative renal function, diabetes, combined valve and coronary operations, and prolonged pump run. Apart from factors mentioned earlier, low perfusion pressure or toxic mediators, such as free iron, may lead to acute tubular necrosis. Among patients who experience renal failure requiring dialysis, the 30-day mortality rate is 30%, and only one-third will recover enough function to become independent of dialysis (120). Patients who are at a high risk of renal failure may benefit from the maintenance of perfusion pressures greater than 80 mmHg and from continuation of "renal" doses of dopamine postoperatively. Evidence of poor renal function should prompt evaluation of cardiac output. Ideally, the administration of vasopressors should be discontinued or minimized. Once renal insufficiency occurs, therapy should be directed at converting the kidneys from oliguric to nonoliguric failure. Administering furosemide as an intravenous bolus (and continuous drip while optimizing filling pressures) and adding renal doses of dopamine may improve renal function among patients with acute tubular necrosis (48). The addition of theophylline may be useful if no response is seen (48). Administering theophylline as a bolus with colloid solutions has been helpful in conjunction with the administration of diuretic drugs, but serious side effects include volume expansion, increased tissue edema, and complications associated with volume overload. Once a diagnosis of renal failure has been established, the choice between hemodialysis and ultrafiltration depends on whether fluid simply needs to be removed or whether other problems exist.

Gastrointestinal Complications

Gastrointestinal complications occur in 2% of patients after cardiopulmonary bypass. The incidence of these complications is increased among patients who have atherosclerotic disease or those who have required perioperative administration of vasopressor agents. Patients whose gastrointestinal complications require laparotomy face a 40% mortality rate (121–123).

Hyperamylasemia has been documented in 35% patients after coronary bypass procedures and frank pancreatitis occurs in 6%. Symptoms of anorexia, nausea, and abdominal pain usually occur on the second or third postoperative day. Treatment is largely supportive because complications requiring surgery rarely occur. Gastrointestinal bleeding occurs in 1% of cases; the risk of peptic ulcer is greatest among elderly patients and those with a history of ulcer. Transient elevation in liver enzymes occurs in 5% of cases, but frank liver failure is uncommon. Patients with right-sided valvular disease, perioperative pulmonary hypertension, mitral insufficiency, or some combination of these conditions are at the greatest risk of hepatic dysfunction. The risk factors for hepatic dysfunction should be considered before anticoagulation is initiated because overanticoagulation can easily occur. Acalculous cholecystitis and intestinal perforation are rare but can occur. Both of these complications are associated with decreased perfusion states. Cholecystitis may be managed by percutaneous drainage or cholecystectomy, depending on the overall condition of the patient.

ACUTE INFECTIOUS COMPLICATIONS
Sternal Infections and Mediastinitis

Superficial sternal infections usually present with serosanguineous drainage, with or without associated cellulitis. The wound should be carefully sterilized topically and cultures should then be taken. If there is any question of sternal instability or deeper infection, the wound should be explored in the operating room. Broad-spectrum antibiotics (covering both gram-positive and gram-negative organisms) should be administered until culture results determine a more specific treatment.

Frank mediastinitis affects 1% to 2% of patients after cardiopulmonary bypass and sternotomy (48). Mortality rates are from 20% to 40%; in many cases, death is due to persistent sepsis or to catastrophic hemorrhage from exposed grafts or the right ventricle (124). A number of risk factors have been determined (Table 8), but a crucial factor is the technique used for sternotomy—whether the division leaves one side too thin or the sternal closure leaves some mobility (125,126). Administration of antibiotics prophylactically is routine and their administration is often continued for 24 to 48 hours postoperatively, but there is no clear evidence that this procedure reliably prevents mediastinitis (48). Most cases develop within two weeks of the initial surgery. Signs and symptoms can vary from mild malaise and low-grade fever to frank sepsis with obvious purulence and drainage of pus from the sternal incision (127). A new sternal "click" is a serious finding that implies new sternal instability (128). Unfortunately, within six weeks of the procedure, no one invasive test can reliably exclude or confirm the diagnosis of mediastinitis in the more indolent cases. Computed tomography (CT) scans of the chest may show fluid collections and minor sternal separation, but these are often normal early findings after bypass. CT-guided needle aspiration may be useful if it excludes the diagnosis of deep infection, thereby allowing treatment of a minor superficial collection. Overall, however, because the role of CT in diagnosing mediastinitis is unclear, its findings are of secondary importance to those of clinical assessment.

If wound drainage is accompanied by sternal instability, or if a diagnosis of mediastinitis is suspected on the basis of clinical findings, the wound should be surgically explored. All necrotic tissue, including bone, must be debrided. If the patient's clinical condition is stable, if fungal or staphylococcal infection has been ruled out, and if the bone and surrounding tissues are pliant and have a relatively normal

Table 8 Risk Factors for Development of Postoperative Mediastinitis

Preoperative risk factors
  Preexisting infection (particularly dental)
  Poorly controlled diabetes
  Immunocompromise
  Preoperative ventilation
  Malnutrition
Intraoperative risk factors
  Contamination
  Prolonged pump run
  Transfusion of more than four units of blood
  Use of both internal mammary arteries (especially if patient has diabetes)
  Thin sternal plates
Postoperative risk factors
  Prolonged ventilator dependence
  Malnutrition

appearance, a reasonable option is to attempt closure over an irrigation system. We prefer to place a Jackson-Pratt drain via a stab wound at the superior aspect of the sternal incision and to drain the wound widely using mediastinal tubes. A number of irrigation solutions have been used, including saline, iodine, and antibiotic solutions (e.g., first-generation cephalosporins, at a total dose of 1–2 g/L given at a rate of 50 cc/hr) (48,129,130). The irrigation can be modified on the basis of subsequent cultures, but this procedure is carried out until all signs of infection are gone and the effluent is clear.

Patients who are immunocompromised, who have grossly purulent infections, who have necrotic bone, or who have staphylococcal or fungal infections should undergo closure with vascularized tissue, usually omentum or pectoralis or rectus flaps. This treatment may also be necessary for all patients with mammary artery grafts and those for whom more conservative measures have failed (131). If sepsis is present, temporization with open dressing and surgical reexploration may be an option, but this method should not be used as a definitive treatment because of the risk of erosion into the right ventricle or into exposed grafts. Many surgeons perform muscle flap closure as primary treatment for almost all patients (132).

Infections at the Site of Vein Harvest

Complications related to the site from which bypass veins are harvested are probably the single most common cause of patients' complaints; these complications affect as many as 30% of patients postoperatively (133,134). The surgeon's preference generally determines which site is used for harvesting; specific complications are associated with each site. Harvesting veins from the thigh may lower the risk of infection (134), but this procedure is associated with an increased risk of hematoma and fat necrosis (135). Harvesting veins from the calf is associated with an increased risk of damage to the saphenous nerve and the lymphatic drainage.

Other risk factors for complications at the site of vein harvest are diabetes, obesity, preoperative anemia, peripheral vascular disease, and low cardiac output; women are more likely to experience these complications than are men. The incidence of complications may be reduced by interrupted or video-assisted harvest. The time of closure (before or after heparin administration) and the technique used (staples or subcuticular suture) do not appear to be important risk factors (133). However, deep wounds and wounds closed over drains are associated with an increased risk of complications (133).

Infection, whether in the form of superficial cellulitis or frank deep infection, can result in serious morbidity after an otherwise successful operation. Cellulitis can be treated with compresses, elevation, and antibiotics, but if deeper infection is suspected the wound must be opened widely. Gram-positive organisms are the most common cause of infection, and antibiotic therapy should be based on this fact. Often, skin grafting is required to treat extensive infection.

Acute Valve Infection

The estimated incidence of prosthetic valve endocarditis is 1% to 2% per patient-year for both tissue and mechanical valves (136). Overall, the risk of prosthetic endocarditis after valve replacement for native endocarditis is 4%, but this risk increases to 15% if valve replacement is performed when native endocarditis is an active infection (137). Native endocarditis generally affects the mitral valve, whereas prosthetic endocarditis generally affects the aortic valve. The incidence of endocarditis is 1.4% after aortic replacement and 0.6% after mitral valve replacement (138). Mechanical valves with smaller sewing rings, such as the St. Jude prosthesis, may be associated with a lower risk of infection than tissue valves (137). More recently, it has been recognized that the treatment of native valve endocarditis may be improved by the use of stentless valves, homografts, the Ross procedure, or some combination of the three (139,140).

Early prosthetic valve endocarditis (occurring within 60 days of surgery) is caused by an intraoperative break in sterile technique, a postoperative infection, or an actively infected surgical field. Organisms that cause this complication include coagulase-negative *Staphylococcus* spp. (52% of infections), fungi (13%), *Staphylococcus aureus* (10%), and enterococci (8%) (138). Patients will exhibit clinical symptoms such as fever, will proceed to experience signs such as new murmur and hemolysis, and will subsequently progress to heart failure, septic emboli, and, in the case of aortic valve infection, even heart block consistent with the formation of annular abscess. Other signs of prosthetic valve endocarditis are perivalvular leak and frank valve dehiscence. Blood cultures that reveal only gram-negative organisms are not definitive. If another potential source of infection is identified, if no murmur is present, and if echocardiography reveals no evidence of infection, empiric therapy for two weeks is appropriate (141). However, gram-positive organisms provide a presumptive diagnosis and require, at the very least, a six-week course of antibiotics.

The overall mortality rate for early prosthetic valve endocarditis is 75%, whereas that for late prosthetic valve endocarditis is 45% (141). The earlier the infection occurs, the higher the mortality rate, especially when infection is not due to streptococcal organisms, when heart failure or systemic emboli are present, and when aortic prostheses are used. Early surgical intervention is warranted but is associated with mortality rates ranging from 10% to 25% (141). Cowgill et al. (136) presented absolute and relative indications for surgery to treat prosthetic valve endocarditis (Table 9). Operative approaches have been likened to cancer surgery because the primary

Table 9 Indications for Surgery for Prosthetic Valve Infection

Absolute indications
Moderate to severe coronary heart failure
Refractory sepsis
Fungal infection
Valve obstruction
Unstable prosthesis
New-onset heart block
Relative indications
Mild coronary heart failure
Infection with organisms other than *Streptococcus* spp.
Embolism
Vegetative state
Perivalvular leak
Relapse
Culture-negative prosthetic valve infection with persistent fever

Source: From Ref. 136.

principle is to excise all infected tissue and spaces. This principle can necessitate wide debridement of the aortic root or the mitral annulus, which can produce such technical challenges as left ventricular–aortic discontinuity. Homograft valve or valved conduit procedures are becoming the optimal choice because they appear to be associated with a reduced incidence of infection and the conduit can be used to rebuild the left ventricular outflow tract (142). The Ross procedure, which uses pulmonary autografts, also appears to be a reasonable option (139).

Pneumonia

Pneumonia occurs in as many as 4% of patients who have undergone cardiac surgery and carries a mortality rate approaching 25% (48). Risk factors for pneumonia include smoking within six weeks of surgery, diminished pulmonary function, and gastroesophageal reflux. Postoperative risk factors include ventilation for more than 48 hours, phrenic nerve injury, and severe pain that limits deep inspiration and coughing. Pneumonia usually develops gradually, with low-grade fever and increased sputum production; chest radiography changes tend to lag behind the clinical picture but eventually demonstrate consolidation. The most common infectious agents are gram-negative rods and gram-positive cocci. Initial therapy consists of appropriate antibiotics, physiotherapy, and regular nasotracheal suctioning. Patients with thick secretions may benefit from a "mini" tracheostomy. If the infection does not respond to antibiotic therapy, bronchoscopy should be considered and quantitative cultures should be examined to determine whether antibiotic resistance has occurred (143).

ACUTE COMPLICATIONS OF VALVE REPLACEMENT OR REPAIR

Each valve has specific anatomic relationships that must be considered when repair or replacement is performed. These relationships include the location of key structures (such as the conduction system) and the role of valve structure in determining overall cardiac function (for example, low cardiac output or frank rupture after mitral valve replacement).

Aortic Valve

The normal three-leaflet valve has a number of crucial relationships to subvalvular structures. The coronary leaflets are in continuity with the anterior mitral leaflet from approximately the midportion of the noncoronary leaflet to a point approximated by the commissure between the noncoronary leaflet and the right coronary leaflet. The bundle of His passes through the ventricular septum near this same commissure. The septum itself lies below the annulus of the right coronary cusp. Portions of the right atrium and the left atrium are in contact with the annulus along the noncoronary cusp.

Complications related to manipulating a calcified aorta have been addressed previously. However, longstanding aortic stenosis can lead to aneurysmal dilatation of the ascending aorta, which can result in friable tissue that can make closure more difficult. In addition, the dilatation can distort the more anterior right coronary anatomy, predominantly by elevating the right coronary ostia (144). The aortotomy is generally oblique, with the right side aimed at the midpoint of the noncoronary cusp, at least 1 cm above the right coronary ostia. If bleeding occurs after closure, and particularly if the aorta is friable, repair should not be attempted unless the aortic pressure can be decreased, either by decreasing pump flow (if the patient is still on bypass) or by temporarily occluding the vena cava (if the patient is off bypass).

Calcification of the valve and annulus is common, and careful debridement is often required. Efforts should be made to prevent embolizing debris from entering the more posterior left coronary ostia, to pack the ventricular cavity with gauze, and to remove any "floaters" by irrigation after debridement. Extensive calcification can extend onto the anterior mitral leaflet and excessive debridement can cause detachment of the anterior leaflet from the "aortic curtain." If detachment occurs, it is managed by resuspending the leaflet with pledgeted sutures placed through the anterior leaflet and then through the annulus, and finally by securing the leaflet to the aortic prosthesis. Annular perforation into adjacent structures, if recognized, is treated similarly. Finally, when valve sutures are placed, taking wider bites on the annular side than on the valve ring can lead to bunching of the annular tissues and to subsequent paravalvular leaks. Paravalvular leaks (without endocarditis) occur in as many as 2% of cases (144), but no specific area of the annulus is at a greater risk of leakage. If leakage is recognized postoperatively and is large or is associated with symptoms or evidence of ventricular strain, early reoperation should be performed

(145). In many instances, only simple sutures will be required, without the need for valve replacement. When surgical procedures are performed for endocarditis, debriding all necrotic tissue is crucial, even if aorto-ventricular discontinuity results. In many (if not most) circumstances, aorto-ventricular discontinuity is anticipated and a homograft is used to reconstruct the aortic root. The coronary "buttons" that are resuspended from the new root should be placed so as not to kink the coronary artery. Acute coronary occlusion may manifest as poor pump function when attempts are made to wean the patient from bypass; however, in the early postoperative period, this complication often causes acute ischemia involving the specific coronary distribution. Acute coronary occlusion requires immediate reevaluation by echocardiography, with a low threshold for reexploration.

The AV conduction system can be damaged by the placement of sutures deep into the septum beneath the commissure of the noncoronary and right coronary cusps or by extensive decalcification in this same area. However, in many instances, such damage is due to edema or mechanical injury and will resolve without surgical treatment. Temporary pacing is usually tried for as long as 10 days before the installation of a permanent pacemaker is recommended.

Mitral Valve

Specific relationships that must be considered when repair or replacement of the mitral valve is performed include the role of the mitral valve apparatus in maintaining cardiac function and preventing ventricular rupture, the risk of injury to the circumflex artery and the noncoronary cusps of the aortic valve, with special attention to the site of the conduction system, and, finally, the risk that mitral valve tissue may prolapse and obstruct the left ventricular outflow tract.

The conduction system, including the AV node, is generally most at risk for injury between the fibrous right trigone and the central tendon areas (146). The midportion of the anterior mitral leaflet marks the commissure between the left coronary and noncoronary cusps and the aortic curtain. The circumflex artery runs parallel along the left side of the heart (as seen by the surgeon), to the annular attachment of the posterior mitral leaflet. If the left coronary artery system is dominant, the circumflex artery may lie parallel to the entire posterior annulus (146). The coronary sinus lies close to the most posterior and right-sided portion of the posterior annulus. Excessively deep sutures in any of these areas can cause damage that usually will manifest itself as low cardiac output, ischemic changes, or both as the patient is weaned from bypass or during the early postoperative period. Injury to the circumflex artery will usually require coronary bypass. Injury to the conduction bundle may respond to removal of the offending sutures.

It is now accepted that the subvalvular apparatus plays a crucial role in preserving left ventricular function. Preservation of one or both mitral attachments to the papillary muscles is associated with decreased ventricular dilation, improved ventricular function, and reduced risk of ventricular rupture (141,147). This knowledge has led to preservation of portions of the mitral leaflets during valve replacement and to increased efforts to supplant replacement with reconstruction whenever possible.

Left ventricular rupture occurs in 1% of cases of mitral valve replacement (148). Patients with small ventricular cavities are at increased risk of this complication. Type I ruptures, which occur along the posterior AV groove, are related to extensive annular resection, forceful traction on the leaflets or the annulus, substantial decalcification, placement of an oversized valve, or elevation of the apex of the heart after valve replacement (141,149). Avoiding elevation of the apex of the heart is the reason that, when combined mitral valve–coronary bypass procedures are performed, the mitral valve replacement is performed after all coronary arteries have been bypassed. Type II ruptures occur at the base of the papillary muscles and are generally attributed to excessive traction on the subvalvular structures. Type III ruptures occur between the base of the papillary muscles and the AV groove and can result from a combination of the causes mentioned above; in particular, however, they are related to perforation of the heart by surgical instruments or to elevation of the heart after valve replacement, which can lead to direct perforation or tearing (150). Type II and III ruptures are probably less common when low-profile prosthetic valves are used for replacement. Ruptures are commonly noted acutely when coronary bypass is terminated (as a jet of blood emanating posteriorly) or within a few hours after the patient's arrival in the intensive care unit (as tamponade, excessive chest tube output, and shock, or as acute low cardiac output). Repair must be performed while the patient is on cardiopulmonary bypass because any attempt to elevate the full, beating heart will result in extension of the injury. External repair with pledgeted strips can be attempted with type II or III ruptures, but repair of type I ruptures (and in many cases also repair of type II and III ruptures) requires removal of the valve, "re-endothelialization" with pericardium and internal repair, and valve replacement (151). No matter which method of repair is chosen, the mortality rate is at least 50% (141).

As another consequence of mitral valve prolapse, the anterior mitral leaflet may be pushed into the left ventricular outflow tract. Mechanisms include a redundant anterior leaflet that is anteriorly displaced by valve replacement or an excessive redundant posterior leaflet that either telescopes into the outflow tract itself or impinges on the anterior leaflet and thus forces it into the outflow tract. Suspected subaortic stenosis (suggested by evidence such as elevated left atrial pressure or poor cardiac output) will be confirmed by echocardiography. In an attempt to reduce the occurrence of this complication after mitral valve repair, various sliding and shortening procedures designed to reduce the redundancy of the posterior leaflet have been described, as have methods of "bunching up" or "trimming" the anterior leaflet during valve replacement (152).

Tricuspid Valve

Three important acute complications of tricuspid valve surgery are right heart failure, conduction block, and coronary sinus injury. Coronary sinus injury should never occur because the coronary sinus is clearly visible when the right atrium is opened. Heart block occurs in as many as 6% of patients after valvuloplasty and in as many as 24% after valve replacement (152). The AV node lies at the midpoint of a line drawn from the coronary sinus to the anteroseptal commissure. The bundle of His travels along this line beneath the septal leaflet base deep to the anteroseptal commissure. Sutures should not be placed in this area. Acute heart block that is recognized at the time of operation should be managed by replacing any potentially offending sutures. Although persistent heart block after tricuspid valve annuloplasty can be managed in a standard fashion, standard ventricular leads cannot be placed after valve replacement; thus, patients undergoing valve replacement will require external placement of the leads through a thoracotomy or attempts at pacing via the coronary sinus.

Determining the benefit of tricuspid valve repair or replacement is difficult when patients have right heart failure and tricuspid regurgitation. If right heart failure is due to essentially irreversible right-sided myocardial damage, then operation for replacement will inevitably result in failure and death. However, persistent pulmonary hypertension that leads to right heart failure— particularly when mitral valve disease is present— may be, to some degree, reversible, and patients can benefit greatly from tricuspid valvuloplasty or replacement of the valve (153).

TRAUMA
Blunt Aortic Injury

The "big three" complications associated with the management of blunt thoracic aortic injury (BAI) are death, rupture (usually fatal), and paralysis. Until the 1980s, the uniformly high mortality rate associated with BAI was sufficient to mandate operative repair as an emergent procedure for all but the most moribund patients. Now that we recognize that as many as three-fourths of patients have confounding extrathoracic injuries that take precedence to BAI and also have intrathoracic injuries that may complicate repair, the emphasis has changed to selective management for BAI, during which a period of nonoperative therapy might be appropriate (4,154–156).

Death

Most patients (more than 70%) with BAI will not reach the hospital alive; of those who do, approximately 5% to 30% will be in a very unstable condition, with expectations of mortality rates being high (as high as 98%) (4). For patients in stable condition, most deaths (approximately 25% overall) are related to associated injuries (4,157). Critical extrathoracic hemorrhage from pelvic or intra-abdominal sources must be treated first. The three serious injuries that have direct impact on the timing of operative repair of BAI are closed head injury, severe pulmonary lacerations, and cardiac risk factors (either "contusion" or coronary ischemia) (4,155,157–159). The operative mortality rate for patients with evidence of cardiac injury is as high as 71%, whereas that for patients without such evidence is 24% (157). The risk of death may not be increased for patients with lung contusion but no deep lacerations; however, these patients exhibit a marked increase in postoperative pulmonary dysfunction (157,160). The risk of such dysfunction has led to the concept of delaying surgical repair or even foregoing it all together for selected patients, assuming that blood pressure can be controlled (154,161). The reported mortality rate associated with urgent repair patients ranges from 33% to 60%, whereas it is only 7% to 25% if surgical repair can be delayed until the patient's condition has stabilized (162,163).

Delayed surgical repair is based on the premise that if the systolic blood pressure can be maintained below 120 mmHg (mean arterial pressure, 80 mmHg), the risk of rupture is very low (4). Whether this premise applies equally to small intimal flaps and to definite pseudoaneurysms is not clear (164). We reviewed our experience (165) with 30 patients with BAI, 15 of whom underwent delayed surgical repair (2–90 days after injury) and 15 of whom did not undergo repair because of advanced age or associated injuries. These 15 patients were followed up with serial helical CT scans every two to three days for the first 10 days after admission. In four patients (including three with intimal flaps), the injury increased in size within seven days of the injury. One patient with an intimal flap experienced rupture on day 7; in retrospect, however, this patient had an injury that was missed on initial angiography, and the patient was not treated with antihypertensive agents. Thus, if nonoperative therapy is chosen, we favor serial evaluation with TEE or helical CT scans for at least the first 7 to 10 days until periaortic fibrosis occurs, thus limiting the risk for expansion and rupture. Intervention should be performed promptly if any injury increases in size.

An alternative, particularly for patients with head injury who might be injured if a lower mean arterial pressure is maintained, is an endovascular stent graft (166,167). Most commercially available devices require a 1-cm "landing zone." Our review of 50 angiograms indicated that in as many as 60% of cases, such a requirement would mean that the graft would be placed across the origin of the left subclavian artery (168). Although flow to the left upper extremity will be diminished, it should be possible to maintain limb viability until a carotid–subclavian bypass can be performed; thus, the endovascular stent graft is still an option.

Rupture

Most patients with BAI (as many as 70%) will die before reaching the hospital (4). Approximately 5% of patients with BAI, or as many as one-third of patients who reach the hospital with detectable vital signs, will become acutely hypotensive, and their mortality rate will approach 98% (4). The remaining patients (as many as 25% of all patients with BAI) will reach the hospital in stable condition, and there will be time to make the diagnosis and develop a treatment plan. Unfortunately, as many as 20% of patients will experience aortic exsanguination while awaiting definitive diagnosis and treatment (108).

Rupture can occur at three distinct periods. The first is during the diagnostic and preoperative stage. The main factor contributing to rupture during this period is hypertension. As noted, the primary intervention for preventing rupture is maintaining systolic blood pressure at or below 120 mmHg (156). This blood pressure can be achieved in most patients with pain medication and beta-blockade, which should be instituted for all patients in stable condition until the diagnosis of BAI has been ruled out or definitive therapy has been established (156). For most patients who arrive at the emergency department with vital signs but whose condition is unstable, the cause of hypotension is something other than free rupture, predominantly pelvic fracture, abdominal hemorrhage, or cardiac causes (157). However, patients with no evidence of pelvic fracture and with negative results from diagnostic lavage or ultrasound but with evidence of large left hemothorax should be rapidly prepared for exploratory thoracotomy, and the surgical team should expect aortic rupture (169). In addition, impending free rupture is suggested by one of the following signs: absence of left radial pulse, pseudocoarctation syndrome, or hemothorax of more than 500 cc without pneumothorax. Clark et al. (170) recommend immediate exploration rather than delay for angiography if one of these signs is detected.

The second period during which rupture can occur is during operation, notably during induction, when wide swings in blood pressure can occur, and when proximal control is attempted. Patients at particular risk of rupture at this time are those whose injury is within 1 cm of the origin of the left subclavian artery. In our series (116), intraoperative rupture occurred in 17% of cases with injury within 1 cm of the left subclavian artery but in only 2% of those with more distal injuries. Reasons for rupture included unrecognized proximal extension of the injury into the arch or inadvertent entry into the hematoma during attempts to encircle the aorta proximally. The best way of avoiding this catastrophe is recognizing its potential, having bypass already in place, and performing the proximal dissection last. Any injury within 1 cm of the left subclavian artery must be managed by obtaining control proximal to the artery. At least 15% of these more proximal tears will be associated with additional injury or extension of injury proximal to the left subclavian artery.

The third period during which rupture may occur is the immediate postoperative period (within 48 hours of the surgical procedure). Blood pressure should be carefully controlled for at least 48 hours in an attempt to prevent graft blowout (108).

Paralysis

The incidence of paralysis after operative repair for BAI ranges from 0% to 35% (108). A number of factors have been studied, most notably cross-clamp times and the use of bypass as opposed to the clamp-and-sew technique. Zeiger et al. (171) noted that the incidence of paralysis increased if cross-clamp times exceeded 35 minutes. In reviewing multiple series, these authors also found that the incidence of paraplegia was 2.9% when bypass was used, 7.9% when Gott shunts were used, and 20.4% when the clamp-and-sew technique was used. In contrast, other authors (157,172) have reported that the clamp-and-sew approach is acceptable and that postoperative paralysis is more closely related to other factors, including preoperative hypotension and associated injuries. In general, however, most authors recommend limiting clamp times to less than 30 minutes and certainly less than 45 minutes; they also favor centrifugal left heart–distal aortic bypass. One procedure that seems to offer potential benefits is direct repair without the placement of grafts. This method may be possible in as many as 75% of cases, although the reported percentage varies widely (173,174). Direct repair appears to reduce cross-clamp times and the incidence of paraplegia (174,175).

A number of other factors should be considered in attempts to avoid paralysis after surgical procedures to repair BAI. The use of sodium nitroprusside either preoperatively or during cross-clamping, as is common when elective aortic resection is performed, has been associated with an increased risk of paralysis, presumably because of a steal phenomenon. For this reason, administering beta-blockers is preferred (4,108). In addition, clamping the subclavian artery, particularly in patients undergoing repair without the support of left heart bypass, appears to be associated with an increased risk of spinal ischemia. When left heart bypass was not employed, paralysis occurred in 28% of cases when the subclavian artery was clamped and in no cases when it was not clamped (116). This finding emphasizes the importance of replacing the proximal clamp distally as soon as the proximal anastomosis is completed so that flow to the spinal collaterals is reestablished.

Cardiac Trauma

In most cases, penetrating cardiac injuries require technically simple repair, whereas blunt injuries are usually managed by supportive measures alone. Complex injuries, usually defined as those involving the coronary arteries, the valves, or the ventricular septum, have been reported in as many as 10% to 20% of clinical reviews (176). Most cardiac injuries are not detected acutely, especially those caused by blunt injury (177,178). The management of these injuries depends upon the overall condition of the patient and on the ability of the heart to provide adequate output. Because, in most cases, the treatment of these injuries will require cardiopulmonary bypass, with its attendant impact on coagulation and the potential for myocardial stunning, a temporizing approach is best until the patient's condition has been stabilized (2,160).

A serious problem that must be avoided is failure to recognize the injury. Patients who arrive at the emergency department in shock may transiently respond to volume expansion, and this response may cause the mistaken belief that severe injury is unlikely (179). If hypotension persists or recurs, CVP increases, or a widened mediastinum is detected, particularly in association with penetrating injury, surgical exploration with a pericardial window or sternotomy is urgently required (180). After either blunt or penetrating injury, patients who are in stable condition with only subtle signs of injury but who require repeated volume boluses should at least undergo urgent transthoracic echocardiography (TTE) (181). Small fluid collections require further investigation, perhaps by means of a pericardial window. Occasionally, patients with blunt injury will exhibit persistent volume requirements, although there is no obvious source of hemorrhage. CT scans of the chest, often performed to determine whether the mediastinum is widened, may show blood totally encircling the heart, which should suggest the diagnosis of cardiac trauma.

Patients who arrive at the emergency department with vital signs and clinical signs of tamponade, but who have not yet undergone intubation, are at risk of acute arrest at the time of intubation. This complication is due to any one or all of the three following factors: venodilation associated with anesthesia and loss of preload, high intrathoracic pressures that are caused by overzealous ventilation and may lead to a further tamponade effect, and systemic vasodilatation due to hyperventilation and anesthetic agents. Draining the pericardium, preferably with ultrasound guidance, just before attempting intubation substantially reduces the risk of acute arrest (182).

If cardiac injury is suspected, sternotomy best exposes the heart and the proximal great vessels. Anterolateral thoracotomy, usually performed in the emergency department, is inadequate in as many as 20% of cases (183). If injury to the great vessel or the ascending aorta is known or suspected, dissection should be started within the pericardium. This method will allow for proximal control before the site of injury is entered. If there is a large injury to the ascending aorta and cardiac arrest and cardiopulmonary bypass are not immediately possible, controlling hemorrhage by performing caval occlusion will allow the heart to beat while it is empty. In this way, visualization of the injury site will be improved so that at least initial sutures can be placed; this procedure also appears to reduce the pulmonary congestion that in many cases is the cause of death for patients who have survived aortic repair (184).

Mural lacerations can be controlled by finger pressure, followed by the placement of sutures. The atria can be clamped and can usually be easily repaired with direct sutures. The ventricle is usually controlled with pledgeted horizontal mattress sutures. In the acute setting, temporary control of hemorrhaging can be achieved with staples (185–188). The wall of the right ventricle is very thin and can easily tear. For this reason, when sutures are placed or when attempts are made to achieve temporary control of hemorrhaging with a Foley catheter, great care must be taken to avoid extending the injury. Injuries to the right atrium adjacent to the ventricle should be approached with caution because the proximal right coronary artery lies in the groove between these chambers and can be inadvertently occluded.

Blunt cardiac injuries ranging from the ill-defined "contusion" to frank rupture usually involve the right ventricle. "Contusion" has been linked to a variety of complications, including cardiogenic shock, life-threatening dysrhythmia, and late rupture, possibly as the result of transitory redistribution of coronary flow, a redistribution that is aggravated by hypovolemia (3,189). Contusion differs from myocardial infarction in that infarction causes cell necrosis, whereas contusion involves various degrees of hemorrhage but does not invariably lead to cell death. Contusion is a nonspecific injury whose clinical significance is not clear. Terms other than contusion, such as blunt cardiac injury with associated specific complications, have been suggested as more specific, and attention has shifted to determining which patients are at risk of these complications (189).

ECG and serial CPK-MB assays vary in sensitivity and specificity for both diagnosis and risk stratification. When patients with cardiac trauma are admitted to the hospital, neither normal nor abnormal findings on ECG reliably predict or preclude the presence of cardiac complications that will require treatment. Serum CPK and MB fractions alone do not predict the likelihood of complications and do not appear to be clinically useful (190). Admitting all asymptomatic patients to the hospital on the basis of CPK or ECG results may produce an undue burden with little defined benefit. Assays for cardiac-specific troponin T or troponin I may be more specific than CPK-MB assays in identifying significant cardiac injury, but these assays require further evaluation (191–194).

TTE is a rapid and noninvasive method of identifying wall motion abnormalities, effusions, or valvular damage. However, its accuracy is limited by chest wall abnormalities and pneumothorax, and an adequate study cannot be obtained for as many as 30% of patients (195). Although TEE is more labor intensive than TTE, its results are more accurate, and it also allows evaluation of the thoracic aorta. TEE is the most accurate method of evaluating cardiac function and injury.

Serious arrhythmias and cardiogenic shock necessitating inotropic support occur in 10% of patients with documented myocardial injury (195). Increases in PEEP and the presence of pulmonary edema or pulmonary contusions can further compromise right ventricular function. Left ventricular function can be affected in as many as one-third of patients. Management of arrhythmia or cardiogenic shock, like that of acute myocardial infarction, includes fluid administration, inotropic support, and pulmonary afterload reduction (3). The IABP or the Biomedicus pump, which are placed by accessing the femoral vein or artery, may provide circulatory support even during urgent noncardiac (usually orthopedic) surgical procedures (4,195,196).

As noted previously, in the best of circumstances after repair of cardiac injury, the patient's condition will be stable enough that a damage control approach, with the primary goal of complete resuscitation and rewarming, will be possible. Later, diagnostic studies can then be used to detect complex injuries that may require intervention. All survivors of penetrating cardiac trauma should undergo early elective TEE or TTE because many (19%) of them will have unrecognized intracardiac injuries (176,197). Delayed complications after blunt trauma, such as valvular dehiscence, myocardial dissection, coronary thrombosis, ventricular aneurysm, septal defect, and intraventricular thrombosis, have been reported to occur as late as six years after the traumatic event, although they usually occur within the first three weeks after injury (179). Follow-up echocardiography should be performed three months after any documented blunt or penetrating injury.

Penetrating coronary artery injuries are usually treated by simple ligation, with cardiac output maintained by an IABP (176). More complex treatment is needed, however, for patients with injuries to the proximal LAD and for patients with any injury to a proximal coronary artery that is clearly associated with substantial myocardial ischemia, even if those patients have minimal associated injuries and are in a relatively stable condition. Off-pump bypass or primary repair may rarely be used, although cardiopulmonary bypass provides the opportunity to rewarm the patient and to correct metabolic derangements

(176). Blunt trauma can rarely lead to coronary thrombosis, which is usually detected by ECG changes that prompt angiography. Acute repair of the coronary injury has been reported in conjunction with repair of aortic injury, but, in general, expectant management is employed (198). Occasionally, angioplasty may be used to reestablish flow through the injured coronary artery (199). Myocardial infarction is a late complication of penetrating cardiac trauma, and there also appears to be an increased association between these injuries and the formation of ventricular aneurysms (200,201).

Although valvular defects have been documented after penetrating injury, they are more often observed after blunt chest trauma (3,176,195,202). Aortic valve rupture is the most common valve injury described in clinical series (203). In general, attempts should be made to stabilize the patient's condition with nonsurgical treatment. However, recalcitrant cardiac decompensation may prompt earlier surgical intervention. Aortic insufficiency will manifest itself acutely as dilation of the left ventricle. IABP is contraindicated. Valve replacement is the best alternative if the patient's condition cannot be stabilized medically (203). Mitral valve rupture can affect any level of the mitral apparatus, from avulsion of papillary muscle to a tear in a leaflet. The clinical presentation of mitral valve rupture varies, but a holosystolic murmur is often identified. When a papillary muscle has ruptured, congestive heart failure usually develops rapidly, whereas rupture of chordae or tearing of the leaflet leads to more insidious decompensation. Again, the best treatment approach is careful volume support, IABP, and interval repair, if the patient's condition responds to such maneuvers. Rupture of the tricuspid valve, which is suggested by distended neck veins with pulsation or hepatomegaly with liver pulsation, is usually well tolerated. Another sign is holosystolic murmur, heard along the left sternal border, which increases with inspiration. Approximately 10% of patients with a ruptured tricuspid valve have a patent foramen ovale. Serious tricuspid regurgitation can lead to clinically significant right-to-left shunt, which will require earlier repair and closure of the foramen (189).

Ventricular septal defects occurring after either blunt or penetrating injuries usually involve the anterior septum. Penetrating septal defects are small and often heal spontaneously, whereas blunt defects tend to involve the apex, are larger, and are less likely to heal. Septal defects that result in severe heart failure require urgent repair. As is true of other complex injuries, rupture of the tricuspid valve can be temporarily treated with IABP, but full cardiopulmonary bypass will be required. If substantial septal defects with left-to-right shunts at a ratio of more than 2:1 persist, repair will be required. Smaller lesions can be managed medically.

Late complications include a variety of cardiovascular fistulae. Most cardiovascular arterio-venous fistulae occur after stab wounds. Virtually all of these fistulae can be detected by the presence of a "machinery" murmur within one week of injury. Innominate arterio-venous fistulae are the most common and require repair or grafting of the artery (4). Coronary artery fistulae, usually to the right ventricle, present with ischemia, cardiomyopathy, subacute bacterial endocarditis, pulmonary hypertension, or some combination of these signs (204). Treatment involves either ligation of the fistula alone or, more commonly, ligation of the coronary artery and coronary bypass. Aorto-cardiac fistulae most commonly involve the aorta just above the right coronary cusp and connect to the right ventricle (4,205). Congestive heart failure is often the presenting picture. Aorto-cardiac fistulae and aorto-pulmonary artery fistulae that can occur just above the aortic valve are closed by patching while the patient is on cardiopulmonary bypass.

Pericardium

Complications involving the pericardium are unpredictable and essentially unavoidable; they are also occasionally difficult to diagnose and life threatening. Physicians need to maintain a high degree of suspicion if they are to recognize the occurrence of these complications. The liberal use of TTE, central monitoring, and early exploration may be required for preventing acute cardiovascular collapse.

Postpericardiotomy Syndrome

The first case of postcardiac injury syndrome was reported to have occurred after a mitral commissurotomy (206). Inflammatory reactions after cardiac surgery have been reported to occur in as many as 18% of adults and 27% of children (207,208). The incidence of pericarditis is as high as 22% among survivors of penetrating cardiac injury (209). The cause of postcardiac injury syndrome is believed to be a postinjury autoimmune reaction that directs antibodies against the myocardium or the pericardium (210). In addition, the introduction of blood into the pericardium may cause a vigorous inflammatory response (211). Dressler reported that the predominant clinical features of postcardiac injury syndrome are recurrent low-grade (38–40°C) fever and pleuropericardial pain (212) that is predominantly precordial but may radiate to the shoulder, neck, or scapula. The pain is aggravated by inspiration, recumbency, and twisting the torso. These symptoms usually occur days or months after the injury. Exudative nonhemorrhagic pericardial effusions leading to tamponade have been reported but are rarely clinically significant (213,214). A pericardial friction rub may be heard until the effusion reaches a volume large enough to cause muffled heart sounds. Large pericardial effusions, with or without tamponade, may result in compression atelectasis of the base of the left lower lobe (215). Echocardiography is the most specific diagnostic method. It will not only document the effusion but may also demonstrate pericardial thickening, a sign consistent with inflammation (215). Progressive tamponade is demonstrated initially by collapse of the right atrium and subsequently by collapse of the right ventricle during diastole. Both findings have a predictive accuracy of 72% for tamponade (215), but this accuracy is affected by volume status and the presence of pulmonary hypertension. In addition, right atrial hypertension may be reflected by inferior vena cava plethora, a condition in which the vena cava no longer demonstrates its normal decrease in diameter of 50% or more during inspiration (216).

In most instances, posttraumatic pericarditis is a self-limiting condition, although recurrences are not uncommon (209). In the elective setting, no specific prophylaxis is recommended, but after open cardiac massage in the trauma setting, initiation of treatment is reasonable if it is not contraindicated (209). Initial treatment, in the absence of tamponade, includes the administration of anti-inflammatory agents. Acetylsalicylic acid is often effective, but if relapses recur, steroids may be required, particularly if a growing effusion is documented (217). Once the effusion causes cardiac decompensation, drainage, either by pericardiocentesis or by operative approaches, is required.

Constrictive Pericarditis

Constrictive pericarditis is quite uncommon after trauma; its occurrence is generally related to the effect of blood in the pericardial cavity (209). This complication may occur weeks after the event, but its occurrence is more common years later (195). Constrictive pericarditis is uncommon after elective cardiac procedures, possibly because the pericardium is widely drained after elective cases. When this complication does occur, especially years after the inciting event, extensive calcification is the rule. The diagnosis of constrictive pericarditis is based on clinical features of systemic venous plethora (including jugular vein distension, pedal edema, and even hepatic engorgement) and is confirmed by echocardiography or by measuring chamber pressures at the time of catheterization. Treatment requires pericardial resection, removing or "cobble-stoning" the pericardium from both phrenic nerves laterally, opening the roots of the pulmonary artery and aorta, and ensuring that both cavae are decompressed. Decompressing these vessels may be limited, in cases of severe calcification, to cracking open the anterior surfaces. The left heart should be decompressed first. This maneuver will prevent acute pulmonary edema that might occur if the right heart was decompressed before the left ventricle was sufficiently freed, to allow it to accept the sudden increase in volume from the pulmonary circuit. If pericardial resection is performed after coronary artery bypass, the status and location of the grafts must be documented, and preparations must be made for possible regrafting in the event that a patent graft is injured. Relative dilation and congestive heart failure may occur postoperatively. These problems can be managed by administering diuretic drugs and digitalis, but the problems may also reflect a degree of underlying cardiomyopathy.

Suppurative Pericarditis

Suppurative pericarditis usually occurs after penetrating injury; its initial symptoms may resemble those of the more typical autoimmune form of postinjury pericarditis. Among children, suppurative pericarditis is often a consequence of pneumonia; the organisms responsible for this condition include *Hemophilus influenza*, *S. aureus*, and *Escherichia coli* (218). The diagnosis should be suggested by a history of penetrating injury or a retained foreign object, coupled with a progressively septic course. Echocardiography, chest radiography, or CT may demonstrate air fluid levels, loculations, or both, with denser fluid levels (219). The diagnosis may be further suggested by evidence of infection at other sites, especially the lungs (219). If the diagnosis is uncertain, pericardiocentesis may confirm it. Operative intervention involves wide debridement, and the procedure should begin with a left anterolateral thoracotomy. Dividing the sternum should be avoided so as to reduce the risk of sternal osteomyelitis (219).

CONCLUSION

During the past two decades, attention has shifted to developing less invasive methods for cardiac operations and prolonging the patency of conduits and grafts. Attempts at minimizing the acute complications related to cardiac operations have focused on ameliorating the inflammatory response to cardiopulmonary bypass, reducing the impact of ischemia–reperfusion, and improving neurological and end-organ preservation. Despite these advances, cardiac surgery is still a complicated technical process fraught with the potential for acute catastrophe. Surgeons must recognize situations in which certain complications are more likely and be prepared to modify approaches accordingly and to react quickly with an organized sequence of efforts when these complications occur.

REFERENCES

1. Bojar R. Coronary artery bypass surgery. In: Bojar R, ed. Adult Cardiac Surgery. Oxford: Blackwell Scientific, 1992:79–152.
2. Karmy-Jones R, van Wijngaarden MH, Talwar MK, Lovoulos C. Penetrating cardiac injuries. Injury 1997; 28(1):57–61.
3. van Wijngaarden MH, Karmy-Jones R, Talwar MK, Simonetti V. Blunt cardiac injury: a 10 year institutional review. Injury 1997; 28(1):51–55.
4. Mattox KL. Red River anthology. J Trauma 1997; 42(3):353–368.
5. Ruchat P, Hurni M, Stumpe F, Fischer AP, von Segesser LK. Acute ascending aortic dissection complicating open heart surgery: cerebral perfusion defines the outcome. Eur J Cardiothorac Surg 1998; 14(5):449–452.
6. Chavanon O, Carrier M, Cartier R, et al. Increased incidence of acute ascending aortic dissection with off-pump aortocoronary bypass surgery? Ann Thorac Surg 2001; 71(1):117–121.
7. Still RJ, Hilgenberg AD, Akins CW, Daggett WM, Buckley MJ. Intraoperative aortic dissection. Ann Thorac Surg 1992; 53(3):374–379.
8. Murphy DA, Craver JM, Jones EL, Bone DK, Guyton RA, Hatcher CR Jr. Recognition and management of ascending aortic dissection complicating cardiac surgical operations. J Thorac Cardiovasc Surg 1983; 85(2):247–256.
9. Salerno TA, Lince DP, White DN, Lynn RB, Charrette EJ. Arch versus femoral artery perfusion during cardiopulmonary bypass. J Thorac Cardiovasc Surg 1978; 76(5):681–684.
10. Weiss SJ. Management of difficult coronary sinus rupture. Ann Thorac Surg 1994; 58(2):548–550.
11. Berger TJ. Coronary sinus rupture. Ann Thorac Surg 1994; 58(4):1214–1215.
12. Kurusz M, Butler B, Katz J, Conti VR. Air embolism during cardiopulmonary bypass. Perfusion 1995; 10(6):361–391.
13. Mills N, Morris J. Air embolism associated with cardiopulmonary bypass. In: Waldhausen J, Orringer M, eds. Complications in Cardiothoracic Surgery. St. Louis: Mosby Year Book, 1991:60–67.
14. Mills NL, Ochsner JL. Massive air embolism during cardiopulmonary bypass. Causes, prevention, and management. J Thorac Cardiovasc Surg 1980; 80(5): 708–717.
15. Blauth CI, Arnold JV, Schulenberg WE, McCartney AC, Taylor KM. Cerebral microembolism during cardiopulmonary bypass. Retinal microvascular studies in vivo with fluorescein angiography. J Thorac Cardiovasc Surg 1988; 95(4):668–676.
16. Brenner W. A battle plan in the event of massive air embolism during open heart surgery. Am J Extracorporeal Tech 1985; 17:133–137.
17. Bruce DA, Gennarelli TA, Langfitt TW. Resuscitation from coma due to head injury. Crit Care Med 1978; 6(4):254–269.
18. Nussmeier NA, Arlund C, Slogoff S. Neuropsychiatric complications after cardiopulmonary bypass: cerebral protection by a barbiturate. Anesthesiology 1986; 64(2):165–170.
19. Mills N, Harmon D. Response to: A battle plan in the vent of massive air embolism during open heart surgery. Am J Extracorporeal Tech 1986; 18:198–199.
20. Armon C, Deschamps C, Adkinson C, Fealey RD, Orszulak TA. Hyperbaric treatment of cerebral air embolism sustained during an open-heart surgical procedure. Mayo Clin Proc 1991; 66(6):565–571.
21. McGoon D. Technics of open-heart surgery for congenital heart disease. Curr Probl Surg 1968:3–42.
22. Horrow JC. Heparin reversal of protamine toxicity: have we come full circle? J Cardiothorac Anesth 1990; 4(5):539–542.

23. Aren C. Heparin and protamine therapy. Semin Thorac Cardiovasc Surg 1990; 2(4):364–372.

24. Bojar R. Cardiopulmonary bypass. In: Adult Cardiac Surgery. Oxford: Blackwell Scientific, 1992:3–36.

25. Horrow J. Protamine allergy. J Cardiothorac Anesth 1988; 2:225–242.

26. Morel DR, Skoskiewicz M, Robinson DR, Bloch KJ, Hoaglin DC, Zapol WM. Leukotrienes, thromboxane A2, and prostaglandins during systemic anaphylaxis in sheep. Am J Physiol 1991; 261(3 Pt 2):H782–H792.

27. Morel DR, Zapol WM, Thomas SJ, et al. C5a and thromboxane generation associated with pulmonary vaso- and broncho-constriction during protamine reversal of heparin. Anesthesiology 1987; 66(5):597–604.

28. Lock R, Hessel EA II. Probable reversal of protamine reactions by heparin administration. J Cardiothorac Anesth 1990; 4(5):604–608.

29. Fullerton DA. Simplified technique for left heart bypass to repair aortic transection. Ann Thorac Surg 1993; 56(3):579–580.

30. Karmy-Jones R, van Wijngaarden MH, Talwar MK, Lovoulos C. Cardiopulmonary bypass for resuscitation after penetrating cardiac trauma. Ann Thorac Surg 1996; 61(4):1244–1245.

31. Cosgrove DM, Loop FD, Lytle BW, et al. Predictors of reoperation after myocardial revascularization. J Thorac Cardiovasc Surg 1986; 92(5):811–821.

32. Lytle B. Coronary reoperations. In: Franco KL, Verrier ED, eds. Advanced Therapy in Cardiac Surgery. Hamilton: B.C. Decker, 1999:84–99.

33. Lytle BW, Cosgrove DM, Taylor PC, et al. Reoperations for valve surgery: perioperative mortality and determinants of risk for 1,000 patients, 1958–1984. Ann Thorac Surg 1986; 42(6):632–643.

34. Lytle BW, Loop FD, Cosgrove DM, et al. Fifteen hundred coronary reoperations. Results and determinants of early and late survival. J Thorac Cardiovasc Surg 1987; 93(6):847–859.

35. Lytle BW, Navia JL, Taylor PC, et al. Third coronary artery bypass operations: risks and costs. Ann Thorac Surg 1997; 64(5):1287–1295.

36. Sabik JF, Lytle BW, McCarthy PM, Cosgrove DM. Axillary artery: an alternative site of arterial cannulation for patients with extensive aortic and peripheral vascular disease. J Thorac Cardiovasc Surg 1995; 109(5):885–890.

37. Gillinov AM, Casselman FP, Lytle BW, et al. Injury to a patent left internal thoracic artery graft at coronary reoperation. Ann Thorac Surg 1999; 67(2):382–386.

38. Mangano DT. Myocardial ischemia following surgery: preliminary findings. Study of Perioperative Ischemia (SPI) Research Group. J Card Surg 1990; 5(3 suppl):288–293.

39. Chaitman BR, Alderman EL, Sheffield LT, et al. Use of survival analysis to determine the clinical significance of new Q waves after coronary bypass surgery. Circulation 1983; 67(2):302–309.

40. Boylan MJ, Lytle BW, Taylor PC, et al. Have PTCA failures requiring emergent bypass operation changed? Ann Thorac Surg 1995; 59(2):283–286.

41. Koshal A, Davies RA, Keen WJ, Beanlands DS, Nair R. Utility of bypass surgery in acute MI. Chest 1990; 97(6):1504.

42. Koshal A, Beanlands DS, Davies RA, Nair RC, Keon WJ. Urgent surgical reperfusion in acute evolving myocardial infarction. A randomized controlled study. Circulation 1988; 78(3 Pt 2):I171–I178.

43. Aldea G. Use of heparin-bonded cardiopulmonary bypass circuits with alternatives to standard anticoagulation. In: Franco KL, Verrier ED, eds. Advanced Therapy in Cardiac Surgery. Hamilton: B.C. Decker, 1999:1–9.

44. Bojar R. Myocardial protection. In: Bojar RM, ed. Adult Cardiac Surgery. Oxford: Blackwell Scientific, 1992:39–76.

45. Houppe JP, Villemot JP, Amrein D, Labourel L, Clavey M, Mathieu P. Early coronary spasm after myocardial revascularization surgery. Presse Med 1983; 12(42):2667–2670.

46. Kopf GS, Riba A, Zito R. Intraoperative use of nifedipine for hemodynamic collapse due to coronary artery spasm following myocardial revascularization. Ann Thorac Surg 1982; 34(4):457–460.

47. Fuse K, Makuuchi H, Konishi T, et al. Coronary artery spasm during coronary artery bypass surgery: its diagnosis, treatment and prevention. Jpn J Surg 1988; 18(6):626–635.

48. Richenbacher W, Kernstine K. Principles of cardiac surgery. In: Corson J, Williamson R, eds. Surgery. London: Mosby, 2001:7:28.1–7:28.11.

49. Mammen EF, Koets MH, Washington BC, et al. Hemostasis changes during cardiopulmonary bypass surgery. Semin Thromb Hemost 1985; 11(3):281–292.

50. Wang JS, Lin CY, Hung WT, et al. Thromboelastogram fails to predict postoperative hemorrhage in cardiac patients. Ann Thorac Surg 1992; 53(3):435–439.

51. Trentalange MJ, Walts LF. A comparison of thromboelastogram and template bleeding time in the evaluation of platelet function after aspirin ingestion. J Clin Anesth 1991; 3(5):377–381.

52. Kondo NI, Maddi R, Ewenstein BM, Goldhaber SZ. Anticoagulation and hemostasis in cardiac surgical patients. J Card Surg 1994; 9(4):443–461.

53. Royston D. The serine antiprotease aprotinin (Trasylol): a novel approach to reducing postoperative bleeding. Blood Coagul Fibrinol 1990; 1(1):55–69.

54. Koshal A, Murphy J, Keon WJ. Pros and cons of urgent exploratory sternotomy after open cardiac surgery. Can J Surg 1986; 29(3):186–189.

55. Stephenson LW, MacVaugh H III, Tomasello DN, Josephson ME. Propranolol for prevention of postoperative cardiac arrhythmias: a randomized study. Ann Thorac Surg 1980; 29(2):113–116.

56. Karmy-Jones R, Hamilton A, Dzavik V, Allegreto M, Finegan BA, Koshal A. Magnesium sulfate prophylaxis after cardiac operations. Ann Thorac Surg 1995; 59(2):502–507.

57. Mullen JC, Khan N, Weisel RD, et al. Atrial activity during cardioplegia and postoperative arrhythmias. J Thorac Cardiovasc Surg 1987; 94(4):558–565.

58. AH Association. 2000 Handbook of Emergency Cardiovascular Care. Salem: American Heart Association, 2000.

59. Lloyd J, Ferguson C. Postcardiac surgical intensive care. In: Webb A, Shapiro M, Singer M, Suter P, eds. Oxford Textbook of Critical Care. Oxford: Oxford Medical Publications, 1999:973–976.

60. Mullen JC, Fremes SE, Weisel RD, et al. Right ventricular function: a comparison between blood and crystalloid cardioplegia. Ann Thorac Surg 1987; 43(1):17–24.

61. Boyle EM Jr., Pohlman TH, Cornejo CJ, Verrier ED. Endothelial cell injury in cardiovascular surgery: ischemia-reperfusion. Ann Thorac Surg 1996; 62(6): 1868–1875.

62. Krishnadasan B, Morgan EN, Boyle ED, Verrier ED. Mechanisms of myocardial injury after cardiac surgery. J Cardiothorac Vasc Anesth 2000; 14(3 suppl 1): 6–10.

63. Rinaldi CA, Hall RJ. Myocardial stunning and hibernation in clinical practice. Int J Clin Pract 2000; 54(10):659–664.

64. Barnes E, Baker CS, Dutka DP, et al. Prolonged left ventricular dysfunction occurs in patients with coronary artery disease after both dobutamine and exercise induced myocardial ischaemia. Heart 2000; 83(3): 283–289.

65. Braunwald E, Rutherford JD. Reversible ischemic left ventricular dysfunction: evidence for the "hibernating myocardium". J Am Coll Cardiol 1986; 8(6):1467–1470.

66. Mahfood S, Higgens T, Loop F. Management of complications related to coronary artery bypass surgery. In: Waldhausen J, Orringer M, eds. Complications in Cardiothoracic Surgery. St. Louis: Mosby Year Book, 1991:265–280.

67. Fowler MB, Alderman EL, Oesterle SN, et al. Dobutamine and dopamine after cardiac surgery: greater augmentation of myocardial blood flow with dobutamine. Circulation 1984; 70(3 Pt 2):I103–I111.

68. Friedel N, Wenzel R, Matheis G, Hetzer R. The use of dopexamine after cardiac surgery: acute and long-term effects in patients with impaired cardiac function. Thorac Cardiovasc Surg 1992; 40(6):378–381.

69. Cosgrove DM III, Petre JH, Waller JL, Roth JV, Shepherd C, Cohn LH. Automated control of postoperative hypertension: a prospective, randomized multicenter study. Ann Thorac Surg 1989; 47(5): 678–682.

70. Novitzky D, Cooper DK, Barton CI, et al. Triiodothyronine as an inotropic agent after open heart surgery. J Thorac Cardiovasc Surg 1989; 98(5 Pt 2):972–977.

71. Bojar R. Circulatory assist devices. In: Bojar RM, ed. Adult Cardiac Surgery. Oxford: Blackwell Scientific, 1992:425–459.

72. Bartlett RH, Roloff DW, Custer JR, Younger JG, Hirschl RB. Extracorporeal life support: the University of Michigan experience. JAMA 2000; 283(7):904–908.

73. Schmid ER, Burki C, Engel MH, Schmidlin D, Tornic M, Seifert B. Inhaled nitric oxide versus intravenous vasodilators in severe pulmonary hypertension after cardiac surgery. Anesth Analg 1999; 89(5):1108–1115.

74. Gold J, Barbut D. Prevention of neurological injury during open heart surgery. In: Franco KL, Verrier ED, eds. Advanced Therapy in Cardiac Surgery. Hamilton: B.C. Decker, 1999:51–61.

75. Libman RB, Wirkowski E, Neystat M, Barr W, Gelb S, Graver M. Stroke associated with cardiac surgery. Determinants, timing, and stroke subtypes. Arch Neurol 1997; 54(1):83–87.

76. Cernaianu AC, Vassilidze TV, Flum DR, et al. Predictors of stroke after cardiac surgery. J Card Surg 1995; 10(4 Pt 1):334–339.

77. Kuroda Y, Uchimoto R, Kaieda R, et al. Central nervous system complications after cardiac surgery: a comparison between coronary artery bypass grafting and valve surgery. Anesth Analg 1993; 76(2):222–227.

78. Llinas R, Barbut D, Caplan LR. Neurologic complications of cardiac surgery. Prog Cardiovasc Dis 2000; 43(2):101–112.

79. Barbut D, Caplan LR. Brain complications of cardiac surgery. Curr Probl Cardiol 1997; 22(9):449–480.

80. Murkin JM, Baird DL, Martzke JS, Yee R. Cognitive dysfunction after ventricular fibrillation during implantable cardiovertor/defibrillator procedures is related to duration of the reperfusion interval. Anesth Analg 1997; 84(6):1186–1192.

81. Taylor KM. Brain damage during cardiopulmonary bypass. Ann Thorac Surg 1998; 65(4 suppl): S20–S26.

82. Wolman RL, Nussmeier NA, Aggarwal A, et al. Cerebral injury after cardiac surgery: identification of a group at extraordinary risk. Multicenter Study of Perioperative Ischemia Research Group (McSPI) and the Ischemia Research Education Foundation (IREF) Investigators. Stroke 1999; 30(3):514–522.

83. Evagelopoulos N, Trenz MT, Beckmann A, Krian A. Simultaneous carotid endarterectomy and coronary artery bypass grafting in 313 patients. Cardiovasc Surg 2000; 8(1):31–40.

84. Wolner E, Deutsch M, Whittlesey D, Geha A. Combined coronary and carotid artery disease. In: Baue A, Geha A, Hammond G, Naunheim K, eds. Glenn's Thoracic and Cardiovascular Surgery. 5th ed. London: Appleton & Lange, 1991:1971–1975.

85. Gillebert T, van de Werf F, Piessens J, de Geest H. Post-traumatic infarction due to blunt chest trauma. Report of two cases. Acta Cardiol 1980; 35(6):445–453.

86. Barbut D, Lo YW, Hartman GS, et al. Aortic atheroma is related to outcome but not numbers of emboli during coronary bypass. Ann Thorac Surg 1997; 64(2):454–459.

87. Barbut D, Hinton RB, Szatrowski TP, et al. Cerebral emboli detected during bypass surgery are associated with clamp removal. Stroke 1994; 25(12):2398–2402.

88. Davila-Roman VG, Phillips KJ, Daily BB, Davila RM, Kouchoukos NT, Barzilai B. Intraoperative transesophageal echocardiography and epiaortic ultrasound for assessment of atherosclerosis of the thoracic aorta. J Am Coll Cardiol 1996; 28(4):942–947.

89. Mizuno T, Toyama M, Tabuchi N, et al. Thickened intima of the aortic arch is a risk factor for stroke with coronary artery bypass grafting. Ann Thorac Surg 2000; 70(5):1565–1570.

90. Taggart DP, Bhattacharya K, Meston N, et al. Serum S-100 protein concentration after cardiac surgery: a randomized trial of arterial line filtration. Eur J Cardiothorac Surg 1997; 11(4):645–649.

91. Swain JA, McDonald TJ Jr., Griffith PK, Balaban RS, Clark RE, Ceckler T. Low-flow hypothermic cardiopulmonary bypass protects the brain. J Thorac Cardiovasc Surg 1991; 102(1):76–83.

92. Ergin M. Principles of cerebral protection during operations on the thoracic aorta. In: Franco KL, Verrier ED, eds. Advanced Therapy in Cardiac Surgery. Hamilton: B.C. Decker, 1999:257–269.

93. Mezrow CK, Midulla PS, Sadeghi AM, et al. Evaluation of cerebral metabolism and quantitative electroencephalography after hypothermic circulatory arrest and low-flow cardiopulmonary bypass at different temperatures. J Thorac Cardiovasc Surg 1994; 107(4):1006–1019.

94. McCullough JN, Zhang N, Reich DL, et al. Cerebral metabolic suppression during hypothermic circulatory arrest in humans. Ann Thorac Surg 1999; 67(6):1895–1899.

95. Ergin MA, Griepp EB, Lansman SL, Galla JD, Levy M, Griepp RB. Hypothermic circulatory arrest and other methods of cerebral protection during operations on the thoracic aorta. J Card Surg 1994; 9(5):525–537.

96. Ueda Y, Miki S, Kusuhara K, Okita Y, Tahata T, Yamanaka K. Surgical treatment of aneurysm or dissection involving the ascending aorta and aortic arch, utilizing circulatory arrest and retrograde cerebral perfusion. J Cardiovasc Surg (Torino) 1990; 31(5):553–558.

97. Juvonen T, Zhang N, Wolfe D, et al. Retrograde cerebral perfusion enhances cerebral protection during prolonged hypothermic circulatory arrest: a study in a chronic porcine model. Ann Thorac Surg 1998; 66(1):38–50.

98. Griepp RB, Juvonen T, Griepp EB, McCollough JN, Ergin MA. Is retrograde cerebral perfusion an effective means of neural support during hypothermic circulatory arrest? Ann Thorac Surg 1998; 64(3):913–916.

99. Pearl JM, Thomas DW, Grist G, Duffy JY, Manning PB. Hyperoxia for management of acid-base status during deep hypothermia with circulatory arrest. Ann Thorac Surg 2000; 70(3):751–755.

100. Hiramatsu T, Miura T, Forbess JM, et al. pH strategies and cerebral energetics before and after circulatory arrest. J Thorac Cardiovasc Surg 1995; 109(5):948–957.

101. Svenson L. New methods of spinal cord protection during operations on the thoracic aorta. In: Franco KL, Verrier ED, eds. Advanced Therapy in Cardiac Surgery. Hamilton: B.C. Decker, 1999:311–318.

102. Svensson LG, Patel V, Robinson MF, Ueda T, Roehm JO Jr., Crawford ES. Influence of preservation or perfusion of intraoperatively identified spinal cord blood supply on spinal motor evoked potentials and paraplegia after aortic surgery. J Vasc Surg 1991; 13(3):355–365.

103. Crawford ES, Crawford JL, Safi HJ, et al. Thoracoabdominal aortic aneurysms: preoperative and intraoperative factors determining immediate and long-term results of operations in 605 patients. J Vasc Surg 1986; 3(3):389–404.

104. Cooley DA, Baldwin RT. Technique of open distal anastomosis for repair of descending thoracic aortic aneurysms. Ann Thorac Surg 1992; 54(5):932–936.

105. Svensson LG, Hess KR, Coselli JS, Safi HJ. Influence of segmental arteries, extent, and atriofemoral bypass on postoperative paraplegia after thoracoabdominal aortic operations. J Vasc Surg 1994; 20(2):255–262.

106. Svensson LG, Crawford ES, Hess KR, Coselli JS, Safi HJ. Variables predictive of outcome in 832 patients undergoing repairs of the descending thoracic aorta. Chest 1993; 104(4):1248–1253.

107. Svensson LG, Crawford ES, Hess KR, Coselli JS, Safi HJ. Experience with 1509 patients undergoing thoracoabdominal aortic operations. J Vasc Surg 1993; 17(2):357–368.

108. Rodriguez A, Chiascone R, Clemens J. Blunt traumatic rupture of the aorta. In: Maull KI, Rodriguez A, Wiles CE III, eds. Complications in Trauma and Critical Care. Philadelphia: W.B. Saunders, 1996:289–305.

109. Safi HJ, Bartoli S, Hess KR, et al. Neurologic deficit in patients at high risk with thoracoabdominal aortic aneurysms: the role of cerebral spinal fluid drainage and distal aortic perfusion. J Vasc Surg 1994; 20(3):434–444.

110. Koudsi B, Yu CD, Ferguson EW Jr., et al. Prevention of spinal cord injury after transient aortic clamping with tissue factor pathway inhibitor. Surgery 1996; 119(3):269–274.

111. Svensson L. Commentary on De Haan and colleagues: efficacy of transcranial motor evoked myogenic potentials to detect spinal cord ischemia during operations for thoracoabdominal aneurysms. J Thorac Cardiovasc Surg 1997; 113:100–101.

112. Vander Salm TJ, Cutler BS, Okike ON. Brachial plexus injury following median sternotomy. Part II. J Thorac Cardiovasc Surg 1982; 83(6):914–917.

113. Morin JE, Long R, Elleker MG, Eisen AA, Wynands E, Ralphs-Thibodeau S. Upper extremity neuropathies following median sternotomy. Ann Thorac Surg 1982; 34(2):181–185.

114. Baisden CE, Greenwald LV, Symbas PN. Occult rib fractures and brachial plexus injury following median sternotomy for open-heart operations. Ann Thorac Surg 1984; 38(3):192–194.

115. Esposito RA, Spencer FC. The effect of pericardial insulation on hypothermic phrenic nerve injury during open-heart surgery. Ann Thorac Surg 1987; 43(3):303–308.

116. Carter Y, Meissner M, Bulger E, et al. Anatomical considerations in the surgical management of blunt thoracic aortic injury. J Vasc Surg 2001; 34:628–633.

117. Chai PJ, Williamson JA, Lodge AJ, et al. Effects of ischemia on pulmonary dysfunction after cardiopulmonary bypass. Ann Thorac Surg 1999; 67(3):731–735.

118. Kollef MH, Wragge T, Pasque C. Determinants of mortality and multiorgan dysfunction in cardiac surgery patients requiring prolonged mechanical ventilation. Chest 1995; 107(5):1395–1401.

119. Weinstein GS, Rao PS, Vretakis G, Tyras DH. Serial changes in renal function in cardiac surgical patients. Ann Thorac Surg 1989; 48(1):72–76.

120. Miedzinski LJ, Keren G. Serious infectious complications of open-heart surgery. Can J Surg 1987; 30(2):103–107.

121. Halm MA. Acute gastrointestinal complications after cardiac surgery. Am J Crit Care 1996; 5(2):109–118.

122. Zacharias A, Schwann TA, Parenteau GL, et al. Predictors of gastrointestinal complications in cardiac surgery. Tex Heart Inst J 2000; 27(2):93–99.

123. Perugini RA, Orr RK, Porter D, Dumas EM, Maini BS. Gastrointestinal complications following cardiac surgery. An analysis of 1477 cardiac surgery patients. Arch Surg 1997; 132(4):352–357.

124. Marggraf G, Splittgerber FH, Knox M, Reidemeister JC. Mediastinitis after cardiac surgery—epidemiology and current treatment. Eur J Surg Suppl 1999; 584:12–16.

125. Newman LS, Szczukowski LC, Bain RP, Perlino CA. Suppurative mediastinitis after open heart surgery. A case control study of risk factors. Chest 1988; 94(3):546–553.

126. Grossi EA, Culliford AT, Krieger KH, et al. A survey of 77 major infectious complications of median

sternotomy: a review of 7,949 consecutive operative procedures. Ann Thorac Surg 1985; 40(3):214–223.

127. Spencer FC, Grossi EA. Mediastinitis after cardiac operations. Ann Thorac Surg 1990; 49(3):506–507.

128. Cuschieri J, Kralovich KA, Patton JH, Horst HM, Obeid FN, Karmy-Jones R. Anterior mediastinal abscess after closed sternal fracture. J Trauma 1999; 47(3):551–554.

129. Nelson RM, Dries DJ. The economic implications of infection in cardiac surgery. Ann Thorac Surg 1986; 42(3):240–246.

130. Berg HF, Brands WG, van Geldorp TR, Kluytmans-VandenBergh FQ, Kluytmans JA. Comparison between closed drainage techniques for the treatment of postoperative mediastinitis. Ann Thorac Surg 2000; 70(3):924–929.

131. Rand RP, Cochran RP, Aziz S, et al. Prospective trial of catheter irrigation and muscle flaps for sternal wound infection. Ann Thorac Surg 1998; 65(4):1046–1049.

132. Levi N, Olsen PS. Primary closure of deep sternal wound infection following open heart surgery: a safe operation? J Cardiovasc Surg (Torino) 2000; 41(2): 241–245.

133. Mullen JC, Bentley MJ, Mong K, et al. Reduction of leg wound infections following coronary artery bypass surgery. Can J Cardiol 1999; 15(1):65–68.

134. Utley JR, Thomason ME, Wallace DJ, et al. Preoperative correlates of impaired wound healing after saphenous vein excision. J Thorac Cardiovasc Surg 1989; 98(1):147–149.

135. DeLaria GA, Hunter JA, Goldin MD, Serry C, Javid H, Najafi H. Leg wound complications associated with coronary revascularization. J Thorac Cardiovasc Surg 1981; 81(3):403–407.

136. Cowgill LD, Addonizio VP, Hopeman AR, Harken AH. A practical approach to prosthetic valve endocarditis. Ann Thorac Surg 1987; 43(4):450–457.

137. Sweeney MS, Reul GJ Jr., Cooley DA, et al. Comparison of bioprosthetic and mechanical valve replacement for active endocarditis. J Thorac Cardiovasc Surg 1985; 90(5):676–680.

138. Gordon SM, Serkey JM, Longworth DL, Lytle BW, Cosgrove DM III. Early onset prosthetic valve endocarditis: the Cleveland Clinic experience 1992–1997. Ann Thorac Surg 2000; 69(5):1388–1392.

139. Joyce F, Tingleff J, Aagaard J, Pettersson G. The Ross operation in the treatment of native and prosthetic aortic valve endocarditis. J Heart Valve Dis 1994; 3(4):371–376.

140. Santini F, Bertolini P, Vecchi B, Borghetti V, Mazzucco A. Results of Biocor stentless valve replacement for infective endocarditis of the native aortic valve. Am J Cardiol 1998; 82(9):1136–1137, A10.

141. Bojar R. Valvular heart disease, including hypertrophic cardiomyopathy. In: Bojar RM, ed. Adult Cardiac Surgery. Oxford: Blackwell Scientific, 1992: 155–240.

142. Kirklin JK, Pacifico AD, Kirklin JW. Surgical treatment of prosthetic valve endocarditis with homograft aortic valve replacement. J Card Surg 1989; 4(4):340–347.

143. Croce MA, Fabian TC, Schurr MJ, et al. Using bronchoalveolar lavage to distinguish nosocomial pneumonia from systemic inflammatory response syndrome: a prospective analysis. J Trauma 1995; 39(6):1134–1139.

144. Wisman C, Waldhausen J. Aortic valve surgery. In: Waldhausen J, Orringer M, eds. Complications in Cardiothoracic Surgery. St. Louis: Mosby Year Book, 1991:237–247.

145. Orszulak TA, Schaff HV, Danielson GK, Pluth JR, Puga FJ, Piehler JM. Results of reoperation for periprosthetic leakage. Ann Thorac Surg 1983; 35(6):584–589.

146. Secomb J, Schaff H. Mitral valve repair: current techniques and indications. In: Franco KL, Verrier ED, eds. Advanced Therapy in Cardiac Surgery. Hamilton: B.C. Decker, 1999:220–231.

147. David TE, Armstrong S, Sun Z. Left ventricular function after mitral valve surgery. J Heart Valve Dis 1995; 4(suppl 2):S175–S180.

148. Karlson KJ, Ashraf MM, Berger RL. Rupture of left ventricle following mitral valve replacement. Ann Thorac Surg 1988; 46(5):590–597.

149. Katske G, Golding LR, Tubbs RR, Loop FD. Posterior midventricular rupture after mitral valve replacement. Ann Thorac Surg 1979; 27(2):130–132.

150. Roberts WC, Isner JM, Virmani R. Left ventricular incision midway between the mitral annulus and the stumps of the papillary muscles during mitral valve excision with or without rupture or aneurysmal formation: analysis of 10 necropsy patients. Am Heart J 1982; 104(6):1278–1287.

151. David TE. Left ventricular rupture after mitral valve replacement: endocardial repair with pericardial patch. J Thorac Cardiovasc Surg 1987; 93(6):935–936.

152. Lee KS, Stewart WJ, Savage RM, Loop FD, Cosgrove DM III. Systolic anterior motion of mitral valve after the posterior leaflet sliding advancement procedure. Ann Thorac Surg 1994; 57(5):1338–1340.

153. Ben-Ismail M, Curran Y, Bousnina A. Long-term results of tricuspid prostheses. Arch Mal Coeur Vaiss 1981; 74(9):1035–1044.

154. Pate JW, Fabian TC, Walker W. Traumatic rupture of the aortic isthmus: an emergency? World J Surg 1995; 19(1):119–125.

155. Fabian TC, Richardson JD, Croce MA, et al. Prospective study of blunt aortic injury: Multicenter Trial of the American Association for the Surgery of Trauma. J Trauma 1997; 42(3):374–380.

156. Fabian TC, Davis KA, Gavant ML, et al. Prospective study of blunt aortic injury: helical CT is diagnostic and antihypertensive therapy reduces rupture. Ann Surg 1998; 227(5):666–676.

157. Karmy-Jones R, Carter YM, Nathens A, et al. Impact of presenting physiology and associated injuries on outcome following traumatic rupture of the thoracic aorta. Am Surg 2001; 67(1):61–66.

158. Camp PC, Shackford SR. Outcome after blunt traumatic thoracic aortic laceration: identification of a high-risk cohort. Western Trauma Association Multicenter Study Group. J Trauma 1997; 43(3):413–422.

159. von Oppell UO, Dunne TT, De Groot MK, Zilla P. Traumatic aortic rupture: twenty-year metaanalysis of mortality and risk of paraplegia. Ann Thorac Surg 1994; 58(2):585–593.

160. Wahl WL, Michaels AJ, Wang SC, Dries DJ, Taheri PA. Blunt thoracic aortic injury: delayed or early repair? J Trauma 1999; 47(2):254–259.

161. Pate JW, Gavant ML, Weiman DS, Fabian TC. Traumatic rupture of the aortic isthmus: program of selective management. World J Surg 1999; 23(1):59–63.

162. Soots G, Warembourg H Jr., Prat A, Roux JP. Acute traumatic rupture of the thoracic aorta: place of delayed surgical repair. J Cardiovasc Surg (Torino) 1989; 30(2):173–177.

163. Blegvad S, Lippert H, Lund O, Hansen OK, Christensen T. Acute or delayed surgical treatment of traumatic rupture of the descending aorta. J Cardiovasc Surg (Torino) 1989; 30(4):559–564.

164. Finkelmeier BA, Mentzer RM Jr., Kaiser DL, Tegtmeyer CJ, Nolan SP. Chronic traumatic thoracic aneurysm. Influence of operative treatment on natural history: an analysis of reported cases, 1950–1980. J Thorac Cardiovasc Surg 1982; 84(2):257–266.

165. Holmes JH IV, Bloch RD, Hall RA, Carter YM, Karmy-Jones RC. Natural history of traumatic rupture of the thoracic aorta managed nonoperatively: a longitudinal analysis. Ann Thorac Surg 2002; 73:1149–1154.

166. Fujikawa T, Yukioka T, Ishimaru S, et al. Endovascular stent grafting for the treatment of blunt thoracic aortic injury. J Trauma 2001; 50(2):223–229.

167. Bruninx G, Wery D, Dubois E, et al. Emergency endovascular treatment of an acute traumatic rupture of the thoracic aorta complicated by a distal low-flow syndrome. Cardiovasc Intervent Radiol 1999; 22(6): 515–518.

168. Borsa JJ, Hoffer EK, Karmy-Jones R, et al. Angiographic description of blunt traumatic injuries to the thoracic aorta with specific reference to endograft repair. J Endovasc Surg 2002:9(S2):II84–II91.

169. Cowley RA, Turney SZ, Hankins JR, Rodriguez A, Attar S, Shankar BS. Rupture of thoracic aorta caused by blunt trauma. A fifteen-year experience. J Thorac Cardiovasc Surg 1990; 100(5):652–660.

170. Clark DE, Zeiger MA, Wallace KL, Packard AB, Nowicki ER. Blunt aortic trauma: signs of high risk. J Trauma 1990; 30(6):701–705.

171. Zeiger MA, Clark DE, Morton JR. Reappraisal of surgical treatment of traumatic transection of the thoracic aorta. J Cardiovasc Surg (Torino) 1990; 31(5):607–610.

172. Mattox KL, Holzman M, Pickard LR, Beall AC Jr., DeBakey ME. Clamp/repair: a safe technique for treatment of blunt injury to the descending thoracic aorta. Ann Thorac Surg 1985; 40(5):456–463.

173. Stothert JC Jr., McBride L, Tidik S, Lewis L, Codd JE. Multiple aortic tears treated by primary suture repair. J Trauma 1987; 27(8):955–956.

174. McBride LR, Tidik S, Stothert JC, et al. Primary repair of traumatic aortic disruption. Ann Thorac Surg 1987; 43(1):65–67.

175. Schmidt CA, Jacobson JG. Thoracic aortic injury. A ten-year experience. Arch Surg 1984; 119(11):1244–1246.

176. Wall MJ Jr., Mattox KL, Chen CD, Baldwin JC. Acute management of complex cardiac injuries. J Trauma 1997; 42(5):905–912.

177. End A, Rodler S, Oturanlar D, et al. Elective surgery for blunt cardiac trauma. J Trauma 1994; 37(5): 798–802.

178. End A, Rodler S, Oturanlar D, et al. Surgery of blunt heart trauma. Chirurg 1992; 63(8):641–646.

179. Ivatury R, Simon R, Rohman M. Cardiac injuries and resuscitative thoracotomy. In: Maull KI, Rodriguez A, Wiles CE III, eds. Complications in Trauma and Critical Care. Philadelphia: W.B. Saunders, 1996:279–288.

180. Knott-Craig CJ, Dalton RP, Rossouw GJ, Barnard PM. Penetrating cardiac trauma: management strategy based on 129 surgical emergencies over 2 years. Ann Thorac Surg 1992; 53(6):1006–1009.

181. Bolton JW, Bynoe RP, Lazar HL, Almond CH. Two-dimensional echocardiography in the evaluation of penetrating intrapericardial injuries. Ann Thorac Surg 1993; 56(3):506–509.

182. Callaham M. Pericardiocentesis in traumatic and nontraumatic cardiac tamponade. Ann Emerg Med 1984; 13(10):924–945.

183. Mitchell ME, Muakkassa FF, Poole GV, Rhodes RS, Griswold JA. Surgical approach of choice for penetrating cardiac wounds. J Trauma 1993; 34(1):17–20.

184. Pate JW, Cole FH Jr., Walker WA, Fabian TC. Penetrating injuries of the aortic arch and its branches. Ann Thorac Surg 1993; 55(3):586–592.

185. Shamoun JM, Barraza KR, Jurkovich GJ, Salley RK. In extremis use of staples for cardiorrhaphy in penetrating cardiac trauma: case report. J Trauma 1989; 29(11):1589–1591.

186. Bowman MR, King RM. Comparison of staples and sutures for cardiorrhaphy in traumatic puncture wounds of the heart. J Emerg Med 1996; 14(5):615–618.

187. Mayrose J, Jehle DV, Moscati R, Lerner EB, Abrams BJ. Comparison of staples versus sutures in the repair of penetrating cardiac wounds. J Trauma 1999; 46(3):441–443.

188. Macho JR, Markison RE, Schecter WP. Cardiac stapling in the management of penetrating injuries of the heart: rapid control of hemorrhage and decreased risk of personal contamination. J Trauma 1993; 34(5):711–715.

189. Pretre R, Bednarkiewicz M, Faidutti B. Blunt cardiac injury: in achieving a practical diagnostic classification. J Trauma 1994; 36(3):462–463.

190. Biffl WL, Moore FA, Moore EE, Sauaia A, Read RA, Burch JM. Cardiac enzymes are irrelevant in the patient with suspected myocardial contusion. Am J Surg 1994; 168(6):523–527.

191. Okubo N, Hombrouck C, Fornes P, et al. Cardiac troponin I and myocardial contusion in the rabbit. Anesthesiology 2000; 93(3):811–817.

192. Ferjani M, Droc G, Dreux S, et al. Circulating cardiac troponin T in myocardial contusion. Chest 1997; 111(2):427–433.

193. Swaanenburg JC, Klaase JM, DeJongste MJ, Zimmerman KW, ten Duis HJ. Troponin I, troponin T, CKMB-activity and CKMB-mass as markers for the detection of myocardial contusion in patients who experienced blunt trauma. Clin Chim Acta 1998; 272(2):171–181.

194. Helm M, Hauke J, Weiss A, Lampl L. Cardiac troponin T as a biochemical marker of myocardial injury early after trauma. Diagnostic value of a qualitative bedside test. Chirurg 1999; 70(11):1347–1352.

195. Pretre R, Chilcott M. Blunt trauma to the heart and great vessels. N Engl J Med 1997; 336(9):626–632.

196. Flancbaum L, Wright J, Siegel JH. Emergency surgery in patients with post-traumatic myocardial contusion. J Trauma 1986; 26(9):795–803.

197. Wall MJ Jr., Soltero E. Damage control for thoracic injuries. Surg Clin North Am 1997; 77(4):863–878.

198. Pretre R, Kursteiner K, Khatchatourian G, Faidutti B. Traumatic occlusion of the left anterior descending artery and rupture of the aortic isthmus. J Trauma 1995; 39(2):388–390.

199. Bokelman TA, Rahko PS, Meany BT, Fausch MD. Traumatic occlusion of the right coronary artery resulting in cardiogenic shock successfully treated with primary angioplasty. Am Heart J 1996; 131(2):411–413.

200. Candell J, Valle V, Paya J, Cortadellas J, Esplugas E, Rius J. Post-traumatic coronary occlusion and early left ventricular aneurysm. Am Heart J 1979; 97(4): 509–512.

201. Cizmarova E, Simkovic I, Zelenay J, Masura J. Post-traumatic coronary occlusion and its consequences in a young child. Pediatr Cardiol 1988; 9(2):117–120.

202. Pretre R, Faidutti B. Aortic valve rupture in closed trauma: the extent of the damage. J Thorac Cardiovasc Surg 1993; 106(2):371–373.

203. Pretre R, Faidutti B. Surgical management of aortic valve injury after nonpenetrating trauma. Ann Thorac Surg 1993; 56(6):1426–1431.

204. Lowe JE, Adams DH, Cummings RG, Wesly RL, Phillips HR. The natural history and recommended management of patients with traumatic coronary artery fistulas. Ann Thorac Surg 1983; 36(3):295–305.

205. Pretre R, LaHarpe R, Cheretakis A, et al. Blunt injury to the ascending aorta: three patterns of presentation. Surgery 1996; 119(6):603–610.

206. Soloff L, Zatuchini J, Janton OH, O'Neill TJ, Blover RP. Reactivation of rheumatic fever following mitral commissurotomy. Circulation 1953; 8:481–497.

207. Engle MA, Gay WA Jr., McCabe J, et al. Postpericardiotomy syndrome in adults: incidence, autoimmunity and virology. Circulation 1981; 64(2 Pt 2): II58–II60.

208. Engle MA, Zabriskie JB, Senterfit LB, Gay WA, O'Loughlin JE Jr., Ehlers KH. Viral illness and the postpericardiotomy syndrome. A prospective study in children. Circulation 1980; 62(6):1151–1158.

209. Symbas P. Traumatic injury of the pericardium. In: Symbas PN, ed. Cardiothoracic Trauma. Philadelphia: WB Saunders, 1989:77–88.

210. McCabe JC, Ebert PA, Engle MA, Zabriskie JB. Circulating heart-reactive antibodies in the postpericardiotomy syndrome. J Surg Res 1973; 14(2): 158–164.

211. Ehrenhaft JL, Taber RE. Hemopericardium and constrictive pericarditis. J Thorac Surg 1952; 24:355–368.

212. Dressler W. A post-myocardial infraction syndrome: preliminary report of a complication resembling idiopathic, recurrent, benign pericarditis. JAMA 1956; 160:1379–1383.

213. Wiegand L, Zwillich CW. The post-cardiac injury syndrome following blunt chest trauma: case report. J Trauma 1993; 34:445–447.

214. Solomon D. Delayed cardiac tamponade after blunt chest trauma: case report. J Trauma 1991; 31:1322–1324.

215. Chong HH, Plotnick GD. Pericardial effusion and tamponade: evaluation, imaging modalities, and management. Compr Ther 1995; (21):378–385.

216. Plotnick GD, Rubin DC, Feliciano Z, Ziskind AA. Pulmonary hypertension decreases the predictive accuracy of echocardiographic clues for cardiac tamponade. Chest 1995; 107:919–924.

217. Bellanger D, Nikas DJ, Freeman JE, Izenberg S. Delayed posttraumatic tamponade. South Med J 1996; 89: 1197–1199.

218. Morgan RJ, Stephenson LW, Woolf PK, Edie RN, Edmunds LH Jr. Surgical treatment of purulent pericarditis in children. J Thorac Cardiovasc Surg 1983; 85(4):527–531.

219. Sato TT, Geary RL, Ashbaugh DG, Jurkovich GJ. Diagnosis and management of pericardial abscess in trauma patients. Am J Surg 1993; 165(5):637–641.

28

Complications of Cardiac Transplantation

Xiao-Shi Qi, Louis B. Louis IV, and Si M. Pham
Division of Cardiothoracic Surgery, DeWitt Daughtry Family Department of Surgery,
University of Miami Miller School of Medicine, Jackson Memorial Hospital,
Miami, Florida, U.S.A.

Cardiac transplantation has become an accepted treatment for patients with an end-stage cardiac disease. Advances during the last five decades have markedly improved the survival rates of cardiac transplant recipients. Currently, the one-year survival rate after cardiac transplantation is approaching 90%, with a subsequent mortality rate of 4% per year (1). Besides the shortage of donors, other important limitations of cardiac transplantation include toxic effects related to the use of nonspecific immunosuppression and allograft vasculopathy (transplant coronary artery disease). This chapter will address the common complications associated with cardiac transplantation.

INDICATIONS FOR CARDIAC TRANSPLANTATION

In general, cardiac transplantation is indicated in patients with an end-stage heart disease that is refractory to medical therapy and not amenable to other surgical treatments (2). The indications and contraindications for cardiac transplantation have evolved over the last four decades and the generally accepted criteria are listed in the Table 1. In recent years, improvement in survival rates has widened the criteria used to select patients for cardiac transplantation. Some centers have increased the upper limit of the recipient's age to 70 years (3,4). Irreversible hepatic or renal dysfunction is no longer considered an absolute contraindication because reasonable survival rates have been achieved by cardiac transplantation combined with either renal (5,6) or hepatic (7–9) transplantation.

OPERATIVE TECHNIQUES
Orthotopic Cardiac Transplantation

Shumway et al. (10) described the classic technique of orthotopic cardiac transplantation using biatrial anastomoses. Briefly, the right atrium of the donor heart is opened posterolaterally, beginning at the junction between the inferior vena cava and the right atrium

and extending to the right-atrial appendage. The donor heart is implanted by sequentially anastomosing the left atrium, the right atrium, the pulmonary artery, and the aorta of the donor heart to the recipient vessels. Recently, more and more surgeons are using the modified technique of bicaval anastomosis; when this procedure is used, the superior vena cava and the inferior vena cava are anastomosed separately. Bicaval anastomosis allows complete excision of the diseased right atrium and is associated with a lower incidence of postoperative sinus node dysfunction and tricuspid regurgitation (11,12). The bicaval technique has been further modified to include separate pulmonary venous anastomoses (13): small left-atrial cuffs from the recipient, which contain the superior and inferior pulmonary veins, are anastomosed to either side of the posterior wall of the donor left atrium to create an almost normal anatomic configuration and to allow synchronous functioning of the atria. This technique is believed to reduce the incidence of atrial arrhythmias and atrioventricular conduction disturbances. However, because of the lack of convincing evidence showing the superiority of this technique and the increased ischemic time it requires, bicaval anastomosis in combination with pulmonary venous anastomosis has not been widely used.

Heterotopic Cardiac Transplantation

Heterotopic cardiac transplantation is indicated when an irreversible increase in pulmonary vascular resistance occurs or when there is a gross mismatch between the weights of the donor and the recipient (14–18). The inferior vena cava and the right pulmonary veins are ligated. The donor left atrium is anastomosed to the recipient's at the interatrial groove; next, the donor superior vena cava is anastomosed to the recipient's right atrium. The donor aorta and pulmonary artery are then connected to those of the recipient in an end-to-side fashion. A short prosthetic graft or aortic homograft is generally used to connect the pulmonary arteries. Compared with orthotopic cardiac

Table 1 Indications and Contraindications for Cardiac Transplantation

Indications
  Severe heart disease (class III–IV symptoms) with limited life expectancy
    and poor responsiveness to medical management
  Age less than approximately 65 yr
  Absence of other life-threatening diseases with limited survival
  Compliance with medical advice
  Psychosocial stability and a supportive social milieu
Potential contraindications
  Significant peripheral vascular or cerebrovascular disease
  Severe pulmonary hypertension
  Active peptic ulcer disease
  Coexisting systemic illness that may limit life expectancy or compromise
    recovery from cardiac transplantation
  Preexisting malignancy
  Moderate or severe chronic obstructive pulmonary disease
  Advanced age (>65 yr)
  Insulin-requiring diabetes mellitus with end-organ complications
  Current or recent diverticulitis
  Active infection
  Recent or unresolved pulmonary infarction
  Cachexia
  Severe osteoporosis
  Psychosocial instability and lack of adequate support systems
  Active substance abuse

transplantation, heterotopic cardiac transplantation is more technically complex, requires a longer ischemic time, and is associated with a greater potential for thrombus formation in the dilated, poorly functioning native heart and with a higher incidence of mitral regurgitation in the donor heart. The procedure is contraindicated for recipients with right-sided heart failure and tricuspid insufficiency.

INTRAOPERATIVE COMPLICATIONS
Immediate Primary Graft Failure

Immediate primary graft failure accounts for approximately 5% of the deaths that occur immediately after cardiac transplantation. Aside from technical errors (which are rare) such as inadvertent occlusion of the coronary arteries or veins with sutures, the main cause of primary graft failure is ischemia-reperfusion injury. The current myocardial preservation technique, which involves hypothermic cardiac arrest (with various cardioplegic solutions) and static hypothermic storage, yields an acceptable total ischemic time of approximately five to six hours. An ischemic time of more than five hours is associated with poor survival rates (19). Primary graft failure is more likely to occur when donors are older than 45 years or have left-ventricular hypertrophy, when ischemic time exceeds five hours, or when the donor-to-recipient weight ratio is less than 0.7 (20,21).

Hyperacute Rejection

Hyperacute rejection occurs within minutes to hours after transplantation and results when preformed antibodies in the recipient are directed against donor human leukocyte antigens (HLAs). Hyperacute rejection may also occur when the donor and recipient blood groups are incompatible (22,23) or when antibodies against donor tissue antigens are present on the vascular endothelial cells (24). When this complication occurs, the graft looks hemorrhagic and edematous, with minimal ventricular contractility, shortly after being reperfused. The patient usually shows signs of disseminated intravascular coagulation. To date, because there is no effective treatment for hyperacute rejection, prevention of the complication is emphasized. Before transplantation, each candidate is tested for the presence of preformed antibodies against a T-lymphocyte panel that represents most HLAs [panel-reactive antibodies (PRA)]. When test results show that the recipient reacts to more than 10% of the T-lymphocytes on the panel (PRA > 10%), most transplant centers prospectively crossmatch donor lymphocytes with recipient serum before transplantation. Because of the dire consequences of hyperacute rejection, positive results from leukocyte crossmatching are generally considered a contraindication to heart transplantation, even though these results are not an accurate predictor of hyperacute rejection (24,25).

EARLY POSTOPERATIVE COMPLICATIONS

In the early postoperative period, recipients of heart transplants are given treatment similar to that given to any patient recovering from cardiac surgery, except for some specific treatment for problems related to the use of immunosuppressive agents. Recipients should be weaned from mechanical ventilatory support and inotropic drugs as quickly as possible. Early mobilization and physical therapy are essential.

Mediastinal Hemorrhage

The management of hemorrhage in heart transplant recipients is similar to the management of this complication in any patient who has undergone open-heart surgery and cardiopulmonary bypass. After cardiopulmonary bypass, approximately 10% to 20% of patients require transfusion of blood components; fewer than 3% require reexploration. Problems such as inadequate heparin reversal, heparin rebound, hypothermia, quantitative or qualitative platelet defects, depletion of coagulation factors, and fibrinolysis should be addressed. Mediastinal exploration will be necessary when bleeding occurs at a rate of 500 cc/hr for one hour, 400 cc/hr for two hours, or 300 cc/hr for three hours, or when there is evidence of cardiac tamponade (26). The importance of early reexploration for mediastinal bleeding cannot be overstated because the morbidity and mortality rates associated with early reexploration are lower than those associated with delayed reexploration (27,28).

Ventricular Dysfunction

Because of reperfusion injury, the function of the transplanted heart is usually depressed in the immediate postoperative period. During the first four to five days after transplantation, the normal inverse relationship between heart rate and stroke volume is not seen (29). Stroke volume remains fixed because of a restrictive hemodynamic pattern. Recipients of cardiac transplants usually require chronotropic support for the first several days after transplantation because of sinoatrial node dysfunction (30). Isoproterenol or dobutamine is commonly used in the immediate posttransplant period to increase inotropy and chronotropy, reduce pulmonary vascular resistance, and improve ventricular diastolic relaxation. Aminophylline also improves heart rate in cardiac transplant recipients (31). Severe pulmonary hypertension may require the concomitant use of inotropic agents and pulmonary vasodilators such as milrinone, nitroglycerine, or inhaled nitric oxide (32–34). Cardiac function and sinoatrial node activity will usually return to normal within seven days. Because the transplanted heart is completely denervated, circulating catecholamines are responsible for the increased chronotropic and inotropic responses to exercise (35,36).

Right-Ventricular Failure

Right-ventricular failure is a frequent cause of early morbidity and mortality after cardiac transplantation. This complication usually results from ischemia-reperfusion injury or from high pulmonary vascular resistance. In recipients with elevated pulmonary vascular pressures, the normal donor right ventricle may be unable to meet the sudden demand of a high afterload. Long ischemic time and a donor-to-recipient size discrepancy (donor body weight lower than recipient body weight) exacerbate this problem. The goal of medical therapy is to increase right-ventricular inotropy, with drugs such as type III phosphodiesterase inhibitors (milrinone, amrinone), isoproterenol, and dobutamine, and to reduce pulmonary vascular resistance, with drugs such as nitroglycerin, prostacyclin, and inhaled nitric oxide. In cases of severe right-heart failure, ventricular-assist device or extracorporeal membrane oxygenation support is needed.

Left-Ventricular Failure

Left-ventricular failure is a rare complication that usually occurs because of prolonged ischemic time and poor myocardial preservation. Occasionally, preexisting coronary artery disease or embolization of air or particulate matter to the coronary arteries may cause ventricular failure. As is true for right-ventricular failure, left-ventricular failure should be treated by increasing ventricular inotropy and reducing ventricular afterload by medical or mechanical means (e.g., intraaortic counterpulsation). For severe cases (approximately 5% of all cases), a ventricular-assist device should be used.

Electrophysiologic Dysfunction

Arrhythmia is common during the early postoperative period and occurs in as many as 70% of patients receiving cardiac transplants (37). Sinus bradycardia, junctional rhythm, and junctional escape rhythms are the most common arrhythmias. These conditions are usually due to injury to the sinus node during surgery but may also herald the onset of acute rejection. Chronic use of beta-blockers and amiodarone before transplantation are associated with prolonged sinus bradycardia, whereas the administration of aminophylline accelerates recovery from sinus bradycardia (31,38). The bicaval technique is reportedly associated with a lower incidence of atrial arrhythmias and sinus node dysfunction than the biatrial approach (39,40). Normal sinus node activity usually returns several weeks after transplantation; therefore, implantation of a permanent pacemaker should be delayed for at least four weeks and after an adequate trial of aminophylline (41,42).

Permanent perioperative right-bundle branch block occurs frequently after cardiac transplantation. However, premature atrial contractions, atrial flutter, and atrial fibrillation usually herald the onset of acute rejection. Premature ventricular contractions occur in more than half of patients during the early posttransplant period and are less frequently associated with acute rejection. However, complex ventricular ectopy can be associated with chronic allograft vasculopathy and is a risk factor for sudden death (30,43).

Because the transplanted heart is denervated, it will not respond to cardiac drugs in the same way the normal heart does. Therefore, it is important to understand the effects of cardiac drugs on the transplanted heart before therapeutic intervention is considered. The following general rules (44) should be observed: (i) the transplanted heart is not affected by drugs that act via the autonomic nervous system; (ii) cardiac receptors on the transplanted heart are more responsive to beta-agonists than those on the native heart; and (iii) drugs with negative inotropic or chronotropic effects are not well tolerated by heart transplant recipients because these effects may not be offset by the autonomically mediated increase in myocardial contractility and sympathetic tones (30,45).

Digoxin exerts its electrophysiologic effect primarily on the autonomically mediated function of sinoatrial and atrioventricular nodes, and therefore this drug has very little therapeutic value in treating supraventricular tachycardia or atrial fibrillation in the denervated transplanted heart. Similarly, atropine, edrophonium, and vagal maneuvers will have no effect on the transplanted heart. Because of their direct electrophysiologic effects, quinidine and procainamide are effective treatments for atrial and ventricular arrhythmias in transplant recipients. The transplanted heart is especially sensitive to adenosine; therefore, this drug must be used carefully and at low doses (one-fifth to one-third the usual dose), if at all (46). Aminophylline can correct sinus bradycardia in transplant recipients by blocking extracellular A1 adenosine receptors and has been used to reverse rejection-induced bradycardia or to treat the bradycardia that may occur in the immediate postoperative period (31,38).

Acute Renal Failure

Cardiac transplant recipients are quite susceptible to acute renal failure. The high incidence of this complication after heart transplantation results from low renal reserve because of hypertension and prolonged congestive heart failure, the nonpulsatile flow produced by cardiopulmonary bypass during transplantation, and toxicity associated with immunosuppressive agents. Nephrotoxicity is one of the common side effects of calcineurin inhibitors (e.g., cyclosporine and tacrolimus) (47) and has both acute and chronic components.

The acute component is the primary cause of acute renal failure in the early postoperative period. Measures that can prevent this toxicity include infusion of a low dose (a renal dose) of dopamine, intravenous infusion of furosemide, hydration, and minimal use of vasoconstrictive agents (48). The incidence of acute renal failure in the early postoperative period may be reduced by using immunosuppressive agents that are not nephrotoxic (e.g., antithymocyte antibodies) and by delaying the administration of calcineurin inhibitors until adequate renal function has returned.

The chronic component of nephrotoxicity results from the long-term use of calcineurin inhibitors and is associated with a gradual increase in the serum creatinine concentration and a decrease in renal function. The severity of renal dysfunction may be reduced by administering a lower dose of cyclosporine or tacrolimus in combination with other immunosuppressive agents. Because nonsteroidal anti-inflammatory agents (e.g., ketorolac tromethamine or ibuprofen) exacerbate the nephrotoxicity of calcineurin inhibitors, heart transplant recipients should not use these agents for pain control, especially in the perioperative period when the incidence of acute renal failure is high.

Stroke

The risk of stroke for cardiac transplant recipients is similar to that of any patient undergoing cardiopulmonary bypass (approximately 2.5%). Stroke may result from low perfusion during cardiopulmonary bypass in a patient with preexisting compromised cerebral circulation (carotid or intracerebral arterial disease) or from embolization of air or particulate matter (fragments of pericardial fat or myocardial tissues, or cholesterol debris from the diseased aorta). Thrombus at the atrial suture line in the transplanted heart is a common source of emboli in the early postoperative period. To minimize thrombus at the suture line, surgeons must take care to evert the atrial

anastomosis and approximate the endocardial layers of the donor and recipient vessels.

Acute Rejection

Despite advances in immunosuppression during the past five decades, acute allograft rejection is still a serious problem after cardiac transplantation. Approximately 70% of recipients will experience an episode of moderate acute rejection (grade 3A) during their lifetime. Acute rejection is mediated by T-lymphocytes and commonly occurs during the first six months after transplantation. Moderate acute rejection may be present without evidence of hemodynamic instability or echocardiographically documented decrease in ventricular function. Therefore, recipients of heart transplants require routinely performed surveillance endomyocardial biopsy for histologic determination of rejection. The standardized grading system for cardiac rejection produces a score ranging from 0 (no rejection) to 4 (severe rejection); treatment of rejection is in part determined by this grade (49,50). Moderate acute rejection (grade 3A or higher) is treated with boluses of methylprednisolone (1 g/day for adults, and 10–20 mg/kg/day for children, for three days); for mild acute rejection, augmenting the level of baseline immunosuppression will usually suffice (grade 1B–2). Lympholytic therapy with antithymocyte globulin or antilymphocyte antibody is reserved for cases of steroid-resistant rejection.

Accelerated Acute Rejection

Accelerated acute rejection usually occurs 24 to 72 hours after transplantation and is mediated by antibodies to donor HLA. It occurs in recipients who have been sensitized to donor antigens but whose level of antidonor antibodies at the time of transplantation is too low to trigger hyperacute rejection. After transplantation, the immune system of a sensitized patient is reexposed to the sensitizing antigens from the donor, resulting in rapid production of high antibody titer to the donor (anamnestic response). The high level of donor-specific antibody will fix complement, and results in deposition of antibody and complement in the vessels of the graft, causing graft dysfunction.

Accelerated acute rejection should be suspected on the basis of clinical findings, including hemodynamic instability, worsening cardiac function, previous history of blood transfusion, or multiple pregnancies. The diagnosis is confirmed by a positive crossmatch between the donor's leukocytes and the recipient's serum (obtained after transplantation), by a rising level of antibody that is specific against donor HLAs, and by the presence of antibodies and complement in endomyocardial biopsy specimens from coronary arteries. Early recognition of this type of rejection is crucial because aggressive therapy with plasmapheresis, high-dose steroids, and antithymocyte globulin may save the graft (51,52).

INFECTIOUS COMPLICATIONS

Bacterial Infections

Infections accounted for most of the postoperative deaths that occurred in the era before cyclosporine (53). The infection rate is now lower than it was earlier, but infection still accounts for 22% of deaths during the first postoperative year (54). After cardiac transplantation, infection is most commonly caused, in decreasing order, by bacteria, viruses, fungi, and protozoans. Of 596 infections that occurred among heart transplant recipients at Stanford University between 1980 and 1989, 42% were bacterial (53). The most common site of infection is the lung; pneumonia occurs in 24% to 40% of patients. The other sites of infection are the bloodstream and the urinary tract. The introduction of cyclosporine to the immunosuppressive regimen for cardiac transplant recipients reduced bacterial and fungal infection; however, viral infection, especially cytomegalovirus (CMV), has emerged as an important cause of morbidity (55).

Viral Infections

The viral agents that commonly cause infection in heart transplant recipients include CMV, herpes simplex virus, and Epstein–Barr virus (EBV). The peak incidence of CMV infection occurs approximately six weeks after transplantation (56). Although the lung is the most common site of CMV infection, the gastrointestinal tract, the liver, and the retina may also be involved. Viral cultures demonstrate CMV infection in 80% to 90% of patients (57). Although most CMV infections are asymptomatic, 15% to 40% of infected patients may develop flu-like symptoms, enteritis, or hepatitis. CMV infection is associated with an increased risk of rejection, and this infection accelerates the development of allograft coronary artery disease (58). Because CMV may be transmitted via the graft, both donor and recipient must be screened for the presence of CMV antibodies. CMV disease is usually mild in a recipient who was seropositive for CMV before transplantation (reactivated CMV infection). However, primary CMV infection, which occurs when a seronegative recipient receives an organ or blood products that are CMV-positive, is quite serious. Therefore, when a seropositive donor heart is implanted into a seronegative recipient, prophylaxis with intravenously administered ganciclovir is recommended (58–60). In addition, if a blood transfusion is required, CMV-negative blood should be used.

The herpes simplex virus is shed postoperatively by half of all transplant recipients. Of these patients, half will experience clinical stomatitis, esophagitis, or genital lesions (54). Most cases of herpes simplex infection occur within the first two to three weeks after transplantation and are treated with orally administered acyclovir. Clinically significant herpetic infections are less common because of prophylactic antiviral regimens. Herpes zoster infection (shingles) occurs in approximately 10% of heart transplant patients and usually follows an uncomplicated course; it should be treated with antiviral therapy to prevent dissemination. However, varicella (chicken pox) is serious and may be fatal; therefore, aggressive antiviral therapy is indicated immediately upon diagnosis. Immunization of seronegative candidates is recommended before transplantation.

Infection with the EBV is common among transplant recipients. EBV infection is associated with the development of posttransplant lymphoproliferative disease (PTLD), and an EBV-seronegative patient receiving a seropositive graft is at substantial risk of PTLD (61).

Other Infections

Pneumocystis carinii pneumonia occurs in 3% to 10% of all cardiac transplant recipients who are not given prophylactic treatment. This infection usually occurs between the 2 and 12 month after transplantation. The common findings are fever, dyspnea, nonproductive cough, and the classic pattern of diffuse interstitial and alveolar infiltrates on chest radiographs. Seventy-five percent of cases will respond to trimethoprim–sulfamethoxazole or pentamidine. Prophylaxis with oral trimethoprim–sulfamethoxazole has markedly decreased the incidence of this infection among transplant recipients (62,63).

Toxoplasma gondii infection is of particular importance for cardiac transplant recipients because this organism often targets the myocardium. This organism is usually transmitted from the donor; therefore, serologic testing should be performed on both the donor and the recipient before the transplant procedure (64). The toxoplasma antibody titers of seronegative recipients who receive a seropositive heart should be carefully checked, and these patients should receive prophylaxis with pyrimethamine and folic acid (65). Acute infection is accompanied by serologic conversion or an increase in antibody titer; however, not all patients will exhibit symptoms. The isolation of tachyzoites from tissue or body fluids is required for diagnosis (65). Autopsy evidence of toxoplasmosis has been found in the heart, lungs, pericardium, and brain of transplant recipients with primary infections (66).

POSTTRANSPLANTATION MALIGNANCY

Chronic immunosuppression is associated with a 100-fold increase in the risk of malignancy (67). In the era before cyclosporine, Krikorian et al. (68) reported that the actuarial probability of developing any type of malignancy (solid tumors and lymphomas) was 2.7% one year after heart transplantation and 25.6% five years after transplantation (68). More recent findings show that malignancy accounts for 18.6% of deaths that occur four years after transplantation (69). After transplantation, the most commonly occurring solid tumor is skin cancer, and the most common malignancy other than solid tumor is PTLD (67,69).

STRATEGIES FOR AVOIDING COMPLICATIONS

- Primary graft failure is usually a result of ischemia-reperfusion injury. This complication is more likely when donors are older than 45 years or have left-ventricular hypertrophy, when ischemic time exceeds five hours, or when the donor-to-recipient weight ratio is less than 0.7. The incidence of primary graft failure can be reduced by closely matching donors' and recipients' weights and by minimizing ischemic time.
- Injury to the right main pulmonary artery at its junction with the main pulmonary artery may occur when the ascending aorta is dissected from the main pulmonary artery, especially in repeated operations. This complication can be avoided by delaying the dissection until after cardiopulmonary bypass has been initiated and the native heart has been removed.
- Stroke is a rare but devastating complication of heart transplantation. In addition to the usual precautions taken to prevent embolism of air and particulate matter during the operation, the endocardium should be meticulously approximated in the left-atrial suture line to avoid thrombus formation and stroke.
- A rare cause of immediate graft failure is the technical complication of catching the circumflex artery or the coronary sinus in the left-atrial suture line. This complication is rare, but requires special vigilance to avoid it, especially when the remnant of the left donor atrium is small, as in the case of concomitant lung retrieval from the same donor.
- Accelerated acute rejection usually occurs 24 to 48 hours after transplantation and results from an anamnestic response to donor antigens. This complication is heralded by increasing hemodynamic instability in a previously sensitized recipient. Plasmapheresis, aggressive immunosuppression, and inotropic or mechanical support may save the patient and the graft.
- Acute renal failure is common in the early postoperative period after heart transplantation. This condition usually responds to hydration, high doses of diuretics, and temporary discontinuation of nephrotoxic drugs. Furosemide is much more effective when administered by continuous infusion (up to 20 mg/hr) than by intermittent bolus. Nonsteroidal anti-inflammatory agents should not be used for pain control because they exacerbate the renal toxicity of calcineurin inhibitors.
- Catastrophic intra-abdominal complications may occur after heart transplantation, but because of the masking effects of immunosuppression, patients may not exhibit the usual signs and symptoms. A high index of suspicion and expedient diagnostic and therapeutic procedures will improve the outcome.

Cumulative findings convincingly suggest that PTLD is related to EBV infection. In immunosuppressed transplant recipients, EBV-infected B-cells undergo malignant transformation into polyclonal or monoclonal EBV-positive lymphomas.

The first line of treatment for these B-cell lymphomas is to reduce the level of immunosuppression (61,70). Chemotherapy, radiation therapy, and gamma-interferon therapy have also been used with limited success. The mortality rate associated with PTLD is high, ranging from 23% to 35%. New treatment strategies that have been developed in recent years have been promising. For bone marrow recipients, adoptive transfer from the donor of cytotoxic, HLA-matched T-cells that are specific for EBV shows encouraging results (71,72). For solid-organ recipients, immunotherapy with autologous lymphokine-activated killer cells has been tried with some success (73). Preliminary studies of the use of humanized anti-CD20 monoclonal antibody against B-cells (rituximab) to treat PTLD have produced promising findings, with an overall response rate of 69% and a one-year survival rate of 73% (74).

Future strategies should focus not only on treating established disease but also on preventing infection by using more specific immunosuppression, vaccination against EBV, and induction of transplantation tolerance.

CARDIAC ALLOGRAFT VASCULOPATHY

Even with the use of potent immunosuppressive agents, the recipient's immune system continues to slowly reject the transplanted organ. This chronic rejection manifests itself as an interstitial fibrosis and as a progressive and diffuse intimal thickening of the graft arteries. For heart transplant recipients, the predominant feature of chronic rejection is the development of an accelerated form of coronary artery disease, which is often called cardiac allograft vasculopathy (CAV). CAV is responsible for more than 50% of late deaths among heart transplant recipients (75). The histologic features of allograft vasculopathy include a diffuse, concentric hyperplasia of the intimal layer of small- and medium-sized arteries; this hyperplasia very rapidly progresses to complete luminal occlusion. It is generally accepted that the intimal hyperplasia is due to the migration and uncontrolled proliferation of vascular smooth muscle cells of the media layer in response to immune-mediated and nonimmune-mediated damage to the graft vessels (76). The cause of CAV is multifactorial and involves immune injury (cellular and humoral rejection), nonimmune injury (graft ischemic injury and CMV infection), and vascular factors (lipid accumulation, thrombosis, and growth factors). Diltiazem (Cardizem®, Biovail Corp., Ontario, Canada) and "statin" drugs reduce the incidence of CAV (77–79). However, because of the diffuse nature of the disease, once CAV is established, there is no effective treatment except retransplantation.

GASTROINTESTINAL COMPLICATIONS

Gastrointestinal complications are common after heart transplantation and occur in approximately 20% of patients (80). The causes of these complications include surgical stress (gastritis, ulceration, and perforation), side effects of medication (steroid-induced gastritis, ulceration, pancreatitis, chemical hepatitis, cholelithiasis, and diverticulitis), and opportunistic infection and malignancy due to immunosuppression (candidiasis, CMV enteritis, and PTLD). Because of the masking effect of immunosuppressive agents, transplant recipients usually do not exhibit the typical systemic and local inflammatory signs and symptoms of gastrointestinal complications. Therefore, physicians must maintain a high index of suspicion for these problems (81,82). Diagnostic procedures, such as endoscopy with biopsy of suspicious lesions, computerized tomography, or exploratory laparotomy, must be initiated expediently to prevent catastrophe (80).

OTHER COMPLICATIONS OF IMMUNOSUPPRESSION

A typical immunosuppressive regimen for heart transplant recipients consists of three agents: corticosteroids (prednisone), an antimetabolite (azathioprine or mycophenolate mofetil), and a calcineurin inhibitor (either cyclosporine or tacrolimus). Lympholytic agents such as rabbit antithymocyte globulin, horse antilymphocyte globulin, and murine monoclonal antibody against the human CD3 T-cell antigen (OK3) are also used as "induction therapy" in the perioperative period and as treatment for steroid-resistant rejection. In addition to their immunosuppressive properties, these agents cause various other toxic effects. Serious side effects of corticosteroids are cushingoid appearance, osteoporosis, diabetes mellitus, hyperlipidemia, peptic ulcer disease, cataracts, and capillary fragility.

Fortunately, now that calcineurin inhibitors are available, the use of steroids has been markedly reduced and a substantial number of heart transplant recipients can be weaned off steroids six months to one year after transplantation (83). Serious side effects of cyclosporine and tacrolimus include nephrotoxicity, hypertension, seizures, tremors, and peripheral neuropathy. Hirsutism and gingival hyperplasia are unique side effects of cyclosporine, whereas alopecia, diabetes mellitus, and hypomagnesemia are more commonly associated with tacrolimus (84). Gout is also a troublesome complication among heart transplant recipients and is associated with both cyclosporine and tacrolimus. Hyperuricemia is a result of decreased renal clearance, which is exaggerated by the use of diuretics to control hypertension (85). As treatment for acute episodes of gout, corticosteroids are the agent of choice because nonsteroidal anti-inflammatory agents frequently potentiate the nephrotoxicity of calcineurin inhibitors. Serious side effects of the antimetabolite drugs are leukopenia, anemia, thrombocytopenia, and gastrointestinal disturbances. Lympholytic agents are associated with cytokine release syndrome, thrombocytopenia, an increased risk of opportunistic infection, and PTLD (86–89).

CONCLUSION

Heart transplantation has matured into an effective treatment for heart failure. Refinements in donor and recipient selection, surgical techniques, perioperative care, and immunosuppression during the past four decades have markedly reduced the rate of postoperative complications. To date, most complications associated with heart transplantation have been related to the use of immunosuppressive agents. Fortunately, during the past two decades, the emergence of new agents with different toxicity profiles has enabled transplant physicians to individualize the immunosuppressive regimen (90). As a result, complications associated with the use of immunosuppression have been manageable and the quality of life after heart transplantation has improved tremendously.

REFERENCES

1. Hosenpud JD, Bennett LE, Keck BM, Boucek MM, Novick RJ. The Registry of the International Society for Heart and Lung Transplantation: Eighteenth Official Report-2001. J Heart Lung Transplant 2001; 20(8): 805–815.
2. Kasper EK, Achuff SC. Clinical evaluation of potential heart transplant recipients. In: Baumgartner WA, Reitz BA, Kasper EK, Theodore J, eds. Heart Heart-Lung Transplantation. 2nd ed. Philadelphia: W.B. Saunders Company, 2002:57–63.
3. Blanche C, Blanche DA, Kearney B, et al. Heart transplantation in patients seventy years of age and older: a comparative analysis of outcome. J Thorac Cardiovasc Surg 2001; 121(3):532–541.

4. Fonarow GC. How old is too old for heart transplantation? Curr Opin Cardiol 2000; 15(2):97–103.

5. Blanche C, Kamlot A, Blanche DA, et al. Combined heart-kidney transplantation with single-donor allografts. J Thorac Cardiovasc Surg 2001; 122(3):495–500.

6. Castillo-Lugo JA, Brinker KR. An overview of combined heart and kidney transplantation. Curr Opin Cardiol 1999; 14(2):121–125.

7. Tazbir JS, Cronin DC II. Indications, evaluations, and postoperative care of the combined liver-heart transplant recipient. AACN Clin Issues 1999; 10(2):240–252.

8. Surakomol S, Olson LJ, Rastogi A, et al. Combined orthotopic heart and liver transplantation for genetic hemochromatosis. J Heart Lung Transplant 1997; 16(5):573–575.

9. Detry O, Honore P, Meurisse M, et al. Advantages of inferior vena caval flow preservation in combined transplantation of the liver and heart. Transpl Int 1997; 10(2):150–151.

10. Shumway NE, Lower RR, Stofer RC. Transplantation of the heart. Adv Surg 1966; 2:265–284.

11. Traversi E, Pozzoli M, Grande A, et al. The bicaval anastomosis technique for orthotopic heart transplantation yields better atrial function than the standard technique: an echocardiographic automatic boundary detection study. J Heart Lung Transplant 1998; 17(11):1065–1074.

12. Beniaminovitz A, Savoia MT, Oz M, et al. Improved atrial function in bicaval versus standard orthotopic techniques in cardiac transplantation. Am J Cardiol 1997; 80(12):1631–1635.

13. Blanche C, Nessim S, Quartel A, et al. Heart transplantation with bicaval and pulmonary venous anastomoses. A hemodynamic analysis of the first 117 patients. J Cardiovasc Surg (Torino) 1997; 38(6):561–566.

14. Barnard CN, Barnard MS, Cooper DK, et al. The present status of heterotopic cardiac transplantation. J Thorac Cardiovasc Surg 1981; 81(3):433–439.

15. Nakatani T, Frazier OH, Lammermeier DE, Macris MP, Radovancevic B. Heterotopic heart transplantation: a reliable option for a select group of high-risk patients. J Heart Transplant 1989; 8(1):40–47.

16. Reichenspurner H, Hildebrandt A, Boehm D, et al. Heterotopic heart transplantation in 1988—recent selective indications and outcome. J Heart Transplant 1989; 8(5):381–386.

17. Ridley PD, Khaghani A, Musumeci F, et al. Heterotopic heart transplantation and recipient heart operation in ischemic heart disease. Ann Thorac Surg 1992; 54(2):333–337.

18. Kawaguchi A, Gandjbakhch I, Pavie A, et al. Cardiac transplant recipients with preoperative pulmonary hypertension. Evolution of pulmonary hemodynamics and surgical options. Circulation 1989; 80(5 Pt 2): III90–III96.

19. Baumgartner WA. Myocardial and pulmonary protection: long-distance transport. Prog Cardiovasc Dis 1990; 33(2):85–96.

20. Anyanwu AC, Rogers CA, Murday AJ. A simple approach to risk stratification in adult heart transplantation. Eur J Cardiothorac Surg 1999; 16(4):424–428.

21. Marelli D, Laks H, Fazio D, Moore S, Moriguchi J, Kobashigawa J. The use of donor hearts with left ventricular hypertrophy. J Heart Lung Transplant 2000; 19(5):496–503.

22. Weil R III, Clarke DR, Iwaki Y, et al. Hyperacute rejection of a transplanted human heart. Transplantation 1981; 32(1):71–72.

23. Cooper DK. Clinical survey of heart transplantation between ABO blood group-incompatible recipients and donors. J Heart Transplant 1990; 9(4):376–381.

24. Trento A, Hardesty RL, Griffith BP, Zerbe T, Kormos RL, Bahnson HT. Role of the antibody to vascular endothelial cells in hyperacute rejection in patients undergoing cardiac transplantation. J Thorac Cardiovasc Surg 1988; 95(1):37–41.

25. Loh E, Bergin JD, Couper GS, Mudge GH Jr. Role of panel-reactive antibody cross-reactivity in predicting survival after orthotopic heart transplantation. J Heart Lung Transplant 1994; 13(2):194–201.

26. Bojar RM, Warner KG. Manual of Perioperative Care in Cardiac Surgery. 3rd ed. Malden, Massachsetts: Blackwell Science, 1998.

27. Unsworth-White MJ, Herriot A, Valencia O, et al. Resternotomy for bleeding after cardiac operation: a marker for increased morbidity and mortality. Ann Thorac Surg 1995; 59(3):664–667.

28. Talamonti MS, LoCicero J III, Hoyne WP, Sanders JH, Michaelis LL. Early reexploration for excessive postoperative bleeding lowers wound complication rates in open-heart surgery. Am Surg 1987; 53(2): 102–104.

29. Tischler MD, Lee RT, Plappert T, Mudge GH, St. John Sutton M, Parker JD. Serial assessment of left ventricular function and mass after orthotopic heart transplantation: a 4-year longitudinal study. J Am Coll Cardiol 1992; 19(1):60–66.

30. Young JB, Winters WL Jr., Bourge R, Uretsky BF. 24th Bethesda conference: cardiac transplantation. Task Force 4: function of the heart transplant recipient. J Am Coll Cardiol 1993; 22(1):31–41.

31. Bertolet BD, Eagle DA, Conti JB, Mills RM, Belardinelli L. Bradycardia after heart transplantation: reversal with theophylline. J Am Coll Cardiol 1996; 28(2): 396–399.

32. Kieler-Jensen N, Lundin S, Ricksten SE. Vasodilator therapy after heart transplantation: effects of inhaled nitric oxide and intravenous prostacyclin, prostaglandin E1, and sodium nitroprusside. J Heart Lung Transplant 1995; 14(3):436–443.

33. Auler Junior JO, Carmona MJ, Bocchi EA, et al. Low doses of inhaled nitric oxide in heart transplant recipients. J Heart Lung Transplant 1996; 15(5):443–450.

34. Ardehali A, Hughes K, Sadeghi A, et al. Inhaled nitric oxide for pulmonary hypertension after heart transplantation. Transplantation 2001; 72(4):638–641.

35. Pope SE, Stinson EB, Daughters GT II, Schroeder JS, Ingels NB Jr, Alderman EL. Exercise response of the denervated heart in long-term cardiac transplant recipients. Am J Cardiol 1980; 46(2):213–218.

36. Stinson EB, Griepp RB, Bieber CP, Shumway NE. Hemodynamic observations after orthotopic transplantation of the canine heart. J Thorac Cardiovasc Surg 1972; 63(3):344–352.

37. Jacquet L, Ziady G, Stein K, et al. Cardiac rhythm disturbances early after orthotopic heart transplantation: prevalence and clinical importance of the observed abnormalities. J Am Coll Cardiol 1990; 16(4): 832–837.

38. Ellenbogen KA, Szentpetery S, Katz MR. Reversibility of prolonged chronotropic dysfunction with theophylline following orthotopic cardiac transplantation. Am Heart J 1988; 116(1 Pt 1):202–206.

39. el Gamel A, Yonan NA, Grant S, et al. Orthotopic cardiac transplantation: a comparison of standard and bicaval techniques. J Thorac Cardiovasc Surg 1995; 109(4):721–730.

40. Trento A, Takkenberg JM, Czer LS, et al. Clinical experience with one hundred consecutive patients undergoing orthotopic heart transplantation with bicaval and pulmonary venous anastomoses. J Thorac Cardiovasc Surg 1996; 112(6):1496–1503.

41. Herre JM, Barnhart GR, Llano A. Cardiac pacemakers in the transplanted heart: short term with the biatrial anastomosis and unnecessary with the bicaval anastomosis. Curr Opin Cardiol 200; 15(2):115–120.

42. Scott CD, Dark JH, McComb JM. Sinus node function after cardiac transplantation. J Am Coll Cardiol 1994; 24(5):1334–1341.

43. Berke DK, Graham AF, Schroeder JS, Harrison DC. Arrhythmias in the denervated transplanted human heart. Circulation 1973; 48(suppl 1):III112–III115.

44. Uretsky BF. Physiology of the transplanted heart. Cardiovasc Clin 1990; 20(2):23–56.

45. Yusuf S, Theodoropoulos S, Dhalla N, et al. Influence of beta blockade on exercise capacity and heart rate response after human orthotopic and heterotopic cardiac transplantation. Am J Cardiol 1989; 64(10): 636–641.

46. Ellenbogen KA, Thames MD, DiMarco JP, Sheehan H, Lerman BB. Electrophysiological effects of adenosine in the transplanted human heart. Evidence of supersensitivity. Circulation 1990; 81(3):821–828.

47. Hunt SA. New immunosuppressive agents in clinical use: mycophenolate mofetil and tacrolimus. Cardiol Rev 2000; 8(3):180–184.

48. Taylor DO, Barr ML, Meiser BM, Pham SM, Mentzer RM, Gass AL. Suggested guidelines for the use of tacrolimus in cardiac transplant recipients. J Heart Lung Transplant 2001; 20(7):734–738.

49. Billingham ME, Cary NR, Hammond ME, et al. A working formulation for the standardization of nomenclature in the diagnosis of heart and lung rejection. Heart Rejection Study Group. The International Society for Heart Transplantation. J Heart Transplant 1990; 9(6):587–593.

50. Billingham ME. Endomyocardial biopsy diagnosis of acute rejection in cardiac allografts. Prog Cardiovasc Dis 1990; 33(1):11–18.

51. Madan AK, Slakey DP, Becker A, et al. Treatment of antibody-mediated accelerated rejection using plasmapheresis. J Clin Apheresis 2000; 15(3):180–183.

52. Woodle ES, Newell KA, Haas M, et al. Reversal of accelerated renal allograft rejection with FK506. Clin Transplant 1997; 11(4):251–254.

53. Pennock JL, Oyer PE, Reitz BA, et al. Cardiac transplantation in perspective for the future. Survival, complications, rehabilitation, and cost. J Thorac Cardiovasc Surg 1982; 83(2):168–177.

54. Dummer JS. Infectious complications of transplantation. Cardiovasc Clin 1990; 20(2):163–178.

55. Hofflin JM, Potasman I, Baldwin JC, Oyer PE, Stinson EB, Remington JS. Infectious complications in heart transplant recipients receiving cyclosporine and corticosteroids. Ann Intern Med 1987; 106(2):209–216.

56. Kirklin JK, Naftel DC, Levine TB, et al. Cytomegalovirus after heart transplantation. Risk factors for infection and death: a multiinstitutional study. The Cardiac Transplant Research Database Group. J Heart Lung Transplant 1994; 13(3):394–404.

57. Dummer JS, White LT, Ho M, Griffith BP, Hardesty RL, Bahnson HT. Morbidity of cytomegalovirus infection in recipients of heart or heart-lung transplants who received cyclosporine. J Infect Dis 1985; 152(6):1182–1191.

58. Valantine HA. Role of CMV in transplant coronary artery disease and survival after heart transplantation. Transpl Infect Dis 1999; 1(suppl 1):25–30.

59. Keay S, Petersen E, Icenogle T, et al. Ganciclovir treatment of serious cytomegalovirus infection in heart and heart-lung transplant recipients. Rev Infect Dis 1988; 10(suppl 3):S563–S572.

60. Balfour HH Jr., Chace BA, Stapleton JT, Simmons RL, Fryd DS. A randomized, placebo-controlled trial of oral acyclovir for the prevention of cytomegalovirus disease in recipients of renal allografts. N Engl J Med 1989; 320(21):1381–1387.

61. Nalesnik MA, Makowka L, Starzl TE. The diagnosis and treatment of posttransplant lymphoproliferative disorders. Curr Probl Surg 1988; 25:367–472.

62. Hughes WT, Kuhn S, Chaudhary S, et al. Successful chemoprophylaxis for *Pneumocystis carinii* pneumonitis. N Engl J Med 1977; 297(26):1419–1426.

63. Dummer JS. *Pneumocystis carinii* infections in transplant recipients. Semin Respir Infect 1990; 5(1):50–57.

64. Hakim M, Wreghitt TG, English TA, Stovin PG, Cory-Pearce R, Wallwork J. Significance of donor transmitted disease in cardiac transplantation. J Heart Transplant 1985; 4(3):302–306.

65. Luft BJ, Naot Y, Araujo FG, Stinson EB, Remington JS. Primary and reactivated toxoplasma infection in patients with cardiac transplants. Clinical spectrum and problems in diagnosis in a defined population. Ann Intern Med 1983; 99(1):27–31.

66. Wreghitt TG, Hakim M, Gray JJ, et al. Toxoplasmosis in heart and heart and lung transplant recipients. J Clin Pathol 1989; 42(2):194–199.

67. Penn I. Tumors after renal and cardiac transplantation. Hematol Oncol Clin North Am 1993; 7(2):431–445.

68. Krikorian JG, Anderson JL, Bieber CP, Penn I, Stinson EB. Malignant neoplasms following cardiac transplantation. JAMA 1978; 240(7):639–643.

69. Hosenpud JD, Bennett LE, Keck BM, Fiol B, Boucek MM, Novick RJ. The Registry of the International Society for Heart and Lung Transplantation: Sixteenth Official Report-1999. J Heart Lung Transplant 1999; 18(7): 611–626.

70. Starzl TE, Nalesnik MA, Porter KA, et al. Reversibility of lymphomas and lymphoproliferative lesions developing under cyclosporin-steroid therapy. Lancet 1984; 1(8377):583–587.

71. O'Reilly RJ, Small TN, Papadopoulos E, Lucas K, Lacerda J, Koulova L. Adoptive immunotherapy for Epstein–Barr virus-associated lymphoproliferative disorders complicating marrow allografts. Springer Semin Immunopathol 1998; 20(3–4):455–491.

72. Papadopoulos EB, Ladanyi M, Emanuel D, et al. Infusions of donor leukocytes to treat Epstein–Barr virus-associated lymphoproliferative disorders after

allogeneic bone marrow transplantation. N Engl J Med 1994; 330(17):1185–1191.

73. Nalesnik MA, Rao AS, Furukawa H, et al. Autologous lymphokine-activated killer cell therapy of Epstein–Barr virus-positive and -negative lymphoproliferative disorders arising in organ transplant recipients. Transplantation 1997; 63(9):1200–1205.

74. Milpied N, Vasseur B, Parquet N, et al. Humanized anti-CD20 monoclonal antibody (Rituximab) in post transplant B-lymphoproliferative disorder: a retrospective analysis on 32 patients. Ann Oncol 2000; 11(suppl 1):113–116.

75. Haverich A. Cyclosporine in heart transplantation. Transplant Proc 1992; 24(4 suppl 2):82–84.

76. Hosenpud JD. Immune mechanisms of cardiac allograft vasculopathy: an update. Transpl Immunol 1993; 1(4):237–249.

77. Schroeder JS, Gao SZ, Alderman EL, et al. A preliminary study of diltiazem in the prevention of coronary artery disease in heart-transplant recipients. N Eng J Med 1993; 328(3):164–170.

78. Wenke K, Meiser B, Thiery J, et al. Simvastatin reduces graft vessel disease and mortality after heart transplantation: a four-year randomized trial. Circulation 1997; 96(5):1398–1402.

79. Kobashigawa JA, Katznelson S, Laks H, et al. Effect of pravastatin on outcomes after cardiac transplantation. N Eng J Med 1995; 333(10):621–627.

80. Mueller XM, Tevaearai HT, Stumpe F, et al. Extramediastinal surgical problems in heart transplant recipients. J Am Coll Surg 1999; 189(4):380–388.

81. Steed DL, Brown B, Reilly JJ, et al. General surgical complications in heart and heart-lung transplantation. Surgery 1985; 98(4):739–745.

82. Johnson R, Peitzman AB, Webster MW, et al. Upper gastrointestinal endoscopy after cardiac transplantation. Surgery 1988; 103(3):300–304.

83. Pham SM, Kormos RL, Hattler BG, et al. A prospective trial of tacrolimus (FK506) in clinical heart transplantation: intermediate term results. J Thorac Cardiovasc Surg 1996; 111(4):764–772.

84. Asante-Korang A, Boyle GJ, Webber SA, Miller SA, Fricker FJ. Experience of FK506 immune suppression in pediatric heart transplantation: a study of long-term adverse effects. J Heart Lung Transplant 1996; 15(4):415–422.

85. Lin HY, Rocher LL, McQuillan MA, Schmaltz S, Palella TD, Fox IH. Cyclosporine-induced hyperuricemia and gout. N Engl J Med 1989; 321(5):287–292.

86. Burk ML, Matuszewski KA. Muromonab-CD3 and antithymocyte globulin in renal transplantation. Ann Pharmacother 1997; 31(11):1370–1377.

87. Taylor DO, Kfoury AG, Pisani B, Hammond EH, Renlund DG. Antilymphocyte-antibody prophylaxis: review of the adult experience in heart transplantation. Transplant Proc 1997; 29(8A):13S–15S.

88. Zuckermann AO, Grimm M, Czerny M, et al. Improved long-term results with thymoglobuline induction therapy after cardiac transplantation: a comparison of two different rabbit-antithymocyte globulines. Transplantation 2000; 69(9):1890–1898.

89. Guttmann RD, Caudrelier P, Alberici G, Touraine JL. Pharmacokinetics, foreign protein immune response, cytokine release, and lymphocyte subsets in patients receiving thymoglobuline and immunosuppression. Transplant Proc 1997; 29(7A):24S–26S.

90. Gummert JF, Ikonen T, Morris RE. Newer immunosuppressive drugs: a review. J Am Soc Nephrol 1999; 10(6):1366–1380.

29

Complications of Mechanical Circulatory Support

Fotios M. Andreopoulos
Departments of Surgery and Biomedical Engineering,
University of Miami School of Medicine, Miami, Florida, U.S.A.

Richard J. Kaplon
Cardiac and Thoracic Surgery Medical Group, Sacramento, California, U.S.A.

During the past 10 years, various modes of mechanical circulatory support have been used clinically to successfully restore homeostasis, improve end-organ function, and serve as a bridge to transplantation or recovery. The true long-term goal, however, once the technology has adequately evolved, is to use cardiac assist devices as destination therapy. Currently available ventricular assist devices (VADs) include extracorporeal membrane oxygenation (ECMO), extracorporeal pulsatile assist devices, implantable assist devices, and the total artificial heart (TAH). Some of these devices provide either univentricular or biventricular support (Thoratec®, ABIOMED®); others provide only left ventricular (LV) assistance [HeartMate® (Thoratec Corporation, Berkley, California, U.S.A.) and Novacor® (WorldHeart Inc., Oakland, California, U.S.A.)]. ECMO and the TAH [CardioWest™ (SynCardia Systems Inc., Tucson, Arizona, U.S.A.)] provide total circulatory support. Current experimental devices include axial flow impeller pumps (Jarvik 2000®, HeartMate II®, NASA/DeBakey VAD™) and a fully implantable electric TAH [AbioCor® (ABIOMED, Inc., Danvers, Massachusetts, U.S.A.)]. This chapter will briefly describe the functional characteristics of ECMO and the various VADs; it will also explain the complications associated with each.

DEVICES

Extracorporeal Membrane Oxygenation

ECMO is used primarily as a therapeutic option for patients suffering from severe acute respiratory distress syndrome or acute cardiogenic shock. This method was introduced in the early 1970s by Hill et al. and has been employed worldwide since the late 1980s (1). ECMO can provide cardiac and pulmonary support for short periods (days to weeks), thereby allowing time for the native heart or lungs to recover. Its basic configuration consists of a venous drainage cannula, a centrifugal pump, an oxygenator, and either a venous or an arterial return cannula. The venous–arterial (V–A) configuration is used primarily for cardiac or cardiorespiratory support, whereas the venous–venous (V–V) mode is used solely for respiratory support (2).

ECMO insertion is typically achieved by peripheral cannulation, either percutaneously or by means of an open cut-down technique; however, central cannulation from the right atrium to the aorta has also been used. Drainage to the pump is typically accomplished from the femoral vein, with return either to the femoral artery (V–A ECMO) or to the right atrium via the femoral vein (V–V ECMO) (2). Alternatively, for V–V ECMO, cannulation may be achieved through the femoral vein or the internal jugular vein (2). In this mode, femoral drainage and atrial reinfusion via the internal jugular vein is preferred to atrial drainage and femoral reinfusion because it provides greater extracorporeal flow and higher pulmonary arterial mixed venous oxygen saturation (3). The main benefits of ECMO include ease of peripheral cannula insertion and effective univentricular or biventricular cardiopulmonary support.

ABIOMED BVS 5000®

The ABIOMED BVS 5000® (ABIOMED Cardiovascular Inc., Danvers, Massachusetts, U.S.A.) is an extracorporeal, pneumatically actuated VAD that can provide short-term left, right, or biventricular support. The device is a dual-chamber pump within a polycarbonate housing. Each chamber contains a seamless polyurethane bladder with a volume of approximately 100 cc. Blood drains by gravity from the native atria of the heart into the upper (atrial) chamber of the pump, which acts as a reservoir for the lower (ventricular) pumping chamber. Two trileaflet polyurethane [Angioflex™ (MicroMed Tech Inc., Houston, Texas, U.S.A.)] valves proximal and distal to the ventricular chamber ensure unidirectional flow. Once the lower chamber has filled with blood, compressed air enters the blood chamber, causing bladder collapse and return of blood to the patient (pump systole). A bedside console that provides self-regulating, pulsatile

---

KEY POINTS

- Bleeding is the most common complication seen with extracorporeal membrane oxygenation (ECMO) and ventricular assist device (VAD) implantation. The use of aprotinin at the time of device placement or the administration of vitamin K can help reduce early bleeding. Postoperative bleeding necessitates blood transfusion, but alloimmunization and elevated panel-reactive antibody levels can complicate organ matching at the time of transplantation.

- The incidence of thromboembolism and stroke is directly related to the type of device used and to the patient's underlying medical condition. Most of the mechanical circulatory assist devices currently used require careful anticoagulation protocols.

- Infection is the leading cause of late mortality for patients treated with assist devices. Causes of infection include the preoperative clinical status of the patient, surgical trauma during device insertion, and exiting cannulae and drivelines. Prevention is the foundation of treatment for infection. Suppressive antibiotic therapy, pump-pocket debridement, device exchange, and explantation are common therapeutic techniques; transplantation is the treatment of choice.

- Right heart failure among patients with left ventricular assist devices (LVADs) is an important cause of perioperative morbidity and may lead to death. Right ventricular dysfunction can be avoided by optimizing patients' clinical condition preoperatively and by administering phosphodiesterase inhibitors and nitric oxide during LVAD implantation.

- Mechanical complications are relatively common in association with ECMO support; these complications necessitate regular exchange of the oxygenator. In contrast, LVADs in general are mechanically resilient; the most common complications are controller malfunctions, inflow valve deterioration, and driveline or outflow kinking.

---

support controls the pump. The console operates asynchronously to the native heart by adjusting pump rate and duration of systole and diastole to compensate for changes in preload and afterload (4).

A number of cannulation options are available for pump insertion (5). Left-sided inflow cannulation sites include the left atrium by means of the interatrial groove, the dome or the left atrial appendage, or the LV apex. Although left dome cannulation may be used for small hearts, the interatrial groove is most frequently used for inflow. LV apical cannulation is associated with higher flows and a lower incidence of LV thrombus formation; this is the site of choice for patients with a prosthetic mitral valve. The right atrial free wall is the site most commonly used for right atrial cannulation, although direct right ventricular (RV) cannulation has also been used successfully. Arterial return is achieved with an end-to-side anastomosis of the outflow grafts to either the ascending aorta or the pulmonary artery. The ABIOMED VAD is approved by the U.S. Food and Drug Administration (FDA) for postcardiotomy support and for short-term bridge-to-recovery therapy. Its use has been expanded to include all forms of reversible heart failure, including myocardial infarction, cardiac trauma, and RV support with an implantable LV assist device (LVAD) as bridge-to-recovery or bridge-to-transplantation therapy.

Thoratec® Ventricular Assist Devices

The Thoratec VAD (Thoratec Corporation, Pleasanton, California, U.S.A.) is also an extracorporeal, pneuma-

tically actuated pump that can provide left, right, or biventricular support. This VAD's rigid polysulfone casing lies on the patient's abdominal wall and contains a diaphragm that separates the air chamber from the polyurethane (Thoralon®) blood sac. An external console provides alternating positive and negative pressure that assists with filling and emptying of the blood sac. Monostrut™ mechanical disc valves in the inflow and outflow conduits of the pump ensure unidirectional flow. The Thoratec VAD can be operated in several modes: fixed-rate (asynchronous) mode, synchronous (timed by the patient's electrocardiogram) mode, or volume mode. The volume mode is recommended for maintaining physiologic blood flow, although it is asynchronous to the heart. Paracorporeal pump placement and right-heart and left-heart cannulation options are similar to those of the ABIOMED BVS 5000.

Once cannulation is complete, air is removed from the pump through the arterial graft. The Thoratec VAD is activated at a slow fixed rate (40 bpm, 20% systolic ejection) with a drive pressure of 100 to 120 mmHg and a vacuum pressure of 0 to −5 mmHg. After the device is checked for leaks, the ejection pressure is gradually increased to 200 mmHg and the vacuum is set between −10 and −20 mmHg. Once the VAD is appropriately filled and emptied, the pump is placed in volume mode. When the chest is closed, full vacuum pressure (−25 to −40 mmHg) is applied, and the ejection pressure is set at 100 mmHg above the systolic blood pressure (6–8).

The paracorporeal position of the device allows for easy inspection of the blood chamber and for easy pump replacement if necessary. The versatility of the Thoratec VAD is due to its multiple cannulation configurations, its biventricular potential, its applicability even for small patients (body surface area of less than 1.5 m^2), and its capability for short-term or long-term support. Additionally, the ability to apply suction to the venous drainage enhances blood return to the pump and helps to maintain adequate flows. The FDA has approved the Thoratec VAD for bridge-to-transplant and bridge-to-recovery purposes. More widespread use of this device is limited because of its large pneumatic driver, which makes outpatient management difficult, and because of the need for aggressive anticoagulation to minimize thromboembolic complications from the mechanical valves and thrombogenic surfaces of the pump.

HeartMate[®]

The HeartMate (Thoratec Corporation, Berkley, California, U.S.A.) is an implantable, pulsatile electric VAD that provides LV support. It is fabricated from sintered titanium and houses a flexible, textured polyurethane diaphragm. The pump is typically implanted in the left upper quadrant and is connected to a controller and a power source by a percutaneous driveline. The blood pump is textured to enable circulating cells to adhere to the pump and form a biological lining that reduces blood–device interaction. This "pseudo-neointima" is responsible for the low thromboembolic risk associated with this device, even without anticoagulation therapy (9). Unidirectional flow is ensured by porcine valves within the inflow and outflow conduits. The vented electric HeartMate device received FDA approval as bridge-to-transplantation therapy in 1998. This device allows patients to be discharged from the hospital and to resume their everyday activities while awaiting heart transplantation. The pump can operate in two different modes: fixed and automatic. The fixed mode allows the pump to operate at set rates ranging from 50 to 120 bpm, whereas the auto mode allows the pump rate to vary according to the physiological filling of the pump. Once the pump chamber has been 90% filled with blood, ejection is initiated. The auto mode is the most common mode of operation and allows the pump to respond to circulatory demand.

The HeartMate may be implanted intraabdominally or in a preperitoneal pocket. Most surgeons experienced with HeartMate implantation favor the preperitoneal location because excessive heat and fluid loss from the abdominal cavity can be avoided, internal organ erosion and bowel obstruction are eliminated, intra-abdominal adhesions are minimized, and infections can be easily managed (10,11). A pocket is created between the peritoneum and the rectus muscle sheath. The pump's driveline exits from the right lower quadrant through a small incision made between the costal margin and the superior iliac crest. Special effort is made to create a subcutaneous tunnel long enough to permit optimal tissue ingrowth around the driveline and to minimize the risk of infection (11). Inflow to the pump is through the LV apex; return is through a Dacron[®] outflow conduit anastomosed end-to-side to the ascending aorta. The inflow conduit is directed away from the interventricular septum to prevent inflow complications associated with sucking the ventricular septal muscle into the cannula. Once the inflow conduit and the arterial outflow graft have been connected, air is removed from the pump with a hand pump to minimize the likelihood of air embolism (11). The presence of air can be monitored by transesophageal echocardiography (TEE). Initially, the HeartMate is activated at a fixed rate of 50 bpm; the rate is then slowly increased as the patient is weaned from cardiopulmonary bypass. Once the patient has been completely weaned from bypass, the device can be fully activated.

The results of Randomized Evaluation of Mechanical Assistance for the Treatment of Congestive Heart Failure (REMATCH), a prospective, multicenter trial, have recently been reported (12). This study, designed to assess the effectiveness of the HeartMate VAD in comparison to the effectiveness of medical therapy for patients with end-stage heart disease, and for whom transplantation is contraindicated, found that the use of implantable VADs enhances survival and improves quality of life. Compared with patients receiving only pharmacologic therapy, patients receiving the HeartMate experienced a 48% reduction in risk of death (12).

Novacor[®] Left Ventricular Assist System

Like the HeartMate, the Novacor LV assist system (LVAS) (World Heart Corporation, Ottawa, Canada) is an implantable, electromechanical device designed for long-term LV support. The integrated blood pump/energy converter is implanted into a preperitoneal pocket in the left upper quadrant (13). During systole, a polyurethane pump sac is compressed by two symmetrical pusher plates that are coupled to a solenoid energy converter; this compression causes blood ejection. Again, unidirectional flow is ensured by bioprosthetic valves attached to the inflow and outflow conduits of the pump chamber. A percutaneous driveline exits the patient's lower right quadrant and is connected to an external control unit. The Novacor device fills passively; upon mechanical actuation of the pusher plate, blood is ejected. As with the Thoratec device, there are three modes of operation: fixed, synchronous, and fill-to-empty. In the fixed mode, the pump rate is set and the device operates asynchronously to the native heart. In the synchronous mode, pump ejection is triggered by the R-wave of the native heart; even though the pump operates synchronously with the native heart, the use of this mode is limited by the dependence of the pump on an external signal. Fill-to-empty is the most common mode of operation, providing sufficient output by responding to variable physiological demands.

Implantation of the Novacor device is accomplished by a procedure similar to that used to implant the HeartMate (13). Briefly, the device itself is assembled by connecting the inflow and outflow valved conduits to the inflow and outflow grafts, respectively. The inflow conduit is tunneled through the diaphragm into the left ventricle through a ventriculotomy at the LV apex. Once the conduits and grafts have been positioned, air is removed from the pump through a needle hole in the outflow graft. The pump is started at a low fixed rate, and the patient is slowly weaned from cardiopulmonary bypass. Once weaning has been completed, the pump can be switched to the fill-to-empty mode. TEE is used to ensure adequate air removal, to assess RV function, and to diagnose aortic insufficiency or to determine the patency of the foramen ovale. Like the HeartMate, the Novacor system because of its wearable configuration, allows the patient to be discharged from the hospital and to resume life outside the hospital.

Initially designed for bridge-to-transplant therapy, the Novacor VAD is now less frequently used because of reports of excessive development of thromboembolism. Recent changes to the inflow conduit appear to have alleviated that problem, and a new trial, Investigation of Non–Transplant-Eligible Patients Who Are Inotrope Dependent, is under way to investigate the use of this device as destination therapy for patients who are not candidates for transplantation.

CardioWest™ Total Artificial Heart

The CardioWest TAH, previously known as the Jarvik 7® or the Symbion® TAH, is a pneumatically driven, biventricular pulsatile pump that provides full circulatory support. It consists of two rigid polyurethane ventricles that are connected to the native atria and great vessels. Each ventricle contains a smooth, flexible polyurethane diaphragm that separates the blood from the air chambers. Compressed air, delivered through a percutaneous driveline that connects each ventricle to an external console, pressurizes the blood chamber, and causes blood ejection. Mechanical valves provide unidirectional flow. The pump has a maximum stroke volume of 70 mL and a maximum pump output of 15 L/min; however, average flow rates range from 6 to 8 L/min. Pump rate, percent systole, and driveline pressures are controlled for each ventricle; the device is operated so that the blood sacs do not fill completely but always empty completely. To ensure full ejection, the drive pressure of the console is set 30 to 40 mmHg higher than the pressure of the great vessels (14).

The CardioWest TAH is implanted in the orthotopic position (15). Because this device does not fit in all patients, sizing guidelines must be followed. Criteria for optimal fit include a body surface area of at least 1.7 m², an appropriate cardiothoracic ratio, and adequate LV diastolic dimensions, anteroposterior distance, and combined ventricular volumes. In smaller patients, the device may not fit well, and left pulmonary vein or inferior vena cava compression may result. Device insertion requires that each ventricle be excised at the atrioventricular groove and that each great vessel be excised at the sinotubular junction. Ventricular tissue is trimmed away to create atrial cuffs, and the TAH "atrial quick connectors" are sewn in place. The great vessels are anastomosed to the outflow conduits, and the ventricles are connected to the atrial quick connectors. After the air has been removed from the ventricles under TEE guidance, the patient is weaned from cardiopulmonary bypass, and pump support is initiated at a slow rate. Once the chest has been closed, vacuum pressure (-10 to -15 cmH$_2$O) is applied to the device during diastole to assist with ventricular filling, and the pump's mode of operation is switched to the more physiological full-eject mode.

Patients who receive the CardioWest TAH must be given anticoagulation therapy to prevent thrombus formation. Patients may ambulate, but their movement is greatly restricted by the large drive console. A smaller portable drive console is being developed for use outside the hospital.

COMPLICATIONS

Complications leading to significant clinical morbidity and mortality are common in association with ECMO, VAD, and TAH support. Despite advances in technology and in our understanding of the physiology of assist devices, the most problematic complications, as expected, are bleeding, thromboembolism, and infection. For patients with left-sided heart support, right heart failure is a unique problem. For all devices, mechanical failure is an underlying concern.

Bleeding

With an incidence as high as 60%, bleeding is the most common complication of ECMO (16–18). Clotting factor deficiency and disseminated intravascular coagulation resulting from hepatic dysfunction are common among patients requiring this type of support. McManus et al. (19) reported that 68% of patients had clotting factor deficiencies before the start of ECMO. Furthermore, the blood–device interface causes mechanical trauma to circulating blood, with resultant activation of platelets, leukocytes, and the clotting and fibrinolytic cascades. Subsequent platelet loss and consumption of clotting factors can lead to hemorrhage, oxygenator obstruction, and system malfunction. The administration of blood products (platelets, fresh frozen plasma, or cryoprecipitate) is often necessary to counter this ECMO-associated blood dyscrasia. Unfortunately, to avoid circuit clotting, anticoagulation is necessary, but this therapy further exacerbates problematic bleeding. Typically, heparin is the anticoagulant of choice; activated clotting times (ACT) of 200 to 220 seconds are recommended. For patients with heparin-induced thrombocytopenia, recombinant hirudin has been used successfully (20). However, for patients with specific contraindications to anticoagulation, heparin-coated circuits (Carmeda®, Medtronic Inc., Minneapolis, Minnesota, U.S.A.) may be used rather than systemic anticoagulation (21,22). As expected, these heparin-bonded circuits have less effect on platelet consumption than uncoated circuits. Promising results have been obtained with selective anticoagulation given directly into the extracorporeal circuit and with new anticoagulants that have a short half-life (23).

As with ECMO, bleeding is the most frequent complication associated with the implantation of VADs or TAHs. The risk of bleeding ranges from 20% to 80% depending upon the device being implanted, the type of support required (univentricular vs. biventricular), and the patient's preexisting conditions (4,24–26). Patients who require VADs, like those who require ECMO, often have underlying clinical or subclinical hepatic dysfunction; in addition, many are already receiving anticoagulants such as heparin or warfarin for ECMO, have been treated with implanted intra-aortic balloon pumps, or have coronary artery disease or underlying poor LV function. According to the Registry of the International Society of Heart and Lung Transplantation, bleeding substantially influences the survival of patients who are supported by mechanical assist devices (27). The incidence of bleeding was lower among bridge-to-transplant patients who were discharged after transplantation than among those patients who died with a VAD in place (28).

Whereas late bleeding is typically associated with leaking at the connection sites and erosion of the device into anatomic structures, early bleeding results from patients' underlying comorbid conditions, cardiopulmonary bypass–induced thrombocytopenia and platelet dysfunction, perioperative hypothermia, and the complexity of the operative technique. Early bleeding is often exacerbated by the need for anticoagulation when certain devices are used (e.g., ABIOMED, Thoratec, Novacor, Cardio-West). One of the advantages of the HeartMate is its textured lining that avoids the need for early anticoagulation. The use of aprotinin, a serine protease inhibitor, has reduced the incidence of early bleeding. Although many surgeons administer aprotinin when the device is placed, some prefer to reserve the use of this agent for the time of device explantation or heart transplantation (29).

The incidence of bleeding is higher for patients who are supported with biventricular devices than for those with LVADs; however, this higher incidence is probably due, at least in part, to the patients' clinical condition before implantation. Most patients require only left-sided heart support; patients who also require right-sided heart support are usually sicker and more malnourished and have experienced more episodes of hepatic congestion and concomitant coagulopathy than patients requiring LVADs. Even for patients who require only LVADs, subclinical hepatic dysfunction is associated with a higher incidence of hemorrhage. Maneuvers as simple as administering vitamin K, even when prothrombin times are normal, can often help to reduce bleeding (30).

Although postoperative hemorrhage is usually not life threatening, it typically necessitates blood transfusion. Platelet use has been associated with alloimmunization and elevated panel-reactive antibody levels among patients receiving VADs; this therapy can complicate organ matching at the time of transplantation and create a need for preoperative crossmatch testing. Massad et al. (31) demonstrated that leukocytes in blood products transfused at the time of device implant increased LVAD recipients' sensitization to human leukocyte antigens. Moazami et al. (32) showed that this sensitization resulted predominantly from platelets. In the Cleveland Clinic experience, LVAD recipients responded to 19% of T-cell panel-reactive antibodies, whereas non-LVAD transplant candidates responded to only 5% (33).

In addition to the immunologic consequences of transfusion, postoperative transfusion requirements can also worsen preexistent pulmonary hypertension. For patients whose transpulmonary gradients are already elevated, this exacerbation of pulmonary hypertension can mean the difference between LVAD or both left and right ventricular assist devices (BiVAD) support and may change a relatively short hospitalization period with discharge on an LVAD to months of in-hospital care on a BiVAD. Furthermore, patients who require multiple units of blood transfusions when the VAD is placed are at increased risk of prolonged ventilatory support and long-term infection. Murphy et al. (34) demonstrated that infection rates are higher (22%) among patients undergoing cardiac surgery who receive six or more units of blood than among patients who receive no more than two units. Given that the predominant long-term cause of death for patients on LVAD support is infection, factors that increase the risk of infection, such as bleeding, must be carefully addressed (12).

ECMO is associated with a substantial risk of intracranial bleeding; in one study, 19% of patients suffered outcome-determining intracranial bleeding while on ECMO support (35). The risk of intracranial hemorrhage is higher among female patients, those taking heparin, those with an elevated serum creatinine concentration (>2.6 mg/mL), and those with thrombocytopenia. The aggressive management of anticoagulation, prevention of renal failure, and correction of thrombocytopenia may reduce the risk of intracranial hemorrhage among adults supported by ECMO.

Thromboembolism and Stroke

The incidence of device-related thromboembolism ranges from 2% to 50%, depending on the type of device used and on the patient's underlying medical condition (4,9,25,26,33). Turbulent flow patterns, platelet damage, and large synthetic blood-contacting surfaces, combined with low blood flow, may predispose patients to the formation of clots and thrombi (36). Although the HeartMate requires no specific anticoagulation and requires only aspirin as antiplatelet therapy, careful anticoagulation protocols must be followed so as to prevent thromboembolic complications with ECMO or the ABIOMED, Thoratec, Novacor, or CardioWest devices.

Patients supported by ECMO are typically treated with heparin for anticoagulation. Once postoperative bleeding has been minimized, heparin is administered to keep ACTs in the range of 200 to 220 seconds. Like patients supported by ECMO, patients supported by the ABIOMED BVS 5000 are treated early with heparin; once their condition has stabilized, antiplatelet therapy in the form of either aspirin or clopidogrel is added. Because the Thoratec and Novacor devices are usually intended for long-term support, after patients with these devices receive early anticoagulation therapy with heparin, they are maintained on a combination of warfarin and aspirin or clopidogrel. To avoid early heparin-related bleeding problems, yet still maintain a low level of anticoagulation, some surgeons use an infusion of dextran to affect rheology and avoid early thromboembolic complications (37). Once the patients are in stable condition, they receive heparin therapy with a target partial thromboplastin time of 60 to 80 seconds, or warfarin with a target international normalized ratio of 2.5 to 3.5. In addition, some patients are treated with dipyridamole.

Whereas the ABIOMED, Thoratec, and Novacor devices use smooth, seamless polyurethane blood-contacting surfaces, the HeartMate has textured interior surfaces. Sintered titanium microspheres are used on the rigid metallic components, and textured polyurethane is used on the flexible pusher-plate diaphragm. The textured surfaces entrap blood elements and form a stable and densely adherent biological lining. This pseudoneointima forms a long-term blood-contacting interface and because the fibrin-based neointima densely adheres to the rough interior surfaces of the pump, it substantially reduces the potential for embolization (9). Patients supported by the HeartMate typically receive only aspirin (325 mg/day).

Despite careful anticoagulation management, the incidence of clinical thromboembolism among patients supported by VADs is substantial. In a report of their experience with the ABIOMED BVS 5000, Samuels et al. (4) noted that of 7 (16%) of 43 patients who underwent device implantation died of thromboembolic events to the central nervous system (4). In a report of their cumulative experience with 111 patients treated with the Thoratec VAD, McBride et al. (25) found thrombus in 14% of devices at the time of explantation, for a complication rate of 19% (25). Similarly, El-Banayosy et al. (26) noted a 15%

incidence of thromboembolism among their 144 patients supported by the Thoratec VAD (26). Reports indicate that the incidence of thromboembolic complications in association with the Novacor LVAS is as high as 48%; the incidence of stroke ranges from 21% to 48% (26,33,38–40). Recent changes in the inflow conduit reduced the stroke rate from 21% to 12% in one series and from 48% to 13% in another (33,40). Whereas the incidence of thromboembolic strokes is 8% among patients supported by a CardioWest TAH despite treatment with anticoagulants, the incidence of thromboembolism among patients supported by the HeartMate is typically 2% to 6% despite a lack of anticoagulation (24,41,42).

In studies comparing outcomes associated with the Thoratec VAD, the Novacor LVAS, and the CardioWest TAH, Copeland et al. found that the incidence of stroke was 34% among patients supported with the Novacor ventricular assist system, 12% among those supported by the Thoratec VAD, and 8% among those supported by the TAH (41). In a similar comparison, Minami et al. (43) found that the incidence of stroke was 22% in the Thoratec group, 39% in the Novacor group, and 16% in the HeartMate group. Notably, this is the highest reported incidence of stroke associated with the HeartMate device; other reports typically document a stroke rate of 2% to 6% (9,24,42). Finally, Kasirajan et al. (33), in their experience with 205 patients, found that the incidence of thromboembolism was 43% among patients supported by the Novacor and 12% among patients supported by the electric HeartMate. In that series, the incidence of early (no more than seven days after device implantation) stroke was the same for the two devices; however, the rate of later ischemic strokes was markedly different (38% for the Novacor and 2% for the HeartMate). As noted above, these researchers found that the rate of neurologic thromboembolism decreased substantially among patients supported by the Novacor LVAS after revision of the inflow conduit (from 48% to 13%).

Infection

Whereas bleeding and thromboembolism account for much of the morbidity associated with VADs, infection leading to sepsis and multisystem organ failure is the primary cause of late mortality for patients treated with these assist devices (12).

Because of the large surface area of synthetic material in ECMO circuits, patients supported by these devices are subject to infections; however, the incidence of sepsis among these patients is lower than among patients supported by other devices. This difference in the incidence of sepsis is most likely due to the short duration of ECMO support (typically <10 days), a time period insufficient for the development of infection. Steiner et al. (44) found that the most reliable predictor of bloodstream infection during ECMO was the duration of support. In their study of 202 neonates supported by ECMO devices, seven patients (3.4%) experienced bloodstream infections. White blood cell counts and absolute neutrophil counts were found to be unreliable markers of infection; whether this unreliability was due to the immune physiology of infants or due to pancytopenia related to the ECMO circuit was not apparent. The median duration of ECMO support before positive blood cultures were obtained was 390 hours. Interestingly, Kawahito et al. (45) demonstrated that the changing pattern of the circulating lymphocytes reliably predicts survival among patients supported with ECMO. Lymphocyte recovery among patients who did not survive was substantially delayed (by 50%) five days after removal from ECMO.

Unlike ECMO recipients, VAD recipients are much more likely to experience infection; the incidence of infection among this group is approximately 50%, and infection contributes to death in many of these cases (46). Findings from the FDA Safety and Efficacy trials for the HeartMate, Thoratec, and Novacor systems, which involved 313 patients, indicated that infection rates ranged from 44% to 66% (46). Studies that included the ABIOMED BVS system demonstrated similar infection rates (47). According to the findings of Kasirajan et al. (33), 83 (55%) of 150 patients undergoing HeartMate placement had positive results from blood cultures, 12 (10%) had pump-pocket infections, and 35 (23%) had driveline infections. Of 55 patients undergoing Novacor LVAS insertion, 23 (42%) had positive results from blood cultures, 4 (7%) had pump-pocket infections, and 10 (18%) had driveline infections. In that series, the overall incidence of VAD-related infection was 85%. Moreover, as shown by data from the REMATCH trial (12), infection is the most common cause of mortality for patients supported by VADs during the two-year study. In that series, 68 patients underwent long-term VAD therapy; after two years, 17 of 41 deaths (41%) were due to sepsis. Unlike studies from the 1980s, which found that the incidence of infection-related death after TAH placement was as high as 40%, recent studies of the CardioWest TAH found that the incidence of infection was 3.7% (48).

Clearly, infection is a constant threat among patients supported with VADs and is associated with a decreased probability of survival. Hermann et al. (49) demonstrated that only 42% of patients with an LVAD infection survived to receive transplants, whereas 85% of patients who did not experience infection survived. The reasons for the high incidence of clinical infections are multifactorial and complicated, but several key issues bear scrutiny. Patients who require support with VADs are typically malnourished and debilitated as a result of end-stage congestive heart failure. Most of these patients have had prolonged hospitalizations, have required multiple indwelling catheters, and have been fairly immobile before VAD placement. Although these factors predispose patients to nosocomial infections, the surgical trauma of device insertion, with its concomitant

hemostatic alterations and suppression of patients' immune mechanisms, also substantially contributes to the high rates of infection experienced by VAD recipients (50). As noted above, the high incidence of perioperative transfusions not only weakens patients' immune systems before eventual transplantation, but also is directly related to the incidence of perioperative infection. Murphy et al. (34) found that the incidence of infection was substantially higher among patients receiving six units of blood or more, than among patients receiving no more than two units. Moreover, the need for reexploration because of bleeding is also associated with a higher incidence of infection among these patients (46). Finally, LVAD support leads to aberrant activation of T cells with impaired cellular immunity, thereby making these patients more susceptible to opportunistic infections (51).

The combination of the patients' preoperative clinical status and the overall insult of assist device insertion probably accounts for the incidence of short-term postoperative infections. However, the presence of a large foreign body with exiting cannulae or drivelines is the most probable source of long-term infections. In most large reported series, the incidence of driveline infections ranges from 14% to 35%. Although this rate underestimates the total incidence of device-related infections, the driveline is clearly a portal for infectious complications (33,52,53). Driveline infections in the absence of pump-pocket collections are typically treated with antibiotics alone. If infected fluid is present around the device, drainage of the pump pocket is usually necessary. With the ABIOMED or Thoratec devices, driveline-related or conduit-related infections may lead to mediastinitis that requires surgical exploration.

Approaches to reducing the incidence of driveline infections have included changes in dressings and driveline placement and alterations in the driveline itself. Anecdotal experience suggests that the use of a new silver-impregnated dressing (Arglaes™, Medline Industries, Inc., Mundelein, Illinois, U.S.A.) decreases the incidence of driveline infections. Choi et al. (54) demonstrated that an LVAD driveline impregnated with chlorhexidine, triclosan, and silver sulfadiazine may prevent early bacterial and fungal driveline infections. Jarvik et al. (55) showed that moving the driveline exit site from the right lower abdominal quadrant to a titanium-pedestal skull mount reduces the incidence of percutaneous infections. These researchers believe that the combination of rigid fixation of the driveline and the high vascularity of the scalp accounts for this improvement. Despite these changes, most experimental device systems now incorporate transcutaneous energy transfer systems that transmit power to the device across the skin to an internal coil and battery, without any breach of the skin barrier (56–59).

The management of infected devices is difficult. For infection-related device malfunctions such as inflow conduit leak, the device must be removed and replaced. However, for patients with systemic infections but normally functioning devices, transplantation is typically the treatment of choice. Prendergast et al. (60) compared 18 patients supported by LVADs, who were undergoing transplantation; 10 patients had infections and eight did not. The researchers found no significant differences between the group with infection and the group without infection with regard to operative death, length of hospitalization, wound complications, or long-term survival rates. Similarly, Sinha et al. (61) demonstrated that infections among LVAD recipients do not adversely affect the rate of successful transplantation; however, other findings from these researchers (62) show that the incidence of LVAD endocarditis is associated with a high mortality rate.

The most common pathogens associated with VAD infections are Staphylococcus, Pseudomonas, Enterococcus, and Candida spp. (63,64). In one study (64) evaluating the relative risk of death associated with each pathogen, fungemia had the highest hazard ratio (10.9), followed by gram-negative bacteria (5.1) and gram-positive bacteria (2.2). LVAD fungal endocarditis, in particular, may be associated with obstruction of the inflow conduit and septic embolization (65,66). Because of the severity of VAD-associated fungal infections, recent findings support the cost-effectiveness of long-term antifungal prophylaxis for these patients (67).

Treatment of device infection begins with attempts at prevention. Meticulous intraoperative sterile technique and careful dressing changes are mainstays of prevention. Patients should be weaned from ventilators and encouraged to walk as soon as possible; nutrition should be maximized. Patients with evidence of infection should be treated with aggressive suppressive antibiotic therapy. If fluid collects in pump pockets, the pocket should be debrided. For patients with infection-related device malfunctions, device exchange or explant may be attempted. However, as noted above, transplantation is the treatment of choice for patients who are on device support and have systemic infections.

Right Heart Failure

Historically, 80% to 90% of patients who require mechanical circulatory support required only left-sided assistance. With improved pharmacologic management of the right side of the heart by phosphodiesterase inhibitors and inhalational nitric oxide, that percentage has declined (24,26,68). Because of the impact of left-sided mechanical unloading, even patients with marginal RV function can usually be treated with only LVAD support (69). LVAD placement results in lower transpulmonary resistance and improved RV ejection fraction (EF); in one series, RV EF increased from 21% to 32% with only Novacor LVAS support (70,71). In addition, left-sided assistance typically increases coronary perfusion, which may in turn improve RV contractility (72). The potential detrimental effects of

LVAD placement on right heart function include increased venous return, which causes elevated central venous and pulmonary artery pressures. Septal bowing due to left-sided unloading with decreased septal systolic function similarly contributes to impaired RV ejection (72).

Right heart failure is a cause of substantial perioperative morbidity and possible mortality in patients undergoing LVAD placement. Farrar et al. (73) reviewed the relative outcomes of 213 patients supported by Thoratec VADs (74 LVADs, 139 BiVADs). The rate of survival to transplantation was significantly higher among patients supported by LVADs (74%) than among those supported by the BiVAD (58%). This difference in survival rate was probably due to the patients' clinical condition before VAD placement. Clinical indices of illness such as fever, pulmonary edema, high-dose inotropic agents, and rising serum creatinine concentrations are better predictors of the need for posttransplant support with LVADs or right ventricular assist devices (RVADs) than are preoperative hemodynamic measures of RV function (74). Smedira et al. (75) have shown that pulmonary hypertension is "not" a risk factor for either RVAD support or death after LVAD placement.

To avoid RV dysfunction, patients' clinical condition should be optimized preoperatively. As noted above, pulmonary vascular unloading may be augmented intraoperatively by phosphodiesterase inhibitors and nitric oxide. Additional maneuvers include optimized oxygenation and avoidance of acidosis or hypercarbia to prevent pulmonary vasoconstriction. Meticulous hemostasis is mandatory to avoid the need for excessive transfusion; both the inflammatory mediators of transfusion and the volume load can lead to exacerbated pulmonary hypertension. Finally, careful attention to removing air from the pump is necessary because air embolism to the right coronary artery is probably the most common cause of early RV dysfunction (33).

Mechanical Complications and Device Malfunctions

Mechanical complications of ECMO are relatively common. In one series, oxygenator failure occurred in 43% of patients (2). The mean time to oxygenator failure was 42 hours; the number of oxygenator changes for each patient while on ECMO support was 2.25. Pump heads were changed in 6% of circuits because a clot was detected. Intracardiac clots occurred in 20% of patients, none of whom were treated with heparin.

Mechanical malfunction is less common with LVAD support than with ECMO support. Laboratory estimates of one-year reliability are 99.9% for the Novacor and 87% for the HeartMate. Catanese et al. (76) found that 14 outpatients with HeartMate LVADs experienced 29 controller malfunctions during 1640 days of support. Also not uncommon with the HeartMate is structural deterioration of the inflow valve over time. This deterioration typically manifests itself as an inflow-conduit leak with high pump flows and clinical signs and symptoms of congestive heart failure. Diagnosis is usually confirmed by TEE, which demonstrates a regurgitant jet; treatment may require replacement of the valve conduit or the entire pump (77). Other reported LVAD malfunctions include kinking of the driveline or the outflow graft and rupture of the inflow conduit (78).

EXPERIMENTAL DEVICES

Because of the limitations of current devices, clinical trials of experimental pumps are under way. Axial flow impeller pumps (Jarvik 2000, HeartMate II, NASA/DeBakey pump) are designed to address the need for smaller, quieter, less invasive mechanical assistance devices. The AbioCor TAH is intended to provide true biventricular support without the tether of a pneumatic controller.

Axial Flow Impeller Pumps

Initially based on the concept of the Archimedes screw, axial flow pumps have fewer moving parts and a smaller surface area that comes into contact with blood. These pumps are also easier to insert than current implantable VADs. The impeller is powered by an electromagnetic field that moves blood across the motor with minimal cell damage. Power may be provided by a small percutaneous driveline; however, a transcutaneous energy delivery system that eliminates existing drivelines is being developed. Early studies with axial flow pumps demonstrated that the left ventricle can be mechanically unloaded and that myocardial oxygen consumption is significantly reduced during axial support (79). Three axial flow devices are nearly ready for clinical use: the Jarvik 2000, the NASA/DeBakey VAD, and the HeartMate II.

Early studies with the Jarvik 2000 documented flow rates of as much as 7 L/min with minimal energy requirements (80). In studies of animals supported for as long as 123 days, Kaplon et al. (80) found no evidence of hemolysis, thromboembolism, or end-organ dysfunction. Westaby et al. (81) reported similar findings in ewes supported for as long as 198 days, and early clinical reports from the Texas Heart Institute (82) confirm these findings in humans.

Early clinical experience with the DeBakey VAD demonstrated safety and effectiveness in providing adequate circulatory support to patients with end-stage congestive heart failure (83,84). A detailed evaluation of the first 32 DeBakey impeller recipients found an 81% probability of survival at 30 days (83). Eleven patients underwent successful transplantation; 10 died while on support. In most instances, death was due to multiorgan failure; there was one device-related death. Bleeding related to anticoagulation was the principal complication; however, few patients experienced pump thrombus.

Like the Jarvik device, the HeartMate II demonstrated reasonable circulatory support with minimal complications in animal studies. After several iterations of pump design, the system has been tested successfully in more than 40 calves; the first human implant occurred in July 2000 (85). Multicenter safety and feasibility trials are expected in the near future.

Early concerns about continuous flow with lack of pulsatility have not been realized. For all of the devices tested both experimentally and clinically, excellent end-organ function has been maintained. This finding may be due in part to flow physiology. Moreover, variable preload to the pump from residual native LV contractility creates a pulse pressure. Although blood elements pass through an impeller, there has been little evidence of hemolysis. However, the need for anticoagulation may continue to pose limitations to device applicability. One problem yet to be addressed with these devices is the lack of a valve for maintaining unidirectional flow. In the event of a device malfunction, open regurgitation of blood into the LV is a possibility. Further clinical trials, particularly with totally implantable versions of these devices, are warranted.

AbioCor® Total Artificial Heart

The AbioCor TAH is a totally implantable electric device intended to function as a replacement heart (86). Although the need for true biventricular support may be limited, patients with fixed pulmonary hypertension and global myocardial dysfunction cannot be adequately supported with LVADs. The evolution from the large pneumatic drivers seen with either the Thoratec BiVAD or the CardioWest TAH to a totally implantable system with internal batteries and a transcutaneous energy delivery system is a tremendous technological advance, particularly for patients who need biventricular support.

The device is electrohydraulically actuated and can provide flows of up to 8 L/min. It consists of an energy converter and two blood pumps that act in unison as the compliance chamber for each other. All blood-contacting surfaces are made from polyurethane (Angioflex™), and unidirectional blood flow is ensured by four trileaflet valves. The TAH is attached to the atria and great vessels of the native heart with Dacron atrial cuffs and outflow grafts. The device is connected to an internal controller, a battery, and the transcutaneous energy delivery coil.

Dowling et al. (86) reported excellent 30-day outcomes in studies of 19 cows supported by the AbioCor TAH. There were no device-related deaths and no significant hemolysis; all animals showed normal hemodynamic function and end-organ function. Similar results were demonstrated by Frazier (87). Moreover, recent clinical studies of implantation into human recipients have confirmed the experimental findings (88,89). Although the first human recipient of the AbioCor TAH eventually died of a thromboembolic complication, he had not been maintained on any anticoagulation while on device support because of a bleeding diathesis. His short-term hemodynamic and clinical improvement was excellent. Future clinical evaluations will be necessary to determine the overall effectiveness of this device; however, the transition to a totally implantable system represents a landmark advancement in mechanical circulatory support.

SUMMARY

Because the supply of donor hearts available for transplantation is limited, mechanical circulatory assist devices are the most immediate and obvious solution to the need for advanced therapy for end-stage heart disease. Currently available devices can provide adequate perfusion to these patients; however, more widespread use of these first-generation VADs has been limited by complications, including bleeding, thromboembolism, infection, and mechanical failure. As the available technology advances, particularly with regard to device size, internal power sources, and remote monitoring capability, future devices will be able to enhance not only survival rates, but also quality of life.

REFERENCES

1. Hill JD, O'Brien TG, Murray JJ, et al. Prolonged extracorporeal oxygenation for acute post-traumatic respiratory failure (shock-lung syndrome). Use of the Bramson membrane lung. N Engl J Med 1972; 286(12):629–634.

2. Kaplon RJ, Smedira NG. Extracorporeal membrane oxygenation in adults. In: Goldstein DS, Oz MC, eds. Cardiac Assist Devices. Armonk, New York: Futura Publishing Company, 2000:263–273.

3. Rich PB, Awad SS, Crotti S, Hirschl RB, Bartlett RH, Schreiner RJ. A prospective comparison of atrio-femoral and femoro-atrial flow in adult venovenous extracorporeal life support. J Thorac Cardiovasc Surg 1998; 116(4):628–632.

4. Samuels LE, Holmes EC, Thomas MP, et al. Management of acute cardiac failure with mechanical assist: experience with the ABIOMED BVS 5000. Ann Thorac Surg 2001; 71(suppl 3):S67–S72.

5. Jett GK, Lazzara RR. Extracorporeal support: The ABIOMED BVS 5000. In: Goldstein DS, Oz MC, eds. Cardiac Assist Devices. Armonk, New York: Futura Publishing Company, 2000:235–250.

6. Ganzel BL, Gray LA Jr., Slater AD, Mavroudis C. Surgical techniques for the implantation of heterotopic prosthetic ventricles. Ann Thorac Surg 1989; 47(1):113–120.

7. Lohmann DP, McBride LR, Pennington DG, Swartz MT. Replacement of paracorporeal ventricular assist devices. Ann Thorac Surg 1992; 54(6):1226–1227.

8. Minami K, Arusoglu L, Koyanagi T, el-Banayosy A, Korner MM, Korfer R. Successful implantation of Thoratec assist device: wrapping of outflow conduit in Hemashield graft. Ann Thorac Surg 1997; 64(3): 861–862.

9. Rose EA, Levin HR, Oz MC, et al. Artificial circulatory support with textured interior surfaces. A counterintuitive approach to minimizing thromboembolism. Circulation 1994; 90(5 Pt 2):II87–II91.

10. McCarthy PM, Wang N, Vargo R. Preperitoneal insertion of the HeartMate 1000 IP implantable left ventricular assist device. Ann Thorac Surg 1994; 57(3):634–637.

11. Oz MC, Goldstein DJ, Rose EA. Preperitoneal placement of ventricular assist devices: an illustrated stepwise approach. J Card Surg 1995; 10:288–294.

12. Rose EA, Gelijns AC, Moskowitz AJ, et al. Randomized Evaluation of Mechanical Assistance for the Treatment of Congestive Heart Failure (REMATCH) Study Group. Long-term mechanical left ventricular assistance for end-stage heart failure. N Engl J Med 2001; 345(20):1435–1443.

13. Pennington DG, McBride LR, Swartz MT. Implantation technique for the Novacor left ventricular assist system. J Thorac Cardiovasc Surg 1994; 108(4):604–608.

14. Copeland J, Arabia F, Smith R, Nolan P. Intracorporeal support: the CardioWest total artificial heart. In: Goldstein DS, Oz MC, eds. Cardiac Assist Devices. Armonk, New York: Futura Publishing Company, 2000: 341–355.

15. Arabia FA, Copeland JG, Pavie A, Smith RG. Implantation technique for the CardioWest total artificial heart. Ann Thorac Surg 1999; 68(2):698–704.

16. Magovern GJ Jr., Magovern JA, Benckart DH, et al. Extracorporeal membrane oxygenation: preliminary results in patients with postcardiotomy cardiogenic shock. Ann Thorac Surg 1994; 57(6):1462–1471.

17. Stallion A, Cofer BR, Rafferty JA, Ziegler MM, Ryckman FC. The significant relationship between platelet count and haemorrhagic complications on ECMO. Perfusion 1994; 9(4):265–269.

18. Smedira NG, Hlozek CC, McCarthy PM. Mechanical support after cardiac surgery. Semin Cardiothor Vasc Anesth 1998; 2(1):66–77.

19. McManus ML, Kevy SV, Bower LK, Hickey PR. Coagulation factor deficiencies during initiation of extracorporeal membrane oxygenation. J Pediatr 1995; 126(6): 900–904.

20. Tandler R, Weyand M, Schmid C, Gradaus R, Schmidt C, Scheld HH. Long-term anticoagulation with recombinant hirudin in a patient on left ventricular assist device support. ASAIO J 2000; 46(6):792–794.

21. Muehrcke DD, McCarthy PM, Stewart RW, et al. Complications of extracorporeal life support systems using heparin-bound surfaces. The risk of intracardiac clot formation. J Thorac Cardiovasc Surg 1995; 110(3):843–851.

22. Muehrcke DD, McCarthy PM, Stewart RW, et al. Extracorporeal membrane oxygenation for postcardiotomy cardiogenic shock. Ann Thorac Surg 1996; 61(2):684–691.

23. Nagaya M, Futamura M, Kato J, Niimi N, Fukuta, S. Application of a new anticoagulant (Nafamostat Mesilate) to control hemorrhagic complications during extracorporeal membrane oxygenation—a preliminary report. J Pediatr Surg 1997; 32(4):531–535.

24. McCarthy PM, Smedira NO, Vargo RL, et al. One hundred patients with the HeartMate left ventricular assist device: evolving concepts and technology. J Thorac Cardiovasc Surg 1998; 115(4):904–912.

25. McBride LR, Naunheim KS, Fiore AC, Moroney DA, Swartz MT. Clinical experience with 111 Thoratec ventricular assist devices. Ann Thorac Surg 1999; 67(5): 1233–1239.

26. El-Banayosy A, Korfer R, Arusoglu L, et al. Device and patient management in a bridge-to-transplant setting. Ann Thorac Surg 2001; 71(suppl 3):S98–S102.

27. Hosenpud JD, Bennett LE, Keck BM, Fiol B, Boucek MM, Novick RJ. The Registry of the International Society for Heart and Lung Transplantation: Sixteenth Official Report—1999. J Heart Lung Transplant 1999; 18(7):611–626.

28. Pavie A, Szefner J, Leger P, Gandjbakhch I. Preventing, minimizing, and managing postoperative bleeding. Ann Thorac Surg 1999; 68:705–710.

29. Goldstein DJ, Seldomridge JA, Chen JM, et al. Use of aprotinin in LVAD recipients reduces blood loss, blood use, and preoperative mortality. Ann Thorac Surg 1995; 59(5):1063–1068.

30. Kaplon RJ, Gillinov MA, Smedira NG, et al. Vitamin K reduces bleeding in left ventricular assist device recipients. J Heart Lung Transplant 1999; 18(4):346–350.

31. Massad MG, Cook DJ, Schmitt SK, et al. Factors influencing HLA sensitization in implantable LVAD recipients. Ann Thorac Surg 1997; 64(4):1120–1125.

32. Moazami N, Itescu S, Williams MR, Argenziano M, Weinberg A, Oz MC. Platelet transfusions are associated with the development of anti-major histocompatibility complex class I antibodies in patients with left ventricular assist support. J Heart Lung Transplant 1998; 17(9):876–880.

33. Kasirajan V, McCarthy PM, Hoercher KJ, et al. Clinical experience with long-term use of implantable left ventricular assist devices: indications, implantation, and outcomes. Semin Thorac Cardiovasc Surg 2000; 12(3): 229–237.

34. Murphy PJ, Connery C, Hicks GL Jr., Blumberg N. Homologous blood transfusion as a risk factor for postoperative infection after coronary artery bypass graft operations. J Thorac Cardiovasc Surg 1992; 104(4):1092–1099.

35. Kasirajan V, Smedira NG, McCarthy JF, Casselman F, Boparai N, McCarthy PM. Risk factors for intracranial hemorrhage in adults on extracorporeal membrane oxygenation. Eur J Cardiothorac Surg 1999; 15(4): 508–514.

36. Pierce WS, Gray LA Jr., McBride LR, Frazier OH. Circulatory Support 1988. Other postoperative complications. Ann Thorac Surg 1989; 47(1):96–101.

37. Swartz MT, Lowdermilk GA, Moroney DA, McBride LR. Ventricular assist device support in patients with mechanical heart valves. Ann Thorac Surg 1999; 68(6): 2248–2251.

38. Schmid C, Weyand M, Nabavi DG, et al. Cerebral and systemic embolization during left ventricular support with the Novacor N100 device. Ann Thorac Surg 1998; 65(6):1703–1710.

39. Thomas CE, Jichici D, Petrucci R, Urrutia VC, Schwartzman RJ. Neurologic complications of the Novacor left ventricular assist device. Ann Thorac Surg 2001; 72(4):1311–1315.

40. Portner PM, Jansen PG, Oyer PE, Weldon DR, Ramasamy N. Improved outcomes with an implantable left ventricular assist system: a multicenter study. Ann Thorac Surg 2001; 71(1):205–209.

41. Copeland JG 3rd, Smith RG, Arabia FA, et al. Comparison of the CardioWest total artificial heart, the Novacor left ventricular assist system and the Thoratec ventricular assist system in bridge to transplantation. Ann Thorac Surg 2001; 71:S92–S97.

42. Frazier OH, Rose EA, Oz MC, et al. HeartMate LVAS Investigators. Left Ventricular Assist System. Multicenter clinical evaluation of the HeartMate vented electric left ventricular assist system in patients awaiting heart transplantation. J Thorac Cardiovasc Surg 2001; 122(6):1186–1195.

43. Minami K, el-Banayosy A, Sezai A, et al. Morbidity and outcome after mechanical ventricular support using Thoratec, Novacor, and HeartMate for bridging to heart transplantation. Artif Organs 2000; 24(6):421–426.

44. Steiner CK, Stewart DL, Bond SJ, Hornung CA, McKay VJ. Predictors of acquiring a nosocomial bloodstream infection on extracorporeal membrane oxygenation. J Pediatr Surg 2001; 36(3):487–492.

45. Kawahito K, Kobayashi E, Misawa Y, et al. Recovery from lymphocytopenia and prognosis after adult extracorporeal membrane oxygenation. Arch Surg 1998; 133(2):216–217.

46. Myers TJ, Khan T, Frazier OH. Infectious complications associated with ventricular assist systems. ASAIO J 2000; 46(6):S28–S36.

47. Korfer R, el-Banayosy A, Posival H, et al. Mechanical circulatory support: the Bad Oeynhausen experience. Ann Thorac Surg 1995; 59(suppl 2):S56–S63.

48. Arabia FA, Copeland JG, Smith RG, et al. Infections with the CardioWest total artificial heart. ASAIO J 1998; 44(5):M336–M339.

49. Hermann M, Weyand M, Greshake B, et al. Left ventricular assist device infection is associated with increased mortality but is not a contraindication to transplantation. Circulation 1997; 95(4):814–817.

50. Goldstein DJ, Oz MC, Rose EA. Implantable left ventricular assist devices. N Engl J Med 1998; 339(21): 1522–1533.

51. Ankersmit HJ, Tugulea S, Spanier T, et al. Activation-induced T-cell death and immune dysfunction after implantation of left-ventricular assist device. Lancet 1999; 354:550–555.

52. Griffith BP, Kormos RL, Nastala CJ, Winowich S, Pristas JM. Results of extended bridge to transplantation: window into the future of permanent ventricular assist devices. Ann Thorac Surg 1996; 61(1):396–398.

53. Springer WE, Wasler A, Radovancevic B, et al. Retrospective analysis of infection in patients undergoing support with left ventricular assist systems. ASAIO J 1996; 42(5):M763–M765.

54. Choi L, Choudri AF, Pillarisetty VG, et al. Development of an infection-resistant LVAD driveline: a novel approach to the prevention of device-related infections. J Heart Lung Transplant 1999; 18(11):1103–1110.

55. Jarvik R, Westaby S, Katsumata T, Pigott D, Evans RD. LVAD power delivery: a percutaneous approach to avoid infection. Ann Thorac Surg 1998; 65(2):470–473.

56. Mussivand T, Hendry PJ, Master RG, Holmes KS, Hum A, Keon WJ. A remotely controlled and powered artificial heart pump. Artif Organs 1996; 20(12): 1314–1319.

57. Marlinski E, Jacobs G, Deirmengian C, Jarvik R. Durability testing of components for the Jarvik 2000 completely implantable axial flow left ventricular assist device. ASAIO J 1998; 44(5):M741–M744.

58. Dowling RD, Etoch SW, Stevens KA, Johnson AC, Gray LA Jr. Current status of the AbioCor implantable replacement heart. Ann Thorac Surg 2001; 71(suppl 3): S147–S149.

59. Burke DJ, Burke E, Parsaie F, et al. The HeartMate II: design and development of a fully sealed axial flow left ventricular assist system. Artif Organs 2001; 25(5):380–385.

60. Prendergast TW, Todd BA, Beyer AF 3rd, et al. Management of left ventricular assist device infection with heart transplantation. Ann Thorac Surg 1997; 64(1):142–147.

61. Sinha P, Chen JM, Flannery M, Scully BE, Oz MC, Edwards NM. Infections during left ventricular assist device support do not affect posttransplant outcomes. Circulation 2000; 102(19 suppl 3):III194–III199.

62. Argenziano M, Catanese K, Moazami N, et al. The influence of infection on survival and successful transplantation in patients with left ventricular assist devices. J Heart Lung Transplant 1997; 16(8):822–831.

63. McCarthy PM, Schmitt SK, Vargo RL, Gordon S, Keys TF, Hobbs RE. Implantable LVAD infections: implications for permanent use of the device. Ann Thorac Surg 1996; 61(1):359–365.

64. Gordon SM, Schmitt SK, Jacobs M, et al. Nosocomial bloodstream infections in patients with implantable left ventricular assist devices. Ann Thorac Surg 2001; 72(3): 725–730.

65. Goldstein DJ, el-Amir NG, Ashton RC Jr., et al. Fungal infections in left ventricular assist device recipients. Incidence, prophylaxis, and treatment. ASAIO J 1995; 41(4):873–875.

66. Goldberg SP, Baddley JW, Aaron MF, Pappas PG, Holman WL. Fungal infections in ventricular assist devices. ASAIO J 2000; 46(6):S37–S40.

67. Skinner JL, Harris C, Aaron MF, et al. Cost-benefit analysis of extended antifungal prophylaxis in ventricular assist devices. ASAIO J 2000; 46(5):587–589.

68. Argenziano M, Choudhri AF, Moazami N, et al. Randomized, double-blind trial of inhaled nitric oxide in LVAD recipients with pulmonary hypertension. Ann Thorac Surg 1998; 65(2):340–345.

69. Kormos RL, Gasior TA, Antaki J, et al. Evaluation of right ventricular function during clinical left ventricular assistance. ASAIO Trans 1989; 35(3):547–550.

70. Gallagher RC, Kormos RL, Gasior TA, Murali S, Griffith BP, Hardesty RL. Univentricular support results in reduction of pulmonary resistance and improved right ventricular function. ASAIO Trans 1991; 37(3):M287–M288.

71. Charron M, Follansbee W, Ziady GM, Kormos RL. Assessment of biventricular cardiac function in patients with a Novacor left ventricular assist device. J Heart Lung Transplant 1994; 13(2):263–267.

72. Farrar D, Compton PG, Hershon JJ, Fonger JD, Hill JD. Right heart interaction with the mechanically assisted left heart. World J Surg 1985; 9(1):89–102.

73. Farrar DJ, Hill JD, Pennington DG, et al. Preoperative and postoperative comparison of patients with univentricular and biventricular support with the Thoratec ventricular assist device as a bridge to cardiac transplantation. J Thorac Cardiovasc Surg 1997; 113(1):202–209.

74. Kormos RL, Gasior TA, Kawai A, et al. Transplant candidate's clinical status rather than right ventricular

function defines need for univentricular versus biventricular support. J Thorac Cardiovasc Surg 1996; 111(4):773–782.

75. Smedira NG, Massad MG, Navia J, et al. Pulmonary hypertension is not a risk factor for RVAD use and death after left ventricular assist system support. ASAIO J 1996; 42(5):M733–M735.

76. Catanese KA, Goldstein DJ, Williams DL, et al. Outpatient left ventricular assist device support: a destination rather than a bridge. Ann Thorac Surg 1996; 62(3): 646–653.

77. Ferns J, Dowling R, Bhat G. Evaluation of a patient with left ventricular assist device dysfunction. ASAIO J 2001; 47(6):696–698.

78. Scheld HH, Soeparwata R, Schmid C, Loick M, Weyand M, Hammel D. Rupture of inflow conduits in the TCI-HeartMate system. J Thorac Cardiovasc Surg 1997; 114(2):287–289.

79. DeRose JJ Jr., Umana JP, Madigan JD, et al. Mechanical unloading with a miniature in-line axial flow pump as an alternative to cardiopulmonary bypass. ASAIO J 1997; 43(5):M421–M426.

80. Kaplon RJ, Oz MC, Kwiatkowski PA, et al. Miniature axial flow pump for ventricular assistance in children and small adults. J Thorac Cardiovasc Surg 1996; 111(1):13–18.

81. Westaby S, Katsumata T, Evans R, Pigott D, Taggart DP, Jarvik RK. The Jarvik 2000 Oxford System: increasing the scope of mechanical circulatory support. J Thorac Cardiovasc Surg 1997; 114(3):467–474.

82. Frazier OH, Myers TJ, Jarvik RK, et al. Research and development of an implantable, axial-flow left ventricular assist device: the Jarvik 2000 Heart. Ann Thorac Surg 2001; 71(suppl 3):S125–S132.

83. Noon GP, Morley DL, Irwin S, Abdelsayed SV, Benkowski RJ, Lynch BE. Clinical experience with the MicroMed DeBakey ventricular assist device. Ann Thorac Surg 2001; 71(suppl 3):S133–S138.

84. Wieselthaler GM, Schima H, Lassnigg AM, et al. Lessons learned from the first clinical implants of the DeBakey ventricular assist device axial pump: a single center report. Ann Thorac Surg 2001; 71(suppl 3): S139–S143.

85. Griffith BP, Kormos RL, Borovetz HS, et al. HeartMate II left ventricular assist system: from concept to first clinical use. Ann Thorac Surg 2001; 71(suppl 3): S116–S120.

86. Dowling RD, Etoch SW, Stevens K, et al. Initial experience with the AbioCor implantable replacement heart at the University of Louisville. ASAIO J 2000; 46(5):579–581.

87. Frazier OH. Future directions of cardiac assistance. Semin Thorac Cardiovasc Surg 2000; 12(3):251–258.

88. SoRelle R. Cardiovascular news. Totally contained AbioCor artificial heart implanted July 3, 2001. Circulation 2001; 104(3):E9005–E9006.

89. SoRelle R. Third Abiocor artificial heart implanted in Houston. Circulation 2001; 104(15):E9033–E9034.

30

Venous Thromboembolism

Yoram Klein

Division of Trauma and Emergency Surgery, Kaplan Medical Center, Rehovot and Department of Surgery, Hadassah EIN, Kerem Medical Center, Jerusalem, Israel

Enrique Ginzburg

Division of Trauma and Surgical Critical Care, DeWitt Daughtry Family Department of Surgery, University of Miami Miller School of Medicine, Miami, Florida, U.S.A.

Venous thromboembolism is a common and potentially lethal complication of trauma and surgery. This entity is composed of two main clinical conditions: deep venous thrombosis (DVT) and acute pulmonary embolism (PE). Because PE is most commonly the result of DVT, it is customary to consider both of these conditions as components of a venous thromboembolism syndrome, with many similarities in pathophysiology, prophylaxis, and treatment. This chapter will summarize current knowledge about the incidence, diagnosis, prophylaxis, and treatment of DVT and PE.

DEEP VENOUS THROMBOSIS
Overview

DVT after surgery or trauma is a serious complication that can occur despite all methods of prophylaxis. Prophylaxis is the key to prevention; however, expeditious diagnosis and management of DVT can prevent the potentially lethal complication of PE.

The components of Virchow's triad—stasis, hypercoagulability, and intimal injury—have been postulated as the main contributors to the formation of thrombus. Stasis occurs in the venous valve sinuses, as demonstrated in contrast studies of supine, immobilized patients. Stasis provides a nidus for the formation of thrombi that can propagate and cause venous obstruction; this obstruction results in edema. In 60% of patients, the thrombus propagates without obstruction; however, it is still susceptible to fragmentation when a long "free-floating tail" forms, and such thrombi result in a PE.

Hypercoagulability also contributes to the formation of DVT. Women who take oral contraceptives are three to six times more likely than other people in general to experience DVT. These women have also been shown to produce less of the inhibitor of factor X

(antithrombin III); it is the binding of antithrombin III to heparin subunits that produces the anticoagulant effect. In the general population, congenital deficiencies in the production of antithrombin III and in the production of protein S, protein C, and factor V-Leiden also result in hypercoagulability defects.

Injuries due to surgery or trauma affect the inherent fibrinolytic pathway that regulates systemic clot formation. After traumatic injuries, the production of antithrombin III decreases; these decreases predispose patients to clot formation in the absence of proper prophylaxis. Obesity, age, and malignancy also increase the risk of DVT because of their effect on one or more of the components of Virchow's triad.

Diagnosis

The choice of tests for diagnosing DVT depends on the clinical state (symptomatic or asymptomatic) of the patient's extremity. Currently, a variety of methods can be used to diagnose DVT: duplex ultrasonography (US), impedance plethysmography (IPG), venography, radioactive-labeled fibrinogen assays, magnetic resonance (MR) imaging, and computed tomographic (CT) venography. Each of these methods has advantages and disadvantages.

Duplex Ultrasonography

Duplex US is currently the most widely available method for diagnosing DVT and is considered the standard of care. It has the advantages of being rapid, cost-effective, and noninvasive. Its primary disadvantage is its relatively low sensitivity in recognizing asymptomatic DVT (1).

The diagnostic principle behind US is simple and is based on the fact that intraluminal thrombi produce an accelerated flow signal in the posterior tibial vein or the common femoral vein (2). Compression of these vessels should alter the flow signal: specifically, distal compression (below the probe) should augment the flow signal and proximal compression (above the probe) should interrupt it. Such alterations can also be produced by the Valsalva maneuver. If distal compression does not augment the flow or if the flow does not resume after release of proximal compression, venous thrombi are probably present.

Prospective studies have shown that compression US is highly sensitive and specific (>90% for both) in diagnosing symptomatic, acute, proximal DVT (3). The usefulness of compression US is limited, however, when patients are obese, when their legs are edematous, or when they suffer from chronic DVT. In addition, US is not reliable in diagnosing thrombi in the iliac veins; in such cases, MR imaging or venography should be used (4). The ultrasound probe can combine gray-scale, duplex, and color Doppler imaging, although a meta-analysis of data from multicenter trials demonstrated that real-time B-mode US, duplex US, and color flow Doppler US are not sensitive enough to diagnose asymptomatic acute proximal DVT (3). This study also emphasized the importance of the competency of the technician (3). Another study, published in the orthopedic literature, used duplex US to screen patients at the time of discharge from the hospital who had undergone an orthopedic procedure; the incidence of DVT was only 1% within 90 days of the procedure, a finding suggesting once again that the sensitivity of duplex US may depend on the skill of the technician (5).

Because it is difficult to distinguish recurrent DVT from chronic DVT, follow-up US performed at three months and six months after an episode of DVT should be used as a baseline for the detection of recurrent DVT.

Most cases of DVT of the upper extremity are caused by indwelling venous catheters. The sensitivity and specificity of US in detecting upper-extremity DVT are similar to those of US in detecting asymptomatic and symptomatic DVT of the lower extremity. PE occurs in as many as 36% of patients with upper-extremity DVT (6).

Impedance Plethysmography

IPG measures the volume response of the extremity to temporary occlusion of the venous system. The diagnosis of DVT depends on the rate of venous emptying of the extremity upon release of the tourniquet. If recording of the outflow wave is prolonged after the inflation cuff or tourniquet is released, the diagnosis of severe venous thrombosis can be made with 95% accuracy. The primary disadvantage of IPG is that it cannot diagnose DVT in the calf vein, nor can it differentiate a new thrombus from old post-thrombotic changes. The role of IPG as a therapeutic decision maker has decreased, but the procedure is still valuable in physiologic research studies.

The sensitivity of IPG in evaluating asymptomatic lower extremities is low, but its accuracy in diagnosing symptomatic DVT is excellent as long as such clinical conditions as pericarditis, cardiac failure, hypotension, and arterial insufficiency are absent.

Venography

Venography with the use of a contrast agent allows direct visualization of the venous system of an extremity. This procedure is the most accurate diagnostic method for DVT and is the standard against which other methods are compared in prospective, randomized studies. The most reliable criterion for the diagnosis of acute DVT is the appearance of a constant intraluminal-filling defect on two or more venographic views (7). False-positive results can be obtained if poor technique causes improper filling or external compression of veins.

One disadvantage of venography is its invasiveness, which may result in contrast-induced phlebitis that leads to thrombosis, allergic reactions, or contrast-induced nephropathy—a complication that occurs most frequently among patients with diabetes. Venography tends to be painful and can be technically difficult when patients are obese or when venous access is poor. In addition, venography is more time consuming and costlier than noninvasive tests. For these reasons, venography is generally not considered the standard of care.

Radioactively Labeled Fibrinogen

Radioactively labeled fibrinogen has been used to diagnose DVT since the advent of portable scintillation counters. When the count in the extremity is 20% higher than that in the heart, the diagnosis of underlying thrombosis is made. Radioactively labeled fibrinogen studies are sensitive in diagnosing DVT of the calf vein but have severe limitations in other applications. Several well-designed orthopedic studies have demonstrated that the use of this method is limited by its low sensitivity (8,9). It cannot detect thrombi in pelvic veins and it cannot be used to study extremities with healing wounds, ulcers, or any other inflammatory process.

D-Dimer Assays

D-dimer assays measure the specific degradation products of fibrin when it undergoes endogenous fibrinolysis. Early trials demonstrated that the various types of D-dimer assays differed in their sensitivity and specificity (10). The enzyme-linked immunosorbent assay is most sensitive, but this assay is costly and cannot be performed rapidly. The latex agglutination tests have the lowest specificity.

Recent studies have shown that D-dimer assays, which can be performed at the bedside, have a high negative predictive value. However, false-positive results are relatively common, and this problem fuels the controversy about the use of D-dimer assays as a first-line screening test. Rapid bedside assays are increasingly available, but additional outcome studies are necessary (11,12). Recently, one study recommended the use of D-dimer assays as the least expensive tests for initial screening and suggested coupling this test with US if the results of the assay were positive (13).

Magnetic Resonance Imaging

The most recent development in the diagnosis of DVT is the use of MR imaging, which can demonstrate occlusive and nonocclusive intraluminal thrombi. Early reports suggested that MR imaging has a sensitivity and specificity of 90% to 100% in detecting symptomatic DVT (1). The value of using MR imaging to screen patients with asymptomatic disease awaits further study.

MR imaging has few promising advantages except for its impressive sensitivity and specificity. It is probably the best test for diagnosing DVT in pelvic veins, especially in the noniliac veins, which can be assessed by no other diagnostic method, including venography. The contour of the vein walls and the appearance of the perivenous tissue may be used as markers to distinguish acute DVT from chronic conditions. Another appealing feature of MR imaging is that it is noninvasive and carries no risk of renal impairment. In addition, MR imaging is unique in that it can diagnose other conditions of the extremity that cause DVT-like symptoms. Pathological conditions such as cellulitis, edema, and joint inflammation are readily demonstrated by MR imaging. The primary disadvantages of MR imaging are its cost and the possibility that it may not be available in remote rural institutions. Because MR imaging is usually not an option for patients with indwelling metallic devices, its use may be precluded for patients in the early postoperative period or those who have been treated with metal instrumentation for fractures.

Summary

At present, no findings support routine screening for DVT when patients exhibit no symptoms. However, each diagnostic center should develop its own algorithm for screening patients with symptoms that suggest a diagnosis of DVT; such algorithms should be based on the institution's available human and technologic resources.

Prophylaxis

Ongoing studies and advances in chemotherapy and technology have resulted in frequent changes in the prophylaxis against DVT among postoperative and trauma patients. Many studies have shown the effectiveness of prophylaxis in preventing thromboembolism. The current effort is directed at finding the optimal method of preventing DVT, with a focus on effectiveness and safety.

Low-Dose Heparin

The time-honored drug heparin is probably still the most commonly used method of prophylaxis against DVT.

Heparin's mechanism of action is based on the potentiation of antithrombin, which, in turn, inhibits a cascade of procoagulation factors, especially IIa and Xa. Heparin has been shown to decrease the risk of DVT by 60% to 70%, although its effectiveness varies according to the specific procedure undergone by the patient (14). The main adverse effects of heparin therapy are bleeding (usually hematoma in the operative wound) and the rare but dangerous occurrence of heparin-induced thrombocytopenia.

Low-Molecular-Weight Heparin

Low-molecular-weight heparin (LMWH) is a fractionated heparin with fewer pentasaccharide chains than other forms of heparin. Several products with slightly different chemical and kinetic properties are commercially available. Because of its reduced molecular weight, LMWH has less effect on factor IIa than do other heparins, although its inhibitory effect on factor Xa is still substantial. Theoretically, this property should increase the effectiveness of LMWH and give it a safer therapeutic profile and better pharmacodynamic properties than unfractionated heparin (UFH). After general surgery, prophylaxis with LMWH offered the same protection against DVT as prophylaxis with heparin (15). LMWH is 2 to 10 times more expensive than heparin, but its pharmacodynamic properties are better; this advantage may reduce the difference in cost between the two treatments. LMWH has been shown to be more effective and safer than UFH for patients undergoing orthopedic procedures and for those who have suffered trauma; thus, it is currently the best treatment choice for these patients (16). The risk of heparin-induced thrombocytopenia is lower with LMWH than with UHF, but LMWH should not be considered an alternative to UFH for patients with this syndrome. This problem will be solved in the future by new investigational chemotherapy agents with heparinoid compounds.

Compression Devices

The fear of postoperative bleeding prompted the implementation of lower-extremity compression devices ranging from simple elastic compression stockings to sophisticated pneumatic compressive devices (PCDs). All of these devices are used in an attempt to minimize the effect of immobilization and blood stasis. After general surgery, the prophylactic effectiveness of PCDs is similar to that of low-dose heparin (14). A recent study has demonstrated no significant difference in DVT between compression devices and LMWH in trauma patients (17). The theory that sequential compression of the extremity may activate the fibrinolysis cascade has not been shown to have clinical significance, and the use of PCDs on the upper extremities of patients with trauma to the lower extremities has not proved to be beneficial.

Summary

For trauma patients, the best prophylaxis against DVT is the use of compression devices. LMWH should be used when casts or hardware on the lower extremities preclude the use of bilateral leg compression devices. If the patient is receiving suboptimal mechanical or chemical anticoagulation, duplex US screening for DVT should be considered (14). When both anticoagulation and mechanical compression are contraindicated, as they are, for example, among patients with spinal cord transection or severe pelvic fractures, PE prophylaxis with an inferior vena cava filter (IVCF) should be considered.

Treatment

The mainstay of DVT treatment is full anticoagulation with intravenously administered adjusted-dose UFH or subcutaneously administered LMWH. Numerous studies and meta-analyses have compared the two methods of treatment. Although most studies have shown no difference in the effectiveness of the two methods of prophylaxis, a meta-analysis of 11 randomized studies found that severe bleeding is less common with LMWH than with UFH (18). Heparin should be the initial treatment for DVT; a bolus of 80 U/kg should be followed by maintenance infusion of 18 U/kg/hr until the patient's partial thromboplastin time is 46 to 70 seconds. Dosages of subcutaneously administered LMWH differ according to the preparations of the individual drugs. Long-term anticoagulation with oral warfarin [adjusted to achieve an international normalized ratio (INR) of 2–3] should be started on the first day after heparin therapy is initiated. After five days, the initial treatment with intravenously administered heparin or LMWH should be discontinued if the INR is higher than 2. LMWH has been used successfully as long-term therapy. Long-term anticoagulation should be continued for 6 to 12 weeks in cases of symptomatic calf-vein thrombosis, for three to six months after the first incidence of proximal DVT, and for life in cases of recurrent venous thromboembolism among patients with chronic risk factors for thromboembolism (19). Although more aggressive treatment with thrombectomy or thrombolytic therapy has been used, it is usually reserved for cases with complicated massive unresolved ileofemoral thrombosis.

Promising New Strategies for Thromboprophylaxis

Recently, new prophylactic medications have been developed. These drugs, known as pentasaccharides, are more effective than LMWH for patients who have undergone hip replacement. The disadvantages of the pentasaccharides are that they cost more than heparin, they are associated with increased bleeding among patients undergoing knee replacement, and their anticoagulant properties cannot be reversed. Several other orally administered prophylactic medications are being investigated.

Complications

The most common complication of DVT is the postphlebitic syndrome (PPS), which will affect as many as 30% of patients with DVT and will cause substantial disability in 7% of patients (20). PPS has a range of symptoms characterized by leg swelling, edema, and skin discoloration leading to ulcers. The syndrome is believed to be the result of venous hypertension caused by outflow obstruction and valvular incompetence. The risk of PPS is highest among patients with recurrent ipsilateral DVT (21). Conservative treatment with graduated compression stockings, weight reduction, and continous nursing care has been shown to reduce the symptoms of 30% of patients, but for approximately two-thirds of patients, the symptoms did not improve or even worsened (22).

Another rare but feared complication of severe venous outflow obstruction is phlegmasia cerulea dolens. This devastating condition results from increased interstitial pressure that compromises tissue perfusion and leads to progressive ischemia. The mortality rate associated with this condition is estimated to be 30% to 40%, with tissue loss appearing in 50% of patients. Aggressive treatment with thrombolysis, fasciotomy, and thrombectomy is necessary once anticoagulation therapy fails (23).

The recurrence of DVT despite adequate treatment depends on the risk factors of each patient. In a study (24) of recurrent DVT, the risk of recurrence approached 30% after eight years. The risk of recurrent DVT was highest among patients with malignancy and lowest among those who had suffered trauma (24).

PULMONARY EMBOLISM
Overview

One of the most devastating experiences for any surgeon is to perform a successful operation or to repair a complex injury, only to have the patient succumb to a massive unexpected PE. The methods of diagnosing PE are constantly evolving and the management of this complication remains controversial.

Incidence

PE most commonly results from thrombi in the popliteal veins and the veins proximal to them in the lower extremity, although half of patients with PE have no detectable DVT. The risk factors for PE are similar to those for DVT because the two conditions occur at different stages of the same disease process. For patients undergoing surgery, those risk factors include increased age, prolonged immobility, malignancy, and trauma. Any thrombophilic condition will also increase the risk of PE and DVT. Rarely, patients undergoing surgery may experience PE in association with the presence of a central venous catheter (25).

Autopsy studies performed before prophylactic measures came into use detected PE in 4% to 16% of patients who had died of traumatic injury, and PE was considered to be the direct cause of death in approximately half of these patients (26,27). Currently, PE occurs in approximately 2% of patients undergoing general surgery without prophylaxis. The use of prophylaxis reduces this overall incidence by more than 50%: with prophylaxis, PE occurs in fewer than 1% of patients undergoing general surgery and in only 0.3% to 2% of patients who have suffered trauma (14). The risk of PE for patients undergoing general surgery is related to each patient's risk factors and to the nature of the procedure. The risk of PE for patients who have suffered trauma is most closely related to the severity of the injury and to the presence of specific injuries involving fractures of the spine, head, pelvis, and long bones (28). For trauma patients, 6% of PEs will occur within the first day after injury and 25% will occur during the first week after injury (29), probably because prophylaxis cannot be administered to these patients early in their treatment course. Thus, PE is the third most common cause of death among trauma patients.

Diagnosis
Physical Examination

The fact that PE is often unsuspected underscores the low sensitivity of the signs and symptoms of this disease. In fact, PE is one of the most common unsuspected causes of death and is often detected only during autopsy. PE should be suspected whenever sudden, unexplained dyspnea occurs. All of the other classic signs, such as pleuritic pain and hemoptysis, are nonspecific for diagnosis. Other signs and symptoms of PE include low-grade fever, pleural rub, and accentuated second heart sound.

Whether hemodynamic-cardiac signs will be evident depends on the extent of the embolus and the degree of acute right heart dysfunction that results. The hemodynamic-cardiac signs can be mild such as tachycardia and lightheadedness but massive obstruction can cause hypotension, cyanosis, neck vein distension, and sudden cardiac arrest (30).

Electrocardiography

The importance of electrocardiography (ECG) in diagnosing PE has declined with the development of high-technology imaging. ECG changes indicative of PE include axis deviation and nonspecific ST-wave and T-wave segment abnormalities in the lateral leads. The diagnostic pattern of the S1Q3T3 sign, right bundle branch block, P pulmonale, and right axis deviation is present in only one-third of patients with massive PE who exhibit clinical signs of acute cor pulmonale. Other nonspecific ECG changes will occur in approximately 87% of patients with proven PE and no underlying cardiac disease (31).

Arterial Blood Gas Analysis

Arterial blood gas analysis is probably the first test ordered by most physicians when PE is suspected because dyspnea and tachycardia are the most common symptoms presented. Hypoxemia is common but is not always present, especially in young patients with no underlying pulmonary pathology. Ten percent of patients with acute PE will have no demonstrable hypoxemia [Prospective Investigation of Pulmonary Embolism Diagnosis (PIOPED) study)] (32).

For approximately one-third of patients with PE who are younger than 40, the partial pressure of oxygen in the plasma phase of arterial blood (PaO_2) will be higher than 80 mmHg (33). For 86% of patients with PE, the alveolar–arterial (a–A) pressure gradient is elevated; thus, the a–A value is considered to be a more sensitive diagnostic indicator than the PaO_2 value, although it can also be normal in patients with PE who do not have underlying lung pathology. In general, hypoxemia or an elevated a–A gradient can indicate the possibility of PE, but normal values cannot rule out the diagnosis (34).

Plain Chest Radiography

The results of plain chest radiography [chest X ray (CXR)] are abnormal but nonspecific for most patients with PE, except for the rare occasion when PE causes lung infarction with its suggestive wedge-shaped consolidation. Other radiographic signs specific for PE include the Westermark sign (decreased vascular marking). CXR is a valuable diagnostic tool because it can detect other pathological conditions that may explain the clinical picture, such as pneumothorax or pneumonia.

D-Dimer Assays

The advantages and disadvantages of D-dimer assays are the same for patients with suspected PE and for patients with suspected DVT. The negative predictive value of a plasma D-dimer value of less than 500 ng/mL is 95%. Unfortunately, D-dimer values are low in 25% of patients who do not have venous thromboembolism. Currently, no published results support the use of D-dimer assays to rule out PE (1).

Ventilation/Perfusion Scans

For many years, the ventilation/perfusion (V/Q) scan has been the cornerstone of the diagnostic work-up for suspected PE. The effort expended in finding other diagnostic methods proves the poor performance of the V/Q scan. The study uses two scans: one after intravenous injection of a radioisotope to evaluate lung perfusion and the other after inhalation of the radioisotope for evaluation of ventilation. The results of the scan are read as normal or as demonstrating low, intermediate, or high probability of PE. The main shortcoming of the test is that most types of coexisting lung disease affect the interpretation of the ventilation scan and, to some extent, that of the perfusion scan. When the results of CXR are normal, approximately 10% of V/Q scans will be interpreted as demonstrating intermediate probability of PE, but this number can be as high as 60% to 70% when CXR demonstrates conditions such as chronic lung disease or pneumonia. Thus, the diagnostic interpretation of V/Q scans is difficult.

Most of the findings associated with the V/Q scan are from the PIOPED. This multicenter study compared the effectiveness of the V/Q scan for diagnosing PE with that of pulmonary angiography and autopsy studies (32). PIOPED demonstrated that better diagnostic accuracy is obtained when the level of clinical suspicion is combined with the results of the V/Q scan. The study showed that 96% of patients for whom the clinical suspicion of PE was high and whose V/Q results indicated a high probability of PE did in fact have a PE. Unfortunately, 40% of the patients for whom the clinical suspicion of PE was high but whose V/Q results indicated a low probability of PE also had a PE. When the clinical suspicion of PE was low, only 56% of patients whose V/Q results indicated a high probability of PE did indeed have a PE. Because CXR often yields abnormal results, especially when patients are being treated with mechanical ventilation, some physicians advocate using only the perfusion scan rather than both parts of the V/Q scan. One study showed that the diagnostic accuracy of the perfusion scan alone was similar to that of the full V/Q scan (35).

The treatment of patients whose V/Q scanning results are inconclusive is controversial. One option is to perform serial noninvasive studies of the lower extremities in an attempt to detect DVT. When the results of V/Q scanning indicate a low probability of PE and the results of DVT studies are negative, the incidence of PE is 25% if the level of clinical suspicion is high (36). The treatment of these patients should be tailored to the clinical situation. All patients whose V/Q scanning results indicate an intermediate or high probability of PE should be treated with anticoagulation measures.

Pulmonary Angiography

Pulmonary angiography is the gold standard for the diagnosis of PE. This study should be performed if other less-invasive tests fail to confirm or rule out a diagnosis of PE. The procedure begins with catheterization of a central vein; the catheter is advanced through the right heart to the pulmonary artery. The lobar or segmental arteries should be injected selectively. The presence of an intraluminal filling defect on two angiographic views is considered diagnostic for PE. Secondary diagnostic criteria are reduced flow, tortuous peripheral vessels, and delayed venous phase (37).

Because pulmonary angiography is the most invasive method of diagnosing PE, it is associated with the highest rate of complications. The risk of serious complications after this study is estimated at approximately 4% (38). Most complications are related to the contrast agent and the cateterization procedures used, but some critically ill patients with pulmonary hypertension and cor pulmonale may experience severe hemodynamic compromise and even cardiac arrest (39).

Helical Computed Tomography

Technological advances in CT scanning during recent years have increased the use of this diagnostic method. During the past decade, the use of helical computed tomography (HCT) as part of the diagnostic work-up for PE has gained increasing popularity. HCT is appealing because it is less invasive than pulmonary angiography and because it can also demonstrate other pathological conditions of the thorax. The main disadvantage of HCT is that it only poorly shows peripheral areas and horizontally oriented vessels. HCT undoubtedly misses some peripheral PEs, but the clinical relevance of these PEs is uncertain. The sensitivity of HCT in detecting PEs in the main, lobar, and segmental (until the fourth order) pulmonary arteries is estimated at more than 90% (40).

Not all studies support the reliability of HCT as a first-line method of diagnosing PE. At least two studies found that HCT was less sensitive than pulmonary angiography in diagnosing PE; disagreement among radiologists about the interpretation of HCT findings, including centrally located PEs, contributed to this lower sensitivity (41,42). In most centers, however, HCT has been adopted as a diagnostic method.

Magnetic Resonance Imaging

The newest method for diagnosing PE is MR imaging. As is true of HCT, MR imaging has not been evaluated in large, controlled studies; thus, we have only limited definitive information about its performance. Only some small pilot studies have shown that the sensitivity and specificity of MR imaging in detecting PE are good (43). Currently, we do not have enough information to support the routine use of this costly method for diagnosing PE.

Echocardiography

Although transthoracic or transesophageal echocardiography has occasionally demonstrated an embolus in the main pulmonary artery, the most common use of these studies is to evaluate right heart dysfunction. Right heart failure is the final cause of death for patients who suffer a massive PE. Although global or regional right ventricle dyskinesia is evident in more than 80% of patients with PE, it is nonspecific for diagnosis and can be associated with other clinically similar conditions such as chronic obstructive pulmonary disease. The role of echocardiography in diagnosing PE remains to be defined.

Summary

Although we have no definitive information about the value of HCT and MR imaging in the diagnosis of PE, these methods are widely used in place of V/Q scans. Prospective studies are currently underway to investigate the accuracy of these modalities.

Prophylaxis and Treatment
Prophylaxis Against Pulmonary Embolism

Prophylaxis is the first line of defense against PE. Administering low-dose heparin reduces the risk of fatal PE from 0.8% to 0.2% (14). Unfortunately, prophylaxis is not perfect: approximately 80% of trauma patients who experience PE received adequate prophylaxis (28).

Treatment for Established Deep Venous Thrombosis or Pulmonary Embolism

Full anticoagulation is the treatment of choice for DVT and PE. This therapy will reduce the risk of proximal thrombus propagation in the deep vein system and in the pulmonary arteries, and will also reduce the risk of recurrent PE.

Inferior Vena Cava Filter

The concept of interrupting the flow through the IVC so as to prevent the passage of emboli from the venous system of the lower extremity was first introduced in 1960. The rationale behind using vena cava interruption is that some form of treatment is needed for the substantial number of patients for whom anticoagulation is not an option or who have experienced complications related to anticoagulation. The first procedure involved ligation of the IVC; however, the high morbidity and mortality rates associated with this procedure prevented it from gaining popularity. Use of the IVCF began in 1967, but this procedure was associated with a nearly 70% risk of IVC thrombosis and occlusion. A breakthrough in this techique occurred in 1973 with the development of the Geenfield–Cimray filter; use of this filter lowered the rate of long-term vena cava occlusion to less than 5%. In the early 1980s, the next technical advance came in the form of percutanous insertion of the IVCF (44). Currently, the two most commonly used filters are the titanium Greenfield filter and the bird's nest filter that has a larger diameter.

Insertion of the IVCF usually takes place in the invasive radiology suite. The first step in the procedure is venographic measurement of the vena cava; the appropriate filter is then placed under the right renal vein. Recently, it has been demonstrated that the filter can be inserted at the bedside with ultrasonographic guidance (45). Experiments indicate that retrievable or temporary filters may offer short-term protection and reduce the incidence of long-term complications (46).

The complications associated with the use of IVCFs can be early or late. The most common early complication is thrombosis of the superficial femoral vein; this complication is related to the size of the introducer. The recent development of introducers with smaller diameters may reduce the incidence of this complication. Other early complications include malpositioning of the filters; this complication occurs in 7% of placement procedures. Late complications include dislodgement of the filter, as a result of erroneous placement in the IVC, and tilting of the filter. IVC thrombosis occurs in 2% to 20% of cases, but recanalization will occur within four years in almost all cases. The most common late complication is DVT. About half of patients with permanent IVCFs will experience DVT, and most of them will exhibit clinical symptoms of venous insufficiency (47). Recurrent PE after insertion of an IVCF has been reported to occur in 3% of patients, mainly those with chronic hypercoagulable conditions such as cancer (48).

There is no universal agreement about some indications for IVCF insertion. Most physicians agree that an IVCF should be placed in patients who have survived a massive PE but whose cardiopulmonary reserve is so limited that another embolic event would be devastating. The same holds true for patients who have undergone pulmonary embolectomy. The primary controversy is related to the use of an IVCF as a prophylactic measure for high-risk patients who have not experienced a documented thromboembolic event. Currently, no studies support the routine use of IVCFs for these patients as prophylaxis against PE.

Thrombolytic Therapy

As described above, the routine treatment for PE is anticoagulation with intravenously administered heparin or subcutaneously administered LMWH. Such treatment will reduce the risk of recurrent emboli and the propogation of the existing thrombi. In most cases, recanalization of the obstructed pulmonary artery will take place. In extreme situations, when massive PE induces significant right heart failure and hemodynamic instability, the increased right heart afterload must be resolved quickly. In these rare situations, thrombolytic therapy with streptokinase, urokinase, or tissue plasminogen activator may be lifesaving. The most serious risk, naturally, is bleeding, but this risk should be weighed against the high mortality rates experienced by patients with massive pulmonary emboli who are in an unstable condition. Although there are reports of the administration of thrombolytic agents to such patients by systemic or local infusion, we do not have sufficient information to determine the success rate and the risks associated with this treatment. However, the use of thrombolytic therapy should be considered when patients are in this desperate situation (19).

Pulmonary Embolectomy

Another treatment option for patients with massive PE whose condition is rapidly deteriorating is surgical pulmonary embolectomy. This procedure is a valid option especially when thrombolysis has failed or is contraindicated. The mortality rate associated with this procedure has been reported to be as high as 75%. Pulmonary embolectomy has not been performed often enough to allow us to evaluate its effectiveness (19). Most authorities recommend the placement of an IVCF after embolectomy.

A few recent reports have described attempts to mechanically fragment and extricate massive PEs by using a percutaneous rotating catheter. Promising results have been achieved with or without follow-up treatment with thrombolytic therapy, and the complication rate is very low (49).

Summary

If possible, every patient who suffers a PE should receive anticoagulation therapy with adjusted-dose intravenously administered heparin or subcutaneously administered LMWH. If anticoagulation therapy is contraindicated, fails, or produces complications, an IVCF should be placed. An IVCF should also be considered for patients with massive PE and low cardiopulmonary reserve or for those who have undergone pulmonary embolectomy. The use of prophylactic IVCFs is sometimes recommended for high-risk patients (e.g., those with spine or head injuries) for whom anticoagulation is contraindicated. When patients are in a hemodynamically unstable condition with acute cor pulmonale resulting from massive PE, decisions about whether to use thrombolytic therapy or surgical (or percutaneous, in the future) pulmonary embolectomy must be made for each case individually.

Outcome

PE is associated with a high mortality rate: 10% to 40% of high-risk patients will die (50). Of those patients who survive the initial event, 1.5% will die of recurrent PE within a year (51).

Occasionally, chronic pulmonary hypertension occurs as a result of recurrent nonfatal PE. This condition is readily diagnosed with V/Q scans. Surgical thrombectomy may be necessary so as to avoid the risk of right heart failure and deteriorating lung function (14).

The Future

Currently, researchers are investigating new pentasaccharides and are studying the use of temporary vena cava occlusion devices. The findings are promising thus far, but further investigation is necessary.

REFERENCES

1. Tapson VF, Carroll BA, Davidson BL, et al. The diagnostic approach to acute venous thromboembolism. Clinical practice guideline. American Thoracic Society. Am J Respir Crit Care Med 1999; 160(3):1043–1066.
2. Greenfield LJ. Complications of venous thrombosis and pulmonary embolism. In: Greenfield LJ, ed. Complications in Surgery and Trauma. 2nd ed. Philadelphia: Lippincott, 1984:406–421.
3. Tapson VF, Carroll BA, Davidson BL, et al. The diagnostic approach to acute venous thromboembolism. Clinical practice guideline. American Thoracic Society. Am J Respir Crit Care Med 1999; 160(3):43, 68, 90.
4. Tapson VF, Carroll BA, Davidson BL, et al. The diagnostic approach to acute venous thromboembolism. Clinical practice guideline. American Thoracic Society. Am J Respir Crit Care Med 1999; 160(3):54.
5. Tapson VF, Carroll BA, Davidson BL, et al. The diagnostic approach to acute venous thromboembolism. Clinical practice guideline. American Thoracic Society. Am J Respir Crit Care Med 1999; 160(3):103.
6. Tapson VF, Carroll BA, Davidson BL, et al. The diagnostic approach to acute venous thromboembolism. Clinical practice guideline. American Thoracic Society. Am J Respir Crit Care Med 1999; 160(3):114.
7. Tapson VF, Carroll BA, Davidson BL, et al. The diagnostic approach to acute venous thromboembolism. Clinical practice guideline. American Thoracic Society. Am J Respir Crit Care Med 1999; 160(3):8.
8. Lensing AW, Hirsh J. 125I-fibrinogen leg scanning: reassessment of its role for the diagnosis of venous thrombosis in postoperative patients. Thromb Haemost 1993; 69:2–7.
9. Cruickshank MK, Levine MN, Hirsh J, et al. An evaluation of impedance plethysmography and 125I-fibrinogen leg scanning in patients following hip surgery. Thromb Haemost 1989; 62:830–834.
10. Elias A, Aptel I, Huc B, et al. D-dimer test and diagnosis of deep vein thrombosis: a comparative study of 7 assays. Thromb Haemost 1996; 76:518–522.
11. Roussi J, Bentolila S, Boudaoud L, et al. Contribution of D-dimer determination in the exclusion of deep venous thrombosis in spinal cord injury patients. Spinal Cord 1999; 37:548–552.
12. Tapson VF, Carroll BA, Davidson BL, et al. The diagnostic approach to acute venous thromboembolism. Clinical practice guideline. American Thoracic Society. Am J Respir Crit Care Med 1999; 160(3):138.
13. Perone N, Bounameaux H, Perrier A. Comparison of four strategies for diagnosing deep vein thrombosis: a cost-effectiveness analysis. Am J Med 2001; 110:33–40.
14. Geerts WH, Heit JA, Clagett GP, et al. Prevention of venous thromboembolism. Chest 2001; 119:132S–175S.
15. Nurmohamed MT, Rosendaal FR, Buller HR, et al. Low-molecular-weight heparin versus standard heparin in general and orthopaedic surgery: a meta-analysis. Lancet 1992; 340:152–156.
16. Hirsh J, Warkentin TE, Shaughnessy SG, et al. Heparin and low-molecular-weight heparin mechanisms of action, pharmacokinetics, dosing, monitoring, efficacy, and safety. Chest 2001; 119:64S–94S.
17. Ginzburg E, Cohn SM, Lopez J, Jackowski J, Brown M, Hameed SM. Randomized clinical trial of intermittent pneumatic compression and low molecular weight heparin in trauma. Br J Surg 2003; 90:1338–1344.
18. Gould MK, Dembitzer AD, Doyle RL, Hastie TJ, Garber AM. Low-molecular-weight heparins compared with unfractionated heparin for the treatment of acute deep

venous thrombosis: a meta-analysis of randomized, controlled trials. Ann Intern Med 1999; 130:800–809.

19. Hyers TM, Agnelli G, Hull RD, et al. Antithrombotic therapy for venous thromboembolic disease. Chest 2001; 119:176S–193S.

20. Hyers TM. Venous thromboembolism. Am J Respir Crit Care Med 1999; 159:1–14.

21. Bernardi E, Prandoni P. The post-thrombotic syndrome. Curr Opin Pulm Med 2000; 6(4):335–342.

22. Milne AA, Ruckley CV. The clinical course of patients following extensive deep venous thrombosis. Eur J Vasc Surg 1994; 8(1):56–59.

23. Patel NH, Plorde JJ, Meissner M. Catheter-directed thrombolysis in the treatment of phlegmasia cerulea dolens. Ann Vasc Surg 1998; 12:471–475.

24. Prandoni P, Villalta S, Bagatella P, et al. The clinical course of deep-vein thrombosis. Prospective long-term follow-up of 528 symptomatic patients. Haematologica 1997; 82(4):423–428.

25. Rogers JZ, Thomas P, Apovian C, Jensen GL. Pulmonary embolus as a complication of a central venous catheter. Nutrition 1996; 12:271–273.

26. McCartney JS. Pulmonary embolism following trauma. Surg Gynecol Obstet 1935; 61:369–379.

27. Sevitt S, Gallagher N. Venous thrombosis and pulmonary embolism: a clinico-pathological study in injured and burned patients. Br J Surg 1961; 48:475–489.

28. Winchell RJ, Hoyt DB, Walsh JC, Simons RK, Eastman AB. Risk factors associated with pulmonary embolism despite routine prophylaxis: implications for improved protection. J Trauma 1994; 37:600–606.

29. Owings JT, Kraut E, Battistella F, Cornelius JT, O'Malley R. Timing of the occurrence of pulmonary embolism in trauma patients. Arch Surg 1997; 132:862–867.

30. Tai NR, Atwal AS, Hamilton G. Modern management of pulmonary embolism. Br J Surg 1999; 86:853–868.

31. The urokinase pulmonary embolism trial: a national cooperative study. Circulation 1973; 47:II1–II108.

32. The PIOPED Investigators. Value of the ventilation/perfusion scan in acute pulmonary embolism. Results of the Prospective Investigation of Pulmonary Embolism Diagnosis (PIOPED). JAMA 1990; 263:2753–2759.

33. Green RM, Meyer TJ, Dunn M, Glassroth J. Pulmonary embolism in younger adults. Chest 1992; 101:1507–1511.

34. Stein PD, Terrin ML, Hales CA, et al. Clinical, laboratory, roentgenographic, and electrocardiographic findings in patients with acute pulmonary embolism and no pre-existing cardiac or pulmonary disease. Chest 1991; 100:598–603.

35. Stein PD, Terrin ML, Gottschalk A, Alavi A, Henry JW. Value of ventilation/perfusion scans versus perfusion scans alone in acute pulmonary embolism. Am J Cardiol 1992; 69:1239–1241.

36. Stein PD, Hull RD, Saltzman HA, Pineo G. Strategy for diagnosis of patients with suspected pulmonary embolism. Chest 1993; 103:1553–1559.

37. Newman GE. Pulmonary angiography in pulmonary embolic disease. J Thorac Imaging 1989; 4:28–39.

38. Stein PD, Athanasoulis C, Alavi A, et al. Complications and validity of pulmonary angiography in acute pulmonary embolism. Circulation 1992; 85:462–468.

39. Mills SR, Jackson DC, Older RA, Heaston DK, Moore AV. The incidence, etiologies, and avoidance of complications of pulmonary angiography in a large series. Radiology 1980; 136:295–299.

40. Remy-Jardin M, Remy J, Artaud D, Deschildre F, Fribourg M, Beregi JP. Spiral CT of pulmonary embolism: technical considerations and interpretive pitfalls. J Thorac Imaging 1997; 12:103–117.

41. Drucker EA, Rivitz SM, Shepard JA, et al. Acute pulmonary embolism: assessment of helical CT for diagnosis. Radiology 1998; 209:235–241.

42. Velmahos GC, Vassiliu P, Wilcox A, et al. Spiral computed tomography for the diagnosis of pulmonary embolism in critically ill surgical patients: a comparison with pulmonary angiography. Arch Surg 2001; 136:505–511.

43. Meaney JF, Weg JG, Chenevert TL, Stafford-Johnson D, Hamilton BH, Prince MR. Diagnosis of pulmonary embolism with magnetic resonance angiography. N Engl J Med 1997; 336:1422–1427.

44. Ferris EJ, McCowan TC, Carver DK, McFarland DR. Percutaneous inferior vena caval filters: follow-up of seven designs in 320 patients. Radiology 1993; 188:851–856.

45. Benjamin ME, Sandager GP, Cohn EJ Jr., et al. Duplex ultrasound insertion of inferior vena cava filters in multitrauma patients. Am J Surg 1999; 178:92–97.

46. Hughes GC, Smith TP, Eachempati SR, Vaslef SN, Reed RL II. The use of temporary vena caval interruption device in high-risk trauma patients unable to receive standard venous thromboembolism prophylaxis. J Trauma 1999; 46:246–249.

47. Patton JH Jr., Fabian TC, Croce MA, Minard G, Pritchard FE, Kudsk KA. Prophylactic Greenfield filters: acute complications and long term follow-up. J Trauma 1996; 41:231–236.

48. David W, Gross WS, Colaiuta E, Gonda R, Osher D, Launti S. Pulmonary embolus after vena cava filter placement. Am Surg 1999; 65:341–346.

49. Schmitz-Rode T, Janssens U, Schild HH, Basche S, Hanrath P, Gunther RW. Fragmentation of massive pulmonary embolism using a pigtail rotation catheter. Chest 1998; 114:1427–1436.

50. O'Malley KF, Ross SE. Pulmonary embolism in major trauma patients. J Trauma 1990; 30:748–750.

51. Douketis JD, Kearon C, Bates S, Duku EK, Ginsberg JS. Risk of fatal pulmonary embolism in patients with treated venous thromboembolism. JAMA 1998; 279:458–462.

31

Epidemiological, Organizational, and Educational Aspects of Trauma Care

Michael E. Ivy

Hartford Hospital, Hartford, and University of Connecticut School of Medicine, Farmington, Connecticut, U.S.A.

Tissues are injured when the energy transferred from the environment to the body exceeds the tolerance of the tissues (1). Any form of energy can result in injury, but the energy transferred usually takes the form of kinetic energy. Examples include the energy transferred during a sudden deceleration to the chest that results in a tear of the thoracic aorta, or the kinetic energy of a knife being transferred to a small area of the body. However, other forms of energy, such as thermal injury, can also cause tissue injury. Much of the credit for our appreciation of this basic concept can be given to Dr. William Haddon, Jr., an engineer and physician who was a pioneer in injury prevention.

Injuries were responsible for 146,941 deaths in the United States in 1998 (2). Motor vehicle crashes (MVCs) were responsible for 28.8% of injury deaths, and firearms accounted for 20.9% (2). It should be noted that the Centers for Disease Control and Prevention (CDC) include poisonings and medical misadventures in this total. In the United States, injuries are the leading cause of death in persons in the age group of 1 to 44 years (2). Consequently, injury is responsible for the loss of more years of productive life (years lost before age 65) than is cancer or heart disease.

The CDC categorizes injuries as intentional or unintentional (Table 1). In 1998, unintentional injuries were responsible for 94,331 deaths (2). The unintentional injuries that are the main causes of mortality are MVCs, falls, drownings, most thermal injuries, and most occupational injuries. Intentional injuries that lead to death are suicides, homicides, and the results of legal interventions. Intentional injuries can result from a variety of mechanisms, including gunshot, piercing, assault, and thermal injuries.

The state of Massachusetts, one of the safest states in the United States, reviewed its experience with injuries in 1989 and estimated that one in four residents is injured every year (3). For every person who died as a result of injury, an estimated 17 were hospitalized and another 535 were injured but not hospitalized.

BACKGROUND

Motor Vehicle Crashes

MVCs are one of the main causes of death and disability in the United States and around the world. In the year 2000 in the United States, 37,338 crashes caused 41,800 fatalities (4). Overall during that year, an estimated 6,266,000 nonfatal crashes occurred and 3,219,000 people were injured. The rates of MVC-associated death vary widely between states. Much of the difference can be explained by the difference in the amount of time that passes before the victims reach a hospital.

Although the overall number of deaths due to MVCs has decreased marginally over the past 35 years, the rates per population and per 100 million vehicle miles traveled (vmt) have dropped substantially (Table 2). Efforts aimed at reducing the rates of deaths and disability due to MVCs have resulted in an important public health triumph. In 1966, 5.5 deaths occurred per 100 million vmt in the United States, for a total of 50,894 deaths that year (5). In response, the U.S. Government, the insurance industry through its proxy the Insurance Institute of Highway Safety, and the auto industry worked together to identify and correct obvious hazards. In 2000, the number of deaths per 100 million vmt had decreased to 1.6, for a total of 41,800 deaths (4). If the fatality rate per 100 million vmt had remained unchanged at 5.5, the year 2000 would have seen approximately 140,000 deaths. This reduction translates into the prevention of more than 100,000 fatalities every year. The impact of motor vehicle fatality prevention programs largely goes unrecognized by the public, but it is important that physicians caring for trauma patients recognize and understand the impact of these interventions on the population.

Falls

Falls are an important cause of loss of life and of hospitalization. In the United States, falls currently

Table 1 Number of Traumatic Deaths for All Age Groups, 1992

	All ages	0–14 yrs	15–44 yrs	45–64 yrs	Over 65 yrs	Age not known
All injuries	146,941	7,537	72,538	29,099	37,560	207
Unintentional	94,331	5,848	40,210	17,568	30,605	109
Suicide	30,575	324	16,337	8,094	5,803	17
Homicide	17,893	1,178	13,327	2,452	881	55
Undetermined	3,746	184	2,362	922	253	25
Other	386	3	311	63	18	1

result in an estimated 13,301 deaths and nearly 783,357 hospitalizations each year (2). The mortality rate associated with falls is highest among the elderly: for Americans older than 85, the mortality rate is 108.7 per 100,000 persons. Consequently, falls may become a more important cause of fatal injuries as the population continues to age. Efforts are beginning to be made to decrease the number of hip fractures that result when elderly persons fall. Potential areas for improvement include better floor surfaces that more effectively absorb energy, as well as padding in clothes for the elderly who are deemed to be at substantial risk of hip fracture with a fall. Kannus et al. (6) recently reported a trial of an effective hip protector for elderly patients; the rate of hip fractures was 46.0 per 1000 person-years for unprotected patients and 21.3 per 1000 person-years for protected patients, a rate that makes this protector remarkably effective.

Gunshot Wounds

The incidence of fatal gunshot wounds has decreased substantially over the past decade. In the United States in 1991, 38,317 people died of gunshot wounds while only 30,242 died in 2002. (6a,6b). Of the deaths in 2002, the majority (17,108) were suicides. Of the remainder, 11,829 were homicides and a much smaller number were either undetermined, unintentional, or the result of legal interventions. Persons at greatest risk of homicide are those aged 15–24 years, and most victims are male (2). The greatest progress in reducing mortality rates seems to have been made for slightly older Americans. For example, the mortality rate for persons aged 25 to 34 declined from 18.2 per 100,000 in 1979 to 11.8 per 100,000 in 1998, a decrease of 35%. The causes of this decline are subject to debate, but may include a decrease in illegal drug use, a decline in the number of persons in the highest-risk age group

Table 2 Numbers and Rates of Fatalities Related to Motor Vehicle Crashes Over Time

Years	Fatalities	Fatalities per 100,000 population	Fatalities per 100 million vmt
1966	50,894	26.02	5.5
1976	45,523	20.92	3.2
1986	46,087	19.19	2.5
2000	41,800	15.20	1.6

Abbreviation: vmt, vehicle miles traveled.

(18–24 years), a healthy economy, better police interventions, the imprisonment of larger numbers of criminal offenders, and the legalization of abortion in 1973.

Burns

For a variety of reasons, the number of fatalities resulting from burns has decreased over the past several decades and this continues to the present. In 1999, an estimated 3910 Americans died of burn injuries, while in 2002, 3,645 died from similar injuries 6b. Some of the decrease is no doubt due to prevention efforts. Specific areas that have been addressed include flame-retardant clothing, elimination of free-standing propane or gas heaters from many homes, improved training of professional firefighters in most major cities across the United States, and the creation of dedicated burn centers to better care for patients with severe thermal injuries.

TRAUMA SYSTEMS

As expected, the development of an organized, systematic approach to the care of injured patients has improved outcomes in this population. A landmark study by West et al. in 1979 compared the preventable injury mortality rates for patients in Orange County with the rates for patients in San Francisco (7). This study documented a marked decrease in preventable trauma deaths in San Francisco and concluded that the trauma system had improved the quality of care. Subsequent studies have confirmed these findings. For example, Shackford et al. reviewed the San Diego County experience and noted that an organized trauma system had improved patient care (8). A recent review of the trauma experience in England and Wales from 1989 to 1997 found that the odds ratio of mortality from injury was 0.72 in 1997; compared to that in 1989, this indicates a decrease in the mortality rate of nearly 30% (9).

The timing of deaths due to injury has been another area of investigation. Baker et al. reviewed all traumatic deaths that occurred in San Francisco in 1977 (10). They noted that the distribution of deaths was trimodal: 53% occurred before arrival at the hospital, 21.5% occurred within 48 hours after arrival at the hospital, and 12.6% occurred more than seven days after injury. Of the late deaths, 78% were due to sepsis and multiple organ failure. Interestingly, only 5% of deaths from penetrating trauma and 8% of deaths from blunt trauma were due to sepsis. On the other hand, burn patients were at substantial risk of death due to sepsis. (At that time, early excision of burn wounds was not routinely practiced.) Overall, 50% of deaths were due to brain injury, 31% were due to exsanguination, and 9.8% were due to sepsis and organ failure.

Sauaia et al. performed a similar study in Denver County in 1992 (11). This study showed that 34% of deaths occurred during the prehospital phase, 53% occurred within 48 hours of arrival at the hospital, and only 9% were classified as late deaths. Most late deaths (61%) resulted from organ failure. Again, late deaths due to organ failure were unusual after penetrating trauma (3%), but were slightly more common after blunt trauma (13%). The authors reported that, overall, 42% of the deaths were due to brain injuries, 39% were due to exsanguination, and 7% were due to organ failure.

These findings show a trend toward improvement in the care of hospitalized trauma patients, with fewer deaths due to late sepsis and organ failure, although improved burn care is at least partly responsible for the decrease in late deaths due to sepsis. The findings also show that because of faster and possibly improved prehospital care, the number of prehospital deaths has decreased, but the number of early hospital deaths has increased. The percentage of deaths due to sepsis and organ failure decreased from 9.8% (10) to 7% (11), a decrease of nearly 30% in the rate of death due to sepsis. Consequently, the distribution of deaths, which was trimodal in earlier studies, appears to be bimodal at present, although the difference in the percentage of late deaths is not great (12% in 1977; 9% in 1992).

In 1991, Davis et al. reviewed the San Diego County Trauma System data from 1985 to 1988 and investigated the importance of errors in critical care delivered to trauma patients (12). Overall, 813 deaths occurred at trauma centers; 62 of these deaths were judged to have been preventable. Of the preventable deaths, nearly half (30 deaths) were due to errors in critical care. Most (67%) of these errors that were related to preventable deaths were errors in management. The authors concluded that errors in critical care are a substantial cause of mortality among trauma patients, and that surgeons caring for trauma patients must be skilled in caring for critically ill patients.

Trauma systems have other important goals besides minimizing the number of preventable deaths; these goals include minimizing morbidity rates and maximizing rehabilitation efforts so that injured persons can return to work and function successfully in society. Rhodes et al. (13) found that 83% of 302 patients who had been admitted to their trauma center had returned to work within six months (13). After three years, 81% of patients who had sustained severe injuries, as defined by an Injury Severity Score (ISS) greater than 15, had returned to work. Documenting the effectiveness of trauma centers and trauma systems is important if we are to justify the continuing investment by society and the medical community in maintaining and improving trauma care. Additionally, these findings and those of related studies are needed if we are to convince governments to expand the funding of trauma systems.

A trauma system encompasses the care of the patient from the scene of the injury, through transport to the initial hospital, through transport to a definitive acute care hospital if necessary, and later through the rehabilitation phase. This level of organization requires the participation of hospital personnel, prehospital personnel, and officials of the local, county, and state governments.

At the trauma center, a coordinated response involves the emergency department (ED), the operating room, the intensive care units, the inpatient floors, the radiology department, the blood bank and laboratory, and eventually the rehabilitation center. Such a coordinated response mandates the availability of skilled physicians who are trained in trauma care. Additionally because of the breadth in the variety of injuries that can occur, a wide range of surgical and nonsurgical specialists must be available. Surgical specialists included in the system are general surgeons, neurosurgeons, orthopedic surgeons, and plastic surgeons. Essential nonsurgical specialists include general internists, cardiologists, gastroenterologists, psychiatrists, radiologists, and pediatricians. A commitment to obtain the resources, talents, and abilities required by a trauma center can raise the overall level of care that a hospital offers, but it also requires an investment of time, money, and effort on the part of the administrators.

PREHOSPITAL CARE
Rapid Prehospital Response

The Emergency Medical Services (EMS) system is in many ways the descendent of the military evacuation systems that have been used for centuries, beginning with Baron Larrey during the Napoleonic Wars. According to McSwain (14), Larrey established the importance of three concepts: (i) rapid arrival of a well-equipped ambulance at the site of the injury; (ii) provision of prehospital care by educated, skilled personnel; and (iii) rapid transport from the scene to a hospital that can care for injured patients. The military continued to develop this concept during World Wars I and II, using mechanized vehicles for transport and mobile hospitals to provide definitive care soon after injury. In Korea, the military began to use helicopters to provide rapid transport to more secure hospitals. The civilian use of these concepts remained limited in the United States until the publication in the 1960s of the National Academy of Sciences report "Accidental Death and Disability: The Neglected Disease of Modern Society." This report called for substantial improvements in the provision of prehospital trauma care.

Education of Prehospital Personnel

It is vital that injured patients receive organized care in the field, where the situation is often chaotic. Bringing order to such a scene and providing a high level of care can be quite difficult. Personnel must be specifically trained to provide this care and, over time, this requirement has mandated the creation of courses for prehospital care providers, from emergency medical technicians (EMTs) to paramedics. In 1969, the Department of Transportation published a manual for prehospital personnel and created a specific curriculum for the Emergency Medical Technician-Ambulance (EMT-A). Further development of prehospital education occurred rapidly as its effectiveness was recognized. The National Association of EMTs created the Prehospital Trauma Life Support Course along guidelines similar to those of the Advanced Trauma Life Support Course that is offered to physicians (14). The American College of Emergency Physicians developed the Basic Trauma Life Support Course. Each of these courses is now regularly offered in locations across the United States to persons interested in providing prehospital care.

Education of prehospital personnel should be and is supported by trauma centers. Such education requires that prehospital personnel participate in standard courses and that opportunities for continuing medical education be created for prehospital personnel.

Communication

Communication between prehospital personnel and hospital physicians is of paramount importance, not only for trauma patients but also for a wide variety of patients with critical illnesses such as myocardial infarctions, arrhythmias, and cerebrovascular accidents. Communication is beneficial in several ways. It allows the physician to direct the care of critically injured patients during transport to the hospital, it allows hospital personnel to prepare for specific types of injuries, and it offers the opportunity to direct the injured patient to a hospital that offers an appropriate level of care.

It is also important to maintain communication between prehospital personnel and physicians after the patient has been transported. Patients can benefit from the development of protocols and standing orders, but such protocols can be appropriately developed only with the collaborative efforts of all parties involved.

Triage

Triage of injured patients occurs at many levels and is a crucial part of the trauma system. Triage began, as did much of the prehospital system of care, as a result of the efforts of Baron Larrey. Two important facets of the epidemiology of trauma combine to make rapid and accurate triage a vital component of any trauma system. The first factor is the recognition that nearly 50% of trauma patients die within the first four hours after injury (11). Most of these deaths are not preventable; however, some of them may be prevented with a fast and accurate assessment of the injuries involved. The second factor is that only 5% to 10% of trauma patients have injuries severe enough to require the services of a trauma center. Consequently, the EMT must triage the remaining 90% of injuries to find the patients who need rapid transport to a trauma center. The alternative is to treat all trauma patients with the same level of urgency, but in such a scenario, most systems would be overwhelmed by the minimally injured, and the care of the seriously injured would be compromised.

Triage in the field is based on mechanism of injury and physiologic parameters. Frequently, a second triage occurs when patients arrive at the ED. Mechanism of injury plays an important role in determining a patient's need for definitive care at a trauma center; triage criteria include MVC with ejection and penetrating injuries of the head, neck, or torso. Examples of physiologic triage criteria include systolic blood pressure below 90 mmHg or a Glasgow Coma Scale (GCS) score of less than 12. Patients can be reassigned to a different triage level on the basis of their initial hospital course while they are still in the ED. For example, a patient whose condition originally appears stable after a fall from a standing position may initially be assigned a low triage level in the field and in the ED, but this triage level may be subsequently upgraded if acute changes in mental status occur.

The evaluation and management of mass casualties is another important component of a well-designed trauma system. Incidents that result in a large number of casualties are relatively infrequent, but unless they are planned and practiced for, can result in a disproportionate number of fatalities. It is important that experienced personnel be present in the field to direct the expeditious triage of victims. Several different triage systems have been used over the years, but all have several features in common. Minimally injured patients are considered walking wounded, and in civilian settings, they are triaged to less urgent care. Patients with very severe injuries are triaged to the expectant category and are given palliative care. Patients with serious injuries who are expected to benefit from relatively minimal interventions are assigned the highest priority. The complexity of the decision-making process, and the need to make the decisions quickly and efficiently make the job very complex. These incidents typically require a coordinated response from area hospitals so that the resources available at any one center will not be completely overwhelmed.

Interventions in the Field

The effectiveness of specific interventions in the prehospital setting has been evaluated. The insertion of an endotracheal tube is clearly beneficial for patients with severe brain injury (26). There is good evidence that hypoxia soon after a severe brain injury greatly increases the risk of death and the risk of a poor outcome (27). Brain-injured patients may retain CO_2, and this retention can result in inappropriate cerebral vasodilation and increased intracranial pressure (ICP). High levels of CO_2 will also cause serious acidosis, which may lead to cerebral vasodilation and even higher ICP. Additionally, unconscious patients may actively aspirate oral and gastric secretions until an endotracheal tube is in place and secured. Stewart et al. (28) studied the ability of prehospital personnel to perform oral intubation of comatose patients in the field. They reported an overall 90% success rate for intubation in the field, although the success rate was only 79% for trauma patients. The complication rate was nearly 10%, although many of the complications, such as vomiting during intubation (0.9%), may well be unavoidable even for more experienced personnel. Attempts by trained hospital personnel to perform intubation on comatose patients in the field are justified.

The effectiveness of administering intravenous fluids to patients before arrival at the hospital is less certain. A retrospective study by Kaweski et al. (29) found no difference in survival rates related to the prehospital administration of fluids. A highly publicized clinical trial in Houston evaluated the intravenous administration of fluids to patients with penetrating trauma to the torso (30). In that study, patients received either standard fluid resuscitation in the field or no fluid resuscitation before arrival in the operating room. The survival rate for patients who received no fluids was significantly higher than that for patients who received standard fluids ($p = 0.04$). Thus, it appears that the prehospital administration of fluids may be harmful to this specific subpopulation of trauma patients. However, random assignment of patients to the groups was not properly carried out, the treatment options were offered on alternate days, the fluid volume regimens were not strictly followed, and the preoperative times were longer than would be acceptable at most centers. These problems lead to concerns about the generalizability of the study's findings. Unfortunately, no properly performed, prospective, randomized controlled trial has been performed to clarify the issue.

Other studies have indicated that the type of fluid given in the prehospital setting may affect the outcome of patients with head injury. A prospective randomized trial was conducted to evaluate the effectiveness of administering hypertonic saline and dextran (HSD) to injured patients in the prehospital setting (31). The rationale behind the study was that HSD is a better plasma volume expander than is isotonic crystalloid solution. Consequently, the small volumes given before arrival at the hospital could rapidly increase the blood pressure of hypotensive trauma patients and improve perfusion to vital organs while the patient is undergoing resuscitation and definitive treatment. The study found that, overall, there were no significant differences in outcome between patients given HSD and those given other types of resuscitation fluids. However, the outcomes were better ($p = 0.068$) for the subgroup of patients with a head Abbreviated Injury Score of 4, 5, or 6 who were treated with HSD.

This finding is consistent with those of other studies that have documented a significantly worse outcome for patients with brain injury, who experience even transient hypotension. In fact, Chesnut et al. (27) reported that a 50% increase in mortality rates was associated with one or more episodes of hypotension experienced in the ED by patients with a GCS score of less than 8. Given the demonstrated importance of hypotension in the ED in determining the outcome of patients with brain injury, it may well be that HSD can better minimize hypotension during the early postinjury period and therefore minimize the risk of secondary brain injury. Additionally, on the basis of numerous studies that began with that by Weed and McKibben in 1919, it has been well established that the sodium concentration of the infused fluid plays a key role in the volume of fluid in the brain (32). It may simply be the case that administering hypertonic saline soon after injury increases the sodium concentration of the plasma and shrinks the extracellular volume of the brain, thereby lowering ICP and increasing cerebral perfusion pressure.

The other important aspect of this study is the finding that aggressive fluid resuscitation administered before bleeding has been controlled may increase bleeding and subsequently put the patient at risk of developing complications and a higher likelihood of mortality. The results of good animal studies demonstrate the adverse consequences of excess fluid resuscitation in the early stages of uncontrolled hemorrhage (33). This adverse consequence of blood pressure restoration in some patients may compensate for the benefit achieved in others and may explain the lack of difference in overall outcomes.

HOSPITAL CARE

To be a successful trauma center, a hospital must be committed as an organization to providing excellent trauma care. A hospital must meet certain standards if it is to be classified as a trauma center. Its ED must be open 24 hours a day and it must be adequately staffed with personnel who have been trained to care for injured patients. These personnel must complete continuing education courses on trauma care. An operating room must be immediately available and appropriately staffed at all times. This requirement is of paramount importance if life-saving operations are to be performed in a timely manner. Because the most severely injured patients will require intensive care after arrival, an intensive care unit must be available and its surgeons must be involved in the care of the patients. As patients recover from their injuries, they must receive physical therapy, occupational therapy, and speech therapy as appropriate for their injuries.

The complexity of the trauma center concept prompted the American College of Surgeons (ACS) to develop a process for verification and consultation in 1987. The Trauma Center Verification program has resulted in an organized approach to the care of injured patients in designated trauma centers. In implicit recognition of the fact that hospitals in some regions of the United States cannot muster the resources to become Level I or Level II trauma centers, the ACS developed guidelines that encompass several levels of care. This approach is based on the belief that care can be improved if a hospital develops an organized trauma system and has a coordinated response to the arrival of a trauma patient. The ACS mandated the creation of quality improvement processes in trauma centers to ensure that cases are reviewed, errors are identified, and, when possible, actions are taken to prevent similar errors in the future.

Trauma Center Volume

Substantial debate persists about the optimal volume of trauma patients that a hospital should care for in a year. It seems intuitively obvious that centers with very low volume will provide less than ideal care, but the exact volume that will allow the best care has not been determined. Three recent studies have examined this issue in depth.

Nathens et al. (15) performed a multivariate analysis of the data from the University Healthsystem Consortium Trauma Benchmarking Study and found that hospital volume was a significant predictor of survival for high-risk patients. Specifically, for patients who arrived at the hospital with hypotension resulting from penetrating abdominal trauma, the odds ratio for mortality was 0.02 at high-volume centers as compared with that at low-volume centers. For comatose patients with multisystem blunt trauma, the odds ratio for mortality was 0.49 at high-volume centers as compared with that at low-volume centers. There was no statistically significant difference in mortality rates for patients with less severe injuries, such as penetrating abdominal trauma without hypotension. In this study, the volume used to distinguish low-volume and high-volume trauma centers was 650 trauma admissions per year.

Pasquale et al. (16) analyzed the Pennsylvania trauma center database and found that, of all factors reviewed, only the trauma center's case volume affected survival rates. The 12 busiest centers were considered high-volume trauma centers, and the 12 slowest centers were considered low-volume trauma centers. The author identified that the transition from low-volume to high-volume center occurred between 607 and 627 trauma admissions per year.

Margulies et al. (17) reviewed the experience at five Level I trauma centers in Los Angeles County. Their analysis of hospital volume was based on the number of patients admitted with ISS higher than 15. Several of the hospitals included in their study are very high volume trauma centers, and all of the centers in the study would probably meet the criteria for high-volume centers in the other two studies discussed above. These authors found that an increasing volume was associated with a statistically significant increase in mortality rates. This association may result from the fact that very high volumes of trauma patients can occasionally overwhelm the available resources at trauma centers.

On the basis of the findings of these studies, it appears that the survival rates of severely injured patients are higher at high-volume trauma centers. Between 600 and 650 trauma admissions are needed annually if trauma centers are to maintain an optimal level of care. However, it is possible that very high volumes may compromise care if hospital resources are overwhelmed.

Physician Involvement

Trauma care is an integral part of general surgery. It is essential that general surgeons be intimately involved in the care of patients at a trauma center. This does not mean that all general surgeons should be caring for trauma patients. There are a number of reasons why surgeons do not want to care for injured patients. Trauma care requires caring for patients who are often uninsured and the care is frequently needed at very inconvenient times. Directing trauma resuscitation can be a very intense experience and many surgeons are simply not interested in providing this kind of care. A separate concern is that having too many surgeons on the call schedule will dilute the trauma experience and could decrease the quality of care being provided. Consequently, in most large hospitals, many of the general surgeons do not take trauma call. However, in smaller communities, it is necessary for all or most of the general surgeons to participate in the care of injured patients. This necessity can and should be viewed as an opportunity to serve the community in a unique and special fashion. Unfortunately, most general surgeons simply do not want to care for trauma patients. When Orange County attempted to organize a trauma system in 1980, only 23 of 225 general surgeons offered to take trauma call (18). A survey by Richardson and Miller found that only 20% of surgery residents wanted to care for trauma patients as part of their practice (19). Those who are willing to take trauma call frequently demand reimbursement for being on the call schedule.

A growing concern in the trauma community is the decreasing number of operative trauma cases and the need for surgeons who are providing trauma care to maintain their operative skills. It is likely that trauma surgeons will need to expand their general surgery practice if they are to perform enough surgical procedures to maintain their operating skills at a high level.

Volume of Trauma Cases for Individual Surgeons

There is debate about the volume of trauma patients that individual surgeons need to treat if they are to provide optimal care. It seems intuitively obvious that, as is the case for trauma centers, surgeons need some volume of patients if they are to maintain their skills. The ACS has essentially declared that surgeons must care for at least 35 trauma patients with an ISS higher than 15 each year if they are to maintain an optimal level of expertise (20). This declaration has been based on the findings of the Pennsylvania study reported by Konvolinka et al. in 1995 (21). This study found that the outcome improved when surgeons treated an average of at least 35 trauma patients with an ISS higher than 12 each year. The study did not examine the case volume of individual surgeons but examined instead the average volume over a system; additionally, it used an ISS higher than 12 instead of an ISS higher than 15 as the definition of serious injury.

Other studies have not found a strong correlation between a trauma surgeon's case volume and patient outcome. A more recent review of the Los Angeles County experience found no link between trauma surgeon volume and survival rates (17). Surgeons in this study treated an annual average of 10 to 20 patients with an ISS higher than 15. It is not clear if this study really addresses the ACS guidelines, but it is remarkable that none of the surgeons in the five Level I trauma centers in Los Angeles County meet the proposed case volume requirements. The debate about case volume will continue, but at present there is no convincing evidence that surgeons need an annual volume of more than 35 injured patients with an ISS higher than 15.

Coverage by In-House Attending Physicians

Another raging debate concerns the need for in-house trauma coverage by attending physicians at trauma centers. The results of several studies are contradictory. The study by Thompson et al. (22) determined that the presence of an in-house trauma-attending physician was irrelevant to patient outcome. However, a study by Rogers et al. (23) at two university Level I trauma centers in the same metropolitan area found that coverage by an in-house attending physician improved outcome. Their study has been criticized because of concerns that other differences between the centers could have confounded its results. Luchette et al. (24) reported that the presence of an in-house surgeon with added qualifications in surgical critical care resulted in more rapid resuscitation but did not decrease mortality rates. The study by Pasquale et al. (16) found no increase in survival in association with the presence of an in-house trauma surgeon.

Training of Surgical Residents

There is a growing concern about the adequacy of training for general surgery residents in trauma care;

this concern is specifically focused on operative volume, which for several reasons is decreasing across the country. Automobiles and roads are safer than in the past, and, although airbags may increase the incidence of orthopedic trauma, they are likely to decrease the incidence of other types of injuries. The increase in the use of nonoperative management for blunt trauma to the liver, spleen, and kidneys has greatly decreased residents' operative experience. Hawkins et al. (25) reviewed the operative trauma experience of their residents and noted a 25% decrease from 1991–1993 to 1994–1996. The rising popularity of angiographic embolization for managing injuries to solid organs will also decrease the operative experience at some centers. A final reason for the decrease in operative volume is the decrease in the incidence of penetrating trauma in almost all cities across the United States. How many operative trauma cases are enough to develop a surgeon's competency in caring for injured patients? How do we ensure that future trauma surgeons perform at least this minimum number of operations? These questions remain unanswered.

Education of Hospital Personnel

The outreach efforts of the ACS have been instrumental in improving the care of injured patients. The creation of the Advanced Trauma Life Support Course has standardized the approach to injured patients and allowed a large number of surgeons and other medical personnel to improve their skills and knowledge. The ACS also requires that surgeons who care for trauma patients at a trauma center obtain continuing medical education credits on topics specifically related to trauma issues. To assure that surgeons can obtain such credits, the ACS annually sponsors several outstanding educational conferences for surgeons interested in trauma care. The ACS manual on the care of the surgical patient includes several sections that deal specifically with the treatment of injured patients. The creation of the field of emergency medicine has increased the number of EDs that are staffed with physicians who have been formally trained in providing trauma care.

RURAL AND URBAN TRAUMA CENTERS

The trauma system approach has been very successful in metropolitan and suburban settings. Unfortunately, much work remains to be done in rural settings. The fatality rates due to all kinds of injuries are much higher in rural settings than in urban or suburban settings. Although the rural population accounts for only one-third of the population of the United States, it accounts for more than 50% of the MVC fatalities (34). Problems include a longer time between an accident and the recognition that an accident has occurred, a longer time before the arrival of prehospital personnel, long transport times to Level II or III trauma centers, and long transport times, often via helicopters or airplanes, to more definitive care centers. Such delays can clearly be life-threatening.

TRIAGE IN THE HOSPITAL

Once the patient has reached the hospital, the value of a well-organized response to trauma has been clearly demonstrated and is widely accepted in the United States. Competing concerns about costs and resource utilization have mandated a graded response to trauma. The highest response should be prompted by several physiologic criteria, including hypotension, a respiratory rate of more than 40 breaths per minute, a GCS of less than 8, and penetrating injury to the head, neck, chest, or abdomen. The ACS recognizes that triage is not an exact science, so it mandates that rates of overtriage and undertriage deficiencies.

MANAGEMENT OF PEDIATRIC TRAUMA

There is ongoing debate about the role of pediatric surgeons in the treatment of injured children. D'Amelio et al. (35) published their experience with pediatric trauma patients treated by surgeons not trained as pediatric surgeons. Their results compared favorably with those obtained by a review of national standards. Consequently, these authors stated that, in areas with a shortage of pediatric surgeons, general surgeons can safely and effectively treat injured children. Tepas et al. (36) analyzed a multi-institutional pediatric trauma registry and reported that mortality rates were higher in very busy pediatric trauma centers. These authors suggested that this fact may reflect the inadequacy of available resources at these particularly busy centers.

PREVENTION OF TRAUMA

The science of injury analysis and prevention began in World War II, largely because of the efforts of Colonel Hugh DeHaven. In 1942, DeHaven published a review of the U.S. military's experience with soldiers who had survived falls from heights of 50 to 150 ft (37). He demonstrated that the forces on the body could be decreased to tolerable levels if the deceleration was extended over a brief but significant time and was spread out over a substantial area of the body.

The implication of this work, that extending the deceleration time spreads out the forces over a greater area of the body, was further investigated. A leading force in the early analysis of injury was Colonel John Stapp. The U.S. Air Force was interested in decreasing the likelihood of injury during airplane crashes. The construction of a rocket sled with controls for speed or deceleration allowed the testing of a variety of innovations in safety equipment. Stapp rode the sled at a speed of 632 mph and stopped it within 1.4 seconds; he sustained only minor injuries, in large part because he was wearing a four-point restraint (38). This type of testing was expanded to include automobile crash testing, and innovations aimed at improving safety soon followed.

Nevertheless, before 1965, the highways in America were exceedingly hazardous and little progress was being made in efforts aimed at reducing the numbers of deaths occurring on the highways. In 1966, the government created the National Highway Transportation Safety Administration (NHTSA) and appointed William Haddon Jr., as its director. Dr. Haddon's approach to injury prevention focused on passive interventions, those that prevent injuries but do not require the active participation of the person at risk of injury (39). For example, the use of restraints had been known since Colonel Stapp's work in injury prevention, but restraints require the active and willing participation of the person at risk and therefore had not been particularly successful in preventing MVC fatalities in the United States. Helmets were known to be effective in preventing brain injuries, but such knowledge was not and still is not a serious consideration for passenger vehicles because of the need for active participation. In contrast, the installation of shatterproof glass in windshields is a very effective way of preventing certain types of injuries.

In 1972, Haddon (40) introduced the Haddon Matrix, a tool used to analyze injury events and to design preventive measures. The matrix is essentially a 3×3 matrix with human, vehicular, and environmental factors on one side and event phases (pre-event, event, and post-event) on the other (Table 3). The effectiveness of the Haddon matrix in decreasing the occurrence of injurious events and in minimizing the consequences of those events when they do occur can be clearly demonstrated by the decline in MVC fatalities over the past three decades. Life-saving interventions have resulted from the use of the Haddon matrix and the combined efforts of the NHTSA, the automobile industry, the construction industry, and the hospital industry, as well as consumer advocacy groups. These interventions include crumple zones in cars, padding of dashboards and steering wheels, better seat belts, three-point restraints, child car seats, air bags in numerous locations, wider highways, breakdown lanes, breakaway light poles, and Jersey barriers, as well as the creation of trauma systems and prehospital emergency care systems.

Table 3 Sample Haddon Matrix for Motor Vehicle Crashes

Phases	Factors		
Pre-event	Driver's education	Center brake light	Speed bumps, street lights
Event	Cell phone use	Air bag; padded dashboard and steering wheel	Guard rails; Jersey barriers
Post-event	Bystander first aid	Measures to decrease incidence of car fires	EMS, trauma center

Abbreviation: EMS, emergency medical services.

It is also important to study innovations to ensure that they are effective. There are several classic examples of ideas that seemed to be effective, but either were not effective in practice or needed modification. Robertson et al. (41) conducted a study evaluating the impact of an intensive advertising campaign on the use of seat belts. Two cities were randomly assigned to receive advertising or no advertising through their cable television system. The intervention had no impact on the rate of seat belt use.

Driver's education programs are commonly believed to be a logical way to save the lives of adolescents. When the State of Connecticut eliminated mandatory driver's education classes, some towns and cities continued to offer driver's education classes, although others did not. Robertson (42) reported that significantly fewer MVC fatalities occurred among teenagers in the towns and cities that did not offer the driver's education classes. The towns that did offer the courses experienced lower rates of MVCs per teenaged driver, but because there were so few teenaged drivers in the areas that did not offer the classes, the rate of MVCs per teenaged driver was much lower in these areas. It is reasonable to conclude that, although driver's education programs are better than no education for individual teenaged drivers, these programs are not as effective in decreasing the overall incidence of MVCs as is delaying licensure for two more years.

Installation of air bags in cars and light trucks was a much anticipated improvement in the safety of automobiles. Air bags are credited with a 16% decrease in driver fatalities and a 23% decrease in deaths due to frontal crashes (43). Even for passengers, air bags are responsible for a 14% decrease in the rate of fatalities due to frontal crashes among passengers wearing seat belts and a 23% decrease in such fatalities among those not wearing belts (44). Unfortunately, air bags are also associated with a 34% increase in the risk of death among children under the age of 10 who ride in the front passenger seat. In an attempt to minimize this risk, important educational efforts have been undertaken and air bags have been modified.

Innovations that reduce the number of deaths due to injury will continue to be introduced. As surgeons caring for the people in our communities, we need to ensure that the innovations are effective. If they are, we need to actively promote their use.

REFERENCES

1. Haddon W Jr. A note concerning accident theory and research with special reference to motor vehicle accidents. Ann N Y Acad Sci 1963; 107:635–646.
2. Murphy SL. National Vital Statistics Reports. Vol. 48, Number 11.
3. Schuster M, Cohen BB, Rodgers CG, Walker DK, Friedman DJ, Ozonoff VV. Overview of causes and costs of injuries in Massachusetts: a methodology for analysis of state data. Public Health Rep 1995; 110:246–250.
4. National Highway Transportation Safety Administration. 1999 Annual Report and 2000 early assessment files. Washington D.C.: U.S. Department of Transportation, 2001.
5. National Highway Traffic Safety Administration. Traffic Safety Facts 1995. Washington D.C.: U.S. Department of Transportation, 1996.
6. Kannus P, Parkkari J, Niemi S, et al. Prevention of hip fracture in elderly people with use of a hip protector. N Engl J Med 2000; 343:1506–1513.
6a. National Center for Health Statistics, Center for Disease Control and Prevention. National Vital Statistics Report 199. Vol 48. 2000.
6b. National Center for Health Statistics, Center for Disease Control and Prevention. National Vital Statistics Report 2002. Vol 54, Number 10. 2006.
7. West JG, Trunkey DD, Lim RC. Systems of trauma care. A study of two counties. Arch Surg 1979; 114:455–460.
8. Shackford SR, Hollingworth-Fridlund P, Cooper GF, Eastman AB. The effect of regionalization upon the quality of trauma care as assessed by concurrent audit before and after institution of a trauma system: a preliminary report. J Trauma 1986; 26:812–820.
9. Lecky F, Woodford, Yates DW. Trends in trauma care in England and Wales 1989–97. UK Trauma Audit and Research Network. Lancet 2000; 355:1771–1775.
10. Baker CC, Oppenheimer L, Stephens B, Lewis FR, Trunkey DD. Epidemiology of trauma deaths. Am J Surg 1980; 140:144–150.
11. Sauaia A, Moore FA, Moore EE, et al. Epidemiology of trauma deaths: a reassessment. J Trauma 1995; 38:185–193.
12. Davis JW, Hoyt DB, McArdle MS, Mackersie RC, Shackford SR, Eastman AB. The significance of critical care errors in causing preventable deaths in trauma patients in a trauma system. J Trauma 1991; 31:813–819.
13. Rhodes M, Aronson J, Moerkirk G, Petrash E. Quality of life after the trauma center. J Trauma 1988; 28:931–938.
14. McSwain NE Jr. Pre-hospital care. In: Feliciano DV, Moore EE, Mattox KL, eds. Trauma. Stamford, CT: Appleton & Lange, 1996:107–122.
15. Nathens AB, Jurkovich GJ, Maier RV, et al. Relationship between trauma center volume and outcomes. JAMA 2001; 285:1164–1171.
16. Pasquale MD, Peitzman AB, Bednarski J, Wasser TE. Outcome analysis of Pennsylvania trauma centers: factors predictive of nonsurvival in seriously injured patients. J Trauma 2001; 50:465–474.
17. Margulies DR, Cryer HG, McArthur DL, Lee SS, Bongard FS, Fleming AW. Patient volume per surgeon does not predict survival in adult level 1 trauma centers. J Trauma 2001; 50:597–603.
18. Trunkey DD. What's wrong with trauma care? Bull Am Coll Surg 1990; 75:10–15.
19. Richardson JD, Miller FB. Will future surgeons be interested in trauma care? Results of a resident survey. J Trauma 1992; 32:229–235.
20. American College of Surgeons Committee on Trauma. Optimal Hospital Resources for Care of the Injured Patient. Chicago: American College of Surgeons, 1999.
21. Konvolinka CW, Copes WS, Sacco WJ. Institution and per-surgeon volume versus survival outcome in Pennsylvania's trauma centers. Am J Surg 1995; 170:333–340.

22. Thompson CT, Bickell WH, Siemens RA, Sacra JC. Community hospital level II trauma center outcome. J Trauma 1992; 32:336–343.

23. Rogers FB, Simons R, Hoyt DB, Shackford SR, Holbrook T, Fortlage D. In-house board-certified surgeons improve outcome for severely injured patients: a comparison of two university centers. J Trauma 1993; 34:871–877.

24. Luchette F, Kelly B, Davis K, Johanningman J, Heink N, James L, Ottaway M, Hurst J. Impact of the in-house trauma surgeon on initial patient care, outcome, and cost. J Trauma 1997; 42:490–497.

25. Hawkins ML, Wynn JJ, Schmacht DC, Medeiros RS, Gadacz TR. Nonoperative management of liver and/or splenic injuries: effect on resident surgical experience. Am Surg 1998; 64:552–557.

26. Winchell RJ, Hoyt DB. Endotracheal intubation in the field improves survival in patients with severe head injury. Trauma Research and Education Foundation of San Diego. Arch Surg 1997; 132:592–597.

27. Chesnut RM, Marshall LF, Klauber MR, et al. The role of secondary brain injury in determining outcome from severe head injury. J Trauma 1993; 34:216–222.

28. Stewart RD, Paris PM, Winter PM, Pelton GH, Cannon GM. Field endotracheal intubation by paramedical personnel. Success rates and complications. Chest 1984; 85:341–345.

29. Kaweski SM, Sise MJ, Virgilio RW. The effect of prehospital fluids on survival in trauma patients. J Trauma 1990; 30:1215–1219.

30. Bickell WH, Wall MJ Jr, Pepe PE, et al. Immediate versus delayed fluid resuscitation for hypotensive patients with penetrating torso injuries. N Engl J Med 1994; 331:1105–1109.

31. Vassar MJ, Perry CA, Gannaway WL, Holcroft JW. 7.5% sodium chloride/dextran for resuscitation of trauma patients undergoing helicopter transport. Arch Surg 1991; 126:1065–1072.

32. Weed LH, McKibben PS. Experimental alteration of brain bulk. Am J Physiol 1919; 48:531–558.

33. Capone AC, Safar P, Stezoski W, Tisherman S, Peitzman AB. Improved outcome with fluid restriction in treatment of uncontrolled hemorrhagic shock. J Am Coll Surg 1995; 180:49–56.

34. Rogers FB, Osler TM, Shackford SR, Martin F, Healey M, Pilcher D. Population-based study of hospital trauma care in a rural state without a formal trauma system. J Trauma 2001; 50:409–414.

35. D'Amelio LF, Hammond JS, Thomasseau J, Sutyak JP. "Adult" trauma surgeons with pediatric commitment: a logical solution to the pediatric manpower problem. Am Surg 1995; 61:968–974.

36. Tepas JJ III, Patel JC, DiScala C, Wears RL, Veldenz HC. Relationship of trauma patient volume to outcome experience: can a relationship be defined? J Trauma 1998; 44:827–831.

37. De Haven H. Mechanical analysis of survival in falls from heights of fifty to one hundred and fifty feet. War Med 1942; 2:586–596.

38. Stapp JP. Effects of mechanical force on living tissues. I. Abrupt deceleration and windblast. J Aviat Med 1955; 26:268–288.

39. Haddon W Jr, Goddard JL. An analysis of highway safety strategies. In: Passenger car design and highway safety. Association for the Aid of Crippled Children and Consumers Union of New York, 1962: 6–11.

40. Haddon W Jr. A logical framework for categorizing highway safety phenomena and activity. J Trauma 1972; 12:193–207.

41. Robertson LS, Kelley AB, O'Neill B, Wixon CW, Eiswirth RS, Haddon W Jr. A controlled study of the effect of television messages on safety belt use. Am J Public Health 1974; 64:1071–1080.

42. Robertson LS. Crash involvement of teenaged drivers when driver education is eliminated from high school. Am J Public Health 1980; 70:599–603.

43. Lund AK, Ferguson SA. Driver fatalities in 1985–1993 cars with airbags. J Trauma 1995; 38:469–475.

44. Braver ER, Ferguson SA, Greene MA, Lund AK. Reductions in deaths in frontal crashes among right front passengers in vehicles equipped with passenger air bags. JAMA 1997; 278:1437–1439.

32

Competing Priorities in the Trauma Patient

Michael E. Ivy

Hartford Hospital, Hartford, and University of Connecticut School of Medicine, Farmington, Connecticut, U.S.A.

Many general surgery residents would prefer that all patients who come to an emergency department (ED) require treatment for gunshot wounds to the anterior abdomen. Because the priorities are clear, the algorithm for such treatment is straightforward, the workup required is minimal, the surgical approach necessitates a laparotomy, and interaction with other services is minimal. Alas, the management of trauma is usually not this simple. At most trauma centers, blunt trauma predominates, injuries regularly require an extensive workup, the management algorithm is complex, and clear supportive evidence for treatment choices is not always found in the medical literature. Optimal care in these situations is achieved only when the general surgeon can interact smoothly with a variety of other specialists, particularly neurosurgeons and orthopedic surgeons. We frequently depend on the services of anesthesiologists, cardiac surgeons, and interventional radiologists. Coordinating the actions of our colleagues, prioritizing treatment for various injuries, and selecting appropriate diagnostic tests in the optimal sequence require an understanding of the complex interactions between different types of injuries and the perspectives of our subspecialty colleagues. Prominent areas of controversy include the evaluation and treatment of patients with combined head and abdominal injuries, combined blunt aortic injury and abdominal injury, and the timing of fracture fixation in patients with severe pulmonary or brain injury.

For many of these issues, there is no single correct approach. Every trauma service needs to develop a system that delivers optimal patient care in their hospital. One example of such a system involves the timing of patient evaluation by subspecialty consultants. This timing is a matter of institutional preference. In some hospitals, the orthopedic surgeons and neurosurgeons are part of the initial trauma response team, whereas in many other hospitals, these specialists respond only when they are called for. In a large university teaching hospital, the presence of neurosurgery and orthopedic surgery residents makes their inclusion in the initial trauma response team more likely. On the other hand, a community hospital trauma center that does not have surgical subspecialty residents would be unlikely to demand that an attending neurosurgeon or orthopedic surgeon participate in the evaluation of every trauma patient. However, the fact that institutional practices are different does not necessarily imply that better care is delivered with one arrangement or the other.

Because all patients are unique and the evaluation and treatment of the multisystem trauma patient will always be challenging, we must do our best to ensure that the care we provide is individualized. It is important to recognize that some combinations of injuries are likely to prompt disagreement about the best way to manage them. Collaborative discussion about these issues and agreement on a treatment protocol can improve the quality of the care provided.

BRAIN AND ABDOMINAL TRAUMA

Each year, roughly 50,000 deaths occur in the United States as a result of traumatic brain injury (1). In some published series, brain injuries have been responsible for 42% of traumatic deaths (2). The combination of brain injury and exsanguination is responsible for another 6% of traumatic deaths (2). The combination of intra-abdominal bleeding and serious brain injury is uncommon but not rare and can present a difficult management problem. This combination of injuries is particularly lethal because bleeding that results in hypotension will render cerebral perfusion inadequate, thereby worsening the brain injury and, ultimately, the chance for recovery. When Chesnut et al. reviewed the Traumatic Coma Databank (TCDB), they defined hypotension as systolic blood pressure (SBP) below 90 mmHg, hypoxia as a partial pressure of arterial oxygen of less than 60 mmHg, and severe brain injury as a Glasgow Coma Scale (GCS) score of less than 8 upon arrival in the ED (3). Patients with hypotension and hypoxia upon arrival had only a 5.8% chance of a good or moderately disabled neurological outcome and 75% of those patients died. Hypotension alone increased the mortality rate from

27% to 65%. The authors reported that 35% of their patients were hypotensive and 46% were hypoxic during the early period after injury; they also emphasized the impact of hypotension and hypoxia on brain-injured patients. These results are particularly discouraging because they imply that the outcome of many of these patients is fixed soon after their arrival in the ED.

General surgeons have interpreted the TCDB study to mean that hypotension in patients with brain injury is to be avoided at all costs. This concept has a sound physiologic basis. An SBP of 90 mmHg roughly corresponds to a mean arterial pressure (MAP) of 60 mmHg. If the patient's intracranial pressure (ICP) is 20 mmHg or more as a result of the injury, the cerebral perfusion pressure (CPP, defined as MAP minus ICP) is below 40 mmHg; this perfusion pressure is inadequate to meet the needs of an injured brain. All efforts should be made to quickly correct fluid deficits, rapidly diagnose, and stop ongoing bleeding. Rarely, neurosurgeons will argue that the need for emergent computed tomography (CT) of the brain takes priority over the need for laparotomy. This argument does not apply to hypotensive patients. Fortunately, the combination of laparotomy and craniotomy is required for only 0.4% of trauma patients who require CT of the head or a neurosurgical procedure (4). The frequency of this combination on injuries may well be decreasing due to the improvements in automobile safety (e.g., air bags) over the past decade.

The clinical presentation of patients with injury to both the brain and the abdomen may vary widely. Therefore, the diagnostic evaluation and treatment must be tailored to each specific patient. Accurate clinical assessment when the patient arrives at the ED is fundamental. Rapid and correct calculation of the GCS score and prompt detection of lateralizing signs are crucial. Lateralizing signs include unilateral dilation of a pupil, hemiplegia, hemiparesis, and asymmetric posturing. The presence of a serious abdominal injury can be suggested by the mechanism of injury. In such cases, clinical clearance of the abdomen is justified only if patients are conscious with an intact sensorium and exhibit no cardiovascular symptoms. Patients with hypotension should immediately undergo diagnostic procedures such as diagnostic peritoneal lavage (DPL) or abdominal ultrasonography (US).

Patients with a GCS score of less than 13 should undergo CT of the head; however, the indications for such scanning when the GCS score is 13 or higher are less clear. Harad and Kerstein (5) reviewed the cases of 302 patients with a GCS score of at least 13 and found that the 18% of patients had abnormal results from CT of the head and that 4% required neurosurgical intervention. Stiell et al. (6) found that 8% of 3121 patients with brain injury and a GCS score of at least 13 had a clinically important brain injury and that 1% required neurosurgical intervention. These authors identified five risk factors that predicted the need for neurosurgical intervention with 100% sensitivity (Table 1). Two other risk factors, along with the five high-risk factors, helped to predict the presence of clinically significant brain injury with a sensitivity of 98.4%. The presence of any one of the risk factors should prompt CT of the head.

Hypotensive patients who have suffered blunt trauma and have a minor head injury should undergo abdominal US during their secondary survey. If the results of US are positive for free intraperitoneal blood and the patients remain hypotensive, laparotomy should be performed without CT of the head. If US is unavailable, DPL is indicated. If the results of DPL are positive, laparotomy is indicated. If the results of DPL are negative, the cause of hypotension should be diagnosed and treated.

A more complex challenge is presented by the hypotensive patient with a GCS score of less than 13. A review of the medical literature demonstrates that no prospective randomized trials have compared the effectiveness of treatment algorithms and that most studies have not considered the role of US in the examination of patients with brain injury whose condition is unstable.

Thomason et al. (7) prospectively studied 14,255 patients from eight trauma centers in North Carolina. Five percent of these patients were alive but hypotensive when they arrived in the ED. Of the hypotensive patients, nearly 10% died in the ED and another 21% required laparotomy. Although 40% of the hypotensive patients were found to have a serious head injury, only 2.5% required emergency craniotomy. Only six hypotensive patients (0.8%) needed both craniotomy and laparotomy. The authors concluded that laparotomy and control of abdominal bleeding are the highest priorities in such patients.

Wisner et al. (4) retrospectively reviewed the cases of 800 consecutive trauma patients who underwent CT of the head or a neurosurgical procedure. In this series, 52 patients (6.5%) required craniotomy, 40 (0.5%) required therapeutic laparotomy, and 63 (7.9%) underwent nontherapeutic laparotomy. Only three patients (0.4%) required both craniotomy

Table 1 Indications for Computed Tomography of the Head for Patients with a GCS Score of 13 or Higher

Factors indicating high risk of head injury
  GCS score less than 15 two hours after injury
  Suspected depressed- or open-skull fracture
  Any sign of basal skull fracture
  Two or more episodes of vomiting
  Age 65 years or more

Factors indicating medium risk of head injury
  Amnesia involving events that took place more than 30 min before the injury
  Mechanism of injury (pedestrian struck by car, ejection from vehicle, fall from a height of more than 3 ft or 5 stairs)

Abbreviation: GCS, Glasgow Coma Scale.

and therapeutic laparotomy. These authors found that only two predictors, intubation in the field (odds ratio, 5.0) and lateralizing findings (odds ratio, 4.0), were significantly associated with the need for craniotomy. Thirty patients in this series exhibited lateralizing signs upon arrival in the emergency room; 10 of these patients required craniotomy.

Wisner et al. (4) recommended a straightforward algorithm for the treatment of patients with trauma to the head and the abdomen (Fig. 1). All hypotensive trauma patients whose condition remains unstable but who have no other obvious cause of cardiovascular instability undergo laparotomy. Hypotensive patients whose conditions stabilize with fluid resuscitation but with peritoneal aspirate grossly positive for blood undergo laparotomy if they do not exhibit lateralizing signs; if they do exhibit lateralizing signs, they undergo CT of the head before celiotomy. Patients whose conditions improve with fluid resuscitation and with peritoneal aspirate negative for blood undergo simultaneous CT of the head and completion of DPL.

Winchell et al. (8) retrospectively reviewed the cases of 212 hypotensive patients with blunt trauma and a suspected head injury. Although most studies define unstable condition as SBP below 90 mmHg, this study defined instability as SBP below 100 mmHg. Patients whose conditions did not respond to fluid resuscitation underwent immediate surgical procedures; those whose conditions did respond to fluid resuscitation underwent CT of the head before operative treatment was performed. For patients whose conditions were unstable, DPL was the primary method of diagnosing abdominal injury. For patients whose conditions continued to be unstable after fluid resuscitation, the intraoperative mortality rate was 70% and the overall hospital mortality rate was 80%. The authors reported that a low GCS score predicts the need for craniotomy: 19% of patients with a GCS score of less than 8 underwent craniotomy, whereas only 9% of those with a GCS score of 8 to 13 required craniotomy.

Although CT scans have revolutionized the management of brain injury, performing them takes time and can delay treatment. Winchell et al. (8) reported that the average time from arrival in the ED to the start of a surgical procedure was 47 minutes for patients in unstable condition and 115 minutes for patients who underwent CT of the head before laparotomy. Because scanners are now faster, the delay should be less than 68 minutes, but much of the delay is unavoidable because of the time required to transport and position patients for the scan.

Huang et al. (9) evaluated the usefulness of US in determining whether these patients should undergo immediate laparotomy or should first undergo CT of the head. These authors used a simple scoring system to calculate the amount of fluid demonstrated by initial US. A US score or 3 or higher was correlated with the presence of at least one liter of free intraperitoneal fluid. All 14 patients in this study with a US score of 3 or higher required therapeutic laparotomy, and all of these patients underwent emergent CT of the head after laparotomy. Two patients required intraoperative placement of an ICP monitor because of evidence of serious brain injury. A more recent study by McKenney and coworkers (10) evaluated a new scoring system for abdominal US after trauma and found that the sensitivity of a US score of 3 or higher in predicting the need for therapeutic laparotomy was 83%.

The algorithm developed by Huang et al. (9) is representative of current actual practice at many trauma centers (Fig. 2). Rapid US is performed as part of the resuscitation procedure in the ED, and laparotomy is performed for patients with continued hypotension and positive US results. Patients with positive US results, persistent unstable conditions persists, and the need neurosurgical monitoring because of low GCS scores or lateralizing signs, undergo placement of an ICP monitor during abdominal exploration. Those patients are taken directly from the operating room to the CT scanner if their physiologic status permits.

At trauma centers where US is not readily available, DPL is used to evaluate abdominal injuries among hypotensive patients. Patients with SBP below 90 mmHg and positive results from paracentesis undergo immediate laparotomy. CT of the head can be performed immediately after the operation if the patient's condition permits. Patients whose conditions respond rapidly and appropriately to fluid resuscitation should undergo CT of the head and abdomen instead of immediate laparotomy.

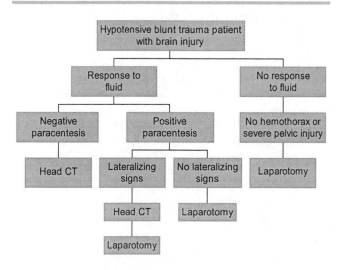

Figure 1 Proposed algorithm using the results of diagnostic peritoneal lavage to guide the management of combined brain and abdominal injuries. *Abbreviation*: CT, computed tomography. *Source*: From Ref. 4.

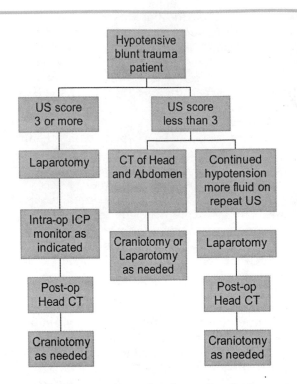

Figure 2 Proposed algorithm using the results of ultrasonography to guide the management of combined brain and abdominal injuries. *Abbreviations*: US, ultrasonography; CT, computed tomography; ICP, intracranial pressure. *Source*: From Ref. 9.

INJURIES TO THE THORACIC AORTA AND THE ABDOMEN

Controversy persists about the evaluation and treatment of patients with abdominal injuries and potential injuries to the thoracic aorta. Tears of the thoracic aorta are the second leading cause of death after blunt injury. Most of these deaths occur in the field very soon after the event. Patients with partial aortic tears who survive to reach the hospital must receive appropriate diagnostic tests and undergo rapid and safe repair of the aorta. General surgeons must understand the controversies surrounding the diagnosis and management of injuries to the thoracic aorta among patients who have suffered blunt trauma. If the care of these patients is to be properly directed, surgeons must be aware of several issues, including the role of CT in diagnosis and screening, the role of transesophageal echocardiography (TEE) in diagnosis, the optimal timing of abdominal and thoracic surgery, and the roles of delayed repair and nonoperative management.

The multicenter American Association for the Surgery of Trauma (AAST) trial (11) reported the status of diagnosis and management of aortic injury in 1997. These researchers enrolled 274 patients from 50 trauma centers over a 30-month period and recorded 86 deaths, for a mortality rate of 31%. Of the injuries, 81% were due to motor vehicle crashes and another 14% were the result of motorcycle crashes or of motor

vehicles striking pedestrians. The mortality rate for hemodynamically stable patients who underwent repair of aortic injury was only 8% (22 patients). Eight of those deaths occurred in the operating room when control of the proximal aorta was lost. Most of the deaths in this study (54 of 86) were due to rupture of the aorta. Other causes of death were head injury (11 deaths), multiple organ failure, or adult respiratory distress syndrome (ARDS; 17 deaths).

Because a substantial amount of energy is required to tear the aorta, it is not surprising that other injuries are frequently associated with such tears. Overall, 51% of the patients in the AAST study had a brain injury, 21% had an abdominal injury, and 34% had a pelvic or long-bone fracture (11). The study reported that 93 laparotomies, 124 orthopedic operations, and eight craniotomies were performed.

In the AAST study (11), the mean time from injury to diagnosis of aortic injury was 4.7 hours, and the time to repair averaged nearly 10 hours after diagnosis and 16 hours after injury. One potential explanation for this delay in treatment is the inclusion in the study of patients who were managed nonoperatively for an extended period of time because of the presence of other injuries or significant comorbid disease. Reporting the median time rather than the mean time to diagnosis and repair might have been more meaningful.

Because most (91%) of the aortic repairs were performed by cardiothoracic surgeons (11), another potential explanation for the prolonged times to diagnosis and repair is a lack of coordination between the trauma service and the cardiac surgery service. Each institution should develop a multidisciplinary protocol for optimizing the diagnosis and management of aortic injury; such protocols should be based on published findings and on the unique resources available at each institution. For example, it can be wasteful and potentially dangerous to spend time performing TEE if the standard practice at the hospital is to perform aortic repair only after angiography.

Any patient who has sustained high-energy impact to the chest is at risk of a partial tear of the aorta. Obtaining a routine chest radiograph (CXR) as part of the initial evaluation when the patient arrives in the ED is important in diagnosing aortic injury. The AAST study (11) found that 85% of patients with blunt chest trauma had a widened mediastinum, 8% had another finding suggestive of aortic injury, and only 7% had normal results from CXR. Radiography of the chest may be a useful screening test; however, for some patients with normal CXR results, an aortic injury will be missed without more extensive evaluation. Unfortunately, the exact indications for obtaining other tests after CXR has yielded normal results have not been well defined. The usefulness of CT of the chest in the diagnosis of aortic injury has been evaluated by large prospective studies. Mirvis et al. (12) reported using contrast-enhanced CT of the chest to screen 1104 of 7826 patients admitted for blunt trauma; an aortic injury was found in 25 of these patients. CT provided direct evidence of aortic injury for all 25 patients; the results of CT were equivocal for three other patients, and angiography was required for these patients. In this series, no aortic injuries were missed by CT of the chest.

TEE can accurately diagnose aortic injuries. Chirillo et al. (13) reported that TEE has a sensitivity of 93% and a specificity of 98% in diagnosing such injuries. However, TEE has several potential drawbacks. First, TEE neither allows good visualization of the aortic arch, nor provides visualization of the proximal great vessels after they branch from the aorta (13). Second, like many US techniques, TEE is an operator-dependent tool; some cardiologists and anesthesiologists who are accustomed to evaluating the heart may not evaluate the aorta with the same sensitivity as that reported in the literature. On the other hand, when TEE is performed by experienced physicians, it may reveal small intimal tears and thrombi that are not clinically significant and require no further intervention (14). The primary advantage of TEE is that it can save time compared to other diagnostic modalities such as angiogram. In the series by Chirillo et al. (13), the procedure saved an average of more than 40 minutes. Such time-savings can be particularly important for the cardiovascularly unstable patient who requires emergent laparotomy. In such cases, TEE can diagnose aortic injury in the operating room and can minimize treatment delays. However, realizing this potential benefit requires the availability of experienced personnel around the clock.

One of the most important controversies related to the treatment of patients with combined abdominal and aortic injuries concerns the timing of surgical procedures. The AAST (11) study found that 66% of patients who needed both laparotomy and aortic repair underwent the abdominal procedure first. That study also demonstrated that patients who are hypotensive because of free rupture of the aorta die before repair can be effected. Another study (15) found that, although as many as 31% of patients with aortic injuries were hypotensive after arrival, as few as 24% of these patients were hypotensive because of the aortic injury. Intra-abdominal injury was a more common cause of cardiovascular instability than was aortic injury. Consequently, the alternative of delaying a therapeutic laparotomy for a hypotensive patient until a thoracotomy and full heparinization can be performed seems unwise. The general recommendation is that laparotomy should be performed first with the goal of preventing exsanguination from abdominal injuries. If there is a sense of urgency about the aortic laceration, it is reasonable to perform a "damage control" laparotomy first so that ongoing bleeding and enteric spillage can be stopped.

Controversy exists about the nonoperative management and the delayed operative management of tears of the thoracic aorta. First because of the increased sensitivity of diagnostic tests, we are diagnosing isolated intimal injuries or small intraluminal thrombi that may not require repair (14). Second, there is a growing recognition that surgery can be delayed for some patients with other life-threatening injuries until they are able to tolerate thoracotomy or until they no longer require operative treatment.

Karmy-Jones et al. (15) reported the results of nonoperative treatment of patients with severe pulmonary injury, symptomatic coronary artery disease, severe brain injury, and comorbid chronic diseases. They noted that three of the patients who received this type of treatment died after free rupture of the aorta. Pate et al. (14) reported the outcomes of 11 patients who underwent nonoperative treatment and 15 patients who underwent delayed treatment. These authors used beta-blockade to maintain a heart rate of less than 90 beats per minute and added vasodilators as necessary to maintain an SBP below 100 mmHg. No patients died of free rupture of the aorta. The authors selected nonoperative therapy for patients with severe head, pulmonary, or abdominal injuries and for patients with preexisting medical conditions such as renal failure or symptomatic coronary artery disease. Follow-up studies showed that patients with small intimal flaps or thrombi had no aortographic evidence of aortic abnormality. It appears that in select circumstances, nonoperative management or delayed repair of the thoracic aorta is acceptable provided that the patient's blood pressure and heart rate are strictly controlled.

TIMING OF FRACTURE FIXATION FOR PATIENTS WITH BRAIN INJURIES

Controversy exists about the optimal timing of fracture fixation for patients with serious brain injury. This scenario involves multiple surgical specialists, including general surgeons, orthopedic surgeons, neurosurgeons, and anesthesiologists. There are essentially two perspectives. Some surgeons strongly believe that fixation within 48 hours of injury reduces the incidence of pulmonary complications, decreases the length of stay, and improves the eventual outcome of rehabilitation. Other surgeons believe that early fixation may worsen brain edema and increase mortality rates and that the benefits related to early mobilization may be lost for comatose patients with head injuries. Several articles pertinent to this controversy have been published, but none of them reports the results of a large, prospective, randomized controlled trial that can help us establish a definitive standard of care. An important problem with all of the studies that have addressed this complex issue is the lack of statistical power because of small sample size.

Fakhry et al. (16) reported the outcome of 87 patients with a brain injury and an Abbreviated Injury Scale (AIS) score of 3 or higher who underwent femur fixation. Early fixation was defined as fixation within 48 hours of arrival in the ED. The mortality rate was 8.5% for patients in the early fixation group and

3.6% for patients in the delayed fixation group; this difference was not statistically significant.

Reynolds et al. (17) prospectively studied 105 patients with brain injury who underwent fixation of femoral fractures. The mean AIS score was 1.96 in the early fixation group and 2.36 in the delayed fixation group; the difference was not statistically significant. The mortality rate was 4.2% for the early fixation group; no deaths occurred in the late fixation group, but this difference was not statistically significant. The number of days spent in the intensive care unit (ICU) and the number of days spent on a ventilator were also nearly identical between groups.

Jaicks et al. at Yale (18) retrospectively reviewed the cases of 33 patients with long-bone fractures and brain injuries. The mean AIS score was 3.3 for patients in the early fixation group and 3.1 for patients in the delayed fixation group. Although 53% of the patients in the early fixation group and only 36% of the patients in the late fixation group had femur fractures, this difference was not statistically significant. The authors reported a mortality rate of 11% in the early fixation group and no deaths occurred in the late fixation group, but this difference was also not statistically significant. The mean number of days spent on a ventilator was 6.4 for patients in the early fixation group and 6.5 for patients in the late fixation group. The most interesting finding of the study was that 16% of the patients in the early fixation group and 7% of the patients in the late fixation group exhibited intraoperative hypotension, defined as SBP below 90 mmHg, and that 11% of the patients in the early fixation group but only 7% of the patients in the late fixation group experienced hypoxia, defined as partial pressure of oxygen below 60 mmHg. Neither of these differences were statistically significant.

Hofman and Goris (19) retrospectively reviewed the cases of 58 patients with severe brain injury and long-bone fractures. The mean GCS score was 4.6 for patients who underwent early fixation and 4.7 for patients who underwent late fixation. These authors reported a statistically significant difference in mortality rates: 13% for patients in the early fixation group and 47% for patients in the late fixation group ($p < 0.02$). On the other hand, Sanker et al. (20) reviewed the cases of patients with a GCS score between 4 and 8; they reported mortality rates of 59% for the early fixation group and 12% for the delayed fixation group ($p < 0.01$). Both of these studies are Level III studies and are not definitive.

The Eastern Association for the Surgery of Trauma (EAST) Practice Management Guidelines Work Group has evaluated all the evidence and has posted its conclusions on their web site (www.east.org). There is no Level I evidence to guide our management practices (21). Because the Level II and Level III evidence are flawed, no strong recommendations can be based on those studies.

Scalea et al. (22) developed a "damage control" approach to the management of long-bone fractures for patients with severe multisystem trauma. These authors retrospectively compared 43 severely injured patients who underwent early external fixation of the femur with 284 patients who were treated with placement of primary intramedullary rods. The patients who underwent external fixation were more severely injured with a mean ISS of 26.8 versus 16.8 ($p = 0.001$). In the external fixation group, 46% of the patients had sustained a head injury with an overall mean GCS of 11 versus 14.2 ($p = 0.001$). Over one-quarter of the external fixation group required ICP monitoring, they had a median opening ICP of 22 mmHg and a median increase up to 27 mmHg. The external fixation procedures were performed either at the bedside or in the operating room and required an average of 35 minutes with an average estimated blood loss of 90 mL. In the cohort managed with external fixation, 9% of the patients died, 65% were discharged to a rehabilitation facility, and 26% were discharged to home a median hospital length of stay of 17.5 days. Less than 1% of the group treated with a primary intramedullary nail died, 51% were discharged to home and 49% were discharged to a rehabilitation facility. Unfortunately, given the variation in severity of injury, it is difficult to determine the effectiveness of the "damage control" approach in this patient population from this study. This innovative procedure may benefit some severely injured patients, but we will need controlled studies before we can state this with confidence.

MANAGEMENT OF LONG-BONE FRACTURES AND PULMONARY INJURIES

Another important controversy surrounds the treatment of patients with fractures and pulmonary injury. Advocates of early fracture fixation believe that outcomes are better and hospital stays are shorter when fracture fixation occurs during the initial 48 hours after injury. Other surgeons argue that early fracture fixation increases the risk of complications and exacerbates the pulmonary disease process.

Fakhry et al. (16) studied 96 patients with a chest injury and an AIS score of at least 3 who underwent delayed or early fixation of femur fractures (16). The mortality rate for patients in the early fixation group was 5%; no deaths occurred in the late fixation group, but the difference was not statistically significant. Reynolds et al. reviewed the impact of chest injury on outcome (17). They reported that the mortality rate was higher for the early fixation group (4.2%) than for the late fixation group (no deaths), but the difference was not statistically significant. Charash et al. (23) performed a nonrandomized, prospective study of 82 patients who underwent fixation of femur fractures. There was no statistically significant difference between the two groups in mortality rates, but pulmonary complications were more likely to occur among patients in the delayed fixation group.

However, it is not clear whether this difference in pulmonary complications is due to differences in injury severity or in patient management. This question arises because 71% of patients in the delayed fixation group were intubated during their initial resuscitation whereas only 24% ($p = 0.01$) of patients of the early fixation group were intubated initially. Thus it is very likely that the delayed fixation patients had sustained more severe pulmonary injuries overall.

The Level II evidence does not demonstrate that a convincing difference in the incidence of ARDS or pneumonia, or the number of days a patient spends on a ventilator or in the ICU, can be clearly attributed to fracture management. The findings of Level III studies are contradictory. Boulanger et al. (24) demonstrated that a delay in fixation was associated with a statistically insignificant increase in the incidence of ARDS (from 4% to 20%; $p > 0.05$). Pape et al. (25) reported that the incidence of ARDS was 33% after early fixation and 8% after late fixation ($p = 0.03$). In light of this contradictory evidence, strong recommendations about the optimal management of femur fractures cannot be made.

The EAST Management Guidelines Work Group has done a superb job of summarizing the evidence obtained to date (21). The Group does not endorse either early or late fixation of fractures for patients with clinically significant pulmonary injuries. It remains to be seen whether the "damage control" approach proposed by Scalea et al. (22) will improve the outcomes of these patients. In the end, we surgeons need to provide each patient with individualized treatment based on the patient's condition.

REFERENCES

1. Sosin DM, Sniezek JE, Waxweiler RJ. Trends in death associated with traumatic brain injury, 1979 through 1992. Success and failure. JAMA 1995; 273:1778–1780.
2. Sauaia A, Moore FA, Moore EE, et al. Epidemiology of trauma deaths: a reassessment. J Trauma 1995; 38: 185–193.
3. Chesnut RM, Marshall LF, Klauber MR, et al. The role of secondary brain injury in determining outcome from severe head injury. J Trauma 1993; 34:216–222.
4. Wisner DH, Victor NS, Holcroft JW. Priorities in the management of multiple trauma: intracranial versus intra-abdominal injury. J Trauma 1993; 35:271–278.
5. Harad FT, Kerstein MD. Inadequacy of bedside clinical indicators in identifying significant intracranial injury in trauma patients. J Trauma 1992; 32:359–363.
6. Stiell IG, Wells GA, Vandemheen K, et al. The Canadian CT Head Rule for patients with minor head injury. Lancet 2001; 357:1391–1396.
7. Thomason M, Messick J, Rutledge R, et al. Head CT scanning versus urgent exploration in the hypotensive blunt trauma patient. J Trauma 1993; 34:40–45.
8. Winchell RJ, Hoyt DB, Simons RK. Use of computed tomography of the head in the hypotensive blunt-trauma patient. Ann Emer Med 1995; 25:737–742.
9. Huang MS, Shih HC, Wu JK, et al. Urgent laparotomy versus emergency craniotomy for multiple trauma with head injury patients. J Trauma 1995; 38:154–157.
10. McKenney KL, McKenney MG, Cohn SM, et al. Hemoperitoneum score helps determine need for therapeutic laparotomy. J Trauma 2001; 50:650–656.
11. Fabian TC, Richardson JD, Croce MA, et al. Prospective study of blunt aortic injury: Multicenter Trial of the American Association for the Surgery of Trauma. J Trauma 1997; 42:374–383.
12. Mirvis SE, Shanmuganathan K, Buell J, Rodriguez A. Use of spiral computed tomography for the assessment of blunt trauma patients with potential aortic injury. J Trauma 1998; 45:922–930.
13. Chirillo F, Totis O, Cavarzerani A, et al. Usefulness of transthoracic and transesophageal echocardiography in recognition and management of cardiovascular injuries after blunt chest trauma. Heart 1996; 75:301–306.
14. Pate JW, Govant ML, Weiman DS, Fabian TC. Traumatic rupture of the aortic isthmus: program of selective management. World J Surg 1999; 23:59–63.
15. Karmy-Jones R, Carter YM, Nathens A, et al. Impact of presenting physiology and associated injuries on outcome following traumatic rupture of the thoracic aorta. Am Surg 2001; 67:61–66.
16. Fakhry SM, Rutledge R, Dahners LE, Kessler D. Incidence, management, and outcome of femoral shaft fracture: a statewide population-based analysis of 2805 adult patients in a rural state. J Trauma 1994; 37:255–261.
17. Reynolds MA, Richardson JD, Spain DA, Seligson D, Wilson MA, Miller FB. Is the timing of fracture fixation important for the patient with multiple trauma? Ann Surg 1995; 222:470–481.
18. Jaicks RR, Cohn SM, Moller BA. Early fracture fixation may be deleterious after head injury. J Trauma 1997; 42:1–6.
19. Hofman PA, Goris RJ. Timing of osteosynthesis of major fractures in patients with severe brain injury. J Trauma 1991; 31:261–263.
20. Sanker P, Frowein RA, Richard KE. Multiple injuries: coma and fractures of the extremities. Neurosurg Rev 1989; 12(suppl 1):51–54.
21. Dunham CM, Bosse MJ, Clancy TV, et al and EAST Practice Management Guidelines Work Group. Practice management guidelines for the optimal timing of long-bone fracture stabilization in polytrauma patients: the EAST Practice Management Guidelines Work Group. J Trauma 2001; 50:958–967.
22. Scalea TM, Boswell SA, Scott JD, Mitchell KA, Kramer ME, Pollak AN. External fixation as a bridge to intramedullary nailing for patients with multiple injuries and with femur fractures: damage control orthopedics. J Trauma 2000; 48:613–623.
23. Charash WE, Fabian TC, Croce MA. Delayed surgical fixation of femur fractures is a risk factor for pulmonary failure independent of thoracic trauma. J Trauma 1994; 37:667–672.
24. Boulanger BR, Stephen D, Brenneman FD. Thoracic trauma and early intramedullary nailing of femur fractures: are we doing harm? J Trauma 1997; 43:24–28.
25. Pape HC, Auf'm'Kolk M, Paffrath T, Regel G, Sturm JA, Tscherne H. Primary intramedullary femur fixation in multiple trauma patients with associated lung contusion—a cause of posttraumatic ARDS? J Trauma 1993; 34:540–548.

33

Complications of Fractures

Bar Ziv Yaron, Kosashvili Yona, Gelfer Yael, and Halperin Nahum
*Department of Orthopedic Surgery, Tel Aviv University, Sackler Faculty of Medicine,
Assaf Harofeh Medical Center, Zeriffin, Israel*

A fracture is a discontinuity of the bone, which is caused by the application of an external force. The amount of energy absorbed by the bone to create the fracture depends on the magnitude of the force and the direction of the load (1). The force required to break a bone depends on the material's properties and the bone's geometry.

Fractures may be classified in a number of ways: by the amount of energy absorbed by the bone (high energy or low energy), by the direction of the force (direct trauma or indirect trauma), or by the extent of the fracture (complete fracture or incomplete greenstick fracture in children). The amount of energy involved in creating a fracture is the most important factor because high-energy trauma causes an open-comminuted fracture with damage to soft tissues, including neurovascular structures. The severity of the soft-tissue injury affects the bone-healing process and the complications associated with the fracture.

The mechanism of injury determines whether the trauma is direct or indirect. In the case of direct trauma, force is applied directly to the fracture site and this direct application causes tapping fractures, crush fractures, and penetrating fractures (2). Tapping fractures typically affect the transverse line in the bone, whereas crush and penetrating injuries results in open-comminuted fractures. A typical result of direct trauma is a fracture of the tibial plateau that results when the tibia is struck directly by an automobile bumper. In the case of an indirect trauma, a force is applied to an area at a distance from the fracture site. A typical result of indirect trauma is a fracture of the upper extremity. For example, falling on an outstretched hand may generate a fracture of the navicular bone, the distal radius, the head of the radius, the humerus, or the clavicle, depending on the point of loading.

Several fracture patterns are produced by indirect force: tension fractures, angulation fractures, rotation fractures, and compression fractures. Fractures are usually produced by a combination of forces rather than by a single force acting alone (3). A typical tension fracture is created when the knee is forcibly flexed while the extensor mechanism is in contraction. Similarly, the deltoid ligament in eversion and external rotation may pull off the medial malleolus. Compression forces may cause impacted fractures such as fractures of the spinal vertebrae. Angulation fractures, rotation fractures, or combinations of indirect forces typically cause spiral and oblique lines; the pattern affects the stability of the fracture.

A pathological fracture occurs when a degree of stress that would leave normal bone intact is applied to a bone weakened by factors such as an underlying tumor, infection, or metabolic disease (4). The most common pathological fractures involve osteoporotic bone in the proximal femur (5), the spine, the proximal humerus, or the distal radius.

A stress fracture results from fatigue brought about by repeated loading. These fractures are seen most frequently among military recruits undergoing strenuous training (6) and among ballet dancers and athletes. Muscle fatigue allows an abnormal concentration of stress, which results in failure of the bone (7).

The incidence of complications may be reduced by careful planning of all treatment aspects, including primary assessment, emergency care, definitive treatment, and rehabilitation.

The complications that may occur after fracture can be acute or chronic. Acute complications are related to injuries to soft tissues, such as vascular, pulmonary, gastrointestinal, and neurological structures. These complications may jeopardize life or limb, depending on the severity of the injury and the systemic response. Long-term complications involve abnormalities of bone healing (malunion, delayed union, and nonunion), posttraumatic osteoarthritis, and avascular necrosis (AVN). The amount of energy and the intensity of the force are responsible for the incidence of early complications after fracture. An unstable fracture of the pelvic ring is very likely to lead to severe systemic complications such as hemorrhagic shock, neurovascular injuries, thromboembolism, and pulmonary embolism (PE). Long-bone fractures resulting from high-energy trauma are often associated with a risk of fat embolism (FE) syndrome and compartment syndrome. Immobility of the limb after a fracture is a risk factor for thromboembolic disease and PE. The risk of complications is substantially increased after a high-energy open fracture.

Stabilizing the fracture is the main goal of emergency care and will reduce the likelihood of early complications. Restoring the bones to a position as close as possible to the *normal anatomical position, by surgical or nonsurgical treatment, is necessary for realigning neurovascular structures, providing optimal circulation to the injured extremity, and minimizing the risk of peripheral nerve compromise. Reestablishing bony length decreases the size of hematomas and the extent of soft-tissue disruption. It also improves venous and lymphatic return and reduces soft-tissue swelling. When soft tissue and neurovascular structures around broken bones are undamaged, later complications such as delayed union, nonunion, malunion, AVN, and heterotopic ossification are less likely.*

ACUTE COMPLICATIONS
Shock

Shock is a clinical condition manifested by poor tissue perfusion with resultant tissue hypoxia, which may damage vital organs. Hemorrhagic (hypovolemic) shock is by far the most common type of shock affecting patients with multiple skeletal injuries. The bone injuries that most commonly produce severe hypovolemic shock are fractures of the pelvis.

Ostrum et al. reported that, of 100 patients with closed, isolated femoral shaft fractures, none experienced class III or IV shock (8). Among these patients, bleeding from the femur fracture was insufficient to produce hypotension. Thus, a meticulous search for a second source of blood loss must be performed when a patient with a closed femoral shaft fracture is hypotensive. More than 90% of pelvic ring injuries are associated with other injuries (9). Although pelvic ring injuries are notorious for hemorrhage, this bleeding is the primary cause of death for only 7% to 18% of fatalities (10). Burgess et al. have shown that hemorrhage from pelvic fractures strongly depends on the type of fracture; fractures associated with complete dissociation of the posterior pelvis (anterior–posterior type III) are associated with the greatest loss of blood, typically more than 20 units of blood in the first 24 hours, and consequently the highest mortality rates related to shock (11). The goal of treating hypovolemic shock is to safely restore adequate intravascular volume and oxygen-carrying capacity.

Hemorrhage and Pelvic Fractures

Approximately 90% of bleeding associated with fractures of the pelvis arises from low venous plexus pressure and fractured cancellous bone surfaces (12–14). The remaining 10% of bleeding originates from named arteries that can be embolized (15). The initial treatment of the fracture is stabilization of the pelvis. Stabilizing the pelvis prevents constant movement during transport and resuscitation (16). It is also believed that decreasing the volume of the pelvis will restore the tamponade effect and lower the volume of bleeding into the retroperitoneum (13,16,17). This stabilization can be achieved by applying an external fixator, which can be used temporarily as an emergency stabilizer or definitively for an open-book fracture. The fixator is applied by inserting pins into the ilium and is held in place with transverse bars that stabilize the pelvis. The patient's condition is considered hemodynamically unstable if the systolic blood pressure upon arrival at the emergency department is below 90 mmHg and remains low after the administration of 2 L of intravenous (IV) crystalloids, or if the pulse rate is greater than 110 beats per minute. Patients whose condition is hemodynamically unstable should undergo suprapubic diagnostic peritoneal lavage (DPL). Negative results from DPL indicate that the bleeding is of retroperitoneal origin and suggest that an external fixator should be applied, if this action has not already been taken (12,13). If the external fixator does not stabilize the patient's hemodynamic condition, the surgeon should be alerted to the possibility that the source of bleeding is arterial and should consider embolization under angiographic guidance (18,19). If the patient's hemodynamic condition is deteriorating, no time should be wasted in transfer to the angiography unit; exploratory laparotomy and retroperitoneal packing (with or without angiographic guidance) should be performed in the operating room (18).

Pearls and Pitfalls

- High grade of suspicion in fracture patterns notorious for hypovolemic shock.
- Ongoing monitoring of hemodynamic status is of outmost importance.

Vascular Injury

The following arterial injuries are commonly associated with fractures. Injury to the brachial artery is associated with proximal fractures of the humeral shaft or with supracondylar fractures of the humerus. Injuries to the deep femoral artery are associated with subtrochanteric fractures of the femur. Injuries to the popliteal artery below the level of Hunter's canal are associated with supracondylar fractures of the femur, whereas injuries to the popliteal artery at the level of trifurcation are associated with metaphyseal fractures of the tibia. Injuries to the anterior tibial artery are associated with fractures to the middle-third of the tibia.

Vascular injuries should also be considered in fracture dislocations, especially of the knee. The rate of arterial injuries ranges between 5% and 30% in anterior and posterior dislocations where the insult results from tethering of the popliteal artery.

Subsequently, the likelihood of arterial injuries must be considered with every fracture or joint dislocation. Injury to a major artery of the extremity may result in histologic changes to nerves and muscles if blood supply is not restored within four to six hours (20). "Hard" signs of vascular injury include massive external bleeding, a rapidly expanding hematoma, and the classic signs of arterial occlusion: lack of pulse, pallor, aesthesia, pain, paralysis, and poikilothermia. When these signs are present, immediate surgical exploration and vascular repair are indicated, particularly if there is substantial external bleeding or the threat of limb loss (21). "Soft" signs of vascular injury include a questionable history of arterial bleeding, proximity of a penetrating wound to an artery, a small nonpulsatile hematoma, or a neurologic deficit. Patients with these signs can be treated with arteriography or observation alone (21). Patients with pulse deficits distal to fractures or dislocation should undergo immediate reduction before any other treatment is undertaken. The presence of normal distal pulses does not rule out a serious vascular injury, and the limb must be repeatedly examined so that an occult lesion is not missed. Lynch and Johansen reported on 100 patients with blunt or penetrating limb trauma; all patients had ankle-brachial indexes (ABIs) measured and were studied by arteriography. ABI less than 0.90 predicted an injury that required intervention with 87% sensitivity and 97% specificity (22).

The treatment of vascular injury requires a complementary team effort by vascular and orthopedic surgeons. The aim of surgery is to shorten the ischemic period as much as possible by promptly restoring the arterial flow to the limb. On the other hand, performing the vascular procedure first puts the repair at risk during the orthopedic manipulation. Priorities in such situations should be jointly established by the vascular and orthopedic surgeons after a complete discussion of the nature of the combined injuries and the duration of the planned repair of both the arterial and the orthopedic injuries (23).

Pearls and Pitfalls

- Fractures of long bones should be stabilized before vascular repair is undertaken.
- If the extremity may be jeopardized by a delay in arterial repair, the vascular injury should be repaired first.
- Fasciotomy is indicated if any of the following has occurred:
  - restoration of blood flow has been delayed
  - the patient has experienced an episode of substantial hypotension
  - considerable swelling is noted
- Specific fractures or dislocations go along with specific neurovascular injuries.

Nerve Injury

Nerve injuries result from direct contusion or laceration by the fracture fragment or by penetrating missiles. Nerves may also be stretched by excessive forces that produce fractures or dislocation about the joint (see Chapters 33, 34). The following nerve injuries are commonly associated with fractures or dislocations: injuries to the axillary nerve are associated with fracture or dislocation of the shoulder; injuries to the radial nerve are commonly associated with fracture of the humeral shaft; injuries to the median nerve at the wrist are commonly associated with displaced fractures of the radius; injuries to the sciatic nerve are commonly associated with fracture or dislocation of the hip; and injuries to the peroneal nerve are commonly associated with fracture of the neck of the fibula.

Fat Embolism Syndrome

FE syndrome is a complex clinical syndrome, consisting of fever, tachycardia, and confusion in association with arterial hypoxemia and other pertinent laboratory findings. Modern techniques for managing respiratory distress have decreased the mortality and morbidity rates associated with this syndrome. Its incidence correlates positively with the number of long bones fractured, with the presence of open fractures and with fractures caused by vehicular accidents (24,25).

The pathogenesis of the FE syndrome is a subject of controversy. Most investigators agree that bone marrow is the source of embolic fat seen in the lungs (26–31). Considerably fewer investigators agree about the exact role of this fat in the production of the clinical FE syndrome (32–39).

Peltier's original hypothesis states that lipase, endogenous to the lung, converts neutral fat to toxic free-fatty acids (40–42). Barie et al. have demonstrated that free-fatty acids are bound rapidly by albumin and transported through the bloodstream and the lymphatic channels in this benign form (32). An abundance of tissue thromboplastin is released with the marrow elements after long-bone fracture. This release activates the complement system and the extrinsic coagulation cascade (35,39) and results in the production of by-products of intravascular coagulation, such as fibrin and fibrin-degradation products. These blood elements, along with leukocytes, platelets, and fat globules, combine to increase pulmonary vascular permeability, both by their direct actions on the endothelial lining and through the release of numerous vasoactive substances (43,44). Suppression of the fibrinolytic system in the injured patient may then aggravate an ongoing accumulation of cellular aggregates, fat macroglobules, and clotting factors that are concentrated in the lung by virtue of its filtering action on venous blood before that blood is recycled to the systemic circulation (43). It has become increasingly apparent that embolic marrow fat and other elements may be only the catalyst for a single early step in a long chain of events that lead to the final common pathway of increased pulmonary vascular permeability in response to many forms of systemic injury.

Clinical Findings

The onset of the clinical symptoms of FE syndrome may be immediate or may not occur for two or three days after the trauma (45). Diagnosing this syndrome is largely a process of exclusion and depends on the clinician's index of suspicion. Symptoms are shortness of breath followed by restlessness and a changing neurologic picture and disorientation, which are followed by marked confusion, stupor, or coma. Arterial hypoxemia is the hallmark of the syndrome. PE should always be excluded by the results of a helical computed tomography scan of the chest before the diagnosis of FE syndrome is considered. Other clinical signs are temperature elevation to 39°C or 40°C; tachypnea, with rates of 30 breaths per minute or higher; and tachycardia, with rates of 140 beats per minute or higher. On the second or third day after injury, petechiae may be seen, characteristically located on the chest, the axilla, the root of the neck, and the conjunctivae. These clinical manifestations result from reduced blood flow to these vital organs. Other clinical signs are blindness and focal neurologic findings, including seizures.

No pathognomonic laboratory test exists for FE syndrome, but arterial hypoxemia is the hallmark of this condition. The measurement of arterial hypoxemia is a sensitive index of the degree of pulmonary FE and monitors the response to treatment. In the early stages, thrombocytopenia may occur with platelet values of less than 150×10^3/mL. The hematocrit often decreases (39). Chest radiographs demonstrate progressive snowstorm-like pulmonary infiltrations. The changes apparent on chest radiographs are characteristic but not specific (38). A cryostat-frozen specimen of clotted blood, which reveals the presence of fat, has been used in identifying FE syndrome; a biopsy of a skin petechial lesion can also demonstrate the presence of embolic intravascular fat (44).

Treatment

The initial (and perhaps the only specific) treatment for FE is aimed at decreasing hypoxemia. Oxygen should be administered immediately upon admission to the emergency department. Accurate monitoring of blood gases is crucial. If the degree of hypoxemia is relatively mild, oxygen can be given by mask; if the degree of hypoxemia is severe and respiratory failure is impending, prompt mechanical ventilatory assistance is mandatory.

A few specific drugs have been suggested as treatment for fat emboli— including ethanol, heparin, and hypertonic glucose— but these drugs are not effective in reducing the incidence of pulmonary failure. Recent clinical research suggests that early administration of corticosteroids may be helpful in treating FE syndrome (44). Another intervention that has been successful is angiographically guided occlusion of a patent foramen ovale in a patient with persistent neurologic sequelae resulting from FE syndrome. Finally, early fracture fixation and patient mobilization can decrease the incidence of FE syndrome and improve pulmonary function (34,46–59).

The prognosis for recovery from FE syndrome is poor for patients who have experienced marked pulmonary failure and coma. The mortality rate associated with these complications is high. Mild cases of this syndrome often go undetected, and mortality rates are low for patients who do not experience severe pulmonary insufficiency or cerebral manifestations.

Pearls and Pitfalls

- When encountered with respiratory or neurological distress, exclude PE and do not forget FE.

Compartment Syndrome

Acute compartment syndrome is a well-recognized complication of various conditions but most commonly of fracture. Compartment syndrome is defined as increased pressure within a fascial space, which compromises oxygen supply to the muscles and nerves within that compartment. The numerous causes of compartment syndrome include complications of open and closed fractures, arterial injury, temporary vascular occlusion, snakebite, drug abuse, burns, physical exertion, and gunshot wounds. Other possible causes are pulsatile lavage and contusion in patients with hemophilia (60).

Pathogenesis

The most common cause of compartment syndrome is muscle injury that leads to muscle edema, which is usually related to the amount of tissue damage. Pressure is increased within a closed space, first by intracellular swelling and then by the formation of a hematoma from the fractured bone. Because the extremities are composed of relatively unyielding fascial compartments, circulatory compromise ultimately occurs as tissue pressure rises, and this condition causes ischemia and tissue damage that result in leakage of intracellular fluid and a further increase in intracompartmental pressure. In the case of arterial injury, the muscle is deprived of its blood supply, and intracellular injury results. When circulation is reestablished, reperfusion injury occurs as the muscle swells, with secondary elevation of tissue pressure and further ischemic damage (60).

When injuries produce complete ischemia, skeletal muscle that is deprived of oxygen may survive for as long as four hours without irreversible damage (60,61). Total ischemia of eight hours duration produces a complete irreversible change. Peripheral nerves conduct impulses for one hour after the onset of total ischemia and can survive for four hours with only neurapraxic damage. After eight hours, axonotmesis and irreversible damage occur (62).

Ischemia caused by reduction or cessation of blood flow to the muscle results when the perfusion gradient in the compartment tissue falls below a critical level. Thus, perfusion is directly related to the patient's blood pressure. Experimentally measured terminal arterial pressure is equal to diastolic pressure, which is therefore used as the crucial measurement (60,61). When the intracompartmental pressure is 20 mmHg below the diastolic pressure, tissue perfusion in injured tissues is substantially decreased.

Fasciotomy should be performed when the intracompartmental pressure approaches 20 mmHg below the diastolic pressure or if an extremity has been completely ischemic for six hours or if the patient's clinical condition is worsening or if substantial tissue injury is present or if the tissue pressure is increasing (63). Prophylactic treatment is important. Fasciotomy will not reverse the changes caused by the initial trauma but can prevent changes that result from secondary ischemia.

Clinical Evaluation

Pain, pallor, paralysis, paresthesia, and pulselessness are the clinical hallmarks of compartment syndrome. It is important to note that these are the signs and symptoms of an established compartment syndrome with ischemic injury; fasciotomy at this stage yields poor results (60).

Pain and aggravation of pain by passive stretching of the muscles in the compartment in doubt are the most sensitive and generally the only clinical findings (60). Because pain is a subjective symptom, it is diagnostically useful only when patients are conscious and can respond cognitively to examination. In unconscious patients at risk of compartment syndrome, tissue-pressure measurements may be the only objective criteria for diagnosis. Lately, several studies have investigated the use of near infrared spectroscopy in the diagnosis of compartment syndrome. Although their results seem promising, clinical data is still required (64–66).

Tissue-Pressure Measurements

The location of the highest tissue pressure can be determined by taking measurements in all of the extremity's compartments, at the level of the fracture and proximal and distal to it (63). The highest pressure noted should serve as a basis for determining the need for fasciotomy. When tissue pressure is increasing, careful follow-up is required with repeated physical examination and pressure measurements every one to two hours until fasciotomy is indicated or pressure has decreased to a safe level and clinical signs and symptoms have improved.

The newer techniques of compartment monitoring allow the introduction of catheters coupled to transducers, which allow continuous monitoring of one or more compartments. However, obtaining repeated measurements at multiple areas in the same compartment is difficult with an indwelling device. Therefore, needle methods are more appropriate for multiple sites and repeated measurements. A number of methods of tissue-pressure measurement have been described. If properly used, all of them are accurate and equally measure the same phenomenon (60). The infusion technique is simple and inexpensive; it requires only mercury, two plastic IV extension tubes, two 18-gauge needles, one 20-mL syringe, one three-way stopcock, and normal saline (Fig. 1).

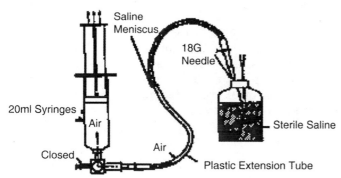

Three-way stopcock open to syringes and one extension tube.

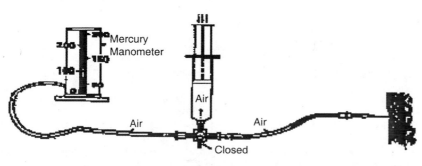

Three-way stopcock open to syringes and both extension tubes.

Figure 1 Infusion techniques.

Pearls and Pitfalls

■ Look for the 5 P's—pain, pallor, paralysis, paresthesia, and pulselessness

Open Fractures

With an open fracture, a break in the skin and the underlying soft tissues leads directly into or communicates with the fracture. The serious consequences of such an injury are contamination and crushing, stripping, and devascularization of soft tissues and the bone they cover (67). A minor injury, managed properly, arouses no great concern; a major injury may necessitate immediate or early amputation (68).

The prognosis of an open fracture is determined primarily by the amount of devitalized soft tissue caused by the injury and by the level and type of bacterial contamination. These two factors working in combination, rather than the configuration of the fracture itself, are the primary determinants of outcome (67). The extent of soft-tissue devitalization is defined by the energy absorbed by the limb at the time of injury. The most important and ultimate goal in the treatment of open fractures is to restore the function of the limb and of the patient as early and as fully as possible. To achieve this goal, the surgeon must prevent infection, restore soft tissues, achieve bone union, avoid malunion, and institute early joint motion and muscle rehabilitation. Of these goals, the most important is avoiding infection because infection is the event that most commonly leads to malunion, nonunion, and loss of function.

Prehospital care is crucial to the outcome of open fractures. The fractures should be aligned and splinted, and sterile dressings should be applied to the wound. In the hospital, all open fractures must be treated as an emergency. Surgery should be initiated as soon as the patient's general condition will allow it. A thorough initial evaluation should be carried out to diagnose other life-threatening injuries, and appropriate antibiotic therapy should be started in the emergency room or, at the latest, in the operating room before the procedure (69,70). The wound should be immediately debrided and the fracture should be stabilized. The wound is then left open for five to seven days.

Classification of open fractures is important because it provides guidelines for prognosis and suggests some methods of treatment. The wound classification system of Gustilo and Anderson (71,72) with subsequent modifications by Gustilo et al. (72–74) is the most widely accepted and quoted system. The crucial factors in this classification system are the degree of soft-tissue injury and the degree of contamination. Table 1 given below is a clarification of that classification (75).

An open fracture should generally be stabilized by using the method that provides adequate stability with a minimum of further damage to the vascularity of the zone of injury and its associated soft tissues (76). For type I wounds, any technique that is suitable for closed fracture management is satisfactory. Treatment of type II and type III wounds is more controversial; investigators have suggested traction, external fixation, nonreamed intramedullary nailing, and, occasionally, plate and screw fixation. Generally, external fixation is preferred for metaphyseal–diaphyseal fractures, with occasional limited internal fixation with screws. For the upper extremity, casting, external fixation, and plate-and-screw fixation are the more popular methods of stabilization. For the lower extremity, open diaphyseal femoral and tibial fractures have been successfully treated with intramedullary nailing, and type I, type II, and type IIIA fractures have been treated with nonreamed intramedullary nails, with encouraging results. External fixation is still the primary method of treatment for salvageable type IIIB and type IIIC fractures (67,68).

After surgery, the extremity must be efficiently immobilized. Gross motion delays wound healing and increases the risk of infection. Edema of the extremity is reduced by elevation and pressure dressings. The patient should be carefully observed so that any impairment in circulation or signs of infection can be promptly discovered.

Pearls and Pitfalls

■ Irrigation and debridement are the mainstay of treatment.
■ Add IV antibiotics.

Table 1 Classification of Open Fractures

Type	Wound	Level of contamination	Soft-tissue injury	Bone
I	<1 cm long	Clean	Minimal	Simple, minimal comminution
II	>1 cm long	Moderate	Moderate, some muscle damage	Moderate comminution
III[a]				
IIIA	Usually >10 cm long	High	Severe with crushing	Usually comminuted; soft-tissue coverage of bone possible
IIIB	Usually >10 cm long	High	Very severe loss of coverage	Bone coverage poor; usually requires soft-tissue reconstructive surgery
IIIC	Usually >10 cm long	High	Very severe loss of coverage plus vascular injury requiring repair	Bone coverage poor; usually requires soft-tissue reconstructive surgery

[a]Segmental fractures, farmyard injuries, fractures occurring in a highly contaminated environment, shotgun wounds, or high-velocity gunshot wounds automatically result in classification as a type III open fracture.
Source: From Ref. 72.

Thromboembolism

Venous thromboembolic disease is the most common complication after trauma to the lower extremities in adults, and PE is the most common fatal complication (77,78). Thrombophlebitis occurs in 40% to 60% of patients older than 40 years after fractures of the femur or tibia (10). Of these patients, 10% are at risk of pulmonary emboli, and, unless adequate protection is provided, 2% will die as a result of this complication (79). Risk factors associated with an increased incidence of venous thrombosis include age, obesity, myocardial infarction, heart failure, malignant disease, and the use of oral contraceptives (70,80–82). A congenital deficiency of antithrombin III and the presence of a lupus anticoagulant are also associated with an increased incidence of venous thrombosis (83).

When diagnosis is based solely on clinical findings such as complaints of pain, swelling, tenderness, Homan's sign, fever, and leukocytosis, thromboembolic disease is markedly underdiagnosed (84). Only 5% to 30% of instances of thrombophlebitis will be detected by physical examination alone (83). Objective testing is mandatory for an accurate diagnosis. Measurement of venous hemodynamics by Doppler ultrasonography can detect obstructions to venous blood flow that are produced by proximal thrombi. These methods are most accurate for thrombi in major veins (thigh) and are less accurate for thrombi in small veins (calf) because of the insignificant difference in outflow (85–87). The diagnostic gold standard is still radiocontrast venography (84,88,89). This is the most precise evaluation technique, with high accuracy in diagnosis of clots in the femoral and calf veins and approximately 70% reliability for clots in the iliac veins. Its disadvantages are that it causes some pain, is difficult to repeat frequently, and may induce thrombophlebitis in 5% of patients and an allergic reaction in 0.02% (83).

Treatment

Prevention is the best treatment for thromboembolic disease. Patients who are at highest risk of this complication are those who are obese, those who are elderly and have undergone multiple injuries or operations, those with a history of associated cardiovascular or pulmonary disease, and those with a prior episode or family history of deep venous thrombosis (DVT) who are about to undergo major musculoskeletal surgery (70,80–82). The prevention methods for venous thrombosis include sodium warfarin [Coumadin® (Bristol-Myers Squibb Company, New York, U.S.A.)], heparin, low-molecular-weight heparin (LMWH), aspirin, dextran, and intermittent pneumatic compression (IPC) devices. The largest clinical comparative study for trauma patients to date found both LMWH and IPC to be equally effective in the prevention of DVT (90).

For established DVT, the treatment is heparin administered by continuous IV infusion to maintain the activated partial thromboplastin time at 1.5 to 2.5 times normal. This treatment is continued for approximately one week. Oral warfarin therapy is usually started approximately three days after the initiation of heparin therapy. This overlap allows the prothrombin time to reach the effective range (1.5 to 2 times normal). Orally administered anticoagulant therapy is continued for four to six months, so that recurrent episodes of DVT can be prevented (83,91).

Pulmonary Embolism

PE occurs after lower extremity trauma in 5% to 19% of patients with DVT, who are unprotected by anticoagulants. Such emboli are fatal in 5% to 10% of patients after hip fracture. Prophylaxis decreases the incidence and mortality rates associated with PE (79).

Diagnosis is based on findings of dyspnea, chest pain, tachypnea, decreased arterial oxygen tension, and changes in the electrocardiogram (S1Q3 pattern of cor pulmonale, axis shift, bundle-branch blocks, and nonspecific ST- and T-wave changes). Each of these changes is nonspecific, but a new appearance in the appropriate clinical setting is highly suggestive of PE. Although 10% of patients with PE never exhibit hypoxemia (92), almost half of trauma patients with sustained hypoxemia experience PE, as demonstrated by pulmonary angiogram (93). Radionuclide ventilation-perfusion scanning is the test most commonly used to obtain an objective diagnosis of PE (94). Scans are considered to indicate a low, intermediate, or high probability of PE on the basis of the degree of conformity to a vascular pattern and the degree of ventilation-perfusion mismatch. Ninety percent of patients with high-probability lesions but only 5% of patients with low-probability lesions will have a PE as demonstrated by angiography (94). Pulmonary angiography is the most accurate method of detecting PE (95). Angiography and lung scanning are complementary studies; both should be performed when necessary and their results should be correlated with those indicated by plain chest radiographs. However, although pulmonary angiography is an invasive procedure, the risks associated with its use for the diagnosis of PE are less than those associated with a severe bleeding episode related to the therapeutic administration of heparin to patients with multiple injuries or those who have undergone surgery (96).

Heparinization is the treatment of choice for PE, followed by oral warfarin therapy for four to six months (91). Full anticoagulation has been shown to be necessary for reducing the risk of recurrent pulmonary emboli. For life-threatening massive emboli, open thoracotomy and embolectomy may be necessary (97,98). In cases of repeated PE, partial obstruction of the inferior vena cava with an inferior vena cava filter may be necessary for avoiding a fatal embolus (91).

- Consider DVT prophylaxis in every immobilizing fracture.

LATE COMPLICATIONS
Malunion

Malunion occurs when a fracture heals in an unsatisfactory position. Surgical correction of the resulting deformity is indicated if it causes unacceptable cosmetic or functional disabilities. Deformities in the weight-bearing bones may cause abnormal stress through the joints and lead to early osteoarthritis. Four main types of malunion occur: angulation, rotation, shortening, and translation.

When malunions are treated, the following facts must be considered. Of the four characteristics that define the acceptability of fracture reduction, the most important is alignment, the second is rotation, the third is restoration of normal length, and the fourth and least important is the actual position of the fragments. A slight deformity can be seriously disabling when a malunion involves a joint or is near a joint. Sometimes, when malunion causes only slight disability, function cannot be improved enough to justify surgery; however, a rotational deformity can be so disabling that surgery is required. Most deformities may correct themselves spontaneously (especially for young patients with immature skeletons) to a functionally satisfying degree during the remodeling phase of fracture healing. Unfortunately, such self-correction will not occur with rotational deformities.

Before surgical correction is attempted, the patient should participate in intensive physical therapy aimed at regaining the maximal range of motion of the joints. Surgical correction creates osteotomies to correct the deformity; either internal or external fixation may be used. Leg length discrepancy can be treated, if indicated, by lengthening the affected limb. For growing children, an epiphysiodesis of the unaffected bone may be performed at an appropriately planned time (99,100).

Nonunion

Nonunion occurs when a fracture has not united within a prescribed period of time, and all healing processes have ceased even though bone continuity has not been restored. The diagnosis is based on clinical and radiographic findings. The amount of time required for a fracture to unite is directly proportional to the amount of energy imparted to the extremity by the injury. The time required for union differs with different bones. Basically, all fractures will unite within four months; a fracture that has not healed within six months may be declared a delayed union and a fracture that has not healed within eight to nine months is defined as a nonunion. Pseudoarthrosis will develop if continued motion occurs at the fracture site and leads to the formation of a pseudocapsule and true synovial lining. Pseudoarthrosis is the final status of nonunion.

There are two types of nonunion. In the first type, the ends of the fragments are hypervascular or hypertrophic and are capable of biological reaction. In the second, the ends of the fragments are avascular or atrophic and are inert and incapable of biological reaction (99,100). The likelihood of nonunion is increased when fractures are open, infected, segmental with an impaired blood supply (usually to the middle fragment), comminuted by severe trauma, uncertainly fixed, immobilized for an insufficient time, treated by ill-advised open reduction, or distracted either by traction or by a plate and screws. Traditional nonsteroidal anti-inflammatory medications have been shown to delay fracture union (101). This effect may be smaller with cyclo-oxygenase-2-specific inhibitors (102).

The treatment of nonunion is individual for each case. In general, hypertrophic (hypervascular) nonunions can be treated by stable fixation of the fragments alone, whereas atrophic (avascular) nonunions require decortication and bone grafting for healing. Improvements in electrical and electromagnetic bone growth stimulators are currently being developed. Bone growth stimulators are usually used in conjunction with cast immobilization and weight bearing. External electrical stimulation is especially advantageous for managing infected nonunion or for treating patients for whom surgical intervention is contraindicated (100).

Avascular Necrosis

AVN or osteonecrosis is the cellular death of bone tissue after a fracture or dislocation; it occurs when the bone is deprived of a sufficient supply of arterial blood during the fracture, the reduction, or the operative fixation (103–107). This condition may be caused by factors other than trauma, but the pathomechanism is the same: intraluminar vascular compression or disruption of a blood vessel. After trauma, AVN occurs most commonly in the femoral head, the carpal scaphoid, and the body of the talus because of the specific retrograde blood supply to these bones (108).

Biopsy is the definitive method of diagnosis. Noninvasive studies include radiography and bone scanning. Advances in magnetic resonance imaging have made earlier diagnosis of AVN of the femoral head possible and have allowed determination of the exact stage and extent of the pathological process, without the use of invasive methods (109,110). Histologically, AVN begins with disappearance of hematopoietic elements and fat cell necrosis, followed by total necrosis of the marrow and osteocytes. The condition is repaired as the body lays new woven bone onto dead trabeculae. As the dead trabeculae are reabsorbed, the remaining unstressed woven bone may fracture, and this fracturing leads to collapse and fragmentation and eventually to an altered joint configuration (108). The main clinical presentation is pain in the involved joint, pain that is aggravated by activity.

The natural history of AVN is unpredictable. The best treatment for osteonecrosis depends on the cause, stage of involvement, symptoms, and location. No method of treatment apart from reducing weight bearing for a period of time has proved effective, but the rate and course of progression are variable, and the radiographic picture may not correlate with the clinical symptoms. The most common site of osteonecrosis requiring surgical treatment is the femoral head. There are several surgical treatment options for a femoral head that has not collapsed, such as core biopsy osteotomies and vascular-free fibular grafts, but these techniques have not consistently produced satisfactory results (111–113). Once osteochondral fracture and collapse occur in the femoral head, most patients require major reconstructive surgery. Osteonecrosis of the talus may also require major surgical reconstruction. When osteonecrosis affects the humeral head, healing may occur without surgical intervention, and many patients will continue to function well, even with moderate deformity. Those who experience severe symptoms can be treated successfully with a prosthetic replacement (108).

Heterotopic Ossification

Bone commonly forms around joints after trauma and surgery. We distinguish between ectopic calcification, heterotopic bone formation (or ossification), and myositis ossificans. Ectopic calcification is the mineralization of soft-tissue structures, areas in which calcification should not occur or is out of place. For example, calcification of the collateral ligaments is very common after elbow dislocation; it presents no functional limitation and requires no treatment (114).

Heterotopic bone formation or ossification refers to the formation of trabecular bone at a location where it does not belong (114,115). Unlike ectopic calcification, this bone forms not necessarily by mineralizing a definable structure but rather by forming new bone in areas of previous hematoma and fibroblast activity. The term "heterotopic ossification" refers to bone that has formed around a joint and is blocking motion. This condition has also been associated with head trauma (116) and burns (117).

Myositis ossificans is a subset of heterotopic bone formation. Myositis ossificans is a specific histopathologic condition that occurs in striated muscle, not simply around the capsule or around the joint. Patients with this condition usually experience swelling, pain, and a decreased range of motion. The most common locations include the thigh (the quadriceps muscle), the arm (the brachialis muscle), the shoulder (the deltoid and scapular muscles), and the hand. Initially, radiographs may show only faint, irregular radiodensities, but as the lesion matures, the radiographic appearance changes to that of more solid bone formation. In most patients, the lesion is not attached to the underlying bone, but it can be attached if it lies near the bone and if the original injury induced an adjacent periosteal reaction. Serial radiographs over a period of years will show that the volume of heterotopic bone gradually decreases (118).

Treatment is aimed at restoring function. Initially, patients are treated with rest and anti-inflammatory agents. Gentle physical therapy is instituted when local heat, edema, and pain subside. Isometric muscle strengthening and gentle, active-assisted range-of-motion exercises (within the limits of pain) are progressively increased until full function has been recovered. Manipulation should be avoided. Excision of the ectopic bone is rarely indicated.

SUMMARY

A fracture is a discontinuity of the bone that is caused by the application of an external force. In most cases, healing of the bone is relatively uneventful, especially in low-energy, closed fractures. However, one has to bear in mind the possible complications that may consequently arise. These complications could be classified into acute and late, each having distinct characteristics and impact.

Acute complications may be life threatening, including hypovolemic shock and fatal PE or FE syndrome. Acute limb threatening complications should be promptly recognized, namely, vascular compromise, neurological deterioration and impending infection. Therefore, an appropriate level of suspicion and alertness may dramatically improve the clinical outcome of these patients.

Late complications such as nonunion, malunion, and AVN mainly influence the long-term life quality of the patient, causing considerable morbidity leading to recurrent surgical interventions. Some of these complications are preventable, whereas others are related to the trauma mechanism. Good clinical practice and effective trauma team cooperation might lower the incidence and severity of undesired complications.

REFERENCES

1. Evans FG. Relation of the physical properties of bone to fractures. Instr Course Lect 1961; 18:110–121.
2. Hipp JA, Hayes WC. Biomechanics of fractures. In: Browner BD, Jupiter JB, Levine AM, Trafton PG, eds. Skeletal Trauma. Vol. 1. 3d ed. Philadelphia: WB Saunders, 2003:90–119.
3. Allum RL, Mowbray MA. A retrospective review of the healing of fractures of the shaft of the tibia with special reference to the mechanism of injury. Injury 1980; 11:304–308.
4. Pentecost RL, Murray RA, Brindley HH. Fatigue, insufficiency, and pathologic fractures. JAMA 1964; 187:1001–1004.
5. Kyle RF, Gustilo RB, Premer RF. Analysis of six hundred and twenty-two intertrochanteric hip fractures. J Bone Joint Surg Am 1979; 61:216–221.
6. Beck TJ, Ruff CB, Shaffer RA, Betsinger K, Trone DW, Brodine SK. Stress fracture in military recruits: gender differences in muscle and bone susceptibility factors. Bone 2000; 27:437–444.

7. Baker J, Frankel VH, Burstein AH. Fatigue fractures: biomechanical considerations [abstr]. J Bone Joint Surg Am 1972; 54:1345–1346.

8. Ostrum RF, Verghese GB, Santner TJ. The lack of association between femoral shaft fractures and hypotensive shock. J Orthop Trauma 1993; 7:338–342.

9. Poole GV, Ward EF. Causes of mortality in patients with pelvic fractures. Orthopedics 1994; 17:691–696.

10. Fox MA, Mangiante EC, Fabian TC, Voeller GR, Kudsk KA. Pelvic fractures: an analysis of factors affecting prehospital triage and patient outcome. South Med J 1990; 83:785–788.

11. Burgess AR, Eastridge BG, Young JW, et al. Pelvic ring disruptions: effective classification system and treatment. J Trauma 1990; 30:848–856.

12. Buckle R, Browner BD, Morandi M. Emergency reduction for pelvic ring disruptions and control of associated hemorrhage using the pelvic stabilizer. Tech Orthop 1995; 9:258–266.

13. Ghanayem AJ, Wilber JH, Lieberman JM, Motta AO. The effect of laparotomy and external fixator stabilization on pelvic volume in an unstable pelvic injury. J Trauma 1995; 38:396–401.

14. Jerrard DA. Pelvic fractures. Emerg Med Clin North Am 1993; 11:147–163.

15. Agnew SG. Hemodynamically unstable pelvic fractures. Orthop Clin North Am 1994; 25:715–721.

16. Sanders R, DiPasquale T. External fixation of the pelvis: application of the resuscitation frame. Tech Orthop 1990; 4:60–64.

17. Ganz R, Krushell RJ, Jakob RP, Kuffer J. The antishock pelvic clamp. Clin Orthop 1991; 267:71–78.

18. Ben-Menachem Y. Pelvic fractures: diagnostic and therapeutic angiography. Instr Course Lect 1988; 37:139–141.

19. Siliski JM. Fractures of the pelvic ring. In: Browner BD, Jupiter JB, Levine AM, Trafton PG, eds. Skeletal Trauma. Vol. 2. 3d ed. Philadelphia: WB Saunders, 1992:2052–2056.

20. Malan E, Tattoni G. Physio-and anatomo-pathology of acute ischemia of the extremities. J Cardiovasc Surg 1963; 4:212–225.

21. Frykberg ER, Dennis JW, Bishop K, Laneve L, Alexander RH. The reliability of physical examination in the evaluation of penetrating extremity trauma for vascular injury: results at one year. J Trauma 1991; 31:502–511.

22. Lynch K, Johansen K. Can Doppler pressure measurement replace "exclusion" arteriography in the diagnosis of occult extremity arterial trauma? Ann Surg 1991; 214:737.

23. Feliciano DV, Moore EE, Mattox KL, eds. Trauma. 3d ed. Publisher, 1996.

24. Collins JA, Gordon WC Jr., Hudson TL, Irvin RW Jr., Kelly T, Hardaway RM III. Inapparent hypoxemia in casualties with wounded limbs: pulmonary fat embolism? Ann Surg 1968; 167:511–520.

25. Collins JA, Hudson TL, Hamacher WR, Rokous J, Williams G, Hardaway RM III. Systemic fat embolism in four combat casualties. Ann Surg 1968; 167:493–499.

26. Armin J, Grant RT. Observations on gross pulmonary fat embolism in man and the rabbit. Clin Sci 1951; 10:441–469.

27. Jacobs RR, Wheeler EJ, Jelenko C III, McDonald TF, Bliven FE. Fat embolism: a microscopic and ultrastructure evaluation of two animal models. J Trauma 1973; 13:980–993.

28. Kerstell J. Pathogenesis of post-traumatic fat embolism. Am J Surg 1971; 121:712–715.

29. Kerstell J, Hallgren B, Rudenstam CM, Svanborg A. The chemical composition of the fat emboli in the post-absorptive dog. Acta Med Scand 1969; suppl 499:3–18.

30. Meek RN, Woodruff B, Allardyce DB. Source of fat macroglobules in fractures of the lower extremity. J Trauma 1972; 12:432–434.

31. Schnaid E, Lamprey JM, Viljoen MJ, Joffe BI, Seftel HC. The early biochemical and hormonal profile of patients with long bone fractures at risk of fat embolism syndrome. J Trauma 1987; 27:309–311.

32. Barie PS, Minnear FL, Malik AB. Increased pulmonary vascular permeability after bone marrow injection in sheep. Am Rev Respir Dis 1981; 123:648–653.

33. Bergentz SE. Studies on the genesis of posttraumatic fat embolism. Acta Chir Scand 1961; suppl 282:1–72.

34. Bone L, Bucholz R. The management of fractures in the patient with multiple trauma. J Bone Joint Surg Am 1986; 68:945–949.

35. Hammerschmidt DE, Weaver LJ, Hudson LD, Craddock PR, Jacob HS. Association of complement activation and elevated plasma-C5a with adult respiratory distress syndrome. Pathophysiological relevance and possible prognostic value. Lancet 1980; 1:947–949.

36. Kaplan JE, Saba TM. Humoral deficiency and reticuloendothelial depression after traumatic shock. Am J Physiol 1976; 230:7–14.

37. LeQuire VS, Shapiro JL, LeQuire CB, Cobb CA Jr., Fleet WF Jr. A study of the pathogenesis of fat embolism based on human necropsy material and animal experiments. Am J Pathol 1959; 35:999–1015.

38. Maruyama Y, Little JB. Roentgen manifestations of traumatic pulmonary fat embolism. Radiology 1962; 79:945–952.

39. Tennenberg SD, Jacobs MF, Solomkin JS. Complement-mediated neutrophil activation in sepsis- and trauma-related adult respiratory distress syndrome. Clarification with radioaerosol lung scans. Arch Surg 1987; 122:26–32.

40. Peltier LF. An appraisal of the problem of fat embolism. Surg Gynecol Obstet 1957; 104:313–324.

41. Peltier LF. The diagnosis and treatment of fat embolism. J Trauma 1971; 11:661–667.

42. Peltier LF, Adler F, Lai SP. Fat embolism: the significance of an elevated serum lipase after trauma to bone. Am J Surg 1960; 99:821–826.

43. Crocker SH, Eddy DO, Obenauf RN, Wismar BL, Lowery BD. Bacteremia: host-specific lung clearance and pulmonary failure. J Trauma 1981; 21:215–220.

44. Gossling HR, Pellegrini VD Jr. Fat embolism syndrome: a review of the pathophysiology and physiological basis of treatment. Clin Orthop 1982; 165: 68–82.

45. Evarts CM. The fat embolism syndrome: a review. Surg Clin North Am 1970; 50:493–507.

46. Whitesides TE, Heckman MM. Acute compartment syndrome: update on diagnosis and treatment. J Am Acad Orthop Surg 1996; 4:209–218.

47. Bone LB, Johnson KD, Weigelt J, Scheinberg R. Early versus delayed stabilization of femoral fractures.

A prospective randomized study. J Bone Joint Surg Am 1989; 71:336–340.

48. Fabian TC, Hoots AV, Stanford DS, Patterson CR, Mangiante EC. Fat embolism syndrome: a prospective evaluation in 92 fracture patients. Crit Care Med 1990; 18:42–45.

49. Goris RJ. The injury severity score. World J Surg 1983; 7:12–18.

50. Goris RJ, Gimbrere JS, Van Niekerk JL, Schoots FJ, Body LH. Early osteosynthesis and prophylactic mechanical ventilation in the multitrauma patient. J Trauma 1982; 22:895–903.

51. Johnson KD, Cadambi A, Seibert GB. Incidence of adult respiratory distress syndrome in patients with multiple musculoskeletal injuries: effect of early operative stabilization of fractures. J Trauma 1985; 25:375–384.

52. Lozman J, Deno DC, Feustel PJ, et al. Pulmonary and cardiovascular consequences of immediate fixation or conservative management of long bone fractures. Arch Surg 1986; 121:992–999.

53. Pipkin G. The early diagnosis and treatment of fat embolism. Clin Orthop 1958; 15:171–182.

54. Riska E, Myllynen P. Fat embolism in patients with multiple injuries. J Trauma 1982; 22:891–894.

55. Riska EB, von Bonsdorff H, Hakkinen S, Jaroma H, Kiviluoto O, Paavilainen T. Primary operative fixation of long bone fractures in patients with multiple injuries. J Trauma 1977; 17:111–121.

56. Rokkanen P, Lahdensuu M, Kataja J, Julkunen H. The syndrome of fat embolism: analysis of thirty consecutive cases compared to trauma patients with similar injuries. J Trauma 1970; 10:299–306.

57. Ruedi T, Wolff G. Vermeidung postraumatischer komplikationen durch fruhe definitive versorgung von polytraumatisierten mit frakturen des bewegungsapparats. [Prevention of post-traumatic complications through immediate therapy of patients with multiple injuries and fractures.]. Helv Chir Acta 1975; 42: 507–512.

58. Seibel R, LaDuca J, Hassett JM, et al. Blunt multiple trauma (ISS 36), femur traction, and the pulmonary failure-septic state. Ann Surg 1985; 202:283–295.

59. Talucci RC, Manning J, Lampard S, Bach A, Carrico CJ. Early intramedullary nailing of femoral shaft fractures: a cause of fat embolism syndrome. Am J Surg 1983; 146:107–111.

60. ten Duis HJ, Nijsten MW, Klasen HJ, Binnendijk B. Fat embolism in patients with an isolated fracture of the femoral shaft. J Trauma 1988; 28:383–390.

61. Whitesides TE, Haney TC, Morimoto K, Harada H. Tissue pressure measurements as a determinant for the need of fasciotomy. Clin Orthop Relat Res 1975; 113:43–51.

62. Worlock P, Slack R, Harvey L, Mawhinney R. The prevention of infection in open fractures. An experimental study of the effect of antibiotic therapy. J Bone Joint Surg Am 1988; 70:1341–1347.

63. Tornetta P III, Templeman D. Compartment syndrome associated with tibial fracture. Instr Course Lect 1997; 46:303–308.

64. Garr JL, Gentilello LM, Cole PA, Mock CN, Matsen FA III. Monitoring for compartmental syndrome using near-infrared spectroscopy: a noninvasive, continuous, transcutaneous monitoring technique. J Trauma 1999; 46(4):613–616.

65. Giannotti G, Cohn SM, Brown M, Varela JE, McKenney MG, Wiseberg JA. Utility of near-infrared spectroscopy in the diagnosis of lower extremity compartment syndrome. J Trauma 2000; 48(3):396–399.

66. Gentilello LM, Sanzone A, Wang L, Liu PY, Robinson L. Near-infrared spectroscopy versus compartment pressure for the diagnosis of lower extremity compartmental syndrome using electromyography-determined measurements of neuromuscular function. J Trauma 2001; 51(1):1–8.

67. Beherens FF, Sirkin MS. Fractures with soft tissue injuries. In: Browner BD, Jupiter JB, LevineAM, Trafton PG, eds. Skeletal Trauma. Vol. 13. 3d ed. Philadelphia: WB Sauders, 2003:293–319.

68. Gustilo RB, Merkow RL, Templeman D. The management of open fractures. J Bone Joint Surg Am 1990; 72:299–304.

69. Waterman NG, Howell RS, Babich M. The effect of a prophylactic antibiotic (cephalothin) on the incidence of wound infection. Arch Surg 1968; 97:365–370.

70. Crandon AJ, Peel KR, Anderson JA, Thompson V, McNicol GP. Postoperative deep vein thrombosis: identifying high-risk patients. Br Med J 1980; 281:343–344.

71. Gustilo RB, Anderson JT. Prevention of infection in the treatment of one thousand and twenty-five open fractures of long bones: retrospective and prospective analyses. J Bone Joint Surg Am 1976; 58:453–458.

72. Gustilo RB, Gruninger RP, Davis T. Classification of type III (severe) open fractures relative to treatment and results. Orthopedics 1987; 10:1781–1788.

73. Gustilo RB. Current concepts in the management of open fractures. Instr Course Lect 1987; 36:359–366.

74. Gustilo RB, Simpson L, Nixon R, Ruiz A, Indeck W. Analysis of 511 open fractures. Clin Orthop 1969; 66:148–154.

75. Chapman MW. The role of intramedullary fixation in open fractures. Clin Orthop 1986; 212:26–34.

76. Worlock P, Slack R, Harvey L, Mawhinney R. The prevention of infection in open fractures: an experimental study of the effect of fracture stability. Injury 1994; 25: 31–38.

77. Tubiana R, Duparc J. Frequency and prevention of thromboembolic complications in orthopaedic and accident surgery. Acta Orthop Belg 1962; 28:605–611.

78. Hamilton HW, Crawford JS, Gardiner JH, Wiley AM. Venous thrombosis in patients with fracture of the upper end of the femur. A phlebographic study of the effect of prophylactic anticoagulation. J Bone Joint Surg Br 1970; 52(2):268–289.

79. Sikorski JM, Hampson WG, Staddon GE. The natural history and aetiology of deep vein thrombosis after total hip replacement. J Bone Joint Surg Br 1981; 63:171–177.

80. Coon WW, Coller FA. Some epidemiologic considerations of thromboembolism. Surg Gynecol Obstet 1959; 109:487–501.

81. Coon WW, Willis PW. Deep venous thrombosis and pulmonary embolism: prediction, prevention and treatment. Am J Cardiol 1959; 4:611–621.

82. Gallus AS, Hirsh J. Prevention of venous thromboembolism. Semin Thromb Hemost 1976; 2:232–290.

83. Aaron RK, Ciombor D. Venous thromboembolism in the orthopedic patient. Surg Clin North Am 1983; 63:529–537.

84. Couch NP. AMA Archives symposium on diagnostic techniques in phlebothrombosis. Arch Surg 1972; 104:132–133.

85. Flinn WR, Sandager GP, Cerullo LJ, Havey RJ, Yao JS. Duplex venous scanning for the prospective surveillance of perioperative venous thrombosis. Arch Surg 1989; 124:901–905.

86. Froehlich JA, Dorfman GS, Cronan JJ, Urbanek PJ, Herndon JH, Aaron RK. Compression ultrasonography for the detection of deep venous thrombosis in patients who have a fracture of the hip. A prospective study. J Bone Joint Surg Am 1989; 71:249–256.

87. Lensing A, Prandoni P, Brandjes D, et al. Detection of deep-vein thrombosis by real-time B-mode ultrasonography. N Engl J Med 1989; 320:342–345.

88. Borow M, Goldson H. Postoperative venous thrombosis. Evaluation of five methods of treatment. Am J Surg 1981; 141:245–251.

89. Culver D, Crawford JS, Gardiner JH, Wiley AM. Venous thrombosis after fractures of the upper end of the femur. A study of incidence and site. J Bone Joint Surg Br 1970; 52:61–69.

90. Ginzburg E, Cohn SM, Lopez J, Jackowski J, Brown M, Hameed SM. Miami Deep Vein Thrombosis Study Group Randomized clinical trial of intermittent pneumatic compression and low molecular weight heparin in trauma. Br J Surg 2003; 90(11):1338–1344.

91. Herndon GH. Chapter 10: Circulatory, respiratory, hematopoietic, gastrointestinal, genitourinary and integumentary systems. In: Fitzgerald RH Jr., ed. Orthopaedic Knowledge Update 2. Park Ridge, Illinois: American Academy of Orthopaedic Surgeons, 1987:107–122.

92. Henry JW, Stein PD, Gottschalk A, Relyea B, Leeper KV Jr. Scintigraphic lung scans and clinical assessment in critically ill patients with suspected acute pulmonary embolism. Chest 1996; 109(2): 462–466.

93. Brathwaite C, O'Malley K, Ross S, Pappas PJ, Alexander JB, Spence RK. Continuous pulse oximetry and the diagnosis of pulmonary embolism in critically ill trauma patients. J Trauma 1992; 33(4):528–531.

94. McBride K, LaMorte WW, Menzoian JO. Can ventilation-perfusion scans accurately diagnose acute pulmonary embolism? Arch Surg 1986; 121:754–757.

95. Bookstein JJ. Segmental arteriography in pulmonary embolism. Radiology 1969; 93:1007–1012.

96. Patterson B, Marchand R, Ranawat C. Complications of heparin therapy after total joint arthroplasty. J Bone Joint Surg Am 1989; 71:1130–1134.

97. Mavor GE, Galloway JM. Iliofemoral venous thrombosis. Pathological considerations and surgical management. Br J Surg 1969; 56:45–49.

98. Miller GA. The diagnosis and management of massive pulmonary embolism. Br J Surg 1972; 59:837–839.

99. Palei D. Principles of deformity correction. In: Browner BD, Jupiter JB, Levine AM, Trafton PG, eds. Skeletal Trauma. Vol. 62. 3d ed. Philadelphia: WB Sauders, 2003:2519–2576.

100. Beaty J. Congenital anomalies of lower extremity. In: Canale ST, ed. Campbell's Operative Orthopedics. Vol. 26. 10th ed. Philadelphia: Mosby, 2003:1048–1054.

101. Giannoudis PV, MacDonald DA, Matthews SJ, Smith RM, Furlong AJ, De Boer P. Nonunion of the femoral diaphysis. The influence of reaming and non-steroidal anti-inflammatory drugs. J Bone Joint Surg Br 2000; 82(5):655–658.

102. Brown KM, Saunders MM, Kirsch T, Donahue HJ, Reid JS. Effect of COX-2-specific inhibition on fracture-healing in the rat femur. J Bone Joint Surg Am 2004; 86-A(1):116–123.

103. Brodetti A. The blood supply of the femoral neck and head in relation to the damaging effects of nails and screws. J Bone Joint Surg Br 1960; 42:794–801.

104. Brodetti A. An experimental study on the use of nails and bolt screws in the fixation of fractures of the femoral neck. Acta Orthop Scand 1961; 31:247–271.

105. Catto M. A histological study of avascular necrosis of the femoral head after transcervical fracture. J Bone Joint Surg Br 1965; 47:749–776.

106. Catto M. The histological appearances of late segmental collapse of the femoral head after transcervical fracture. J Bone Joint Surg Br 1965; 47:777–791.

107. Rizzo PF, Gould ES, Lyden JP, Asnis SE. Diagnosis of occult fractures about the hip. Magnetic resonance imaging compared with bone-scanning. J Bone Joint Surg Am 1993; 73:395–401.

108. Levine M. In: Beaty JH, ed. Orthopaedic Knowledge Update 6: Home Study Syllabus. Rosemont, Illinois: American Academy of Orthopaedic Surgeons, 1999; 38:455–492.

109. Greenspan A. Radiologic evaluation of trauma. In: Greenspan A, ed. Orthopedic Radiology. 3d ed. Philadelphia: Lippincot Williams and Wilkins, 1999:71–76.

110. Lang P, Jergesen HE, Genant HK, Moseley ME, Schulte-Monting J. Magnetic resonance imaging of the ischemic femoral head in pigs. Dependency of signal intensities and relaxation times on elapsed time. Clin Orthop 1989; 244:272–280.

111. Brunelli G, Brunelli G. Free microvascular fibular transfer for idiopathic femoral head necrosis: long-term follow-up. J Reconstr Microsurg 1991; 7:285–295.

112. Fujimaki A, Yamauchi Y. Vascularized fibular grafting for treatment of aseptic necrosis of the femoral head—preliminary results in four cases. Microsurgery 1983; 4:17–22.

113. Urbaniak JR. Aseptic necrosis of the femoral head treated by vascularized fibular graft. In: Urbaniak JR, ed. Microsurgery for Major Limb Reconstruction. St. Louis: Mosby, 1987:178–184.

114. Ackerman LV. Extra-osseous localized non-neoplastic bone and cartilage formation (so-called myositis ossificans): clinical and pathological confusion with malignant neoplasms. J Bone Joint Surg Am 1958; 40:279–298.

115. Coventry MB. Ectopic ossification about the elbow. In: Morrey BF, ed. The Elbow and Its Disorders. Philadelphia: WB Saunders, 1985:464–471.

116. Garland DE, Hanscom DA, Keenan MA, Smith C, Moore T. Resection of heterotopic ossification in the adult with head trauma. J Bone Joint Surg Am 1985; 67:1261–1269.

117. Seth MK, Khurana JK. Bony ankylosis of the elbow after burns. J Bone Joint Surg Br 1985; 67:747–749.

118. Greenspan A. Radiologic evaluation of trauma. In: Greenspan A, ed. Orthopedic Radiology. 3d. Philadelphia: Lippincot Williams and Wilkins, 1999:63–80.

34

Complications of Dislocations

Howard Richter and Gregory A. Zych
*Department of Orthopedics and Rehabilitation, University of Miami, Miller School of Medicine,
Miami, Florida, U.S.A.*

A dislocation is a complete disruption of a joint so that the articular surfaces are no longer in contact. Most often, the cause of the dislocation is a traumatic event and the result is a loss of structural stability of the joint. Traumatic dislocation usually causes pain, deformity of the involved extremity, and marked limitation of joint motion. Appropriate treatment of a dislocation involves careful neurovascular evaluation, radiographic studies, and prompt reduction of the involved joint. Complications and long-term sequelae of traumatic dislocation include neurovascular injuries, avascular necrosis, heterotopic bone formation, posttraumatic arthritis, musculotendinous injuries, joint instability, and joint stiffness.

VASCULAR INJURIES ASSOCIATED WITH DISLOCATION

Vascular injury can occur in the involved extremity because the joint is forcibly displaced from its anatomic location. The medical literature contains reports of 200 cases of vascular injury after shoulder dislocations (1). Most of these cases involved elderly patients, whose vessels are stiffer and more fragile. The axillary artery consists of three sections that lie medial to, behind, and lateral to the pectoralis minor muscle. The second section of the artery is most commonly injured when the thoracoacromial trunk is avulsed, and the third section is most commonly injured when the subscapular and circumflex branches are avulsed (2). The mechanism of injury is believed to be the forced abduction and external rotation of the shoulder. Because the humeral head dislocates anteriorly, the artery becomes taut and is displaced forward. Because the artery is relatively fixed at the lateral margin of the pectoralis minor muscle, this forward displacement causes the pectoralis minor muscle to act as a fulcrum over which the artery is deformed and ruptured. Patients with axillary artery injuries resulting from shoulder dislocation experience pain, an expanding hematoma, pulse deficit, peripheral cyanosis, pallor, and neurologic dysfunction. Treatment requires emergent vascular repair.

Vascular injuries have also been reported after elbow dislocations. Approximately 30 cases of brachial artery disruption have been reported after elbow dislocations (3). Brachial artery injury occurs most often with open dislocations and in the presence of associated fractures.

The most common dislocation resulting in vascular injury is dislocation of the knee (Fig. 1). Green and Allen, in a review of 245 knee dislocations, found a 32% incidence of popliteal artery injury in association with traumatic dislocation of the tibiofemoral

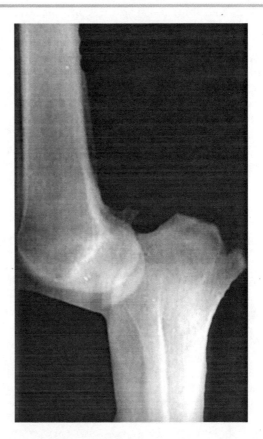

Figure 1 Posterior dislocation of a knee. The direction of the dislocation is determined by the position of the tibia relative to that of the femur.

(A) **(B)**

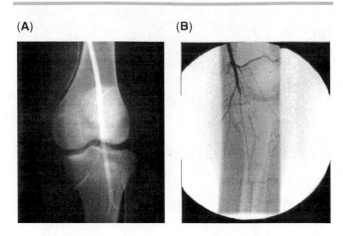

Figure 2 Angiogram of a knee after dislocation. Note the beading of the vessel just proximal to the knee joint. This finding indicates intimal damage to the popliteal artery.

joint (4). Anatomically, the popliteal artery is tethered proximally to the femur in the adductor hiatus and distally to the fibula by the fibrous bands of the soleus fascia. This tethering of the artery explains the high incidence of vascular injury in association with disruption and subsequent displacement of the knee joint (Fig. 2). Posterior dislocations (posterior displacement of the tibia) can result in complete transection of the artery because the vessel impacts the posterior rim of the tibial plateau. Anterior dislocations (anterior displacement of the tibia) typically cause a contusion of the vessel with intimal injury. Popliteal artery injuries are a surgical emergency requiring immediate repair. Consensus exists among traumatologists that circulation to the extremity needs to be restored within six to eight hours if the risk of amputation is to be minimized because an amputation rate of 85% has been reported for cases in which the popliteal artery injury was left untreated or was not repaired within eight hours (5).

NEURAL INJURIES ASSOCIATED WITH DISLOCATION

In the event of the joint being dislocated, the surrounding neural structures can be contused, stretched, or even lacerated. The sciatic nerve, specifically the peroneal component, is injured in 8% to 19% of patients who sustain a posterior dislocation of the hip (6). Epstein et al. (7) postulated that one of the most important factors in the production of sciatic nerve injury is the marked internal rotation of the hip that occurs at the time of dislocation. The internal rotation causes a winding and tightening of the sciatic nerve. As the hip dislocates posteriorly, it directly contuses or entraps the nerve, and this contusion or entrapment often results in peroneal nerve palsy. These nerve injuries must be recognized early because nerve tissue does not tolerate pressure well

and permanent ischemic changes occur quickly. Treatment again involves a thorough physical and radiographic examination followed by a prompt reduction. Most reports of series of patients show that 60% to 70% of patients with sciatic nerve palsy eventually experience functional recovery (8).

The axillary nerve is the neural structure most commonly injured in association with shoulder dislocations. Axillary nerve injury has been reported to occur with 5% to 33% of all shoulder dislocations; it is most common among elderly patients, after high-energy trauma, and in association with long-standing dislocations (9). The axillary nerve lies directly across the anterior surface of the subscapularis muscle. As the humeral head displaces the subscapularis muscle and tendon forward and anterior in glenohumeral dislocations, traction and direct pressure are produced on the axillary nerve and result in injury to the neural structures. The diagnosis of nerve injury is made on the basis of neurologic signs such as weakness or numbness after dislocation. Blom and Dahlback demonstrated that the usual sensory testing of the axillary nerve on the skin of the lateral arm just above the deltoid insertion yields unreliable diagnostic findings (10). Most axillary nerve injuries are traction neuropraxias and will recover completely.

Common peroneal nerve palsies can result after knee dislocations. Typically, 20% to 40% of knee dislocations, primarily those involving lateral and posterolateral dislocations of the tibia, result in peroneal nerve palsies (11). Approximately half of these palsies are permanent. Treatment involves symptomatic care with the use of assistive ambulation devices, possible surgical exploration, tendon transfers, or nerve grafting.

AVASCULAR NECROSIS AFTER DISLOCATION

Avascular necrosis of the femoral head is a well-recognized complication after posterior dislocation of the hip. The incidence of avascular necrosis varies from 6% to 40% after posterior dislocation of the hip (12). The cause of the avascular change is believed to be ischemia caused by damage to the vessels of the ligamentum teres and the retinaculum of Weitbrecht. Both the degree of initial trauma and the time during which the hip remains dislocated have been found to directly correlate with the likelihood of avascular necrosis. Hougaard and Thomsen reported that reduction within six hours of injury substantially decreased the incidence of avascular necrosis (13). Therefore, prompt reduction is mandated in all cases of hip dislocation. Avascular necrosis has been reported to occur as long as two to five years after posterior dislocation of the hip. Thus, careful monitoring and follow-up must be maintained after reduction if possible avascular changes are to be detected. If avascular necrosis is not diagnosed early, femoral head collapse and traumatic arthritis will result.

HETEROTOPIC BONE FORMATION AFTER DISLOCATION

Heterotopic ossification of the surrounding soft tissue can occur as a result of traumatic joint dislocation. This condition is most frequently noted after elbow dislocation and occurs in as many as 75% of cases (14). The most common sites of periarticular calcification are the anterior elbow region and the collateral ligaments. Ectopic bone formation is associated with delayed surgical intervention, closed head injury, and aggressive passive elbow joint manipulation after dislocation. If heterotopic bone formation is limiting joint motion, resection of the involved bone should be delayed until the ossification appears mature on plain radiographs, typically six months after the initial trauma. Radiographic maturation is characterized by well-defined cortical margins with linear trabeculations.

Ectopic bone formation has also been reported after hip dislocation (Fig. 3). Epstein reported a 2% incidence of myositis ossificans after hip dislocation (15). The ectopic bone formation is believed to result from the initial muscle damage, the formation of hematoma, and the influx of inflammatory mediators. The severity of the traumatic dislocation seems to be the best predicator of the occurrence of bone formation in the surrounding tissue. Restriction of motion is not common; therefore, treatment is based on symptoms and the recommended excision time of the extraosseous tissue correlates with the maturity of the ectopic bone.

POSTTRAUMATIC ARTHRITIS AFTER DISLOCATION

The traumatic process of a joint dislocation can permanently and irreversibly injure the articular cartilage

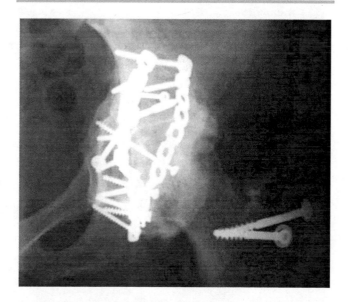

Figure 3 Heterotopic ossification of the soft tissues surrounding the hip joint after posterior dislocation of the hip.

lining the involved joint. This injury to the cartilage can lead to the development of osteoarthritis. The severity of the initial trauma and the structural damage to the articular surface are the primary factors in determining the later development of posttraumatic arthritis. Hip and ankle dislocations are most commonly associated with the later development of arthritic changes.

MUSCULOTENDINOUS INJURY AFTER DISLOCATION

Dislocation may disrupt surrounding muscles and tendons and cause a functional disability. Anterior and inferior glenohumeral dislocations can injure the rotator cuff of the shoulder. Tijmes et al. (16) reported rotator cuff tears in association with 28% of anterior dislocations. The frequency of this complication increases with the age of the patient. Thirty percent of patients older than 40 years and 80% of patients older than 60 years typically sustain rotator cuff tears with dislocations (16). Injury to the rotator cuff causes pain and weakness with external rotation and abduction of the shoulder. Treatment involves appropriate radiographic studies to assess the extent of the rotator cuff tear, conservative therapy, and possibly surgical repair.

INSTABILITY AFTER DISLOCATION

Traumatic dislocations can seriously injure the supportive structures of the joint, thus rendering it unstable during physiologic motion. This instability is most common after glenohumeral dislocations in young patients. McLaughlin and MacLellan (17) observed recurrence of 95% of 181 primary traumatic dislocations of the shoulder in teenagers. Most of the secondary dislocations occurred within two years of the initial traumatic dislocation. This increased rate of instability is linked to the high incidence of disruption of the labral attachment of the anterior inferior glenohumeral ligament and of fracture of the anterior inferior glenoid rim (Bankart lesion) after dislocations. Disruption of the anterior inferior glenohumeral ligament, which is the primary static restraint to anterior shoulder dislocation, increases the patient's susceptibility to repeated dislocation during abduction and external rotation. Treatment involves sling immobilization and possibly surgical intervention.

Hip dislocation can also result in persistent joint instability. Lutter reported the occurrence of repeated dislocations after approximately 1% of hip dislocations (18). Instability is believed to be linked to repeated injury, a shallow acetabulum or deficient posterior rim, and massive soft-tissue injury. Treatment typically involves some form of capsular plication.

After traumatic elbow dislocation, insufficiency of the lateral elbow ligaments can lead to elbow instability. Injury to the ulnar lateral collateral ligament is primarily responsible for this lack of stability. With injury to the ulnar collateral ligament, the elbow subluxates with elbow supination and flexion. Typically, nonoperative treatment with elbow immobilization is adequate to allow regaining the stability of the joint.

Most dislocations of the knee involve tears of the central pivot, including both the posterior cruciate ligament and the anterior cruciate ligament. The collateral ligaments are also frequently disrupted in dislocations of the tibiofemoral joint. Incompetence of these ligaments— which are the primary stabilizers to anterior, posterior, varus, and valgus stresses— makes the knee quite unstable and severely limits the patient's ability to ambulate. Current treatment guidelines recommend early (within one to two weeks) surgical reconstruction or repair of all involved ligamentous structures so that stability and mobility of the knee can be maximized.

JOINT STIFFNESS AFTER DISLOCATION

Stiffness of the elbow joint is very common after traumatic dislocation. Most patients will lose the terminal 10° to 15° of elbow extension after elbow dislocation. The stiffness is frequently caused by thickening and fibrosis of the anterior joint capsule. Early active mobilization, usually within two weeks of injury, is necessary if this complication is to be minimized. Elbow capsular release can be considered if an elbow contracture of more than 30° persists after six months of therapy.

REFERENCES

1. Gugenheim S, Sanders RJ. Axillary artery rupture caused by shoulder dislocation. Surgery 1984; 95:55–58.
2. Beeson M. Complications of shoulder dislocation. Am J Emerg Med 1999; 17:288–295.
3. Cohen MS, Hastings H II. Acute elbow dislocation: evaluation and management. J Am Acad Orthop Surg 1998; 6:15–23.
4. Green NE, Allen BL. Vascular injuries associated with dislocation of the knee. J Bone Joint Surg Am 1977; 59:236–239.
5. Good L, Johnson RJ. The dislocated knee. J Am Acad Orthop Surg 1995; 3:284–292.
6. Stewart MJ, McCarroll HR Jr., Mulhollan JS. Fracture-dislocation of the hip. Acta Orthop Scand 1975; 46:507–525.
7. Epstein HC, Wiss DA, Cozen L. Posterior fracture dislocation of the hip with fractures of the femoral head. Clin Orthop 1985; 201:9–17.
8. Epstein HC. Traumatic Dislocation of the Hip. Baltimore: Williams & Wilkins, 1980.
9. Rockwood C, Wirth M. Subluxations and dislocations about the glenohumeral joint. In: Bucholz, Heckman, eds. Rockwood and Green's Fractures in Adults. Vol. 2. 5th ed. Philadelphia: Lippincott-Raven Publishers, 2001:1109–1201.
10. Blom S, Dahlback LO. Nerve injuries in dislocations of the shoulder joint and fractures of the neck of the humerus. A clinical and electromyographical study. Acta Chir Scand 1970; 136:461–466.
11. Siliski JM, Plancher K. Dislocation of the knee. Presented at the Annual Meeting of the American Academy of Orthopedic Surgeons, 1989. Proceedings of the American Academy of Orthopedic Surgeons, 1989.
12. Upadhyay SS, Moulton A. The long-term results of traumatic posterior dislocation of the hip. J Bone Joint Surg Br 1981; 63:548–551.
13. Hougaard K, Thomsen PB. Coxarthrosis following traumatic posterior dislocation of the hip. J Bone Joint Surg Am 1987; 69:679–683.
14. Josefsson PO, Johnell O, Gentz CF. Long-term sequelae of simple dislocation of the elbow. J Bone Joint Surg Am 1984; 66:927–930.
15. Epstein HC. Traumatic dislocations of the hip. Clin Orthop 1973; 92:116–142.
16. Tijmes J, Loyd HM, Tullos HS. Arthrography in acute shoulder dislocations. South Med J 1979; 72:564–567.
17. McLaughlin HL, MacLellan DI. Recurrent anterior dislocation of the shoulder. II. A comparative study. J Trauma 1967; 7:191–201.
18. Lutter LD. Post-traumatic hip redislocation. J Bone Joint Surg Am 1973; 55:391–394.

35

Complications of Amputations

Yoram Klein
Division of Trauma and Emergency Surgery, Kaplan Medical Center, Rehovot and Department of Surgery, Hadassah EIN, Kerem Medical Center, Jerusalem, Israel

Mauricio Lynn
Division of Trauma and Surgical Critical Care, DeWitt Daughtry Family Department of Surgery, University of Miami, Miller School of Medicine, Miami, Florida, U.S.A.

Amputation is one of the earliest recorded operative procedures in the history of mankind. There is evidence that amputations were preformed as early as the Neolithic era. Hammurabi, King of Babylon (1792–1750 B.C.), dictated the use of amputation as a punishment for offenders, including surgeons who killed or blinded their patients during treatment (1). A few cultures still use amputation as a punishment today, mainly for thieves. The most important year in the history of amputation was probably 1338, the year in which gunpowder was introduced. Subsequently, surgery evolved along with the history of war, and military surgeons led the way in improving surgical techniques and perioperative care.

Surgical complications changed over the years, as did indications for amputation, surgical techniques, and perioperative care. Hemorrhage, which was the most deadly complication in the early era, was treated with hot oil coagulation and by amputating through devitalized tissue, as advised by Hippocrates. In the Middle Ages, pressure bandages made of ox bladder were used to control postoperative bleeding. In the 16th century, the tourniquet was introduced and hemostatic ligature was accepted as the preferred means of controlling bleeding. Intraoperative pain was another problem. The most common technique for minimizing pain was to perform the procedure as quickly as possible; most surgeons performed amputations within only a few minutes. Other methods of pain control were cooling with ice and administering opium and alcohol, until general anesthesia was introduced in the 19th century. Lister's 1867 discovery of the value of antisepsis had a tremendous impact on the postoperative infection rate and the indications for amputation. Before antisepsis techniques were introduced, almost every limb with a compound fracture was amputated because of gas gangrene. Other milestones in the evolution of war amputation were the development of antibiotics and transfusion therapy, which decreased mortality rates related to amputation from 8% during World War I to 2.5% during the Korean conflict.

GENERAL CONSIDERATIONS

Amputation is considered one of the most common surgical procedures (1); more than 100,000 amputations are performed each year in the United States (3). During the first half of the 20th century, military trauma was by far the leading reason for amputation. Since then, peripheral vascular disease and diabetes mellitus have become the most common indications for amputation. Peripheral vascular occlusive disease is responsible for approximately 60% to 70% of extremity amputations, diabetes mellitus for 10% to 20%, and trauma for 10% to 20% (4). Other indications are acute or chronic infections, tumors, nondiabetic neuropathic disorders, congenital anomalies, and iatrogenic complications (i.e., intra-arterial catheterization, extravasation of intravenous drugs, etc.).

Most of the information in this chapter addresses lower-extremity amputations because they are much more common than upper-extremity amputations, which account for only 15% of all amputations. The accepted levels of amputation are illustrated in Figure 1.

PREOPERATIVE CONSIDERATIONS

Before surgery, the clinician should optimize the patient's general condition in an effort to increase the chances for uncomplicated healing. The need for emergent amputation may limit preoperative diagnostic and therapeutic efforts.

Several conditions may increase the likelihood of complications. As is true with any other surgical procedure, amputation is more likely to be associated with complications when the patient has cardiovascular (e.g., myocardial ischemia, congestive heart failure, or malignant dysrhythmias) or respiratory disease.

Conditions that interfere with wound healing, such as diabetes mellitus, malnutrition, or steroid treatment, are associated with a higher rate of wound

---

KEY POINTS

- The most common reasons for amputation are peripheral vascular disease and diabetes mellitus.
- A delay in amputation after its indication has been determined to be correlated with an increased risk of perioperative complications.
- The level of amputation substantially affects the likelihood of wound complications and the potential for successful rehabilitation. This decision should be based on clinical judgment and the results of preoperative studies.
- Meticulous surgical technique should be maintained so that the fitting of a prosthesis can be optimized.
- Primary closure may shorten healing time, but revision amputation is required in 10% of cases of wound healing failure.
- Appropriate application of rigid dressings and early physical therapy will minimize the risk of contractures and chronic pain syndrome.
- Thirty percent of patients will die within two years of the amputation.

---

infections, dehiscence, and repeated amputation. Patients with chronic renal failure have a higher mortality rate (24% vs. 7%) and a higher complication rate (61% vs. 9%) than patients without renal failure (5). Smoking also has a deleterious effect on this group of patients. The higher rate of infection (42% vs. 22%) and wound dehiscence among active smokers is attributed to the nicotine-induced release of catecholamine, which reduces cutaneous blood flow, and to the procoagulation effect of nicotine, which increases the occurrence of microthrombi (6). Patients should stop smoking at least one week before amputation so that platelet aggregation and fibrinogen levels can return to normal (7).

The influence of prior vascular reconstruction on the complication rate associated with amputation is still controversial. Several laboratory abnormalities have been shown to be correlated with increased rates of postoperative complications, especially infection. These abnormalities include hypoalbuminemia, hypocalcemia, hyperglycemia, and azotemia (8). One of the most important preoperative determinants of postoperative complications is the delay between admission and amputation (8). Amputation early in the hospital course will limit suffering (both preoperative and chronic postoperative pain), disorientation, uncontrolled diabetes, and ascending venous thrombosis (9). Minimizing the delay in definitive management will also reduce the risk of wound infection and increase the likelihood of success with the use of more distal amputation sites (10). The only reason to delay a necessary amputation is the assumption that the patient will not survive the surgical stress. In this case, a "physiological amputation" by placing dry ice on the diseased limb should be considered (11). Sepsis caused by an ischemic, infected limb is also a tremendous physiological stressor for the critically ill patient in unstable condition.

The decision about the level of amputation is a crucial preoperative step that has a tremendous impact on the rate of complications. Several authors have identified the choice of the level of amputation as the most important cause of repeated amputation and wound infection (12,13). It is known that a lower level of amputation is better for the outcome of rehabilitation efforts. On the other hand, amputation through compromised tissue without adequate blood supply will lead to an increased rate of wound dehiscence and infection, a longer hospitalization, and an increased incidence of repeated amputation at a higher level.

Several invasive and noninvasive methods have been recommended for determining the optimal level of amputation. Doppler ultrasonography, angiography, scintigraphy, and photoplethysmography have all been used to predict healing with varying degrees of success. Clinical judgment based on the findings of physical examination, especially the location of the most distal pulse, is still very useful (14,15), although some authors state that this method is not satisfactory in and of itself (16). Another determinant of the level of amputation is the anticipated success of postoperative rehabilitation efforts. A patient with no chance of being able to use prosthesis because of physiological status (severe heart or lung insufficiency) or neurological condition (stroke with complications and spinal injury with paralysis) should undergo an amputation at the level associated with the lowest risk of postoperative wound complications. Preexisting local limb pathology, such as proximal joint deformities and contractures, will usually prevent the surgeon from performing amputation at a lower level because these conditions will preclude the use of prosthesis.

INTRAOPERATIVE CONSIDERATIONS

Technical details of the surgical procedure are outside the scope of this chapter. Nevertheless, a few common operative considerations for avoiding complications must be emphasized. The process of evaluation for the best level of amputation must continue in the

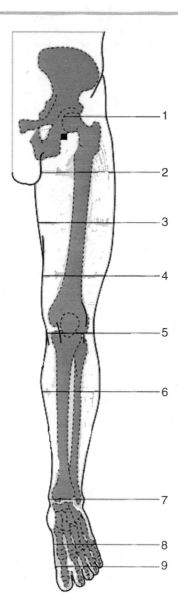

Figure 1 Accepted levels of amputation.

operating room. If the skin and muscle do not seem to bleed or to contract to electrical stimuli, as would be expected of viable tissue, the level of amputation must be reconsidered and amputation should probably be performed at a higher level. The future interface between stump and prosthesis should be considered when skin, muscle, and bone are excised. An excessively long fibula, inadequate beveling of the tibia, or an excessively long femur will interfere with the comfortable fit of the prosthesis, as will excessive soft tissue at the end of the stump. Although a more distal amputation offers superior potential for rehabilitation, an excessively long stump below the knee will cause alignment problems, impaired cosmesis, and discomfort with no functional advantage. On the other hand, if the remaining soft tissue and muscle are inadequate to cover the bony stump (especially

the posterior flap in a below-knee amputation), further shortening of bone may be required, with the risk of compromising future function. General rules of good surgical technique— such as minimizing the use of electrocautery, avoiding extensive debridement of devitalized tissue, and avoiding unnecessary tension during suturing—must be followed religiously because the tissue is already compromised and susceptible to infection.

The next decision to be made is whether to close the wound primarily, to leave it to secondary healing, or to use a delayed primary closure. The most important factor in this decision is the clinical circumstances. The failure rate of primary healing in an extremity with vascular compromise is approximately 20% (16). Nevertheless, primary closure, when successful, is associated with the shortest healing time and hospitalization time. The rehabilitation process may also be facilitated by primary closure (17). The advantages of primary closure must be weighed against the 10% rate of stump revision in the case of failure (18). Even in the case of amputation due to mine explosion, which was traditionally treated with an open technique for secondary healing, the success rates are as high as 87% for primary closure (19) and 84% for delayed primary closure (20). Placing a drain in a stump that has been closed primarily is still a controversial practice, although it is commonly performed in an effort to avoid retained hematoma, which may become secondarily infected. Flexion contracture of the knee after a below-knee amputation is best avoided by using a rigid plaster dressing or a posterior plaster splint.

POSTOPERATIVE COMPLICATIONS

The average amputee is older and has several comorbid conditions, especially advanced atherosclerosis; therefore, the likelihood of potential complications after amputation is higher than that for younger, healthier patients who undergo other surgical procedures. Although amputation surgery is usually perceived as a failure, its goal is to improve the patient's quality of life, and it may sometimes be life-saving. Any postoperative complication experienced by amputees may decrease the chances of successful rehabilitation. Postoperative complications may be categorized as those related to the operative wound, those related to the prosthesis, and those related to pain syndromes.

Wound Complications

Wound infection and wound breakdown are the most common complications after amputation surgery. The incidence of wound infection is directly related to the indication for amputation. The general incidence of wound infection is 10% to 30% but may be as high as 60% when the limb is infected (21). The use of prophylactic antibiotics is routine at most centers.

Infections caused by gram-positive or gram-negative bacteria are usually treated with second- or third-generation cephalosporins; coverage for anaerobes is added for patients with diabetes. The use of prophylactic antibiotics has been found to reduce the rates of wound infection and repeated amputation by as much as 50% (22). The question of whether antibiotics can adequately penetrate ischemic tissue has been answered by several studies that showed sufficient levels of antibiotics in the stump wound (22,23). In fact, in cases in which the level of antibiotics in the stump was not adequate, the rate of failed stump and the necessity for repeated amputation was much higher that for cases in which the antibiotic level was sufficient. This fact suggests that the problem was an incorrect choice of amputation level rather than antibiotic bioavailability (25). In cases of preexisting infection, antibiotic treatment should be guided by the specific preoperative cultures. If cultures are not available, treatment with broad-spectrum antibiotics against gram-positive, gram-negative, and anaerobic bacteria should be initiated. In severe cases of purulent infection, surgical drainage of the infected collection should be considered before the amputation is performed. In extreme situations, in which severe infection requires an emergent amputation, a guillotine procedure may be performed as a lifesaving procedure.

Failure to heal is another common wound complication after amputation, especially among patients with a devascularized limb. In this situation, primary healing can be anticipated in only 20% to 50% of cases, and as many as 35% of those cases will require secondary amputation at a higher level (16,18,26,27). The most common reason for failure to heal is low oxygen delivery to the wound (28), primarily because of primary vascular insufficiency related to an incorrect choice of the level of amputation. The more distal the amputation level, the more limited the oxygen delivery to the tissues, and the greater the likelihood of wound breakdown (29). Other reasons for healing failure are increased pressure in the wound caused by undrained hematoma, compromised venous or lymphatic drainage, or sutures that are too tight, infection, immunosuppressive medications such as corticosteroids and metabolic disorders such as hypoalbuminemia or malnutrition.

Problems with Function or with the Prosthesis

When evaluating the outcome of amputations, one must remember the general physical condition of the patient who requires amputation. Amputation is usually necessitated by diffuse atherosclerosis or poorly controlled diabetes. In 40% to 50% of cases, the patient will require a contralateral amputation within two years (8,30). Functional outcome after amputation depends on certain commonly measured variables. Although some series identify ability to independently perform activities of daily living as the main factor contributing to quality of life after

amputation (8), the most common variable measured for determining quality of life is independent ambulation. Successful fitting of prosthesis should be expected after 75% of below-knee amputations and after 50% of above-knee amputations (31). More than 60% of those patients will still be able to use prosthesis three years after amputation (32).

The main reason for failure in fitting a primary prosthesis is a technical problem related to inadequate shaping of the distal stump during the operation. Another reason is flexion contracture of the proximal joint, which is usually the result of a technical error (i.e., leaving a femur stump that is too short), failure to maintain the proper postoperative position of the stump, or failure to provide adequate physical therapy. Flexion contracture of more than 9° at the hip or 15° at the knee is considered a contraindication for the use of prosthesis. Inability to use the prosthesis after a successful primary fitting is usually due to stump shrinkage. Less common complications that might interfere with prosthesis use are calluses over weight-bearing bony prominences (usually because of the lack of soft-tissue coverage), bone spur of the distal stump, bone overgrowth in children, and osteoporosis of the stump bone caused by disuse. The combination of pressure and friction within the prosthesis socket can cause skin complications such as epidermoid cysts, which might become infected and are very likely to recur, even after a surgical removal. The most dramatic skin complication is verrucous hyperplasia. Proximal constriction in the socket without adequate distal tissue support causes extreme skin edema with wart-like appearance and occasional exudation. Surgical reshaping of the distal stump will gradually correct this problem.

The general health of the patient can also affect independent ambulation. Cardiac, lung, or neurological pathology can result in inability to use the prosthesis because the patient cannot endure the excessive physical strain. A patient who has undergone unilateral below-knee amputation will require 10% more energy for ambulation than will a man of the same age who has not undergone amputation. The energy requirement for ambulation is increased by 50% for unilateral above-knee amputation and by 200% for bilateral above-knee amputation (33).

Pain

Although amputation may be the treatment for severe chronic and ischemic pain, several types of pain syndromes can affect the patient after amputation. The first and most common of these is immediate postoperative pain, which is no different from the pain that follows any other major surgical procedure. Usually, this pain is nonspecific and subsides during the first postoperative week. Carefully applied rigid dressings may decrease this pain by reducing local edema.

Neuroma of the stump can cause severe localized pain during the weeks or months after amputation. Neuroma is a universal nerve repair phenomenon and cannot be prevented. Usually, neuroma does not cause discomfort unless the area is subjected to excessive pressure or is not covered or supported by sufficient soft tissue. The pain is deep and dull in nature and may be resistant to conventional analgesic therapy (34). The best strategy for minimizing the clinical manifestations of neuroma is cutting the nerve deep in the muscle tissue during the primary operation. The tradition of ligating a mass of major nerves is of no value because it will not prevent the formation of neuroma.

When amputations are performed after trauma, imbalanced sympathetic tone can cause reflex sympathetic dystrophy. This syndrome, originally termed causalgia, may cause burning pain along with mottled, cool skin and osteopenic bone in the stump. Lumbar sympathectomy for lower-extremity amputation and thoracic sympathectomy for upper-extremity amputation may offer some relief, but the success rate varies.

The most common postamputation pain syndrome is phantom pain. Almost all amputees experience phantom limb sensation, which is the feeling that the missing limb is still present. Some patients will experience phantom pain, which is a poorly localized pain that is burning, cramping, aching, or stabbing in nature (35). Three major characteristics define this syndrome: (i) pain that lasts for some time after the wound has healed; (ii) pain elicited by the activation of trigger zones; and (iii) pain that resembles the pain experienced preoperatively. Changes in somatic input, such as massaging the stump or treating it with ultrasound, may affect this pain (36).

The likelihood of phantom pain is correlated with the site of the amputation; the higher the level of amputation, the more likely the phantom pain. Phantom pain is more likely after upper-extremity amputations than after lower-extremity amputations.

No single therapy or combination of therapies, medical or surgical, has proved successful in treating this disabling syndrome. The incidence of severe stump pain or phantom pain is reported to range from 30% to 85% (35,37,38), but some authors report that the likelihood of this disabling postamputation complication can be reduced to less than 5% by an early, aggressive rehabilitation program (39).

MORTALITY

The high mortality rate after major amputation reflects the fact that most patients who require amputation suffer from multiple diseases. The estimation is that one-third of patients who undergo lower-limb amputation will die by the second postoperative year and two-thirds will die within five years (40). The immediate operative and postoperative mortality rates range from 10% to 30%. The level of amputation is highly correlated with the mortality rate. The lower the level of amputation, the lower the mortality rate. Recent studies showed mortality rates of 2% for below-knee amputation and 9% for above-knee amputation (41,42). The mortality rate after bilateral amputation is 18%, and the mortality rate after above-knee amputation that followed a failed below-knee amputation is 21% (5). The reason that the mortality rate is higher after a higher-level amputation is probably related to the fact that these patients generally have more severe general atherosclerosis and an increased rate of cardiac complications. The amputation associated with the highest mortality rate (44%) is hip disarticulation. The mortality rate associated with this procedure is as high as 60% when it is required after trauma, probably because the victim has sustained a devastating amount of energy (43).

SUMMARY

Since the end of the global military conflicts that characterized the 20th century, the most common indications for amputation have been peripheral vascular disease and diabetes. Patients undergoing amputation usually suffer from diffuse atherosclerosis or diabetes and from the end-organ dysfunction that accompanies these diseases. Thus, a high rate of postoperative complications can be anticipated. The surgeon must often make a difficult choice between the procedure that provides the best chance for rehabilitation and the procedure that carries the lowest complication rate. A judicious choice of the level of amputation, together with meticulous surgical technique and aggressive postoperative physical therapy, will give the patient the best chance for timely and successful rehabilitation. No other surgical procedure better illustrates the important rule of surgery: it is easier to prevent a complication than to treat it.

REFERENCES

1. Johns CHW. The Code of Hammurabi. 11th ed. Encyclopaedia Britannica, 1910–1911.
2. Wheeler HB. Myth and reality in general surgery. Bull Am Coll Surg 1993; 78:21–27.
3. Krupski WC, Nehler MR. Amputation. In: Way LW, Doherty GM, eds. Current Surgical Diagnosis and Treatment. 11th ed. Boston: McGraw-Hill, 2002:859–870.
4. Hansson J. The leg amputee. A clinical follow-up study. Acta Orthop Scand 1964; 10(suppl 69):1–104.
5. Dossa CD, Shepard AD, Amos AM, et al. Results of lower extremity amputations in patients with end-stage renal disease. J Vasc Surg 1994; 20:14–19.
6. Lind J, Kramhoft M, Bodtker S. The influence of smoking on complications after primary amputations of the lower extremity. Clin Orthop 1991; 267:211–217.
7. Cryer PE, Haymond MW, Santiago JV, Shah SD. Norepinephrine and epinephrine release and adrenergic

mediation of smoking-associated hemodynamic and metabolic events. N Engl J Med 1976; 295:573–577.

8. Weiss GN, Gorton TA, Read RC, Neal LA. Outcomes of lower extremity amputations. J Am Geriatr Soc 1990; 38:877–883.

9. Rosenberg N, Adiarte E, Bujdoso L, Backwinkel KD. Mortality factors in major limb amputations for vascular disease: a study of 176 procedures. Surgery 1970; 67:437–441.

10. Bunt TJ, Manship LL, Bynoe RP, Haynes JL. Lower extremity amputation for peripheral vascular disease. A low-risk operation. Am Surg 1984; 50:580–584.

11. Bunt TJ. Physiologic amputation for acute pedal sepsis. Am Surg 1990; 56(9):530–532.

12. Harris JP, Page S, Englund R, May J. Is the outlook for the vascular amputee improved by striving to preserve the knee? J Cardiovasc Surg (Torino) 1988; 29:741–745.

13. Ebskov B, Josephsen P. Incidence of reamputation and death after gangrene of the lower extremity. Prosthet Orthot Int 1980; 4:77–80.

14. O'Dwyer KJ, Edwards MH. The association between lowest palpable pulse and wound healing in below knee amputations. Ann R Coll Surg Engl 1985; 67:232–234.

15. Clyne CA. Selection of level for lower limb amputation in patients with severe peripheral vascular disease. Ann R Coll Surg Engl 1991; 73:148–151.

16. van den Broek TA, Dwars BJ, Rauwerda JA, Bakker FC. A multivariate analysis of determinants of wound healing in patients after amputation for peripheral vascular disease. Eur J Vasc Surg 1990; 4:291–295.

17. Aligne C, Farcot M, Favre JP, Alnashawati G, De Simone F, Barral X. Primary closure of below-knee amputation stumps: a prospective study of sixty-two cases. Ann Vasc Surg 1990; 4:143–146.

18. Senkowsky J, Money MK, Kerstein MD. Lower extremity amputation: open versus closed. Angiology 1990; 41:221–227.

19. Atesalp AS, Erler K, Gur E, Solakoglu C. Below-knee amputations as a result of land-mine injuries: comparison of primary closure versus delayed primary closure. J Trauma 1999; 47:724–727.

20. Simper LB. Below knee amputation in war surgery: a review of 111 amputations with delayed primary closure. J Trauma 1993; 34:96–98.

21. Desai Y, Robbs JV, Keenan JP. Staged below-knee amputations for septic peripheral lesions due to ischemia. Br J Surg 1986; 73:392–394.

22. Norlin R, Fryden A, Nilsson L, Ansehn S. Short-term cefotaxime prophylaxis reduces the failure rate in lower limb amputations. Acta Orthop Scand 1990; 61:460–462.

23. Kerin MJ, Greenstein D, Chisholm EM, Sheehan SJ, Kester RC. Is antiobiotic penetration compromised in the ischaemic tissues of patients undergoing amputation? Ann R Coll Surg Engl 1992; 74:274–276.

24. Sonne-Holm S, Boeckstyns M, Menck H, et al. Prophylactic antibiotics in amputation of the lower extremity for ischemia. A placebo-controlled, randomized trial of cefoxitin. J Bone Joint Surg Am 1985; 67:800–803.

25. Mars M, Elson KI, Salisbury RT, Robbs JV. Do preoperative antibiotics reach the operative field in amputation surgery for peripheral vascular disease? A pilot study. S Afr J Surg 1990; 28:58–61.

26. Finch DR, Macdougal M, Tibbs DJ, Morris PJ. Amputation for vascular disease: the experience of a peripheral vascular unit. Br J Surg 1980; 67:233–237.

27. Keagy BA, Scwartz JA, Kotb M, Burnham SJ, Johnson G Jr. Lower extremity amputation: the control series. J Vasc Surg 1986; 4:321–326.

28. Kuhne HH, Ullmann U, Kuhne FW. New aspects on the pathophysiology of wound infection and wound healing—the problem of lowered oxygen pressure in the tissue. Infection 1985; 13:52–56.

29. Burgess EM, Matsen FA III, Wyss CR, Simmons CW. Segmental transcutaneous measurements of PO2 in patients requiring below-the-knee amputation for peripheral vascular insufficiency. J Bone Joint Surg Am 1982; 64:378–382.

30. Bodily RC, Burgess EM. Contralateral limb and patient survival after leg amputation. Am J Surg 1983; 146:280–282.

31. Steinberg FU, Sunwoo I, Roettger F. Prosthetic rehabilitation of geriatric amputee patients: a follow-up study. Arch Phys Med Rehabil 1985; 66:742–745.

32. De Luccia N, Pinto MA, Guedes JP, Albers MT. Rehabilitation after amputation for vascular disease: a follow-up study. Prosthet Orthot Int 1992; 16:124–128.

33. Huang CT, Jackson JR, Moore NB, et al. Amputation: energy cost of ambulation. Arch Phys Med Rehabil 1979; 60:18–24.

34. Fisher GT, Boswick JA Jr. Neuroma formation following digital amputations. J Trauma 1983; 23:136–142.

35. Abramson AS, Feibel A. The phantom phenomenon: its use and disuse. Bull N Y Acad Med 1981; 57:99–112.

36. Melzack R. Phantom limb pain: implications for treatment of pathological pain. Anesthesiology 1971; 35:409–419.

37. Sherman RA. Published treatment of phantom pain. Am J Phys Med 1980; 59:232–244.

38. Sherman RA, Sherman CJ, Parker L. Chronic phantom and stump pain among American veterans: results of a survey. Pain 1984; 18:83–95.

39. Malone JM, Moore WS, Leal JM, Childers SJ. Rehabilitation for lower extremity amputation. Arch Surg 1981; 116:93–98.

40. Potts JR III, Wendelken JR, Elkins RC, Peyton MD. Lower extremity amputation: review of 110 cases. Am J Surg 1979; 138:924–928.

41. Rush DS, Huston, CC, Bivins BA, Hyde GL. Operative and late mortality rates of above-knee and below-knee amputations. Am Surg 1981; 47:36–39.

42. Kald A, Carlsson R, Nilsson E. Major amputation in a defined population: incidence, mortality and results of treatment. Br J Surg 1989; 76:308–310.

43. Endean ED, Scwarcz TH, Barker DE, Munfakh NA, Wilson-Neely R, Hyde GL. Hip disarticulation: factors affecting outcome. J Vasc Surg 1991; 14:398–404.

36

Complications of Hand Surgery

Charles Eaton
The Hand Center, Jupiter, Florida, U.S.A.

The primary goal of treating hand trauma is simply to avoid complications.

In this chapter, complications are grouped as complications of missed diagnoses, complications of treatment, and complications of injuries.

COMPLICATIONS OF MISSED DIAGNOSES
Missed Hand Injuries

The best insurance against missed diagnoses related to hand injuries is eliciting an adequate history and performing a thorough physical examination.

History

Because severe upper extremity injuries are frequently dramatic and are attended by emotional factors, it is usually best to elicit a history in a deliberate, orderly way. If possible, after hearing the story, the examiner should physically demonstrate the scenario of injury so that the patient can confirm the examiner's understanding of the details, including the position of the extremity at the time of injury. If an injury involves machinery, the machinery should be described in enough detail to allow the examiner to visualize it. In simple mechanical terms, was the mechanism sharp or dull? Did it involve rotating blades, belts, or chains; heat, cold, or chemicals? Did the patient land on the palm with the wrist extended or on the dorsum of the wrist? Was the patient able to pull the hand out or was it trapped, requiring extrication? Was the bleeding pulsatile? One should not assume that all problems with the hand resulted from a single reported injury. Did the pain or numbness start immediately after the event or later? Has the hand been injured previously? Did these injuries occur recently or a long time ago? Were there prior problems with numbness, weakness, or pain? Attention to such details from the onset can avoid misguided treatment and false expectations. Additionally, hand injuries are a common starting point for personal injury litigation, and clear initial documentation of these points will prevent needless difficulties later when an attorney becomes involved.

Physical Examination

A working knowledge of anatomy usually allows assessment of an acute injury without touching the obvious site of injury. Sensory, motor, and vascular function distal to the injury can provide clues about the status of more proximal wounds. This gentle approach is clearly preferable to attempting to define the injury by probing or applying an instrument to a wound in the emergency room.

Rapid Survey of the Hand

A focused, informative survey of the injured hand can be performed in approximately one minute. It is best to use a systems checklist (Table 1) when examining an injured hand. Such a checklist will review both objective and subjective findings. A focused examination of the median, ulnar, and radial nerves can be performed within a few seconds (Fig. 1). Indirect tenderness or pain that occurs when gentle percussion, traction, torsion, or bending stress is applied to the skeleton at a distance from the area of injury will occur when there is pathologic skeletal micromotion caused by fracture or ligament injury. Active unresisted motion may be limited but can confirm that tendons are in continuity and that innervation of the proximal muscles is intact.

Table 1 Subjective and Objective Findings Obtained by a Rapid Survey of the Hand

Objective findings
  Skin: wounds, texture, turgor
  Vasculature: color, temperature, turgor, capillary refill, pulses
  Bone and joint: deformity, instability
  Muscle and tendon: posture, compartment turgor
Subjective findings
  Perception of injury: pain, tenderness, apprehension of pain, weakness
  Peripheral nerve function: nerve-specific sensory islands; muscles with unique innervation
  Skeleton: tenderness at the site of injury
  Muscle and tendon: strength

Rapid Hand Survey

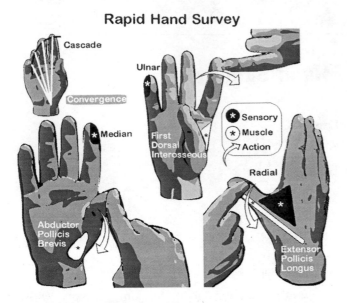

Figure 1 Rapid assessment of the hand includes color, temperature, range of motion, tenderness convergence of fingertips toward the distal pole of the scaphoid to assess fracture malrotation, sensory and motor assessment of the median (radial index fingertip/abductor pollicis brevis), ulnar (ulnar small fingertip/first dorsal interosseous), and radial (dorsal first web space/extensor pollicis longus) nerves.

Tips for Examining the Hand of an Unconscious Patient

Much information can be obtained in the absence of subjective findings by using the four categories of assessment listed below.

Vascular Assessment. Comparing the color of the skin and nail beds of the injured hand to the color of those sites on the other hand can indicate arterial insufficiency (if the injured hand is paler) or venous insufficiency (if the injured hand is dark or purple). Allen's test can be performed without patient participation by gently squeezing the palm while occluding the radial and ulnar arteries at the wrist, and then releasing one artery to assess the patency of the two main arteries and of the palmar arch. The digital Allen's test is performed similarly; the examiner uses his or her fingertips to exsanguinate a finger from distal to proximal points and then releases one or the other side at the base of the finger (Fig. 2). Forearm compartment pressures can be measured with commercial kits or with materials available in any emergency room.

Muscle and Tendon Assessment. The posture of the fingers can indicate specific tendon injuries. Even if the patient is unconscious, if the tendons and phalanges are intact, the fingers should assume a cascade position of progressively more flexion of both proximal and distal interphalangeal joints, from the index to the small finger (Figs. 1 and 3). Tenodesis-induced motion of the fingers can be

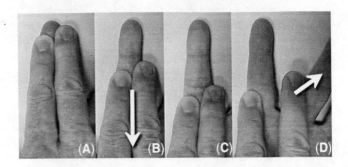

Figure 2 Allen's type of testing may be performed on each digit to confirm patency of each digital artery. The finger is exsanguinated with distal to proximal massage (**A, B, C**), and then one of the digital arteries is released (**D**) and pattern of refill observed. This can be helpful as an adjunct test for evaluation of possible digital nerve injuries, because digital nerves are superficial to digital arteries and digital artery injury from a penetrating wound has a high likelihood of associated digital nerve injury.

used to check relative finger posture during passive wrist flexion and extension (Figs. 4 and 5). Squeezing the mid-forearm will tighten the finger flexor tendons and mimic their active action.

Bone and Joint Assessment. Rotation of the fingers may be suspected if the tips overlap, but if the fingertips are not adjacent during flexion, it is normal for all of them to converge toward the distal pole of the scaphoid, where the flexor carpi radialis tendon intersects the wrist flexion crease (Figs. 6 and 7). Contour abnormalities at joints or along long bones may indicate fractures or dislocations. Common contour changes resulting from displaced fractures include those due to distal radius fractures (Fig. 8), metacarpal neck fractures, and proximal phalanx fractures. Metacarpophalangeal or proximal interphalangeal joint dislocations alter flexor–extensor tendon tension balance and may cause unusual posture or positioning of the joints distal to the injury (Fig. 9). Bruising

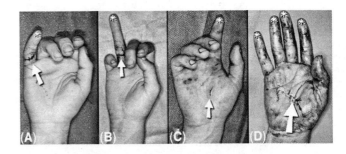

Figure 3 Finger posture changes following flexor tendon injury. Fingers at rest follow a natural flexion cascade, which is altered when either one or both flexor tendons have been cut. These patients show characteristic abnormal straightening of digits (∗) due to proximal flexor tendon injuries (*arrows*): small finger superficialis (**A**), both tendons of ring finger (**B**), index profundus tendon (**C**), all tendons of all fingers, thumb spared (**D**).

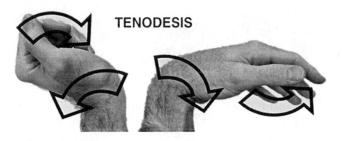

Figure 4 Wrist tenodesis normally results in passive changes in finger posture: finger extension when the wrist is flexed, and finger flexion when the wrist is extended.

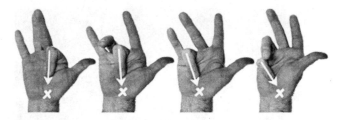

Figure 6 In flexion, the fingertips converge toward a common point in the proximal palm, approximately the distal pole of the scaphoid (X). This can be helpful in quickly assessing for rotational malalignment of a metacarpal or phalangeal fracture in an unconscious patient.

at a site away from an area of impact, such as bruising of the dorsal wrist after a fall on the outstretched palm, strongly suggests an underlying skeletal injury even when radiographic results are normal. Passive range-of-motion examination of the elbow, wrist, and fingers can be used to assess crepitation (which indicates an injury to the joint surface), resistance (which indicates swelling, subluxation, or dislocation), and instability (which indicates ligament injury).

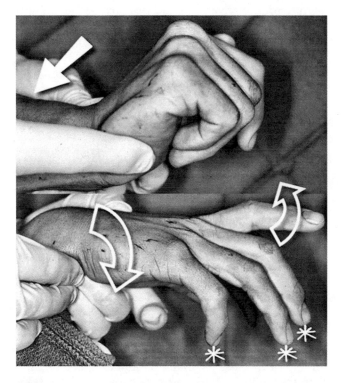

Figure 5 This unconscious patient had a dorsal forearm laceration (*straight arrow*), which appeared superficial, but wrist tenodesis (*curved arrows*) demonstrated injury to the extensor tendons of the middle, ring, and small fingers (*asterisks*), which had incomplete extension with passive wrist flexion. This was confirmed in the operating room. Because of the obliquity of the laceration, the injury could not have been demonstrated by simple wound exploration in the emergency room.

Nerve Assessment. The digital nerves are superficial to the digital arteries. Thus, an abnormal finding on a digital Allen test (Fig. 2) in the context of any palmar finger laceration strongly suggests an associated digital nerve injury because the zone of external injury must pass through the nerve before reaching the artery. *Tactile adherence* is assessed by sliding an object with a smooth surface across the palmar skin. A smooth surface such as a glass slide or the barrel of a shiny, smooth plastic pen will slide with much less resistance (adherence) over skin affected by nerve injury than over normal skin because recently denervated skin does not sweat. Normally, microscopic sweat droplets on the palmar skin create resistance to this motion. The *wrinkle test* makes use of the finding that recently denervated skin does not wrinkle upon prolonged

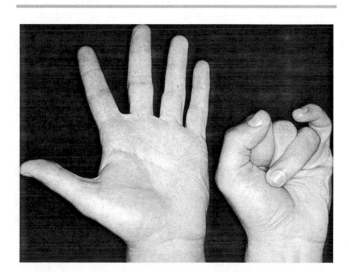

Figure 7 Rotational malalignment of metacarpal fractures may not be apparent with the fingers in extension. The rotation of this patient's ring and small finger malunions is much less obvious with his fingers extended (*left*) than with attempted full flexion (*right*). Reduction of rotational malalignment should be checked in the acute setting by placing the fingers in full flexion.

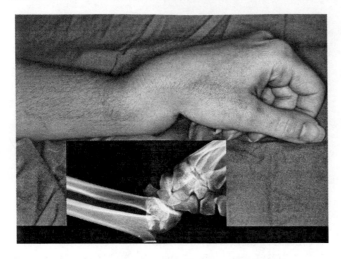

Figure 8 Acute deformity. The angulation of this fracture is obvious even in an unconscious patient. The fracture (*above*); The X–ray (*below*).

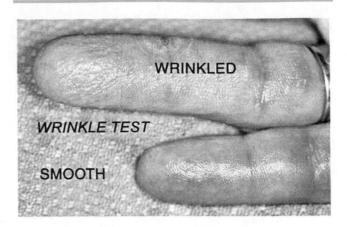

Figure 10 The wrinkle test may be used to assess sensory nerve function in the unreliable patient. For a period of months after nerve injury, denervated skin loses its ability to wrinkle when immersed in water. Here, failure of the small finger skin to wrinkle when immersed in water for 10 minutes (compared to normal adjacent ring finger) strongly suggests injury of both digital nerves of the small finger.

contact with water. In this test, the fingers are immersed in water (not in saline or another salt solution) for five minutes and are then inspected for wrinkling. The absence of wrinkling indicates denervation (Fig. 10). The mechanism behind this phenomenon is unknown.

Missed Problems Elsewhere

A dramatic hand injury can divert attention from a standard trauma systems evaluation. Life-threatening complications resulting from missed injuries are most

likely when a patient has sustained a traumatic amputation in a blunt trauma scenario, such as a traffic accident or a fall. Life-threatening central nervous system or thoracoabdominal injuries may be missed, as may proximal skeletal and brachial plexus injuries. An occult medical condition commonly accompanying hand injury is substance abuse; in one report, nearly half of patients requiring emergency room treatment for hand trauma tested positive for alcohol or another substance (1).

COMPLICATIONS OF TREATMENT

The most common complication of any hand injury is *stiffness*, which results from the collaborative effects of inflammation, swelling, and immobility. Attempts at preventing stiffness are much more effective and worthwhile than later attempts at correcting established stiffness. Stiffness and other complications are less likely when the treatment follows priority-based guidelines.

Priorities

Management priorities are the same for severe and minor injuries: establish the extent of injury, remove the bad, reconstruct the good, involve the patient, and tailor the surgery to the patient (63). Severe upper extremity injuries with soft tissue loss result in shorter hospitalization periods and more rapid recovery when primary reconstruction is performed, even if such treatment requires primary microvascular free-flap surgery (76). One conceptual approach to organizing the initial management of severe hand injuries is to break down priorities as they relate to either healing or function.

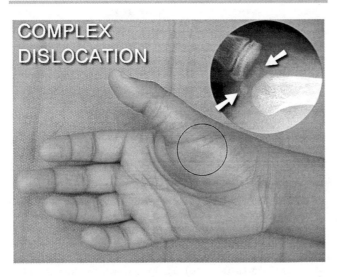

Figure 9 Complex dislocations of the thumb metacarpophalangeal joint present with an extended posture of the thumb, and occasionally a dimple or bruising at the palmar metacarpal head level. X-rays may show sesamoid interposition as is seen here. Such a finding increases the likelihood that open reduction will be necessary.

Healing Priorities: Circulation, Skeleton, Closure

Inadequate blood supply is the single most likely explanation for complications of delayed healing, fibrosis, and infection. Adequate blood supply is achieved by aggressive debridement, revascularization, and the use of vascularized flaps. Edema indicates inadequate lymphatic circulation and has the same ultimate effects as inadequate blood supply. Edema is best treated with elevation and active range-of-motion exercises, when possible. Optimum bone and joint reconstruction goals are prompt anatomic reduction of injury and stable skeletal fixation with the least amount of additional soft-tissue disruption. Wounds should be closed and covered with mobile, well-vascularized soft tissue as quickly as possible. In the hand, stiffness, difficulty with use, and ultimate disability are directly related to the length of time required for wound healing.

Functional Priorities: Nerve, Joint, Muscle

Nerve injuries should be approached aggressively because there is never a better time to evaluate injuries and to perform repairs, and the only satisfactory time at which partial nerve lacerations can be repaired is in the acute setting (Figs. 11 and 12). Passive range-of-motion exercises have two purposes. The first purpose is preservation of the gliding function of the surfaces of the joints and tendons. This is achieved by early protected motion: all moving parts that can be moved safely are moved frequently, against no resistance and at the earliest opportunity. The second

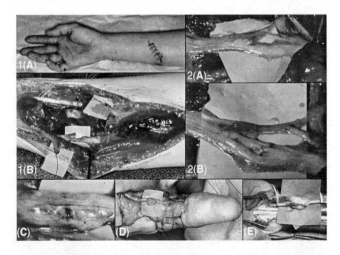

Figure 11 Forearm laceration (**1A**) with complete ulnar artery and partial ulnar nerve laceration (**1B**). Partial forearm posterior interosseous nerve laceration (**2A**) with primary fascicular repair (**2B**). (**C**) Local crush injury of proximal median nerve with central disruption, epineurium intact; excellent recovery after primary debridement and epineural repair. Exploration of digital (**D**) and median (**E**) neuromas late after partial injuries. When partial nerve function remains, resection and grafting is an unpredictable solution, and primary repair is preferable for partial nerve injuries.

purpose is maintenance of the physiological length of capsuloligamentous and muscular tissues. This is achieved by splinting the hand between exercises in the "protective position": interphalangeal joint extension, metacarpophalangeal joint flexion, and preservation of the thumb–index finger web space span (Fig. 13). Active range-of-motion exercises have the additional benefits of reducing edema, building strength, promoting bone healing, preventing dysfunctional patterns of disuse, and probably reducing the incidence of complex regional pain syndrome.

Complications of Bandaging
Tight Dressings

Finger dressings made from tubular gauze may produce ischemic pressure complications. Technical errors in application that can result in tubular gauze pressure complications include excessive longitudinal traction during application, a twist of more than a 90° during application, and rolled proximal edges of the dressing (21). Even minimally tight elastic dressings applied as part of a circumferential bandage may lead to progressive swelling, thereby aggravating all of the previously described ill effects of swelling of the injured hand. Swelling may hinder assessment and may delay surgery until it has been reduced by elevation and changed to a noncompressive dressing. A useful technique is to place multiple layers of circumferential gauze as the deepest portion of the bandage and then split them longitudinally before completing the bandage. This technique ensures that at least the deepest layer of bandage cannot exert circumferential pressure. Tight casts may result in local pressure sores, discomfort, and, in the worst scenario, vascular compromise and compartment syndrome. The risk of complications is highest when circumferential casts are applied after closed reduction of an elbow or forearm fracture on the day of injury. In this situation, the risk may be reduced by splitting ("bivalving") the cast into two separate longitudinal sections immediately after application.

Inadequate Positioning

Splints and other supportive dressings maintain a posture that may be helpful or detrimental. Often, splints fabricated for comfort in the emergency room restrain joints in positions that promote stiffness. Even splints intended to maintain the generic "protective position" may actually do just the opposite, a problem that may be confirmed only by radiography (Fig. 14).

Complications of Wound Care

The goal of wound care is to maintain an environment that discourages excessive bacterial growth and encourages normal healing. Excessive bacterial growth occurs on moist, undisturbed surfaces and is a common problem in the interdigital web spaces of the

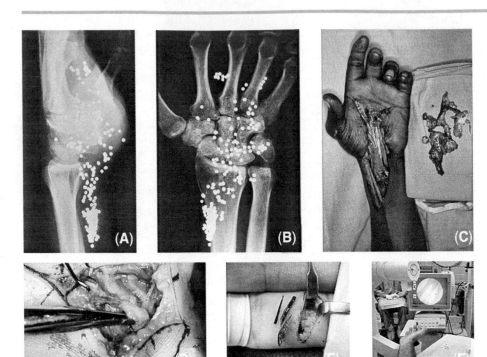

Figure 12 Complications of foreign bodies. **(A, B, C)** A close-range shotgun blast of the palm, treated with local wound care, resulted in median neuropathy and finger stiffness. At exploration for reconstruction a year later, the entire plastic shotgun casing was found embedded in the proximal carpal tunnel. **(D)** Wood impaling the index finger ulnar digital nerve one month following injury. **(E)** Wood splinters lodged in the flexor tendon sheath. **(F)** Intraoperative fluoroscopy is essential for removal of radiopaque foreign bodies. The small piece of shrapnel lodged within the finger flexor tendon moved over a 1 in. excursion with finger motion.

immobilized hand and beneath occlusive bandages. Eventually, unchecked surface growth produces such high concentrations of organisms that the skin is invaded directly, producing maceration dermatitis. This condition may progress to cellulitis, but it can be stopped in the early stages by increasing the frequency of dressing changes and, when possible, allowing the affected skin to dry. Allergic contact dermatitis may develop over the course of treatment with topical antibiotics or skin preparation formulas such as Mastisol® (Fernade Laboratories, Inc., Michigan, U.S.A.) (Fig. 15). This complication can produce a confusing picture because inflammation associated with the reaction may be confused with infection.

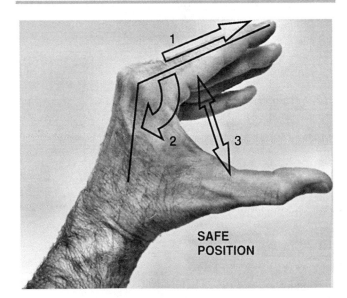

Figure 13 The generic "safe position" for hand immobilization is intended to prevent the usual pattern of stiffness after hand disuse. The three features are maintenance of interphalangeal joint extension (1), metacarpophalangeal joint flexion (2), and first web-space span (3).

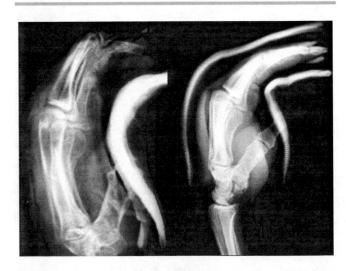

Figure 14 Safe hand position is sometimes difficult to maintain with splinting. The thickly padded palmar plaster splint applied in the emergency room is usually totally inadequate (*left*), but even a cast that appears correct may not be if the palmar flexion point is constructed distal to the center of the palm (*right*).

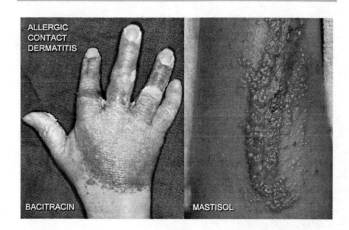

Figure 15 Allergic contact dermatitis. Sensitivity to topical agents may develop after an initial exposure of 7 to 14 days, or earlier in patients who had been previously sensitized. (*Left*) Dermatitis developing from bacitracin was used to treat a superficial burn. As is frequently the case in application of topical antibiotics to treat or prevent infection, the allergic reaction was confused with infection, prompting further use of the offending agent. (*Right*) [Mastisol® (Ferndale Laboratories, Inc., Michigan, U.S.A.)] was used to improve the attachment of surgical skin closure tape. Appearance seven days after surgery. Symptoms from severe reactions are best controlled with short-course high-dose systemic steroids.

The early hallmarks of contact dermatitis are itching and tiny blisters accompanying the reaction.

Complications of Hand Procedures
Tourniquet Palsy

Tourniquet palsy occurs postoperatively in an average of 1 in 5000 cases; it is more commonly associated with microsurgical procedures than with other procedures (22). All nerves are usually affected to some degree, but the radial nerve is usually the most affected. Tourniquet palsy is more likely among patients with coagulation disorders or preexisting neuropathy, those who are thin and malnourished, those with systemic lupus erythematosus (22), and those with unintentionally high tourniquet pressures due to gauge failure (36).

Toxic Shock Syndrome

Toxic shock syndrome is a rare complication but has been reported after elective reconstructive hand surgery (32).

Needlestick or Vascular Cannulation Injuries
Radial Artery Catheterization

Acute ischemia of the hand may occur after radial artery catheterization if there is inadequate perfusion through the ulnar artery (42). This problem is more likely when ulnar artery perfusion is not confirmed by Allen's test before catheterization, when cannulas of relatively large diameter (18 gauge as opposed to

20 gauge) are used (45), during prolonged periods of cannulation, and when hypercoagulability is present (42). In the presence of ulnar artery occlusion, even a single radial artery needlestick for arterial blood gas determination, can precipitate acute hand ischemia (Fig. 16). Although uncommon, ischemia resulting in finger amputation has been reported after arterial monitoring of infants (60).

Cutaneous Nerve Injury

The cephalic vein is frequently cannulated for intravenous access. It is closely related to the antebrachial cutaneous nerve in the proximal forearm and the branches of the superficial radial nerve in the distal forearm. Needlestick injuries can affect either of these nerves (33) and can lead to prolonged morbidity, although this complication is uncommon. Patients report a strong electrical paresthesia at the time of injury; this symptom should be taken as a sign of possible injury. Numbness or tingling lasting more than a day may indicate partial nerve injury and should lead to consideration of early exploration. Treatment options for chronic cases are the same as for any cutaneous neuroma and lingering symptoms are common.

Extravasation Injuries

Extravasation injuries (96–102) of the hand are common because the hand is commonly used for intravenous access. Local tissue necrosis has been reported after subcutaneous extravasation of chemotherapeutic agents, osmotically active substances, and tissue-toxic preparations such as injectable phenytoin. These injuries often exhibit delayed presentation, delayed healing, and prolonged morbidity, requiring reconstructive surgery if treated late. Serious limb growth disturbances may occur after extravasation or thrombosis in the neonatal period. Although not well described in the literature, tense hematomas associated with intravenous access of the wrist or dorsal hand may also result in tissue loss (Fig. 17). The outcome of extravasation injuries is best when they are recognized and treated early. Unfortunately, delayed presentation is still common because of the typically slow development of visible signs of injury. Treatment recommendations have varied over the years, but early treatment with soft-tissue infiltration and irrigation has the most consistent history of effectiveness. Local injection with hyaluronidase is helpful, but this drug is no longer available for use. Prevention appears to be the best approach; avoid the dorsal hand, anterior wrist, and antecubital fossa for infusion of tissue-toxic solutions because these locations are most likely to develop complications associated with extravasation.

Prior Axillary Lymphadenectomy

Although it is common practice to instruct patients who have undergone mastectomy and axillary dissection to

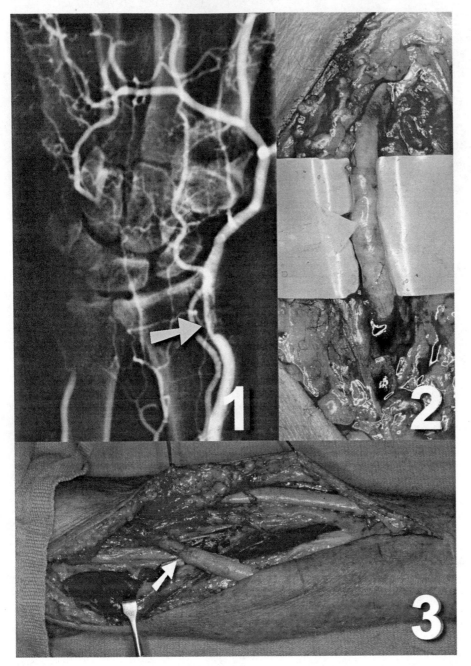

Figure 16 Iatrogenic vascular problems. Hand ischemia due to radial artery thrombus from blood gas puncture in a patient with undiagnosed ulnar artery occlusion (**A, B**). Median nerve compression from dialysis shunt crossing directly over the median nerve (**C**).

avoid manipulation or instrumentation of the hand, the risk of complications in this context has not been documented (88). Hand surgery ipsilateral to previous axillary dissection is probably safe.

Complications of Anesthesia
Epinephrine in Digital Block

Although traditional wisdom holds that the use of epinephrine in digital nerve blocks may result in digital gangrene, there are no reported cases of finger gangrene resulting specifically from the use of epinephrine with lidocaine for digital block, and the safe use of epinephrine has been reported (12).

Postoperative Ulnar Nerve Palsy

Palsy of the ulnar nerve due to ulnar neuropathy at the level of the elbow is a recognized but poorly understood complication of surgery involving general anesthesia (15). The exact mechanism of this process remains unknown. Preventative measures—including protective positioning of the arm on the operative table, use of elbow pads, and avoidance of abduction, pronation, and elbow flexion—may reduce the incidence of this complication. Final outcome is unpredictable; both conservative and operative treatments have yielded mixed results.

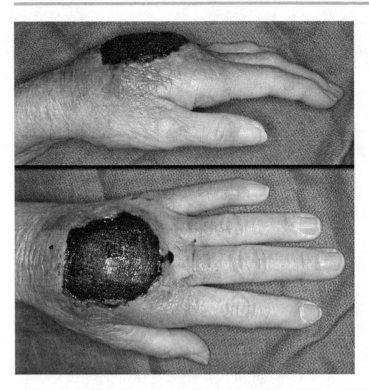

Figure 17 Tense dorsal hand hematomas may result in necrosis of the overlying skin. This problem occurs most often in the context of anticoagulation. Emergent surgical evacuation may limit the extent of soft tissue loss, but the extent of the problem may be impossible to determine in the acutely ill and unstable patient. Skin graft or flap coverage is usually required and hand stiffness is a common outcome.

Brachial Plexus Block Anesthesia

The incidence of postoperative dysesthesias after brachial plexus block anesthesia ranges from less than 2% (91,92) to 12% (17,89). Although rare, perineural fibrosis (90) and permanent neurologic injury (18) have also been reported after axillary block anesthesia.

COMPLICATIONS OF INJURY
General Complications of Hand Injury

Severe hand injuries are most often the result of crush or rotating blade mechanisms and are best treated by a hand surgery specialist (63). Such injuries usually involve all organ systems of the hand and are always associated with complications. The treatment principles and initial management that may be adequate for lesser injuries may be inadequate for a mangled hand (81). Intervention by a specialist reduces the duration and extent of disability and reduces the overall care requirements and cost of care associated with severe trauma to the extremity.

Scar Contracture

Contractures resulting from skin scarring are more likely to be a problem if the scars extend longitudinally across the flexor surface of a joint. In severe cases, scar contractures may develop over the first few weeks after injury, but in many cases they progress over the course of months. In the growing child, scar contractures may lead to progressive growth disturbances. Stiffness and contractures due to mechanical changes in joints and tendons, as discussed above, may develop independently.

Cosmetic Deformity

The immature scar may be hypertrophic: thick, red, and raised. These changes usually resolve gradually over the course of a year, although the process may take longer for young children. Permanent visible deformity from hyperpigmentation, thin stretched scars over extensor surfaces, and tight scar bands across flexor surfaces may all be troublesome. Fingernail deformities are common after lacerations and crush injuries in the area of the nail bed. The most common problems are split nail resulting from nail bed injury and hook nail deformity resulting from loss of the tuft of the distal phalanx by a fingertip amputation. Such problems are sometimes unavoidable, but the best prevention is meticulous anatomic repair of nail bed lacerations. Once established, fingernail deformities may be difficult or impossible to correct.

Complex Regional Pain Syndrome

Complex regional pain syndrome (Figs. 18 and 19)— previously known as reflex sympathetic dystrophy, algodystrophy, sympathetic maintained pain, and Sudeck's atrophy—may develop after any hand injury, but is particularly common in association with nerve injury or irritation. This problem may occur spontaneously after major or minor injury. It may

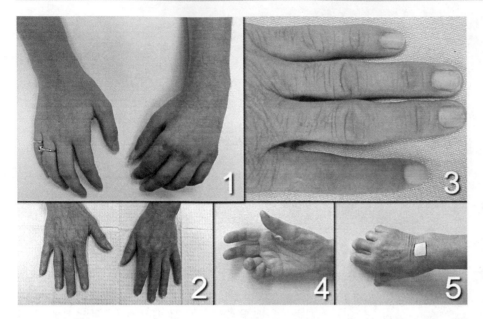

Figure 18 Reflex sympathetic dystrophy usually results in swelling, stiffness, disuse, and color and temperature changes. The entire hand is usually affected (**A, B**), less commonly a single digit (**C**). Dupuytren's type contractures are common (**D**). This may follow elective surgery, but is most often seen after injury, such as a distal radius fracture (**E**).

cause spontaneous burning pain, hyperalgesia, swelling, vasomotor disturbances, and disuse, and it may be exacerbated by movement. Although there may be spontaneous resolution, most patients experience some degree of chronic symptoms such as pain, stiffness, and difficulty with normal use of the hand, despite all available treatment (103). The best treatment results require early recognition, aggressive medical therapy, and elimination of triggering phenomena. Medical therapy may involve sympathetic nerve blocks, gabapentin or other medications, and biofeedback. Triggers known to aggravate the condition include peripheral nerve irritation due to neuroma or compressive neuropathy, aggressive passive range-of-motion therapy, and dynamic hand splinting. The effects of complex regional pain syndrome may be far more disabling than the initial injury.

Dysfunction

Patients may develop maladaptive patterns of use after injury, ranging from awkward positioning to

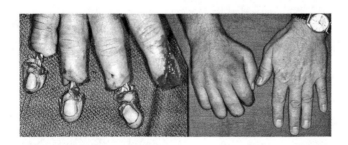

Figure 19 Reflex sympathetic dystrophy following multiple traumatic finger amputations.

complete disuse of the hand. This complication is often due to unconscious reflex protective mechanisms and may be difficult to correct. Extensor habitus refers to the tendency for the injured index finger or small finger to be held in extension. This unconscious posturing is powered by the independent extensor of the finger and is best treated by early recognition and buddy taping. Alien hand syndrome refers to complete disuse of the hand accompanied by the patient's perception that the hand is "not mine." Such problems may also be factitious, but labeling them as such does not improve the patient's overall outcome.

Compartment Syndrome

Compartment syndrome of the hand may develop after crush injury, reperfusion after fracture-related ischemia, intravenous injections, crush or blast injury (25), bleeding after fracture, arterial cannulation or regional surgery, or prolonged pressure on the hand or arm. The forearm is the most common site of compartment syndrome in the upper extremity. Compartment syndrome of the upper extremity is more likely to develop among patients with obtundation. Seriously ill children who receive multiple venous and arterial injections are also at particular risk. Treatment requires prompt recognition and decompression of intrinsic muscle compartments, as well as carpal tunnel release in selected cases (16). The late consequence of compartment syndrome of the upper extremity is Volkmann's contracture (5,67), which involves both muscle contracture and local ischemic neuropathy. Ischemic muscle contractures respond poorly to nonoperative measures such as splinting; this condition requires an aggressive surgical approach using muscle slides, tendon lengthening, and tendon transfers similar to those used in the treatment of upper extremity spasticity. Neurolysis is indicated for persistent nerve symptoms, but the outcome is unpredictable.

Complications of Specific Injuries
Complications of Missed Complex Wounds

Complex wounds are those that require additional procedures, such as radical debridement or flap wound closure.

Severe Contamination

Severe contamination is common with missed complex wounds of the hand because the hand is so often physically exposed to contaminated mechanisms of injury.

Bite Injuries
Human Bite Injuries. Human bite injuries to the hand most often occur as clenched-fist bite injuries, sustained when the fist strikes the mouth of another person during an altercation. The most common constellation of injuries is a skin laceration at the level of the metacarpal head accompanied by injury to the extensor tendon and the metacarpal head. This injury is usually sustained when the hand is in a clenched-fist position, but the patient frequently does not present for treatment until the metacarpophalangeal joint is pulled into extension by dorsal hand swelling. This change in positioning places the soft tissue and bone injuries at an offset, giving the appearance that the injury is more superficial than it is (Figs. 20 and 21). Treatment requires a high level of suspicion, aggressive debridement, and intravenous antibiotics appropriate for a bite injury.

Animal Bite Injuries. Animal bites to the hand are most often dog or cat bites. These bites can lead to prolonged morbidity, particularly when there is a delay between injury and initial treatment (66). Dog bites are associated with soft-tissue crush injury and fractures. Cat bites are particularly dangerous in hand because the cat's needlelike teeth can easily penetrate into joint spaces, tendon sheaths, and other deep compartments of the hand through a relatively innocuous skin wound.

Insect Bites. Bites to the hand from insects such as brown recluse spiders may cause painful, slow-healing wounds, resulting in chronic functional deficits. The initial bite injury may be painless. When surgical excision is indicated, the results appear to be better when surgery is delayed until after the acute inflammatory process has subsided (103).

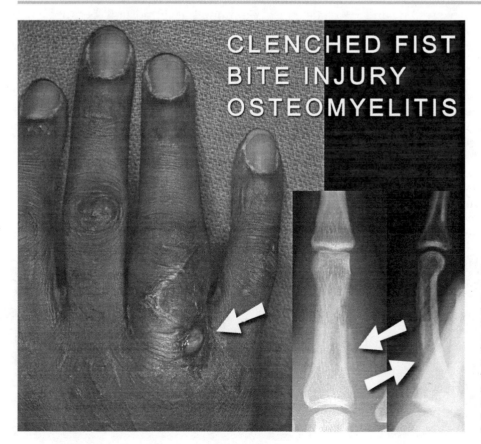

CLENCHED FIST BITE INJURY OSTEOMYELITIS

Figure 20 Clenched fist bite injuries of the metacarpal head or proximal phalanx are highly contaminated, often deeply penetrating wounds with bone involvement. They are at particular risk for the development of septic arthritis and osteomyelitis. This patient developed osteomyelitis of the proximal phalanx following such an injury, and received inadequate surgical and antibiotic treatment due to neglect. The image on the left shows a healed wound and a draining sinus, and arrows on the right show periosteal bone formation and erosions due to osteomyelitis. This eventually resulted in amputation.

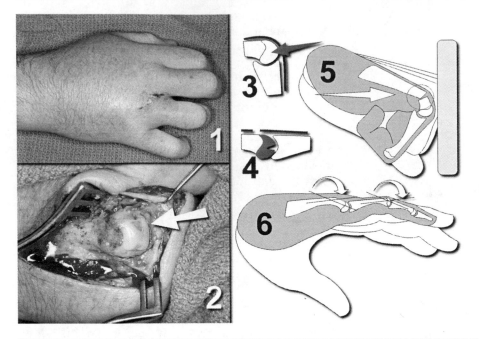

Figure 21 Complications of boxer's fractures. Penetrating injuries of the metacarpal head from clenched fist bite injury mechanism are frequently delayed in presentation, and may rapidly progress to pyarthrosis and osteomyelitis. The patient may present with infection and a trivial appearing wound (**A**), masking a direct injury of the metacarpal head (**B**). Casual inspection of the wound in the emergency room may be misleading because the offset of soft tissue and joint penetration at the time of injury (**C**) is different than at the time of presentation when swelling results in metacarpophalangeal joint extension (**D**). Palmar angulation of the distal fracture fragment (**E**) may result in tendon imbalance and secondary flexion contracture of the proximal interphalangeal joint, usually to the same extent as angulation of the fracture malunion (**F**).

Rattlesnake Bites. Rattlesnake bites to the upper extremity are associated with serious complications; at least one-third of patients experience complication such as local soft-tissue necrosis (the most common complication), coagulopathy, stiffness, loss of sensibility, and Volkmann's contracture (43). Antivenin and steroids reduce the degree of swelling and hemorrhage but do not affect or prevent tissue necrosis, which may require operative treatment.

Chemical Burns

Industrial Acid Burns. The hand may suffer industrial acid burns when an inexperienced or careless worker splashes even small amounts of acid onto the fingers or hand. This type of injury can go undetected upon initial evaluation unless a careful history is obtained because visible signs of injury are often delayed (Fig. 22). Hydrochloric and hydrofluoric acids are used in industrial processing and may cause severe burns that do not manifest themselves for a day after exposure. Early recognition and treatment with topical, intravenous, or intra-arterial calcium gluconate can reduce both pain and the extent of tissue loss.

White Phosphorus Burns. Workers may sustain white phosphorus burns as the result of handling military munitions, fireworks, and other industrial and agricultural products. Such injuries may result in deep, progressive burns and the systemic effects of multiple organ system failure. Although copper sulfate has been recommended as a specific antidote, the safest and most effective treatment is copious irrigation with water (105). Again, recognition of the nature of injury and immediate treatment are essential for reducing long-term complications.

Injection Injuries

High-pressure Injection Injuries. High-pressure injection of paint, sand, lubricating fluid, or other materials is uncommon, but important because such injuries are often missed in the accident ward. Typically, the patient has briefly placed the hand or fingertip over a pressure spray nozzle, thereby sustaining an injection of material into the soft tissues. Under pressure, this material tracks up tissue planes next to flexor tendons, nerves, and arteries

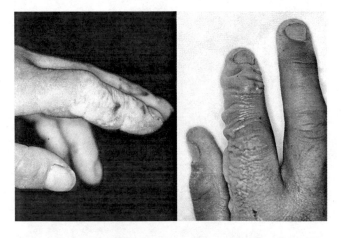

Figure 22 Topical hydrofluoric acid burns typically do not show visible evidence of injury for a day or two after exposure. By then, effectiveness of topical or systemic calcium treatment is diminished.

and through the named bursae and compartments of the hand and arm. Debris may be driven from the fingertip to the chest wall. The examiner may be misled by a small visible wound and (depending on the material injected) relatively few physical findings, and the patient may be discharged only to return within 24 hours because of worsening symptoms. Radiographs may show the presence of air, particulate debris, or pigment (in certain types of paint) in soft tissues.

Treatment is emergency radical debridement (62). The pressure-injected material tends to track through the loose areolar tissue along longitudinal structures, and only careful debridement may allow preservation of all vital structures (Fig. 23). In contrast, late surgical treatment may require *en bloc* tumor-like excision of contaminated zones, or even amputation. Late results are worst when the injected material is either a petroleum-based solvent or a particulate material (sandblasting), when the tendon sheath is involved, and when there is wide proximal spread of the injected material (80). The injected material is not sterile and prophylactic antibiotic treatment is indicated. Poor perfusion in association with such injuries should be treated with primary amputation (80). Injection of pressurized aerosol fluorocarbon liquids such as that used in refrigerants may also result in deep frostbite injury.

Intentional Injection Injuries. Injuries associated with the intentional injection of household cleaners, solvents, mercury, or illicit drugs may be difficult to evaluate because of the delusional or drug-seeking

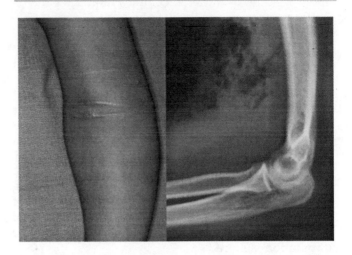

Figure 24 Soft-tissue gas is a frequent benign finding accompanying open wounds immediately after injury, but in the presence of infection should always be assumed to be due to gas-forming organisms. Multiple organisms were isolated from the necrotizing infection in the antecubital area of this intravenous drug abuser.

nature of the patient. Radiographs may show particulate or metallic debris or evidence of gas-forming infection (Fig. 24).

Factitious or Intentional Wounds

Factitious or intentional wounds to the hand are uncommon, but successful treatment is very difficult because of recurrence. Swelling, ulceration, and recurrent wound breakdown are common. Such wounds are most typical on the dorsum of the nondominant hand. Narcotic-seeking behavior may be part of the overall picture. The most important aspect of treatment is recognition, so that unnecessary, unsuccessful, or mutilating procedures may be avoided. Although the problem is psychiatric, psychiatric intervention may or may not be helpful, and confrontation or intervention is generally ineffective. Such patients may jump from doctor to doctor within a community, and it is wise to notify local colleagues when such problems with a patient are identified.

Complications of Obvious Complex Wounds

Complex wounds are, by definition, prone to complications, even with ideal management. Common complex injuries of the hand are associated with predictable types of complications, which are listed below.

Traumatic Amputations

Hand injuries involving traumatic amputation most often affect the fingers. The associated nerve injury always forms a neuroma, and the treating surgeon should trim the digital nerve ends away from the distal wound so as to lessen the chance of disabling scar

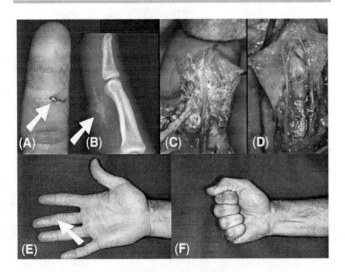

Figure 23 Paint pressure injection injury. This patient presented with a relatively low pressure–injection injury of the middle finger with a small entrance wound (**A**). Titanium pigment in the paint was visible on X ray (**B**). Optimum treatment involved emergency meticulous radical debridement of all stained or damaged tissues, aided by use of the operating microscope (**C, D**). Late result with recovery of full sensation and range of motion (**E, F**).

tenderness. Dysesthesia is common and all patients should be provided with an early desensitization program that can be performed at home. Complex regional pain syndrome may be triggered and then maintained by tender finger stumps (Fig. 19); at first it may be difficult to distinguish this condition from the swelling, stiffness, tenderness, and avoidance that are always associated with the injury. Sensitivity to or intolerance of cold is a problem for most patients, but this condition usually improves after the first year. When more than the distal third of the phalanx is lost, a hook nail deformity will result, with the fingernail curving toward the palm and covering the distal fingertip. This and other variations of retained nail remnant may be avoided by careful total excision of the entire germinal matrix when the amputation is closed.

Fingertip amputations are no less problematic than more proximal amputations, particularly when the critical contact areas used in pinching and fine manipulation are involved (Fig. 25). Amputations through the proximal phalanx often result in extensor habitus, described in the section General Complications of Hand Injury/Dysfunction. Metacarpophalangeal joint disarticulation of the index or small finger results in an easily traumatized and visibly prominent metacarpal head. Metacarpophalangeal joint disarticulation of the middle or ring finger results in a "hole in the hand," through which small objects held in the cupped palm can fall. Treatment of either of these scenarios with removal of a metacarpal replaces the original problem with a narrowed palm and reduced torque grip strength.

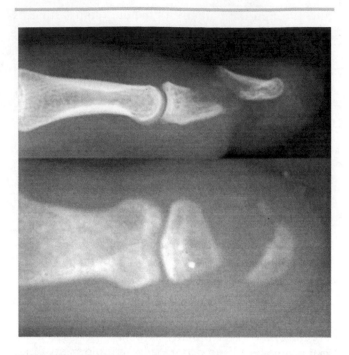

Figure 26 Distal phalanx nonunions are uncommon and usually follow open injuries. Risk factors include inadequate reduction of displaced fragments, soft-tissue interposition, or bone loss, including bone loss due to surgical debridement. The *top* image shows the type of acute displaced fracture that is best treated with internal fixation. The *bottom* image shows an established nonunion following bone debridement and wound closure. Most fractures that require bone debridement would benefit from internal fixation. Late salvage of distal phalanx nonunions is technically demanding and requires precision bone grafting techniques.

Fingertip Injuries

Fingertip injuries other than amputation are associated with all of the painful and otherwise disabling complications of finger amputations. Nail deformities, tender scars, and nonunion (Fig. 26) are difficult treatment issues. Pediatric fingertip crush injuries are common, and severe injuries involving a sterile matrix laceration with a tuft fracture are frequently missed in children (78). These injuries require meticulous nail bed repair so as to avoid deformity.

Foreign Bodies

Foreign bodies in the hand are likely to cause symptoms when they involve the distal phalanx (34). Removal of foreign bodies that are lodged entirely beneath the surface of the skin should be performed with tourniquet control and surgical anesthesia. Otherwise, a common result is that the area where the foreign body is lodged is incised, attempts at retrieval are unsuccessful, and the problem is compounded by the inflammation and scarring resulting from instrumentation. Foreign bodies are most likely to give rise to problems when they are composed either of organic materials (wood, plant thorn, etc.) or of highly contaminated materials. Phoenix date palm thorns frequently produce a chronic sterile

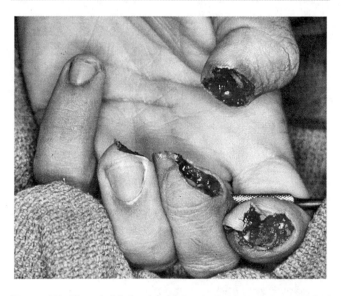

Figure 25 Fingertip injuries that involve the "critical contact areas" of the thumb, index, and middle fingers pose particularly difficult challenges for reconstruction. Rotating blade saws commonly result in combined injuries such as shown here, impairing the ability to use the hand for fine manipulation.

inflammatory reaction and require primary treatment with radical debridement and extensive synovectomy (93). Foreign-body entry points at the dorsal surfaces of the metacarpophalangeal or interphalangeal joints or at the palmar flexion creases of the fingers are at particular risk for contamination of tendons and deep-space infections. Chronic symptomatic foreign-body problems require tumor-like excision and synovectomy, not incision and removal (Fig. 12).

Thermal Burn Injuries

Thermal burns to the upper extremity result in stiffness of the hand; this complication is best prevented by early active motion within two weeks of injury (65). This goal is difficult to achieve reliably because the depth of the burn may be difficult to assess, and areas that require skin grafting must be immobilized for at least one week after surgery. When possible, the goal is early definitive wound closure with full-thickness or tangential excision and skin grafts or flaps, followed by motion at the earliest possible opportunity. The ultimate disability in hand function is thought to relate to the time required to achieve wound closure, although this point is controversial (72).

Burn injuries can cause lifetime problems that cannot be cured by any amount of surgery and therapy, and the surgeon must strive to promote realistic, achievable goals (70). Common complications are compartment syndrome (6,25); contractures (68) of web spaces and extensor and flexor surfaces; and hypertrophic scars and heterotopic ossification. Surface contact burns over the course of the brachial artery are rare but may lead to ischemic limb loss (4). Among children, burns to the hand more commonly involve an isolated contact burn to the palm, particularly among infants, that is sustained when a child grasps a hot object such as a curling iron and then grips even more tightly in response to pain. As for burns in other areas, excision and grafting are indicated if healing is expected to take more than three weeks, but in this instance contractures requiring additional reconstructive procedures are common (68). Pediatric hand burns have the most favorable outcome when managed in a specialty treatment program (77).

Frostbite

A wide variety of early treatments are recommended for frostbite (106), but rapid rewarming is standard. Traditional management is observation and delayed amputation (Fig. 27). A bone scan may help distinguish unsalvageable from potentially salvageable regions. Early surgery may provide marginal tissue with a new blood supply and may preserve both the function and the length of the upper extremity.

Electrical Injuries

Electrical injuries to the upper extremity may produce extensive deep-tissue injury, compartment syndrome,

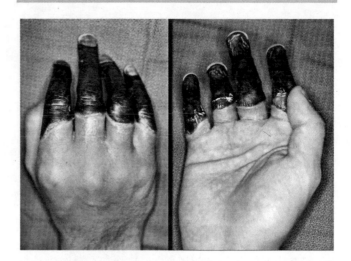

Figure 27 Frostbite injuries most commonly affect the face, fingers, and toes. Viability may be estimated from bone scan, but even with this information, it is best to wait until a line of demarcation is clear. In the absence of infection, this process may take months.

delayed tissue necrosis, and delayed vascular thrombosis (110). Early exploration and decompression of deep compartments, vascular graft reconstruction of segmental defects, and early free microvascular flap reconstruction reduce the likelihood of amputation and shorten recovery times (85,108,109,111). Even with optimum treatment, however, long-term sensory loss is common and is an unsolved problem (107).

Degloving Injuries

When the hand is caught in moving machinery, degloving injuries often result. If microvascular replantation of the degloved tissues is possible, this treatment approach probably yields the best final result, although achieving sensory recovery is difficult even with this technique (51). If replantation is not possible, efforts to salvage a crushed avulsed flap are usually unrewarding, and primary excision and resurfacing with a graft or flap (Fig. 28) are indicated so as to avoid a prolonged course of progressive flap loss, delayed healing, infection, and stiffness.

Mangling Hand Injuries

The hand can be mangled by a wide range of mechanical injuries, usually involving all tissue components of the hand. Mechanisms include crush, blast, ballistic, traction, and avulsion injuries. All complications are possible and patients with these injuries are at particular risk of delayed healing, marginal wound necrosis (Fig. 29), infection (Fig. 30), delayed thrombosis, prolonged swelling, compartment syndrome (16,25), intrinsic muscle contractures (Fig. 31), nonunion (Figs. 32 and 33), stiffness, and lack of sensory

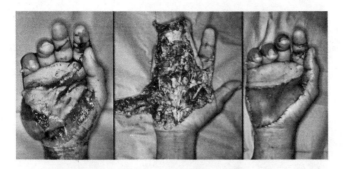

Figure 28 Traumatic flaps have unpredictable vascularity, particularly when they are distally based, involve a crush mechanism, and involve the skin of the palm. This patient sustained a crush injury of the hand, resulting in distally based long, thin, palmar flaps (*left, center*). Primary wound healing and early recovery are most reliably achieved with excision and resurfacing areas of indeterminate viability. In this case, a full-thickness graft was applied to the palm (*right*).

recovery (51). The initial management plan is crucial, as outlined in the next section.

Complications Associated with the Treatment of Severe Hand Wounds

Severe hand wounds may lead to many different complications that can add additional trouble to an already difficult situation.

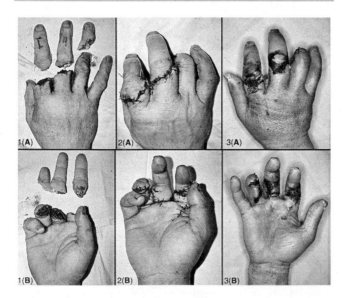

Figure 29 This series demonstrates marginal necrosis in a complex wound. This patient sustained multiple amputations in a power saw accident and underwent replantation of two of his fingers. Figures **1A** and **1B** show the original injury, and **2A** and **2B** show the appearance immediately after replantation. Figures **3A** and **3B** show peripheral necrosis of both proximal and distal wound margins. In this case, such conditions may lead to late failure of replantation due to thrombosis of the vascular repairs due to an inhospitable wound environment. Fortunately, secondary healing was uneventful and the replanted digits survived.

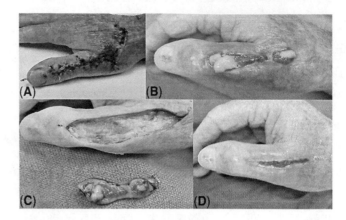

Figure 30 Crush and avulsion wounds typically have combined effects of indeterminate or inadequate vascularity and widespread contamination. Infection following such wounds is due to inadequate debridement, and primary wound closure increases the chance of marginal wound necrosis. This patient presented after primary closure of a dorsal hand crush–avulsion injury in which the extensor pollicis longus had been repaired. The wound margins became necrotic (**A**) and the extensor pollicis longus tendon underwent a progressive septic liquefaction necrosis (**B**). He was treated with wide debridement (**C**), and then was lost to follow-up. He performed his own wound care and healed uneventfully with the wound nearly closed one month after debridement (**D**).

Failure to Proceed with Primary Amputation

It is difficult and emotionally stressful to decide when or whether to amputate a severely injured hand or digit, particularly when the part in question has at least the appearance of an existing blood supply.

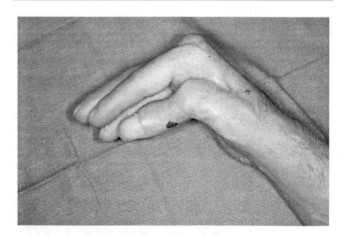

Figure 31 Intrinsic contractures. This patient sustained a crush injury of the hand, resulting in direct damage and late fibrosis of all of the intrinsic muscles. The thumb intrinsic muscles were extruded through burst wounds. Intrinsic contractures produce metacarpophalangeal joint flexion contractures, first web space contracture, and extension contractures of the interphalangeal joints, all evident here. Secondary swan-neck deformity of the fingers is also common. Correction requires extensive release of the intrinsic muscles, and then in cases such as this, first web reconstruction with a flap and opponensplasty.

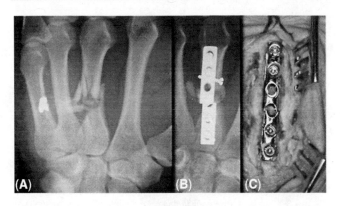

Figure 32 High-velocity gunshot wounds result in a wide zone of soft-tissue injury. Fractures associated with high-energy injuries (**A**) are more likely to have complications of delayed union, nonunion, and hardware failure (**B, C**).

"Saving" a mangled hand may simply burden the patient with a painful, useless extremity, resulting in a triumph of technique over judgment. One guide to making this decision is to ask the following question: If this injured extremity looked like this but involved complete amputation, would replantation be indicated? If the answer is clearly no, primary amputation should be strongly considered (Fig. 34). The best time to proceed with primary amputation for a mangled extremity is at the very first operation. If the surgeon realizes at the time of the first operation that the hand is unsalvageable but does not amputate, a precedent is set for false expectations and even greater disappointment than would otherwise be endured. The patient and the family see the bandage, conclude that the

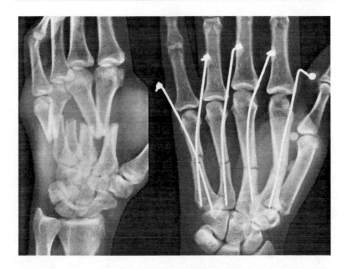

Figure 33 Crush injuries are prone to delayed wound healing and stiffness with standard open reduction and internal fixation techniques. Percutaneous fracture pinning allows fracture stabilization without the addition of additional trauma from fracture site exposure.

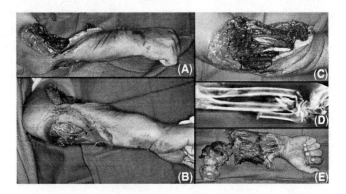

Figure 34 The decision to proceed with primary amputation is the most emotionally difficult when there are apparently salvageable parts. This patient's arm was trapped in a rotating wheel mechanism, resulting in combined crush and burn injuries of the forearm from above the elbow to below the wrist, and six hours of complete ischemic time prior to arrival at the trauma center. The hand was relatively spared. While technically possible to replant the hand at the level of the distal humerus, a prosthesis would be expected to provide better function and appearance, and the injury was converted to an above elbow amputation.

hand has been "saved," and will find it much more difficult later to accept the fact that it has not. Although some patients with a saved mangled extremity may decide later to undergo elective amputation (59), most will be unable to make this decision even if the hand is a burden and is clearly inferior to a prosthesis.

Inadequate Debridement

The single common denominator of wound healing complications such as infection, delayed healing, marginal necrosis, and wound breakdown is inadequate debridement. If the zone of injury can be determined with reasonable certainty, severe wounds should be radically débrided with anticipation of the potential need for complex flap closure. Debridement should remove severely contaminated tissues and all ischemic tissues that cannot be revascularized, including crushed flaps, distally based flaps with a length-to-width ratio of more than one to two, and flaps that are obviously ischemic. Initial debridement should be performed under tourniquet control, and proper initial debridement of severe wounds involves en bloc tumor-like excision with a scalpel and saw, not a curette or irrigation, although these techniques may be used later. The skin of the palm has a primarily perpendicular rather than tangential vascular pattern, and traumatic palmar flaps should be considered for primary excision and alternate resurfacing because their vascularity is quite unreliable (Fig. 28).

Poor Timing of Wound Closure

Traditionally, the timing of closure of severe hand wounds has been classified as primary (immediate), delayed primary (within two weeks), and secondary (after two weeks). Historically, delayed primary closure was recommended for military and other severe hand injuries. This recommendation is still appropriate when the only available wound closure technique is direct closure or closure with local flaps. However, the timing of wound closure using distant or microvascular free flaps follows different guidelines. The status of severe open wounds that are candidates for flap closure is classified as acute (before the appearance of granulation tissue; usually less than one week), subacute (after the appearance of granulation tissue but before dense scarring; usually one to four weeks), or chronic (usually after one month). Wounds that require flap closure are associated with the lowest complication rate (fewer flap failures, fewer postoperative infections, shorter hospitalization periods, fewer operations, and shorter overall period of disability) when closure is performed during the acute phase, and with the highest complication rate when surgery is performed during the subacute phase (27,76,83,84,86,87). Free flap reconstruction of burn injuries is associated with the lowest complication rate when it is used for the reexploration and reconstruction of healed, closed burn injuries (85).

Technical Failure of Complex Wound Closure

Even with adequate debridement, avoidance of local flaps from the potential zone of injury, and careful planning, wound closure may fail. Skin grafts to the hand may be lost because of inability to provide adequate immobilization, and flaps may be lost when the complex wound dimensions exceed the capacity of the flap. Although free flaps tend to be successful or to be lost on an "all or none" basis, partial loss of a free flap may occur. Loss of a pedicled flap usually occurs at the exact point at which flap coverage is crucially needed (Fig. 35). However, even a perfectly designed and executed flap cannot obviate the effects of inadequate debridement or poor timing of wound closure.

Complications of Replantation

All complications of complex hand wounds can occur after replantation, including tendon adhesions, tendon rupture, neuroma, and delayed healing. In addition, however, replantation carries the risk of a number of additional problems. Early vascular failure (Fig. 36) of replantation is influenced by the mechanism of injury and patient selection. Early failure is more common among smokers (69), when replantation occurs at a more distal level, and when the injury has involved crush or avulsion (79). After successful revascularization, venous problems are more likely than arterial thrombosis to result in loss of the replanted extremity (14,20). The crucial time for failure or successful salvage is the first four postoperative days (20).

As is true for other wounds, replantation can result in marginal necrosis or interval gangrene

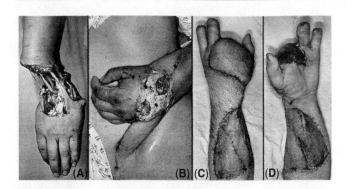

Figure 35 Loss of axial pedicle flaps. Axial flaps, although generally reliable, still have a peninsular vascular anatomy, and the most distal extent of the flap may fail if the blood supply is compromised either by kinking or by tension of the flap. This last problem is most likely when a flap has been placed in a circumferential geometry, where swelling produces progressive tension along the circumference of the flap. **(A, B)** Pedicled inferior epigastric flap used to resurface the hand dorsum following hand replantation. The flap tip was lost, most likely due to unprotected tension and kinking at the juncture of the flap and the recipient site. **(C, D)** Reversed pedicled radial forearm flap tip lost due to combination of extension of flap harvest out of the most vascular zone and tension from circumferential wrapping of the flap around the hand.

(Fig. 29) if debridement is inadequate or if the surgeon in unable to distinguish viable from nonviable tissues in a wide zone of injury. The most common complication of successful replantation is stiffness due to tendon adhesions (14). Cold intolerance is uncommon after pediatric replantation but occurs after most adult replantations (14). Aesthetically disturbing fingertip atrophy occurs with nearly half of all replanted digits (14) because of the effects

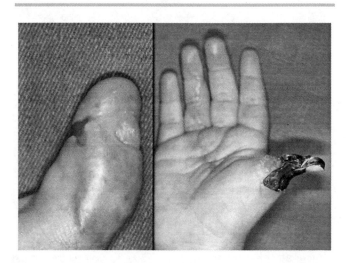

Figure 36 Digital replantation may fail in part due to damage from long periods of ischemia (left), or more commonly fail completely because of inability to maintain revascularization (right).

of incomplete reinnervation and, in some cases, the late effects of prolonged ischemia (Fig. 36). Lack of sensory recovery is more common when the patient is an adult, when both arteries have not been repaired (51), and when the injury involves avulsion (79).

As with any other vascular repair, replantation may be associated with local vascular complications such as pseudoaneurysm (5), arteriovenous fistula (37), stricture, and late thrombosis. Delayed union, nonunion, or avascular necrosis may occur, particularly when the replantation is performed at the level of the phalangeal neck (44) because the phalangeal head is covered with cartilage and has a primarily intramedullary blood supply. Fractures or osteotomies through this level are prone to these complications even after procedures other than replantation (61). Prolonged incapacitation and multiple operations are typical; the average patient requires two or more additional procedures after replantation (52). Judgment as to the indications for replantation must include the realization that the poor results after replantation may be much more disabling than primary amputation. Functional outcome is significantly worse when replantation involves prolonged ischemia (Fig. 36) or injury in flexor tendon zone II (69).

Complications of Vascular Injuries
Missed Vascular Hand Injuries
Ring Avulsion Injuries

Ring avulsion injuries range from trivial skin lacerations to arterial or venous disruption to combined injuries in continuity to complete amputation. The zone of injury is usually greater than would be detected by casual inspection, and extremities with combined vascular and skeletal disruption injuries are often not salvageable despite the external appearance of a simple laceration (Fig. 37). When the ring is completely pulled off the finger in association with a circumferential finger wound, the distal soft-tissue envelope is usually severely injured, effectively turning the soft tissue sleeve inside out and irreparably damaging the distal part. For all but the most minor injuries, successful salvage with vein grafts and flaps is unlikely and, even when successful, often results in a stiff, insensate digit.

Partial Vascular Laceration

Partial vascular laceration is the most likely cause of persistent uncontrolled hemorrhage; such an injury may result in substantial bleeding. Persistent bleeding is better controlled by local pressure than by blind clamping, which may result in iatrogenic nerve injuries (Fig. 38). Late effects of partial vessel laceration include pseudoaneurysm, delayed hemorrhage, and delayed thrombosis.

Iatrogenic Hand Injuries Related to Vascular Surgery
Graft Harvest. Harvesting the radial artery for coronary artery bypass procedures may result in hand

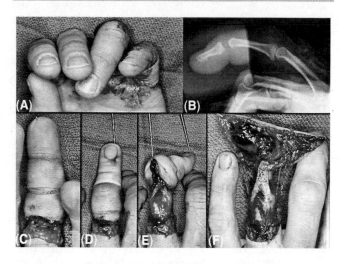

Figure 37 Ring avulsion injuries may appear deceptively normal because of color from blood trapped in the digit and active range of motion maintained by the long tendons. In this example, the finger appeared viable (**A**), despite a long zone of tissue disruption from the distal interphalangeal joint (**B**) to the base of the finger (**C, D, E**). In fact, the finger was only attached by the flexor tendons and digital nerves (**F**) and was unsalvageable.

ischemia or injury to the superficial radial nerve (7,41). The incidence of hand ischemia after radial artery harvest may be reduced by the use of preoperative color duplex scanning in addition to careful physical examination.

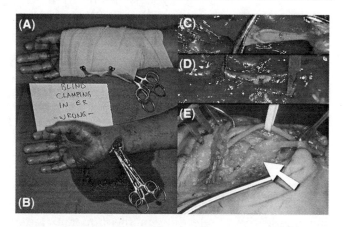

Figure 38 The drama of hemorrhage may lead to unwise maneuvers in the emergency room. Blind clamping of bleeding structures without proximal tourniquet control is risky and may compound injury. (**A, B**) This patient had inadequate control of bleeding despite multiple clamps placed by an inexperienced physician, who was successful in clamping the ulnar nerve and flexor carpi ulnaris tendon, but failed to control the large subcutaneous vein that was actually responsible for the bleeding. Continued hemorrhage is often due to partial vessel lacerations, as in this partial laceration of the cephalic vein (**C**) and this partial laceration of the radial artery (**D**). Ligation of structures without adequate visualization in the emergency room is also problematic, as in this patient who had inadvertent ligation of the ulnar nerve within Guyon's canal (**E**).

Dialysis Access. Nearly 2% of patients undergoing new angio-access procedures experience severe hand ischemia (11). This problem is more common among diabetic patients who have undergone multiple angio-access procedures (9) or who have diabetic neuropathy (24). Prompt recognition and treatment are crucial if tissue loss and permanent nerve injury are to be avoided. This problem should be suspected when finger pain, numbness, or nerve symptoms arise immediately after angio-access surgery. Optimum treatment options include ligation of the fistula, intraoperative duplex scanning–guided banding (10), or distal revascularization–interval ligation. Neurologic symptoms may arise even if critical ischemia cannot be demonstrated, and recovery of nerve function is unpredictable (24). Direct nerve compression may result from adjacent access materials (Fig. 16) or from hematoma around the side of a vascular suture line (35).

Bypass Surgery. Upper extremity ischemia has been reported as a steal phenomenon after axillofemoral bypass grafting, and as the result of emboli after thrombosis of an axillofemoral bypass graft (9,40).

General Complications of Upper Extremity Vascular Injuries

After vascular injury to the hand, as elsewhere, ischemic gangrene, chronic ischemia, intrinsic contracture, traumatic aneurysm, arteriovenous fistula, thrombosis, and embolism may occur. Supracondylar fractures of the humerus may result in brachial artery compression or disruption, and postischemic reperfusion compartment syndrome of the forearm can follow restoration of arterial flow after either closed reduction or vascular repair. Fasciotomy should be considered if ischemic time exceeds two hours and should be performed if compartment pressures are elevated.

Complications of Treatment of Vascular Injuries
Inappropriate Use of Techniques to Control Bleeding

The use of inappropriate techniques to control bleeding in the emergency room can add substantial injury. Nearly all bleeding in the upper extremity can be controlled by elevation and direct pressure. In the emergency room, the use of tourniquets should be limited to a few minutes at most, and tourniquets should ideally be used only by the surgeon who will provide the definitive surgical care. Inflating a tourniquet and then waiting for the hand surgeon to arrive in the emergency room is inappropriate and dangerous, and it limits future treatment options. Similarly, the use of local destructive intervention with clamps, ligature, or cautery (Fig. 38) by anyone other than the surgical specialist assuming final care of the patient should be strongly discouraged.

Inappropriate Primary Call to the Vascular Surgeon

A common problem with hand injuries is an inappropriate primary call to the vascular surgeon. Upper extremity hemorrhage is usually best managed by an upper extremity surgeon. Time permitting, the ideal order of repair of the severely injured upper extremity is debridement, skeletal stabilization, musculotendinous repairs, nerve repairs, and *then* vascular repairs (Fig. 39), all under tourniquet control. Such an approach minimizes hemorrhage and allows the most precise primary repairs. Unfortunately, a common scenario is that the bleeding arm is first managed by a vascular surgeon, who does not provide definitive care of adjacent nerve and musculoskeletal injuries.

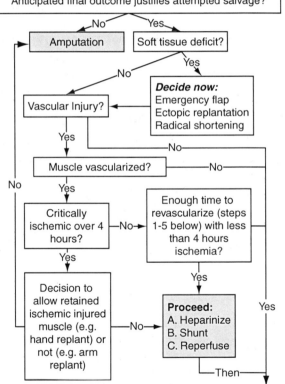

Severe Trauma: Order of Procedures

Anticipated final outcome justifies attempted salvage?

No → Amputation
Yes → Soft tissue deficit?

Soft tissue deficit? Yes → **Decide now:** Emergency flap / Ectopic replantation / Radical shortening

No → Vascular Injury?

Vascular Injury? Yes → Muscle vascularized?

Muscle vascularized? Yes → Critically ischemic over 4 hours?
No →

Critically ischemic over 4 hours? No → Enough time to revascularize (steps 1-5 below) with less than 4 hours ischemia?

Critically ischemic over 4 hours? Yes → Decision to allow retained ischemic injured muscle (e.g. hand replant) or not (e.g. arm replant)

Enough time to revascularize... Yes → **Proceed:** A. Heparinize B. Shunt C. Reperfuse

Decision to allow retained ischemic injured muscle... No → **Proceed:** A. Heparinize B. Shunt C. Reperfuse

Then →

Proceed as applicable, *in this order*:
1. Debride under tourniquet control, extensile incisions
2. Wound irrigation/lavage
3. Skeletal realignment and stabilization
4. Fasciotomies if muscle ischemia time over 2 hours
5. Musculotendinous repairs adjacent to vascular injuries
6. Definitve vascular repairs
7. Confirm final plan for wound closure
8. Remaining deep soft issue repairs
9. Wound closure

Figure 39 Optimum management of severe extremity trauma involves an organized approach to avoid useless attempts at salvage, maximize the potential success of salvage, and minimize iatrogenic complications such as excessive blood loss.

In this situation, the vascular injury is repaired, often with a graft, and then the extremity surgeon is called in to complete the work. When the adjacent nerve and muscles are then repaired, the vascular "gap" that was thought to require a graft disappears, and the graft may need to be removed to avoid kinking due to redundancy. Similarly, performing only vascular repair, closing the wound, and referring the patient for secondary repair of adjacent structures may sacrifice the best opportunity for a precise primary repair of all structures in the most safe and efficient manner.

Complications of Tendon Injuries
Complications of Missed Tendon Injuries

Tendon injuries can be missed when either the patient or the initial examining physician fails to appreciate subtle findings.

Partial Tendon Lacerations

A partial tendon laceration (Fig. 40) should be suspected when the patient apparently has full motion, but has pain when attempting to use the tendon against resistance. Consequences of partial tendon lacerations include delayed rupture, scarring with tendon adhesions, triggering, and weakness.

Missed Injuries to the Extensor Mechanism of the Finger

Injuries to the extensor mechanism of the finger may be missed because the broad expanse of the extensor mechanism can initially maintain posture until softening from the healing process allows the remnants of support to give way. Terminal tendon injuries at the distal interphalangeal joint and central slip injuries

at the proximal interphalangeal joint should be suspected when the patient has suffered a regional injury and has pain upon attempted extension against resistance, even if the patient has full, active motion without resistance.

Missed Injuries to the Flexor Tendon of the Finger

Missed flexor tendon injuries are less common than missed extensor tendon injuries because of the change in the resting posture of the hand (Fig. 3). Isolated superficialis tendon injury with an intact profundus tendon produces only a subtle change in finger posture and is easily missed. Profundus tendon avulsion injuries (Fig. 41) are often unappreciated by the patient, who believes that the finger is simply "jammed" and delays medical evaluation until the best window of opportunity for treatment has passed. If there is substantial proximal retraction after profundus avulsion, the flexor tendon sheath fills with blood and within a matter of days shrinks enough so that reinsertion is either impossible or does not result in functional movement.

Missed Injuries to the Extensor Tendon Injuries of the Dorsal Hand

Injuries to the extensor tendon of the dorsal hand may be missed because they often cause little initial functional deficit, either because of the action of adjacent

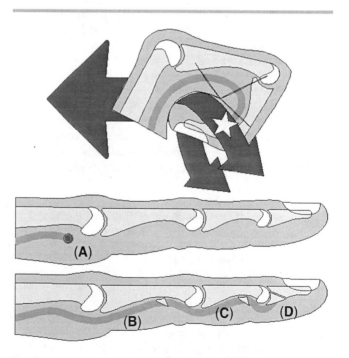

Figure 41 Flexor profundus tendon avulsion injuries occur when the fingertip is suddenly pulled into extension while being actively flexed. The tendon may retract all the way into the palm at the metacarpal neck level (**A**). Lesser degrees of tendon retraction are more likely when the injury results in an avulsion fracture, which may lodge at the A2 or A4 flexor tendon pulley (**B, C**) or be minimally displaced (**D**). Retraction proximal to the proximal interphalangeal joint disrupts the vincular arteries, ischemic tendon damage, and a worse outcome.

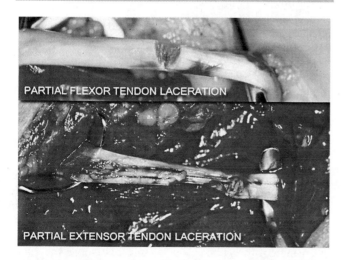

PARTIAL FLEXOR TENDON LACERATION

PARTIAL EXTENSOR TENDON LACERATION

Figure 40 Partial tendon lacerations should be suspected after penetrating wound injury when the muscle tendon unit functions with pain, or when there is pain when attempting motion against resistance. Missed partial tendon injuries may result in triggering, loss of motion from adhesions, or delayed tendon rupture.

tendinous junctures or because only one of two (proprius and communis) tendons in the index or small fingers have been cut. Extensor pollicis longus tendon injuries may be missed because of trick motion through the action of the thumb intrinsic muscles on the thumb extensor mechanism; this action may allow interphalangeal joint extension to neutral despite a divided extensor pollicis longus tendon.

Common Complications of Tendon Injuries of the Hand

Injuries to the tendons of the hand can result in complications such as stiffness, contractures, tendon rupture, recurrent adhesions, and weakness. The number and degree of complications depend on the exact level of injury.

The worst results of flexor tendon injuries occur when the injuries are located in the flexor tendon sheath extending from the metacarpal head to the middle portion of the middle phalanx, referred to as "Zone II" or "no man's land." Even with ideal treatment, only about half of the patients with injuries at this level recover to experience good-to-excellent function, and fewer have a satisfactory outcome after staged flexor tendon reconstruction with a tendon graft (58). Quadrigia syndrome, or limited excursion of the middle, ring, and small fingers, occurs because of tethering connections between the profundus tendons of these fingers. This condition may follow a simple flexor tendon injury or may be the result of adhesions after amputation.

The worst results of extensor tendon injuries occur when the injuries are located over the dorsum of the proximal phalanx or the proximal interphalangeal joint. Loss of proximal interphalangeal joint motion may take the form of a fixed contracture, a swan-neck deformity, or a boutonniere finger. Thin soft-tissue coverage and poor tolerance of any change in length contribute to the poor results associated with injuries at this level.

Complications of the Treatment of Tendon Injuries
Tendon Adhesions

Adhesions are the most common problem after tendon repair. Rupture of a flexor tendon repair occurs in at least 4% of cases after primary flexor tendon repair in Zone II with postoperative controlled passive motion (58). Stiffness may be due to either adhesions or rupture, and it may be impossible to determine the nature of loss of motion, even with magnetic resonance imaging.

Mallet Finger

Nearly half of the patients treated for mallet finger experience some type of treatment complication. Complications after surgery are more common, more serious (e.g., deep infection), and more frequently permanent than those arising from splinting alone (30).

Bowstringing

Bowstringing due to incompetence of the flexor tendon pulley system may follow injury or iatrogenic injury during efforts to expose, retrieve, and repair the tendon. External ring splints are commonly used to support the tendon pulley system, but have not been shown to be mechanically effective in preventing bowstringing.

Staged Reconstruction of the Flexor Tendon

Reconstructing the flexor tendon in stages by using temporary silastic tendon spacers followed by tendon grafts carries all of the risks of primary tendon repair. In addition, staged reconstruction is more likely to result in flexion contractures and greatly extend the length of the necessary incapacitation.

Complications of Nerve Injuries
Missed Nerve Injuries
Partial Nerve Lacerations

Partial nerve lacerations may be missed because their presentation does not provide a full-blown picture of anesthesia or paralysis. Such injuries are best treated by primary repair (Fig. 11). Delayed or secondary exploration may result in additional nerve injury because it may be impossible to distinguish between healing tissue, scar tissue, and nerve tissue that is either functioning or has the capacity to heal. Late exploration of a healed partial nerve injury usually reveals an amorphous neuroma in continuity, and the only practical option may be to completely divide the nerve, excise the neuroma, and reconstruct the nerve with nerve grafts. This procedure may be difficult to justify when the patient has either retained or recovered partial nerve function.

Motor Branch Injuries

Motor branch injuries are most often missed after wounds with a small entry site but deep penetration. The ulnar motor branch in the palm, the median motor branch in the palm, and the posterior interosseous nerve in the forearm may be injured without producing sensory loss, and these injuries may be missed by a casual survey.

Complications of Common Nerve Injuries

Nerve injuries in the hand can lead to complications such as tender neuroma, paralysis, and incomplete sensory recovery. In addition, upper extremity nerve injuries usually produce some degree of cold intolerance and are a common trigger of complex regional pain syndrome. Dysesthesia and disuse of the hand may occur and are best treated with an aggressive desensitization and sensory reeducation program under the supervision of a hand therapist. Median nerve injuries result in a greater loss of hand function than ulnar nerve injuries because the critical contact areas of the hand are affected.

Complications of the Treatment of Nerve Injuries

The treatment of nerve injuries may also result in complications, including failure due to repair under tension or repair within a poorly vascularized soft-tissue bed and contractures due to splinting for the relief of tension on a tight repair. Patients who have a wide zone of anesthesia must be instructed about self-protection from cuts and burns. Contractures resulting from paralysis are avoidable but must be anticipated and prevented with splinting: if median nerve palsy is left untreated, a contracture of the first web space will result, and ulnar nerve palsy will result in proximal interphalangeal joint contractures of the ring and small fingers.

Complications of Fractures and Joint Injuries
Missed Fractures and Joint Injuries
Scaphoid and Hook of Hamate

Scaphoid and hook of hamate fractures are commonly missed. These fractures are discussed below.

Reversed Bennett's Fracture

A reversed Bennett's fracture is an intra-articular fracture of the base of the small finger metacarpal. This injury is usually associated with dorsal and proximal subluxation of the metacarpal shaft, which is caused by the unresisted action of the extensor carpi ulnaris tendon. In contrast to intra-articular fractures of the thumb metacarpal base (Bennett's and Rolando's fractures), which have a similar pathologic anatomy (Fig. 42) and good outcome with a variety of treatment techniques (64), reversed Bennett's fractures are prone to chronic symptoms related to post-traumatic arthritis. These fractures are easily missed on plain anteroposterior and lateral radiographs, and their presentation is frequently delayed when they are sustained as boxing injuries.

Phalangeal Neck Fractures

Fractures of the phalangeal neck may go unrecognized despite rotation or dorsal translation of the distal fracture fragments because alignment may look deceptively normal on routine posteroanterior radiographs. The rotated phalangeal neck fracture is unstable, prone to nonunion (61), and sometimes referred to as a "hangman's fracture" (Fig. 43), not only because it involves the "neck," but also because it is easy to miss in children and difficult to treat late.

Missed Ligament Injuries

When ligament injuries are missed, it is usually because the patient downplays the extent of injury, only to seek evaluation later because of persistent symptoms. The most common missed ligament injuries are gamekeeper's thumb and scapholunate ligament injuries, both of which are discussed below.

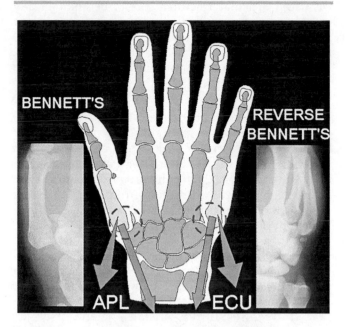

Figure 42 Bennett's and reverse Bennett's fractures. These are fracture dislocations of the thumb and small metacarpal bases, respectively. They are each inherently unstable because of the resultant unopposed distracting forces of remaining muscle tendon attachments on the larger fracture fragment. The abductor pollicis longus displaces the thumb Bennett's fracture, and the extensor carpi ulnaris displaces the small finger reverse Bennett's fracture. Each of these requires at least temporary internal fixation to reliably maintain reduction.

Complications of Common Fractures and Joint Injuries
Intra-Articular Fractures

Intra-articular fractures of the fingers frequently result in stiffness and functional impairment, particularly when they are sustained during childhood (49).

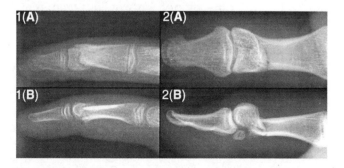

Figure 43 Phalangeal neck fractures are sometimes referred to as "hangman's fracture," either because the break is through the "neck" of the bone, or more importantly because the posterioranterior X-ray may be deceptively normal (**1A, 2A**), despite extension rotation of the distal fragment, as in these cases, rotated 30° (**1B**) and 70° (**2B**). Ninety-degree rotation may occur with little change on the PA view. Such fractures are prone to avascular necrosis of the distal part, even more so following later attempts at corrective osteotomy.

Displaced articular fractures should be anatomically reduced and fixed whenever possible. Even minor degrees of malalignment are usually unacceptable. Long-term problems, including degenerative arthritis, are common, even with optimum initial care.

Pathologic Fractures

Pathologic fractures of the hand are most commonly due to enchondroma involving one of the tubular bones. Complications of treatment are more likely in association with immediate rather than delayed treatment of the tumor (2), and the preferred management of pathologic fracture resulting from a benign tumor is to let the fracture heal and then initiate definitive treatment of the tumor.

Complications of Phalangeal Fracture

Distal Phalanx Fractures.   Fractures of the distal phalanx carry all of the complications associated with fingertip injuries, as previously discussed. Displaced fractures of the distal phalanx (Fig. 26) may give rise to nonunion if they are not reduced and provided with adequate internal fixation. Phalangeal neck fractures are discussed above. Phalangeal shaft fractures are affected to a much greater degree by associated soft-tissue damage and have an overall worse outcome than metacarpal fractures of similar magnitude. Poor functional outcome is common with phalangeal fractures that are open, comminuted, or associated with either significant soft-tissue injury or periosteal stripping, including periosteal stripping performed during open reduction (56,95) when there is associated nerve or tendon injury. Only about one in six displaced phalangeal fractures is stable after closed reduction (56), and redisplacement may occur after temporary fixation with Kirschner wires. Angulation causes a zigzag posture because of tendon imbalance, which results in joint contracture to a degree similar to the degree of proximal angulation (Fig. 44). Outcome is not improved when plate-and-screw fixation is used instead of Kirschner wire fixation (54). On the basis of outcome studies, a strong argument can be made that all finger fractures should be referred to a surgeon with specialty training in hand surgery (55).

Phalangeal Joint Injuries Prone to Complications.   Essentially all interphalangeal joint injuries are prone to complications because of the precision nature of the interphalangeal joints. It is common for the sprained proximal interphalangeal joint to be stiff, tender, painful, and swollen for 6 to 12 months after injury. Permanent joint enlargement and flexion contractures are common consequences of even a minor sprain or "jammed finger." Mallet fracture dislocations (Fig. 45) of the distal interphalangeal joint should be distinguished from simple stable displaced mallet fractures because outcome after conservative management of such dislocations is

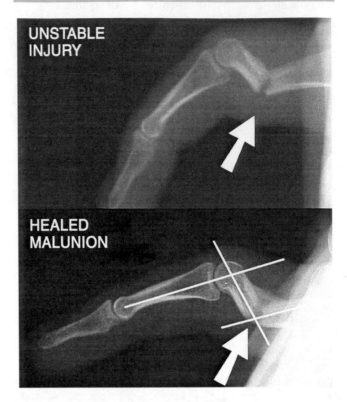

Figure 44 Unstable phalangeal fractures follow a predictable course regarding three complications. First, dorsal-palmar angulation of mid-shaft phalangeal fractures occurs due to asymmetric pull of muscle tendon units. Proximal phalanx fractures typically fall into a dorsal concave ("apex volar") angulation. Second, failure of reduction often results in complete recurrence of fracture deformity. Third, tendon imbalance due to malunion in angulation results in joint contractures distal to the fracture equal in magnitude and opposite in direction as the malunion. The *top* radiograph demonstrates initial angulation of such a fracture. The fracture was reduced and stabilized with Kirschner wires, but redisplaced after the original surgeon removed the fixation. The *bottom* radiograph demonstrates the healed malunion, complete recurrence of the initial deformity, with a flexion contracture of the proximal interphalangeal joint equal in degree to the angle of malunion.

poor as the result of joint incongruity. Pure dislocations of the proximal interphalangeal joint (Fig. 46) are most commonly dorsal, are usually stable after reduction, and carry about the same outlook as a bad sprain of this joint. In contrast, palmar dislocations or dislocations with a lateral component are frequently unstable after reduction and are more prone to progressive contractures, angulation, and degenerative joint changes.

Fracture dislocations of the proximal interphalangeal joint are usually dorsal with a small volar plate avulsion fracture. These dislocations are usually stable if the volar fracture fragment comprises less than one-third of the articular surface. In contrast, dorsal fracture dislocations in which the palmar fragment involves more than one-third of the joint surface, palmar fracture dislocations, and combined dorsal and palmar fractures ("pilon fractures") are intrinsically unstable and cause persistent subluxation

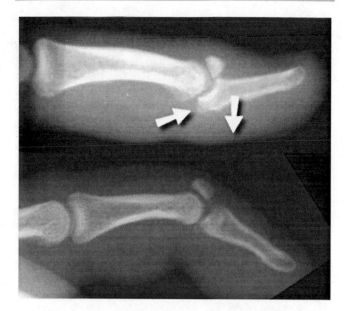

Figure 45 Mallet fractures in which the smaller fracture fragment includes half or more of the joint surface may be unstable, resulting in palmar subluxation of the distal phalanx (*top*). However, this is not always the case, and the joint may remain stable despite a large avulsion fragment (*bottom*).

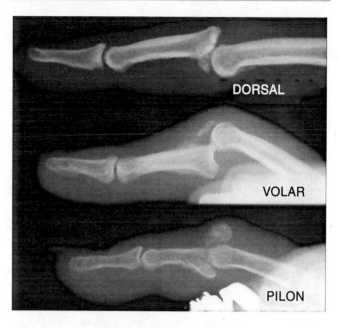

Figure 47 Proximal interphalangeal joint fracture-dislocations are always unstable. Internal and/or external fixation are usually appropriate. Stiffness, flexion contracture, and posttraumatic arthritis are common consequences.

(Fig. 47). These injuries are extremely difficult to treat and may require internal and external fixation and cancellous or osteochondral grafting. In fact, these injuries may be unsalvageable.

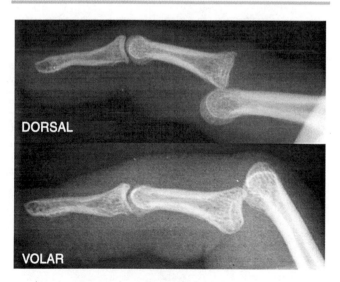

Figure 46 Proximal interphalangeal (PIP) joint "simple" dislocations are usually dorsal, and may be reduced by extending the finger to reproduce the deformity and then dorsal pressure on the base of the middle phalanx. These are usually stable following reduction. Volar dislocations represent a more serious injury, are less commonly easily reduced, and more commonly unstable following reduction. Although often passed off as a "jammed finger," PIP dislocations commonly result in 6 to 12 months of swelling, PIP flexion contracture, and permanent joint enlargement.

Metacarpal Fractures Prone to Complications. Metacarpal fractures heal in a fairly predictable manner, but nonunion is more likely when injuries involve a crush or blast mechanism. Gunshot injuries of the fingers frequently result in amputation, but similar injuries in the metacarpal area may produce surprisingly little nerve and tendon damage despite severe skeletal injury and risk of nonunion (Fig. 32). Multiple metacarpal fractures are often sustained in association with crush injuries, and the treating surgeon must decide between compartment decompression with wide exposure for open reduction and internal fixation or percutaneous fixation that can minimize additional injury (Fig. 33).

Metacarpal Joint Injuries Prone to Complications. Complex dislocations are those in which intra-articular soft tissue interposition provides a block to reduction; they are also referred to as irreducible dislocations. These injuries most often involve the metacarpophalangeal joint of the thumb, and are usually associated with sesamoid interposition (Fig. 9). These dislocations usually require open reduction and must be recognized so that additional injury from overzealous attempts at closed reduction can be avoided. Rupture of the ulnar collateral ligament of the metacarpophalangeal joint of the thumb, also known as ski pole thumb or gamekeeper's thumb, occurs when the thumb is forced into radial deviation. The extent of injury is frequently not appreciated by the patient, and delayed presentation is common. The results are better with

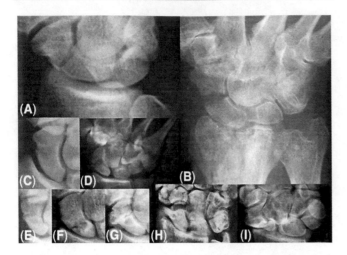

Figure 48 Scaphoid fractures usually occur as an isolated fracture (**A**) but may be part of a larger injury complex (**B**). Oblique (**C**), comminuted (**D**), and proximal (**I**) fracture lines are prone to nonunion. Nonunion may be radiographically subtle (**E**), cystic (**F**), or hypertrophic (**G**). The majority of scaphoid nonunions progress to a pattern of radioscaphoid and mid-carpal arthritis referred to as scaphoid nonunion advanced collapse or "SNAC wrist" (**H, I**).

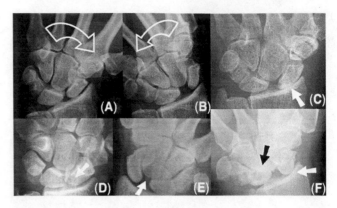

Figure 49 Scapholunate dissociation may require dynamic stress views to demonstrate (**A, B**). The natural progression of scapholunate dissociation is a pattern of wrist arthritis involving the radioscaphoid and capitolunate joints, referred to as scapholunate advanced collapse or "SLAC wrist" (**C, F**). Very proximal scaphoid avulsion fractures (**D, E**) are mechanically similar to scapholunate ligament injuries.

acute ligament repair than with late reconstruction (53), and arthrodesis may be indicated.

Carpal Injuries Prone to Complications. *Scaphoid Fractures.* Scaphoid fractures (Fig. 48) are prone to healing problems because of the combination of poor perfusion of the proximal fracture fragment and strong forces across the fracture site because of normal wrist mechanics. Scaphoid fractures may heal in malunion ("humpback deformity"), but delayed union and nonunion are much more common and difficult problems. Left untreated, scaphoid nonunions naturally progress to a characteristic pattern of wrist arthritis, initially involving the radioscaphoid and capitolunate joints, referred to as scaphoid nonunion advanced collapse, or "SNAC wrist." Unstable, displaced, or proximal fractures are prone to nonunion even with prolonged casting and should be considered for early open reduction because the outcome of surgery is more likely to be satisfactory for acute unstable or displaced fractures than for unstable or displaced nonunions. For unstable or displaced nonunions, open reduction and fixation with bone graft and screws is associated with a failure rate as high as 40% (46).

Scapholunate Ligament Injuries. Injuries to the scapholunate ligament result from the same mechanism of injury as scaphoid fractures. Like scaphoid fractures, these injuries may not be apparent on initial radiographs. Dynamic scapholunate dissociation may be obvious only on kinematic or stress-deviation radiographs. Conversely, bilateral benign congenital scapholunate diastasis may be confused

with an acute injury if both sides are not compared. Left untreated, scapholunate dissociation naturally progresses to a characteristic pattern of wrist arthritis, initially involving the radioscaphoid and capitolunate joints, referred to as scapholunate advanced collapse, or "SLAC wrist" (Fig. 49) (94). Treatment options include partial wrist fusion, proximal row carpectomy, and a variety of soft-tissue ligament reconstruction procedures. Capsulodesis procedures appear to be more successful than tendon graft procedures, although no current soft-tissue procedure reliably corrects scapholunate diastasis that is visible on radiographs (48). The outcome of injuries associated with scapholunate dissociation or partial ligament disruption is better than that for injuries resulting in complete disruption with a static instability pattern (48).

Perilunate Dislocations and Fracture Dislocations. Perilunate dislocations and fracture dislocations (Figs. 50 and 51) are severe wrist injuries that usually result in some degree of permanent wrist stiffness, even with ideal management. These injuries may not be appreciated on casual inspection; the most common report of inadequate evaluation is "something just isn't right." These injuries require open reduction and internal fixation and frequently require carpal tunnel release for acute traumatic neuritis.

Hook of Hamate Fractures. Hook of hamate fractures are often difficult to demonstrate on plain radiographs, and additional evaluation and management may be indicated on the basis of clinical suspicion (Fig. 52). Fractures of the hook of the hamate rarely heal with conservative treatment. The problem may mimic a variety of other problems, including carpometacarpal or capitohamate joint disorders.

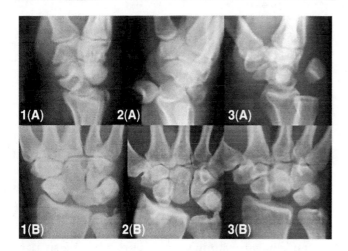

Figure 50 Lunate dislocations may be missed in the emergency room through failure to recognize the typical states such as the "spilled teacup" sign on the lateral wrist X-ray (**1A**), and hand abnormalities that are not dramatic on the PA film (**1B**). It is unusual for the lunate to be displaced enough to be obvious to the untrained eye as in these examples of complete volar (**2A**, **2B**) and dorsal (**3A**, **3B**) lunate dislocations.

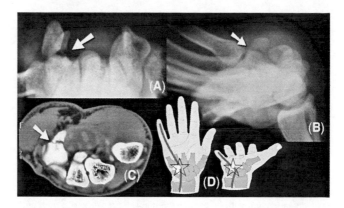

Figure 52 Hook of hamate fractures have a high incidence of nonunion (**A, B, C**). The hook acts as a pulley for the profundus tendon to the small finger, and rough surfaces created by nonunion may result in tendon rupture (**D**).

Problems with this fracture include flexor tendon rupture because of abrasion against the fractured hook area. Tendon rupture is a serious complication, often resulting in permanent disability despite multiple operations and extensive therapy. Surgery to remove the fractured hook and inspect the tendons and nerves is indicated to minimize the risk of complications.

Forearm Fractures Prone to Complications. Distal radius fractures account for about one of every six fractures and three of four forearm fractures seen in the emergency room. They are most common in children of both sexes between the ages of 6 and 10 years and in women between the ages of 60 and 69 years. These fractures may be classified according to a number of schemes, but no existing scheme correlates well with final functional outcome (73).

A large number of operative and nonoperative treatment options have been recommended, many of which appear to give comparable results. Operative treatments include external fixation, percutaneous pinning, open reduction, and any combination of these. Poor final outcome is more likely when the fracture is initially very displaced, when the distal radioulnar joint is involved, when the radiocarpal joint is comminuted, when there is residual shortening of more than 2 mm, or when there is dorsal angulation of more than 15°. The outcome of closed reduction of intra-articular distal radius fractures is satisfactory in about four of five cases (47). However, redisplacement will occur with about one of three closed reductions, and the final outcome when redisplacement occurs and repeated closed manipulations are required will be good or excellent for only one of three fractures (47).

There are conflicting reports regarding the importance of final fracture alignment on function, but one can make the argument that malunion should

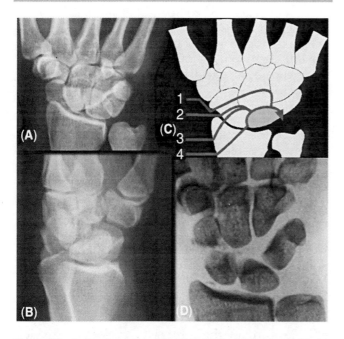

Figure 51 Perilunate fracture-dislocations represent high-energy injuries, which are usually best treated with provisional closed reduction and then definitive open repair. Unreduced radiographs (**A, B**) are usually difficult to interpret. Many variations exist, including trans-scaphoid transcapitate perilunate fracture-dislocation (**C1**), trans-scaphoid perilunate fracture-dislocation (**C2**), transradial trans-scaphoid perilunate fracture-dislocation (**C3**), and transradial perilunate fracture-dislocation (**C4**). Traction films are helpful in defining the exact pathology, as in this trans-scaphoid perilunate fracture-dislocation (**D**).

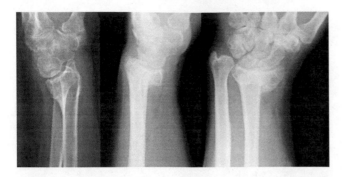

Figure 53 Distal radius malunions are common after closed reduction of an unstable fracture pattern, resulting in dorsal (*left*) or volar (*center*) angulation, shortening and loss of radial inclination (*right*). Functional outcome correlates poorly with radiographic changes.

be avoided (Fig. 53) because secondary surgery for distal radius malunion is successful in only three of four cases (71). Nonunion (Fig. 54) is uncommon but is more likely after severely displaced fractures because of the possibility of pronator quadratus or other soft-tissue interposition. Complex regional pain syndrome (Fig. 18) and finger stiffness occur to some degree in as many as one of three patients. Loss of motion is also common but unpredictable. Tendon rupture (19) may occur early or late, with either open or closed reduction, and may be related to fracture displacement, hardware irritation (Fig. 54) (13), or ulnar head prominence. Median or ulnar nerve compression may develop early or late after this fracture.

Posttraumatic arthritis is most common among young adults and is seen on radiographs of two out of three young patients, years after injury. Fortunately, the evidence on radiographs does not correlate well with the degree of symptoms, and many of these patients have no symptoms. Compartment syndrome of the forearm may develop in association with emergency reduction and stabilization of a distal radius fracture with a circumferential cast. However, compartment syndrome of the forearm may develop after a high-energy injury distal radius fracture even in the absence of circumferential cast or bandages (26) and may develop up to 48 hours after the initial injury (23). Men less than 50 years old are at particular risk of distal radius fractures (31), probably because they are more likely to suffer high-energy injuries.

If clinical examination is unreliable, as in patients with obtundation or those whose symptoms may be masked by narcotics in hospital observation, repeated measurement of compartment pressures may be indicated during the first two days after injury. Carpal instability may develop, either as a discrete ligament injury or as a result of changes in the angle of the radiocarpal joint. Nonunion of associated ulnar styloid fractures is common and is usually painless. Prolonged recovery (6–12 months) is typical, as are long-term subjective symptoms such as pain, fatigue, and loss of grip strength. Such symptoms are reported by about half of the patients with an injury not related to compensation, in about four of five adult patients under the age of 45, and in essentially all patients with a compensation-related injury. Nevertheless, on average, three of four patients experience a satisfactory functional result after distal radius fracture.

Fractures of Both Forearm Bones. Fractures of both bones of the forearm in an adult may result in a variety of problems. Complications are more common and prognosis is worse for displaced fractures and for open fractures. On the average, nondisplaced fractures take six to eight weeks to heal, and displaced fractures take three to five months. Satisfactory functional end results may be expected in about 8 of 10 patients with nondisplaced fractures and in about half of those with displaced fractures. As many as half of the patients will have obvious loss of forearm pronation, which may or may not be functionally significant. Loss of forearm rotation is most likely when fractures occur in the middle third of the forearm. Synostosis may lock the forearm in a fixed position of rotation.

Nonunion occurs in as many as one of 10 patients (Fig. 55). Nonunion related to technique is more likely when semitubular plates are used, or when fewer than six cortices are engaged on each side of the fracture. Early protected motion appears to improve the odds of satisfactory final motion. Internal or external fixation is usually indicated for open or very unstable fractures; the surgeon must accept the

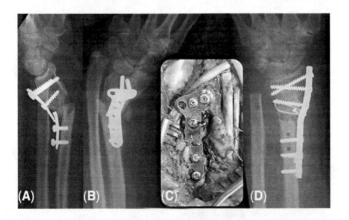

Figure 54 Distal radius nonunions are uncommon, but usually symptomatic due to progress of angulation and symptoms from distal radioulnar joint disruption. This patient developed progressive angulation and hardware failure following dorsal plating of a Galeazzi type metaphyseal distal radius fracture-dislocation (**A, B**). The original surgeon should have used a more sturdy plate and should have captured more cortices proximally. At exploration, soft-tissue interposition was found in the fracture line, and the extensor pollicis longus tendon was on its way to an attritional rupture, positioned behind the plate (**C**). The fracture was reduced, stabilized with a 3.5-mm plate and cerclage, and the distal ulna was used as bone graft (**D**).

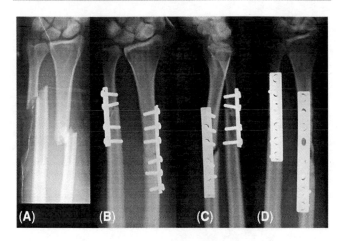

Figure 55 Example of inadequate fixation. This patient underwent open reduction and internal fixation of a displaced both bone forearm fracture (**A**). Technical errors by the first surgeon include use of semitubular plates, which have inadequate rigidity for this type of fracture, and failure to achieve purchase of at least four cortices on each side of the fracture (**B**). Each of these errors increases the chance of nonunion. This patient developed nonunion with progressive angulation of the radius (**C**), which required repeat fixation with bone graft and compression plates (**D**).

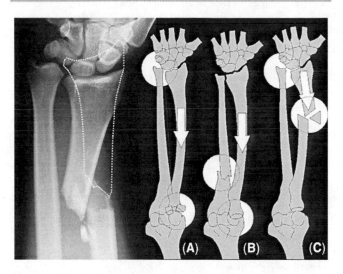

Figure 56 Combined fractures include three special combinations of injury: the Essex-Lopresti lesion (**A**), Monteggia fracture-dislocation (**B**), and Galeazzi fracture-dislocation (*left* and **C**). Galeazzi fracture-dislocation refers to a fracture of the shaft of the radius associated with dislocation of the distal radioulnar joint. Monteggia fracture-dislocation refers to fracture of the ulna with dislocation of the radial head. Each of these fracture-dislocation patterns is best treated with open fracture reduction and closed treatment of the dislocation. Essex-Lopresti lesion refers to longitudinal disruption of the radioulnar interosseous membrane and proximal migration of the radius, associated with fractures involving the proximal radioulnar joint, the distal radioulnar joint, or both sites. The most common presentation of Essex-Lopresti is associated with radial head excision for fracture, resulting in ulnocarpal impingement syndrome. Treatment is controversial. When diagnosed acutely in the context of an unreconstructable radial head fracture, Essex-Lopresti justifies use of a temporary radial head implant. Late surgical options include ulnar shortening osteotomy or the developing technique of ligament reconstruction with a tendon graft.

risk that postsurgical infection may occur in as many as 1 of 20 patients.

Proximal forearm fractures are associated with a variety of problems, including nonunion, nerve and tendon injuries, and synostosis. One-fifth to one-half of the patients can be expected to have significant permanent loss of forearm rotation. Open treatment of acute fracture or nonunion may be complicated by additional nerve injury or synostosis, more likely when injuries are open or classified as high energy. Synostosis, or cross-union between the radius and ulna, is much more common with proximal than with distal forearm fractures, occurring in about 1 of 15 patients with proximal fractures. Synostosis is more likely among children, when fractures are open fractures, when surgical access to both forearm bones is achieved with a single incision, and when the injuries are high energy. The results of surgery for correction of synostosis are poor when surgery is performed less than one year or more than three years after injury; even under ideal conditions, only one in five patients can be expected to regain as much as 50° of forearm rotation.

Longitudinal Forearm Fracture Dislocations. Fracture dislocations of the longitudinal forearm (Fig. 56) include three special combinations of injury: Galeazzi fracture-dislocation, Monteggia fracture-dislocation, and the Essex-Lopresti lesion (52). Galeazzi fracture-dislocation refers to a fracture of the shaft of the radius associated with dislocation of the distal radioulnar joint. Monteggia fracture-dislocation refers to fracture of the ulna with dislocation of the radial head. Each of these fracture-dislocation patterns is best treated with open fracture reduction and closed treatment of the dislocation. Essex-Lopresti lesion refers to longitudinal disruption of the radioulnar interosseous membrane and proximal migration of the radius; this lesion is associated with fractures involving the proximal radioulnar joint, the distal radioulnar joint, or both sites. The most common presentation of Essex-Lopresti lesion is associated with radial head excision for fracture, which results in ulnocarpal impingement syndrome. Treatment is controversial. When diagnosed acutely in the context of an unreconstructable radial head fracture, Essex-Lopresti lesion justifies the use of a temporary radial head implant. Late surgical options include ulnar shortening osteotomy or the developing technique of ligament reconstruction with a tendon graft.

Radial Head Fractures. Fractures of the radial head often appear to be isolated injuries but are associated with distal radial ulnar joint pathology due to proximal migration of the radius, elbow arthritis, and loss of elbow motion. Early excision of radial head fractures is associated with a substantial complication rate, including proximal migration of the radius, which occurs to some degree in most patients (3). Efforts should be made to reconstruct rather than excise a fractured radial head.

Skeletally Immature Forearm Fractures and Dislocations. "Isolated" radial head fractures in children are often associated with some degree of plastic deformation of the ulna, or "plastic" Monteggia fracture. Chronic pediatric radial head dislocation associated with plastic deformation of the ulna is frequently unrecognized, and late treatment requires open reduction and ulna osteotomy (74).

Complications of the Treatment of Fractures and Joint Injuries

The complications associated with the treatment of fractures and joint injuries have been covered in previous sections. The most common of these are nonunion (Figs. 32, 55, and 57); infection or fracture related to external fixation (Fig. 57); arthrofibrosis and capsuloligamentous contractures; osteomyelitis (Fig. 58); tendon adhesions or rupture (Fig. 54); hardware prominence, exposure, or related fracture (Figs. 59 and 60); and complex regional pain syndrome (Fig. 18).

Complications of Infection

Missed Diagnosis of Infection

Herpetic whitlow, a viral skin infection of the finger pulp, is commonly misdiagnosed as an abscess, felon, or paronychia. Diagnosis is suggested by a prodrome of pain and early signs of tiny vesicles and itching. Treatment by incision and drainage only prolongs recovery and should be avoided if possible. Missed deep infections (Fig. 61) of the hand are possible

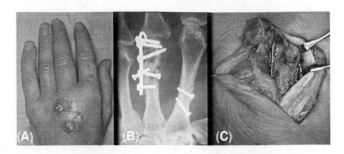

Figure 58 Osteomyelitis is uncommon in the hand, usually requiring the combination of severe contamination and crush injury as in this patient who was kicked by a horse and developed osteomyelitis after being treated for open metacarpal fractures. Draining wound (**A**) radiographs suggestive of septic non union (**B**), gross pus found at exploration (**C**).

because the dense fibrous compartments within the hand mask swelling and contour changes associated with a deep abscess. The diagnosis is based on suspicion, with the caveat that throbbing hand pain that keeps the patient awake at night and is associated with any other signs of infection indicates deep hand abscess until proven otherwise. Missed severe contamination has been discussed in the previous section on complications of missed complex wounds.

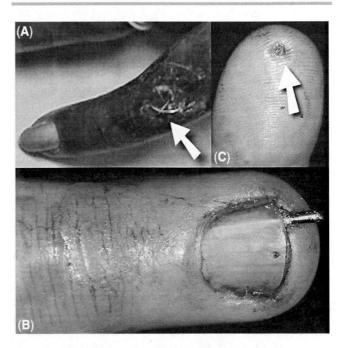

Figure 59 Complications of hardware exposure. (**A**) Exposed tension band wire years following proximal interphalangeal joint arthrodesis. (**B**) Kirschner wire penetration of nail bed. The original surgeon should not have accepted this pin position, which resulted in a permanent split-nail deformity. (**C**) Improper choice of length for the Kirschner wire. Hardware should be either placed entirely beneath the skin or allowed to protrude well beyond the skin entrance site. Cutting pins off at skin level greatly increases the chance of pin tract infection.

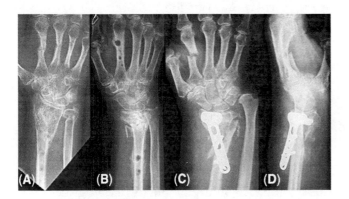

Figure 57 Complications of external fixation. External fixers used for distal radius fracture fixation may result in sensory nerve injury and symptomatic neuroma, pin tract infections, osteomyelitis, and fracture through the pin site. (**A**) Healed index of metacarpal fracture following external fixation in a patient with osteogenesis imperfecta. (**B**) Pin loosening and periosteal reaction in another patient. (**C, D**) Index metacarpal fracture through pin site and complete loss of reduction in another patient.

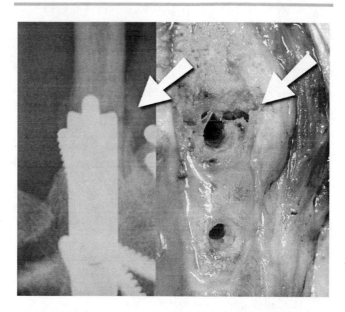

Figure 60 Following wrist arthrodesis, the distal screw hole securing the plate to the metacarpal (left) formed a stress riser which resulted in a symptomatic metacarpal fracture (right).

Complications of Infections and Infections Prone to Complications

Unsatisfactory results are more likely when hand infections involve anaerobes, *Eikenella corrodens*, or human bites (57). Quantitative cultures are the single most sensitive and specific predictor of infection after microvascular free-flap reconstruction of complex extremity injuries and should be a routine part of this form of treatment. Complex wounds that contain more than 1000 organisms per cubic centimeter at the time of free-flap closure should be treated with a second surgical procedure involving flap elevation, repeated debridement, and closure (82). Atypical infections (57) may involve subcutaneous tissues or, more commonly, tendon sheath spaces. Mycobacteria species, most commonly *Mycobacterium marinum*, produce slowly progressing hand infections. Deep-space involvements with either typical or atypical infection usually follow puncture wounds that contaminate tendon sheath compartments or joint spaces.

The most vulnerable areas in which apparently trivial wounds can contaminate deep spaces are the flexion creases of the fingers and the extension creases on the dorsum of the fingers. Diabetic hand infections, particularly in patients with diabetic chronic renal failure, are common, are frequently severe, and often result in tissue loss. Hand infections among such patients are frequently more severe than clinical examination indicates, and the surgeon must consider early extensive surgical debridement of the entire zone of inflammation (50). Gram-negative infections are common, and amputation is a common consequence. Pyarthrosis and septic arthritis of the small joints of the hand are more likely to be associated with a poor outcome if they occur more than 10 days after injury or are associated with severe trauma (75). The

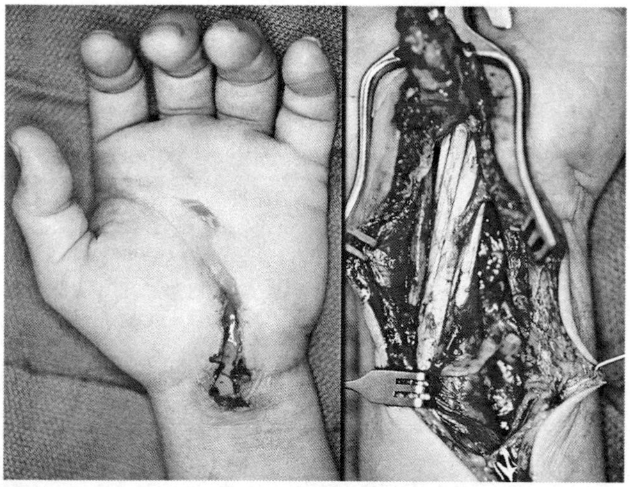

Figure 61 Wound infection following carpal tunnel surgery. This patient developed worsening pain one week after opening carpal tunnel release. She was seen by her original surgeon, who was unimpressed by her physical findings and dismissed her as being narcotic seeking. She sought a second opinion, and at exploration later that day, was found to have pus throughout the carpal tunnel and tracking deep to the flexor tendons into the retroflexor space (Parona's space). Deep wound infections are uncommon following elective clean hand surgery, and the signs of a deep-space infection may be subtle, requiring a high degree of suspicion for diagnosis.

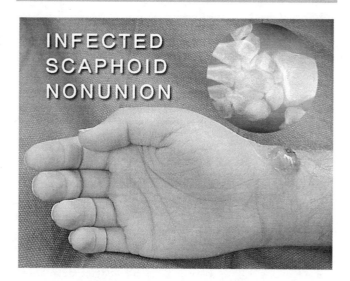

Figure 62 Scaphoid nonunion eventually leads to progressive wrist arthritis in many patients. Uncommonly, nonunion may be the site of infection. This patient had undergone open reduction of a scaphoid fracture, and by history had a pin tract infection of one of the Kirschner wires used for scaphoid fixation, requiring early removal by the first surgeon. He presented over a year later with an abscess at the site of the prior pin tract infection, tracking deep to an infected scaphoid nonunion. Infection control involved radical debridement, including a proximal row carpectomy.

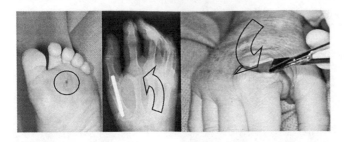

Figure 63 Infection of implants may arise late due to hematogenous seeding from distant infection. This patient with diabetes and rheumatoid arthritis on immunosuppressive therapy developed a plantar abscess following an unrecognized injury (*left*). She presented with infection of a long-standing functioning index metacarpophalangeal silastic joint spacer (*middle*). Organisms cultured from the site (*right*) were the same as those present in the foot. Implant infection is more likely when there is a permanent space where motion occurs adjacent to the implant, as is the case with silicone rubber joint replacements.

most common scenario for small-joint infection of the hand involves clenched fist bite injury (Fig. 21).

Hematogenous seeding resulting in implant infection (Figs. 62 and 63) is an uncommon but catastrophic problem justifying the administration of prophylactic antibiotics during high-risk procedures for patients who have implants such as silastic joint spacers, which maintain a permanent open space around the implants. Tetanus may develop after hand injuries (38) and is most common in the context of parenteral drug abuse. More commonly, deep soft-tissue infections from parenteral drug abuse are polymicrobial and may present as gas-forming infection (Fig. 24), necrotizing infection, or suppurative thrombophlebitis (39). Treatment requires excision of the involved area, wide drainage, repeated debridement, and appropriate parenteral antibiotics.

REFERENCES

1. Hutchinson DT, McClinton MA, Wilgis EF, Frisk-Millner N. Drug and alcohol use in emergency hand patients. J Hand Surg (Am) 1992; 17(3):576–577.
2. Ablove RH, Moy OJ, Peimer CA, Wheeler DR. Early versus delayed treatment of enchondroma. Am J Orthop 2000; 29(10):771–772.
3. Leppilahti J, Jalovaara P. Early excision of the radial head for fracture. Int Orthop 2000; 24(3):160–162.
4. Colville RJ, Berry RB. A small contact burn injury requiring upper limb amputation. Burns 2000; 26(7): 656–658.
5. Gerard F, Obert L, Garbuio P, Tropet Y. An unusual complication of reimplantation of the hand: a false aneurysm of the radial artery anastomosis. Apropos of a treated case. Chir Main 1999; 18(2):149–152.
6. Gundes H, Cirpici Y, Sarlak A, Muezzinoglu S. Prognosis of wrist ganglion operations. Acta Orthop Belg 2000; 66(4):363–367.
7. Arons JA, Collins N, Arons MS. Permanent nerve injury in the forearm following radial artery harvest: a report of two cases. Ann Plast Surg Sep 1999; 43(3):299–301.
8. Rijbroek A, Vermeulen EG, Slotman BJ, Wisselink W, Rauwerda JA. Radiation-induced arterial disease. Ned Tijdschr Geneeskd 2000; 144(8):353–356.
9. Sessa C, Pecher M, Maurizi-Balzan J, et al. Critical hand ischemia after angioaccess surgery: diagnosis and treatment. Ann Vasc Surg 2000; 14(6):583–593.
10. Shemesh D, Mabjeesh NJ, Abramowitz HB. Management of dialysis access-associated steal syndrome: use of intraoperative duplex ultrasound scanning for optimal flow reduction. J Vasc Surg 1999; 30(1):193–195.
11. Tordoir JH, Leunissen KM. Arterial perfusion disorders of the hand in 9 patients with arteriovenous fistula for hemodialysis. Ned Tijdschr Geneeskd 1999; 143(21):1093–1098.
12. Wilhelmi BJ, Blackwell SJ, Miller J, Mancoll JS, Phillips LG. Epinephrine in digital blocks: revisited. Ann Plast Surg 1998; 41(4):410–414.
13. Bell JS, Wollstein R, Citron ND. Rupture of flexor pollicis longus tendon: a complication of volar plating of the distal radius. J Bone Joint Surg Br 1998; 80(2):225–226.
14. Schwabegger AH, Hussl H, Ninkovic MM, Anderl H. Replantation in childhood and adolescence. Long-term outcome. Unfallchirurg 1997; 100(8):652–657.
15. Stahl S, Norman D, Zinman C. Postoperative ulnar nerve palsy of the elbow. Harefuah 1997; 133(11):533–535, 590.
16. Ouellette EA, Kelly R. Compartment syndromes of the hand. J Bone Joint Surg Am 1996; 78(10):1515–1522.
17. Pearce H, Lindsay D, Leslie K. Axillary brachial plexus block in two hundred consecutive patients. Anaesth Intensive Care 1996; 24(4):453–458.
18. Stark RH. Neurologic injury from axillary block anesthesia. J Hand Surg (Am) 1996; 21(3):391–396.
19. Bonatz E, Kramer TD, Masear VR. Rupture of the extensor pollicis longus tendon. Am J Orthop 1996; 25(2):118–122.
20. Janezic TF, Arnez ZM, Solinc M, Zaletel-Kragelj L. One hundred sixty-seven thumb replantations and revascularisations: early microvascular results. Microsurgery 1996; 17(5):259–263.
21. Giandoni MB, Vinson RP, Grabski WJ. Ischemic complications of tubular gauze dressings. Dermatol Surg 1995; 21(8):716–718.
22. Landi A, Saracino A, Pinelli M, Caserta G, Facchini MC. Tourniquet paralysis in microsurgery. Ann Acad Med Singapore 1995; 24(4 suppl):89–93.
23. Simpson NS, Jupiter JB. Delayed onset of forearm compartment syndrome: a complication of distal radius fracture in young adults. J Orthop Trauma 1995; 9(5):411–418.
24. Hye RJ, Wolf YG. Ischemic monomelic neuropathy: an under-recognized complication of hemodialysis access. Ann Vasc Surg 1994; 8(6):578–582.
25. Naidu SH, Heppenstall RB. Compartment syndrome of the forearm and hand. Hand Clin 1994; 10(1):13–27.
26. Denolf F, Roos J, Feyen J. Compartment syndrome after fracture of the distal radius. Acta Orthop Belg 1994; 60(3):339–342.
27. Stanec Z, Skrbic S, Dzepina I, et al. High-energy war wounds: flap reconstruction. Ann Plast Surg 1993; 31(2):97–102.
28. Atabek U, Spence RK, Alexander JB, Pello MJ, Camishion RC. Upper extremity occlusive arterial

disease after radiotherapy for breast cancer. J Surg Oncol 1992; 49(3):205–207.

29. Farina C, Schultz RD, Feldhaus RJ. Late upper limb acute ischemia in a patient with an occluded axillo-femoral bypass graft. J Cardiovasc Surg (Torino) 1990; 31(2):178–181.

30. Stern PJ, Kastrup JJ. Complications and prognosis of treatment of mallet finger. J Hand Surg (Am) 1988; 13(3):329–334.

31. Stockley I, Harvey IA, Getty CJ. Acute volar compartment syndrome of the forearm secondary to fractures of the distal radius. Injury 1988; 19(2):101–104.

32. Smith PA, Hankin FM, Louis DS. Postoperative toxic shock syndrome after reconstructive surgery of the hand. J Hand Surg (Am) 1986; 11(3):399–402.

33. Yuan RT, Cohen MJ. Lateral antebrachial cutaneous nerve injury as a complication of phlebotomy. Plast Reconstr Surg 1985; 76(2):299–300.

34. Morgan WJ, Leopold T, Evans R. Foreign bodies in the hand. J Hand Surg (Br) 1984; 9(2):194–196.

35. Reinstein L, Reed WP, Sadler JH, Baugher WH. Peripheral nerve compression by brachial artery-basilic vein vascular access in long-term hemodialysis. Arch Phys Med Rehabil 1984; 65(3):142–144.

36. Aho K, Sainio K, Kianta M, Varpanen E. Pneumatic tourniquet paralysis. Case report. J Bone Joint Surg Br 1983; 65(4):441–443.

37. Matsubara J, Seko T, Ohta T, et al. Arterio-venous fistula formation after hand replantation. Jpn J Surg 1983; 13(3):207–210.

38. Thorne FL, Kropp RJ. Wound botulism: a life-threatening complication of hand injuries. Plast Reconstr Surg 1983; 71(4):548–551.

39. Sears N, Grosfeld JL, Weber TR, Kleiman MB. Suppurative thrombophlebitis in childhood. Pediatrics 1981; 68(5):630–632.

40. Bandyk DF, Thiele BL, Radke HM. Upper-extremity emboli secondary to axillofemoral graft thrombosis. Arch Surg 1981; 116(4):393–395.

41. Nunoo-Mensah J. An unexpected complication after harvesting of the radial artery for coronary artery bypass grafting. Ann Thorac Surg 1998; 66(3):929–931.

42. Rodriguez Montalban R, Martinez de Guerenu Alonso MA, et al. Acute ischemia of the hand as a complication of radial artery catheterization. Apropos of 2 cases following abdominal sarcoma surgery. Rev Esp Anestesiol Reanim 2000; 47(10):480–484.

43. Grace TG, Omer GE. The management of upper extremity pit viper wounds. J Hand Surg (Am) 1980; 5(2):168–177.

44. Snelling CF, Hendel PM. Avascular necrosis of bone following revascularization of the thumb. Ann Plast Surg 1979; 3(1):77–87.

45. Davis FM. Radial artery cannulation: influence of catheter size and material on arterial occlusion. Anaesth Intensive Care 1978; 6(1):49–53.

46. Gupta A, Risitano G, Crawford RJ, Burke FD. The ununited scaphoid: prognostic factors in delayed and nonunions of the scaphoid. Hand Surg 1999; 4(1):11–19.

47. Leung F, Ozkan M, Chow SP. Conservative treatment of intra-articular fractures of the distal radius -factors affecting functional outcome. Hand Surg 2000; 5(2):145–153.

48. Saffar P, Sokolow C, Duclos L. Soft tissue stabilization in the management of chronic scapholunate instability without osteoarthritis. A 15-year series. Acta Orthop Belg 1999; 65(4):424–433.

49. Leclercq C, Korn W. Articular fractures of the fingers in children. Hand Clin 2000; 16(4):523–534.

50. Gunther SF, Gunther SB. Diabetic hand infections. Hand Clin 1998; 14(4):647–656.

51. Adani R, Busa R, Castagnetti C, Castagnini L, Caroli A. Replantation of degloved skin of the hand. Plast Reconstr Surg 1998; 101(6):1544–1551.

52. Idler RS, Steichen JB. Complications of replantation surgery. Hand Clin 1992; 8(3):427–451.

53. Arnold DM, Cooney WP, Wood MB. Surgical management of chronic ulnar collateral ligament insufficiency of the thumb metacarpophalangeal joint. Orthop Rev 1992; 21(5):583–588.

54. Pun WK, Chow SP, So YC, et al. Unstable phalangeal fractures: treatment by A.O. screw and plate fixation. J Hand Surg (Am)1991; 16(1):113–117.

55. Davis TR, Stothard J. Why all finger fractures should be referred to a hand surgery service: a prospective study of primary management. J Hand Surg (Br) 1990; 15(3):299–302.

56. Pun WK, Chow SP, So YC, et al. A prospective study on 284 digital fractures of the hand. J Hand Surg (Am)1989; 14(3):474–481.

57. Dellinger EP, Wertz MJ, Miller SD, Coyle MB. Hand infections. Bacteriology and treatment: a prospective study. Arch Surg 1988; 123(6):745–750.

58. Strickland JW. Results of flexor tendon surgery in zone II. Hand Clin 1985; 1(1):167–179.

59. Brown PW. Sacrifice of the unsatisfactory hand. J Hand Surg (Am) 1979; 4(5):417–423.

60. Green JA, Tonkin MA. Ischaemia of the hand in infants following radial or ulnar artery catheterisation. Hand Surg 1999; 4(2):151–157.

61. Al-Qattan MM. Phalangeal neck fractures in children: classification and outcome in 66 cases. J Hand Surg (Br) 2001; 26(2):112–121.

62. Zyluk A, Walaszek I. Results of treatment for high-pressure injection hand injuries. Chir Narzadow Ruchu Ortop Pol 2000; 65(4):367–374.

63. Germann G, Karle B, Bruner S, Menke H. Treatment strategy in complex hand injuries. Unfallchirurg 2000; 103(5):342–347.

64. Bartelmann U, Dietsch V, Landsleitner B. Fractures near the base of the first metacarpal bone–clinical outcome of 21 patients. Handchir Mikrochir Plast Chir 2000; 32(2):93–101.

65. Tredget EE. Management of the acutely burned upper extremity. Hand Clin 2000; 16(2):187–203.

66. Grant I, Belcher HJ. Injuries to the hand from dog bites. J Hand Surg (Br) 2000; 25(1):26–28.

67. Lanz U, Felderhoff J. Ischemic contractures of the forearm and hand. Handchir Mikrochir Plast Chir 2000; 32(1):6–25.

68. Barret JP, Desai MH, Herndon DN. The isolated burned palm in children: epidemiology and long-term sequelae. Plast Reconstr Surg 2000; 105(3):949–952.

69. Waikakul S, Sakkarnkosol S, Vanadurongwan V, Unnanuntana A. Results of 1018 digital replantations in 552 patients. Injury 2000; 31(1):33–40.

70. Salisbury RE. Reconstruction of the burned hand. Clin Plast Surg 2000; 27(1):65–69.

71. Flinkkila T, Raatikainen T, Kaarela O, Hamalainen M. Corrective osteotomy for malunion of the distal radius. Arch Orthop Trauma Surg 2000; 120(1–2):23–26.

72. van Zuijlen PP, Kreis RW, Vloemans AF, Groenevelt F, Mackie DP. The prognostic factors regarding long-term functional outcome of full-thickness hand burns. Burns 1999; 25(8):709–714.

73. Gliatis JD, Plessas SJ, Davis TR. Outcome of distal radial fractures in young adults. J Hand Surg (Br) 2000; 25(6):535–543.

74. Kemnitz S, De Schrijver F, De Smet L. Radial head dislocation with plastic deformation of the ulna in children. A rare and frequently missed condition. Acta Orthop Belg 2000; 66(4):359–362.

75. Boustred AM, Singer M, Hudson DA, Bolitho GE. Septic arthritis of the metacarpophalangeal and interphalangeal joints of the hand. Ann Plast Surg 1999; 42(6):623–628.

76. Schwabegger AH, Anderl H, Hussl H, Ninkovic MM. Complex hand injuries. Importance of primary repair with free flaps. Unfallchirurg 1999; 102(4):292–297.

77. Sheridan RL, Baryza MJ, Pessina MA, et al. Acute hand burns in children: management and long-term outcome based on a 10-year experience with 698 injured hands. Ann Surg 1999; 229(4):558–564.

78. Giddins GE, Hill RA. Late diagnosis and treatment of crush injuries of the fingertip in children. Injury 1998; 29(6):447–450.

79. Aziz W, Noojin F, Arakaki A, Kutz JE. Avulsion injuries of the thumb: survival factors and functional results of replantation. Orthopedics 1998; 21(10):1113–1117.

80. Lewis HG, Clarke P, Kneafsey B, Brennen MD. A 10-year review of high-pressure injection injuries to the hand. J Hand Surg (Br) 1998; 23(4):479–481.

81. Pechlaner S, Hussl H. Complex trauma of the hand. Orthopade 1998; 27(1):11–16.

82. Breidenbach WC, Trager S. Quantitative culture technique and infection in complex wounds of the extremities closed with free flaps. Plast Reconstr Surg 1995; 95(5):860–865.

83. Godina M. Early microsurgical reconstruction of complex trauma of the extremities. Plast Reconstr Surg 1986; 78(3):285–292.

84. Melissinos EG, Parks DH. Post-trauma reconstruction with free tissue transfer—analysis of 442 consecutive cases. J Trauma 1989; 29(8):1095–102; (discussion 1102–1103).

85. Shen TY, Sun YH, Cao DX, Wang NZ. The use of free flaps in burn patients: experiences with 70 flaps in 65 patients. Plast Reconstr Surg 1988; 81(3):352–357.

86. Arnez ZM. Immediate reconstruction of the lower extremity—an update. Clin Plast Surg 1991; 18(3):449–457.

87. Scheker LR, Langley SJ, Martin DL, Julliard KN. Primary extensor tendon reconstruction in dorsal hand defects requiring free flaps. J Hand Surg (Br) 1993; 18(5):568–575.

88. Dawson WJ, Elenz DR, Winchester DP, Feldman JL. Elective hand surgery in the breast cancer patient with prior ipsilateral axillary dissection. Ann Surg Oncol 1995; 2(2):132–137.

89. Hartung HJ, Rupprecht A. The axillary brachial plexus block. A study of 178 patients. Reg Anaesth 1989; 12(1):21–24.

90. Regnard PJ, Soichot P, Ringuier JP. Local complications after axillary block anesthesia. Ann Chir Main Memb Super 1990; 9(1):59–64.

91. Stan TC, Krantz MA, Solomon DL, Poulos JG, Chaouki K. The incidence of neurovascular complications following axillary brachial plexus block using a transarterial approach. A prospective study of 1,000 consecutive patients. Reg Anesth 1995; 20(6):486–492.

92. Fanelli G, Casati A, Garancini P, Torri G. Nerve stimulator and multiple injection technique for upper and lower limb blockade: failure rate, patient acceptance, and neurologic complications. Anesth Analg 1999; 88(4):847–852.

93. Cahill N, King JD. Palm thorn synovitis. J Pediatr Orthop 1984; 4(2):175–179.

94. Watson HK, Ballet FL. The SLAC wrist: scapholunate advanced collapse pattern of degenerative arthritis. J Hand Surg (Am). 1984; 9(3):358–365.

95. Duncan RW, Freeland AE, Jabaley ME, Meydrech EF. Open hand fractures: an analysis of the recovery of active motion and of complications. J Hand Surg (Am) 1993; 18(3):387–394.

96. Kumar RJ, Pegg SP, Kimble RM. Management of extravasation injuries. Aust N Z J Surg 2001; 71(5):285–289.

97. Cicchetti S, Jemec B, Gault DT. Two case reports of vinorelbine extravasation: management and review of the literature. Tumori 2000; 86(4):289–292.

98. Raley J, Geisler JP, Buekers TE, Sorosky JI. Docetaxel extravasation causing significant delayed tissue injury. Gynecol Oncol 2000; 78(2):259–260.

99. von Heimburg D, Pallua N. Early and late treatment of iatrogenic injection damage. Chirurg 1998; 69(12):1378–1382.

100. Fullilove S, Fixsen J. Major limb deformities as complications of vascular access in neonates. Paediatr Anaesth 1997; 7(3):247–250.

101. Hayes AG, Chesney TM. Necrosis of the hand after extravasation of intravenously administered phenytoin. J Am Acad Dermatol 1993; 28(2 Pt 2):360–363.

102. Loth TS, Eversmann WW Jr. Extravasation injuries in the upper extremity. Clin Orthop 1991; (272):248–254.

103. Zyluk A. The sequelae of reflex sympathetic dystrophy. J Hand Surg Br 2001; 26(2):151–154.

104. DeLozier JB, Reaves L, King LE Jr., Rees RS. Brown recluse spider bites of the upper extremity. South Med J 1988; 81(2):181–184.

105. Eldad A, Wisoki M, Cohen H, et al. Phosphorous burns: evaluation of various modalities for primary treatment. J Burn Care Rehabil 1995; 16(1):49–55.

106. Su CW, Lohman R, Gottlieb LJ. Frostbite of the upper extremity. Hand Clin 2000; 16(2):235–247.

107. Tredget EE, Shankowsky HA, Tilley WA. Electrical injuries in Canadian burn care. Identification of unsolved problems. Ann N Y Acad Sci 1999; 888: 75–87.

108. d'Amato TA, Kaplan IB, Britt LD. High-voltage electrical injury: a role for mandatory exploration of deep muscle compartments. J Natl Med Assoc 1994; 86(7): 535–537.

109. Teot L, Griffe O, Brabet M, Gavroy JP, Thaury M. Severe electric injuries of the hand and forearm. Ann Chir Main Memb Super 1992; 11(3):207–216.

110. Bongard O, Fagrell B. Delayed arterial thrombosis following an apparently trivial low-voltage electric injury. Vasa 1989; 18(2):162–166.

111. Wang XW, Bartle EJ, Roberts BB. Early vascular grafting to prevent upper extremity necrosis after electric burns: additional commentary on indications for surgery. J Burn Care Rehabil 1987; 8(5):391–394.

37

Postoperative Pain Management

Edward Lubin, Michael J. Robbins, and Raymond S. Sinatra

*Department of Anesthesiology, Yale University School of Medicine, New Haven,
Connecticut, U.S.A.*

*Pain is among the most common of complaints that
patients make to health practitioners, and yet it
remains poorly treated. Patients in pain historically
have been victimized by disdain, underdosing of
analgesics, and unnecessary physical and emotional
suffering.*

*We, practitioners, must exercise our responsibility
to control pain most especially in the care of those
patients recovering from major surgery and trauma. Why
is this so? First, here we know pain is bound to occur,
and yet in no case is pain control more frequently neglected.
This irony is compounded insofar as persistent pain in
these acute settings is by and large preventable. It is
certainly more easily managed at this stage than at any
other. Moreover, the costs of not treating are too high:
the experience of pain sets off a cascade of physiologic
and emotional events, the impact of which is felt by the
patients and their family well beyond the passing of
the acute stimulus (1,2). This cascade of events may
facilitate the development of a chronic pain syndrome, a
condition about which we have incomplete knowledge,
and for which in many instances we have little to offer.
Finally, the memory of pain often overshadows the
initial insult in its long-term impact on the patient, a
phenomenon that has led to the worldwide application of
techniques to preempt both the experience and the memory
of pain (3).*

*The purpose of this chapter, then, is to present the
current thinking about management of pain in the care
of the trauma patient in the acute postoperative setting,
and to describe our most recent breakthroughs in the
treatment of chronic pain that may well develop later.
The new treatments in both these phases include the
introduction of more potent analgesics, more efficient
means of their administration, and neuroaugmentative
techniques based on a clearer picture of the mechanism
of the development of chronic pain. All these efforts
have dramatically improved the safety and efficacy of
postoperative pain management, and have reduced the
incidence and severity of persistent pain.*

PATIENT AND CAREGIVER VARIABLES INFLUENCING PERIOPERATIVE ANALGESIC EFFECT

The clinical inadequacy of traditional pain management is a continuing problem. More than 75% of adult
patients, treated with on-demand doses of narcotic,
continue to experience moderate to severe pain (4). What
are we doing wrong? Analgesic underadministration
has been related to a variety of factors, foremost of
which is the physicians' inadequate or erroneous pain
assessment, likely stemming from their general lack of
clinical experience and training in pain management.
Few physicians have detailed knowledge of opioid
pharmacology; the majority of them commonly underestimate the range of effective doses while, at the same
time, overestimate analgesic duration and the risk of
overdose. That nurses generally administer as little
as 25% of the prescribed dose compounds the patient's
problem further (5).

Practitioners, as a rule, administer opioid analgesics on a milligram per kilogram basis, and yet there is
no evidence linking body weight to individual dose
requirement. Age appears to be one of the most important variables in determining dose response and the
degree of pain relief achieved following administration of opioid analgesics. Advancing age is generally
associated with greater risk of unrelieved pain (6).
While earlier studies (7) show reductions in pain perception in the elderly, more recent work shows little
difference in pain intensity and perception with age
(8). Thus, despite our knowledge of enhanced opioid
sensitivity and decreases in opioid consumption with
advancing age, these concepts must be viewed with
healthy skepticism when treating the elderly in the
postoperative period (9).

The site, extent, and duration of surgery have a
dramatic influence on both the intensity of postoperative pain and analgesic requirements. Thoracotomy,
upper abdominal, and flank procedures require the
most painful incisions, while laparoscopic, breast, and
pelvic surgery are associated with lower pain intensity. The importance of the role of sex upon opioid

dose requirements is unclear. Epidemiologic studies show that many painful states parse out with greater female than male prevalence, particularly head and neck, musculoskeletal, and autoimmune diseases, and visceral conditions, while males show prevalence in complaints related to, for example, pancreatic disease, paratrigeminal syndrome (Raeder's syndrome), brachial plexus neuropathy, and posttraumatic and cluster headaches (10). Merskey and Bogduk (10) have compiled an exhaustive epidemiologic list of sex differences in painful states; the neurobiological underpinnings of these remain unclear. Bias is known to exist insofar as women are more likely to report pain as a symptom, and in general are more eager to seek medical care (11). Sex hormonal influence, gender roles, and tools for clinical assessment may all play a part in these differences.

Let us look at pain from the patient's perspective. Pain is defined by the International Association for the Study of Pain as "an unpleasant sensory and emotional experience associated with actual or potential tissue damage, or described in terms of such damage" (12). It is foremost an *experience*, with all of the personal and subjective character this implies. It is *emotional*, which at once defines it out of the realm of average practitioners' expertise, unless they are particularly sensitive to the patient or have some psychiatric training. Finally, it is *unpleasant*, and therefore its relief, above other medical or surgical problems that may be present, takes primacy in the patient's mind.

Much of our knowledge of the neurophysiologic basis of pain is derived from animal studies. However, by our definition mentioned above and for clinical purposes, pain is an individual, and a human, phenomenon. Reaction to pain is arguably a conditioned behavior that reflects the values of a given individual and culture. The patient's coping strategies must therefore not be ignored when fashioning postoperative pain treatment. These strategies are rooted in cultural differences, learned behavior, and one's unique perception of pain and disability. It is difficult, and occasionally unwise, to generalize about the pain response of an individual or an entire group of people. On the other hand, an appreciation of such conditioning is in order, if it will help us understand someone's pain, and thereby deliver better care. Responses to pain will vary, but may be divided into two very broad categories: stoic, which are those responses in which the patient expresses minimal discomfort verbally; and emotive, which are those we associate with patients who are vocal in their response to, and their demands to be relieved from, pain. Highly aggressive and angry patients also tend to get, and consume, more medication than patients whose coping styles are more passive. The phenomenon of "catastrophizing," wherein patients focus on excessively negative thoughts, is a potent example of such a cognitive coping strategy with important ramifications for care (13,14). The successful clinician will treat pain based on the patient's informed self-report,

carefully factoring in subjective variables, and thus foster an atmosphere of mutual trust.

We have noted that undertreatment of pain is rooted in lack of knowledge. A more insidious cause for both undertreatment and lack of familiarity with appropriate treatment of pain is the clinician's hesitancy to use opioids, out of both concern for the development of addiction, and the (not unwarranted) fear of recrimination by oversight agencies such as the federal government. This issue has been taken up with great care by Portenoy (15,16) with respect to cancer pain. It is regrettable that the relatively freer use of opioids in the postoperative period, as well in the emergency room setting, is based on our expectation of short-term use of these agents by the patient, or, as a manifestation of further disingenuousness, the brevity of the encounter between the practitioner and the patient. Many of our colleagues are only too happy to leave matters of addiction, diversion, or social stigma of opioid prescription use to those health care personnel with a more protracted relationship with the patient. This approach skirts our responsibility to understand the neurobiologic bases of pain and addiction, and to familiarize ourselves with the advantages and dangers of the drugs we use on a daily basis.

Physicians also tend to limit opioid administration in patients with an ongoing history of substance abuse. However, more recent and enlightened thinking has helped to deliver well-supervised opioid and nonopioid analgesic therapy to patients with alcohol, cocaine, and heroin addictions (17,18). Patients with a history of chronic pain and opioid dependence often require larger amounts of opioid to compensate for the development of *tolerance*. Tolerance is a normal and predictable change of physiologic state, probably due to opioid receptor downregulation and enhanced drug metabolism and elimination, in which higher doses are needed to produce effects formerly achieved at lower doses. Physicians must therefore take into account both baseline opioid requirements, as well as that needed to control acute postsurgical pain.

Just as neglecting aspects of the patient's cultural, social, and medical history may lead to opioid underdose, underestimating the patient's compromised physiologic state may lead to overdose. Decrements in cardiac, hepatic, and renal function are often associated with significant alterations in the volume of distribution, clearance, and excretion of most analgesic agents. For analgesics having high hepatic uptake and clearance, reductions in hepatic blood flow are accompanied by proportional decrements in the overall extraction rate and prolonged pharmacological effects. Agents that undergo biotransformation or are eliminated by the kidneys may produce serious adverse events in patients with renal failure unless dose adjustments are made (19).

In the postsurgical setting, the physical and emotional responses to poorly controlled pain are undesirable (Table 1). In addition to ethical and humanitarian concerns for minimizing pain and suffering,

Table 1 The Acute Injury Response: Potential Benefits After Traumatic Injury Vs. Disadvantages in Controlled Postsurgical Settings

Beneficial effects after traumatic injury	Adverse effects in patients recovering from surgery
Maintenance of intravascular volume and mean	Hypertension, hypervolemia, increased risk of arterial pressure hemorrhage, stroke
Maintenance of cardiac output and cerebral perfusion	Tachycardia, arrhythmias, myocardial ischemia, perfusion congestive heart failure
Enhanced hemostasis	Hypercoagulable state, increased risk of arterial and deep venous thromboses
Substrate mobilization, enhanced energy	Hyperglycemia, negative nitrogen balance production
Immobilization, minimizing further tissue injury	Reduction in respiratory volume and flow rates
Learned avoidance hypoxia, pneumonia	Anxiety, fear, demoralization, prolonged convalescence

the physician wishes to avoid the pain-related anxiety, sleeplessness, and release of catecholamines and other stress hormones, all of which may have deleterious effects upon postsurgical outcome. This is particularly true in elderly or critically ill populations (19,20).

ANATOMY AND PATHOPHYSIOLOGY

Pain may be defined as the conscious awareness of tissue injury (20,21). Therefore, understanding the basic anatomy and physiology of how this injury is translated to conscious awareness of pain is essential to effective management.

Pain perception can be divided into two major components. The sensory-discriminative component describes the location and quality of the stimulus. The affective-motivational component underlies suffering and emotional components of pain and is responsible for learned avoidance and other behavioral responses (21,22). This latter component will be discussed in the clinical sections throughout the chapter. The first component is pain perception (nociception), which reflects the activation of nociceptors following thermal, mechanical, or chemical tissue injury, afferent transmission to the spinal cord, and relay via dorsal horn to higher cortical centers.

Tissue injury causes cellular disruption, resulting in escape of intracellular potassium ions (K^+) and the release of bradykinin (BK), serotonin (5-HT), and prostaglandin (PG), all of which are potent activators of the peripheral endings of nociceptive neurons (23). BK and PG stimulate release of substance P, which in turn sensitizes additional nociceptive neurons at sites adjacent to the injury (23). This process of recruitment and sensitization of peripheral nerve endings underlies hyperalgesia, an altered state of sensibility in which the intensity of pain sensation induced by noxious stimulation is greatly increased.

Peripheral nerve endings are for the most part free nerve endings of myelinated A-delta and unmyelinated C-fibers (20). These fibers are the peripheral extension of bipolar sensory neurons, and are

classified according to their responses to mechanical, thermal, and chemical stimulation, and to the conduction velocity of their axonal fiber (21). The cell bodies of these peripheral afferents are found in the dorsal root ganglia. The central component projects to the dorsal horn of the spinal cord, where they synapse upon the second-order sensory neurons, the majority of which coalesce to form the spinothalamic tract, the principal ascending spinal pathway for pain.

There are three types of this dorsal horn neuron, based on its location in the dorsal horn and on the source of its input. Wide–dynamic range neurons are found in laminae I to VI (principally in IV–VI) and receive signals from low- and high-threshold mechanoreceptors and polymodal C-fibers (23). As their name implies, these neurons receive multiple inputs and increase their signal frequency (intensity) over a wide range of externally applied mechanical deformation and heat.

The other two types of dorsal horn spinothalamic neuron are both called nociceptive specific (21). Both types are found mainly in the marginal layer of the dorsal horn. The first of these receives input from mechano- and thermoreceptors and responds primarily to firm pressure or pinch, while the second, receiving input exclusively from A-delta high-threshold mechanoreceptors, fires in response only to noxious cutaneous mechanical stimulation (21,22).

The spinothalamic tract synapses primarily in the thalamus, in its ventral portion, but sends branches to the spinal reticular formation and the periaqueductal gray matter (20). Third-order sensory neurons carry nociceptive information from the thalamus to cortex.

Because of the numerous synapses and areas of connection, there is potential for the nervous system to modulate the transmission of the painful stimulus at many levels. This modulation can take the form of molecular memory, peripheral and central sensitization, descending pain inhibitory pathways, the neuroendocrine response, and the elaboration of endogenous opioid transmitters.

Molecular Memory

Molecular memory began as a concept in the study of memory function in *Aplysia* in the 1980s, when it was discovered that oncogenes could be found in stimulated neurons. We can now expand this concept to include a wide variety of changes in the environment of the neuron, including protein-binding characteristics, receptor surface density, intracellular calcium concentration, and *N*-methyl-D-aspartate (NMDA) receptor function. These molecular changes lead to changes in the firing pattern which individual neurons demonstrate in response to pain stimulation.

Central Sensitization

Central sensitization can in turn be defined as the result of modulation of molecular memory. In general, it is the "priming" of the central nervous system (CNS), such that incoming pain messages to the system generate subsequent responses out of proportion to the original stimulus, and non-nociceptive stimuli thus generate "pain" responses.

The phenomenon of central sensitization was hypothesized by Woolf and Chong (25), who developed an animal model in 1983 to investigate and subsequently prove the hypothesis. Following the discovery, central sensitization has been documented as a cause of somatosensory hypersensitivity observed in patients after surgical trauma (26).

Central sensitization begins with the induction of activity in peripheral C-fibers, which can be activated by mechanical, thermal, or chemical stimuli. During the initiation phase of central sensitization, pain is induced by a variety of peripheral substances such as potassium and hydrogen ions, histamine, 5-HT, BK, and PG E_2, all found in the "inflammatory soup" in peripheral tissue after trauma.

Glutamate is the most ubiquitous of the CNS neurotransmitters; thus as was inevitable, its role in the transmission of pain has been elucidated (24). The NMDA receptor, one of glutamate's principal binding sites, in turn has been found to play a crucial role in the development of central sensitization. Indeed, the principal component of central sensitization is mediated by the activation of presynaptic NMDA receptors, located on the central terminals of C-fibers. This component of central sensitization is marked by increased intracellular levels of calcium, which promote excitability of dorsal horn neurons. Theoretically, then, central sensitization can be forestalled by NMDA receptor antagonism, voltage-dependent calcium ion channels, as well as G-protein–coupled receptors such as P NK1 and mGluR (25,26). This exciting lead in pain relief, examined in detail in animal studies, has not panned out in the treatment of pain in humans. Those NMDA blockers currently available in clinical practice, such as ketamine, amantadine, memantine, and dextromethorphan, and the experimental drug CHF3381, all show some clinical effect, but their efficacy is far less than that which would be predicted by theoretical and experimental work (27).

Peripheral Sensitization and Neuroendocrine Responses

Nociceptive mediators, released during tissue injury, activate primary afferent neuronal endings, and increase regional nociceptive sensitivity to further tissue damage and painful stimulus. This primary *hyperalgesia* is worsened by ambulation, incentive spirometry, or physical therapy and leads to an increased dynamic or "effort-dependent" pain.

Nociceptive impulses also impact upon and alter the activity of hypothalamus and adrenal cortex and medulla. These changes, termed the neuroendocrine or "stress" response to injury, are characterized by an increased secretion of catabolic hormones such as cortisol, glucagon, growth hormone, and catecholamines. Innumerable chemical mediators participate in this response, and many novel mediators recently have been discovered. Nerve growth factor, first purified by Levi-Montalcini and colleagues in 1987, is the prototypical neurotrophic factor, and has been shown to play an exciting functional role as neuromodulator, coordinating inflammatory and neuroendocrine responses, with increased endogenous levels in acute inflammation as well as chronic pain states (28). Such alterations mediate enhanced mobilization of substrate, hyperglycemia, and a negative nitrogen balance. This catabolic response leads to muscle wasting, impaired immunocompetence, and decreased resistance to infection. Related to this is the concept of *sympathoadrenal activation*. Surgical injury is associated with marked increases in plasma epinephrine and norepinephrine concentrations. Increased sympathetic tone has been associated with an increased risk of perioperative myocardial ischemia in patients with poorly compensated coronary artery disease. Severe pain is commonly associated with an impaired ability to ambulate and decreased venous flow. Catecholamines, angiotensin, and other factors associated with surgical stress increase platelet–fibrinogen activation, while surgical manipulation in and around the pelvis may damage venous conduits, diminishing blood return from the lower extremity. These factors underlie Virchow's triad of venous stasis, hypercoagulability, and endothelial injury, which increases the risk of clot formation, deep vein thrombosis, and pulmonary embolus (28).

Humoral and neurologic alterations in and around the site of injury may be responsible for increased postoperative discomfort and disability. Continued activation of nociceptors secondary to neural compression, stretch, infection, hematoma, and edema can explain ongoing or progressive worsening of acute pain as well as prolonged disability and impaired rehabilitation. In these settings, continued periosteal and muscle irritation may initiate reflex motor responses leading to spasm and myofascial pain. Heightened reflex activity in sympathetic efferent fibers results in vasoconstriction and continued nociceptor sensitization. Alterations in blood flow and efferent outflow may be responsible for persistent pain syndromes.

PAIN SERVICES AND THERAPEUTIC OPTIONS FOR POSTOPERATIVE ANALGESIA

Nearly 25 million surgeries are performed annually in the United States, and most require some form of pain management. Major goals in pain management are to (i) reduce the severity of acute postoperative or posttraumatic pain in both adult and pediatric populations; (ii) introduce new and potentially more effective methods of providing analgesia; (iii) educate patients to effectively communicate increases in pain intensity; (iv) teach caregivers about the need for prompt evaluation and treatment; and (v) by these efforts reduce the number of pain-associated complications, improve outcome, and shorten hospital stay.

Postsurgical pain service is generally multidisciplinary, with anesthesiologists, surgeons, nurses, pharmacists, and nursing assistants playing important roles. Pain intensity has increasingly become recognized as the "fifth vital sign": that is, a variable (approaching zero) associated with homeostasis, to be measured frequently and maintained at a predetermined optimized value. Pain intensity may be reliably measured using visual analog scale scores, verbal pain scores, or "Oucher" type picture scales for very young, elderly, and mentally impaired patients (29). These scores are incorporated in the patient's chart on a regular basis to gauge overall analgesic effectiveness and quality assurance. Continued staff education and the use of standardized orders significantly reduce the number of nurse calls for assistance.

PARENTERALLY AND ORALLY ADMINISTERED ANALGESICS

A cautionary note on PRN: although "as-needed" (or PRN) intramuscularly and orally administered analgesic regimens remain the mainstay of acute pain management, a large number of papers have documented inadequacies associated with such therapy (3). A major deficiency relates to the timing of the analgesic dose because patients often wait too long to seek pain relief and request medication, and staff may not be able to immediately deliver it. A second problem associated with PRN dosing relates to its ineffectiveness in maintaining therapeutic plasma concentrations (30). When intramuscular (IM) analgesics are administered every three to four hours, concentrations in plasma may equal or exceed minimal effective analgesic concentration only 30% of the intervening time. The provision of pain medication on a traditional PRN every-three-to-four-hour dosing schedule involves an elaborate sequence of events, which inevitably delays administration, resulting in repetitive cycles of increasing pain. Because pain is usually not treated as an emergency, the length of time that the patient waits for an analgesic is dependent principally upon the nursing workload at the time of the request. Once the level of pain is deemed significant to warrant treatment, the nurse must then take the time-consuming steps (i.e., medication sign-out, preparation, etc.) necessary to administer the dose. These steps delay the onset of effective relief and worsen pain-induced anxiety, helplessness, and sleep deprivation. Because the dose administered is often relatively large and absorption is erratic and prolonged, the initial analgesic effect is often followed by sedation and some degree of respiratory depression (31).

Oral Analgesics

Oral administration of analgesics offers a safe, simple, and cost-effective method of controlling postoperative pain that should always be considered in patients tolerating oral diet and experiencing moderate discomfort. Oral dosing is best employed during the rehabilitation phase following surgery; however, alterations in gastrointestinal function and perfusion that follow exposure to general anesthesia and traumatic injury markedly reduce the reliability and effectiveness of such therapy, particularly during the emergent phase (29).

Oral opioids, including morphine, meperidine, hydrocodone, and oxycodone, and compounded opioid preparations containing acetaminophen, aspirin, or ibuprofen (e.g., oxycodone in Percocet®, Tylox®, Percodan®, and Combunox®; hydrocodone in Vicodin®, Lortab®, and Lorcet®), provide effective relief for patients complaining of moderate to severe pain. (While oxycodone is available as an uncompounded oral product, hydrocodone is not; an upward titration of hydrocodone is therefore limited by associated acetaminophen increase.) Orally administered morphine and meperidine are poorly absorbed and undergo significant enterohepatic metabolism. For this reason, onset is delayed, duration is less predictable, and dose requirements are high, perhaps two to three times higher than parenteral requirements. Oxycodone and hydrocodone have higher oral effectiveness, as they are more reliably absorbed and are less likely to undergo first-pass hepatic metabolism. Sustained-release oral opioid preparations are available for morphine (MS-Contin®) and oxycodone (Oxycontin®). These offer wider dosing schedules, which is convenient for the patient and can reduce hospital labor. These preparations avoid the frequent peaks and trough plasma levels that lead to the cycles of euphoria, dysphoria, and sedation at the peak, and discomfort at the trough. This greater analgesic uniformity allows for 8 to 12 hours of pain relief per dose, and is ideally suited for patients who have opioid-responsive chronic pain, or who are engaged in prolonged physical rehabilitation. Over the last few years, Oxycontin has been increasingly prescribed for pain control in acute postsurgical settings. Personal communication to R. Sinatra determined the dose relationship between oral Oxycontin and intravenous (IV) patient-controlled analgesia (PCA) morphine in patients recovering from general, gynecological, and orthopedic surgery. They found that the initial dose of Oxycontin needed to maintain effective pain control was only 1.3 times higher than the prior day's dose of morphine. We have found that the relationship is closer to 1:1; that is, if, on the previous day, the patient required 40 mg of morphine, the initial dose of Oxycontin is 40 mg/day, or 20 mg every 12 hours. Oxycontin 20 to 40 mg every 12 hours may also be utilized as an effective transitional analgesic in patients previously treated with epidural analgesics during the first 24 to 48 hours following surgery (16). Oral Oxycontin is started either one to two hours following discontinuation of the epidural infusion or as soon as the patient notices a slight increase in pain intensity. Onset of analgesia is noted within 30 to 60 minutes, and highly uniform pain relief is maintained for 10 to 12 hours. The early introduction of Oxycontin is generally well tolerated, and allows the duration of epidural therapy to be shortened from 72 hours to 24 to 48 hours, all the while minimizing the need for parenteral analgesics (32).

The safety and effectiveness of Oxycontin versus doses of immediate-release oxycodone given PRN and "by the clock" was evaluated in patients recovering from anterior cruciate ligament repair (31). Patients treated with sustained-release formulation required less drug and experienced superior pain control than individuals treated with oxycodone. They also benefited from a reduction in opioid-related side effects such as nausea, vomiting, sedation, and sleep disturbance. Patients treated with oral immediate- and sustained-release opioid preparations are always at risk for ileus and constipation, mandating that such therapy be supplemented with a bowel regimen that includes stool softeners, bulk laxatives, and occasional enemas.

Less potent analgesics may be prescribed in patients with mild to moderate pain, and may be given alone, or as supplements to opioid therapy or regional neural blockade. These include tramadol, a weak noncontrolled opioid, Ultram ER, a tramadol extended-release oral preparation, tramadol compounded with acetaminophen (Ultram®), and a variety of nonsteroidal anti-inflammatory drugs (NSAIDs). Rofecoxib (Vioxx®), celecoxib (Celebrex®), and valdecoxib (Bextra®) represent a newer, and potentially safer, class of NSAID, termed the cyclooxygenase-2 (COX-2) inhibitors. These agents selectively block COX-2, thereby inhibiting PG synthesis following tissue injury. Unlike other NSAIDs, however, they do not block COX-1, which constitutively maintains platelet function and gastric mucosal integrity. (In the fall of 2005, both Vioxx and Bextra became unavailable in the United States; Vioxx was removed by the Food and Drug Administration (FDA) over concerns of excessive cardiovascular risk; Bextra was withdrawn voluntarily by its manufacturer over concerns related to the very uncommon occurrence of Stevens–Johnson syndrome. The degree of hazard posed to the public by these drugs, compared to their potential benefit, is yet unclear; it is entirely possible that by publication of this writing, both agents would have returned, at some recommended dose level, to the American market.) Meloxicam (Mobic®) is another NSAID, which is similar in this regard, as it has relative specificity to the COX-2 isoform. Following long-term use of these drugs, the incidence of gastric ulcer is similar to that observed with placebo, and significantly lower than that observed with nonselective NSAIDs. Despite this increase in safety, the

COX-2 inhibitors should not be given to patients with active bleeding ulcer. COX-2 is also expressed in the kidney: here the enzyme is inducible in response to salt restriction and hypovolemia, and participates in renin release. Thus, COX-2–specific agents are contraindicated in prerenal azotemia. The COX-2 inhibitors have no effect on bleeding time, and their safety and effectiveness have been demonstrated in several post-orthopedic surgical models. For example, rofecoxib 50 mg/day for five days is as effective as naproxen sodium in reducing pain intensity and opioid dose requirements in patients recovering from orthopedic surgery (26). There has been only one comparison of rofecoxib versus celecoxib for postoperative pain management (28). In this study, rofecoxib 50 mg was associated with a more prolonged duration and greater reduction in morphine consumption than was Celecoxib® 200 mg (31).

Parenteral Analgesics

Morphine remains the standard opioid analgesic for control of orthopedic injuries, as it effectively blocks musculoskeletal and visceral pain. Onset of analgesia occurs within five minutes after IV, and 15 minutes following IM administration, while duration ranges from two to four hours, depending upon dose and site of administration. Administration of morphine may release histamine and has been associated with hypotension and biliary colic. Meperidine (Demerol®) and hydromorphone (Dilaudid®) are useful alternatives in patients intolerant of morphine's adverse effects. Meperidine's parenteral potency is one-tenth that of morphine, while its duration of effect is only two-thirds as long. Doses exceeding 600 mg/day may result in seizures secondary to accumulation of its metabolite, normeperidine. Hydromorphone is approximately five times as potent as morphine, but has a more rapid onset of analgesia and lower incidence of adverse effects. Fentanyl is a potent analgesic advocated for use in patients with marked hemodynamic instability or individuals highly tolerant to opioid analgesics. Bolus doses (50–200 µg) and IV infusions (50–200 µg/hr) of fentanyl are particularly useful in patients who remain intubated. The most serious complications associated with parenteral opioids, as with oral preparations, include constipation, increasing sedation, and progressive respiratory depression. The rapid onset and increased potency of parenterally delivered opioids, however, mean that the practitioner must be more vigilant in their use.

Ketorolac (Toradol®) is a potent NSAID available in parenteral form (32). Ketorolac reduces pain intensity by nonselectively reducing PG synthesis at the peripheral site of injury, as well as in pain-processing circuits in the CNS (32,33). Ketorolac in doses of 30 to 60 mg is as potent as 10 mg of morphine, and is particularly useful in managing posttraumatic musculoskeletal pain. Although it is not associated with excessive sedation or respiratory depression, major side effects, including increased risk of hemorrhage, gastric ulceration, and renal toxicity, limit its usefulness during the acute and emergent phases following injury. To minimize these complications, ketorolac dose should be limited to 7.5 to 15 mg every 6 hours for a maximum of 48 hours. Injectable COX-2 inhibitors and IV acetaminophen derivatives that offer greater safety and equivalent analgesic effects as ketorolac will soon be available for perioperative use.

INTRAVENOUS PATIENT-CONTROLLED ANALGESIA

PCA allows patients to titrate small doses of pain medication in amounts proportional to a perceived pain stimulus. The technique avoids cycles of excessive sedation and ineffective pain control observed with "by the clock" and PRN IM dosing, and limits variation related to inappropriate pain assessment on the one hand and unpredictable drug absorption on the other (32). Patients control the dose frequency (within prescribed time limits) and thereby correct for individual differences in pain perception and pharmacokinetics and delays in administration. It must always be borne in mind that while the patient is titrating the drug, it is being done within the careful limits set by the administering physician; i.e., patient self-titration should not be confused with self-administration. Furthermore, PCA prescription is not an alibi for inadequate patient assessment and monitoring.

Commercially developed PCA systems incorporate microprocessors that allow the patient to interact with an infusion pump connected to the established IV line. A patient activates the pump by pressing a button connected to the apparatus. A preprogrammed amount of opioid (incremental bolus dose) is then administered over 10 to 30 seconds, and a preset "lockout" time interval begins, within which a second dose will not be delivered. A prolonged lockout interval or inadequate incremental bolus may diminish analgesic effectiveness (34). Conversely, too large incremental dose increases the number of treatment failures related to intolerable side effects. Patients inevitably find themselves titrating pain against sedation, excessive nausea, or other side effects. Interestingly, patients report that they are usually willing to accept some amount of pain in order to have a clear sensorium (30,32,34).

One of the keys to successful initiation of PCA is the administration of an opioid "loading" dose. This first dose provides baseline plasma concentrations of analgesic, which can then be augmented by patient-initiated boluses. In general, morphine (5–15 mg) or hydromorphone (0.5–3 mg) is titrated to patient comfort for this purpose. While morphine remains the standard and most widely administered PCA analgesic, it does have drawbacks, including delay to peak analgesic effect, sedation, and histamine release (35). Other opioids employed for IV-PCA, and suggested dosage and lockout intervals, are presented in Table 4.

More sophisticated PCA devices incorporate a continuous (basal) rate infusion in addition to patient-activated bolus doses on demand. Patients receiving basal opioid infusions should be monitored carefully, as the continuous delivery of opioid bypasses the inherent safety of PCA, and may result in progressive sedation. Conversely, some newer PCA devices incorporate a "safety setting," whereby a three- or four-hour limit on total drug delivery may be set. While superficially appealing, this "safety setting" technique reincorporates all the drawbacks of PRN, i.e., cyclical blood levels of opioids, while eliminating the very advantage of the PCA technique: that is, patient self-titration of the drug. Using a "safety setting" encourages lax dose, lockout interval, and basal adjustments in an environment of false security, and does nothing to establish a PCA dose schedule that can be converted to a postoperative oral (P.O.) regimen. Furthermore, safety, as has been stated, is established in patient assessment and monitoring. The most appealing advances in PCA technology are those which allow the nurse and physician to record the number and times of dose demand against the doses delivered. This provides the most useful data in adjusting delivery parameters to steady opioid blood levels and thereby optimizes therapy (32,34).

The two most common reasons for patient dissatisfaction and failure of the PCA method of treatment are *inadequate analgesia* and *nausea and vomiting*. In large measure, both of these complications can be treated well with patient education. It must be said that PCA therapy must begin with the patient's complete understanding of the self-titration method. Countless cases of poor results with PCA therapy stem from patients simply not understanding how to push the button, and when. Patients must be trained to treat their pain before it overwhelms them, for example, just prior to physical therapy, or before any form of movement that might increase discomfort. Similarly, the patient should know to avoid the button during periods of relative comfort. If the patients have intolerable side effects, they may call the nurse or the pain service to ask for help or another medication; they should be instructed not to abandon the PCA device in the meantime. Finally, concerned relatives (and nurses!) should never push the PCA button for the patient (32,34).

SPINAL OPIOID ANALGESIA

The administration of opioid analgesics into the intrathecal or epidural space, termed *spinal opioid analgesia*, is perhaps the most powerful method of controlling pain in many clinical settings (35,36). Following an epidural injection, a portion of the analgesic crosses the dura to enter the cerebrospinal fluid (CSF). Intrathecal (or "spinal") injection administers this medicine directly to the CSF. Opioid molecules then only bind to receptors in dorsal horn, effectively blocking pain transmission at the first synapse in the CNS. Intrathecal and epidural opioids provide greater analgesic potency than similar doses administered parenterally. In general, epidural doses of hydrophilic opioids such as morphine and hydromorphone exhibit the greatest potency, while doses of highly lipophilic opioids behave similar to IV (37–39). A second advantage noted with spinal opioids is the "selectivity" of analgesic effect, which is maintained in the absence of motor or sympathetic blockade (38,39).

A single intrathecal bolus (0.25–0.5 mg) or multiple epidural boluses (2.5–5 mg) of morphine are commonly used for the control of pain following trauma and lower extremity orthopedic surgery (34). Doses are usually administered via spinal needles or epidural catheters inserted at lumbar interspaces. In general, analgesic onset is appreciated after 30 to 60 minutes, and peak effect at 90 to 120 minutes. Duration ranges from 12 to 24 hours. Twenty-four hour milligram analgesic requirements are reduced to about one-tenth the parenteral dose. While this method is effective and simple, the major drawback is the abrupt rise in CSF opioid concentrations following each epidural or spinal bolus, which may result in a high incidence of occasionally serious adverse effects.

Continuous Epidural Analgesia

Infusions of epidural opioids, opioids diluted in local anesthetics, and local anesthetics alone have been advocated as methods to control postoperative pain (40,41). Continuous infusion permits analgesia to be more precisely titrated to the level of pain stimulus and rapidly terminated if problems arise. This avoids the high peak concentrations that follow intermittent epidural boluses and reduces the risk of delayed respiratory depression (39–41). Continuous infusion technique also provides greater therapeutic versatility because shorter-acting opioids and dilute local anesthetic solutions may be administered.

Continuous infusions of morphine (Duramorph®, Astramorph®) and hydromorphone offer effective epidural analgesia for patients recovering from a variety of surgical procedures (39–41). Epidural infusions of morphine mixed with dilute bupivacaine provide excellent analgesia, are associated with an extremely low incidence of serious adverse events, and may be safely administered to patients recovering on routine postsurgical wards (42). Hydromorphone infusion compares favorably with morphine. Over 90% of patients receiving continuous lumbar epidural infusions of low-dose hydromorphone for postthoracotomy analgesia report either no pain or only mild discomfort. Hypoventilation, pruritus, and nausea are milder than that observed with equipotent doses of epidural morphine. Patients on continuous epidural infusions of hydromorphone experience effective pain relief, with less sedation and pruritus, than patients on continuous infusions of morphine at equivalent doses (43).

Fentanyl is commonly administered as continuous epidural infusion because of its rapid onset, and short duration facilitates analgesic titration. Epidural fentanyl dose requirements are high (40–70 mcg/hr) and are often equivalent to that required with IV infusions of fentanyl. Improved analgesic effectiveness may be achieved by combining epidural fentanyl with dilute solutions of bupivacaine (44,47).

Epidural infusion of local anesthetics, especially bupivacaine and ropivacaine, offers reliable and effective analgesia in a segmental fashion for patients recovering from lower extremity vascular and orthopedic surgery or trauma. Local anesthetic infusions are particularly useful in patients who are sensitive to the side effects of opioid analgesics. Local anesthetic therapy is associated with sensory-motor and sympathetic blockade. Hypotension and impaired micturation, however, occur more frequently with epidural local anesthetics than with opioids.

Patient-Controlled Epidural Analgesia

Patient-controlled epidural analgesia (PCEA) offers higher analgesic efficacy and lower dose requirement than IV-PCA, while providing greater control and patient satisfaction than either single doses or continuous infusions of epidural opioids. This technique combines the control and titratability of patient-controlled administration with the higher analgesic efficacy associated with neuraxial analgesia (45).

Morphine's latency to peak effect and risk of delayed onset respiratory depression represent undesirable characteristics for PCEA, therefore hydromorphone and more lipophilic opioids such as fentanyl, which offer rapid onset and greater titratability, have become the agents of choice in this setting (46,48). Epidural dose requirements for single bolus techniques, continuous epidural infusion, and patient-controlled epidural infusion are presented in Table 9.

ADVERSE EVENTS AND CONTRAINDICATIONS OF NEUROAXIAL ANALGESIC TECHNIQUES

Epidural and intrathecally administered opioids are associated with a number of annoying and occasionally serious adverse effects including pruritus, nausea, urinary retention, somnolence, and respiratory depression (41,42,45). Treatment protocols have been developed which can decrease the incidence and severity of side effects and improve patient safety while maintaining effective analgesia. The presence of side effects should be assessed frequently and treated quickly in order to minimize morbidity and patient dissatisfaction.

Pruritus and nausea are the most common side effects associated with epidural or spinal opioids; however, respiratory depression is the most feared complication (41–43,45,46,49). Respiratory depression following epidural or intrathecal morphine occurs at two different intervals (46,49). An early mild phase observed soon after administration is followed by delayed depression occurring between 8 and 12 hours later. Risk factors for respiratory depression are listed in Table 8. The speed with which epidural opioid-induced respiratory depression develops is not sudden, but slowly progressive, and is generally preceded by nausea, vomiting, and increased sedation (46). Vigilant nursing observation, and documentation of inadequate respiratory effort, slow respiratory rate, or unusual somnolence represent the best form of monitoring (46). Prophylactic naloxone infusions (400 µg/L) at 100 to 125 ml/hr have been advocated to reduce the risk of opioid-induced respiratory depression in elderly or debilitated patients while maintaining effective analgesia (47,48,51). Naloxone infusions effectively reduce the incidence and severity of other adverse effects including pruritus, nausea, and urinary retention (47).

Relative contraindications to neuraxial opioid analgesia include spinal fracture, infection at the insertion site, septicemia, coagulopathy, and treatment with low-molecular weight heparinoids. Epidural placement requires assessment of coagulation status, and the absence vertebral fractures, instability, and neural deficit. Catheters should not be inserted in patients with consumptive or drug-induced coagulopathy unless the underlying cause is corrected. There is concern about the safety of epidural catheter placement in patients receiving using anticoagulant-based prophylaxis of deep venous thrombosis. In 1997, the FDA issued an advisory about the potential risk of epidural hematoma in patients receiving regional (spinal or epidural) anesthesia and low-molecular weight heparin. The American Society of Regional Anesthesia and Pain Medicine has published guidelines regarding safe use of anticoagulants in patients undergoing neuraxial anesthesia and analgesia.

NEURAL BLOCKADE FOR ACUTE PAIN MANAGEMENT

Peripheral neural blockade minimizes exposure to opioids and are ideally suited for patients sensitive to opioid-induced ileus and bowel obstruction. Other indications include avoidance of opioid-induced ventilatory depression, particularly in patients with underlying pulmonary disease.

Infiltration techniques employ injections of local anesthetic at the site of surgery and offer up to 12 hours of postoperative analgesia. These techniques require surgical infiltration of concentrated local anesthetic solutions into skin, subcutaneous tissues, and into the joint capsule. Continuous infiltration techniques typically employ 20-gauge multiport catheters to deliver local anesthetic (usually dilute bupivacaine) under the skin and muscle layers of an incision. In addition, catheters may be placed in the iliac crest (donor bone graft site), pleural space, femoral nerve fascial compartment, and brachial plexus. Additional analgesia may be safely provided with IV-PCA (32,34).

POSTTRAUMATIC PAIN

Pain management in the trauma patient has been divided into three phases: emergent, acute, and rehabilitative. During the *emergent phase*, primary attention must be given to stabilizing the patient's respiratory and cardiovascular status; thereafter the intensity of pain may be assessed and carefully controlled. Primary analgesic therapy includes IV titration of opioids in doses that provide pain relief while not compromising the patient's hemodynamic status or obscuring the diagnostic process.

The *acute phase* begins with admission to the intensive care facility and ends with transfer to the medical/surgical ward. Acute phase pain management is determined not only by the primary injury, but also by associated medical-procedural interventions. For instance, not only does the noxious periosteal and ligamentous pain of a rib fracture need to be addressed, but also that associated with chest tube insertion or thoracotomy. The same premise is evident in the following upper abdominal injuries; patients suffering blunt abdominal trauma may require an exploratory laparotomy for diagnosis and treatment of acute abdomen. IV-PCA provides useful pain control following major orthopedic trauma and extensive soft-tissue injuries. If there are no contraindications to regional analgesia, IV-PCA may be supplemented with intercostal, brachial plexus, or interpleural blocks. Continuous epidural analgesia should be considered the technique of choice in patients recovering from multiple rib fractures and flail chest. In general, epidural morphine may be administered at lumbar sites while hydromorphone and fentanyl are infused via thoracic catheters. Dilute concentrations of bupivacaine (0.03–0.1%) are added to the epidural infusate in hemodynamically stable patients. Manipulative procedures including external bone fixation, wound debridement, burn eschar excision, and dressing changes are quite painful pain and generally require greater amounts of analgesic than is routinely prescribed. During these procedures, IV-PCA may be supplemented with rapid-acting, short-duration opioids (fentanyl 1–5 µg/kg or equivalent doses of alfentanil), or ketamine (1–3 mg/kg) (32,34).

The *rehabilitative phase* begins when the patient is transferred from the intensive care unit to the medical/surgical ward and ends with full recovery. Patients are expected to move out of bed, ambulate with increasing frequency, and participate in physical therapy. As gastrointestinal (GI) function returns and diet is advanced, IV-PCA and epidural analgesia may be discontinued and oral pain medications substituted. Baseline (resting) pain may be relieved with timed-release preparations of morphine and oxycodone, or methadone. Increases in pain intensity associated with physical therapy may be controlled with morphine or oxycodone given immediately prior to the procedure. During the rehabilitative phase, NSAID may be used to augment timed-release oral opioids, while tricyclic antidepressants, clonidine, and sympathetic blockade may be employed to control persistent neuropathic and sympathetically mediated pain (32,34).

NEW IDEAS IN PAIN MANAGEMENT
Preemptive Analgesia

In the late 1980s, Wall (52) proposed the concept of "preemptive preoperative analgesia," suggesting that analgesic intervention is most effective when it is made in advance of the pain stimulus rather than in reaction to it. The possibility that preemptive intervention produces analgesic effects that long outlast the pharmacological duration of the agents or techniques employed, suggests important new avenues of treatment of the trauma and postsurgical patient (53). Patients treated with femoral nerve block prior to arthroscopic knee surgery require 50% less opioid analgesic during the first 24 hours of recovery than individuals receiving a similar block at completion of the procedure. Preemptive analgesic benefits have also been observed with epidural opioids. A single dose of epidural fentanyl (4 mcg/kg), administered prior to thoracotomy incision, is more effective in reducing postoperative pain scores and IV-PCA morphine requirements in the day following surgery than a similar epidural fentanyl dose administered during surgery (54).

Conversely, Figure 25 illustrates why single-treatment preemptive therapy may be insufficient for the management of surgical pain beyond the immediate postoperative period. Woolf et al. (1,2) has proposed that optimal preemptive analgesia should be continuous and perioperative in nature, and should include preoperative initiation as well as intra- and postoperative maintenance of therapy. To date, only a few studies have compared pre- and postoperative initiation of continuous preemptive treatment (55). In one study (55), there was no clinically significant difference in postoperative pain during continuous epidural bupivacaine–morphine infusion initiated either before or following completion of colon surgery. Its authors speculate that the study protocol may not have prevented central sensitization because complete preemptive afferent blockade was not achieved. While the majority of clinical studies have examined relief of postsurgical pain and acute disability, preemptive analgesia may also provide longer term convalescent-rehabilitative benefits and prevent or minimize the severity of persistent pain syndromes (56). Patients recovering from back-fusion surgery, in which donor bone is taken from the iliac crest, may develop chronic periosteal pain that persists for months to years after the operation. Infusion of bupivacaine via an iliac crest catheter attenuates the intensity of acute postoperative pain and appears to minimize development of chronic sensitivity (56). Neuralgias, phantom limb pain, and deafferentation syndromes are common after amputation. Recent evidence indicates that preemptive analgesia provided by perioperative epidural conduction blockade can prevent the development of chronic stump and phantom limb pain in patients recovering from below the knee amputation (Fig. 26) (56).

Multimodal Analgesia

Complete abolition of postsurgical pain (pain prevention) is difficult to achieve with a single drug or analgesic technique (55). In an effort to minimize single agent dose requirements and the potential toxicity associated with reliance on one agent, "balanced" or multimodal analgesic regimens have been advocated. It is thought that effective pain relief may be achieved by the additive or synergistic activity of two or more analgesics. By reducing the amount of each drug administered, the incidence and severity of potentially serious side effects may be diminished. Multimodal analgesic therapy employs a variety of agents which interfere with noxious transmission and pain perception at different levels within the peripheral and CNS. Recommendations for multimodal anesthetic and perioperative analgesic dosing are presented in Table 2.

PAIN CONTROL AND POSTSURGICAL OUTCOME

Do efforts to minimize postoperative pain and associated stress responses result in improved postsurgical outcome? The cost of PCA and epidural infusion devices is considerably higher than traditional forms of analgesia. Studies are under way to determine whether optimal postsurgical analgesia can decrease morbidity and duration of hospital stay, thus offsetting cost.

Patients who benefit most from intraspinal opioid analgesia are those recovering from extensive surgical procedures where parenteral opioid dose requirements are high. Therapeutic gains are dramatic in patients with underlying cardiovascular and pulmonary disease, whereas they are less obvious in healthy individuals recovering from minimally invasive procedures. Optimally administered epidural analgesia can suppress release of catecholamines, maintain hemodynamic stability, reduce myocardial oxygen requirements, improve respiratory function, and facilitate physical therapy. Such therapy has also been shown to reduce mortality, hospital stay, and overall cost. These desirable outcomes outweigh the greater invasiveness and potential side effects associated with epidural placement and indwelling catheters (32).

Epidural infusions of local anesthetic (0.25–0.5% bupivacaine) can suppress sympathoadrenal and neuroendocrine responses accompanying surgical trauma. Suppression is most effective after lower abdominal and extremity procedures (56). Epidural conduction blockade has been shown to significantly reduce thromboembolic complications in patients

Table 2 Dosing Guidelines for Intravenous Patient-Controlled Analgesia

Opioid	Concentration	Dose	Bolus	Dose Interval (min)	Rate	Comments
Morphine	1 mg/m	3–10 mg	0.5–1.5 mg	6–8	0.5–1.5 mg/hr	Major abdominal/orthopedic surgical pain; slow onset
Meperidine	10 mg/ml	25–50mg	5–15 mg	6–8		Not recommended Useful for visceral pain, limit dose to 600 mg/24hrs
Hydromorphone	0.2 mg/ml	0.5–1 mg	0.1–0.3 mg	6–8	0.1–0.3 mg/hr	Rapid onset, minimal side effects
Oxymorphone	0.1 mg/ml	0.3–1 mg	0.1–0.2 mg	6–8	0.1–0.2 mg/hr	Rapid onset, best for severe pain, high incidence of nausea/vomiting
Fentanyl	20 mcg/ml	30–100 mcg	10–20 mcg	5–6	10–20 mcg/hr	Rapid onset, short duration of effect,

recovering from hip surgery (57). In a study of critically ill patients recovering from major surgery, Yeager et al. (58) noted that patients treated with epidural morphine benefited from significant reductions in cardiac and respiratory failure and incidence of major infections when compared with individuals administered IV opioids. Seventy-six percent of patients in the general anesthesia parenteral opioid group (19/25) developed some form of organ failure versus 32% (9/28) in the epidural anesthesia–analgesia group. Similar results were reported in patients undergoing major vascular surgery and randomized to receive epidural anesthesia–analgesia or general anesthesia with parenteral opioids for postoperative pain relief. Patients in the general group experienced greater postsurgical morbidity, in particular cardiovascular and infectious complications (32,34,56).

CHRONIC PAIN

Despite our best efforts at controlling pain in the perioperative period, the patient's discomfort may linger long past the resolution of the initial physical trauma. *Chronic pain* (pain lasting more than three to six months beyond the initial insult) is one of the greatest challenges in medical practice today. It may be the result of inadequate treatment of the acute pain, or the peculiar physical and emotional makeup of the patient. In some instances, the pain is due to traumatic or perioperative nerve injury, with the subsequent development of *neuropathic pain*, a type of chronic pain that is singularly resistant to common therapies. The following sections include a description of the common perioperative neuropathies, and a brief discussion of the development and treatment of neuropathic pain.

Perioperative Neuropathies

Perioperative nerve injury is a considerable source of patient injury and liability in both anesthesia and surgical practice.

Neuropathies secondary to surgery are infrequent, however, they can be potentially debilitating in surgical patients. According to the American Society of Anesthesiologists Closed Claims Project, perioperative nerve injury is the second most common class of injury, accounting for 15% of all claims

(60). Many of these neuropathies are avoidable and are usually associated with inappropriate patient positioning in the operating room. The most common nerves affected are the peripheral nerves such as the ulnar and sciatic nerves. However, more centrally located nerves, such as the brachial plexus and the lumbosacral nerve roots, can also be affected. Additionally, and of particular interest, there are epidemiologic and anatomic studies to suggest that factors other than intraoperative malpositioning may contribute to the development of neuropathies.

Nevertheless, the occurrence of mechanical nerve injury in connection with anesthesia and surgery is probably more common than generally believed, and by no means all cases are reported to the patient injury claims department. Both incorrect positioning of the patient on the operating table and pressure from retractors and other instruments can contribute to the occurrence of such injuries. Both neurological and neuropsychological procedures should be used to localize the injury, particularly for the purpose of insurance assessment. Most important of all, however, is prevention of injury. Risk minimization is dependent on the observation of meticulous routines in surgery units, and clear division of staff responsibilities.

Common Perioperative Neuropathies

Upper Extremity

Carpal Tunnel Syndrome. Median neuropathy at the wrist is the most common nerve entrapment syndrome. Hundreds of papers have been written to describe the condition and its diagnosis and treat-

Table 3 Factors Which Increase the Risk of Spinal Opioid-Induced Respiratory Depression

Drug-related factors
  Hydrophilic opioids
  Excessive dose
  Large volume of injectate
  Excessive dose frequency
  Intrathecal administration
  Concomitant administration of parenteral opioids
Patient-related factors
  Age greater than 60 years
  Debilitated individuals
  Coexisting respiratory disease
  Raised intrathoracic pressure
  Shock-wave lithotripsy
  Trendelenberg position

Table 4 Dosing Guidelines for Epidural Opioid Analgesia

Morphine Lumbar catheters: Administer 3–8 mg bolus 2–4 mg bolus followed by 2–4 mg bolus followed Ketorolac 15–30 mg q 6 hr
incisions below T8 in 10 ml preservative infusion (50 mcg/ml at 10–15 infusion (50 mcg/ml at 8–Epidural bupivacaine
Thoracic catheters free saline every 8–24 ml/hr, lumbar catheters), 10 ml/hr, lumbar; 4 ml/hr 0.1% or less
for upper abdominal hours as clinically 4–8 ml/hr, thoracic catheters) thoracic) PCEA bolus dose
and thoracic surgery indicated 1–2 q 15 min, 4 hr limit
30–50

Hydromorphone Lumbar catheters: 0.5–1.5 mg bolus every 0.5–1.5 mg bolus followed 0.5–1.5 mg bolus followed by Ketorolac 15–30 mg q 6 hr
incisions below T8, 6–10 hours infusion (10 mcg/ml at 10–15, infusion (10–20 mcg/ml at 8–10 Epidural bupivacaine
thoracic catheters for lumbar catheters), (20 mcg/ml ml/hr, lumbar; 4–6/hr 0.1–0.05% or less
upper abdominal and at 4–8 ml/hr, thoracic thoracic) PCEA bolus dose
thoracic surgery catheters) 1–2 q 15 min, 4 hr limit
30–50 ml

Meperidine Lumbar catheters: 50–75 mg bolus every 50–75 mg bolus followed 50–75 mg bolus followed by Ketorolac 15–30 mg q 6 hr
incisions below T8, 4–6 hours infusion (100 mcg/ml at 10–15, infusion (100 mcg/ml at 8–10 Epidural bupivacaine 0.1%
thoracic catheters for lumbar catheters), (4–8 ml/hr ml/hr, lumbar; 4–6/hr
upper abdominal and thoracic catheters. thoracic) PCEA bolus dose
thoracic surgery 1–2 q 6–10 min, 4 hr limit
30–50

Fentanyl Lumbar catheters: 50–100 mcg bolus 50–100 mcg bolus followed 50–100 mcg bolus followed by Ketorolac 15–30 mg q 6 hr
incisions below T12, every 2–4 hr infusion (5 mcg/ml at 10–15, infusion (5mcg/ml at 8–10 Epidural bupivacaine 0.05–
thoracic catheters for (not recommended) lumbar catheters), (4–8 ml/hr ml/hr, lumbar; 4–6/hr 0.1% or less
almost everything else thoracic catheters. thoracic) PCEA bolus dose
30–50

Sufentanil Lumbar catheters: 20–30 mcg bolus 20–30 mcg bolus followed 20–40 mcg bolus followed by Ketorolac 15–30 mg q 6 hr
incisions below T12, every 2–4 hr infusion (1–2 mcg/ml at 10–15, infusion (1–2 mcg/ml at 8–10 Epidural bupivacaine 0.05–
thoracic catheters for (not recommended) lumbar catheters), (4–8 ml/hr ml/hr, lumbar; 4–6/hr 0.1% or less
almost everything else thoracic catheters. thoracic) PCEA bolus dose
30–50

∗Dependent on age, physical status, height, extent of surgical dissection, and so on.

Note: The bolus amount for each agent may be used as a starting hourly basal infusion rate.

ment (61). While it is a common outpatient nerve disorder, its prevalence as a perioperative injury is low in comparison.

Ulnar Neuropathy. The ulnar nerve is the single most common site of perioperative peripheral nerve injury, constituting 28% of all perioperative nerve claims. Approximately 50% of all patients with ulnar neuropathy have deficits that persist for more than a year. External compression of the ulnar nerve in the cubital tunnel is usually regarded as the most important cause of anesthesia-related injury; however, detailed study of individual cases has not provided strong correlation. In a large-scale multivariate analysis, Warner et al. (69) isolated several independent risk factors for ulnar neuropathy, including male gender, high or low body mass, and prolonged hospital stay. How these factors spe-

cifically relate to intraoperative mechanisms of injury still remain unclear. Anatomic studies reveal differences in the elbow anatomy of men and women (degree of adipose tissue and thickness of the retinaculum in the cubital tunnel). However, the current understanding of the role that these differences play in the genesis of nerve injury has not evolved beyond speculation. An identifiable mechanism of injury has been reported in only 9% of cases in the Closed Claims Project database.

Although the true mechanisms of anesthesia-related ulnar neuropathy remain undefined, it has been assumed that external pressure exerted against the nerve is the likely etiologic factor. Several reports suggest that the ulnar nerve is more susceptible to ischemia than the radial or median nerve. Many authors acknowledge that ulnar neuropathy remains a clinical entity for which we still have minimal understanding of cause-and-effect relationships (62), nor whether it is always a preventable complication (64). Accumulating evidence suggests ulnar nerve injury can occur at any time during the course of hospitalization.

Prielipp et al. made an important breakthrough in the current study of perioperative or old or nerve injury using a pressure-sensitive mat to determine how changes in arm position affect the external pressure transmitted to the ulnar groove. Supination of the forearm produces the least amount of pressure at the ulnar groove, pronation produces the most, and

Table 5 Advantages of Epidural Patient Controlled Analgesia

Vs. intravenous patient-controlled analgesia
    Superior pain relief
    Reduced drug requirement
    Reduction in drug-related side effects
    Shorter hospitalization
Vs. continuous epidural opioid infusion
    Patient self-adjustment
    Reduced hourly infusion requirement
    Accommodation for changes in pain intensity (i.e., ambulation)
    Reduced anxiety, increased patient control

a neutral forearm precision results in an intermediate value. The findings of this study are consistent with inferences from basic anatomic considerations. Their study also used somatosensory-evoked potentials to explore the relationship between sensory changes and the electrophysiologic changes that occur when external pressure is applied to the ulnar nerve. Interestingly, half of other volunteers failed to perceive any sensory changes despite marked abnormal changes in somatosensory-evoked potential signal strength. Therefore, this suggests that the patient's report is of limited value for the early detection of compressive nerve injury. Although a humbling reminder that we have limited understanding of the relationship between perioperative care and the generation of peripheral nerve injury, the study has practical application for clinical decision-making.

Brachial Plexus Neuropathy. Stretch of the brachial plexus is particularly induced by arm abduction, external rotation, and posterior shoulder displacement (60). Conditions that may predispose to this include extension and lateral flexion of the head to one side with the patient in the supine position, in addition to abduction and external rotation of the arm by allowing it to drop away from the side of the body. Considerable stretch of the brachial plexus roots can also occur from extreme in abduction of the arm with the hand resting above the head. Patients who are placed in the prone position may also be vulnerable to stretch of the brachial plexus (67).

Stretch or compression of the brachial plexus has also been described with upward movement of the clavicle secondary to sternal retraction and median sternotomy (63,64). Brachial plexus nerve injury during the sternal retraction is most common during the internal mammary artery dissection (65,66). The mechanism is assumed to be an asymmetric retraction of the rib cage displacing the upper rib cage that may stretch or compress the C8 through T1 nerve trunks. The trunks form the major contribution to the ulnar nerve and therefore brachial plexus neuropathy may

be difficult to distinguish from a peripheral ulnar neuropathy. In the lateral decubitus position, compression plays a predominant role in injury when the plexus is compressed against the thorax by the humeral head. Anatomical variations of the thoracic outlet and the presence of an extra rib on the seventh cervical vertebrae can also be predisposing factors.

Brachial plexus neuropathy associated with procedures that are performed on patients in a steep head-down position and who are restrained with shoulder braces can be caused by direct compression or stretch of the brachial plexus. Theoretically, stretch of the plexus may occur when the head is turned contralateral and when the ipsilateral arm is abducted with elbow flexion. Fortunately, the frequency of perioperative brachial plexus neuropathy seems to be low in patients who are positioned prone.

Trunk

Postherniorrhaphy Pain/Ilioinguinal Neuropathy. Chronic pain after inguinal herniorrhaphy is a well-known complication that can be debilitating. The reported incidence of chronic groin or inguinal pain after hernia repair varies from 0% to 62% after one year depending on the studies reviewed (70–72). Between 6% and 16% of patients across the studies report moderate to severe pain one year after surgery with a greater incidence in those with recurrent repair. Eleven to sixty-two percent report some degree of pain in the groin area with 10% reporting persistent pain that interferes with activity two years postoperatively. Several distinct types of chronic pain have been reported. The most common pain appears to be somatic and localized to the common ligamentous insertion to the pubic tubercle. The second is neuropathic and referable to possible injury to the ilioinguinal or genitofemoral nerves either at the site of surgery or due to encroachment of scar tissue. The third pain type is visceral and related to ejaculatory pain. Persistent numbness can be common in the distribution of the branches of the ilioinguinal or iliohypogastric nerves in up to 24% of patients.

Table 6 Multimodal Analgesia: Clinical Applications

In the setting of General Anesthesia:

Premedication-analgesic base consisting of moderate to long duration opioid such as morphine (0.05–0.1 mg/kg) or hydromorphone 2. An additional 0.1–0.2 mg/kg morphine dose administered immediately prior to anesthetic induction (the administration of preoperative and induction doses of benzodiazepines, and induction agents should be reduced), 3. Preincisional administration of ketamine (0.2 mg/kg and NSAID (rofecoxib 50 mg, Celecoxib 200 mg or ketorolac 15–30 mg) unless contraindicated by patient status or surgical procedure) 4. preincisional neural blockade; either wound and fascial infiltration, peripheral nerve block or plexus block, 5. IV PCA started in the PACU as soon as the patient is considered alert enough to appropriately utilize such therapy, 6. Maintenance oral rofecoxib 50 mg/day X5days, ketorolac 7.5–15 mg slow IV q 6 hr for 24–48 hrs.

In the setting of epidural/spinal anesthesia or epidural-light general anesthetics : 1. To reduce local anesthetic-opioid doses requirements (increase neuroaxial specificity) epidural catheters should be inserted at interspaces adjacent to the site of surgery. 2. Epidural induction with 2% lidocaine or 0.5–0.75% bupivacaine in doses sufficient to block afferent input from dermatomal sites of surgical incision and deeper dissection. Utilize lower concentrations and total dose of local anesthetic in elderly patients or individuals at risk for intraoperative hypovolemia. 2. Preincisional administration of epidural opioid (morphine, hydromorphone, fentanyl) prior to incision, 3. Preincisional administration of NSAID (ketorolac 15–30 mg) and ketamine (0.2 mg/kg for epidural-light general patients) if not clinically contraindicated, 4. Opioid-bupivacaine infusion initiated during surgical closure or upon arrival in the PACU, 5. Addition of Patient controlled epidural dosing when deemed appropriate (refer to Table 26-5), 6. Maintenance of ketorolac 7.5–15 mg IV q6hr for 24–48 hrs.

Treatments for persistent pain range from local anesthetic injection to remedial surgery and appear to have varying results. Heise and Starling (73) report that remedial surgery with coincident neurectomy affords more favorable results in 60% of patients than mesh removal alone. En bloc resection of the scar tissue has also been suggested by some authors as a potential treatment.

The true incidence of chronic pain after hernia repair remains to be documented. Patients treated for recurrent hernia and those with a high initial pain score and persistent pain four weeks after repair are more likely to report chronic pain one year postoperatively. Mesh repair has become very popular. Its tension-free properties should lead to less acute postoperative pain, however, in randomized studies it has not proven superior to other open repair techniques with respect to acute pain or the use of analgesics (74,75). Nerve injury at the time of operation may be an important mechanism and it appears that remedial surgery with neurectomy may afford acceptable results.

Lower Extremity

Vascular, general surgical, orthopedic, or gynecologic procedures performed either inside the abdominal cavity or on the lower extremities may result in nerve injury. Motor and sensory neuropathy in the lower extremity is a well-recognized potential complication of procedures that can either be related to the surgery itself or to surgical positioning of the patient. Injury resulting in lower extremity neuropathy can virtually occur after any invasive procedure outside of the spinal column from the L1 vertebral level down. The true incidence of neurologic injury is likely underreported and one can imagine that anywhere a surgical scalpel crosses a nerve, where retractors are held, and any position that results in direct pressure or vascular compromise to a peripheral nerve can lead to neurologic consequences.

Common Peroneal Nerve Injury.

Sciatica. The sciatic nerve is especially at risk if the patient is thin, the operating room table hard, the operation long, and when the opposite buttock is elevated as in the hip-pinning position. Smoking during the preoperative period has also been associated with the development of neuropathies. External rotation of the flexed thigh in the lithotomy position may damage the nerve by stretch (76). Several studies have suggested that many factors other than inappropriate intraoperative care and positioning may contribute to the risk of lower extremity nerve injuries (77–79). In a retrospective review of the frequency and type of motor neuropathies that occurred in 198,461 consecutive patients who underwent procedures in the lithotomy position, it was found that the nerves most often involved are the common peroneal nerve (81%), sciatic nerve (15%), and femoral nerve (4%) (80).

In view of the fact that prolonged duration in the lithotomy position as well as patient-specific factors is involved in the development of neuropathy, use findings suggest that not all neuropathies should be assumed to be the result of inappropriate positioning.

Femoral Neuropathy. Unlike many other neuropathies in which the anesthesia provider or inappropriate positioning is implicated, those injuries that involve the femoral nerve and its branches are thought to result from inappropriate placement of abdominal wall retractors and direct compression of the nerve during surgery (81). Here, it is assumed that the retractor used for an abdominal surgical approach to the pelvis places continuous pressure on the iliopsoas muscle, thereby stretching the nerve. An alternate explanation is that retractor compression causes nerve ischemia by occluding the external iliac artery or its branches that penetrate the nerve as it passes through the muscle. It has also been speculated by Rosenblum et al. (82) that self-retaining retractors placed in the abdomen are more likely than hand-held retractors to result in femoral neuropathy, as these devices exert a continuous pressure against the tissues and the surrounding structures.

In addition to retractors, certain patient factors may be associated with femoral neuropathy in the perioperative period. An extremely thin body habitus and smoking are associated with lower extremity neuropathy after surgery. Additionally, type II diabetic patients are susceptible to compression neuropathy, as they are insulin resistant and the nerve tissue is dependent on glycolysis.

Identification of Neuropathic Pain

The symptomatic complaint of nerve-related pain in the face of a new motor deficit makes for easy diagnosis. Identification of neuropathic pain may not be straightforward. First, neuropathic pain may take on a variety of characteristics, many of which may be difficult for the patient to describe. This further confuses the clinician and delays the correct diagnosis. Second, when faced with the complaint of neuralgia without accompanying motor deficit, the physician must entertain a higher index of clinical suspicion. Reliance on knowledge of the anatomy of nerve contributions from the various dermatomes and myotomes is the key when taking a detailed history of the patient's symptomatic complaint in order to correctly identify where the pathology lies. Frequently, this will require serial examinations of the patient. The subjective complaints on these occasions will include new descriptive characteristics if central sensitization or *wind-up* occurs.

Patients with neuropathic pain may exhibit persistent or paroxysmal pain that is independent of an inciting stimulus. This stimulus-independent pain is usually described as shooting, lancinating, and burning, and may depend on activity of the sympathetic nervous system. The pain complaint may also take on the characteristic of a deep ache, constriction, or band-like sensation, or the feeling of tissue expansion or swelling. Stimulus-evoked pain is a common component of peripheral nerve injury and has two key features which we have previously encountered: *hyperalgesia* and *allodynia*. Hyperalgesia is an increased response to a suprathreshold noxious stimulus and is the result of abnormal processing of nociceptor input. Allodynia is the sensation of pain elicited by a typically non-noxious stimulus.

The treatment of neuropathic pain can be difficult as multiple etiologic mechanisms may be involved. These mechanisms can include an alteration in the number and type of sodium channel receptors along the axon, expression of alpha-adrenergic receptors that renders the nerve sensitive to circulating catecholamines and norepinephrine released from postganglionic sympathetic nerve terminals, disruption of the fiber input into the dorsal horn of the spinal cord responsible for inhibitory pathways, and a myriad of additional mechanisms responsible for chemical and receptor changes in the spinal cord. Unfortunately, there is no treatment known which can neither prevent the development of neuropathic pain nor reliably control established neuropathic pain. Although laboratory investigation and quantitative sensory testing in patients have advanced our knowledge of the mechanisms that produce neuropathic pain, we are lacking in the sensitive and specific diagnostic tools that are needed to reveal the particular pathologic process that is responsible for pain in a particular patient. The responsibility rests with the physician to use the techniques of history, physical examination, and extant diagnostic tools in an appropriate way to identify and treat neuropathic pain.

Diagnosis of Neuropathic Pain

The diagnosis of neuropathic pain lies completely in the patient's subjective complaint of pain, the physical examination, and the clinical suspicion of the physician. Electromyographic (EMG) testing is unreliable for the diagnosis of neuropathic pain, as it tests the integrity only of A-beta fibers, and does not test the function of A-delta or C-fibers, the elements that are responsible for pain transmission. However, as the A-beta fibers are involved in the activation of segmental inhibitory pathways, an abnormal EMG may signify loss of inhibitory control by this pain fiber population. It bears emphasizing that a "normal EMG" does not exclude the diagnosis of neuropathic pain. Other clues, such as the minimal response to opioid medications or a clinical response to empiric therapy with medications directed at the treatment of nerve pain, make the diagnosis in retrospect.

The physical examination of the patient complaining of pain, as is true for any neurologic investigation, should be conducted in a thorough, logical manner. Therefore, it should begin with light touch or stroke of the physician's palpating hand over the affected body region, and progress in a layer-by-layer palpatory fashion; i.e., by subsequently applying more pressure so as to palpate the deeper structures. If pain is elicited by light stroke or mild deformation of the overlying skin, the physical examination should be conducted to identify the total surface area involved that may represent a dermatomal or an irregular shaped peripheral nerve distribution. A stocking-glove distribution may signify a more central neurologic process. An underlying mechanism of injury such as local soft-tissue trauma or more central neurologic process should be sought after. In many cases, the exact cause will go unidentified. Physicians skilled in anatomy and regional anesthesia have the option of "compartmentalizing" a particular nerve or group of nerves with the administration of local anesthetic to aid in the diagnosis. This can be performed as a simple office procedure, or may require the use of fluoroscopy in an operating suite. The underlying cause should be identified and treated accordingly; however, medication management directed toward palliation of symptoms should not be withheld in the meantime.

Treatments for Neuropathic Pain

As a general rule, if neuropathic pain is suspected, medications known to be effective in the treatment of nerve pain should be considered. Strategically selecting any particular agent that would benefit the patient can be difficult due to multiple factors (2,3). However, each situation is different and necessitates a careful assessment and identification of the particular neuropathy involved. Neuropathy may be sensory or motor and, in general, sensory lesions are more frequently transient when compared with motor lesions.

If the symptoms consist of numbness or tingling only (that is, without pain), conservative management would be appropriate, and treatment would not require the use of any medications. It is important both to inform the patient that such neuropathy often resolves postoperatively (84) and to instruct the patient to avoid positions that might compress or stretch the involved nerve. A full neurological examination should be performed and documented in the medical record. If the neuropathy has a motor component, a neurologist should be consulted immediately. EMG studies may not be revealing within the first 14 to 21 days after the initial injury.

Medication Trials
Tricyclic Antidepressants. The tricyclic antidepressants were so named because they are all three-ringed structures with more or less substitution at the middle ring. They are further classified as secondary or tertiary amines based on the terminal substitution of the side chain.

The antidepressant medications are generally well absorbed after oral administration. They undergo extensive first-pass hepatic metabolism and are highly bound to serum proteins. Their elimination half-lives are long and they frequently have active metabolites. These drugs are generally oxidized by hepatic system and conjugated for excretion. Elimination occurs via urine and feces.

The antidepressant medications exert their actions by altering monoamine neurotransmitter activity at the level of the synapse; specifically, they block presynaptic uptake of 5-HT and norepinephrine. It appears that neurotransmitter modulation is the probable mechanism. Review of multiple studies indicates that the antidepressants alone or in combination with other medications can be beneficial to the patient suffering from neuropathic conditions. Therapy with antidepressant medications should begin with the lowest dose, to be taken one to two hours before sleep. The medication can be titrated to clinical effect, and any sign of toxicity should prompt a serum level determination.

Antidepressants can cause a number of side effects such as sedation, dry mouth, and orthostatic hypotension. Abrupt discontinuation of antidepressants can lead to sleep disruption, characterized by vivid and colorful dreams that are usually not dysphoric. The presenting signs of antidepressant overdose are related to the extremes of their sedative effects and their influence on the cardiac conduction system. This is frequently accompanied by significant hypotension that may be unresponsive to IV fluid management.

These medications are used as one part of a comprehensive approach to chronic pain. They have demonstrated analgesic activity, are nonaddicting, and have a myriad of beneficial pharmacologic actions.

Anticonvulsants. The anticonvulsants are a heterogeneous group of drugs used in pain management. Numerous agents, including valproic acid, carbamazepine, clonazepam, gabapentin, topiramate, and tiagabine, have been used in the treatment of neuropathic pain. The mechanisms of action of the drugs for this purpose are not well understood and are probably unique to each drug. They are generally believed to have effects on sodium, calcium, and potassium flux, and some have effects on gamma-amino-butyric acid (GABA) activity. Anticonvulsant medications, and in particular carbamazepine, are considered to be the treatment of choice in trigeminal neuralgia; however, they are used in a variety of neuropathic conditions, with varying levels of success. Newer agents such as topiramate, tiagabine, and zonisamide are receiving clinical attention in antineuralgic therapy because as a group they are more easily titrated (frequent blood levels are not necessary) and have more favorable side effect profiles. Unfortunately, apart from trigeminal neuralgia and its responsiveness to carbamazepine, pharmacotherapy for neuropathic pain has been less than ideal, and it effects are unpredictable due to the multiple underlying mechanisms that may be involved.

Opioids. Although effective for most pain, oral opioids may be only partially effective in the treatment of neuropathic pain. As a result, many patients self-medicate in a desperate attempt to obtain pain relief, with limited success and much grief. Patients often finish their opioid medication prescriptions early, running the risk of becoming unwelcome and stigmatized by the medical profession.

Unremitting pain of this sort has emotional, psychological, and behavioral consequences, and the administration of opioids in these circumstances may be useless or worse. Because of this, and because of the practitioner's confusion and incomplete understanding of neurologic anatomy and the process of central sensitization, the patient is frequently regarded as malingering or somatisizing.

This is not to say that there is no place for opioids in the treatment of chronic, nonmalignant pain. Interestingly, opioids given via the epidural or subarachnoid route behave very differently with respect to onset, duration, and side effects than the same drugs given systemically. Therefore, pain unresponsive to systemic opioids may respond to those same opioids given centrally. In addition, by administering the agent centrally, the dose of opioid can be reduced a 100- or a 1000-fold, reducing many unwanted effects that were unavoidable in doses given systemically.

Advanced Pain Therapies

Spinal cord stimulation for the clinical control of pain was introduced in 1967 by Shealy et al. (89), based on the expectation of effect predicted by the *gate control theory of pain*, published in 1965 by Melzack and Wall (90). The basic premise of Melzack and Wall's theory is that the stimulation of sensory input carried by the large myelinated A-beta fibers, by their earlier arrival at the spinal "gate," suppress or modify information carried by the carrying nerve fibers carrying nociceptive information, such as A-delta and C-fibers. Shealy et al. speculated that if the A-beta fibers of the dorsal columns were electrically stimulated, reception of painful information would be inhibited. They presented the first clinical evidence for electrical stimulation in the treatment of pain. Many theories subsequently have been presented in the literature that postulate the mechanisms underlying the efficacy of spinal cord stimulation. Basically, spinal cord stimulation appears to influence the release of neurotransmitters and neuromodulators, and to play an inhibitory role at sympathetic efferent neurons, which have been shown to promote the maintenance of neuropathic pain. These effects of spinal cord stimulation are seen at both spinal and supraspinal sites. While the exact mechanism of spinal cord stimulation's effects remains obscure, it is clear that the treatment

Table 7 Pain Amenable to Spinal Cord Stimulation

Sympathetically maintained pain
   Causalgia
   Reflex sympathetic dystrophy
Arachnoiditis
Perineural fibrosis/failed back surgery
Radicular pain
Peripheral vascular insufficiency
Phantom limb pain
Deafferentation pain
   Postherpetic neuralgia
   Peripheral neuropathies
   Spinal cord injury
Angina

is effective for a variety of painful neuropathic conditions. Spinal cord stimulation, a form of *neuroaugmentation*, appears to be in favor by pain specialists nowadays, as opposed to older, destructive procedures such as neurolysis. Table 7 illustrates the types of pain amenable to spinal cord stimulation.

Intrathecal Pump

Radiofrequency ablation and *cryodenervation* are methods of applying thermal destruction to a nerve for the treatment of a variety of painful conditions involving peripheral nerves and sympathetic fibers. Both these techniques have had varying degrees of success in the treatment of intercostal neuralgia, painful neuroma, biomechanical spinal pain, peripheral neuropathies, and a variety of cranial and facial pain syndromes. It is essential that the provider of these techniques be fully aware of the regional anatomy required for any specific procedure. These techniques are generally applied to sensory nerve fibers, and not mixed fibers carrying motor and sensory information, as lesioning of the latter can produce profound motor weakness of an extremity or important muscular structure.

Chemical Neurolysis. The provision of neurolytic blockade in patients with chronic nonmalignant pain is controversial. The reappearance of causalgic pain is a feature common to most ablative procedures (85,86). This can be minimized by limiting the selection of patients to those with a short-life expectancy. Here, the patient is unlikely to outlive the duration of pain relief. A potential for damage to nontargeted tissue is of concern with any destructive procedure, though it is less likely to occur when peripheral neurolysis, as opposed to central or deep sympathetic neurolytic blockade, is undertaken. This is particularly true when localization is facilitated by diagnostic electrical stimulation, radiographic guidance, or administration of test doses of local anesthetic (87,88). Peripheral neurolysis has specific but important indications in the management of intractable cancer pain syndromes. It is generally thought inappropriate and inadequate for benign intractable nonmalignant pain.

Summary

Poorly controlled pain following major surgery incites several pathophysiological responses that increase postoperative morbidity, increase the incidence of prolonged rehabilitative pain, and may lead to persistent pain. The development of chronic pain is a tragedy that must be prevented. By assessing the severity and character of the pain stimulus, optimum pain control may be provided at each phase of the recovery process. Analgesic regimens in the acute phase, including opioid infusions, IV- and epidural-PCA, and continuous regional blockade, not only provide effective pain relief and high patient satisfaction, but also lead to improved function, decreased recovery time, and shortened hospitalization. Diagnosis and effective treatment of chronic pain are still in their infancy, but the development of new, creative techniques and the simple application of good medicine are making headway in the care of these disabled patients.

REFERENCES

1. Woolf CJ, Max MB. Mechanism-based pain diagnosis: issues for analgesic drug development. Anesthesiology 2001; 95:241–249.
2. Woolf CJ, Thompson SW. The induction and maintenance of central sensitization is depedent on N-methyl D-aspartic acid receptor activation; implications for the treatment of post-injury pain hypersensitivity states. Pain 1991; 44:293–299.
3. Carr DB. JAMA 1998; 279:1114–1115.
4. Apfelbaum JL, Chen C, Mehta S, et al. Postoperative pain experiences: results from a national survey suggest postoperative pain continues to be undermanaged. Anesth Analg 2003; 97:534–540.
5. Dolin SJ, Cashman JN, Bland JM. Effectiveness of acute postoperative pain management: I: evidence from published data. Br J Anaesth 2002; 89:409–423.
6. Melzack R, Abbott FV, Zackon W, et al. Pain on a surgical ward: a survey of the duration and intensity of pain and the effectiveness of medication. Pain 1987; 29: W67–W72.
7. Belville JW, Forrest WH, Miller E, et al. Influence of age on pain relief from analgesics. J Am Med Assoc 1971; 217:1835–1841.
8. Gagliese L, Jackson M, Ritvo P, et al. Age is not an impediment to effective use of patient controlled analgesia by surgical patients. Anesthesiology 2000; 93:601–610.
9. Macintyre PE, Jarvis DA. Age is the best predictor of postoperative morphine requirements. Pain 64:357–364.
10. Merskey H, Bogduk N, eds. Classification of Chronic Pain: Descriptions of Chronic Pain Syndromes and Definitions of Pain Terms. 2nd ed. Seattle: IASP Press, 1994.
11. Isacson D, Bingefors K. Epidemiology of analgesic use: a gender perspective. Eur J Anesth Suppl 2002; 26:5–15.
12. Merskey H, Bogduk N, eds. Classification of Chronic Pain. 2nd ed. Seattle: IASP Press, 1994.
13. Sullivan MJ, Thorn B, Haythornthwaite JA, et al. Theoretical perspectives on the relation between catastrophizing and pain. Clin J Pain 2001; 17:52–64.

14. Butler RW, Damarin FL, Beaulieu C, et al. Assessing cognitive strategies for acute postsurgical pain. Psychol Assess 1989; 1:41–45.

15. Portenoy RK. Appropriate use of opioids for persistent non-cancer pain. Lancet 2004; 364(9436):739–740.

16. Portenoy RK. Current pharmacotherapy of chronic pain. J Pain Symptom Manage 2000; 19(suppl 1): S16–S20.

17. Portenoy RK. The effect of drug regulation on the management of cancer pain. NYS J Med 1991; 91(suppl 11): 13S–18S.

18. Portenoy RK. Management of common opioid side effects during long term therapy of cancer pain. Ann Acad Med (Singapore) 1994; 23(2):160–170.

19. McMahon SB, Koltzenburg M. Opioids: clinical use. Wall and Melzack's Textbook of Pain. 5th ed. London: Elsevier, 2006:443–457.

20. Lubenow TR, McCarthy RJ, Ivankovich AD. Management of acute postoperative pain. In: Barash PG, Cullen BF, Stoelting RK, eds. Clinical Anesthesia. Philadelphia: JB Lippincott, 1992:1547–1577.

21. Price DD, Dubner R. Neurons that subserve the sensory discriminative aspects of pain. Pain 1977; 3:307.

22. Willis WD. The pain system: the neural basis of nociceptive transmission in the mammalian nervous system. In: Gildenberg PL, ed. Pain and Headache. Vol. 8. Basel: S. Karger, 1985:1547–1577.

23. Price DD, Hayes RL, Ruda M, Dubner R. Spatial and temporal transformations of input to spinothalamic tract neurons and their relation to somatic sensations. J Neurophysiol 1980; 41:933.

24. Salt TE, Hill RG. Transmitter candidates of somatosensory primary afferent fibres. Neuroscience 1983; 10:1083–1103.

25. Woolf CJ, Chong MS. Preemptive analgesia-treating postoperative pain by preventing the establishment of central sensitization. Anesth Analg 1993; 77:362–379.

26. Mannion RJ, Woolf C. Pain mechanisms and management: a central perspective. Clin J Pain 2000; 16(suppl 3): S144–S156.

27. Sang CN. Clinically available glutamate receptor antagonists in neuropathic pain states. In: Sirinathsinghji DJS, Hill RG, eds. NMDA Antagonists as Potential Analgesic Drugs. Basel: Birkhauser, 2002:165–180.

28. McMahon SB, Bennett DLH, Bevan S. Inflammatory mediators and modulators of pain. In: Wall and Melzack's Textbook of Pain. 5th ed. London: Elsevier, 2006:49–71.

29. Berde CB. Pediatric postoperative pain management. Pediatr Clin North Am 1989; 36:921–940.

30. Brown DL, Carpenter RL. Perioperative analgesia: a review of risks and benefits. J Cardiothorac Anesth 1990; 4:368–383.

31. Ali J, Weisel RD, Layug AB, et al. Consequences of postoperative alterations in respiratory mechanics. Am J Surg 1974; 128:376–382.

32. Sinatra RS: Unpublished Observations, 1994–1996, Yale University Acute Pain Service.

33. Grass JA, Sakima NT, Valley M, et al. Assessment of ketorolac as an adjuvant to fentanyl patient-controlled epidural analgesia after radical retropubic prostatectomy. Anesthesiology 1993; 78:642–648.

34. Lubin E. Unpublished Observations, 2000–2001, Yale University Acute and Chronic Pain Service.

35. Abboud TK, Dror A, Mosaad P, et al. Minidose intrathecal morphine for the relief of post-cesarean section pain: safety and efficacy, and ventilatory responses to carbon dioxide. Anesth Analg 1988; 67:137–141.

36. Anand KJS, Hickey PR. Halothane-morphine compared with high dose sufentanil for anesthesia and postoperative analgesia in neonatal cardiac surgery. N Engl J Med 1992; 326:1–9.

37. Beattie WS, Buckley DN, Forrest JB. Epidural morphine reduces the risk of postoperative myocardial ischemia in patients with cardiac risk factors. Can J Anaesth 1993; 40:523–541.

38. Breslow MJ, Jordan DA, Christopherson R, et al. Epidural morphine decreases postoperative hypertension by attenuating sympathetic nervous system hyperactivity. JAMA 1989; 261:3577–3581.

39. Brodsky JB, Chaplan SR, Brose WG, Mark JBD. Continuous epidural hydromorphone for postthoracotomy pain relief. Ann Thorac Surg 1990; 50:888–893.

40. Bromage PR, Camporesi EM, Durant PAC, et al. Nonrespiratory side effects of epidural morphine. Anesth Analg 1982; 61:490–495.

41. Christopherson R, Beattie C, Meinert CL, et al. Perioperative morbidity in patients randomized to epidural or general anesthesia for lower extremity vascular surgery. Anesthesiology 1993; 79:1–12.

42. de Leon-Casasola OA, Parker B, Lema MJ, et al. Postoperative epidural-bupivacaine-morphine therapy: experience with 4,227 surgical cancer patients. Anesthesiology 1994; 81:368–375.

43. Chaplan SR, Duncan SR, Brodsky JB, Brose WG. Morphine and hydromorphone epidural analgesia: a prospective, randomized comparison. Anesthesiology 1992; 77:1090–1094.

44. Ferrante FM, Covino BG. Patient-controlled analgesia: a historical perspective. In: Ferrante FM, Ostheimer GW, Covino BG, eds. Patient-Controlled Analgesia. Boston: Blackwell Scientific, 1990.

45. El-Baz NMI, Faber LP, Jensik RJ. Continuous epidural infusion of morphine for treatment of pain after thoracic surgery: a new technique. Anesth Analg 1984; 63:757–764.

46. Geller E, Chrubasik J, Graf R, et al. A randomized double-blind comparison of epidural sufentanil versus intravenous sufentanil or epidural fentanyl analgesia after major abdominal surgery. Anesth Analg 1993; 76:1243–1250.

47. Glass PSA, Estok P, Ginsberg B, et al. Use of patient-controlled analgesia to compare the efficacy of epidural to intravenous fentanyl administration. Anesth Analg 1992; 74:345–351.

48. Grass JA, Zuckerman RL, Sakima NT, Harris AP. Patient controlled analgesia after cesarean delivery-epidural sufentanil versus intravenous morphine. Reg Anesth 1994; 19:90–97.

49. Gwirtz KH, Young JV, Walker SG, et al. Intrathecal opioid analgesia for acute postoperative pain: experience with 4,134 surgical patients. Anesthesiology 1995; 83:A780.

50. Parker RK, White PF. Epidural patient-controlled analgesia: an alternative to intravenous patient-controlled analgesia for pain relief after cesarean delivery. Anesth Analg 1992; 75:245–251.

51. Sinatra RS, Sevarino FB, Paige D, et al. Patient-controlled analgesia with sufentanil: a comparison of

epidural versus intravenous administration. J Clin Anesth 1996; 8:123–129.

52. Woolf CJ, Chong MS. Preemptive analgesia-treating postoperative pain by preventing the establishment of central sensitization. Anesth Analg 1993; 77:362–379.

53. Cousins MJ. Acute pain and the injury response: immediate and prolonged effects. Reg Anesth 1989; 16:162–176.

54. Kehlet H. Modification of responses to surgery by neural blockade: clinical implications. In: Cousins MJ, Bridenbaugh PO, eds. Neural Blockade in Clinical Anesthesia and Management of Pain. Philadelphia: Lippincott, 1987.

55. Liu S, Carpenter RL, Mackey DC, et al. Effects of perioperative analgesic technique on rate of recovery after colon surgery. Anesthesiology 1995; 83:757–765.

56. Stevens DS, Dunn WT. Acute pain management for the trauma patient. In: Sinatra RS, Hord AH, Ginsberg B, Preble LM, eds. Acute Pain Mechanisms and Management. St Louis: Mosby Yearbook, 1992.

57. Modig J, Malmberg P, Karlstrom G. Effect of epidural versus general anesthesia on calf blood flow. Acta Anesthesiol Scand 1980; 24:305–311.

58. Scott DA, Beilby DS, McClymont C. Postoperative analgesia using epidural infusions of fentanyl with bupivacaine. Anesthesiology 1995; 83:727–737.

59. Yeager MP, Glass DG, Neff RK. Epidural anesthesia and analgesia in high-risk surgical patients. Anesthesiology 1987; 66:729–736.

60. Dhuner KG. Nerve injury following operations: survey of cases and occurring during a 6-year period. Anesthesiology 1950; 11:202–207.

61. Kroll DA, Caplan RA, Posner K, Ward RJ, Cheney FW. Nerve injury associated with anesthesia. Anesthesiology 1990; 73:202–207.

62. Cousins M, Mather L. Intrathecal and epidural administration of opioids. Anesthesiology 1984; 1:276–310.

63. Seyfer AE, Grammar NY, Bogumill GP, Provost JM, Chaudry U. Upper extremity neuropathies after cardiac surgery. J Hand Surg 1985; 10:16–19.

64. Casscells CD, Lindsey RW, Ebersole J, Li B. Ulnar neuropathy after median sternotomy. Clin Orth Rel Res 1993; 291:259–265.

65. Vahl CF, Carl I, Muller-Vahl H, Struck E. Brachial plexus injury after cardiac surgery: the role of internal mammary artery preparation: a prospective study of 1,000 consecutive patients. J Thoracic Cardiovasc Surg 1991; 102:724–729.

66. Roy RC, Stafford MA, Charlton JE. Nerve injury and musculoskeletal complaints after cardiac surgery: influence the internal mammary artery dissection and left arm position. Anesth Analg 1998; 67:277–279.

67. Martin JT. The ventral decubitus (prone) positions. Positioning in Anesthesia and Surgery. 3rd ed. Philadelphia: Saunders, 1997:155–195.

68. Kroll DA, Caplan RA, Posner K, Ward RJ, Cheney FW. Nerve injury associated with ancsthesia. Anesthesiology 1990; 73:202–207.

69. Warner MA, Warner ME, Martin JT. Ulnar neuropathy: incidence, outcome, and risk factors in sedated or anesthetized patients. Anesthesiology 1994; 81: 1332–1340.

70. Cunningham J, Temple WJ, Mitchell P, Nixon JA, Preshaw RM, Hagen NA. Cooperative hernia study. Pain in the postoperative patient. Ann Surg 1996; 224:598–602.

71. Lichtenstein IL, Shulman AG, Amid PK, Montlor MM. Cause and prevention of post herniorrhaphy neuralgia: a proposed protocol for treatment. Am J Surg 1998; 155:786–790.

72. Kark AE, Kurzer M, Waters KJ. Tension-free mesh hernia repair: review of 1098 cases effect local anesthesia in a day unit. Ann R Coll Surg Engl 1995; 77: 299–304.

73. Heise CP, Starling JR. Mesh inguinodynia: a new clinical syndrome after inguinal herniorrhaphy? J Am Coll Surg 1998; 187:514–518.

74. Callesen T, Bech K, Neilsen R, et al. Pain after groin hernia repair. Br J Surg 1998; 85:1412–1414.

75. Barth RJ Jr, Burchard KW, Tosteson A, et al. Short term outcome after mesh or shouldice herniorrhaphy: a randomized, prospective study. Surgery 1998; 123:121–126.

76. Buckhart FL, Daly JW. Sciatic and peroneal nerve injury: a complication of vaginal operations. Obstet Gynecol 1966; 28:99–102.

77. Rose HA, Hood RW, Otis JC, Ranawat CS, Insall JN. Peroneal nerve palsy following total knee arthroplasty: a review of the Hospital for Special Surgery experience. J Bone Joint Surg Am 1982; 64:347–351.

78. James SE, Wade PJ. Lateral popliteal nerve palsy as a complication of the use of a continuous passive motion knee machine-a case report. Injury 1987; 18:72–73.

79. Weber ER, Daube JR, Coventry MB. Peripheral neuropathies associated with total hip arthroplasty. J Bone Joint Surg Am 1976; 58:66–69.

80. Warner MA, Martin JT, Schroeder DR. Offord KP, Chute CG. Lower extremity motor neuropathy associated with surgery performed on patients a lithotomy position. Anesthesiology 1994; 81:6–12.

81. Dornette WH. Compression neuropathies: medical aspects and legal implications. Int Anesthesiol Clin 1986 (Winter); 24:201–229.

82. Rosenblum J, Schwartz GA, Bendler E. Femoral neuropathy-a neurological complication of hysterectomy. JAMA 1966; 195:409–414.

83. X-femoral neuropathy and type II diabetics.

84. Warner MA, Warner DO, Matsumoto JY, Schroeder DR, Offord KP, Maxson PM. Ulnar neuropathy in surgical patients [abstract]. Anesthesiology 1996; 85(suppl):A921.

85. Patt R. Neurosurgical interventions for chronic pain problems. Anesth Clin N Am 1987; 5:609.

86. Ramamurthy S, Walsh NE, Schoenfeld LS, et al. Evaluation of neurolytic blocks using phenol and cryogenic block in the management of chronic pain. J Pain Symptom Manage 1989; 4(2):72–75.

87. Pender JW, Pugh DG. Diagnostic and therapeutic nerve blocks: necessity for roentgenograms. JAMA 1951; 146:798.

88. Raj PP, Rosenblatt R, Montgomery S. Uses of the nerve stimulator for peripheral blocks. Reg Anesth 1980; 5:14.

89. Shealy CN, Mortimer JT, Reswick J. Electrical inhibition of pain by stimulation of the dorsal column: preliminary clinical reports. Anesth Analg 1967; 46:489–491.

90. Melzack R, Wall P. Pain mechanisms: a new theory. Science 1965; 150:971–978.

91. Graves DA et al. Ann Intern Med 1983; 99:360–366.

92. Bach S, Noreng MF, Tjellden NU. Phantom limb pain in amputees during the first 12 months following limb amputation after preoperative lumbar epidural blockade. Pain 1988; 33:297–301.

38

Complications After Craniotomy

Andrew Jea and Nizam Razack

*Department of Neurological Surgery, University of Miami Miller School of Medicine,
Miami, Florida, U.S.A.*

The care of a patient with head injury can be particularly intimidating to the uninitiated physician. The severe nature of an extensive neurologic insult requires that the patient receive care in the intensive care unit. This chapter will describe the most common complications that occur after a patient undergoes a craniotomy: mass lesions, central nervous system infections, cerebral infarctions, and neurogenic metabolic imbalances. The chapter will also include an algorithm for managing complications after craniotomy.

MASS LESIONS
Hematoma

Before patients undergo intracranial procedures, their clotting ability should be carefully evaluated. Platelet counts should exceed 100,000 and the platelets should be functional. Essential screening tests include prothrombin time, partial thromboplastin, and international normalized ratio. It is essential that dissemination intravascular coagulation, if present, be detected during or prior to surgery (1,2).

A postoperative hematoma may be extra-axial, occurring in the epidural or subdural space (Fig. 1), or intra-axial, occurring within the parenchyma of the brain (3,4). The clinical presentation of these lesions is not specific, and both should be included in the differential diagnosis for postoperative patients who become increasingly lethargic and exhibit focal signs such as hemiparesis, aphasia, cranial nerve palsy (5), or seizure. Changes in vital signs, such as Cushing's triad (hypertension, bradycardia, and abnormal respiratory pattern), may reflect increasing intracranial pressure (ICP) (6,7).

The routine technical use of tack-up sutures to surrounding bone structures reduces the occurrence of epidural hematoma. Waxing the bone edges is also fundamental. Follow-up computed tomography (CT) scans after surgery should not show depression of the dura. In ideal circumstances, the goal of closure is to reduce the dead space in the epidural compartment.

Achieving hemostasis before closing the dura is essential. Occasionally a subdural drain is necessary when oozing cannot be controlled despite all efforts. Some subdural hematomas resolve spontaneously after surgery, but others may cause significant mass effect and require reexploration and drainage.

Intraparenchymal hematomas develop at the point of maximal dissection or retraction (8). These hematomas are common after biopsy or resection of tumors (Fig. 2). Increasing the patient's blood pressure intraoperatively may help identify potential sources of hemorrhage.

Hematomas are usually treated by reexploration and evacuation of the mass lesion. Their development is usually recognized by bedside evaluation. Determining the anatomic location of the hematoma—epidural,

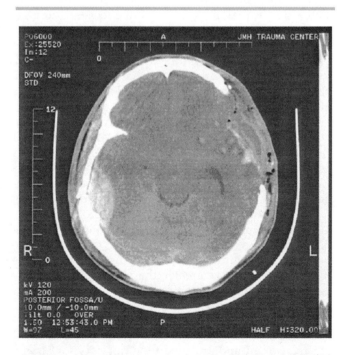

Figure 1 Development of right temporoparietal epidural hematoma after evacuation of left subdural hematoma and decompressive craniectomy.

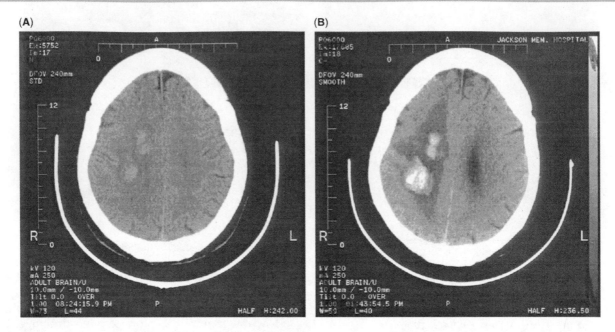

Figure 2   **(A)** Computed tomography scan of brain immediately after stereotactic biopsy of right parietal high-grade glioma. **(B)** Blossoming of intraparenchymal hematoma two hours after stereotactic biopsy of right parietal high-grade glioma.

subdural, or intracerebral—is unimportant during the initial examination (8–11). A CT scan should be obtained if a developing hematoma is suspected and the patient's condition is stable enough to permit a rapid work-up (12). However, if the patient's condition is rapidly deteriorating, the more prudent course may be immediate exploration after localization of the lesion by a brief but precise neurologic examination.

Regardless of whether the patient has to undergo CT scanning or emergent reexploration, some steps can be taken immediately to increase the patient's tolerance of the suspected mass lesion (13). Mannitol is an effective osmotic agent and will rapidly decrease ICP (14–20). It is given as an initial intravenous bolus of 1 to 1.5 g/kg body weight with subsequent doses of 0.5 g/kg body weight every four hours (9). Measuring serum osmolarity is important for avoiding a hyperosmolar state with the potential for severe metabolic derangements and acute renal failure. Because of this danger, mannitol should be infused through a central line to allow rapid resuscitation should the effects of mannitol become supratherapeutic (21). Mannitol should be discontinued if the serum osmolarity is greater than 320 mOsm because the effect of mannitol, as an osmotic agent, plateaus when the serum osmolarity exceeds this level (22).

Patients whose neurological condition is deteriorating and whose level of consciousness is decreasing require an endotracheal tube not only for airway protection, but also for allowing hyperventilation (9,16,23–26). Monitoring arterial blood gases is essential, and the ventilator setting should be adjusted to keep the patient hyperventilated with a partial pressure of carbon dioxide level between 30 and 35 torr (15,24,27,28).

If an extraventricular drain is in place, it may be opened to allow cerebrospinal fluid (CSF) to drain at a constant height above the ear (5 to 10 cm should suffice). This procedure will result in decompression but not in overdrainage (29–41).

Although postoperatively the patient's condition may deteriorate as the result of a hematoma, such deterioration may also be caused by brain edema or infarct, neither of which requires or responds to reexploration. For this reason, CT scanning is valuable when the patient's condition is stable enough to allow it.

The patient whose condition deteriorates many days or weeks after craniotomy may have a chronic subdural hematoma (9,42). This lesion appears on CT scan as a lucent, subdural mass lesion and can be drained by burr holes with gentle aspiration, provided that the collection is not associated with enclosing membranes, which may be detected on a CT scan with contrast (43). A chronic subdural hematoma with membranes can be evacuated only by full craniotomy. If the subdural hematoma appears isodense on CT scan, the dense, acute clot is at an intermediate stage of liquefaction before acquiring the final lucent, liquid appearance of the chronic subdural hematoma (29). The presence of a chronic subdural hematoma is suggested by clinical changes and by the appearance on a CT scan of a mass effect, i.e., a midline shift with ventricular collapse and sulcus effacement. Such a hematoma can usually be evacuated by burr holes (44).

Brain Edema

When brain edema (45) occurs during the postoperative period, its cause may be excessive retraction or intraoperative trauma (46). On CT scan, brain edema appears as an area of decreased density associated with brain shift. Brain edema is commonly associated with intracerebral hemorrhage and contusion. Edema associated with cerebral infarction generally indicates a severe stroke and may lead to herniation. All of these causes may be seen during the postoperative period. Edema often accompanies neoplastic lesions and is more commonly associated with metastatic tumors.

The treatment of brain edema depends on the cause of the lesion. Lesions caused by neoplasia or inflammation respond to treatment with steroids. The role of steroids in treating edema caused by trauma, infarction, or anoxia is unproven (47–50). In fact, using steroids in these settings may actually increase morbidity and mortality by increasing risk of septic complications or gastrointestinal hemorrhage. Brain edema that occurs after surgery for trauma, infarction, or hemorrhage represents increased tissue water. It exerts a mass effect and will usually be accompanied by an increase in ICP. This vasogenic edema is best treated with an intravenous infusion of mannitol. The typical dosage is an initial bolus of 1 g/kg followed by a maintenance dose of 0.5 g/kg every four hours, not to exceed a serum osmolarity of 320 mOsm (51).

Pneumocephalus

Pneumocephalus is simply the accumulation of air in the intracranial spaces. It commonly occurs after craniotomy if the air is not completely evacuated before the bone flap is replaced. It may also occur after a traumatic basilar skull fracture when air is introduced into the subarachnoid space by communication with the exterior environment, usually through the ethmoid, sphenoid, or frontal sinuses. Pneumocephalus may cause a patient to become lethargic and confused (52). A CT scan may show the accumulation of air beneath a bone flap or in communication with one of the sinuses (53). Most cases of pneumocephalus are treated with 100% oxygen by a non-rebreather mask, followed by keeping the patient in a completely flat position. Tension pneumocephalus marked by an enlarging pocket of air causing mass effect (midline shift, sulcal effacement, or both) demands more aggressive and invasive intervention. Emergency surgery is necessary to resolve the mass effect.

Pneumocephalus indicates communication between the exterior environment and the intracranial cavity. This condition can be a precursor of CSF leakage. CSF may drain through the ethmoid or sphenoid sinus complex, causing rhinorrhea, or through the mastoid air cells, causing otorrhea. Although pneumocephalus indicates a tear in the dura, a CSF leak indicates a relatively large dural tear allowing a stream of CSF to flow. CSF may also leak from the scalp suture line; the flow of CSF to the external environment should stop after a watertight closure has been established by oversewing the suture line. When rhinorrhea or otorrhea occurs postoperatively, it should be treated conservatively with a lumbar drain. The drain should be opened and the height should be adjusted to allow a flow of 10 to 15 cc/hr for three to five days. Before the lumbar drain is removed, it should be clamped for 24 hours to determine whether any further drainage from the nose or ear will occur. If a seal is not accomplished after 10 to 14 days of conservative treatment, surgical intervention is necessary. The use of antibiotics to treat pneumocephalus alone or pneumocephalus with subsequent CSF leak is controversial. Treatment with antibiotics should not be initiated unless signs and symptoms of CSF infection develop. Prophylactic treatment with antibiotics should be initiated only if the patient has sinusitis.

Hydrocephalus

Hydrocephalus or a loculated ("trapped") ventricle may cause symptoms resembling those caused by focal, expanding mass lesions. A loculated ventricle occurs when the drainage pathway from one lateral ventricle into the third ventricle is blocked. In the postoperative period, this blockage typically results from unilateral intraventricular hemorrhage, which causes a blood clot at the foramen of Monro, or from a midline shift, which causes a block at the foramen of Monro by obliteration. The patient will become lethargic and will demonstrate progressive signs of hemiparesis consistent with that caused by a hemispheric mass lesion. Hydrocephalus can be diagnosed by CT scan; diagnosis must be followed by permanent drainage of the loculus. The treatment of choice is emergent ventriculostomy and placement of a shunt.

There are two primary types of hydrocephalus: communicating and noncommunicating. Communicating hydrocephalus blocks the reabsorption of CSF downstream from the foramen of Luschka to its point of reabsorption through the arachnoid villi into the major venous sinuses. The point of obstruction may be at the tentorial incisure as the result of scarring from meningitis or damage to the arachnoid granulations. The most common cause of communicating hydrocephalus in the postoperative period is the blockage of absorption pathways by subarachnoid blood. Communicating hydrocephalus causes the patient's condition to deteriorate slowly, generally over a period of days. No focal signs are usually present; the patient may exhibit gait ataxia, difficulty with memory, or urinary incontinence. A CT scan shows universal dilation of all ventricles. Lumbar puncture may demonstrate a high opening pressure. The CSF may be xanthochromic with a high protein level, indicating the viscous nature of the fluid and the potential problem in filtering it through the arachnoid villi. Serial lumbar punctures may be performed as a temporizing measure to diagnose and treat communicating hydrocephalus. If the patient's neurological condition improves after lumbar puncture, definitive treatment by shunting may be required.

Any lesion that causes an obstruction at the narrow fourth-ventricular inflow or outflow track can create noncommunicating or obstructive hydrocephalus. Such lesions include cerebellar edema or infarct after surgery to the posterior fossa or an intraventricular blood clot in the fourth ventricle. It is often difficult to determine the pathophysiologic cause of hydrocephalus; however, resolution is the primary focus of treatment. Noncommunicating hydrocephalus usually causes rapid deterioration of the patient's condition. The patient may at first be agitated but then enters a comatose state. Sedating a patient who is agitated after craniotomy without first ruling out hydrocephalus as the cause of this alteration in mental status is a common fatal mistake because sedation masks the increase in ICP and the eventual herniation. Therefore, patients at risk of blockage of CSF flow, such as those who have recently undergone surgery to the posterior fossa or those with intraventricular hemorrhage, require more careful, anticipatory observation for the signs of deterioration caused by acute hydrocephalus. A ventriculostomy kit should be placed at the bedside of the patient so that immediate decompression can be provided if necessary. In contrast to patients who have a communicating hydrocephalus, patients with an obstructive hydrocephalus can never be safely treated with lumbar puncture because the pressure gradient created by this procedure places the patient at risk of tonsillar herniation and sudden death. The patient may be temporarily stabilized with a ventriculostomy to provide decompression by draining CSF out of the intracranial cavity. Permanent shunt placement is the definitive treatment for obstructive hydrocephalus.

Obstructive hydrocephalus is commonly associated with lesions of the posterior fossa and is a dreaded complication of surgical procedures to this area of the brain. After surgery to the posterior fossa, obstructive hydrocephalus must be considered as dangerous a complication as postoperative hematoma.

INFECTION
Meningitis

Meningitis is an infection of the leptomeninges (the pia and the arachnoid) and thus of the subarachnoid space (54). This space is continuous from the hemispheric convexities to the lumbosacral subarachnoid space. Infection of the subarachnoid space can be diagnosed by sampling the CSF through a lumbar puncture. Infection localized to the subdural space (subdural empyema) may leave the ventricular and lumbar fluids sterile with little more than a parameningeal

reaction or reactive pleocytosis. The same is true of cerebritis and brain abscess, unless there is erosion into the ventricular system or the subarachnoid space.

Meningitis typically causes high fever, meningismus, positive Kernig's and Brudzinski's signs, headache, a depressed level of consciousness, seizures, syndrome of inappropriate antidiuretic hormone (SIADH) secretion, and, in severe advanced cases, diabetes insipidus (DI). Meningitis may occur as late as four weeks after surgery because of violation of mastoid air cells in the face of a CSF leak. After craniotomy, the patient's preoperative depressed level of consciousness may persist, rendering the patient unable to complain of headaches; the patient may also be predisposed to seizures or meningeal irritation as the result of blood in the subarachnoid spaces after the surgical procedure. Unfortunately, after craniotomy the patient may exhibit all of the clinical signs of an aseptic meningitis, including fever; therefore, the diagnosis may depend entirely upon examination of CSF and careful observation.

The manifestations of postoperative meningitis are often much more subtle than those of the typical pneumococcal or meningococcal variety. If signs of meningeal irritation should occur in isolation or in association with any other changes, neurologic or metabolic, examination of the CSF is mandatory before any antibiotics are administered. Because cell count, glucose concentration, and protein concentration are abnormal after craniotomy, an absolute diagnosis must await the result of CSF culture or the demonstration of bacteria on gram stain. Empiric treatment with broad-spectrum intravenous antibiotics should be started while the results of culture are awaited. Therapy directed at gram-positive cocci and gram-negative organisms must be instituted. The antibiotic regimen should then be tailored once the final culture results and sensitivities have been obtained.

Ventriculitis

The clinical picture of ventriculitis differs little from that of meningitis, although the presentation is usually much more subtle. Meningeal symptoms may be minimal and fever variable, whereas alteration in mental status and neurologic function predominate. Diagnosis requires careful observation; the only diagnostic test is microscopic and bacteriologic examination of the ventricular fluid.

Both meningitis and ventriculitis tend to occur in the postoperative period more than three days after violation and contamination of the subarachnoid or ventricular space. The usual postoperative effects of operative trauma and brain edema begin to resolve during this period. Any reversal in this pattern of healing should alert the clinician to infection in one of these spaces. Both meningitis and ventriculitis may be associated with elevated ICP, and infection should be considered in a patient with increasing ICP, especially if the elevation has no clear or reasonable cause and if no mass effect is visible on CT scan.

Again, selecting a treatment regimen depends on the results of CSF cultures and sensitivities. In the meantime, the intrathecal administration of antibiotics may be considered so as to provide broad-spectrum coverage. The antibiotic regimen can be tailored once the results of final cultures and sensitivities have been obtained.

Abscess

Brain abscess (55)—or its immediate precursor, cerebritis—is relatively rare in the postoperative period. The development of meningeal signs or infected CSF in the face of focal deficits suggests that this process must be ruled out. The absence of focal deficit does not rule out the presence of abscess.

If an abscess does not communicate with the ventricular or subarachnoid space, meningeal signs will usually be absent. In 95% of cases of cerebral abscesses, the CSF may be completely normal and the patient can be afebrile. As is the case with meningitis or ventriculitis, steroids may suppress or delay neurologic change in the developing abscess; therefore, abscess must be considered when a patient's condition worsens after discontinuation of steroids.

The treatment (55) of brain abscess is the same as that of any other abscess: incision and drainage. This procedure is also diagnostic. Needle aspiration combined with the administration of high-dose antibiotics will clear approximately 80% to 85% of abscesses. The remainder will require craniotomy for complete cure. If infection also involves the craniotomy flap, then reoperation, bone flap removal, and drainage of the abscess should be carried out for definitive therapy. The increased use of intraventricular antibiotics in the past decade has provided an effective means of treating certain forms of infection, especially meningitis and ventriculitis caused by highly resistant gram-positive and gram-negative organisms.

Subdural Empyema

Subdural empyema is a specific form of abscess (56,57). This entity is also marked by neurologic deterioration, with the development of focal signs of hemiparesis, seizures, or both. The seizures associated with subdural empyema tend to begin focally, then become generalized, and then quickly progress to status epilepticus. These neurologic findings are related to mass effect from edema. Unlike subdural hematomas, subdural empyemas are associated with edema that is out of proportion to the volume of fluid in the subdural space.

Subdural empyema is rare after craniotomy but may follow burr hole drainage of a chronic subdural hematoma. Most subdural empyemas are associated with chronic sinusitis in adults or with middle ear infections in young children and infants.

Diagnosis by CT scan may be difficult and a high index of suspicion is required. However, a parafalcine subdural collection, which can be seen on CT scan, is pathognomonic of subdural abscess.

Inflammatory effects are predominant and treatment with drainage and antibiotics are the gold standard. The drugs and doses are the same as those recommended for meningitis, which may also be present. Drainage may be accomplished by reoperation or burr holes, and many surgeons recommend placing subdural catheters for irrigation of this space with antibiotic solutions such as concentrated bacitracin.

INFARCTIONS
Arterial Infarcts

Infarctions resulting from occlusion of the arterial vascular supply are most commonly associated with atherosclerotic disease. Arterial infarct is a rare complication after craniotomy but may occur if there has been substantial intraoperative manipulation of cerebral vessels (7,16,58–60). Intraoperative coagulation or ligation of bleeding vessels in patients without good collateral circulation leads to postoperative infarction. An intraoperative angiogram may be obtained to predict the deficits that the patient is expected to have in the postoperative period as the result of the arterial territory loss. A CT scan performed in the immediate postoperative period may not show areas of infarct; however, a second CT scan 24 to 48 hours later will show areas of hypodensity representing infarct (61). Clinically, the patient will usually exhibit focal neurological deficits. If a large area or bilateral areas of the brain are involved, the patient may experience a global decrease in level of consciousness and more extensive neurologic deficits. If the stroke is detected early, an attempt to save the penumbra should be made by improving blood flow through collateral vessels to keep the patient euvolemic, hypertensive, and anticoagulated.

Any involvement of the arteries serving the cerebellum may lead to a cerebellar infarct; thus, immediate neurosurgical attention is necessary. Cerebellar infarction places the patient at high risk of obstructive hydrocephalus as the cerebellar swelling continues to deform and occlude the fourth ventricle. In the conscious patient, there is an orderly progression of clinical signs and symptoms. Symptoms and signs related to cerebellar dysfunction, such as dizziness, vertigo, nausea, vomiting, truncal ataxia, nystagmus, and dysarthria, appear first. Next, the patient may suffer from the onset of hydrocephalus with symptoms of headaches, agitation, and finally obtundation. The patient suffers a palsy of the sixth cranial nerve that cannot be overcome by doll's eye maneuver, followed by a peripheral deficit of the seventh cranial nerve, resulting in hemifacial weakness. The development of cranial dysfunction necessitates neurosurgical intervention for decompression of the posterior fossa.

Venous Infarcts

Venous infarcts are generally seen after craniotomy, especially if the venous sinuses are involved in the surgical field. Repair of dural sinus lacerations or prolonged compression of a sinus by an extrinsic force places the patient at risk of venous sinus thrombosis and infarction postoperatively (62).

In the conscious patient, thrombosis results in symptoms that include headache, nausea, vomiting, seizures, and symptoms resembling those caused by pseudotumor cerebri. Cerebral venous thrombosis and/or dural sinus thrombosis can lead to venous infarction (63). This infarction may be hemorrhagic and often involves the subcortical white matter and traverses the typical arteriovascular boundaries seen on CT scan. In the absence of hemorrhage, the patient should be kept euvolemic to hypervolemic to prevent further exacerbation of thrombosis in the dehydrated state.

The component of hemorrhage or significant mass effect resulting from edema becomes a neurosurgical emergency. Evacuation of the clot may be necessary, as may decompressive craniectomy to reduce the increase of ICP in a patient whose condition is deteriorating.

METABOLIC IMBALANCES
Hyponatremia

Sodium imbalance is the most common metabolic disturbance experienced by a neurosurgical patient. Electrolyte levels should be checked daily after craniotomy until the levels are stable. Sodium concentrations outside the normal physiological range lead to a decreased level of consciousness, disorientation, seizures, and global encephalopathy. After craniotomy, low sodium concentrations may be attributable to cerebral salt wasting (CSW) or SIADH.

CSW is a condition in which an unknown mechanism, currently believed to be a signal for overproduction of atrial natriuretic protein (ANP), causes a natriuresis or overexcretion of sodium into the urine. This condition causes the body to respond to hypovolemia by increasing the secretion of antidiuretic hormone (ADH). Water is reabsorbed from the effects of ADH, whereas sodium continues to be excreted under the influence of ANP, thus resulting in a hyponatremic state. In contrast, SIADH causes water to be reabsorbed despite a euvolemic or hypervolemic state, thus also resulting in hyponatremia.

It is important to differentiate between the two mechanisms of hyponatremia because they require different treatments. CSW causes the urine electrolytes to show an inappropriately high content of sodium. The patient may have clinical signs and symptoms of dehydration, along with a high serum osmolality. Treatment of this condition involves a combination of fluid restriction and replacement of intravascular volume with a colloid solution high in sodium content, most commonly albumin. Replacing the intravascular volume with colloid breaks the vicious cycle of ADH secretion.

SIADH (7,9) causes a hypervolemic state and may produce the clinical signs and symptoms of low serum osmolality. Urine electrolyte levels will show a high sodium concentration, but not as high as that seen with CSW. The treatment is strict restriction of parenterally and enterally administered fluids.

The use of hypertonic saline should be considered for cases in which hyponatremia continues to progress despite the initiation of fluid restriction, the infusion of colloid, or both. The crystalloid solution should be administered at a rate of 20 to 30 cc/hr, and sodium levels should be checked frequently. A too rapid correction of sodium levels may lead to the devastating complication of central pontine myelinolysis. Sodium concentrations should be corrected to 126 mEq/L with hypertonic saline.

Hyponatremia after craniotomy is usually temporary. It is important to support the patient until his own physiologic mechanisms of dealing with sodium balance return to full function.

Hypernatremia

After craniotomy, hypernatremia frequently occurs with dysfunction of the hypothalamic or pituitary axis resulting from inadvertent manipulation of these areas during surgery. This dysfunction results in DI (64), which causes too much water to be lost in the urine and produces a high serum sodium concentration as the result of inadequate production of ADH. Postoperatively, DI may be diagnosed by using three criteria: (i) urine output of more than 250 cc/hr for two consecutive hours; (ii) an increasing serum sodium concentration higher than 145 mEq/L; and (iii) specific gravity of the urine below 1.005. Continued DI should be managed by administering a hypotonic saline solution delivered at a rate higher than that used for maintenance intravenous fluids. The urine output should be replaced cubic centimeter per cubic centimeter hourly up to a maximum of 250 cc. A conscious patient should be allowed to drink water in an amount equaling that of the urine output.

Aqueous pitressin should be used only if the DI is refractory to intravenous fluid therapy or if the patient gets tired of drinking large volumes of water and is unable to keep up with the urine output. A one-time subcutaneous injection of five units of aqueous pitressin should be administered with continued close monitoring of sodium concentrations and urine output. If the DI continues, another injection of aqueous pitressin may be administered. The goal is a slow, gradual correction of the serum sodium concentration. Correcting hypernatremia too rapidly may result in lethal brain edema.

After craniotomy, patients are expected to experience only a temporary problem with hypernatremia unless the pituitary stalk or posterior lobe of the pituitary has been completely destroyed. Once the stunned pituitary recovers function, the hypernatremia is expected to resolve.

REFERENCES

1. Clark JA, Finelli RE, Netsky MG. Disseminated intravascular coagulation following cranial trauma. Case report. J Neurosurg 1980; 52:266–269.
2. Pitts LH. Comment on "The incidence and significance of hemostatic abnormalities in patients with head injuries." Neurosurgery 1989; 24:832.
3. Ribas GC, Jane JA. Traumatic contusions and intracerebral hematomas. J Neurotrauma 1992; 9:S265–S278.
4. Miller JD, Murray LS, Teasdale GM. Development of a traumatic intracerebral hematoma after a "minor" head injury. Neurosurgery 1990; 27:669–673.
5. Marshall LF, Barba D, Toold BM, Bowers SA. The oval pupil: clinical significance and relationship to intracranial hypertension. J Neurosurg 1983; 58:566–568.
6. Savitz SI. Cushing's contributions to neuroscience, part 1: through the looking glass. Neuroscientist 2000; 6:411–414.
7. Savitz SI. Cushing's contributions to neuroscience, part 2: Cushing and several dwarfs. Neuroscientist 2001; 7:469–473.
8. Lobato RD, Rivas JJ, Gomez PA, et al. Head-injured patients who talk and deteriorate into coma. Analysis of 211 cases studied with computerized tomography. J Neurosurg 1991; 75:256–261.
9. Miller SM. Management of central nervous system injuries. In: Turndorf H, Capan LM, Miller SM, eds. Trauma: Anesthesia and Intensive Care. Philadelphia: JB Lippincott Co., 1991;321–355.
10. Rockswold GL, Pheley PJ. Patients who talk and deteriorate. Ann Emerg Med 1993; 22:1004–1007.
11. Andrews BT. Management of delayed posttraumatic intracerebral hemorrhage. Contemp Neurosurg 1988; 10:1.
12. Wilberger JE Jr, Rothfus WE, Tabas J, Goldberg AL, Deeb ZL. Acute tissue tear hemorrhages of the brain: computed tomography and clinicopathological correlations. Neurosurgery 1990; 27:208–213.
13. Woster PS, LeBlanc KL. Management of elevated intracranial pressure. Clin Pharm 1990; 9:762–772.
14. Muizelaar JP, Lutz HA, Becker DP. Effect of mannitol on ICP and CBF and correlation with pressure autoregulation in severely head-injured patients. J Neurosurg 1984; 61:700–706.
15. Rosner MJ, Daughton S. Cerebral perfusion pressure management in head injury. J Trauma 1990; 30:933–940.
16. Rosner MJ, Coley I. Cerebral perfusion pressure: a hemodynamic mechanism of mannitol and the postmannitol hemogram. Neurosurgery 1987; 21:147–156.
17. Bouma GJ, Muizelaar JP, Bandoh K, Marmarou A. Blood pressure and intracranial pressure-volume dynamic in severe head injury: relationship with cerebral blood flow. J Neurosurg 1992; 77:15–19.
18. Cruz J, Minoja G, Okuchi K, Facco E. Successful use of the new high-dose mannitol treatment in patients with Glasgow Coma Scale scores of 3 and bilateral abnormal papillary widening: a randomized trial. J Neurosurg 2004; 100:376–383.
19. Muizelaar JP, Wei EP, Kantos HA, Becker DP. Mannitol causes compensatory cerebral vasoconstriction and vasodilation in response to blood viscosity changes. J Neurosurg 1983; 59:822–828.
20. Schrot RJ, Muizelaar JP. Mannitol in acute traumatic brain injury. Lancet 2002; 359:1633–1634.

21. Burke AM, Quest DO, Chien S, Cerri C. The effects of mannitol on blood viscosity. J Neurosurg 1981; 55:550–553.
22. Marshall LF, Smith RW, Rauscher LA, Shapiro HM. Mannitol dose requirements in brain-injured patients. J Neurosurg 1978; 48:169–172.
23. Diringer MN, Videen TO, Yundt K, et al. Regional cerebrovascular and metabolic effects of hyperventilation after severe traumatic brain injury. J Neurosurg 2002; 96:103–108.
24. Fessler RD, Diaz FG. The management of cerebral perfusion pressure and intracranial pressure after severe head injury. Ann Emerg Med 1993; 22:998–1003.
25. Oertel M, Kelly DF, Lee JH, et al. Efficacy of hyperventilation, blood pressure elevation, and metabolic suppression therapy in controlling intracranial pressure after head injury. J Neurosurg 2002; 97:1045–1053.
26. Lee JH, Kelly DF, Oertel M, et al. Carbon dioxide reactivity, pressure autoregulation, and metabolic suppression reactivity after head injury: a transcranial Doppler study. J Neursurg 2001; 95:222–232.
27. Artru AA. Reduction of cerebrospinal fluid pressure by hypocapnia: changes in cerebral blood volume, cerebrospinal fluid volume, and brain tissue water and electrolytes. J Cereb Blood Flow Metab 1987; 7:471–479.
28. Newell DW, Weber JP, Watson R, Aaslid R, Winn HR. Effect of transient moderate hyperventilation on dynamic cerebral autoregulation after severe head injury. Neurosurgery 1996; 39:35–43.
29. Stern WE. Intracranial fluid dynamics: the relationship of intracranial pressure to the Monro-Kellie doctrine and the reliability of pressure assessment. J R Coll Surg Edinb 1963; 168:18–36.
30. Kosteljanetz M. Intracranial pressure: cerebrospinal fluid dynamics and pressure-volume relations. Acta Neurol Scand Suppl 1987; 111:1–23.
31. Maset AL, Marmarou A, Ward JD, et al. Pressure-volume index in head injury. J Neurosurg 1987; 67:832–840.
32. Lundberg N. Continuous recording and control of ventricular fluid pressure in neurosurgical practice. Acta Psychiatr Scand 1960; 36(suppl 149):1–193.
33. Neff S, Subramaniam RP. Monro-Kellie doctrine. J Neurosurg 1996; 85:1195.
34. The Brain Trauma Foundation. The American Association of Neurological Surgeons. The joint section on neurotrauma and critical care. Recommendations for intracranial pressure monitoring technology. J Neurotrauma 2000; 17:497–506.
35. Narayan RK, Kishore DR, Becker DP, et al. Intracranial pressure: to monitor or not to monitor? A review of our experience with severe head injury. J Neurosurg 1982; 56:650–659.
36. Yano M, Kobayashi S, Otsuka T. Useful ICP monitoring with subarachnoid catheter method in severe head injuries. J Trauma 1988; 28:476–480.
37. The Brain Trauma Foundation. The American Association of Neurological Surgeons. The joint section on neurotrauma and critical care. Indications for intracranial pressure monitoring. J Neurotrauma 2000; 17:479–491.
38. Zentner J, Duffner F, Behrens E. Percutaneous needle trephination for external CSF drainage: experience with 226 punctures. Neurosurg Rev 1995; 18:31–34.
39. Caruselli G, Recchioni MA, Occhipinti C, Bernardini M, Caruselli M. The role of CSF ventricular drainage in

controlling intracranial hypertension in patients with brain lesions. Comparison of three methods. Preliminary results. J Neurosurg Sci 1992; 36:219–225.

40. Gudeman SK, Young HF, Miller JD, Ward JD, Becker DP. Indications for operative treatment and operative technique in closed head injury. In: Becker DP, Miller JD, Povlishock J, Selhorst J, Young H, eds. Textbook of Head Injury. Philadelphia: WB Saunders, 1989:138–181.

41. Marmarou A, Maset AL, Ward JD, et al. Contribution of CSF and vascular factors to elevation of ICP in severely head-injured patients. J Neurosurg 1987; 66:883–890.

42. Yamashima T, Friede RL. Why do bridging veins rupture into the virtual subdural space? J Neurol Neurosurg Psychiatr 1984; 47:121–127.

43. Markwalder TM. Chronic subdural hematomas: a review. J Neurosurg 1981; 54:637–645.

44. Lee JY, Ebel H, Ernestus RI, Klug N. Various surgical treatments of chronic subdural hematoma and outcome in 172 patients: is membranectomy necessary? Surg Neurol 2004; 61:523–527.

45. Durward QJ, Del Maestro RF, Amacher A, Farrar JK. The influence of systemic arterial pressure and intracranial pressure on the development of cerebral vasogenic edema. J Neurosurg 1983; 59:803–809.

46. Yoshino E, Yamaki T, Higuchi T, Horikawa Y, Hirakawa K. Acute brain edema in fatal head injury: analysis by dynamic CT scanning. J Neurosurg 1985; 63:830–839.

47. Gudeman SK, Miller JD, Becker DP. Failure of high dose steroid therapy to influence intracranial pressure in patients with severe head injury. J Neurosurg 1979; 51:301–306.

48. Dearden NM, Gibson JS, MacDowall DG, Gibson RM, Cameron MM. Effect of high dose dexamethasone on outcome from severe head injury. J Neurosurg 1986; 64:81–88.

49. Braakman R, Schouten HJ, Blaauw-van Dishoeck M, Minderhoud JM. Megadose steroids in severe head injury. Results of a prospective double-blind trial. J Neurosurg 1983; 58:326–330.

50. Giannotta SL, Weiss H, Apuzzo ML, Martin E. High dose glucocorticoids in the management of severe head injury. Neurosurgery 1984; 15:497–501.

51. Miller JD, Leech P. Effects of mannitol and steroid therapy on intracranial volume-pressure relationships in patients. J Neurosurg 1975; 42:274–281.

52. Markham JW. The clinical features of pneumocephalus based upon a survey of 284 cases with report of 11 additional cases. Acta Neurochir (Wien) 1967; 16:1–78.

53. Osborn AG, Daines JH, Wing SD, Anderson RE. Intracranial air on computerized tomography. J Neurosurg 1978; 48:355–359.

54. Baltas I, Tsoulfa S, Sakellariou P, Vogas V, Fylaktakis M, Kondodimou A. Posttraumatic meningitis: bacteriology, hydrocephalus, and outcome. Neurosurgery 1994; 35:422–427.

55. Stephanov S. Surgical treatment of brain abscess. Neurosurgery 1988; 22:724–730.

56. Kubik CS, Adams RD. Subdural empyema. Brain 1943; 66:18–42.

57. Dill SR, Cobbs CG, McDonald CK. Subdural empyema: analysis of 32 cases and review. Clin Infect Dis 1995; 20:372–386.

58. Martin NA, Doberstein C, Zane C, Caron MJ, Thomas K, Becker DP. Posttraumatic cerebral arterial spasm: transcranial Doppler ultrasound, cerebral blood flow, and angiographic findings. J Neurosurg 1992; 77:575–583.

59. Hoh BL, Topcuoglu MA, Singhal AB, et al. Effect of clipping, craniotomy, or intravascular coiling on cerebral vasospasm and patient outcome after aneurysmal subarachnoid hemorrhage. Neurosurgery 2004; 55:779–786.

60. Suwanwela C, Suwanwela N. Intracranial arterial narrowing and spasm in acute head injury. J Neurosurg 1972; 36:314–323.

61. Krause GS, White BC, Aust SD, Nayini NR, Kumar K. Brain cell death after ischemia and reperfusion: a proposed biochemical sequence. Crit Care Med 1988; 16:714–726.

62. Ferrera PC, Pauze DR, Chan L. Sagittal sinus thrombosis after closed head injury. Am J Emerg Med 1998; 16:382–385.

63. Stefini R, Latronico N, Cornali C, Rasulo F, Bollati A. Emergent decompressive craniectomy in patients with fixed dilated pupils due to cerebral venous and dural sinus thrombosis: report of three cases. Neurosurgery 1999; 45:626–629.

64. Griffin JM, Hartley JH Jr, Crow RW, Schatten WE. Diabetes insipidus caused by craniofacial trauma. J Trauma 1976; 16:979–984.

39

Spinal Cord Trauma

Michael Y. Wang, Iftikharul Haq, and Barth A. Green
Department of Neurological Surgery & The Miami Project to Cure Paralysis,
University of Miami School of Medicine, Miami, Florida, U.S.A.

Accounts of spinal cord injury date back more than four millennia to the Edwin Smith Papyrus (1,2). The record of a case managed by Imhotep, physician to Pharoh Zoser III, describes incontinence, paralysis, and loss of sensation. Imhotep's recommendation that cervical spine injuries were "an ailment not to be treated" persisted until the last half-century. Until the advent of modern nursing care and antibiotics, even young patients were quick to succumb to pneumonia, sepsis, and thromboembolism after spinal cord injuries. Indeed, as recently as 1924, the British Medical Council stated, "the paraplegic may live a few years in a state of more or less ill-health" (3).

Sir Ludwig Guttman established the Spinal Injuries Centre of Stoke Mandeville Hospital in 1944. This center was established in part in response to the devastating casualties of World War II; it focused on providing aggressive medical care for paraplegic patients. Physical therapy, occupational therapy, and nursing services targeted at returning these patients to independent living were successful in prolonging the life expectancy and improving the quality of life of these patients (3). Since that time, the proliferation of spinal cord injury centers, particularly in the Veterans Administration Medical Centers in America, has substantially improved the outlook for paraplegic and quadriplegic patients. The patient with spinal cord injury now has a life expectancy approximating that of uninjured adults.

The past half-century has seen remarkable advances in spinal instrumentation technology. Restoring spinal stability through internal fixation has obviated the need for prolonged immobilization, thereby reducing the risk of medical complications; the increasing safety of general anesthesia and improvements in microsurgical technique raise the question of whether emergent surgery to relieve compressed neural structures may be beneficial even after the loss of neurologic function; and the advent of effective pharmacologic interventions to limit secondary injury offers the hope of finding a cure for this ailment.

EPIDEMIOLOGY

Traumatic spinal cord injuries are a serious public health problem in North America. Each year an estimated 11,000 new cases occur, but the tragedy of spinal cord injury lies in its devastating effect on predominantly young, healthy adults between 15 and 35 years of age (4). Because of improvements in prehospital care and post-trauma medical and surgical management, survival even after severe injuries is commonplace. As a consequence, it is estimated that more than 200,000 patients with spinal cord injury are currently alive in the United States at an annual financial cost of roughly $4 billion (3).

Motor vehicle accidents are the most common mechanism of injury (55%), followed by occupation-related trauma (22%), sports injuries (18%), and assault 5% (4). Most injuries are due to blunt trauma resulting in fracture, dislocation, or subluxation of the vertebrae, although penetrating injuries from gunshots and stabbings do occur. Injuries are most common at the transitional regions of the spine at the junction where a more mobile segment meets a less mobile one (i.e., craniovertebral, cervicothoracic, and thoracolumbar regions).

The cervical spine is the most commonly affected region, followed by the thoracic and lumbar regions (5). When all spinal levels are considered, a fracture or dislocation of the vertebral column carries a 14% chance of neural injury. However, the spinal level of involvement will influence the likelihood of neurological impairment: 40% in the cervical region, 10% in the thoracic region, 35% in the thoracolumbar area, and 3% in the lumbar region.

BIOMECHANICS OF INJURY

The neural and musculoskeletal components of the human spine are intimately associated. Thus, any discussion of blunt traumatic spinal cord injury requires an understanding of the vertebral column. Motion occurs between the 25 distinct vertebrae, and although these motion segments are stereotyped, variabilities exist in each spinal region. Rotatory motion in the axial plane occurs primarily at the occipitocervical and thoracic regions. Flexion and extension in the sagittal plane occur at the cervical and lumbar levels. The orientation and configuration of the facet joints determine to a large extent the degree of mobility at each motion segment. The thoracic spine is also made less mobile because of its articulations with the rib cage.

Concepts of stability in the vertebral column are complex and frequently confusing. The vertebral column serves to transmit loads, permit motion, and protect the spinal cord. Instability of the spinal column may then be defined as its failure to perform any of these functions under physiologic levels of mechanical loading. This failure may occur either acutely or in a progressive, delayed manner. In cases of traumatic spinal cord injury, the vertebral column acutely fails to shield the neural elements from external forces as a result of being stressed beyond its mechanical tolerances.

Numerous classification schemes have been devised to predict whether the spine is unstable. The most common of these is the three-column theory introduced by Denis (6). Although this theory was originally based on studies of thoracolumbar fractures, its principles have also been applied to other regions of the spine (Fig. 1). This classification system divides the spine into anterior, middle, and posterior columns. The anterior column consists of the anterior half of the vertebral body, the anterior half of the intervertebral disk, and the anterior longitudinal ligament. The middle column consists of the posterior half of vertebral body, the posterior half of the intervertebral disk, and the posterior longitudinal ligament. The posterior column consists of the posterior arch, the facet joint

complex, the interspinous ligament, the supraspinous ligament, and the ligament flavum. The diagnosis of instability is made if two or more of the columns are compromised.

External forces placed upon the spine include axial compression, distraction, flexion, extension, and translation. Axial compression in the cervical spine results in disruptions of the ring of C1 and in burst fractures of the remaining vertebrae. Axial compression in the thoracolumbar spine results in burst fractures. When compressive forces are applied anterior to the spinal column and result in a component of flexion, anterior compression fractures result. Severe flexion is the most common mechanism of injury in the cervical spine. This motion can cause odontoid fractures, teardrop fractures of the vertebral bodies, dislocations of the vertebral bodies, and jumped facets. In the thoracolumbar spine, severe flexion results in compression of the anterior vertebral body. If the fulcrum of force is anterior to the vertebral column, as occurs when a seat-belted passenger is involved in a motor vehicle accident, a flexion-distraction injury of the thoracolumbar junction may result.

PATHOPHYSIOLOGY

The pathological outcome of trauma to the spinal cord is related to a *primary* mechanical injury at the epicenter of the damage. Direct crush, stretch, and shear injuries to neurons and axons within the spinal cord lead to immediate cell death. However, delayed cascades of cellular and molecular events known as *secondary* spinal cord injury occur in the hours and days after the traumatic event and lead to further cell death. The release of excitotoxic amino acids such as glutamate disturbs ionic homeostasis in neural tissues. The resulting increases in intracellular calcium ions, cellular energy failure, and accumulation of free radicals lead to local cell death in a delayed fashion (7,8).

Because patients with spinal cord injury frequently suffer polytrauma, they are susceptible to derangements of systemic homeostasis. Cardiovascular and pulmonary compromise may affect perfusion and oxygen delivery to the spinal cord, thereby exacerbating the damage. Vasoactive substances released by injured cells and endothelin released by damaged capillaries may also disrupt the microcirculation of the spinal cord. Ischemia may thus cause neurologic deficits to extend rostrally beyond the initially injured area (9,10). Because cell death due to secondary injury and ischemia occurs after the patient has reached a medical treatment facility, it is hoped that early pharmacologic intervention and maintenance of adequate tissue perfusion can salvage these neurons.

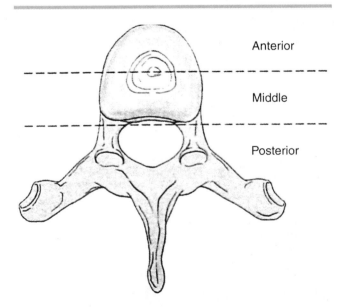

Figure 1 Three-column theory of spinal stability as proposed by F. Denis.

Anterior

Middle

Posterior

CLINICAL FEATURES

The neurological examination is of paramount importance in localizing the probable site of injury.

Particular attention should be paid to the motor, sensory, reflex, and rectal examinations. On the basis of the degree of functional impairment, the American Spinal Injury Association (ASIA) has proposed an easily used scoring system (Table 1). The ASIA score, in conjunction with the lowest normal segmental level, defines the neurologic injury in simple terms. In this classification scheme, grade "A" denotes a complete injury, and grades "B" through "D" denote incomplete injuries (11). Complete recovery of function after an ASIA "A" injury is exceedingly rare; however, improvement of one or two ASIA grades is seen in more than 10% of patients. Recovery is most likely after grade "D" injuries (12).

Neural compression typically results from acute displacement of bone fragments, ligaments, and herniated discs. Delayed spinal cord compression may also result from a hematoma within the spinal canal or from movement of bone or prolapsed disc in a spine that is not properly immobilized. The characteristic clinical picture is that of a patient without neurologic deficits or with an incomplete injury who then experiences complete paralysis, particularly after intubation or transportation. Deterioration can also occur in the chronic setting weeks to months after injury. Post-traumatic syringomyelia and progressive bony deformity are the most frequent causes. Overall, loss of neurologic function occurs in roughly 3% of patients who are admitted for spinal cord trauma (12).

Specific neurological syndromes have been described for particular partial cord injuries. The *anterior cord syndrome* is characterized by complete paralysis and hypoalgesia (anterior and anterolateral column function) below the level of injury with preservation of the senses of position, vibration, and light touch (posterior column function). This syndrome occurs most commonly after ischemia in the territory supplied by the anterior spinal artery, which supplies the corticospinal and spinothalamic tracts. The *central cord syndrome* is characterized by more pronounced motor dysfunction in the distal upper extremities, accompanied by various degrees of sensory loss and bladder dysfunction. This injury characteristically occurs after a hyperextension injury in elderly patients and can occur even in the absence of any clear radiographic evidence of disruption of the bones or ligaments. Most patients recover the ability to walk, with partial restoration of upper extremity strength. The *posterior cord syndrome* is uncommon; the senses

of position and vibration are impaired because of injury to the dorsal columns. The *Brown-Sequard syndrome* or hemisection cord syndrome causes ipsilateral paresis and loss of proprioception below the level of the lesion and contralateral loss of pain and temperature sensations. This syndrome can be the result of penetrating injuries or tumor compression and is usually not seen in a pure form. The *conus medullaris syndrome* occurs with injuries at the thoracolumbar junction. This syndrome has components of both spinal cord injury and nerve root injury because of the dense population of lower nerve roots emerging from the caudal end of the spinal cord. Symmetrical lower extremity motor impairment and anesthesia with bowel and bladder dysfunction are typical. Recovery from this syndrome is unlikely. In contrast, partial recovery after *cauda equina syndrome* is possible with early decompression. Cauda equina injuries occur at spinal levels below the termination of the cord at L1 or L2.

Cord concussions exhibit fleeting neurologic symptoms followed by rapid resolution. These injuries, also called "stingers," occur most commonly among athletes with low-velocity hyperflexion or extension injuries of the cervical spine. Complete recovery is the rule; however, patients should be evaluated meticulously for occult spinal instability and intraspinal hematomas.

EVALUATION OF SUSPECTED INJURY

The current medicolegal environment in the United States is intolerant of missed spinal injuries. Indeed, failure to detect spinal instability can cause delayed loss of neurologic function. In the most extreme case, a patient who is not paralyzed by the traumatic event may become quadriplegic after inappropriate mobilization by the medical team. Thus, it is not surprising that tremendous resources and efforts are directed at detecting spinal injuries.

The diagnosis of a spinal column injury is based on the findings of clinical and radiological examinations. In a conscious, nonintoxicated patient, the absence of pain along the spinal axis is useful in ruling out injury. In these patients, diagnosis of a low-velocity injury may require no radiography, and diagnosis of a high-velocity injury may require only limited plain films. It is essential that radiographic evidence of spinal column injury be correlated with the findings of the clinical examination because 10% of patients will have injuries at multiple spinal segments. Radiography, computed tomography (CT), and magnetic resonance imaging (MRI) are needed when patients are not able to cooperate fully with the neurologic examination.

Radiographs are useful not only for detecting but also for classifying injuries. The fracture type and the degree of cord compression are particularly important aspects of the injury that will determine the

Table 1 American Spinal Injury Association Grading Scale for Spinal Cord Injury

Clinical grade	Results of neurological examination
A	No motor or sensory function preserved
B	Sensory but no motor function preserved
C	Nonuseful motor function preserved (< antigravity strength)
D	Motor function preserved but weak
E	Normal motor and sensory function

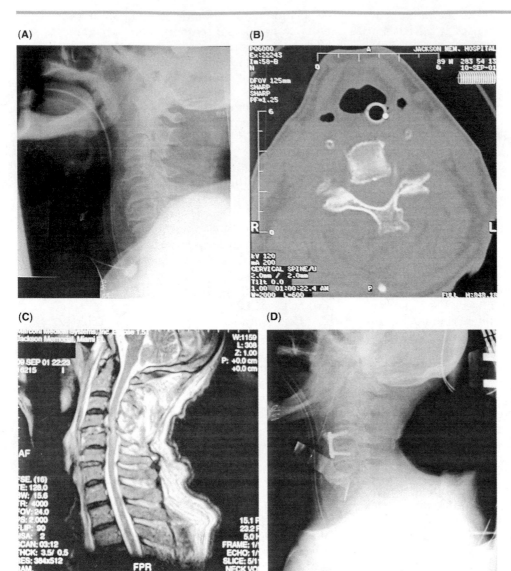

Figure 2 Cervical subluxation with unilateral jumped facet and acute disk herniation causing quadriplegia after a rollover motor vehicle accident. (**A**) Lateral radiograph showing subluxation at C. (**B**) Computed tomography scan showing "reverse hamburger sign" of jumped facets on one side. (**C**) Magnetic resonance image showing a herniated disk compressing the cervical spinal cord. (**D**) Postoperative radiograph after diskectomy for decompression and fusion with plating.

management strategy. For the cervical spine, plain lateral radiographs must include the C7–T1 junction because 31% of injuries occur between C6 and T1 (Fig. 2). When patients are large and bulky, downward traction on the shoulders, a swimmer's view, or CT scanning may be needed to properly visualize the cervicothoracic junction. Lateral radiographs allow evaluation of vertebral alignment, canal diameter (normal is >12 mm), angulation of the intervertebral space (normal is <11°), interspinous gap, and atlantodental interval (the distance between the anterior margin of the dens and the closest point on the anterior arch of C1 should be ≤3 mm in adults). Soft-tissue swelling in the prevertebral space is an indirect indicator of cervical spine injury (maximum prevertebral space in adults is 10 mm at C1, 5–7 mm at C2–C4, and 22 mm at C5–C7).

In the thoracic and lumbar spine, anterior compression fractures and fracture dislocations are usually clearly visible on lateral radiographs. Splaying of the interspinous ligaments indicates disruption of the posterior tension band, composed of the spinous processes and the interspinous ligament. Burst fractures may be difficult to detect on a lateral radiograph but are indicated when one interpedicular space is abnormally larger than that at adjacent levels (Fig. 3). After burst fractures, CT scanning is particularly useful for assessing the degree of canal compromise by retropulsed bone fragments from the vertebral body.

ACUTE MANAGEMENT

Care of the patient with spinal injury begins in the field with Emergency Medical Services personnel. Maintaining a patent airway and managing shock take precedence. The patient is immobilized with a rigid cervical collar and backboard for transportation to a trauma center. Intubation and helmet removal should be attempted only with strict attention to

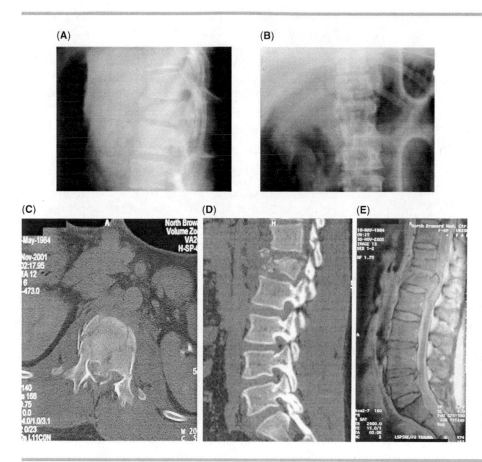

Figure 3 Burst fracture of the L1 vertebra after a 20-foot fall resulting in complete loss of neurological function (Grade A injury). **(A)** Lateral and **(B)** anteroposterior radiograph showing widening of the interpedicular distance characteristic of a burst fracture. **(C)** Axial computed tomography (CT) image showing 75% compromise of the spinal canal by bone fragments. CT sagittal reconstruction showing vertebral displacement **(D)** and injury at the level of the conus medullaris **(E)**.

maintaining neck alignment, particularly when patients are unresponsive because 3% to 5% of comatose patients have a cervical spine injury.

In the trauma center, the priority remains the maintenance of tissue oxygenation and perfusion, with particular attention to maintaining an adequate mean arterial blood pressure. In this regard, the patient with spinal injury presents particular challenges. Immobilization of the cervical spine during intubation is essential and is best accomplished with awake nasotracheal maneuvers with or without fiberoptic assistance. However, mechanical respiratory efforts may be minimal when the injury occurs at the C5 level or higher. In these patients, muscular expansion of the rib cage is absent and diaphragmatic breathing may be weakened. Thus, intubation with in-line stabilization using two physicians may be the only option for quickly establishing airway control and ventilation. Caution should be exercised in suctioning the oropharynx because this action may stimulate autonomic reflex arcs, thereby causing profound bradycardia and even cardiac arrest.

Cervical and high-thoracic injuries may result in neurogenic shock, which can severely complicate the management of a patient already in hypovolemic shock. Neurogenic shock results from the loss of sympathetic vasoregulatory tone. The clinical picture is hypotension with an associated bradycardia.

Treatment involves mild fluid resuscitation and continuous intravenous infusions of inotropic agents possessing alpha-adrenergic properties; these medications increase heart rate, cardiac output, and vasomotor tone. Dopamine because of its mixed alpha- and beta-adrenergic effects, is useful in treating neurogenic shock. Acutely symptomatic bradycardia should be treated with intravenously administered atropine.

Associated extraspinal injuries are common and must also be ruled out. Because spinal column injuries are typically the result of severe traumatic mechanisms, the incidence of cranial, thoracic, abdominal, and orthopedic injuries is high. Priority must be given to the most life-threatening injuries.

Cervical traction with either a halo frame or Gardner-Wells tongs may be used to restore alignment of the spine and to reduce neural compression. However, traction must be initiated with caution because neurologic deterioration can result from overdistraction or from movement of acutely herniated disk material (13). Before traction is initiated, a full set of radiographs and MR images will be helpful in reducing the likelihood of worsening deficits. For injuries in the subaxial spine, it is prudent to begin traction with 10 pounds and to add weight either until reduction has been achieved or until a total of five pounds per cervical level has been applied. Serial lateral radiographs or fluoroscopic images should be taken after each addition of weight to ensure that the neck has not been overdistracted.

PHARMACOLOGIC THERAPY FOR SPINAL CORD INJURY

Animal models of spinal cord injury have offered the hope that damage caused by secondary injury can be mitigated by early pharmacologic intervention. Three large, randomized, multicenter clinical trials have investigated the usefulness of high doses of methylprednisolone for spinal cord injury (14). These studies National Acute Spinal Cord Injury Study (NASCIS I–III) found that a bolus dose of 30 mg/kg followed by doses of 5.4 mg/kg each hour mildly improved the functional outcome of some patients with either complete or incomplete injuries. If steroid is administered within four hours of injury, the infusion should be continued for 24 hours; if it is administered within four to eight hours after injury, the infusion should be continued for 48 hours (15). High doses of steroids are not likely to be useful in treating penetrating spinal cord injuries, and the systemic effects of steroids on polytraumatized and pediatric patients have not been fully assessed. Although some controversy surrounds the effectiveness of high doses of methylprednisolone, this drug is the only widely available pharmacologic agent that has demonstrated some effectiveness in large clinical trials.

Trials of other pharmacologic interventions for spinal cord injury are currently under way. Initial studies of GM-1 gangliosides and the 21-aminosteroid tirilazad are promising, but the results are preliminary (16). Opiate opioid antagonists, *N*-methyl-D-aspartate receptor blockers, calcium channel blockers, and antioxidants have shown promise in animal models of spinal cord injury but remain unproven in humans.

SURGICAL MANAGEMENT

Radiologically proven compression of the spinal cord and nerve roots in patients with incomplete spinal cord injuries mandates surgical intervention for decompression and stabilization. Surgical treatment for patients with complete loss of neurologic function remains controversial. Early surgical stabilization within the first few days after injury has more recently become popular because of the increasing safety of general anesthesia. Early stabilization allows for safe mobilization of the patient, for physical and occupational therapy, and for improved pulmonary toilet. Surgery may have to be delayed for patients who have suffered severe injuries to vital organs. In these cases, maintenance of spinal precautions with a cervical collar and strict "log rolling" for nursing care should prevent any neurologic deterioration.

Whether emergent surgery to decompress the spinal cord will improve neurologic outcome remains controversial (17). To date, all studies showing that early surgery or traction reduction of the spine improves neurological outcome fall within Class III levels of evidence (18). In contrast, three Class II studies have demonstrated no advantage with early surgery. No definitive studies have been performed to resolve this issue, but plans for a randomized, prospective, multicenter study to compare early and late surgery are currently under way (13).

PREVENTION OF COMPLICATIONS
Cutaneous and Musculoskeletal Complications

Pressure ulcers occur in 25% to 30% of patients with spinal cord injury (19). Because of transport on hard backboards, prolonged immobilization, and loss of cutaneous sensation, these patients are at extremely high risk of skin breakdown. The most common sites of involvement are the sacrum, heels, ischium, and occiput.

Prevention of pressure ulcers begins in the emergency room. During the secondary trauma survey, all of the patient's clothes should be removed to allow inspection of the body for bruising and abrasion. The patient should be removed from the backboard as soon as possible because pressure necrosis of the skin can occur within as little as one hour when the patient is on a hard surface. In the acute care setting, the patient should be turned by "log rolling" every two hours until the spine has been proved to be stable or has been stabilized surgically. An alternative to this manual turning is the use of an electrically driven kinetic bed such as the Roto-Rest® (Midmark Corporation, Versailles, Ohio, U.S.A.) (20).

The best treatment for pressure and decubitus ulcers is prevention and early detection. Stage I lesions can be managed with aggressive mobilization and adhesive barrier dressings. However, once the dermis has been compromised, daily sterile dressing changes may be needed for wound debridement. Deeper lesions may require debridement and skin grafting in the operating room. Proper management of even mild lesions will prevent devastating late sequelae such as sepsis from infected ulcers.

In the subacute and chronic settings, muscle denervation leads to atrophy, spasticity, and contracture formation. Passive range of motion exercises and splinting forestall the formation of deformities and contracture. Administering etidronate sodium and increasing mobility may reduce heterotopic ossifications (21).

Thromboembolism

Paralyzed patients are at high risk of deep venous thrombosis and pulmonary embolism. The incidence of lower extremity venous thrombosis is as high as 79% if fibrinogen scanning, impedance plethysmography, and venography are used (22,23). Pulmonary embolism occurs in 2% to 3% of patients and is responsible for roughly 10% of all deaths after spinal cord trauma (5). The risk of thromboembolism peaks two to three weeks after injury.

The early use of pneumatic compression devices and subcutaneously administered heparin can reduce the risk of thromboembolism (24). In the absence of any medical or surgical contraindication to anticoagulation, 5000 units of heparin should be administered subcutaneously twice each day, starting within the first two days after injury. Low-molecular-weight heparin can also be used for anticoagulation and may be associated with a lower incidence of hemorrhagic side effects (25). The prophylactic use of a vena cava filter may reduce the risk of potentially fatal pulmonary embolism (26).

Genitourinary and Lower Gastrointestinal Complications

The aim of bladder management is to preserve renal function and to prevent urinary tract infections. Immediately after a complete spinal cord injury, the bladder is acontractile. Indwelling catheters will allow bladder drainage and measurements of fluid balance. Intermittent catheterization every four to six hours should commence as soon as possible under strict aseptic technique. Paraplegic patients should be taught to self-catheterize as soon as they are able to sit up.

Urinary tract infections are common and should be treated aggressively so as to prevent urosepsis. Urea-splitting bacteria such as *Proteus* spp. are associated with a high incidence of renal calculus formation, which should be vigorously treated. Renal calculi are found in approximately 1% of patients (19).

After severe spinal injury, rectal tone is absent. Constipation can easily occur unless manual evacuation is carried out regularly. The judicious use of rectal suppositories stimulates bowel emptying, and regular doses of a stool softener should also be administered.

Upper Gastrointestinal Complications

Post-traumatic ileus is common among patients with spinal cord injury. A nasogastric tube should be placed in the emergency room to suction drainage. Tube placement will help prevent the aspiration of any regurgitated stomach contents and will minimize the distension caused by ileus. Nutritional support is crucial after trauma. Patients with spinal cord injury require a caloric intake of roughly 150% of their basal requirement, and special attention must also be directed at meeting increased protein requirements. Proper nutritional support prevents catabolism, supplements wound healing, and maximizes immune protection (27). Parenteral nutrition is appropriate until the ileus resolves, but tube feeding should begin as early as possible. Even small amounts of enteral nutrition given through a nasogastric tube may reduce the risk of sepsis.

Gastric ulcers are common among patients with spinal cord injury, and the risk of this complication is increased by the use of high doses of methylprednisolone. Gastrointestinal hemorrhage is less common;

it occurs in 3% of patients (19). H_2 blockers, proton pump inhibitors, and sucralfate appear to be similarly effective in reducing the risk of gastrointestinal hemorrhage. Pancreatitis and acalculous cholecystitis can also occur, especially if parenteral nutrition is administered for prolonged periods of time. Pancreatitis can be diagnosed by elevated amylase activity, and acalculous cholecystitis can be diagnosed by elevated bilirubin concentrations. Early recognition of these disorders requires a heightened level of suspicion.

Pulmonary Complications

Respiratory diseases account for 28% of deaths and are the leading cause of mortality in the first year after spinal cord injury (5). For a number of reasons, patients with spinal injury are at high risk of pulmonary infection. Prolonged mechanical ventilation, poor pulmonary toilet, an inability to clear upper airway secretions, poor respiratory capacity, nosocomial exposure, weakened immune responses, or any accompanying chest trauma increases the risk of pneumonia. The judicious use of aggressive suctioning, chest physiotherapy, bronchodilators, positive pressure ventilation, and bronchoscopic airway clearance helps prevent infection. Severe atelectasis can also cause respiratory distress in the absence of infection.

The risk of pulmonary complications clearly increases with injuries at higher levels of the spinal column. For patients with injuries at C1 to C4, tracheostomy and prolonged mechanical ventilation will probably be required. However, when injuries occur at lower levels, all attempts should be made to avoid a tracheostomy.

SPINAL CORD INJURY IN CHILDREN

By the time a person reaches adolescence, the spine is well developed and the patterns of injury resemble those of adults. Perhaps because of the increased mobility of the developing spine, pediatric spinal cord injuries are rare (28). However because the head composes a greater proportion of the body mass of children than of adults, children are more susceptible to atlanto-occipital injuries. The hypermobility of the pediatric spine also accounts for cases of spinal cord injury without radiographic abnormality (SCIWORA). Approximately 15% to 20% of all pediatric spinal cord injuries are classified as SCIWORA (29).

The principles of managing pediatric spinal cord injuries are similar to those of managing such injuries in adults. However because children cannot cooperate fully with the physical examination, it is important to recognize subtle physical and radiological signs, and an increased reliance must often be placed on radiographic studies. Many of the standard measurements used to evaluate cervical radiographs need to be adjusted for the pediatric spine.

The relatively large size of the head in comparison to the body will result in neck flexion when children are placed on a rigid backboard. This malalignment can accentuate deformity of the cervical spine and should be avoided. Equipment tailored for pediatric spine immobilization should be used whenever possible. Unlike spine injuries in adults, most such injuries in children can be treated nonsurgically with bracing (30).

FUTURE ADVANCES

Future advances in the science of treating spinal cord injury will provide the hope of improved quality of life for patients with such injuries. The past decade has already seen an explosion of knowledge about the mechanisms that underlie primary and secondary spinal cord injury. Numerous drugs have shown promise in limiting nerve cell death resulting from secondary injury, and the results of a number of human trials of these medications should be available within the next decade.

Future studies will also demonstrate whether early surgery will be beneficial for these patients, and, if so, in which subpopulation. The timing of surgery and the best approach (anterior or posterior) will be more clearly delineated. Advances in the science of spinal fusion and instrumentation will allow stabilization surgery to be performed with less morbidity and tissue trauma, and early surgery will also provide the opportunity for direct drug delivery to the site of injury.

Advances will also come from other related fields of medicine. The specialty of intensive care medicine continues to make strides in preventing and treating the complications of prolonged hospitalization. Patients with spinal cord injury will no doubt benefit from decreased risks of pneumonia, infection, wound breakdown, and thromboembolism. Improvements in imaging science will enable treating physicians to detect instability quickly and reliably. Rehabilitation of the patient with spinal cord injury will integrate robotic technology that will offer the plegic patient increased mobility.

The Holy Grail of spinal cord injury is neural restoration. Whether through the transplantation of stem cells, molecular manipulation with transfection techniques, or modulation of the local cytokine milieu, the hope is to restore function to cells and axons that have already been destroyed. Because reinnervation of the spinal cord is the only way to restore neurologic function, research in this area remains the primary goal of the Miami Project to Cure Paralysis.

Despite all of the advances forthcoming in the field of spinal cord injury, prevention of injury remains a top priority. Programs such as the Think First initiative in Florida have already dramatically reduced the incidence of diving-related injuries to the cervical spine. Physicians, who are most acutely aware of the devastating consequences of spinal cord injury, must assume a key role in educating the public about how to avoid these catastrophic injuries.

REFERENCES

1. Breasted J. The Edwin Smith Papyrus. Chicago: Chicago University Press, 1930.
2. Elsberg C. The Edwin Smith surgical papyrus and the diagnosis and treatment of injuries to the skull. Ann Med Hist 1931; 3:271–279.
3. Guttman L. Spinal Cord Injuries: Comprehensive Management and Research. Oxford: Blackwell Scientific, 1973.
4. Nobunaga AI, Go BK, Karunas RB. Recent demographic and injury trends in people served by the Model Spinal Cord Injury Care Systems. Arch Phys Med Rehabil 1999; 80:1372–1382.
5. DeVivo MJ, Krause JS, Lammertse DP. Recent trends in mortality and causes of death among persons with spinal cord injury. Arch Phys Med Rehabil 1999; 80:1411–1419.
6. Denis F. The three column spine and its significance in the classification of acute thoracolumbar spinal injuries. Spine 1983; 8:817–831.
7. Amar AP, Levy ML. Pathogenesis and pharmacological strategies for mitigating secondary damage in acute spinal injury. Neurosurgery 1999; 44:1027–1040.
8. Lu J, Ashwell KW, Waite P. Advances in secondary spinal cord injury. Spine 2000; 25:1859–1866.
9. Tator C, Fehlings M. Review of the secondary injury theory of acute spinal cord injury with emphasis on vascular mechanisms. J Neurosurg 1991; 75:15–26.
10. Harrop JS, Sharan AD, Vaccaro AR, Przybylski GJ. The cause of neurologic deterioration after acute cervical spinal cord injury. Spine 2001; 26:340–346.
11. Maynard FM Jr., Bracken MB, Creasey G, et al. International standards for neurological and functional classification of spinal cord injury. Spinal Cord 1997; 35:266–274.
12. Marino RJ, Ditunno JF Jr., Donovan WH, Maynard F Jr. Neurologic recovery after traumatic spinal cord injury: data from the Model Spinal Cord Injury Systems. Arch Phys Med Rehabil 1999; 80:1391–1396.
13. Tator CH, Fehlings MG, Thorpe K, Taylor W. Current use and timing of spinal surgery for management of acute spinal cord injury in North America: results of a retrospective multicenter study. J Neurosurg 1999; 91(suppl 1):12–18.
14. Bracken MB, Shepard MJ, Collins WF Jr., et al. Methylprednisolone or naloxone treatment after acute spinal cord injury: 1-year follow-up data. Results of the Second National Acute Spinal Cord Injury Study. J Neurosurg 1992; 76:23–31.
15. Bracken MB, Shepard MJ, Holford TR, et al. Administration of methylprednisolone for 24 or 48 hours or tirilizad mesylate for 48 hours in the treatment of acute spinal cord injury. Results of the Third National Acute Spinal Cord Injury Randomized Controlled Trial. National Acute Spinal Cord Injury Survey. JAMA 1997; 277:1597–1604.
16. Geisler FH, Dorsey FC, Coleman WP. Recovery of motor function after spinal-cord injury—a randomized, placebo-controlled trial with GM-1 ganglioside. N Engl J Med 1991; 324:1829–1838.
17. Waters RL, Meyer PR Jr., Adkins RH, Felton D. Emergency, acute, and surgical management of spine trauma. Arch Phys Med Rehabil 1999; 80:1383–1390.
18. Fehlings MG, Tator CH. An evidence-based review of decompressive surgery in acute spinal cord

injury: rationale, indications, and timing based on experimental and clinical studies. J Neurosurg 1999; 91(suppl 1):1–11.

19. Chen D, Apple DF Jr., Hudson LM, Bode R. Medical complications during acute rehabilitation following spinal cord injury—current experience of the Model Systems. Arch Phys Med Rehabil 1999; 80:1397–1401.

20. Green BA, Green KL, Klose KJ. Kinetic nursing for acute spinal cord injury patients. Paraplegia 1980; 18:181–186.

21. Stover S. Heterotopic ossification. In: Bloch R, Basbaum M, eds. Management of Spinal Cord Injuries. Baltimore: Williams & Wilkins, 1986:284–301.

22. Weingarden SI. Deep venous thrombosis in spinal cord injury. Overview of the problem. Chest 1992; 102: 636S–639S.

23. Harris S, Chen D, Green D. Enoxaparin for thromboembolism prophylaxis in spinal injury: preliminary report on experience with 105 patients. Am J Phys Med Rehabil 1996; 75:326–327.

24. Nicolaides AN, Fernandes e Fernandes J, Pollock AV. Intermittent sequential pneumatic compression of the legs in the prevention of venous stasis and deep venous thrombosis. Surgery 1980; 87:69–76.

25. Deep K, Jigajinni MV, McLean AN, Fraser MH. Prophylaxis of thromboembolism in spinal injuries—results of enoxaparin used in 276 patients. Spinal Cord 2001; 39:88–91.

26. Velmahos GC, Kern J, Chan LS, Older D, Murray JA, Schekelle P. Prevention of venous thromboembolism after injury: an evidence-based report—part II. Analysis of risk factors and evaluation of the role of vena caval filters. J Trauma 2000; 49:140–144.

27. Apelgren KN, Wilmore DW. Nutritional care of the critically ill patient. Surg Clin North Am 1983; 63: 497–507.

28. Durkin MS, Olsen S, Barlow B, Virella A, Connolly ES Jr. The epidemiology of urban pediatric neurological trauma: evaluation of, and implication for, injury prevention programs. Neurosurgery 1998; 42:300–310.

29. Grabb P, Pang D. Magnetic resonance imaging in the evaluation of spinal cord injury without radiographic abnormality in children. Neurosurgery 1994; 35:406–414.

30. Eleraky MA, Theodore N, Adams M, Rekate HL, Sonntag VK. Pediatric cervical spine injuries: report of 102 cases and review of the literature. J Neurosurg 2000; 92(suppl 1):12–17.

40

Complications of Nerve Injury and Repair

Patrick W. Owens

Department of Orthopedics and Rehabilitation, University of Miami, Miami, Florida, U.S.A.

Because of its proximity to tendons, bones, and neurovascular structures, the peripheral nervous system is vulnerable to injury due to trauma or to complications of surgical procedures. Prevention or early recognition of these nerve injuries is vital for optimal outcome. Unfortunately, many patients with nerve injuries experience only limited recovery, even when the injuries are promptly diagnosed and treated.

Most injuries to major peripheral nerves result from trauma. The prevalence of major peripheral nerve injuries among trauma patients at one institution was 2.8%, and 54% of these patients required surgery for these injuries (1). However, iatrogenic injuries also account for a substantial number of nerve injuries. A study of a series of 2000 major nerve injuries at two hospitals found that 10% of the injuries were the result of medical treatment (2).

DIAGNOSIS OF NERVE INJURIES

Nerve injuries can be diagnosed by an adequate neurologic examination. Because nerve damage is possible among patients with fractures, lacerations, and other forms of trauma, a neurologic examination of the extremity should be performed as soon as possible after the injury. Simple soft-tissue lacerations are frequently repaired without neurologic examination, and in such cases, a nerve injury may not be detected. Missing an injury may result in a delay in treatment and may sometimes preclude the possibility of primary repair because the nerve ends retract. Long delays adversely affect the outcome of nerve injuries.

Detailed neurologic examinations are often impractical for patients with multiple traumatic or life-threatening injuries. An attempt should be made to examine at least the distal sensation and motor function of the extremities. Assessing distal function is a quick way to determine whether an injury to the nerve has occurred. Physicians at all levels of training should be familiar with and adept at performing these examinations. In the upper extremity, the median, radial, and ulnar nerves can be evaluated quickly and simply. Motor function of all three nerves can be tested by asking the patient to extend the thumb ("hitch-hiking" or "thumbs-up" maneuver), to separate the index and long fingers (the "peace sign"), and to touch the tip of the thumb with the tip of the small finger. Sensation can be tested at three autonomous sensory areas: the tip of the index finger, the tip of the small finger, and the dorsal web space between the thumb and index fingers. For the lower extremity, flexing and extending the great toe tests the motor component of the terminal portions of the tibial and peroneal nerves. Sensation can be assessed on the plantar surface and in the first web space of the foot.

When patients have signs of nerve injury due to penetrating trauma, immediate exploration and repair are indicated. Repairing nerve injuries shortly after they occur has been shown to improve outcome (3). When patients are believed to have a nerve injury as the result of closed trauma, electromyography (EMG) should be performed if complete recovery has not occurred after three to four weeks. Such testing will help to confirm the diagnosis, localize the lesion, and provide a baseline for monitoring recovery. EMG should be repeated three months later if recovery is not yet complete. By this time, reinnervation can often be detected. If EMG shows no recovery of the nerve, surgery for neurolysis or excision of the damaged nerve with repair or grafting should be considered.

ANATOMY

A knowledge of the general anatomy of peripheral nerves is important for an understanding of nerve injuries and their potential for regeneration. The epineurium is the connective tissue that forms the outer layer of the nerve and runs around and between the nerve fascicles. It forms a dense layer around the periphery of the nerve to protect and support the fascicles. The perineurium is the connective tissue layer that surrounds each fascicle and gives the nerve most of its tensile strength. The endoneurium is the loose connective tissue within the fascicle. Each fascicle contains numerous axons surrounded by Schwann cells and their myelin sheath.

The primary vascular supply to each nerve runs longitudinally in the epineurium. These vessels interconnect with the vessels of the perineurium and endoneurium, forming a rich anastomotic plexus.

CLASSIFICATION OF NERVE INJURIES

Sunderland developed the most commonly used system for classifying nerve injuries (4). This system describes lesions that fall into "pure" categories, in which all parts of the nerve undergo the same level of injury; unfortunately, most nerve injuries fall into a mixed category. Nevertheless, the system works fairly well in explaining why lesions differ in regeneration potential.

According to the Sunderland classification, a type 1 injury, also called neuropraxia, is characterized by local myelin damage; the axons remain in continuity. These lesions are usually caused by nerve compression. Because the axons remain in continuity, complete recovery occurs, although it may take weeks to months.

In Sunderland type 2 injuries, the axons are physiologically disrupted but all of the supporting tissues are intact. Because these tissues remain intact, the axons are guided along their normal course and full recovery can be expected. When the axons are disrupted, the distal ends undergo degeneration and the axon must regrow toward its target. Recovery from such lesions often takes many months, and the time taken for recovery depends on the level of the injury.

Because each additional connective tissue layer is damaged, the Sunderland grade goes up. For example, in Sunderland type 3 injuries, the axons and the endoneurium are disrupted but the perineurium and epineurium remain intact. When the endoneurium is damaged, axonal regeneration is blocked by intrafascicular fibrosis and recovery is incomplete.

In Sunderland type 4 injuries, only the epineurium is intact. Increased damage within the nerve leads to increased scarring. Very little useful recovery can be expected and surgical excision with repair or grafting is required. Complete disruption of the nerve is a type 5 injury, from which spontaneous recovery is rarely seen.

COMPLICATIONS OF NERVE REPAIR

Most nerve injuries leave nerves in gross continuity. The most common causes of such injuries are compression, blunt trauma, and traction. The main problem in treating these injuries is deciding when to intervene operatively. When nerve injuries fail to resolve within three months, disruption of the axons has most likely occurred. With proximal nerve injuries, clinical recovery of even lower grade injuries may not be evident for up to three months because of the distance of axons from the distal target. EMG is useful in these situations to confirm whether recovery is occurring. Four main factors have consistently been shown to adversely affect the results of nerve repair: gaps greater than 5 cm between axons, delay of repair for more than three months, the patient's age being more than 20 years, and blunt (as opposed to penetrating) injury (5).

After nerve transection or resection of a nerve lesion in continuity, the nerve must be sutured; the surgeon whose task it is to repair injured nerves may encounter a number of pitfalls. These problems may include failure to recognize the extent of the nerve injury, excessive tension on the repair, failure of sutures, malalignment of the repair, and suture of the nerve to a nonneural structure.

One of the most common problems associated with nerve repair is failing to recognize the extent of injury to the nerve and attempting to repair unhealthy nerve ends. Unless a patient has sharp lacerations in the acute setting, it is often difficult to assess the full extent of nerve injury. When nerve injuries result from blunt force or gunshot wounds, the architecture of the internal nerve is often disrupted beyond the obvious severed ends of the nerve. Intraneural scarring increases and leads to poor axonal regeneration. When a nerve lesion in continuity is resected, the same problems can be encountered and a neuroma can form. A longer nerve graft is more likely to succeed than a shorter graft between two scarred nerve ends.

Nerve repair may also fail if there is too much tension on the repair site. Tension can cause gaps that may fill in with scar tissue, thereby blocking axonal regeneration. Even in the absence of gapping, excess tension at the repair site can impede nerve healing by reducing intraneural circulation. When the nerve length is increased by 15%, the blood flow to the nerve decreases by approximately 80%, with little recovery over time (6). When a gap exists between the nerve ends, some mobilization of the nerve ends can help reduce tension, but excessive dissection may further strip the nerve of blood supply. If the gap is too large, a nerve graft should be performed. However, in most situations, a repair under modest tension is more likely to recover than is a nerve graft (7).

Suturing a nerve to another anatomical structure is not uncommon. Such problems most often occur during treatment of lacerations to the volar wrist because the median nerve can be mistaken for the palmaris longus or flexor tendon. Tourniquet control and loupe magnification are useful in avoiding this problem. Malalignment can also be decreased with loupe magnification to identify and match the epineural vessels and the fascicles. Recent advances in intraoperative nerve staining techniques have also made it possible to align motor and sensory fascicles more accurately. Nerves should be repaired with 9-0 nylon suture because it is easy to use and does not tend to cause foreign-body reaction or nerve gapping. Smaller suture fails under tension and larger suture fails by pull-out (8).

With lesions in continuity, the decision to perform neurolysis or excision with repair, grafting, or both may be a difficult one. Sparing of intact or regenerating portions of the nerve is ideal but is often technically demanding. A nerve stimulator may be of help, but relatively spared portions of the nerve may still be resected (9).

Other problems associated with nerve grafting are poor harvesting technique, graft-size mismatch, graft tension, graft necrosis, and failure to recognize multilevel nerve injury.

INJURIES ASSOCIATED WITH NERVE INJURIES

Because of the proximity of nerves to bones and blood vessels, nerve trauma often accompanies injuries to these structures; therefore patients with such injuries should always be evaluated for nerve injuries. Depending on the regional anatomy, each fracture or dislocation is associated with a unique pattern of potential nerve injuries. For example, shoulder girdle injuries are often associated with brachial plexus lesions. Patients with shoulder dislocations should be evaluated for axillary nerve injuries because of the high incidence of traumatic dysfunction (10). Approximately 10% of humeral shaft fractures are associated with injury to the radial nerve in the spiral groove (11). Elbow injuries, especially dislocations and displaced fractures of the distal humerus, frequently involve the ulnar nerve, the median nerve, or both (12,13). Wrist fractures can be accompanied by injuries to the median nerve; acute carpal tunnel syndrome occurs in as many as 17% of patients with such injuries (14). The reported incidence of nerve injuries in association with severe injuries to the pelvis is 34% (15), and 10% of fractures or dislocations of the hip are accompanied by nerve injuries, usually to the peroneal branch of the sciatic nerve (16). Knee dislocations and fractures of the fibular head can injure the peroneal nerve. Open fractures and high-energy fractures are more likely than other injuries to be associated with nerve damage. The callus of a healing fracture can also entrap or compress nerves; such compression can cause progressive gradual loss of function.

Soft-tissue swelling resulting from fractures can cause nerves to be secondarily entrapped in fixed positions. The ulnar nerve can be compressed in the cubital tunnel; this nerve should be transposed during surgical procedures for most severe fractures of the distal humerus or proximal ulna. Acute carpal tunnel syndrome or compression of the ulnar nerve in Guyon's canal at the wrist can occur after wrist fractures, even when there has been no direct trauma to the nerve; division of the transverse carpal ligament should be strongly considered.

Vascular injuries are also common in association with nerve trauma. Two published studies found that 40% of patients with traumatic vascular injuries also had nerve damage (17,18). Vessel injuries are often associated with aneurysms, arteriovenous fistulae, and bleeding, all of which can lead to nerve compression. Injury to the axillary artery or the subclavian artery may result in aneurysms that can compress the brachial plexus, causing progressive neurologic deficit or even a complex regional-pain syndrome (19). Hematoma formation in a confined space can cause progressive neurologic deterioration even without direct neural injury.

Patients with traumatic brain injuries have been found to have a 10% to 34% incidence of peripheral nerve injuries (20,21). Because the patients often do not complain of problems associated with the nerve injury, physicians caring for them should have a high index of suspicion for nerve lesions. Thorough neurologic examination with EMG can be helpful in diagnosing these injuries. As many as 10% of patients with traumatic brain injuries will also have brachial plexus lesions (20). Thus, in addition to brain injury, patients with brachial plexus palsy may also have injuries to the cervical spine, clavicle, scapula, or proximal humerus.

Compartment syndrome of the extremity is another important cause of neurologic loss, even without intrinsic nerve injury. Acute compartment syndrome can be caused by a number of different conditions that affect local blood flow, such as fractures, shock, crush injuries, tight dressings, vascular injuries, severe swelling, or bleeding into a compartment. The local blood flow to the tissues is diminished by a decrease in arterial inflow pressure, an increase in venous pressure, or a combination of both. Pain with passive stretch and pain out of proportion to the patient's injury are the most important clinical findings in the conscious patient with suspected compartment syndrome. Splitting of casts or other circumferential dressings down to the skin (22) has been shown to significantly decrease compartment pressure. Circumferential casts should not be used for obtunded patients because the conditions of these patients cannot be reliably monitored. The diagnosis can be confirmed by measuring compartmental pressures with intravenous tubing attached to an arterial line transducer, a handheld pressure monitor, or another technique. When intracompartmental pressures are higher than 30 mmHg, decompressive fasciotomy is indicated. Prompt recognition of compartment syndrome is essential because permanent damage may occur after no more than three to four hours, and certainly after six to eight hours, of prolonged muscle ischemia (23).

Volkmann's ischemic contracture occurs when an acute compartment syndrome is left untreated. Nerve dysfunction occurs for two main reasons. The initial nerve problem results from nerve ischemia. Later, the nerves are entrapped by tight, constricting bands of fibrotic muscle that had been injured by ischemia in the initial phase of the compartment syndrome. Volkmann's contracture can be devastating, with loss of function of the muscles, joint contractures, and diminished sensation. In general, this problem can be avoided by prompt diagnosis and treatment of compartment syndromes (24).

INJURIES TO NERVES FROM OPERATIONS OR OTHER MEDICAL PROCEDURES

As stated previously, as many as 10% of nerve injuries are iatrogenic. Although most of these injuries will resolve spontaneously, deficits will occasionally linger and may require surgery. Every effort should be made to prevent potentially avoidable lesions and to minimize complications when a nerve injury has occurred.

Lower Cranial Nerves and Cervical Nerves

The vagus nerve and its branches are susceptible to injury when neck surgery is performed; these injuries are most often associated with carotid endarterectomy (CEA) or cardiac surgery. The reported incidence of nerve injury is approximately 1% for primary CEA (25) and as high as 12% for repeat CEA (26). After coronary artery bypass grafting (CABG), vocal cord dysfunction is seen in 1.9% to 7.8% of patients (27,28). Injury to the vagus nerve or its branches may cause hoarseness or dysphagia and can lead to aspiration. Diagnosis is made by laryngoscopy. More than 90% of these injuries will resolve with time, although some patients will require treatments such as Teflon injection into the vocal cords to obtain a satisfactory result (29). In one reported case, chest tube insertion caused hemorrhage around the vagus nerve, which led to severe bradycardia and death (30).

The hypoglossal nerve can also be damaged during surgery to the neck; damage to this nerve has been reported with CEA and with anterior cervical spine surgery (26,31). Most of these lesions will resolve spontaneously.

The spinal accessory nerve is the sole motor innervation of the trapezius muscle. Damage to this nerve causes weakness of the trapezius, drooping of the shoulder, and even winging of the scapula. Spinal accessory nerve palsies are not common, but approximately 10% of these injuries are accounted for by iatrogenic injury (32). The nerve is most susceptible to injury in the posterior triangle of the neck, where it lies in a superficial position. Injury can be caused by a wide variety of surgical procedures, including radical neck dissection, lymph node biopsy, and CEA, and can also result from irradiation or even from prolonged use of a sling (33). Occasionally, the spinal accessory nerve is deliberately cut and used in nerve transfer to treat severe brachial plexus injuries. Patients who experience complete nerve palsies after surgery or penetrating trauma should be treated with neurolysis, nerve repair, or grafting. Although recommendations state that surgery should be performed within the first three months after injury, useful recovery has been seen in patients undergoing surgery as long as 14 months after injury (34). Patients with chronic trapezius palsy lasting more than one year may benefit from transfer of the levator scapulae and rhomboid muscles (35).

The phrenic nerve arises from the third, fourth, and fifth cervical nerve roots, travels through the neck and chest, and innervates the diaphragm. The nerve may be injured at any level along its course, but intrathoracic lesions are most common. The left phrenic nerve is more frequently affected because of its close association with the pericardium. Cases of bilateral damage are rare. Although any thoracic surgical procedure may damage the phrenic nerve, injuries are most common after open heart surgery. Two mechanisms by which the nerve can be damaged may play a role alone or in combination: topical myocardial cooling and phrenic ischemia after dissection of the internal mammary artery (IMA). Topical hypothermia is routine during cardiac surgery, and because of the proximity of the phrenic nerve to myocardial tissue, the nerve also undergoes substantial cooling. In a prospective study, postoperative fluoroscopy showed diminished motion of the left hemidiaphragm in nearly 60% of patients who underwent cardiac cooling (36). The other proposed mechanism of injury to the phrenic nerve is damage to the nerve's vascular supply during IMA dissection; ligation of the pericardiophrenic artery may potentiate the effects of hypothermic damage (37). There is no gold standard for the diagnosis of phrenic nerve dysfunction. The most commonly used tests at present are phrenic nerve conduction studies, fluoroscopy, and ultrasonography (38). Symptoms may range from none to difficulty in weaning from mechanical ventilation and may vary according to the patient's underlying pulmonary function. Most phrenic nerve injuries resolve within three to six months (39). Pediatric patients do not recover as well from phrenic nerve paralysis as do adult patients, and they are also more likely to experience difficulty in weaning from mechanical ventilation (38). When the effects of phrenic nerve dysfunction are severe, treatment with diaphragmatic plication is sometimes performed (40).

The long thoracic nerve is seldom injured, but it may be damaged during radical mastectomy, first-rib resection, and transaxillary sympathectomy (41). The long thoracic nerve provides the only innervation of the serratus anterior muscle; damage to this nerve leads to winging of the scapula. Exploration with early neurolysis, repair, or grafting should be considered for patients with iatrogenic injuries or penetrating trauma, but few published studies have documented the results of this treatment (42). Patients with persistent winging of the scapula after prolonged conservative treatment or failure of surgery may be candidates for transfer of the sternal portion of the pectoralis major to the scapula (42).

Brachial Plexus and Shoulder Level

Brachial plexus injuries are among the most common iatrogenic injuries to the peripheral nervous system. Postoperative brachial plexopathy is associated with median sternotomy, transaxillary first-rib resection, radical mastectomy, surgery for shoulder instability, shoulder arthroscopy, injuries from regional anesthesia, and poor positioning (38,43–45). The brachial plexus may also be injured by irradiation, usually after surgery for breast cancer.

The incidence of postoperative brachial plexus palsy in association with open heart surgery ranges from 2.7% to 10% (46,47). Key factors associated with brachial plexopathy after median sternotomy are sternal retraction and IMA dissection. With sternal retraction, the first rib rotates superiorly and the clavicle pushes into the retroclavicular space, thereby stretching the brachial plexus (48). Fracture of the posterior first rib by sternal retraction can cause direct injury to the plexus; neurologic complaints are associated with the fracture site of the first rib. Vander et al. found that a more caudal placement of the sternal retractor decreased the incidence of first-rib fracture, and they also recommended that the retractor be opened as little as possible to decrease the likelihood of rib fractures (49). Other investigators found that removing the uppermost pair of blades from an Ankeney-type retractor reduced the incidence of first-rib fracture from 50% to 16% (50).

Brachial plexus lesions have also been associated with dissection of the IMA for use as a graft. In a prospective study of 1000 patients, Vahl et al. found that the incidence of neuropathies was 1% for patients who had not received IMA grafts but 10.6% for those who had received IMA grafts (46). It is believed that these lesions are caused by the asymmetric sternal retraction required for harvesting the graft.

The only patient characteristic associated with increased risk of postoperative brachial plexopathy is advanced age (49,51). Other characteristics such as diabetes mellitus, sex, height, weight, and smoking status are not significant risk factors (52).

The lower roots of the brachial plexus (C8–T1) are most commonly affected by plexopathies after sternotomy. Patients typically exhibit symptoms in the distribution of the ulnar nerve. Ulnar nerve dysfunction at the elbow can coexist with brachial plexopathies; this dysfunction may be a preexisting but subclinical condition or may be related to positioning during surgery (53). Thorough physical examination can often help to determine whether a lesion exists and its severity because the muscles innervated by the C8 to T1 contributions of the median (flexor pollicis longus) and radial nerves (extensor pollicis longus) will also be affected. EMG may also be useful in localizing the lesion (53). Fortunately, only approximately 1% of patients will have symptoms that persist for more than three to four months (46,52).

The infraclavicular portions of the brachial plexus (cords and terminal branches) are at risk during surgical procedures to the shoulder and axilla. Complete transection of the brachial plexus has been seen in association with axillary dissection during radical mastectomy (45). Injuries to several nerves about the shoulder, most commonly to branches of the axillary nerve, have been reported after shoulder arthroscopy. The incidence of nerve injury after anterior reconstruction for glenohumeral instability has been reported to be approximately 8% (54). Eighty-seven percent of patients with these lesions experienced full recovery within six months, and all were believed to have traction-type lesions. Another study of eight patients with iatrogenic nerve injuries after surgery for shoulder instability found that seven had visible structural damage (nerve lacerations or suturing) (55). In both studies, the musculocutaneous nerve was most frequently involved.

Radiation-induced brachial plexus injuries can be a devastating complication of radiation therapy after mastectomy for breast cancer. Symptoms usually develop months to years after treatment; symptoms usually begin with sensory loss but may progress to complete plexopathy with a flaccid, insensate arm. Pathologically, the nerves are often entrapped in dense scar tissue, but damage to the vasculature of the nerves probably plays an important role in nerve damage (56). Unfortunately, there is no effective treatment for this type of lesion (44).

Arm and Forearm Level

Using tourniquets during surgery to the extremities causes nerve injuries in approximately 1 in 5000 cases (57). The usual clinical picture is involvement of all major nerves in the extremity, with greater involvement of motor nerves than sensory nerves. Conservative treatment is the rule because nearly all patients will experience a complete recovery.

Ulnar nerve injuries at the elbow have been reported as a complication of surgical repair of elbow fractures and of ulnar nerve transposition. Displaced fractures of the distal humerus in children are usually treated with closed reduction and percutaneous pinning of the fracture. Postoperative ulnar nerve palsy develops in approximately 5% of patients after crossed pinning (58). Although some authors recommend observation alone for this problem, others advocate pin removal with exploration of the nerve because of the possibility of direct penetration of the nerve by the pin (59). Whether treated surgically or not, most patients with ulnar nerve palsy will experience complete recovery, although resolution may take several months. Patients who suffer malunion of the distal humerus with progressive deformity may also experience late ulnar nerve palsy.

The median nerve is most often injured at either the elbow or the wrist. Injuries around the elbow are usually due to venipuncture or arterial catheterization. At the wrist level, the median nerve is most frequently injured during carpal tunnel release. Both the endoscopic and the open technique have been reported to be associated with lacerations of the main trunk of the median nerve, the palmar cutaneous branch, the median motor branch, the common and proper digital nerves, the main trunk of the ulnar nerve, or the motor branch of the ulnar nerve (60). By far, the most common nerve lesion is neuropraxia, which is self-limited and resolves completely. The median nerve may also be injured during corticosteroid injections to treat carpal tunnel syndrome if these injections are inadvertently administered intraneurally (61). There are also several reported cases of mistaken removal of the median nerve during attempts to harvest the palmaris longus tendon for use as a graft (62). This mistake is often not recognized until it is too late, and the nerve must be reconstructed with nerve grafting.

The radial nerve can be injured during surgical treatment of fractures or nonunions of the humeral shaft, during surgical approaches to the elbow (anterior or lateral approaches), by the placement of external fixation pins, by surgery for de Quervain's tenosynovitis, or by surgical procedures on the radial artery. Awareness of neurologic complications resulting from harvesting the radial artery for CABG has increased. A survey of patients who underwent such harvesting showed that 30% subsequently reported some type of neurologic complaint (sensation abnormality or thumb weakness) (63). Because of the nature of this study, it is difficult to determine whether the median nerve, the radial nerve, or both were involved or whether the problems were due to nerve traction or insufficient vascularity. A recent report described the cases of two patients with longstanding dysesthesias resulting from radial sensory nerve injury after radial artery harvest (64).

Pelvis and Hip Level

Injuries to the ilioinguinal, iliohypogastric, and genitofemoral nerves can cause pain in the inguinal region. These nerves are most commonly injured during inguinal herniorrhaphy but can also be damaged during inguinal lymph node dissection, abdominal hysterectomy, abdominoplasty, and harvest of iliac crest bone grafts (65). The incidence of nerve entrapment after herniorrhaphy has been reported to be 4.2% with laparoscopic techniques and 1.8% with conventional surgery (66). The nerve most commonly entrapped was the genitofemoral nerve (2% of patients) (66). The best results of surgical treatment were achieved for patients with lesions of the ilioinguinal nerve or the iliohypogastric nerve, and the worst results were in patients with injuries to the genitofemoral nerve (67).

The lateral femoral cutaneous nerve (LFCN) is vulnerable to injuries during herniorrhaphy, during surgical procedures to the pelvis, especially those using the ilioinguinal approach, and during spine surgery. Injury to this nerve causes pain, numbness, or both to the anterolateral thigh; such injury is also called meralgia paresthetica. An anatomical study of the LFCN showed that 25% of patients in an autopsy series had an anatomically variant course of the nerve (68). The reported incidence of nerve entrapment in association with hernia repair is approximately 1% (66). During spine surgery, placing the patient on the Hall–Relton frame may cause external pressure on the nerve at the anterior superior iliac spine (69). The nerve can also be injured by retroperitoneal hematoma or during harvest of iliac crest bone grafts (69,70). Almost 90% of patients experienced complete recovery within three months, and more than 90% of those requiring surgical decompression experienced good to excellent outcomes (69,70).

The femoral nerve forms within the substance of the psoas muscle, emerging along the lateral border to run between the psoas and iliacus muscles. It then enters the thigh after passing beneath the inguinal ligament, branches out to supply motor input to the quadriceps, and continues as the saphenous nerve. The nerve can be injured in either its intrapelvic portions or its extrapelvic portions. Symptoms range from mild paresthesias to profound motor and sensory deficits. Motor weakness is usually manifested by buckling of the knee as the result of weakness of the quadriceps. Most femoral nerve lesions are iatrogenic. Causes include compression from self-retaining retractors, transection or suture during herniorrhaphy, infrainguinal vascular procedures, ischemia, cement entrapment in hip arthroplasty, traction, and positioning (71–74). Probably the most common cause is compression by self-retaining retractors, most often during pelvic surgery. The reported incidence of femoral nerve lesions in association with total abdominal hysterectomy is 11% (75). Anatomical studies have shown that the lateral blade of the retractor can directly compress the nerve or can trap the nerve and the psoas muscle between the retractor and the pelvic wall (71). Most authors recommend using smaller blades on the self-retaining retractors to prevent this problem (75,76).

The saphenous nerve is the sensory continuation of the femoral nerve; it provides sensory supply to the anteromedial aspect of the leg and the medial side of the foot. Patients can experience anesthesia, hyperesthesia, or pain in its distribution when the nerve is damaged. The nerve is commonly injured during harvest of vein grafts for CABG. One study showed that 90% of patients experienced some anesthesia after vein harvest, and 72% were still experiencing these symptoms 20 months after harvest (77).

Because of its proximity to the hip joint, the sciatic nerve is most commonly injured during hip arthroplasty. The incidence of such injuries in association with primary hip arthroplasty is 1% and increases to 3% in association with revision surgery (78). Although intraoperative traction of the nerve is believed to be the most common cause of injury, the nerve may also be injured by postoperative dislocation (79), by heat damage from cement (80), or by nerve laceration. The prognosis is best for patients who can walk immediately after surgery or who regain motor function within two weeks (74). However, only 44% of patients experience full recovery (74). Whether patients undergo neurolysis, nerve repair or grafting, or conservative treatment, recovery is more likely in the tibial nerve distribution than in the peroneal division of the nerve (81). Other causes of iatrogenic sciatic injury include ischemia after prolonged intra-aortic balloon pump therapy (82), improper patient positioning during surgical procedures, and injection injuries.

The peroneal nerve is susceptible to injury because it winds around the posterolateral corner of the knee joint. Damage to this nerve causes footdrop, a weakness of dorsiflexion of the ankle. Peroneal nerve palsies have been reported as a complication of knee arthroplasty, tibial osteotomy, knee arthroscopy, lower-extremity casts, positioning during surgery, and the use of pneumatic compression devices (83–86). As with most iatrogenic nerve lesions, most injuries to the peroneal nerve will resolve with time. If surgery is performed, only 40% of patients will recover sufficient strength to prevent footdrop, and approximately half will regain protective sensation in the foot (87).

Injection and Catheterization Injuries

Peripheral nerves are at risk of injury during all invasive procedures, including intramuscular injections, arterial and venous catheterization, and even routine venipuncture. A review of sciatic nerve injuries at the level of the buttocks reported that more than half were the result of misplaced gluteal muscle injections. Not all injection palsies resolve spontaneously (81). Published reports have described brachial plexus neuropathy after subclavian catheterization and median neuropathy after brachial artery catheterization (88,89). Many reports describe peripheral nerve injury leading to complex regional-pain syndrome after routine venipuncture (90).

Anesthesia-Related Nerve Injuries

Peripheral nerve damage associated with anesthesia may result from injury to the nerves themselves by administration of regional anesthesia or may be related to patient positioning. Regional anesthesia for upper-extremity surgery is associated with a number of serious neurologic complications, although most of these complications are minor and transient (91). Injury may result from direct needle trauma to nerves or from hematomas that form after transarterial techniques.

Although in this chapter injuries related to patient positioning are treated as anesthesia-related complications, it is imperative that every surgeon be aware of these complications and know how to avoid them. Analysis of the American Society of Anesthesiologists Closed Claims Database showed that 16% of claims were for anesthesia-related nerve injuries and that nearly 30% of those claims were for injuries to the ulnar nerve (92). The most commonly affected nerves are the ulnar nerve and the peroneal nerve, probably because of their superficial course in the extremities. The ulnar nerve can be injured by compression against the operating table or by excessive flexion of the elbow. The

peroneal nerve is vulnerable to injury because it winds around the fibular head, and it may be compressed against the lithotomy pole or by placing the patient in the lateral position. If the patient's arm rests on a hard edge, the radial nerve can be compressed against the posterior part of the humerus. The sciatic nerve is at risk of compression when patients are thin; other risk factors are lengthy procedures and hard tables. The nerve can also suffer traction injury when patients are placed in the lithotomy position with the hip flexed and in maximal external rotation. The lithotomy position can also cause femoral nerve palsies by entrapping the nerve against the inguinal ligament when the hip is hyperflexed. The brachial plexus can also undergo traction injury as the result of positioning, particularly when the arms are placed in abduction with external rotation and posterior shoulder displacement.

REFERENCES

1. Noble J, Munro CA, Prasad VS, Midha R. Analysis of upper and lower extremity peripheral nerve injuries in a population of patients with multiple injuries. J Trauma 1998; 45(1):116–122.
2. Birch R, Bonney G, Dowell J, Hollingdale J. Iatrogenic injuries of peripheral nerves. J Bone Joint Surg Br 1991; 73:280–282.
3. Mackinnon SE. New directions in peripheral nerve surgery. Ann Plast Surg 1989; 22:257–273.
4. Sunderland S. Nerve Injuries and Repair. A Critical Appraisal. Oxford: Churchill Livingstone, 1990.
5. Frykman GK, Gramyk K. Results of nerve grafting. In: Gelberman RH, ed. Operative Nerve Repair and Reconstruction. Philadelphia: JB Lippincott, 1991:553–567.
6. Clark WL, Trumble TE, Swiontkowski MF, Tencer AF. Nerve tension and blood flow in a rat model of immediate and delayed repairs. J Hand Surg [Am] 1992; 17(4):677–687.
7. Hentz VR, Rosen JM, Xiao SJ, McGill KC, Abraham G. The nerve gap dilemma: a comparison of nerves repaired end to end under tension with nerve grafts in a primate model. J Hand Surg [Am] 1993; 18: 417–425.
8. Giddins GE, Wade PJ, Amis AA. Primary nerve repair: strength of repair with different gauges of nylon suture material. J Hand Surg [Br] 1989; 14:301–302.
9. Spinner RJ, Kline DG. Surgery for peripheral nerve and brachial plexus injuries or other nerve lesions. Muscle Nerve 2000; 23(5):680–695.
10. Visser CP, Coene LN, Brand R, Tavy DL. The incidence of nerve injury in anterior dislocation of the shoulder and its influence on functional recovery. A prospective clinical and EMG study. J Bone Joint Surg Br 1999; 81(4):679–685.
11. Samardzic M, Grujicic D, Milinkovic ZB. Radial nerve lesions associated with fractures of the humeral shaft. Injury 1990; 21:220–222.
12. Lyons ST, Quinn M, Stanitski CL. Neurovascular injuries in type III humeral supracondylar fractures in children. Clin Orthop 2000; 376:62–67.
13. Galbraith KA, McCullough CJ. Acute nerve injury as a complication of closed fractures or dislocations of the elbow. Injury 1979; 11(2):159–164.

14. Stewart HD, Innes AR, Burke FD. The hand complications of Colles' fractures. J Hand Surg [Br] 1985; 10:103–106.

15. Majeed SA. Neurologic deficits in major pelvic injuries. Clin Orthop 1992; 282:222–228.

16. Cornwall R, Radomisli TE. Nerve injury in traumatic dislocation of the hip. Clin Orthop 2000; 377:84–91.

17. Pillai L, Luchette FA, Romano KS, Ricotta JJ. Upper-extremity arterial injury. Am Surg 1997; 63(3):224–227.

18. Stanec S, Tonkovic I, Stanec Z, Tonkovic D, Dzepina I. Treatment of upper limb nerve war injuries associated with vascular trauma. Injury 1997; 28(7):463–468.

19. Tripp HF, Cook JW. Axillary artery aneurysms. Mil Med 1998; 163(9):653–655.

20. Stone L, Keenan MA. Peripheral nerve injuries in the adult with traumatic brain injury. Clin Orthop 1988; 233:136–144.

21. Cosgrove JL, Vargo M, Reidy ME. A prospective study of peripheral nerve lesions occurring in traumatic brain-injured patients. Am J Phys Med Rehabil 1989; 68(1):15–17.

22. Garfin SR, Mubarak SJ, Evans KL, Hargens AR, Akeson WH. Quantification of intracompartmental pressure and volume under plaster casts. J Bone Joint Surg Am 1981; 63:449–453.

23. Trumble TE. Compartment syndrome and Volkmann's contracture. In: Trumble TE, ed. Principles of Hand Surgery and Therapy. Philadelphia: WB Saunders, 2000:179–191.

24. Hovius SE, Ultee J. Volkmann's ischemic contracture. Prevention and treatment. Hand Clin 2000; 16(4):647–657.

25. Johna S, Gaw F, Berten R, Miro J. Carotid endarterectomy for severe asymptomatic carotid stenosis: a perioperative experience at a community hospital. Am Surg 2000; 66(11):1046–1048.

26. AbuRahma AF, Choueiri MA. Cranial and cervical nerve injuries after repeat carotid endarterectomy. J Vasc Surg 2000; 32:649–654.

27. Shafei H, el-Kholy A, Azmy S, Ebrahim M, al-Ebrahim K. Vocal cord dysfunction after cardiac surgery: an overlooked complication. Eur J Cardiothorac Surg 1997; 11:564–566.

28. Kawahito S, Kitahata H, Kimura H, Tanaka K, Oshita S. Recurrent laryngeal nerve palsy after cardiovascular surgery: relationship to the placement of a transesophageal echocardiographic probe. J Cardiothorac Vasc Anesth 1999; 13:528–531.

29. AbuRahma AF, Lim RY. Management of vagus nerve injury after carotid endarterectomy. Surgery 1996; 119(3):245–247.

30. Ward EW, Hughes TE. Sudden death following chest tube insertion: an unusual case of vagus nerve irritation. J Trauma 1994; 36(2):258–259.

31. Sengupta DK, Grevitt MP, Mehdian SM. Hypoglossal nerve injury as a complication of anterior surgery to the upper cervical spine. Eur Spine J 1999; 8(1):78–80.

32. Kim D, Cho YJ, Tiel RL, Kline DG. Surgical outcomes of 111 spinal accessory nerve injuries. Neurosurgery 2003; 53(5):1106–1112.

33. Wiater JM, Bigliani LU. Spinal accessory nerve injury. Clin Orthop 1999; 368:5–16.

34. Nakamichi K, Tachibana S. Iatrogenic injury of the spinal accessory nerve. Results of repair. J Bone Joint Surg Am 1998; 80(11):1616–1621.

35. Bigliani LU, Compito CA, Duralde XA, Wolfe IN. Transfer of the levator scapulae, rhomboid major and rhomboid minor for paralysis of the trapezius. J Bone Joint Surg [Am] 1996; 78:1534–1540.

36. Benjamin JJ, Cascade PN, Rubenfire M, Wajszczuk W, Kerin NZ. Left lower lobe atelectasis and consolidation following cardiac surgery: the effect of topical cooling on the phrenic nerve. Radiology 1982; 142(1):11–14.

37. O'Brien JW, Johnson SH, VanSteyn SJ, et al. Effects of internal mammary artery dissection on phrenic nerve perfusion and function. Ann Thorac Surg 1991; 52(2):182–188.

38. Sharma AD, Parmley CL, Sreeram G, Grocott HP. Peripheral nerve injuries during cardiac surgery: risk factors, diagnosis, prognosis, and prevention. Anesth Analg 2000; 91:1358–1369.

39. DeVita MA, Robinson LR, Rehder J, Hattler B, Cohen C. Incidence and natural history of phrenic neuropathy occurring during open-heart surgery. Chest 1993; 103(3):850–856.

40. Tripp HF, Bolton JW. Phrenic nerve injury following cardiac surgery: a review. J Card Surg 1998; 13(3):218–223.

41. Kauppila LI, Vastamaki M. Iatrogenic serratus anterior paralysis. Long-term outcome in 26 patients. Chest 1996; 109:31–34.

42. Wiater JM, Flatow EL. Long thoracic nerve injury. Clin Orthop 1999; 368:17–27.

43. Boardman ND III, Cofield RH. Neurologic complications of shoulder surgery. Clin Orthop 1999; 368:44–53.

44. Wilbourn AJ. Iatrogenic nerve injuries. Neurol Clin 1998; 16(1):55–82.

45. Kline DG, Hackett ER. Reappraisal of timing for exploration of civilian peripheral nerve injuries. Surgery 1975; 78:54–65.

46. Vahl CF, Carl I, Muller-Vahl H, Struck E. Brachial plexus injury after cardiac surgery. The role of internal mammary artery preparation: a prospective study on 1000 consecutive patients. J Thorac Cardiovasc Surg 1991; 102(5):724–729.

47. Seyfer AE, Grammer NY, Bogumill GP, Provost JM, Chandry U. Upper extremity neuropathies after cardiac surgery. J Hand Surg [Am] 1985; 10(1):16–19.

48. Kirsh MM, Magee KR, Gago O, Kahn DR, Sloan H. Brachial plexus injury following median sternotomy incision. Ann Thorac Surg 1971; 11(4):315–319.

49. Vander Salm TJ, Cereda JM, Cutler BS. Brachial plexus injury following median sternotomy. J Thorac Cardiovasc Surg 1980; 80(3):447–452.

50. Baisden CE, Greenwald LV, Symbas PN. Occult rib fractures and brachial plexus injury following median sternotomy for open-heart operations. Ann Thorac Surg 1984; 38(3):192–194.

51. Vander Salm TJ, Cutler BS, Okike ON. Brachial plexus injury following median sternotomy. Part II. J Thorac Cardiovasc Surg 1982; 83(6):914–917.

52. Hanson MR, Breuer AC, Furlan AJ, et al. Mechanism and frequency of brachial plexus injury in open-heart surgery: a prospective analysis. Ann Thorac Surg 1983; 36(6):675–679.

53. Morin JE, Long R, Elleker MG, Eisen AA, Wynands E, Ralphs-Thibodeau S. Upper extremity neuropathies following median sternotomy. Ann Thorac Surg 1982; 34(2):181–185.

54. Ho E, Cofield RH, Balm MR, Hattrup SJ, Rowland CM. Neurologic complications of surgery for anterior

shoulder instability. J Shoulder Elbow Surg 1999; 8(3):266–270.

55. Richards RR, Hudson AR, Bertoia JT, Urbaniak JR, Waddell JP. Injury to the brachial plexus during Putti-Platt and Bristow procedures. A report of eight cases. Am J Sports Med 1987; 15(4):374–380.

56. Vujaskovic Z. Structural and physiological properties of peripheral nerves after intraoperative irradiation. J Peripher Nerv Syst 1997; 2(4):343–349.

57. Landi A, Saracino A, Pinelli M, Caserta G, Facchini MC. Tourniquet paralysis in microsurgery. Ann Acad Med Singapore 1995; 24(suppl 4):89–93.

58. Lyons JP, Ashley E, Hoffer MM. Ulnar nerve palsies after percutaneous cross-pinning of supracondylar fractures in children's elbows. J Pediatr Orthop 1998; 18(1):43–45.

59. Rasool MN. Ulnar nerve injury after K-wire fixation of supracondylar humerus fractures in children. J Pediatr Orthop 1998; 18(5):686–690.

60. Palmer AK, Toivonen DA. Complications of endoscopic and open carpal tunnel release. J Hand Surg [Am] 1999; 24(3):561–565.

61. McConnell JR, Bush DC. Intraneural steroid injection as a complication in the management of carpal tunnel syndrome. A report of three cases. Clin Orthop 1990; 250:181–184.

62. Vastamaki M. Median nerve as free tendon graft. J Hand Surg [Br] 1987; 12(2):187–188.

63. Denton TA, Trento L, Cohen M, et al. Radial artery harvesting for coronary bypass operations: neurologic complications and their potential mechanisms. J Thorac Cardiovasc Surg 2001; 121(5):951–956.

64. Arons JA, Collins N, Arons MS. Permanent nerve injury in the forearm following radial artery harvest: a report of two cases. Ann Plast Surg 1999; 43(3):299–301.

65. Nahabedian MY, Dellon AL. Outcome of the operative management of nerve injuries in the ilioinguinal region. J Am Coll Surg 1997; 184(3):265–268.

66. Stark E, Oestreich K, Wendl K, Rumstadt B, Hagmuller E. Nerve irritation after laparoscopic hernia repair. Surg Endosc 1999; 13(9):878–881.

67. Lee CH, Dellon AL. Surgical management of groin pain of neural origin. J Am Coll Surg 2000; 191(2):137–142.

68. de Ridder VA, de Lange S, Popta JV. Anatomical variations of the lateral femoral cutaneous nerve and the consequences for surgery. J Orthop Trauma 1999; 13(3):207–211.

69. Mirovsky Y, Neuwirth M. Injuries to the lateral femoral cutaneous nerve during spine surgery. Spine 2000; 25(10):1266–1269.

70. Nahabedian MY, Dellon AL. Meralgia paresthetica: etiology, diagnosis, and outcome of surgical decompression. Ann Plast Surg 1995; 35(6):590–594.

71. Walsh C, Walsh A. Postoperative femoral neuropathy. Surg Gynecol Obstet 1992; 174(3):255–263.

72. Busch T, Strauch J, Aleksic I, Sirbu H, Dalichau H. Incidence and importance of lower extremity nerve lesions after infrainguinal vascular surgical interventions. Eur J Vasc Endovasc Surg 1999; 17(4):290–293.

73. Jerosch J. Femoral nerve palsy in hip replacement due to pelvic cement extrusion. Arch Orthop Trauma Surg 2000; 120(9):499–501.

74. Schmalzried TP, Noordin S, Amstutz HC. Update on nerve palsy associated with total hip replacement. Clin Orthop 1997; 344:188–206.

75. Kvist-Poulsen H, Borel J. Iatrogenic femoral neuropathy subsequent to abdominal hysterectomy: incidence and prevention. Obstet Gynecol 1982; 60(4):516–520.

76. Dillavou ED, Anderson LR, Bernert RA, et al. Lower extremity iatrogenic nerve injury due to compression during intraabdominal surgery. Am J Surg 1997; 173(6):504–508.

77. Mountney J, Wilkinson GA. Saphenous neuralgia after coronary artery bypass grafting. Eur J Cardiothorac Surg 1999; 16(4):440–443.

78. Schmalzried TP, Amstutz HC, Dorey FJ. Nerve palsy associated with total hip replacement. Risk factors and prognosis. J Bone Joint Surg Am 1991; 73(7):1074–1080.

79. Johanson NA, Pellicci PM, Tsairis P, Salvati EA. Nerve injury in total hip arthroplasty. Clin Orthop 1983; 179:214–222.

80. Birch R, Wilkinson MC, Vijayan KP, Gschmeissner S. Cement burn of the sciatic nerve. J Bone Joint Surg Br 1992; 74(5):731–733.

81. Kline DG, Kim D, Midha R, Harsh C, Tiel R. Management and results of sciatic nerve injuries: a 24-year experience. J Neurosurg 1998; 89(1):13–23.

82. McManis PG. Sciatic nerve lesions during cardiac surgery. Neurology 1994; 44(4):684–687.

83. Idusuyi OB, Morrey BF. Peroneal nerve palsy after total knee arthroplasty. Assessment of predisposing and prognostic factors. J Bone Joint Surg Am 1996; 78(2):177–184.

84. Marti RK, Verhagen RA, Kerkhoffs GM, Moojen TM. Proximal tibial varus osteotomy. Indications, technique, and five to twenty-one-year results. J Bone Joint Surg Am 2001; 83(2):164–170.

85. McGrory BJ, Burke DW. Peroneal nerve palsy following intermittent sequential pneumatic compression. Orthopedics 2000; 23(10):1103–1105.

86. Rodeo SA, Sobel M, Weiland AJ. Deep peroneal-nerve injury as a result of arthroscopic meniscectomy. A case report and review of the literature. J Bone Joint Surg Am 1993; 75(8):1221–1224.

87. Wilkinson MC, Birch R. Repair of the common peroneal nerve. J Bone Joint Surg Br 1995; 77(3):501–503.

88. Kennedy AM, Grocott M, Schwartz MS, Modarres H, Scott M, Schon F. Median nerve injury: an underrecognised complication of brachial artery cardiac catheterisation? J Neurol Neurosurg Psychiatr 1997; 63(4):542–546.

89. Trentman TL, Rome JD, Messick JM Jr. Brachial plexus neuropathy following attempt at subclavian vein catheterization. Case report. Reg Anesth 1996; 21(2):163–165.

90. Horowitz SH. Venipuncture-induced causalgia: anatomic relations of upper extremity superficial veins and nerves, and clinical considerations. Transfusion 2000; 40(9):1036–1040.

91. Stark RH. Neurologic injury from axillary block anesthesia. J Hand Surg [Am] 1996; 21(3):391–396.

92. Cheney FW, Domino KB, Caplan RA, Posner KL. Nerve injury associated with anesthesia: a closed claims analysis. Anesthesiology 1999; 90(4):1062–1069.

Psychological and Behavioral Complications of Trauma

Thomas Mellman
*Dartmouth Hitchcock Medical Center, Dartmouth Medical School, Lebanon,
New Hampshire, U.S.A.*

Gillian Hotz
Department of Surgery, University of Miami Miller School of Medicine, Miami, Florida, U.S.A.

If complications of trauma are to be approached comprehensively, the cognitive, emotional, and behavioral domains must be considered. Brain structure and function are commonly affected by physical injury. In addition to the more overt changes in level of consciousness or behavior, which can result from moderate to severe brain injury, physical trauma to the head can also lead to more subtle alterations of cognition and mood that nonetheless can have a profound impact on functioning and quality of life. One category of trauma complications that warrants specific consideration is traumatic brain injury (TBI).

It is also increasingly recognized that a substantial number of patients who survive life-threatening experiences will develop emotional and behavioral consequences that sometimes persist and can be associated with substantial distress and dysfunction. The most specific manifestations are subsumed under the psychiatric diagnosis posttraumatic stress disorder (PTSD). Both TBI and PTSD overlap a number of other conditions, most notably depression. These two conditions seem to be the most salient to a discussion of psychological and behavioral complications of traumatic injury. Finally, it is recognized that a focus on complications of surgery would require discussion of a number of other issues, ranging from delirium to adjustment to pain and loss of function. This chapter will focus on trauma sequelae, specifically following TBI and PTSD, conditions that we believe are generally under-recognized and that can contribute profoundly to the outcomes of patients with trauma. We will present information on these conditions separately; however, the issue of their coexistence is of interest. One report considered the occurrence of PTSD to be incompatible with an event associated with TBI because of impaired memory consolidation (1). However, a substantial incidence of PTSD has been reported among patients who have experienced TBI (2). The issue of how these conditions can interrelate is an important matter for clinical attention and future studies.

TRAUMATIC BRAIN INJURY
Severity and Prognostic Indicators

Trauma is a common cause of brain injury, and TBI is a leading cause of death and disability in the United States. Each year, an estimated 1.5 million Americans sustain a TBI. Of these, 50,000 die; 230,000 are hospitalized and survive; and approximately 80,000 to 90,000 experience long-term disability (3). Advances in prehospital care, classifications of injury severity and outcome, imaging, critical care, and rehabilitation have contributed to a reduction in mortality and to improved outcomes for patients with TBI (4–6). The health care costs of TBI are estimated at approximately US $35 billion per year (7).

Computed tomography has revolutionized the early diagnosis and treatment of patients with TBI (8). The immediate detection of intracranial mass lesions has made a significant difference in the outcome of patients with brain injury. Indications for intracranial pressure monitoring, the role of glucocorticoids, the role of prophylactic antiseizure medications, the use of hyperventilation, and the importance of cerebral perfusion pressure in the care of patients with severe TBI have all made an impact. In 1996, the Guidelines for the Management of Severe Head Injury (9) were distributed to all Board-certified neurosurgeons in the United States and Canada. The document provided evidence-based standards, guidelines, or options regarding the role of neurosurgeons in trauma systems. Several other elements of the treatment of patients with head injury were also included. With these guidelines, the management of severe TBI and its outcomes is now more consistent across North America.

The duration of coma and the period of posttraumatic amnesia (PTA) are important predictors of outcome. The patient's condition during the first few hours after injury is an important early index of severity and is measured by the Glasgow Coma Scale (GCS) (4), which serves as an objective measure of level of consciousness. This scale allows for the best assessment of verbal, motor, and visual response with a corresponding classification of brain injury as mild (GCS score, 13–15), moderate (GCS score, 9–12), or severe (GCS score, 3–8). The period of PTA was first described by Russell (10) and refers to the duration of time from the point of injury to until the patient has continuous memory of ongoing events and is able to retain new information. Cognitive function during PTA is highly variable and difficult to evaluate. Those patients who remain in coma longer and experience longer periods of PTA suffer significant neurological and behavioral deficits that are often irreversible.

The effect of age at the time of injury to the brain is also an important variable that should not be ignored. Many clinicians assume that because of brain plasticity, children will have a better prognosis for neurobehavioral recovery after TBI than will adults (11). Studies have reported that an early injury to the brain in younger children may limit the brain's ability to develop normally or may interfere with the timing of neural development (12). In addition, new deficits may emerge at later stages after injury. Therefore, from the mildest of injuries to the most catastrophic injury, patients may demonstrate different severities of brain injury, which results in different types of cognitive and behavioral impairments.

Pathophysiology

An understanding of cognitive and behavioral deficits first requires an understanding of the neuropathology of diffuse and focal injuries and the different patterns of recovery associated with them. Damage to the frontal and temporal lobes is considered to be responsible for most of the cognitive and behavioral deficits associated with TBI. The pathophysiology of head trauma includes both the immediate impact (primary injury) and delayed brain injury (secondary injury). The result of mechanical forces applied to the skull and transmitted to the brain is focal brain damage, diffuse brain damage, or both. Focal lesions result from a direct blow to the head and include brain laceration, contusion, intracerebral hemorrhage, subarachnoid or subdural hemorrhage, and ischemic infarct. The mechanism of injury involves a rapid acceleration and deceleration of the head, such as that typically produced by motor vehicle crashes or falls. The areas most commonly affected are the orbitofrontal area and the temporal area (13). Also, the differential motion of the brain within the skull causes shearing and stretching of axons (14). The widespread spectrum of injuries, ranging from brief physiological disruption to widespread axonal tearing, is called diffuse axonal injury (15).

In addition to damage occurring at the time of impact, secondary damage may occur during the recovery period. Secondary damage can include hypoxia, anemia, metabolic abnormalities, infection, hydrocephalus, intracranial hypertension, fat embolism, and subarachnoid hemorrhage. Other delayed effects include release of excitatory amino acids, production of oxidative free radicals, release of arachidonic acid metabolites, and disruption of neurotransmitters such as monoamines and serotonin (16–18).

Most trauma surgeons are familiar with the early stages of brain recovery and, in most cases, do not observe (or follow up) the patient in the postacute or rehabilitation stages. Once the condition of the more severely injured patients becomes medically and surgically stable, they are usually transferred to an acute-care setting, a rehabilitation facility, or a subacute-care setting. Most of the cognitive and behavioral problems that occur after TBI emerge during the rehabilitation phase. It is because of these deficits that patients remain unable to return to work or school or to become functional members of their communities (19).

After mild TBI, most deficits resolve within three months (20). The most common postconcussive complaints are headaches, dizziness, fatigue, irritability, anxiety, insomnia, memory problems, and noise sensitivity (21). These symptoms usually follow mild TBI, but are also seen after all other degrees of TBI (22,23). After moderate or severe TBI, patients are left with a combination of physical, cognitive, and behavioral deficits that may persist for months or years after the injury. These deficits are best treated by a multidisciplinary team of experts that includes a physician with expertise in brain injury rehabilitation, nurses, a physical therapist, an occupational therapist, a speech pathologist, a neuropsychologist, a recreational therapist, a dietician, a social worker, and the patient's family.

Cognitive Sequelae

Cognition is defined by Neisser as the processes by which sensory input is transformed, reduced, elaborated, stored, recovered, and used (24). Cognitive deficits are caused by the effects of focal and diffuse brain damage (15). Despite the variability in the severity of brain injury and the cognitive deficits associated with it, certain common patterns exist because of the typical damage to the frontal and temporal lobes (gray matter), the midbrain, and the corpus callosum (white matter) (24). Cognitive outcome depends on a number of factors, including degree of diffuse axonal injury, age, duration of loss of consciousness, duration of PTA, brain stem dysfunction at the time of injury, and presence and size of focal hemispheric injury (25).

The cognitive disorders typically experienced by patients with TBI include impairment of arousal, attention, concentration, memory, language, visuospatial and perceptual function, and executive function (26). Deficits in attention and memory are among the most commonly reported disorders after TBI. Attention is not a single entity, but is rather a finite set of brain processes that interact with other brain processes in the performance of different perceptual, cognitive, and motor tasks (27). Components of attention include vigilance (attending to a task over time), selection (attending to different targets), and executive attention (planning and coordination of multiple tasks). Attention is the basis for information processing, learning, and execution of the activities of daily living.

Memory is a complex process that includes the ability to encode (analyze and restructure information into storable forms), store (maintain stored memories), and retrieve (locate stored information and return it to awareness) information (26). Patients with head injury demonstrate a combination of retrograde (inability to recall events preceding the injury) and anterograde (difficulty in acquiring new information) amnesia, caused by damage to the medial temporal lobes and the hippocampus or to portions of the thalamus (28). Schacter and Tulving (29) describe three types of memory that are regarded as cognitive in that they require contemplation and conscious awareness: working memory, semantic memory, and episodic memory. Working memory is used in performing tasks that require short-term storage and manipulation of new or previously learned information. Semantic memory is based on factual and conceptual knowledge of the world. Episodic memory is memory of personal past and present experiences. All of these types of memory may be impaired after TBI.

Disorders of communication and language may take many forms depending on the site and extent of the lesion. It has been reported that language disorders associated with TBI are a manifestation of underlying cognitive disorganization (30). Patients demonstrate reduced word fluency, impaired visual naming, impaired auditory comprehension, anomia, paraphasias, and problems with reading and writing. The most commonly reported deficit is anomia, or problems with finding words or naming objects. Anomia is described as the inability to generate names on visual confrontation or in spontaneous speech, with damage to the dominant parietal area (31). Heilman et al. (32) report that anomia is often accompanied by signs of dysgraphia, dyslexia, and dyscalculia. Verbal fluency may be affected by left frontal or bifrontal lesions (33). Executive function problems include poor planning, organizing, sequencing, and set-shifting abilities, with impaired judgment and impulse control (34).

Visuospatial and perceptual deficits are not as common as other deficits because the posterior areas of the brain are less often damaged than the frontal and temporal areas. Prosopagnosia (inability to recognize familiar faces) is associated with lesions of the right inferior occipitotemporal region (35,36). Other visuospatial deficits include problems with neglect, motor planning, perception of forms, spatial relations, color, and figure–ground relationships (37). Patients with hemispatial neglect have difficulty attending to either the right or the left half of space. Such deficits can be quite devastating because of their functional consequences, which limit the patients' ability to perform activities of daily living such as dressing, feeding, and grooming themselves. Treatment for neglect is limited to environmental and behavioral manipulations.

It is important to screen patients during the acute phase of brain injury to assess a wide range of cognitive, memory, and language deficits that are first seen in the early stages of recovery. In the acute stage, the patient is usually disoriented and confused. The Galveston Orientation Amnesia Test (38) should be administered daily to track the patients' progress through PTA. The Brief Test of Head Injury (39) is a standardized cognitive–linguistic screening tool designed to quickly identify and measure a variety of deficits in patients with TBI. A full neuropsychological assessment should be administered to patients during the rehabilitation phase. A scale commonly used to follow a patient's progress through cognitive recovery is the Rancho Los Amigos Scale (40), which describes the patient's current level of cognitive functioning. The scale ranges from Level I (no response) to Level VIII (purposeful, appropriate). Various treatment techniques have been developed and used at different stages of recovery. Patients recover at different rates depending on the severity of the brain injury.

The rehabilitation of cognitive deficits may be referred to as cognitive retraining, cognitive remediation, or cognitive rehabilitation (25). Cognitive rehabilitation is a set of therapies used to help improve damaged intellectual, perceptual, psychomotor, and behavioral skills. Approaches may vary from the use of computer programs to paper-and-pencil and traditional therapy tasks, may focus on single components of cognition or on cognitive aspects embedded in functional tasks, or may be aimed directly at improving impaired cognitive processes or at developing compensatory strategies. Cognitive retraining involves using techniques to retrain the patient in specific cognitive domains by providing a series and a hierarchy of mental stimuli, tests, and activities. This therapy consists of task repetition and assistance provided by cueing techniques (41). Therapeutic strategies of cognitive rehabilitation have been classified in the literature as either restorative (repetitive exercise with the goal of restoring lost function) or compensatory (development of internal strategies or external prosthetic assistance for dysfunction) (42,43).

Neuropharmacological management involving psychostimulants and other dopaminergic agents has been reported to be beneficial in improving deficits of arousal, poor attention, concentration, and memory (44–47). Recently, the use of cholinergic agents has been reported to be promising in treating these deficits (48,49).

Behavioral Sequelae

Frequently reported behavioral sequelae after TBI include agitation, disinhibition, depression, apathy, mania, and psychosis. These behavioral problems have been mostly associated with injury to the frontal and temporal lobes (50).

Agitation

Impaired cognitive processes, such as problems with attention and language comprehension or expression, may contribute to agitated and aggressive behavior problems by increasing confusion and misunderstanding. Patients may demonstrate behaviors such as screaming, restlessness, and hitting. Damage to the frontolimbic structures plays a role in this impulsive and inappropriate behavior.

Focal damage to the orbitofrontal area causes disinhibition, whereas injury to the dorsal convexity of the frontal lobe causes attentional and organizational problems. Damage to the temporal lobe causes memory problems and emotional lability (51). Treatment should include a combination of environmental, behavioral, and vocational retraining. Psychotherapy and family therapy programs are also recommended. The use of psychostimulants, opioid antagonists, selective serotonin reuptake inhibitors (SSRIs), high-dose beta-blockers, buspirone, trazodone, and anticonvulsants has been suggested to be beneficial for subgroups of patients (52).

Depression

Approximately 25% of patients with TBI experience depression (53,54). Depression has been associated with impaired cognitive functioning, exacerbation of existing neurological deficits, and diminished motivation to complete the rehabilitation process (55,56). The patient and family report feelings of loss, demoralization, and discouragement. Many patients may experience fatigue, irritability, suicidal thoughts, disinterest and initiation problems, and insomnia many years after TBI (44,45).

A poor premorbid level of functioning and a past history of psychiatric illness are important risk factors for depression after TBI (53). A mechanism of depression after TBI may be disruption of biogenic amine–containing neurons as they pass through the basal ganglia or the frontal subcortical white matter (57). The presence of left dorsolateral frontal and left basal ganglia lesions is associated with an increased likelihood of severe depression (53).

Patients with depression resulting from brain injury seem to respond to serotonergic agents such as fluoxetine and sertraline, but they do not respond to tricyclic antidepressants. The reasons for this response pattern are not clear. Observations strongly indicate that the neurochemical mechanism responsible for depression after brain injury is related to serotonin (58).

Apathy

Approximately 60% of patients with TBI experience some degree of apathy or depression (59). They demonstrate symptoms of disinterest, disengagement, lack of motivation, and absence of emotional responsivity. Apathy may result from damage to the mesial frontal lobes (60). Neuropharmacological treatment may include psychostimulants, dextroamphetamine, amantadine, or bromocriptine (45).

Mania

Mania is less common than depression after TBI, but has been reported to occur in 9% of patients (61). Changes in mood, sleep patterns, and activity level can include irritability, euphoria, insomnia, agitation, aggression, impulsivity, and violent behavior (62). These behaviors have been associated with right-hemispheric limbic lesions (61). Treatment with anticonvulsants such as carbamazepine or valproate may be more effective than treatment with lithium, which is not specific to the neuropathology of TBI and may worsen cognitive impairment (50).

Anxiety

Many kinds of anxiety disorders have been reported after TBI, such as generalized anxiety disorder, panic disorder, phobic disorders, PTSD, and obsessive-compulsive disorder. Patients with TBI often experience anxiety associated with persistent worry, tension, and fearfulness (63). Increased activity of the aminergic system and decreased activity of the gamma-amino butyric acid inhibitory network is the proposed mechanism for the clinical manifestation of anxiety. Right-hemispheric lesions are more often associated with anxiety disorder than are left-hemispheric lesions (64). Treatment includes antidepressants such as SSRIs, opioid antagonists (such as naltrexone), and buspirone. Benzodiazepine and antipsychotic agents should be avoided because they can cause memory impairment, disinhibition, and delayed neuronal recovery (65). Behavioral therapy and psychotherapy are also important in the treatment of anxiety.

Psychosis

A review of the literature (66) found that approximately 7% to 10% of patients with TBI develop a schizophrenia-like psychosis. Reported psychotic symptoms include delusions, hallucinations, illogical thinking, agitation, grimacing, disinhibition, regression, and impulsive aggressiveness (67,68). These features may be transient or persistent. Anticonvulsants are not effective in treating psychosis, and dopamine agonists may exacerbate psychosis (69).

Conclusion

With the recognition that most psychiatric disorders have a neurochemical basis, we will be able to use new advances in neurobiological research methods, such as positron emission tomography, magnetic resonance spectroscopy, and other new imaging techniques, to learn more about the neurochemical basis of the sequelae of TBI. The assessment and treatment of patients with TBI are most beneficial when a multidisciplinary approach is taken. The premorbid education, life skills, and personality of the patient must be taken into consideration when treatment programs are set up. In most cases, not only does the patient demonstrate cognitive and behavioral deficits, but also the family frequently develops substantial psychosocial dysfunction because of the abrupt change in family relationships and the role change of the injured family member. Another difficulty to be faced is the frustration and stress of dealing with the injured family member, whose condition may improve, but who demonstrates residual cognitive and behavioral problems. There is great need for support and intervention along the entire continuum of care after TBI.

POSTTRAUMATIC STRESS DISORDER
Prevalence: Community and Risk Factors After Traumatic Injury

According to a large epidemiological study (70), more than half of the adults in the United States have undergone experiences that would be considered traumatic and capable of engendering PTSD. Eight percent of those surveyed met the criteria for PTSD during their lifetimes (70). The development of PTSD in some (a significant minority) but not all of those exposed to trauma has become an important issue for psychiatrists and psychologists, and attempts have been made to define risk factors that could have implications for preventative interventions. When PTSD develops and persists, it is frequently associated with other psychiatric disorders, most commonly depression and substance-abuse disorders. The relationship of PTSD to other psychiatric comorbidities is complex. Equally often, these other disorders precede or follow the onset of PTSD (70). Prior mental health problems probably contribute to the risk of PTSD. On the other hand, chronic PTSD is often complicated by the secondary development of depression, other anxiety disorders, and substance-abuse disorders, and it can exacerbate these conditions if they are preexisting. The course of PTSD often becomes chronic, continuing over many years in one-third of cases. The National Comorbidity Study further found that remission was unusual when the duration of PTSD exceeded one year (70). Chronic PTSD is associated with considerable distress and impairment (71).

Traumatic injury is a common antecedent of PTSD and related psychiatric morbidities such as depression (72–76). Michels et al. (76) found that PTSD and depression were important (negative) predictors of functional status, and satisfaction with recovery after the analysis was controlled for severity of injury. Motor vehicle accidents (MVAs) are the most common cause of injury in the general community

and carry a low to moderate risk of PTSD in community studies. The incidence of PTSD is higher after intentionally inflicted violence and serious accidents not related to transportation (72). MVAs sampled in the community, however, represent a range of incident severity. Studies of clinically recruited cohorts of MVA victims have found PTSD rates ranging from 10% to 38% (73–76).

Diagnostic Features of Posttraumatic Stress Disorder

PTSD is unique among psychiatric disorders because it is defined as a specific syndrome and is diagnosed only in association with severely stressful life events. In contrast, the onset of an episode of depression or panic disorder may or may not be preceded by a stressful event. Adjustment disorders are not very specifically defined as syndromes.

The stressor definition for diagnosing PTSD has gone through several iterations since the diagnosis became official with the publication of the third revision of American Psychiatric Association Diagnostic and Statistics Manual [(DSM)-III] in 1978. The initial definition of a trauma "out of the range of normal human experience" was challenged by subsequent studies' findings of high rates of exposure to events that can engender PTSD in community samples (70,72). The current definition (DSM-IV) (77) has two components. The first is objective: experiencing or witnessing an event "that involved actual or threatened death or serious injury, or a threat to the physical integrity of self or others." The second criterion is subjective: a requirement that "the person's response involved intense fear, helplessness, or horror."

The syndrome of PTSD involves three main components that are delineated in DSM-IV: reexperiencing the trauma, avoidance and emotional numbing, and symptoms of heightened arousal. Reexperiencing symptoms most often takes the form of intrusive and distressing memories of the trauma. PTSD is also often associated with distressing dreams in which the trauma is replayed or otherwise represented. A less common but potentially dramatic and distressing form of reexperiencing is referred to as flashbacks and involves the person's perceiving or feeling as if he or she is back in the traumatic situation. The second diagnostic cluster includes both behavioral (places and situations) and cognitive (thoughts) avoidance of reminders of the trauma. Numbing symptoms include diminished emotional reactivity, interpersonal detachment, and a sense of foreshortened future. Heightened arousal symptoms can be understood as being related to psychophysiological reactions that can enhance survival during a time of threat, but that persist maladaptively in the form of disrupted sleep, heightened vigilance, and an exaggerated startle response.

A certain number of these symptoms from each cluster must persist if the diagnosis of PTSD is to be made. The disorder is considered chronic if it continues for more than three months because a substantial naturalistic waning of PTSD symptoms can occur during the early aftermath of trauma. The potential downside of a duration criterion is the possible discouragement of early identification of persons exposed to trauma who may be at risk of PTSD. The DSM-IV attempted to remedy this situation by creating a new category called acute stress disorder (ASD). This condition can be diagnosed within a month of a traumatic event; if the condition has not resolved after this time period, the diagnosis becomes PTSD. In addition to the presence of PTSD-like symptoms, the diagnosis of ASD requires the presence of dissociative symptoms, which often manifest during or immediately after the trauma. Dissociative reactions or symptoms can include marked detachment, reduced awareness of one's surroundings (a state of shock), feelings of unreality, and lack of memory for an important aspect of the trauma. These symptoms have been included because several studies demonstrated relationships between early dissociative reactions and subsequent PTSD (78–80). A number of recent and ongoing investigations are continuing to evaluate and refine our understanding of how persisting distress and psychopathology (PTSD) are related to dissociation and other early clinical manifestations and initial reactions to a traumatic stressor.

As previously mentioned, once PTSD becomes established, it can become chronic and is typically part of a more complex diagnostic picture with frequent comorbidity. Chronic PTSD, other anxiety disorders, severe depression, and substance-use disorders often coexist and present diagnostic and therapeutic challenges.

Risk Factors for Posttraumatic Stress Disorder

Risk factors for PTSD have been identified in epidemiological studies. One is the nature or severity of the traumatic experience. The most prevalent antecedent of PTSD among adult women in the United States is sexual assault; for men, it is military combat. Sexual assault and military combat are associated with higher rates of PTSD than are most other categories of trauma (70). Individual risk factors identified in cross-sectional community-based studies include female sex, past personal and familial psychopathology, and multiple episodes of traumatization (72).

Although an understanding of the risk factors for PTSD is important in our understanding of the disorder and has some clinical relevance, we remain limited in our ability to adequately direct therapeutic or monitoring resources on the basis of a prediction of which persons will develop PTSD after trauma. A number of recent prospective studies have focused on early posttraumatic reactions. The findings tend to support the relationship between early dissociation and subsequent PTSD that was previously referred to and that underlies the criteria for ASD (80). Other

factors that have been identified in these studies include elevated heart rate within hours of the trauma (81), the overall intensity of early PTSD symptoms (80,82), and avoidant styles of coping (82).

Therapeutic Approaches to Posttraumatic Stress Disorder

Recently, substantial advances have been made in the understanding of how to treat PTSD optimally. These advances form the basis of the first comprehensive and authoritative set of recently published treatment guidelines for the disorder (83). Interventions may be psychotherapeutic or pharmacological. Among the available psychotherapies, cognitive-behavioral therapy (CBT) has the best-established effectiveness. One effective form of CBT, prolonged exposure, includes sessions during which the memory of the traumatic experience is recounted in the first person, in as much detail as possible, over multiple sessions. Related strategies can incorporate cognitive restructuring and anxiety-management techniques. When successful, these approaches facilitate "emotional processing," which allows the person to habituate to the fear-inducing aspect of a trauma memory and to develop a more adaptive set of associations and beliefs. Although CBT is the most established treatment, there is evidence that other approaches, including a variant of exposure that also uses eye movements (eye movement desensitization reprocessing), psychodynamic therapy, and group therapy, can be beneficial (84).

Medications are also established therapeutic options for PTSD. Sertraline, an antidepressant medication from the SSRI class, is the first and so far the only medication to be specifically approved for the indication of PTSD by labeling from the Food and Drug Administration. Sertraline and other SSRIs have been well studied for the treatment of PTSD in randomized, controlled clinical trials, in which most but not all of the results have supported effectiveness. Other psychotropic medications, although less established, are often used to treat PTSD because of intolerance, partial response, or lack of response to SSRIs, or because of the need to target various comorbid conditions. Categories of agents include other types of antidepressants, mood stabilizers, noradrenergic blocking agents, and novel types of antipsychotic medications (83).

There is little established support for preventing the development of PTSD by intervening during the acute aftermath of trauma. Critical incident debriefing has been a popular approach; however, comparative studies have not supported its overall effectiveness in preventing PTSD (85). Preliminary emerging evidence from a trial that enrolled patients within a month after MVA suggests that a briefer adaptation of CBT is associated with a lower incidence of development of PTSD (86). It is not presently known whether the medications effective for treating established PTSD are effective when prescribed early. One study suggests that early and sustained treatment with benzodiazepines after trauma is not associated with improved outcomes (87).

Considerations for the Setting of Acute Trauma Care

Synthesis of the information given above presents dilemmas in conceptualizing optimal care systems with respect to managing PTSD issues in the setting of acute trauma care. PTSD will develop in a substantial minority of severely injured patients. When PTSD develops and persists, it compromises functional recovery and quality of life and becomes increasingly difficult to treat over time. Thus, the acute trauma setting would seem to present an important opportunity for preventive intervention. As discussed, there are limitations to the current state of knowledge with regard to early identification of cases at risk and effectiveness of early interventions. These limitations being acknowledged, we do know enough to make some sensible recommendations that can be refined as the field progresses.

Providers in acute trauma settings should have a general awareness of issues related to PTSD so that they can optimally assess and manage risks for complications of injury. Educating injured patients about the possibility of PTSD symptoms could provide a useful and cost-effective intervention. Patients who begin to experience nightmares or flashbacks are often confused and frightened by their symptoms and benefit from having a frame of reference for understanding them. A brief routine screening assessment could help to serve this purpose. Although our current ability to predict longer-term PTSD is limited, important signs of risk can be readily ascertained in an acute trauma care setting. An injured person who manifests some combination of signs or symptoms, including intense reexperiencing, anxiety, sleep disturbance, or dissociation, and who appears to be trying hard not to think about what happened or not to be reminded of it, is probably at high risk of continuing problems. At this point, definitive recommendations regarding medication treatment cannot be made; however, treatment is warranted for severe anxiety or sleep problems and for persisting or worsening depression. CBT approaches have yielded the most promising findings for early intervention with patients at risk. This is a somewhat specialized approach; however, support for such expertise clearly seems to be justified for comprehensive care and prevention of morbidity. In the absence of the availability of formal CBT, it is reasonable to extrapolate that its key components (education about the nature of PTSD symptoms and coping methods and facilitation of expression of memories, thoughts, and feelings related to the trauma) should be provided to injured patients who are manifesting acute psychological distress.

REFERENCES

1. Sbordone RJ, Liter JC. Mild traumatic brain injury does not produce post-traumatic stress disorder. Brain Inj 1995; 9:405–412.
2. Harvey AG, Bryant RA. Two-year prospective evaluation of the relationship between acute stress disorder and posttraumatic stress disorder following mild traumatic brain injury. Am J Psychiatry 2000; 157:626–628.
3. Thurman DJ, Alverson C, Dunn KA, Guerrero J, Sniezek JE. Traumatic brain injury in the United States: a public health perspective. J Head Trauma Rehabil 1999; 14(6):602–615.
4. Teasdale G, Jennett B. Assessment of coma and impaired consciousness. A practical scale. Lancet 1974; 2:81–84.
5. Marshall LF, Marshall SB, Klauber MR, et al. The diagnosis of head injury requires a classification based on computed axial tomography. J Neurotrauma 1991; 9(suppl 1):S287–S292.
6. Jennett B, Bond M. Assessment of outcome after severe brain damage: a practical scale. Lancet 1975; 1:480–484.
7. Max W, Mackenzie E, Rice DP. Head injuries: cost and consequences. J Head Trauma Rehabil 1991; 6(2):76–91.
8. Marion DW. Management of traumatic brain injury: past, present, and future. Clin Neurosurg 1999; 45:184–191.
9. Guidelines for the management of severe head injury. Brain Trauma Foundation, American Association of Neurological Surgeons, Joint Section on Neurotrauma and Critical Care. J Neurotrauma 1996; 13:641–734.
10. Russell WR. Cerebral involvement in head injury. Brain 1932; 35:549–603.
11. Buchwald JS. Comparison of plasticity in sensory and cognitive processing systems. Clin Perinatol 1990; 17:57–66.
12. Dennis MB, Barnes M. Developmental aspects of neuropsychology: childhood. In: Zaidel D, ed. Handbook of Perception and Cognition. Vol. 15. Neuropsychology. New York: Academic Press, 1994:210–246.
13. Gennarelli TA. Cerebral concussion and diffuse brain injuries. In: Cooper PK, ed. Head Injury. Vol. 2. Baltimore: Williams and Wilkins, 1987:108–124.
14. McAllister TW. Neuropsychiatric sequelae of head injuries. Psychiatr Clin North Am 1992; 15:395–413.
15. Auerbach SH. The pathophysiology of traumatic brain injury. In: Horn L, Cope DN, eds. Physical Medicine and Rehabilitation: State of the Art Review, Traumatic Brain Injury. Vol. 3. Philadelphia: Hanley and Belfus, 1989:1–11.
16. Palmer AM, Marion DW, Botscheller ML, Swedlow PE, Styren SD, DeKosky ST. Traumatic brain injury-induced excitotoxicity assessed in a controlled cortical impact model. J Neurochem 1993; 61:2015–2024.
17. Hamill RW, Woolf PD, McDonald JV, Lee LA, Kelly M. Catecholamines predict outcome in traumatic brain injury. Ann Neurol 1987; 21:438–443.
18. Vecht CJ, van Woerkom CA, Teelken AW, Minderhoud JM. Homovanillic acid and 5-hydroxyindoleacetic acid cerebrospinal fluid levels. A study with and without probenecid administration of their relationship to the state of consciousness after head injury. Arch Neurol 1975; 32:792–797.
19. Dikmen SS, Temkin NR, Machamer JE, Holubkov AL, Fraser RT, Winn HR. Employment following traumatic head injuries. Arch Neurol 1994; 51:177–186.

20. Levin HS, Mattis S, Ruff RM, et al. Neurobehavioral outcome following minor head injury: a three-center study. J Neurosurg 1987; 66:234–243.

21. Evans RW. The postconcussion syndrome and the sequelae of mild head injury. Neurol Clin 1992; 10:815–847.

22. Rutherford WH, Merrett JD, McDonald JR. Symptoms at one year following concussion from minor head injuries. Injury 1979; 10:225–230.

23. McLean A Jr., Temkin NR, Dikmen S, Wyler AR. The behavioral sequelae of head injury. J Clin Neuropsychol 1983; 5:361–376.

24. Neisser U. Cognitive Psychology. New York: Appleton-Century-Crofts, 1967.

25. Whyte J, Rosenthal M. Rehabilitation of the patient with head injury. In: DeLisa JA, Gans BM, eds. Rehabilitation Medicine, Principles and Practice. Philadelphia: J.B. Lippincott, 1998:585–611.

26. Levin HS, Benton AL, Grossman RG. Neurobehavioral Consequences of Closed Head Injury. New York: Oxford University Press, 1982.

27. Parasuraman R, ed. The Attentive Brain. Cambridge: MIT Press, 1998.

28. Auerbach SH. Neuroanatomical correlates of attention and memory disorders in traumatic brain injury: an application of behavioral subtypes. J Head Trauma Rehabil 1986; 1(3):1–12.

29. Schacter DL, Tulving E, eds. Memory Systems 1994. Cambridge: The MIT Press, 1994.

30. Hagen C. Language disorders in head trauma. In: Holland A, ed. Language Disorders in Adults: Recent Advances. San Diego: College Hill Press, 1983:245–281.

31. Albert M, Goodglass H, Helm N, Rubens A, Alexander M. Clinical Aspects of Dysphasia. New York: Springer-Verlag, 1981.

32. Heilman KM, Safran A, Geschwind N. Closed head trauma and aphasia. J Neurol Neurosurg Psychiatry 1971; 34:265–269.

33. Benton AL. Differential behavioral effects of frontal lobe disease. Neuropsychologia 1968; 5:53–60.

34. Rao V, Lyketsos C. Neuropsychiatric sequelae of traumatic brain injury. Psychosomatics 2000; 41:95–103.

35. Benton AL. Behavioral consequences of closed head injury. In: Odom GL, ed. Central Nervous System Trauma Research Status Report. Bethesda: NINCDS, 1979:220–231.

36. Meadows JC. The anatomical basis of prosopagnosia. J Neurol Neurosurg Psychiatry 1974; 37:489–501.

37. Wahlstrom PE. Occupational therapy evaluation. In: Rosenthal M, Griffith ER, Bond MR, Miller JD, eds. Rehabilitation of the Head Injured Adult. Philadelphia: FA Davis, 1983.

38. Levin HS, O'Donnell VM, Grossman RG. The Galveston Orientation and Amnesia Test. A practical scale to assess cognition after head injury. J Nerv Ment Dis 1979; 167:675–684.

39. Helm-Estabrooks N, Hotz G. The Brief Test of Head Injury (BTHI). Chicago: Riverside Publishing Company, 1990.

40. Malkmus D, Booth BJ, Kodimer C. Rehabilitation of the head-injured adult: comprehensive cognitive management. (Professional Staff Association of Ranch Los Amigos Hospital, Downey, California), 1980.

41. Wilson BA. Cognitive rehabilitation: how it is and how it might be. J Int Neuropsychol Soc 1997; 3:487–496.

42. Coelho CA, DeRuyter F, Stein M. Treatment efficacy: cognitive-communicative disorders resulting from traumatic brain injury in adults. J Speech Hear Res 1996; 39(5):S5–S17.

43. Wehman P, Kreutzer J, Sale P, et al. Cognitive impairment and remediation: implications for employment following traumatic brain injury. J Head Trauma Rehabil 1989; 4(3);66–75.

44. Karli DC, Burke TD, Kim HJ, et al. Effects of dopaminergic combination therapy for frontal lobe dysfunction in traumatic brain injury rehabilitation. Brain Inj 1999; 13:63–68.

45. Van Reekum R, Bayley M, Garner S, et al. N of 1 study: amantadine for the amotivational syndrome in a patient with traumatic brain injury. Brain Inj 1995; 9:49–53.

46. Bleiberg J, Garmoe W, Cederquist J, et al. Effects of dexedrine on performance consistency following brain injury. Brain Inj 1993; 6:245–248.

47. Kraus MF, Maki P. The combined use of amantadine and l-dopa/carbidopa in the treatment of chronic brain injury. Brain Inj 1997; 11:455–460.

48. Taverni JP, Seliger G, Lichtman SW. Donepezil-mediated memory improvement in traumatic brain injury during post-acute rehabilitation. Brain Inj 1998; 12:77–80.

49. Goldberg E, Gerstman LJ, Mattis S, Hughes JE, Bilder RM Jr., Sirio CA. Effects of cholinergic treatment on posttraumatic anterograde amnesia. Arch Neurol 1982; 39:581.

50. Kraus MF. Neuropsychiatric sequelae: assessment and pharmacologic intervention. In: Marion DW, ed. Traumatic Brain Injury. New York: Thieme Medicine Publishers, 1998:173–185.

51. Gualtieri CT. Neuropsychiatry and Behavioral Pharmacology. New York: Springer-Verlag, 1990.

52. Silver JM, Yudofsky SC. In: Silver JM, Yudofsky SC, Hales RE, eds. Psychopharmacology in Neuropsychiatry of Traumatic Brain Injury. Washington, D.C.: American Psychiatric Press, 1994:631–670.

53. Fedoroff JP, Starkstein SE, Forrester AW, et al. Depression in patients with traumatic brain injury. Am J Psychiatry 1992; 149:918–923.

54. Jorge RE, Robinson RG, Arndt SV, Forrester AW, Geisler F, Starkstein SE. Comparison between acute- and delayed-onset depression following traumatic brain injury. J Neuropsychiatry Clin Neurosci 1993; 5:43–49.

55. Silver JM, Hales RE, Yudovsky SC. Psychopahrmacology of depression in neurologic disorders. J Clin Psychiatry 1990; 51:33–39.

56. Binder LM, Rattock J. Assessment of postconcussive syndrome after mild head trauma. In: Lezak MD, ed. Assessment of the Behavioral Consequences of Head Trauma. New York: John Wiley and Sons, 1989:37–48.

57. Starkstein SE, Robinson RG, Price TR. Comparison of cortical and subcortical lesions in the production of poststroke mood disorders. Brain 1987; 110:1045–1059.

58. Marshall LF. Head injury: recent past, present, and future. Neurosurgery 2000; 47:546–561.

59. Kant R, Duffy JD, Pivovarnik A. Prevalence of apathy following head injury. Brain Inj 1998; 12:87–92.

60. Duffy JD, Campbell JJ. The regional prefrontal syndromes: a theoretical and clinical overview. J Neuropsychiatry Clin Neurosci 1994; 6:379–387.

61. Jorge RE, Robinson RG, Starksein SE, Arndt SV, Forrester AW, Geisler FH. Secondary mania following traumatic brain injury. Am J Psychiatry 1993; 150: 916–921.

62. Stewart JW, Hemsath RH. Bipolar illness following traumatic brain injury: treatment with lithium and carbamazepine. J Clin Psychiatry 1988; 49:74–75.

63. Lewis L, Rosenberg SJ. Psychoanalytic psychotherapy with brain-injured adult psychiatric patients. J Nerv Ment Dis 1990; 178:69–77.

64. Paul SM. Anxiety and depression: a common neurobiological substrate? J Clin Psychiatry 1988; 49(suppl):13–16.

65. Preston GC, Ward CE, Broks P, Traub M, Stahl SM. Effects of lorazepam on memory attention and sedation in man: antagonism by Ro 15–1788. Psychopharmacology (Berl) 1989; 91:222–227.

66. Davison K, Bagley CK. Schizophrenia-like psychosis associated with organic disorder of the CNS. Br J Psychiatry 1969; 4(suppl):113–184.

67. Brown G, Chadwick O, Shaffer D, Rutter M, Traub M. A prospective study of children with head injuries: III. Psychiatric sequelae. Psychol Med 1981; 11:63–78.

68. Thomsen IV. Late outcome of very severe blunt head trauma: a 10–15-year follow-up. J Neurol Neurosurg Psychiatry 1984; 47:260–268.

69. Feeney DM, Sutton RL. Pharmacotherapy for recovery of function after brain injury. Crit Rev Neurobiol 1987; 3:135–197.

70. Kessler RC, Sonnega A, Bromet E, Hughes M, Nelson CB. Posttraumatic stress disorder in the National Comorbidity Survey. Arch Gen Psychiatry 1995; 52:1048–1060.

71. Zatzick DF, Marmar CR, Weiss DS, et al. Posttraumatic stress disorder and functioning and quality of life outcomes in a nationally representative sample of male Vietnam veterans. Am J Psychiatry 1997; 154(12): 1690–1695.

72. Breslau N, Kessler RC, Chilcoat HD, Schultz LR, Davis GC, Andreski P. Trauma and posttraumatic stress disorder in the community: the 1996 Detroit Area Survey of Trauma. Arch Gen Psychiatry 1998; 55(7):626–632.

73. Mayou R, Bryant B, Duthie R. Psychiatric consequences of road traffic accidents. BMJ 1993; 307:647–651.

74. Ursano RJ, Fullerton CS, Epstein RS, et al. Acute and chronic posttraumatic stress disorder in motor vehicle accident victims. Am J Psychiatry 1999; 156(4):589–595.

75. Blanchard EB, Hickling EJ, Barton KA, Taylor AE, Loos WR, Jones-Alexander J. One-year prospective follow-up of motor vehicle accident victims. Behav Res Ther 1996; 34(10):775–786.

76. Michels AJ, Michaels CE, Moon CH, Zimmerman MA, Peterson C, Rodriguez JL. Psychosocial factors limit outcomes after trauma. J Trauma 1998; 44(4):644–648.

77. American Psychiatric Association. DSM-IV: Diagnostic and Statistical Manual of Mental Disorders. 4th ed. Washington, D.C.: American Psychiatric Association, 1994.

78. Marmar CR, Weiss DS, Schlenger WE, et al. Peritraumatic dissociation and posttraumatic stress in male Vietnam theater veterans. Am J Psychiatry 1994; 151: 902–907.

79. Classen C, Koopman C, Hales R, Spiegel D. Acute stress disorder as a predictor of posttraumatic stress symptoms. Am J Psychiatry 1998; 155:620–624.

80. Harvey AG, Bryant RA. The relationship between acute stress disorder and posttraumatic stress disorder: a prospective evaluation of motor vehicle accident survivors. J Consult Clin Psychol 1998; 66(3):507–512.

81. Shalev AY, Sahar T, Freedman S, et al. A prospective study of heart rate response following trauma and the subsequent development of posttraumatic stress disorder. Arch Gen Psychiatry 1998; 55(6):553–559.

82. Bryant RA, Harvey AG. Avoidant coping style and post-traumatic stress following motor vehicle accidents. Behav Res Ther 1995; 33:631–635.

83. Friedman MJ, Davidson JRT, Mellman TA, Southwick SM. Pharmacotherapy. In: Foa EB, Keane TM, Friedman TM, Friedman MJ, eds. Effective Treatments for PTSD: Practice Guidelines from the International Society for Traumatic Stress Studies. New York: Guilford Press, 2000.

84. Rothbaum BO, Meadows EA, Resick P, Foy DW. Cognitive-behavioral therapy. In: Foa EB, Keane TM, Friedman MJ, eds. Effective Treatments for PTSD: Practice Guidelines from the International Society for Traumatic Stress Studies. New York: Guilford Press, 2000:60–83.

85. Bisson J, McFarlane A, Rose S. Psychological debriefing. In: Foa E, Keane T, Friedman M, eds. Effective treatments for PTSD. Practice guidelines from the International Society for Traumatic Stress Studies. New York: Guilford Press, 2000.

86. Bryant RA, Harvey AG, Dang ST, Sackville T, Basten C. Treatment of acute stress disorder: a comparison of cognitive-behavioral therapy and supportive counseling. J Consult Clin Psychol 1998; 66(5):862–866.

87. Gelpin E, Bonne O, Peri T, Brandes D, Shalev AY. Treatment of recent trauma survivors with benzodiazepenes: a prospective study. J Clin Psychiatry 1996; 57:390–394.

42

Complications of Wound Repair

Nicole S. Gibran and F. Frank Isik
Department of Surgery, University of Washington, Seattle, Washington, U.S.A.

"For truly, if a man had a dangerous wound, the longer he waited to cure himself the more would it fester and hasten him toward his death; and also the wound would be but the harder to heal."

Geoffrey Chaucer (Canterbury Tales, The Parson's Tale; ~1400)

Wound repair is a common theme for all surgical subspecialties. The principles of wound closure and tissue handling that are practiced by a plastic surgeon should be no different from those practiced by a cardiac or laparoscopic surgeon. Because we know very little about the cellular and molecular processes required for normal wound repair, controlling the response to injury has not yet been clinically successful. As surgeons, we must use clinical judgment and good technique to optimize our patients' results. This chapter presents a brief outline of what is known about concepts related to normal wound healing and addresses a few of the complications and failures associated with the repair processes.

CONTINUUM OF NORMAL WOUND REPAIR PROCESSES

Tissue repair begins immediately after injury. The immediate hemostatic response involves microvasculature constriction coupled with coagulation. Extrinsic and intrinsic coagulation pathways combine with platelet accumulation to complete hemostasis and to provide the matrix scaffolding for cellular migration.

The coagulation cascade is initiated by tissue factor and results in thrombin-mediated cleavage of fibrinogen to fibrin. Factor XIII, the enzyme known to cross-link fibrin and other matrix molecules, stabilizes the provisional wound matrix (1,2). The activated enzymes of the plasminogen system, secreted by inflammatory and resident cells in the wound, cleave plasminogen to plasmin. Plasminogen activator inhibitors regulate the plasminogen system and assure that the clot is not resolved too rapidly. Exogenous plasminogen activator may promote the conversion of the zone of stasis in an acute burn wound to a zone of hyperemia (3).

Vasodilation and capillary leak with neutrophil infiltration into the tissue follow the transient vascular constriction. Neuropeptides derived from sensory nerves contribute to microvascular dilatation and capillary leak. Neuropeptides indirectly induce mast cell degranulation of histamine (4), induction of cytokines and adhesion molecules by keratinocytes and endothelial cells, chemotaxis of neutrophils, and proliferation of fibroblasts (5). Serotonin, histamine, bradykinin, and the arachidonic acid–pathway products (prostacyclin and leukotrienes) prolong vasodilation and capillary permeability (6).

Endogenous cells may be the most important contributors to cutaneous inflammation. "Skin-associated lymphoid tissue" includes cells derived from bone marrow, such as Langerhan's cells, dermal dendrocytes, keratinocytes, and microvascular endothelial cells (7). Keratinocytes synthesize cytokines, including interleukin-1 (8,9), interleukin-8 (10), interleukin-6 (11), monocyte chemoattractant protein–1 (12), and tumor necrosis factor (13,14). Dermal microvascular endothelial cells not only synthesize interleukin-6 (15) and monocyte chemoattractant protein–1 (12,16), but also regulate neutrophil migration by increasing the production of cell surface adhesion molecules ICAM-1 (17,18), VCAM, and E-selectin (19). These adhesion molecules bind to circulating neutrophils and facilitate neutrophil margination into the wound (20).

Prior to margination into the extravascular space, neutrophils plug the capillaries, thereby increasing inflammation and potential tissue ischemia. In burn wounds, neutrophil-mediated reperfusion injury may cause the zone of stasis to convert to a zone of coagulation, which will not heal. Inhibition of the neutrophil–endothelial adherence in contact burns in rabbits improves healing kinetics (21); whether humans respond similarly must be determined.

The interaction of inflammatory mediators after tissue injury is at best complicated. The arachidonic acid pathway, the kinin system, the complement system, and oxidative processes potentiate microvascular permeability, activate neutrophils, and contribute to matrix degradation. Oxidative byproducts and tumor necrosis factor contribute to the antimicrobial activity at wound sites. Each of these pathways has been targeted as a potential site at which the inflammatory response could be limited. Although in vitro studies and animal studies have been promising, the disappointing results of clinical trials attest to the complexity and probable redundancy in the inflammatory web.

Angiogenesis is widely thought to be mandatory for normal wound repair. Granulation tissue provides clinical evidence that a wound is healthy and is ready for closure. However, no study has demonstrated that angiogenesis is necessary; two recent reports suggest that angioinhibition does not prevent excisional wound closure (22,23). Grafts and tissue flaps require angiogenesis for engraftment. Delivery of oxygen and nutrients to the wound occurs for a few days by imbibition—or diffusion; however, graft take requires neovascularization, which occurs by connection between existent capillaries in the graft and in the wound bed—a process known as inosculation. Soluble growth factors including vascular endothelial cell growth factor, fibroblast growth factor (FGF), platelet-derived growth factor (PDGF)-BB, and transforming growth factor (TGF)-α induce endothelial cell proliferation and migration. Growth factor receptors are tightly regulated and may be influenced by endothelial cell interactions with extracellular matrix molecules (25).

Epithelialization restores the protective barrier with fluid maintenance, temperature regulation, and prevention of microbial invasion. It may also represent a transition in the inflammatory state of the wound. Many studies have demonstrated that epidermal–dermal interactions regulate morphogenetic processes such as fetal skin development and wound repair (26,27). The epidermis responds to mesenchyme-derived mediators (28), and migrating keratinocytes in the advancing epidermal tongue appear to promote dermal inflammation by secreting cytokines and growth factors (10,29). Once the wound has epithelialized, release of the inflammatory mediators may decrease. Evidence for an epidermal influence on the inflammatory response includes not only experimental data about keratinocyte biology in culture and in wound models (30) but also clinical observations that partial thickness wound coverage with a viable biological dressing such as allograft eliminates granulation tissue formation and promotes healing (31).

Clinicians know that full-thickness wounds heal from the edges and that partial thickness wounds heal from the remnants of epidermal appendages in the wound bed. The advancing epithelial tongue can migrate for approximately 1 cm before it stops migrating and heaps up at the edge of the wound. Keratinocyte migration is dependent on the underlying matrix, which may promote migration or anchorage. Compton et al. have determined that cultured epithelial grafts display poorly formed anchoring fibers comprising immature collagen VII fibrils for approximately 12 months after grafting (32), which correlated with the time that the patient stopped blistering. Therefore,

manipulation of the underlying matrix or keratinocyte receptors may constitute a treatment approach to a long-term rehabilitative problem.

Application of exogenous PDGF, FGF, and TGF-α increases epithelialization in diabetic mice with abnormal healing responses (33–35). However, administration of exogenous growth factors to chronic wounds in human clinical trials has had limited success (36). Studies about the temporal and spatial relationships of growth factors and growth factor receptors in normal and impaired wounds are essential before we can ethically treat human burns with costly recombinant growth factors.

Whereas an epithelialized wound is considered to be healed, fibrogenesis is critical for long-term wound appearance and strength. From the time of the initial injury, the extracellular matrix is undergoing constant change. Remodeling occurs as a continuum in healing wounds—beginning with dissolution of the fibrin clot and ending with the mature wound, 12 to 24 months later. The provisional matrix molecules fibrin, thrombin, fibronectin, and vitronectin promote cellular migration and proliferation for angiogenesis and fibrogenesis in the early wound. As fibroblasts migrate into the wound from the margins, they synthesize collagen. Deposition of collagen III and subsequently collagen I results in a basket-weave distribution that typifies dermal scar (37). As the wound matures, collagen I fibrils are cross-linked into cables, thereby increasing the dermal breaking strength. Regardless, the tensile strength of a wound never meets that of uninjured skin.

Centrifugal forces in the center of the wound cause wound contraction, which significantly contributes to wound closure. Myofibroblasts—highly differentiated fibroblasts characterized by intracellular smooth muscle actin filaments (42)—may be involved in the contractile mechanism. The extreme of wound contraction is contracture—a scarring process that negatively impacts joint motion. Whereas constant attention to stretching, exercising, and splinting diminishes contracture development, surgical release to restore normal function may be necessary.

With scar maturation, the epidermis continues to undergo changes with time. Melanocytes migrate from the wound edge and from the epidermal appendages soon after the keratinocytes. Repigmentation can be unpredictable and may result in either increased or decreased melanin in partial-thickness wounds. Clinicians must advise patients that exposure to ultraviolet rays exacerbates pigmentation changes in the wound and that topical bleaching agents may cause chemical burns to the recently injured skin.

Patients with healing partial-thickness wounds complain of pruritis. Histologically, there is an increased number of nerve fibers in human burn wounds, two weeks after injury, compared to normal skin (43). Hypertrophic scars, which are classically very pruritic, also have increased numbers of sensory nerves compared to normal scars and uninjured skin (44).

TYPES OF WOUNDS

Incisional wounds or lacerations involve linear separation of the epidermis, the dermis, and sometimes the subcutaneous tissue. Primary closure of these wounds can generally be performed surgically. In the event of a traumatic laceration, the wound edges should be trimmed; the wound should then be closely inspected for foreign bodies and irrigated liberally.

Partial-thickness wounds involve removal of the epithelium and the superficial dermis (papillary dermis). Most of the dermis and the epithelial appendages remain in the wound bed. Wound closure occurs by epithelial proliferation and migration from the hair follicles and sweat glands. Examples of partial-thickness wounds are scald burns and donor sites for split-thickness skin grafts.

Full-thickness wounds involve destruction of all layers of the skin. These wounds close by contraction and by epithelial proliferation and migration from the wound edge. An advancing epithelial tongue generally can migrate 1 cm; thus, a quarter-sized wound is roughly the largest wound that can heal by epithelialization alone. Examples of full-thickness wounds are avulsion injuries and electrical injuries.

Chronic nonhealing wounds are those that do not heal within three months after injury. They usually involve impairment in epithelial migration coupled with poor dermal regeneration. Epithelial proliferation appears to be adequate in many chronic wounds because the epithelial tongue at the wound edge heaps up with a raised rim of epithelium. Whereas no single cause of the impaired healing response has been identified, infection, impaired vascular supply, and inadequate oxygen delivery have been implicated.

WOUND CLOSURE AND COVERAGE

Whether a wound can be closed by suturing or requires alternative wound coverage depends on the type of wound, the level of contamination, and the size of the wound.

Primary wound closure involves surgical wound closure with direct approximation of the wound edges using sutures, staples, glue, or tape soon after the wound has been created. Wounds amenable to primary closure include most surgical incisions and fresh lacerations. Lacerations on the face can be safely closed primarily within six hours after injury. Lacerations in other anatomic sites with less vascular supply should be closed sooner.

Delayed primary wound closure involves surgical closure of a wound one to five days after injury. Indications for delayed primary closure include grossly contaminated surgical wounds (abdominal wounds with intraoperative fecal spillage) and lacerations contaminated with foreign matter or bacteria. The closure of human bite wounds should be delayed unless the wounds are on the face. A recent advance in the treatment of wounds is the introduction of the Wound Vac®. This negative-pressure system promotes cellular ingrowth into the deeper wound and reduces tissue edema. The sponge attached to a vacuum pump can be applied to a granulating deep wound to promote closure of dead spaces (45); it can also be applied directly to a skin graft to increase graft adherence to the wound bed (46).

Closure by secondary intention involves spontaneous healing of the wound without surgical closure. Generally, the wound granulates and contracts with limited epithelialization; a skin graft is often required. Infected abdominal wounds with dehiscence of the rectus abdominus fascia and evisceration of the bowel benefit from closure of the fascia and secondary skin closure.

SURGICAL TECHNICAL PRINCIPLES

Incision orientation should follow the natural skin creases to minimize tension on the scar. Incisions along tension lines subsequently minimize contracture and are hidden in the natural body contours. This concept also applies to skin graft placement. The outcome of grafts can be superior when the junctures are placed parallel to the skin lines rather than at angles to the lines; placement at angles accentuates the appearance of an abnormal surface marking. Incisions on the extremities should zigzag across a joint to break up a linear scar and avoid joint contracture.

Hemostasis must be meticulous so as to prevent the development of hematomas, which increase the likelihood of healing complications by increasing the risk of infection and causing a fibroplastic reaction. Hematomas prevent vascularization of flaps or skin by mechanically separating the wound bed from the graft.

Biological dressings and skin substitutes are important means of closing wounds that will not epithelialize. Different types of permanent or temporary dressings exist; several are discussed below.

Autograft, a sheet of the patient's own skin, is the gold standard for coverage of a nonhealing wound. For burns, early excision and autografting of deep dermal or full-thickness burns decrease the hospital stay and the time away from work or school; this procedure also reduces scarring (47). Thicker grafts contract less and are more durable than thinner grafts but do not "take" as well. The optimal thickness of the graft and the need for meshing to expand the size of the graft depend on the site of the wound. Whereas thicker grafts may be ideal, they are not always practical because of lack of donor sites or donor site complications. Planning a surgical approach to wound coverage must include deciding when covering the wound is important enough to risk donor site complications. Like other wounds, deep donor sites result in deep dermal injury, which can lead to scarring complications. Wounds on the palm are ideally treated with full-thickness grafts. Likewise, wounds on the face or the dorsal side of the hands benefit from thick partial-thickness grafts. Sites that are cosmetically or functionally less important can be treated with thinner grafts.

Allograft or homograft is a graft from one person to another. This "cadaver skin" is harvested just as are other tissues from organ donors. In general, allograft is available as frozen sheet grafts. Because the sheets have been frozen, cellular viability is limited (48). The tissue is viable enough to engraft, but the keratinocytes do not proliferate or migrate across a wound bed. Because the grafts do "take," they undergo rejection, which leads to a substantial inflammatory response. Indications for the use of allograft include temporary wound coverage until a donor site can be found and testing a wound bed to determine whether an autograft would engraft.

Xenograft is harvested from a different species. In the United States, the most commonly used xenograft is pig skin, which is available as frozen sheet grafts. Xenograft adheres to the wound but does not engraft. Appropriate use of xenografts includes application to uniformly shallow wounds in patients with toxic epidermolysis necrosis. As the wound epithelializes, the xenograft lifts off the surface of the wound.

Integra® is a commercially available dermal substitute with a temporary outer silastic layer that "closes" the wound while autologous fibroblasts migrate into the matrix formed by synthetic collagen I and chondroitin-6-sulfate. Once the dermal layer has vascularized, the silastic layer can be removed and an ultrathin autograft can be applied. The advantages of Integra are the creation of a pliable neodermis and the use of thinner grafts; these thinner grafts result in shallower donor sites that heal quickly and scar less (49). Integra requires fastidious surgical excision and perioperative wound care.

AlloDerm® (BMI, Florida, U.S.A.) is a commercially available dermal substitute derived from allografts that have been processed to remove the epidermis at the basement membrane and to remove all dermal cells. Because this material is composed of uninjured human dermis, it is conceptually attractive. The use of AlloDerm requires simultaneous application of a thin skin graft or cultured epithelial cells.

Apligraft® (Organogenesis, Inc., Canton, Massachusetts, U.S.A.) is a construct of collagen I with allogeneic human neonatal foreskin keratinocytes and fibroblasts. The fibroblasts are interspersed into prealigned collagen fibrils to create a dermis-like synthetic layer. Keratinocytes are seeded on the surface of the graft to create a multilayered skin substitute. Apligraft has been primarily marketed and successfully used for the treatment of nonhealing ulcers.

Tissue transfer of vascularized tissue may be necessary to cover tissue defects that will not take a skin graft because of exposed, poorly vascularized vital structures—such as nerves, tendons, vessels, or bones—and that are not amenable to other closure techniques. The ability to transfer complex and vascularized tissues, whether skin, fat, fascia, muscle, or bone, singly or in various combinations, allows for optimal tissue restoration. The size and location of the defect dictate the source of the tissue, which should have form and function similar to those of the missing tissue. When the donor tissue is available adjacent to the wound, advancement or rotation flaps provide a reliable method of closing both the defect and the donor site. When local tissue availability is limited, as in the head and neck, or when the defect is large, as with the extirpation of large recurrent cancers, distant tissues must be used. In the past two decades, numerous free flaps containing combinations of skin, fascia, fat, muscle, and bone have been created; the territories of these flaps can be completely perfused by a single artery and vein. The transfer is accomplished by microsurgical anastomosis of pedicle arteries and veins that may be 1 to 2 mm in diameter. The use of local and distant free flaps has favorably affected the treatment of patients with chronic wounds and has facilitated reconstruction after trauma and extirpative surgery.

RISK FACTORS FOR ABNORMAL WOUND REPAIR

Every medical student learns the acronym "FRIEND" with regard to nonclosing fistulas. The words whose initial letters compose this term also apply in some respects to wound complications: foreign body; radiation; inflammation; epithelialization; neoplasia; and distal obstruction (although for wounds, "diabetes mellitus" might be a more appropriate term).

Foreign bodies, whether small (glass fragments) or large (sutures and drains), disrupt wound closure (Fig. 1A). Removal of large foreign bodies (such as bullets) in the deep tissue may be contraindicated if the dissection would cause excessive injury to the tissues. On the other hand, aggressive efforts should be made to remove superficial dirt or tar from skin abrasions because these foreign bodies can cause infections or permanent pigmented tattoos in the healed wounds.

Radiation kills the rapidly proliferating cells that repopulate the wound bed; killing these cells leads to an impaired response to injury. Decreased angiogenesis results in tissue ischemia, and reduced keratinocyte proliferation and migration lead to inadequate epithelialization. Dense collagen production, combined with decreased cellular proliferation, results in a hard yet fragile wound that is easily disrupted. Incisional wound strength is markedly diminished, and secondary closure of an open wound may be delayed or may lead to a chronic wound. Patients with rectal cancers that have been treated with preoperative radiation followed by abdominoperineal resection are at a particularly high risk of chronic draining perineal wounds and may benefit from tissue transfer of viable rectus abdominus muscle flaps into the wound bed.

Infection complicates healing of preexisting wounds such as burn wounds or donor sites (50) or can be the direct cause of wounds such as carbuncles and

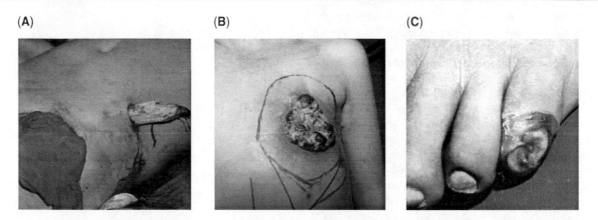

Figure 1 Risk factors for wound complications. **(A)** Foreign bodies protruding through the skin not only prevent healing of the entrance site, but also constitute a risk for infection. Intraoperative removal of foreign bodies should involve not only evaluation of the deep tissues, but also aggressive irrigation and debridement of the wound track. This wound should not be closed primarily. **(B)** Neglected breast cancer may present as a fungating, open, draining wound. Debridement of a chronic wound should include pathologic evaluation of the tissue to rule out neoplasm. **(C)** Diabetic ulcers have multifactorial causes, including microangiopathy and neuropathy. Twenty percent of patients with these chronic nonhealing wounds undergo amputation of the extremity.

hidradenitis. Bacteria colonize the skin under normal conditions. To guide clinical management, surgeons have traditionally classified wounds as clean (surgical incisions and simple lacerations), contaminated (bites, bowel injuries, and open fractures), or dirty (abscesses). Whereas quantitative bacterial counts less than 10^5 bacterial colonies per gram of tissue do not affect the response to acute injury, higher counts will invariably lead to wound breakdown (51). Osteomyelitis, or bony infection, often follows traumatic injury such as open fractures of the tibula or fibula; this condition causes substantial morbidity. After cardiac bypass surgery, sternal osteomyelitis can complicate surgical results when the left internal mammary artery is used to revascularize the heart. In approximately 2% to 4% of the population, this condition results in inadequate vascular supply to the remaining inferior sternum. Without bacterial seeding, the result is limited to sterile nonunion of the sternal wound. However, bacterial infection of the wound results in life-threatening mediastinitis, which requires immediate debridement of the devitalized sternum followed by coverage with healthy vascularized tissue.

Neoplasia should always be suspected when there is no known cause for chronic nonhealing wounds. Debridement of chronic wound should include pathologic evaluation to rule out neoplasm. Marjolin's ulcer in an old burn wound is the classic example of an aggressive squamous cell cancer in a nonhealing wound. Alternatively, neglected breast cancer or squamous cell cancer can result in fungating, open, draining wounds (Fig. 1B).

Diabetes mellitus is an important risk factor for wound healing. Not only do sensory neuropathy and microangiopathy increase the incidence of nonhealing wounds in the lower extremities (Fig. 1C), but

hyperglycemia also increases the risk of wound infection, which contributes to wound breakdown.

In addition to these commonly recognized causes of delayed healing, other important risk factors and comorbidities can affect the response to injury. Details about these factors should be collected during history taking and physical examination.

Nutrition can often be overlooked because so many persons eat well-balanced diets. Nevertheless, according to the Centers for Disease Control and Prevention, the incidence of rickets increased in the United States in 2001 because of vitamin D deficiency; therefore, we need to remain cognizant of our patients' nutritional status. Essentially, all vitamins, minerals, and trace elements play some cellular or enzymatic role that makes them crucial for normal wound healing processes. Vitamin C deficiency leads to dermal scar degeneration during the remodeling stage because prolyl hydroxylation, a necessary step in collagen synthesis, is dependent on vitamin C. Vitamin A is also involved in collagen synthesis and is essential for keratinocyte differentiation. Vitamin E deficiency leads to immune dysfunction. Vitamin K deficiency should be suspected in patients with fat malabsorption because a deficiency in this vitamin can lead to bleeding and wound hematomas. Zinc deficiency leads to delayed epithelialization, reduced tensile strength, and increased infection.

Vascularity is crucial insofar as oxygen delivery is necessary for normal wound healing. Revascularization can aid and abet the closure of wounds on ischemic limbs. Recent studies have observed normal wound closure in the face of angioinhibition (22,23); thus, the ultimate role of wound microvascularity may require reevaluation. Increased vascularity in granulation tissue probably contributes to excessive scar formation.

Genetic conditions are rare but should be considered when patients have fragile skin, poor wound strength, easy wound disruption, or spontaneous large-vessel nonatherosclerotic aneurysms. The most common genetic disturbances that alter dermal response to injury are the seven distinct variants of Ehlers–Danlos syndrome and Marfan's syndrome. Patients with Ehlers–Danlos syndrome have very thin skin with marked diminution of the dermis; extra caution must be taken with these patients to ensure careful tissue handling and wound closure. Proper testing should be undertaken if there is any clinical suspicion of a previously undiagnosed genetic connective tissue disorder. Blistering disorders such as epidermolysis bullosa may be more clinically obvious, and special attention should be paid to wound care.

Pharmacologic agents are notorious for altering the response to injury.

Corticosteroids inhibit the inflammatory response that is crucial for normal wound repair. Corticosteroids also repress the action of the enzyme prolyl hydroxylase; this repression leads to decreased collagen cross-linking and weaker incisional wounds.

Colchicine, a common antirheumatologic agent known for its anti-inflammatory effects, decreases wound contraction and wound strength. Clinical reports of delayed healing in patients treated with colchicine abound (52). This agent has been touted as an effective treatment for keloids. However, in a prospective randomized study of keloid treatments, postoperative colchicine prevented recurrence in only 32% of cases (53). At the cellular and molecular level, the recognized effects of this agent include inhibition of cell proliferation and migration, microtubule disruption, and altered collagen synthesis. However, at best, our knowledge about the effects of colchicine on collagen metabolism is muddy. Most findings support the idea that colchicine suppresses the production of type I collagen but stimulates the production of collagenase (54). Conversely, colchicine has been found to decrease the production of macrophage-derived collagenase (55). The direct effects of colchicine on wound repair processes must be clarified.

Anticoagulants can often be associated with postoperative formation of hematomas, a formidable and easily preventable complication. Patients taking therapeutic Coumadin® are especially at risk of perioperative bleeding because the effect of Coumadin is not quickly reversible. These patients should be switched to heparin treatment preoperatively to facilitate correction of the coagulation diathesis in the event of perioperative bleeding. Other agents that interfere with platelet adhesion include aspirin, nonsteroidal anti-inflammatory drugs, and the long-chain carbohydrates such as dextran, which are commonly used by microvascular surgeons for tissue transfers.

Naturopathic agents present an increasingly confounding variable in treating patients (56). Whereas surgeons routinely obtain a list of the medications their patients are taking before surgery and instruct patients

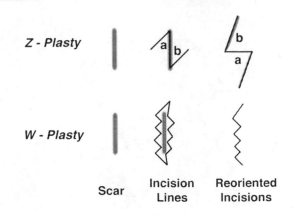

Figure 2 Scar revisions can be used either to lengthen a contracted incision (Z-plasty) or to break up the appearance of an unsightly scar (W-plasty).

to hold medications that may interfere with hemostasis, nonprescription drugs may not be captured in the history. Knowing that a patient takes naturopathic medications such as *Gingko biloba* may be essential. This particular medication, which is used to treat a wide variety of symptoms including dementia, memory loss, headache, sexual dysfunction, depression, and premenstrual syndrome, has been associated with spontaneous (57) and perioperative bleeding (58), possibly because of inhibition of platelet-activating factor and reduced platelet aggregation.

Pressure and other mechanical forces such as shear and friction frequently compromise skin integrity for patients with neuropathy, including diabetes mellitus, spinal cord injuries, and head injuries. Education about the methods to avoid pressure ulcers, such as frequent repositioning, and the catastrophic consequences of lesions are essential preventative measures.

SURGICAL TISSUE INJURY

Crush injury should be avoided during surgical procedures by gentle tissue handling and the use of non-crushing instruments. To avoid ischemia of the outer layer of the skin, the surgeon should take care to

Table 1 Pearls for Avoiding Wound Complications

Preoperative management
  Optimize nutrition
  Review all medications
  Control serum glucose concentrations
  Verify adequate vascularity
Intraoperative management
  Use skin lines to plan incisions
  Avoid surgical tissue injury or excessive tension
  Debride all nonviable tissue
  Achieve hemostasis
Postoperative management
  Avoid pressure from casts and dressings
  Diagnose and treat infection early

avoid picking up the subcutaneous tissue or the dermis rather than the epidermal layer.

Tension can be excessive, especially when running sutures are used. The temptation to pull tightly on the suture to approximate the wound edges will probably result in tissue ischemia and may lead to wound dehiscence, especially on fascia closures. An appropriate motto should be, "approximate, don't strangulate" (59). Sutures or staples left in for too long lead to permanent scarring because of both the crushing effect and the tension on the skin.

Dog ears, often encountered when elliptical incisions are being closed, result from excess skin and subcutaneous fat at the two edges of the closure. Removal involves upward traction with a single skin hook perpendicular to the skin at the end of the incision. In upward traction, a semicircular incision (180°)

is made around the base of the excess skin down to the subcutaneous fat. The cut skin margin is rotated and pulled away from the initial incision at a 90° angle, until the dog-ear deformity has been resolved. The remaining upper edge of the excess skin is transected to provide optimal resection of the dog ear. Removal of a dog ear leads to a longer final incision.

Scar revision should not be undertaken earlier than one year after the injury. The reason for this delay derives from the observation that tissue remodeling occurs for as long as one to two years after closure of the wound. Often, the incision looks worst (raised and hyperemic) two to three months after closure. With time, most of these raised and red wounds recede and fade without intervention. Whereas waiting for a wound to mature is the widely used therapeutic approach for normally healing wounds,

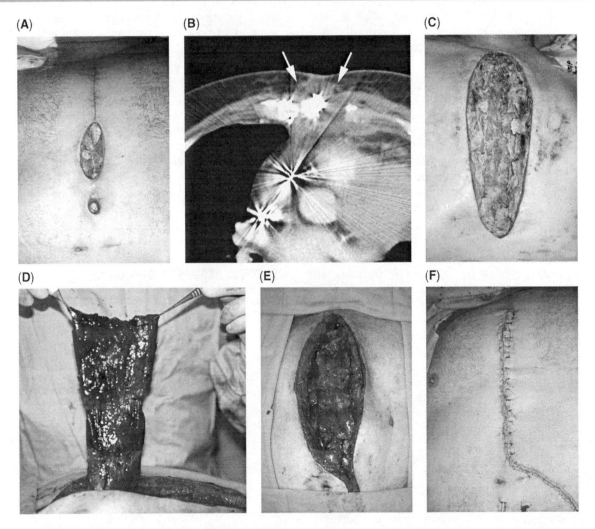

Figure 3 Case report. **(A)** Postoperative mediastinitis presents as a small, draining, incisional wound infection, but the underlying process extends into and beneath the sternal wound. **(B)** Computed tomography scan may confirm the clinical diagnosis but is generally not necessary for the clinical management of this complication. **(C)** Debridement of the wound verifies that the entire mediastinum is purulent with necrotic tissues both subcutaneously and deep. **(D)** The hallmark of therapy is rotation of viable tissue into the wound bed to protect the underlying vital structure; in this case, the rectus abdominus muscle has been mobilized. **(E)** The muscle flap is laid into the wound bed to provide coverage with viable tissue. **(F)** The skin incision is closed primarily over drains.

WOUND HEALING COMPLICATION CASE REPORT

A 60-year-old man with diabetes, who is a smoker, undergoes coronary artery bypass grafting using the left internal mammary artery. His initial recovery is uneventful and he is discharged from the hospital. On postoperative day 12, the patient experiences fever and chills and notes drainage coming from the inferior aspect of his sternal wound (Fig. 3A). Accompanying erythema surrounds the entire incision. A computed tomography scan of the chest confirms the diagnosis of mediastinitis (Fig. 3B). The fluid coming from the wound is cultured, the patient is treated with systemic antibiotics, and the entire incision is opened at the bedside (Fig. 3C), revealing a separated sternal edge with exposure of the wires and the right ventricle. Pus fills the entire cavity.

In the operating room, with the patient under general anesthesia and with good surgical exposure, the entire wound edge is excised until healthy bleeding tissues remain, and the sternal wires are removed. Copious irrigation of the entire wound bed and the exposed heart is performed. Debridement of the right sternal edge reveals healthy bleeding marrow, but the left sternal edge has minimal bleeding because of ischemia resulting from harvest of the left internal mammary artery. This situation mandates debridement of the sternum to viable and vascularized bone. The removal of the bone leaves a potential dead space above the heart. To obliterate the potential dead space and provide the protection of an additional layer of tissue over the right ventricle, a pedicled local pectoralis major or rectus abdominis muscle (Fig. 3C) is transferred into the wound (Fig. 3D), and the skin incision is closed primarily (Fig. 3E). The patient is discharged from the hospital on the seventh postoperative day.

This case illustrates several important principles in wound management: foreign bodies (sternal wires), diabetes, devitalized tissue, and wound contamination placed this patient at an increased risk of a chronic nonhealing wound over a vital structure. Treatment must include debridement of all necrotic tissue and wound coverage with vascularized, viable tissue. New findings suggest that patients at risk of sternal wound infections benefit from preoperative prophylaxis with intranasally administered mupirocin (60).

---

early scar revision may be justified if patients are miserable because of wound pruritus and cosmetic unsightliness, especially after deep dermal wounds. For hypertrophic scars, intralesional excision and primary closure are widely performed.

Z-plasty wound closure is one method of lengthening shortened, contracted scars. When linear scars contract, shortening of skin and subcutaneous tissues may limit motion, especially across joints such as the volar aspect of a digit. The Z-plasty requires the presence of adjacent mobile unscarred tissue to advance into the scar; this procedure lengthens the wound proportionate to the amount of advanced tissue (Fig. 2). A second objective in the use of a Z-plasty is to reorient a scar so that it is in the lines of skin tension; such reorientation will render the scar less noticeable and often narrower.

W-plasty reorients and breaks up a scar to minimize contraction. Unlike Z-plasty, W-plasty does not lengthen a scar. A long linear scar that runs perpendicular to the lines of skin tension may be quite visible and wide and can be revised by using a small, repeating up-and-down pattern, hence the name W-plasty (Fig. 2).

SPECIFIC EXAMPLES OF WOUND COMPLICATIONS

Keloids are scars that extend beyond the boundaries of the original wound with an excessive amount of dermal collagen. These cauliflower-like wounds tend to be increased in more darkly pigmented individuals and are commonly located on earlobes and presternal skin. No treatment is uniformly successful for all patients. Some therapeutic choices include intralesional steroid injection, pressure therapy, or surgical debulking with or without postoperative radiation.

Hypertrophic scars resemble keloids clinically, but they never extend beyond the boundaries of the original wound and they often resolve over a period of 12 to 24 months without intervention. They are raised scars characterized by pruritus, hyperemia, and warmth. Years of research has found that hypertrophic scars are associated with extracellular matrix molecules, growth factors, and enzymes, but no cellular or molecular cause of this undesirable response to injury has been identified. Hypertrophic scars occur at the same body sites where contraction prevails, such as the presternal skin. Hypertrophic scars uniformly develop in deep dermal wounds that take a long time to heal; this fact suggests that the deep dermis or subcutaneous tissue may hold the answer to the cause of this scarring. As is true for keloids, therapeutic options often provide unsatisfactory results.

REFERENCES

1. Sane DC, Moser TL, Pippen AM, Parker CJ, Achyuthan KE, Greenberg CS. Vitronectin is a substrate for transglutaminases. Biochem Biophys Res Commun 1988; 157: 115–120.

2. Prince CW, Dickie D, Krumdieck CL. Osteopontin, a substrate for transglutaminase and factor XIII activity. Biochem Biophys Res Commun 1991; 177:1205–1210.

3. Isik S, Sahin U, Ilgan S, Guler M, Gunalp B, Selmanpakoglu N. Saving the zone of stasis in burns with recombinant tissue-type plasminogen activator (r-tPA): an experimental study in rats. Burns 1998; 24:217–223.

4. Payan DG, Levine JD, Goetzl EJ. Modulation of immunity and hypersensitivity by sensory neuropeptides. J Immunol 1984; 132:1601–1604.

5. Ansel JC, Kaynard AH, Armstrong CA, Olerud J, Bunnett N, Payan D. Skin-nervous system interactions. J Invest Dermatol 1996; 106:198–204.

6. Arturson G. Pathophysiology of the burn wound. Ann Chir Gynaecol 1980; 69:178–190.

7. Streilein J, Tigelaar R. SALT: skin-associated lymphoid tissue. In: Daynes R, Spikes J, eds. Experimental and Clinical Photoimmunology. Vol. 1. Boca Raton: CRC Press, 1983:151–172.

8. Kupper TS, Deitch EA, Baker CC, Wong WC. The human burn wound as a primary source of interleukin-1 activity. Surgery 1986; 100:409–415.

9. Kupper TS. Interleukin-1 and other human keratinocyte cytokines: molecular and functional characterization. Adv Dermatol 1988; 3:293–307.

10. Nickoloff BJ, Karabin GD, Barker JN, et al. Cellular localization of interleukin-8 and its inducer, tumor necrosis factor-alpha in psoriasis. Am J Pathol 1991; 138:129–140.

11. Sehgal PB. Interleukin-6: molecular pathophysiology. J Invest Dermatol 1990; 94:2S–6S.

12. Gibran NS, Ferguson M, Heimbach DM, Isik FF. Monocyte chemoattractant protein-1 mRNA expression in the human burn wound. J Surg Res 1997; 70:1–6.

13. Kock A, Schwarz T, Kirnbauer R, et al. Human keratinocytes are a source for tumor necrosis factor alpha: evidence for synthesis and release upon stimulation with endotoxin or ultraviolet light. J Exp Med 1990; 172:1609–1614.

14. Rodriguez JL, Miller CG, Garner WL, et al. Correlation of the local and systemic cytokine response with clinical outcome following thermal injury. J Trauma 1993; 34:684–695.

15. Nijsten MW, Hack CE, Helle M, ten Duis HJ, Klasen HJ, Aarden LA. Interleukin-6 and its relation to the humoral immune response and clinical parameters in burned patients. Surgery 1991; 109:761–767.

16. Strieter RM, Wiggins R, Phan SH, et al. Monocyte chemotactic protein gene expression by cytokine-treated human fibroblasts and endothelial cells. Biochem Biophys Res Commun 1989; 162:694–700.

17. Nakagawa N, Sano H, Iwamoto I. Substance P induces the expression of intercellular adhesion molecule-1 on vascular endothelial cells and enhances neutrophil transendothelial migration. Peptides 1995; 16:721–725.

18. Quinlan KL, Song IS, Bunnett NW, et al. Neuropeptide regulation of human dermal microvascular endothelial cell ICAM-1 expression and function. Am J Physiol 1998; 275:C1580–C1590.

19. Kraling BM, Razon MJ, Boon LM, et al. E-selectin is present in proliferating endothelial cells in human hemangiomas. Am J Pathol 1996; 148:1181–1191.

20. Winn RK, Ramamoorthy C, Vedder NB, Sharar SR, Harlan JM. Leukocyte-endothelial cell interactions in ischemia-reperfusion injury. Ann N Y Acad Sci 1997; 832:311–321.

21. Bucky LP, Vedder NB, Hong HZ, et al. Reduction of burn injury by inhibiting CD18-mediated leukocyte adherence in rabbits. Plast Reconstr Surg 1994; 93: 1473–1480.

22. Jang YC, Arumugam S, Gibran NS, Isik FF. Role of alpha (v) integrins and angiogenesis during wound repair. Wound Repair Regen 1999; 7:375–380.

23. Bloch W, Huggel K, Sasaki T, et al. The angiogenesis inhibitor endostatin impairs blood vessel maturation during wound healing. FASEB J 2000; 14:2373–2376.

24. Gibran NS, Isik F, Heimbach D, Gordan D. Basic fibroblast growth factor in the early human burn wound. J Surg Res 1994; 56:226–234.

25. Jang YC, Arumugam S, Ferguson M, Gibran NS, Isik FF. Changes in matrix composition during the growth and regression of human hemangiomas. J Surg Res 1998; 80: 9–15.

26. Wu L, Pierce GF, Galiano RD, Mustoe TA. Keratinocyte growth factor induces granulation tissue in ischemic dermal wounds. Importance of epithelial-mesenchymal cell interactions. Arch Surg 1996; 131:660–666.

27. Kaplan ED, Holbrook KA. Dynamic expression patterns of tenascin, proteoglycans, and cell adhesion molecules during human hair follicle morphogenesis. Dev Dyn 1994; 199:141–155.

28. Bohnert A, Hornung J, Mackenzie IC, Fusenig NE. Epithelial-mesenchymal interactions control basement membrane production and differentiation in cultured and transplanted mouse keratinocytes. Cell Tissue Res 1986; 244:413–429.

29. Ehrlich HP, Buttle DJ. Epidermis promotion of collagenase in hypertrophic scar organ culture. Exp Mol Pathol 1984; 40:223–234.

30. Detmar M, Yeo KT, Nagy JA, et al. Keratinocyte-derived vascular permeability factor (vascular endothelial growth factor) is a potent mitogen for dermal microvascular endothelial cells. J Invest Dermatol 1995; 105:44–50.

31. Kirsner RS, Falanga V, Eaglstein WH. The biology of skin grafts. Skin grafts as pharmacologic agents. Arch Dermatol 1993; 129:481–483.

32. Compton CC, Gill JM, Bradford DA, Regauer S, Gallico GG, OConnor NE. Skin regenerated from cultured epithelial autografts on full-thickness burn wounds from 6 days to 5 years after grafting. A light, electron microscopic and immunohistochemical study. Lab Invest 1989; 60:600–612.

33. Phillips LG, Abdullah KM, Geldner PD, et al. Application of basic fibroblast growth factor may reverse diabetic wound healing impairment. Ann Plast Surg 1993; 31:331–334.

34. Greenhalgh DG, Sprugel KH, Murray MJ, Ross R. PDGF and FGF stimulate wound healing in the genetically diabetic mouse. Am J Pathol 1990; 136:1235–1246.

35. Brown RL, Breeden MP, Greenhalgh DG. PDGF and TGF-alpha act synergistically to improve wound healing in the genetically diabetic mouse. J Surg Res 1994; 56:562–570.

36. Steed DL. The role of growth factors in wound healing. Surg Clin North Am 1997; 77:575–586.

37. Ashcroft GS, Horan MA, Ferguson MW. Aging is associated with reduced deposition of specific extracellular matrix components, an upregulation of angiogenesis, and an altered inflammatory response in a murine incisional wound healing model. J Invest Dermatol 1997; 108:430–437.

38. Stricklin GP, Li L, Jancic V, Wenczak BA, Nanney LB. Localization of mRNAs representing collagenase and TIMP in sections of healing human burn wounds. Am J Pathol 1993; 143:1657–1666.

39. Vernon RB, Sage EH. Contraction of fibrillar type I collagen by endothelial cells: a study in vitro. J Cell Biochem 1996; 60:185–197.

40. Hembry RM, Ehrlich HP. Immunolocalization of collagenase and tissue inhibitor of metalloproteinases (TIMP) in hypertrophic scar tissue. Br J Dermatol 1986; 115:409–420.

41. Nwomeh BC, Liang HX, Cohen IK, Yager DR. MMP-8 is the predominant collagenase in healing wounds and nonhealing ulcers. J Surg Res 1999; 81:189–195.

42. Doillon CJ, Hembry RM, Ehrlich HP, Burke JF. Actin filaments in normal dermis and during wound healing. Am J Pathol 1987; 126:164–170.

43. Dunnick CA, Gibran NS, Heimbach DM. Substance P has a role in neurogenic mediation of human burn wound healing. J Burn Care Rehabil 1996; 17:390–396.

44. Crowe R, Parkhouse N, McGrouther D, Burnstock G. Neuropeptide-containing nerves in painful hypertrophic human scar tissue. Br J Dermatol 1994; 130: 444–452.

45. Greer SE, Duthie E, Cartolano B, Koehler KM, Maydick-Youngberg D, Longaker MT. Techniques for applying subatmospheric pressure dressing to wounds in difficult regions of anatomy. J Wound Ostomy Continence Nurs 1999; 26:250–253.

46. Blackburn JH II, Boemi L, Hall WW, et al. Negative-pressure dressings as a bolster for skin grafts. Ann Plast Surg 1998; 40:453–457.

47. Engrav LH, Heimbach DM, Reus JL, Harner TJ, Marvin JA. Early excision and grafting versus nonoperative treatment of burns of indeterminant depth: a randomized prospective study. J Trauma 1983; 23: 1001–1004.

48. Bravo D, Rigley TH, Gibran N, Strong DM, Newman-Gage H. Effect of storage and preservation methods on viability in transplantable human skin allografts. Burns 2000; 26:367–378.

49. Heimbach D, Luterman A, Burke J, et al. Artificial dermis for major burns. A multi-center randomized clinical trial. Ann Surg 1988; 208:313–320.

50. Matsumura H, Meyer NA, Mann R, Heimbach DM. Melting graft-wound syndrome. J Burn Care Rehabil 1998; 19:292–295.

51. Robson MC, Heggers JP. Delayed wound closure based on bacterial counts. J Surg Oncol 1970; 2:379–383.

52. Alster Y, Varssano D, Loewenstein A, Lazar M. Delay of corneal wound healing in patients treated with colchicine. Ophthalmology 1997; 104:118–119.

53. Lawrence WT. In search of the optimal treatment of keloids: report of a series and a review of the literature. Ann Plast Surg 1991; 27:164–178.

54. Chung KY, Kang DS. Regulation of type I collagen and interstitial collagenase mRNA expression in human dermal fibroblasts by colchicine and D-penicillamine. Yonsei Med J 1999; 40:490–495.

55. Wahl LM, Lampel LL. Regulation of human peripheral blood monocyte collagenase by prostaglandins and anti-inflammatory drugs. Cell Immunol 1987; 105:411–422.

56. Tsen LC, Segal S, Pothier M, Bader AM. Alternative medicine use in presurgical patients. Anesthesiology 2000; 93:148–151.

57. Rowin J, Lewis SL. Spontaneous bilateral subdural hematomas associated with chronic Ginkgo biloba ingestion. Neurology 1996; 46:1775–1776.

58. Fessenden JM, Wittenborn W, Clarke L. Gingko biloba: a case report of herbal medicine and bleeding postoperatively from a laparoscopic cholecystectomy. Am Surg 2001; 67:33–35.

59. Mullikan J. Management of wounds. In: May HL, ed. Emergency Medicine. New York: John Wiley & Sons Inc, 1984:283–298.

60. Cimochowski GE, Harostock MD, Brown R, Bernardi M, Alonzo N, Coyle K. Intranasal mupirocin reduces sternal wound infection after open heart surgery in diabetics and nondiabetics. Ann Thorac Surg 2001; 71:1572–1579.

43

Complications of Thermal Injuries

Mark Cockburn
*Department of Surgery, Miller School of Medicine at the University of Miami, Miami,
Florida, U.S.A.*

Nicholas Namias
Miller School of Medicine at the University of Miami, Miami, Florida, U.S.A.

Burn injuries present great metabolic, immunologic, and mechanical challenges to the human body. Additionally, burn injuries are associated with a variety of complications (Table 1). In this chapter, we will discuss the prevention, diagnosis, and treatment of many of these associated complications.

COMPLICATIONS OF BURN INJURIES
Definitions

Burns are categorized by the depth of injury. Burns involving only the epidermis are first-degree burns and require no specific therapy. Burns involving part of but not the entire thickness of the dermis are second-degree burns. There is a high degree of variability within the class of second-degree burns. Superficial second-degree burns can be expected to heal spontaneously in as little as a few days or in as much as two to three weeks, with minimal risk of hypertrophic scarring or functional disability. Deeper second-degree burns can also close spontaneously over longer periods of time but can be expected to be associated with significant hypertrophic scarring and unstable overlying epithelium, which is prone to blisters and injuries from minor trauma. Indeterminate second-degree burns are those whose appearance defies classification by the trained observer, or those that are of mixed depth and require longer periods of observation before the wounds can be clearly defined as deep or superficial burns. Burns involving the entire thickness of the dermis are classified as third-degree or full-thickness burns. All of the dermal elements are destroyed and the wound can close only by contraction from its perimeter. This type of closure may be acceptable when the burns are very small, depending on their location, but when such burns occur in important functional or cosmetic areas, closure by contraction leads to unacceptable functional outcomes and cosmetic deformities. Excision and grafting are generally required for the treatment of third-degree burns. Burns involving the muscle fascia and deeper structures are sometimes referred to as fourth-degree burns, but this is not a widely used term.

Immediate Complications

The risk of complications begins at the time of burning. Maneuvers performed to extinguish flames, such as rolling on the ground or immersing the wound in standing water, may contaminate the wound. Aeromonas infection can occur when the wound is immersed in a natural body of water. If water or ice is applied to large burns, systemic hypothermia can occur. For this reason, cooling maneuvers are recommended only for small burns. Efforts to neutralize chemical burns can lead to further injury due to the neutralizing agent. However, the conventional belief that neutralization is an exothermic reaction that will cause further burning has recently been challenged in animal studies (unpublished data). Failure to recognize the depth of burning can lead either to incorrect triage or to delay of appropriate therapy. Immersion burns may have a moist red appearance suggestive of a superficial scald; careful observation will reveal that these wounds do not blanch and that the redness is caused by fixed hemoglobin in a deep wound. Some deep-contact burns may have an intact epidermis that can easily be rubbed away to reveal the deep underlying dermal burn. If this epidermis is left undisturbed, the presence of the burn may be unappreciated. If medical care is not obtained within 24 hours after burning, the burns may have a coat of proteinaceous exudates, which can confound the determination of burn depth.

Burn wounds exist in three dimensions. The area of direct exposure to heat will contain the zone of coagulation, i.e., the area of the burn that has undergone coagulation necrosis. Surrounding this zone in every direction is the zone of stasis, a zone of variable protein coagulation and impaired circulation that results from endothelial injury. This zone is at risk

Table 1   Overview of Complications of Thermal Injuries

Immediate complications
Contamination
Infection
  Immune suppression
  Cellulitis
  Burn-wound infection
Hypothermia
Misdiagnosis/mistriage
Inadequate pain relief
Under-resuscitation/over-resuscitation
Complications of topical antimicrobial agents
Silver nitrate solution 0.5%
  Hyponatremia
  Hypochloremia
  Hypothermia
Silver sulfadiazine
  Cutaneous hypersensitivity
  Transient leukopenia
Mafenide acetate
  Cutaneous hypersensitivity
  Metabolic acidosis
Pulmonary
Pneumonia
ARDS
Tracheobronchitis
Gastrointestinal
Paralytic ileus
Mucosal ulceration
Perforation
Renal
Acute tubular necrosis
Renal failure secondary to myoglobinuria
Complications of reconstruction
Donor site conversion to full-thickness injury
Skin graft loss
Graft contraction
Sponge deformity
Contracture across joints
Psychological
Posttraumatic stress disorder
Anxiety
Depression
Complications of electrical injury
Neurologic
  Loss of consciousness
  Paresthesia
Cardiac
  Ventricular fibrillation
  S-T segment changes
  Sinus tachycardia
Musculoskeletal
  Compartment syndrome
  Post-tetanic fractures

Abbreviation: ARDS, adult respiratory distress syndrome.

of becoming part of the zone of coagulation if the patient is inadequately resuscitated or if the wound becomes infected (1).

Commonly, burn patients suffer unnecessarily because of inadequate pain control. Effective relief of burn pain generally requires opioids; commonly prescribed non-narcotic analgesics are generally inadequate. Inadequate pain control may prevent the patient from performing adequate wound care and participating in rehabilitation.

Both early under-resuscitation and over-resuscitation are common complications for burn patients. The Advanced Burn Life Support program of the American College of Surgeons recommends resuscitation with 2 to 4 cc of fluid/kg body weight times the percentage of the body surface area that is burned; this amount of fluid should be administered over a 24-hour period, half during the first eight hours. Those unfamiliar with burns may not appreciate the large volumes of fluid required to resuscitate a burn patient, and this lack of knowledge can lead to under-resuscitation and its consequences of renal failure and multiple organ system failure. Conversely, those loosely familiar with the need for fluid resuscitation of burn patients are likely to injudiciously over-resuscitate, and this problem leads to unnecessary degrees of edema that can cause local tissue hypoxia in the edematous areas or airway obstruction in severe cases.

Infectious Complications

The burn patient is at risk of infection because of impaired mechanical, cellular, and humoral host defenses. This break in the defensive barrier, coupled with contamination, nutritional difficulties, and gut effects (bacterial translocation through an already compromised, hypoxic mucosal barrier) (2), accounts for the incidence of infectious complications.

Both cell-mediated and humoral responses (2) are adversely affected in the burn patient. It is thought that defects in the lysosomal enzymes and a decrease in the production of oxygen radicals account for the decrease in the intracellular bacterial killing capacity of neutrophils despite normal phagocytic ability (3,4). Activation of the complement system also creates a condition of relative immunosuppression in burn patients (5). The levels of certain cytokines, interleukin-1-beta, interleukin-6, interleukin-10, and tumor necrosis factor alpha are elevated in severely burned patients. These changes appear to increase susceptibility to infection.

Historically, gram-positive organisms (*Streptococci* and *Staphylococci* spp.) have been most frequently associated with septic death among burn patients. Since the advent of penicillin antibiotics and the use of topical antimicrobial agents, these organisms are rarely the cause of death. However, when *Streptococci* cause burn wound infection, there is an increase in pain, erythema, and induration (2). Classically, in these cases, erythema originates at the burn wound margin, and progression of the infection to the lymphatics may occur. Penicillin is the antibiotic of choice for *Streptococcal* cellulitis. A dreaded complication of *Streptococcal* infection is the conversion of donor sites to full-thickness injury. *Streptococcal* infection can also result in skin-graft loss (2). *Staphylococcal* infection of burn wounds has also been treated with nafcillin, oxacillin, or methicillin. Recent years have seen the development of infection due to methicillin-resistant *Staphylococcus aureus* (MRSA). Vancomycin is the drug of choice for treating this infection (2). The development of toxic shock syndrome, although rare, requires aggressive management with antibiotics, intravenous human immunoglobulin, and circulatory support. *Clostridial* infections are rare but must be watched for in patients with deep-tissue injury. Intravenous antibiotics and early aggressive debridement of nonviable tissue are the mainstay of infection management.

More recently, the cause of burn-wound infections has been predominantly gram-negative bacteria. One of the primary pathogens involved in these infections is *Pseudomonas aeruginosa*; these bacteria can invade the burn wound locally and cause sepsis. Early infection with *Pseudomonas* can be detected by the classic fruity smell of the wound and its dressing and by the characteristic green pigment produced by the bacteria. Visualization of fluorescence under a Woods lamp can also be helpful. Using Dakin's solution (0.25%) in topical dressings has been helpful in the control of *Pseudomonas* infection in burn wounds. Subeschar clysis of antibiotics has been used in the past to treat invasive burn-wound sepsis, but this procedure is rarely used currently in the developed world, where proper antisepsis, topical antimicrobial agents, and early excision of the burn wounds make burn-wound sepsis a preventable complication. The keys to early recognition of pathogens and the use of appropriate antibiotics are the microbial prevalence patterns and the antibiotic susceptibility reports of individual burn units and centers.

The emergence and increasing incidence of fungal infections among burn patients have resulted from the increasing use of systemic antibacterial agents and effective topical antibacterial burn-wound regimens (2). Although silver sulfadiazine (SSD) is effective against *Candida*, another commonly used topical agent, mafenide acetate, allows *Candida* to overgrow the margins of the burn wound (6). *Candida* species are the most common fungal organisms causing burn-wound infections (2). Commonly, *Candida* may be a wound contaminant, but when *Candida* causes a local wound infection, nystatin can be used locally. When systemic infection with *Candida* organisms occurs, systemic antifungal therapy is necessary. The administration of systemic antibacterial agents should be discontinued if possible. Early aggressive surgical debridement with rapid coverage has also been beneficial in controlling systemic fungal infections (2).

Complications of Topical Antimicrobials

A number of topical agents are used in the care of burn patients. Some of these agents are used in wound-cleansing procedures and others as part of the wound dressing. Certain complications are related to the use of these agents.

Silver nitrate can cause hyponatremia and hypochloremia, and thus serum electrolyte levels must be carefully monitored while this agent is being administered.

SSD 1% cream, formulated in 1967, has excellent activity against *P. aeruginosa*, *S. aureus*, and other organisms, including yeast. Mild cutaneous hypersensitivity reactions may occur in fewer than 5% of patients (7,8). A transient leukopenia may occur, typically within two to three days after the institution of therapy; however, no increased susceptibility to infectious complications has been identified (6). Some bacteria, such as all *Enterobacter cloacae* strains and some *Pseudomonas* strains, are not susceptible to SSD (Silvadene®, King Pharmaceuticals, Inc., Bristol, Tennessee, U.S.A.).

Sulfamylon® (mafenide acetate 0.5% cream), introduced in the mid-1960s, is readily absorbed through the eschar. It is available in both a 10% water-soluble cream and a 5% solution. It has a wide antibacterial spectrum against most gram-positive bacteria, including *Clostridia*, and most gram-negative bacteria (6,7). Cutaneous hypersensitivity reactions may be seen in as many as 50% of patients. Mafenide is a potent carbonic anhydrase inhibitor, and its use can result in metabolic acidosis. A compensatory hyperventilation may occur; minute ventilation as high as 50 L has been reported (9). Consequently, when mafenide is used, the patient's respiratory status, pH levels, and blood gases must be frequently monitored. Because of its ability to inhibit human keratinocytes and fibroblasts in vitro and to suppress the activity of polymorphonuclear leukocytes (PMNs) and lymphocytes, mafenide inhibits re-epithelialization more than SSD does (7).

Cerium nitrate–SSD was developed by adding the lanthanide salt cerium nitrate to SSD. This agent has excellent bacteriostatic activity on wounds. Methemoglobinemia has occurred in some patients treated with this agent and is caused by the absorption of reduced nitrates. No other electrolyte abnormalities have been noted when cerium nitrate–SSD is used (6).

Povidone-iodine, as a 10% ointment, has a wide spectrum of antibacterial and antifungal activity and is effective against protozoa. Its systemic absorption through the wound is associated with decreased renal function or renal failure. Patients using povidone-iodine dressings for prolonged periods of time should be monitored for symptoms of iodine toxicity, which include hypercalcemic metabolic acidosis, cardiovascular instability (bradycardia, hypertension), elevation of hepatic enzymes, and central nervous and progressive renal dysfunction (10).

Dakin's solution (sodium hypochlorite 0.5% or 0.25% solution) is bactericidal, fungicidal, and virucidal. It is effective against MRSA, methicillin-resistant *Staphylococcus epidermidis*, and *Enterococci* (6). Sodium hypochlorite dissolves clots and may cause bleeding. At concentrations higher than 0.025%, it is toxic to fibroblasts, keratinocytes, and PMNs (7).

The aforementioned complications of topical antimicrobial agents, of course, can be eliminated if these agents are not used. It is possible not to use them in some circumstances, if an occlusive wound dressing can be applied. Types of these dressings include simple clear adhesive dressings for small wounds and Biobrane® (UDL Laboratories, Inc., Rockford, Illinois, U.S.A.), xenograft, and allograft for larger wounds. These dressings can be left in place, thereby obviating the need for frequent painful dressing changes and avoiding the complications that may accompany the use of topical antimicrobial agents. However, the occlusive dressings introduce their own complications. Primary among these is the chance that definitive treatment of the wound may be delayed. Such delay may occur if the depth of the wound was underestimated when the dressing was applied, particularly if the dressing remains adherent and the underlying wound is not examined. Acticoat® and other silver-containing occlusive dressings combine the advantages of the topical antimicrobial agents and those of the occlusive dressings. However, Acticoat can cause a burning sensation on application and can temporarily limit range of motion if allowed to desiccate.

The complications associated with the topical antimicrobial agents and the occlusive dressings can be avoided with early definitive excision and grafting. Pediatric patients treated with immediate excision and grafting have experienced less blood loss and shorter hospital stays than similar patients who were not treated in this way (11,12). Preliminary data from our institution suggest that we can decrease the length of stay for adults by 50% if burn wounds are excised as an emergency, that is, at the time of presentation. We have performed such excision with no increase in the mortality rates, the number of transfusions needed, or the occurrence of infectious complications. We have excised as much as 60% of the entire burn in a single sitting without the occurrence of hemodynamic instability or hypothermia and without excessive need for transfusions.

Pulmonary Complications

Historically, wound infection was the most common infection suffered by burn patients. Since the development of topical antimicrobials and intravenous antibiotics, however, the infection most frequently suffered by burn patients is pneumonia (13). In fact, for burn patients, the leading cause of death is respiratory failure. Early diagnosis with sputum assessment and chest radiographs is necessary when respiratory failure occurs. The results of cultures should guide the use of antibiotic therapy, and aggressive pulmonary toilet should be instituted. Before culture results are ready, empiric therapy against the organisms that predominate in the unit should be used.

Some patients who suffer thermal injury experience inhalation injury. Inhalation injury is a chemical tracheobronchitis and acute pneumonitis caused by inhalation of smoke and other irritative products of incomplete combustion. The mortality rates for burn patients with inhalation injury are greater overall than that for patients with burns of similar size but with no inhalation injury (14). Chest radiography is insensitive in making the diagnosis (15); fiberoptic bronchoscopy (FOB) and Xenon-133 scans are more reliable. FOB evidence of mucosal inflammation or ulceration and deposition of carbon particles indicate inhalation injury. Therapy depends on the severity of the injury. For mild cases, humidified oxygen–enriched air and incentive spirometry may be the only treatment required. However, for impaired mucociliary function, repeated FOB may be necessary. For the patient with progressive respiratory difficulty, endotracheal intubation and mechanical ventilation must be undertaken (16). Because of the increased mortality rates associated with inhalation injury, the appearance of a new infiltrate on the chest radiograph of a patient with progressive respiratory difficulty should prompt the clinician to obtain endobronchial cultures and to begin treatment with intravenously administered antibiotics for presumptive bronchopneumonia.

Patients with inhalation injury are at a significant risk of carbon monoxide poisoning, particularly if they are burned in an enclosed space. Treatment involves endotracheal intubation (in cases of severe respiratory distress) and administration of oxygen-enriched air mixtures. Hyperbaric oxygen therapy can be used, especially for those patients who are comatose and have carbon monoxide poisoning (14).

Both severe pneumonia and inhalation injury can lead to the development of adult respiratory distress syndrome. Patients with this disease may require prolonged mechanical ventilatory assistance, and the use of this treatment further increases the incidence of ventilator-associated pneumonia.

Gastrointestinal Complications

Patients sustaining burns over more than 25% of the body are likely to experience paralytic ileus. With adequate resuscitation, the return of gastrointestinal motility occurs around the third to fifth postburn day. Thus, the initiation of enteral nutrition is delayed. Because of this delay and the development of focal ischemia (which can occur as early as three to five hours after the burn), there is a great risk of mucosal ulcerations and perforation (14). The burn patient with sepsis is also at an increased risk of mucosal ulceration. Histamine-2 blockers have been shown to be more effective than sucralfate in preventing gastric mucosal ulceration among critically ill patients without burns (17). Additionally, antacids are effective and are used at the author's institution in an effort to prevent erosive gastritis (Curling's ulcer). Vitamin A supplementation may help prevent ulceration by assisting in mucin production. Cholestyramine can be used to prevent bile reflux gastritis. Today we rarely see massive hemorrhage from mucosal ulcers, but when they occur the patient's likelihood of mortality is increased. It is unclear whether very sick patients with an already poor prognosis are more likely to experience these massive gastrointestinal bleeds or whether the massive hemorrhage by itself increases the patient's likelihood of mortality.

Renal Complications

Adequate fluid resuscitation of burn patients cannot be sufficiently stressed. Of concern is the fact that, as the patient's blood pressure falls, there is progressive vasoconstriction of the afferent arterioles. The efferent arterioles may also undergo vasoconstriction as the result of the administration of norepinephrine and angiotensin. The net result is hypoxia at the level of the glomerulus and the tubules. The potential for muscle necrosis with resulting myoglobinuria or hemoglobinuria, coupled with a decrease in blood flow to the tubules, further potentiates the acute tubular necrosis. When myoglobinuria is suspected, alkalinization of the urine (18) by adding sodium bicarbonate to the intravenous fluid and maintenance of urine output of 100 cc/hr or greater are recommended.

Complications of Reconstruction

Skin grafting has shortened recovery time and has decreased the rate of infectious complications among burn patients (11,19). However, skin grafting is also associated with complications. Of particular importance is the contraction of skin grafts. It has been noted that full-thickness skin grafts suffer less contraction than split-thickness skin grafts. In addition, the interval of time between the initial release of contraction and subsequent releases was longer with full-thickness grafts than with split-thickness grafts (20).

"Graft take" is affected by infection and may be delayed in the malnourished patient. Thus, various degrees of graft loss can be experienced. Sponge deformity is a complication of skin grafting that usually occurs around the periphery of the excised area where the excision was shallower or with thicker skin grafts (21). It may be that the bed beneath the graft epithelializes from residual epithelial elements before vascularization of the autografts develops (18).

Psychological Complications

Victims of burn injuries suffer from a variety of psychological disorders. The equivocal findings of some studies suggest a relationship between total body surface area of the burn and the incidence of posttraumatic stress disorder (PTSD) (22). However, other studies suggest a correlation between the occurrence of PTSD and previous psychological adjustment, preburn affective disorder, delirium or severe pain during acute treatment, and weaker perceptions of social support (23). It has been noted that patients are at risk of PTSD both at the time of hospitalization and after discharge. Thus, it is important for clinicians to provide all patients with education and psychological intervention during hospitalization, and with aggressive follow-up after discharge (19). Some patients experience anticipatory anxiety as a result of unavoidable, painful wound dressing changes (24). Adequate premedication before dressing changes can minimize the likelihood that aversion reactions will occur. Depressive symptoms may develop as the result of changes in body image and excessive pain. One would expect that the degree of disfigurement would correlate with the degree of depressive symptoms. However, no such correlation has been shown in previous studies.

COMPLICATIONS OF ELECTRICAL INJURIES

Electrical injuries depend on the source of the current, the voltage, the amperage, the duration of contact, and the surface area through which the current flows. Certainly, the greater the voltage and amperage and the greater the duration of contact (25), the more energy delivered to the victim and the more severe the potential injury. The complications can be categorized as acute or early, ongoing, and late.

Early Complications

Neurological sequelae, when they occur, can be early or late and can affect both the central and the peripheral nervous systems. Up to 70% of patients who sustain a high-voltage injury are rendered unconscious (26), particularly if current passes through the head. All patients who have not sustained a fatal injury regain consciousness. Patients who fall after being electrocuted can experience closed head injuries, which must be managed in much the same way as they are managed in the regular trauma setting. The tetanic contractions that occur at the time of electrocution can produce vertebral fractures that can result in paralysis and other neurological deficits (27). Thus, maintaining spinal precautions when examining the electrocuted victims and completely evaluating these patients for associated injuries are very important.

Ventricular fibrillation can occur with electrical injury and can be fatal. However, sinus tachycardia and nonspecific ST-T segment changes are the most common cardiac findings (28,29). Most of these disturbances resolve spontaneously within a few hours. Patients who are burned by either low-voltage current or high-voltage current but who reach the emergency room without evidence of cardiac abnormalities rarely experience these abnormalities later. If the patient suffers arrhythmia or demonstrates electrocardiogram evidence of acute myocardial infarction, then cardiac monitoring is necessary. These are key points because such patients usually require multiple surgical procedures, which should not be delayed because of questionable findings (30).

Patients who are apneic at the time of injury should undergo full cardiopulmonary resuscitation and support. Chest radiographs of patients who have fallen should be obtained and examined for evidence of pneumothorax or hemothorax. Effusions and pneumonitis may occur near entrance and exit wounds. Effusions can be treated by tube thoracostomy.

Ongoing Complications

The fluid requirements of patients with thermal burns can be estimated more accurately than can those of the electrically burned patient. Because current has passed through the tissue between the entrance and exit sites, it is difficult to gauge the fluid requirement strictly by outward evidence of injury. Thus, one must be hypervigilant so that ongoing injuries and consequent fluid requirements are not overlooked. Adequate urine output can still be used as a guide to resuscitation. Muscle tissue can become edematous when injured. The muscles lie within compartments, and as the muscle swells the pressure within the compartment increases. At a certain critical value, the blood flow to the muscle decreases, and further muscle damage is produced. The five symptoms of pain, pallor, paresthesias, paralysis, and pulselessness are all evidences of compartment syndrome. However, the earliest sign of this syndrome is paresthesia. The consequences of muscle injury include limb loss with the need for extensive rehabilitation and acute renal failure caused by myoglobin deposition within the renal tubules.

Determining the extent of tissue damage and viability is difficult. The resistance of bone is high; thus, heat is produced deep within the limb (25). Consequently, the superficial muscles may be viable although the deeper muscles are necrotic. There is no good test to determine the viability of the muscles short of exploring the compartments to determine whether the muscle bleeds or contracts (31). The problem caused by failure to detect necrotic muscle is that this tissue provides a focus for the development of infection and sepsis. When necrotic muscle is detected, debridement is mandatory. Subsequent reexploration and additional debridement may be required.

When rhabdomyolysis is suspected, the urinary output should be maintained at 100 cc/hr. Mannitol has been used to enhance excretion of hemochromogens. Alkalinization of the urine may be helpful in preventing crystallization of myoglobin within the renal tubules (22). Because of the large fluid shifts that take place, shock can occur. It is essential to administer large volumes of fluid because under-resuscitation is the most common cause of acute renal failure among these patients.

The direct passage of current through the abdominal wall may injure both the wall and the underlying intestines. Injury to intra-abdominal viscera can occur even when the entrance and exit sites are not on the abdomen. A high index of suspicion is necessary to make the diagnosis, particularly if patients have other severe injuries. Bowel perforation (32), pancreatitis, and gallbladder necrosis (33) have been reported. Exploratory laparotomy may be necessary

Table 2 Tips for Avoiding Complications of Thermal Injury

Use aseptic technique at all times
Maintain warm environment
Titrate fluids carefully
Control pain adequately
Wean patients from ventilator as rapidly as is safely possible
Administer enteral feedings early, but stop feeding if tolerance is in question
Err on the side of grafting in areas where contractures is a concern
Remain cognizant of concomitant injury and the potential for compartment syndrome
Provide emotional and psychological support

when suspicion is high. Curling ulcers may also occur (25). This complication was discussed earlier under gastrointestinal complications of thermal injuries.

Late Complications

Fibrosis and scarring of locally damaged tissue in and around peripheral nerves may result in late compression and decreased conductance. The perineural tissue may undergo vascular inflammation, thrombosis, or fibrosis. Causalgia, motor weakness, paresthesias, and hyperesthesia have been reported. With regard to the central nervous system, cortical encephalopathy, hemiplegia with or without aphasia, striatal syndrome, and brain stem dysfunction can occur (34). Seizure disorders can also occur late. Spinal cord symptoms similar to those of progressive muscular atrophy, amyotrophic lateral sclerosis, or transverse myelitis may develop later (35).

Cataracts may occur in 5% to 7% of patients and frequently are bilateral (24). The onset of blurred vision usually begins about six months after injury (36). Because of the possibility of such a devastating complication, patients should undergo ophthalmologic examination as part of their acute care and should be made aware of the potential for cataracts (28).

Complications of thermal injuries clearly can involve any of the body's systems (Table 2). Although prevention is the goal, knowledge of the potential pitfalls may help to mitigate the detrimental effects of the complications when they do occur. Careful attention and a high index of vigilance can help to prevent some, but not all, of these complications.

REFERENCES

1. Jackson DM. The diagnosis of the depth of burning. Br J Surg 1953; 40:588–596.
2. Treat RC. Infectious complications. In: Maull KI, ed. Complications in Trauma and Critical Care. Philadelphia: Saunders, 1996:505–512.
3. Cole WQ, Cook JJ, Grogan JB. In vitro neutrophil function and lysosomal enzyme levels in patients with sepsis. Surg Forum 1975; 26:79–81.
4. Curreri PW, Heck EL, Browne L, Baxter CR. Stimulated nitroblue tetrazolium test to assess neutrophil

antibacterial function: prediction of wound sepsis in burned patients. Surgery 1973; 74(1):6–13.

5. Gelfand JA. How do complement components and fragments affect cellular immunological function? J Trauma 1984; 24(9 suppl):S118–S124.

6. Heggers J, Linares HA, Edgar P, Villareal C, Herndon DN. Treatment of infections in burns. In: Herndon DN, ed. Total Burn Care. Philadelphia: Saunders, 1997: 120–169.

7. Ward RS, Saffle JR. Topical agents in burn and wound care. Phys Ther 1995; 75(6):525–538.

8. Kaye ET. Topical antibacterial agents. Infect Dis Clin North Am 2000; 14(2):321–339.

9. Monafo WW, West MA. Current treatment recommendations for topical burn therapy. Drugs 1990; 40:364–373.

10. Burks RI. Povidone-iodine solution in wound treatment. Phys Ther 1998; 78(2):212–218.

11. Xiao-Wu W, Herndon DN, Spies M, Sanford AP, Wolf SE. Effects of delayed wound excision and grafting in severely burned children. Arch Surg 2002; 137(9): 1049–1054.

12. Desai MH, Herndon DN, Broemeling L, Barrow RE, Nichols RJ Jr., Rutan RL. Early burn wound excision significantly reduces blood loss. Ann Surg 1990; 211(6): 753–762.

13. Pruitt BA Jr. Infection and the burn patient. Br J Surg 1990; 77(10):1081–1082.

14. Shirani KZ, Pruitt BA Jr., Mason AD Jr. The influence of inhalation injury and pneumonia on burn mortality. Ann Surg 1987; 205:82–87.

15. Clark WR, Bonaventura M, Myers W. Smoke inhalation and airway management at a regional burn unit: 1974–1983: part I. Diagnosis and consequences of smoke inhalation. J Burn Care Rehabil 1989; 10:52–62.

16. Wolf SE, Herndon DN. Burns. In: Townsend CM, ed. Sabiston Textbook of Surgery. Philadelphia: Saunders, 2001:345–63.

17. Cook D, Guyatt G, Marshall J, et al. A comparison of sucralfate and ranitidine for the prevention of upper gastrointestinal bleeding in patients requiring mechanical ventilation. Canadian Critical Care Trials Group. N Engl J Med 1998; 338(12):791–797.

18. Ron D, Taitelman U, Michaelson M, Bar-Joseph G, Bursztin S, Better OS. Prevention of acute renal failure in traumatic rhabdomyolysis. Arch Intern Med 1984; 144:277–280.

19. Echinard CE, Sajdel-Sulkowska E, Burke PA, Burke JF. The beneficial effect of early excision on clinical response and thymic activity after burn injury. J Trauma 1982; 22:560–565.

20. Iwuagwu FC, Wilson D, Bailie F. The use of skin grafts in postburn contracture release: a 10-year review. Plast Reconstr Surg 1999; 103:1198–1204.

21. Engrav LH, Gottlieb JR, Walkinshaw MD, Heimbach DM, Grube B. The "sponge deformity" after tangential excision and grafting of burns. Plast Reconstr Surg 1989; 83:468–470.

22. Baur KM, Hardy PE, Van Dorsten B. Posttraumatic stress disorder in burn populations: a critical review of the literature. J Burn Care Rehabil 1998; 19(3):230–234.

23. Yu BH, Dimsdale JE. Posttraumatic stress disorder in patient with burn injuries. J Burn Care Rehabil 1999; 20(5):426–433.

24. Taal LA, Faber AW. Posttraumatic stress and maladjustment among adult burn survivors 1–2 years postburn. Burns 1998; 24:285–292.

25. Briggs SM. Electrical complications. In: Maull KI, ed. Complications in Trauma and Critical Care. Philadelphia: Saunders, 1996:521–528.

26. Skoog T. Electrical injuries. J Trauma 1970; 10:816–830.

27. Warden GD, Heimbach DM. Burns. In: Schwartz SI, ed. Principles of Surgery. New York: McGraw-Hill, 1998:223–262.

28. Baxter CR. Present concepts in the management of major electrical injury. Surg Clin North Am 1970; 50:1401–1418.

29. Hartford CE, Ziffren SE. Electrical injury. J Trauma 1971; 11:331–336.

30. Housinger TA, Green L, Shahangian S, Saffle JR, Warden GD. A prospective study of myocardial damage in electrical injuries. J Trauma 1985; 25: 122–124.

31. Robson MC, Smith DJ. Care of the thermally injured victim. In: Jurkwicz MJ, Krize TJ, Mathes SJ, Ariyan S, eds. Plastic Surgery: Principles and Practice. St. Louis: CV Mosby Company, 1990:1355–1410.

32. Frank DH, Fisher JC. Complications of electrical injury. In: Greenfield LJ, ed. Complication in Surgery and Trauma. Philadelphia: Lippincott, 1990:26–36.

33. Smith J, Rank BK. A case of severe electrical burns with an unusual sequence of complications. Br J Surg 1946; 33:365–368.

34. Christensen JA, Sherman RT, Balis GA, Waumett JD. Delayed neurologic injury secondary to high-voltage current, with recovery. J Trauma 1980; 20:166–168.

35. Farrell DF, Starr A. Delayed neurological sequelae of electrical injuries. Neurology 1968; 18:601–606.

36. Monafo WW, Freedman BM. Electrical and lightning injury. In: Boswick JA, ed. The Art and Science of Burn Care. Rockville: Aspen Publishers Inc., 1987: 241–254.

44

Complications of Skin Grafting

Raquel Garcia-Roca and David S. Lasko
University of Miami School of Medicine/Jackson Memorial Hospital, Miami, Florida, U.S.A.

Nicholas Namias
Miller School of Medicine at the University of Miami, Miami, Florida, U.S.A.

The skin is the body's largest organ and consists of two layers with different embryologic origins. The epidermis is derived from ectoderm; it consists of layers of epithelial cells that mature from the basal layer to the surface and finally desquamate, a process taking two to four weeks. The dermis originates from the mesoderm and is on an average 10 times thicker than the epidermis. The dermis consists primarily of fibroblasts that produce the extracellular matrix, especially collagen and elastin; cells of this type confer elasticity to the skin.

Because the skin has multiple functions and plays an important role in homeostasis, the loss of a substantial amount of skin (most commonly as the result of severe burns or immune disorders such as Stevens–Johnson Syndrome) often results in significant derangements in homeostasis, thermoregulation, immune function, and metabolism. Advances in critical care and in surgical treatment of large skin wounds have greatly improved outcomes for patients with extensive skin injury or loss. The primary surgical advance in treating large skin wounds (mainly burns) has been the development and improvement of skin and skin-substitute grafting techniques. Despite these advances, however, treating patients with large skin wounds is challenging and fraught with potential complications.

TYPES OF SKIN GRAFTS

Skin grafts can be either partial (split-thickness) grafts or full-thickness grafts. Split-thickness skin grafts contain epidermis and variable amounts of dermis, whereas full-thickness skin grafts include epidermis and the entire dermal layer. Split-thickness grafts contain less tissue than full-thickness grafts and therefore require less revascularization after transfer, a factor that increases their chances for successful engraftment. Compared to split-thickness grafts, full-thickness grafts are more resistant to trauma, result in substantially less wound contraction, and often provide better cosmetic results.

Grafts are also categorized on the basis of the source of the donor skin. Autografts take skin from a donor site on the patient's own body, whereas allografts take skin from another human donor and xenografts take skin from a nonhuman donor. One newer source of skin-graft tissue is the cultured autograft, which consists of epithelium grown in vitro and processed into a graftable form. This technique is used to increase the amount of available donor tissue when the patient has extensive skin loss and potential donor areas are limited.

Cultured epidermal skin-autograft techniques were introduced by Rheinwald and Green in 1975 (1,2). A full-thickness skin biopsy of the patient is processed, and epithelial cells are separated and plated in a culture medium that allows the epithelium to expand into sheets. The cells can be transferred to other culture plates and expanded, thereby creating large surfaces of autogenic epithelial sheets for permanent wound coverage. Experience has proved that when full-thickness excised wounds are closed with epithelial cells alone, graft survival rates and long-term durability are less than optimal. However, in the face of large wounds with minimal availability of donor skin, epithelial cell wound closure is a valuable adjunct to the overall treatment of the patient.

GRAFT-WOUND HEALING

Skin grafts heal in three phases. Initially, the graft survives by diffusion of nutrients from the wound bed, a process known as imbibition. Any barrier that forms between the wound bed and the graft (including hematomas, seromas, or necrotic tissue resulting from incomplete debridement) prevents the graft from obtaining the required nutrients and decreases the likelihood of graft survival. The second stage of healing occurs two to three days after grafting. New blood vessels form in the wound bed and grow to join the native graft vessels by a process called inosculation. Any shearing forces at this time will lead to hematoma formation, interrupt neovascularization, and cause graft loss. The final stage of graft healing is maturation, in which new collagen bridges form between the bed and the graft. This process takes months; the graft initially thickens and becomes more vascular and erythematous over the first three to four months and subsequently thins and fades in color. The maturation process is similar to that associated with healing of other wounds and requires a total of one to two years for completion (3).

TECHNIQUES OF SKIN GRAFTING

Donor skin can be harvested by using a freehand technique, in which the skin thickness is unpredictable, or by using a dermatome, which can precisely measure the depth of the graft. Various techniques have been described for freehand harvesting; the advantages of the procedure are that it can be performed with the use of local anesthesia and does not require any special equipment. Freehand harvesting is infrequently used in most centers, however because the inconsistency in graft thickness results in inferior cosmetic outcome of the donor site and reduces the likelihood of graft survival (4). The freehand technique requires a certain level of expertise because the depth of the graft varies depending on the actions of the operator. The use of a freehand knife (e.g., Goulian, Humby, or Watson) on tensely edematous tissue, if the blade is held at an excessively acute angle, can cause a skin laceration, and underlying structures (e.g., tendons) can be rapidly forced into the field and lacerated. The freehand knife should be used only by trained, experienced surgeons.

Harvesting a skin graft with a dermatome is a fast and easy method of obtaining a graft with a uniform, precise thickness. However, the procedure is also associated with certain complications. Care must be taken to ensure that the equipment is properly fixed. It is the surgeon's responsibility to verify that the blade and the guards if any are installed appropriately, that the depth is set appropriately, and that the air pressure or electric motor used to drive the dermatome is driving the blade at an appropriate speed. Once harvested, the skin may be meshed by passing it through a device that creates slits; these slits allow the graft to expand to cover large recipient areas. Meshing a graft is especially helpful when the number of accessible donor sites is reduced because of the degree of the injury. The graft can be expanded from 1.5 to 9 times its original size. The final cosmetic outcome of meshed grafts is less than optimal, but the perforations can be narrowed to slits and cosmetic imperfections can be minimized by using a low-ratio mesh. Meshed grafts also allow free drainage of any fluid that accumulates between the graft and the recipient bed. Draining this fluid prevents seromas or hematomas, which can separate the graft from the recipient area; such separations are a common cause of graft loss. Technical problems associated with meshing should be avoided. When crushing meshers (i.e., those whose ratio is set by use of a plastic card) are used, the grooved side must face the cutting wheels or the skin will be cut into strips rather than meshed. When noncrushing meshers (generally fixed-ratio devices used without plastic cards) are used, care must be taken to ensure that all components are appropriately assembled. A loose or bent comb, which removes the graft from the cutting wheel, can cause the graft to circulate repetitively around the cutting wheel, thereby destroying the graft.

Thought must be given to choosing and caring for autograft donor sites because graft harvest generates an iatrogenic wound with the potential for complications. Obtaining an even split-thickness graft requires the use of a flat, supported surface such as the thighs, buttocks, abdomen, arm, or inner forearm. Unstable surfaces yield poor grafts. The dermatome can skip areas if contact is lost between the skin and the instrument because of laxity of the skin or lack of firm resistance from the underlying anatomy. Having assistants apply traction to the skin in front of and behind the dermatome is helpful; skin harvesting is difficult when the skin oscillates with the blade. Lack of firm resistance from the underlying anatomy of the abdomen can be overcome by pulling up on the abdominal wall with penetrating towel clamps. Skin can be harvested more easily from irregular surfaces, such as areas over bony prominences or concave areas, with the help of tumescent technique. The authors prefer to inject normal saline subdermally to even the surface. We do not inject epinephrine solutions for tumescence. Others (5) have described the safe use of solutions containing diluted epinephrine to minimize bleeding, but we have found that bleeding from the donor site usually stops spontaneously before any meaningful blood loss occurs. Serious hemodynamic consequences can occur if large volumes of epinephrine are inadvertently injected.

Once appropriate donor sites have been chosen, perioperative preparation and postoperative care are very important for maximizing graft survival. The recipient wound surface should be freshly debrided of necrotic tissue and should be free of infection, good hemostasis should be obtained before the graft is applied so as to avoid hematoma collection between the graft and the wound bed, and the grafted area should be immobilized for about five days postoperatively to avoid shearing forces. If the recipient wound has granulation tissue, the graft should be thin (0.15–0.2 mm) to allow better chances of survival.

COMPLICATIONS OF SKIN GRAFTING

Both early and late complications occur after skin grafting. Early complications relate primarily to graft failure resulting from hematoma or seroma formation, infection, or shearing forces. Late complications can be cosmetic or functional. Long-term cosmetic morbidity results from mismatches of the color and texture of the graft with those of the surrounding skin, hypopigmentation and hyperpigmentation, and prolonged erythema. Hypertrophic scarring may also occur at both the graft site and the donor site, in addition to fragility and breakdown in areas of constant trauma. Functional complications are the main long-term concerns with split-thickness grafts because they tend to contract more than full-thickness grafts. The amount of contraction increases inversely with the thickness of the graft and can lead to significant cosmetic and functional deformities.

Graft Failure

Skin graft failure is a serious complication that increases the patient's morbidity and hospital stay and requires further surgical intervention for regrafting. Early failure, seen during the first week after grafting, results from the absence of revascularization between the wound bed and the graft. Proper surgical technique is essential to minimizing graft failure. All necrotic tissue must be debrided to the level of viable, bleeding tissue. Granulation tissue should also be excised to the level of the fibrous bed beneath the friable erythematous tissue.

Any increase in the interface between the graft and the wound bed increases the distance that blood and vital nutrients must travel to reach the graft and decreases the likelihood of graft survival. Therefore, a fluid collection under the graft (hematoma or seroma) can be a potential cause of graft loss. When full-thickness skin grafts are used, the distance from the wound bed to the graft's dermis and epidermis is greater; these grafts are usually applied as unmeshed sheet grafts. Therefore, when applying full-thickness grafts, surgeons must be particularly careful to achieve meticulous hemostasis and to avoid seroma formation.

Hematoma formation can be avoided by using appropriate hemostatic techniques during debridement and excision. Applying sponges soaked in diluted epinephrine to the wound bed causes vasoconstriction of the small arterioles and capillary beds, which have been exposed during the debridement or tangential excision of the wound. One disadvantage of this wide application of vasopressors is that it may produce relative ischemia of the wound, and this condition may compromise the surgeon's ability to judge the adequacy of excision after the sponges have been removed. Limb tourniquets have also been used to minimize blood loss, but tourniquets also impair the surgeon's ability to judge the adequacy of excision of a wound bed and can lead to ischemic complications if they are applied for too long. The dermis of the graft is a good hemostatic agent once applied and accumulated blood can be evacuated

once the graft has been applied and secured in place. Pressure dressings also aid in hemostasis beneath the graft.

Accumulations of fluid other than blood can also prevent the graft from adhering to the wound. Seromas are infrequent when split-thickness grafts are expanded by meshing techniques because fluid can drain through the interstices of the meshed graft. It is important to examine the dressing during the first 48 postoperative hours so that the quantity of fluid drainage can be determined; excessive fluid accumulation should be avoided, and the dressing may need to be left open.

In addition to an increased interface between the graft and the wound bed, shearing forces during the postoperative period can lead to graft failure. Initially, the graft is attached to the wound by newly forming vessels, which constitute very frail, easily disrupted attachments. Therefore, grafts should remain immobilized for the first five postoperative days. When grafts are applied over joints, the extremity should be immobilized and splinted to avoid the shearing forces that can compromise graft adhesion. Patients with truncal grafts are kept on bed rest and are instructed to minimize friction against the bed. It is important to reduce the manipulation of the dressings on the grafted area so as to avoid dislodging the underlying graft. Physical therapy involving the grafted area is avoided during this period of graft immobilization. Once the graft is adherent, the dressing can be removed, and the patient can resume normal activity and physical therapy.

An uncommon cause of early failure of split-thickness grafts is inverted placement of the graft. The dermal layer of the graft, which is shiny and smooth, should always be the side that is in contact with the recipient wound bed.

Graft loss can also result from late complications, particularly local skin infection (6,7). Grafting procedures should be delayed until infection of the recipient wound site has been controlled; such a control is defined as the resolution of symptoms such as local erythema, edema, skin warmth and tenderness, leukocytosis, and fever. Topical antimicrobial therapy or systemic treatment may be required to eradicate infection, and perioperative antibiotics have been shown to decrease donor-site and graft-site infections in patients with small or moderate burns (8). More recent studies have shown that perioperative antibiotic prophylaxis does not decrease the incidence of bacteremia in clean burn surgery and therefore is theoretically unnecessary (9–11). These studies do not directly address the incidence of wound infection; however, the issue of whether perioperative antibiotics should be used in such cases has not been fully resolved. The risk of infection seems to increase with the length of delay between injury and excision.

Some clinicians advocate performing a biopsy for culture of the wound before a graft is applied so as to obtain a quantitative assessment of infection.

If the results of such cultures show less than 10,000 colonies/cm^2 of tissue, successful grafting can be expected. Another approach to treating infected wounds that require grafting is to excise the wound to the deep dermal tissue or to the level of the fascia. This technique removes all infected tissue and allows for immediate grafting.

Melting Graft Syndrome

Epithelial loss from a previously adherent graft, a healed burn wound, or a donor site, without clinical signs of local or systemic infection, is known as melting graft syndrome. This condition must be distinguished from trauma or excoriation of the healed epithelium, in which the wound edges are sharp and well demarcated. This complication causes prolonged healing time, increases the time between harvesting procedures, and, most importantly, may advance to wound sepsis and death.

Historically, the cause of melting graft syndrome, without other clinical signs of infection, was believed to be growth of Streptococcus spp., especially the group A beta-hemolytic variety. Groups B, C, and G Streptococci have also been implicated in the destruction of epithelializing skin grafts. Matsumura et al. (12) reported a series of cases in which Staphylococcus aureus, including the methicillin-resistant type, was the suspected microbial pathogen. The pathophysiology of the melting graft syndrome remains unclear, as does its prevention. Treatment is eradication of wound infection and regrafting.

Sponge Deformity

Improvement in the systemic treatment of severely burned patients has resulted in their prolonged survival, thus creating a new group of patients who require sequential burn excision and grafting. The sequential procedures have led to a new complication, termed sponge deformity, which was described by Engrav et al. in 1989 (13). The deformity occurs around the periphery of tangentially excised areas. The periphery of the excised bed is shallow and heals without sloughing of the overlying graft, thereby creating a bridge of scar tissue. Other areas of the bed heal, but the overlying graft sloughs. One hypothesis for the cause of this process is that the debrided bed has enough epithelial remnants to allow it to heal before the union between graft and bed heals. The part of the overlying graft that has adequate vascular support (particular at the periphery) does not slough and a bridge is formed. In more central areas with an insufficient vascular supply, the graft sloughs and a pockmark is created.

This process results in a very irregular healed surface, which is often very difficult to wash. These wounds also tend to catch on clothing, bleed as the result of frequent trauma, and have a poor aesthetic outcome. Sponge deformity occurs in meshed and unmeshed grafts with thicknesses ranging from 0.010 to 0.015 in. The grafts appear to adhere well initially, but after approximately two weeks small foci of inflammation develop on their periphery. Local wound care is often used to control the inflammation, but bridges and pockmarks characteristic of sponge deformity may still appear after several weeks.

Treatment of sponge deformity consists of simple excision of the edges and bridges of the graft by using curved iris scissors with the patient under local or general anesthesia. The results obtained by dermabrasion or by excision with the Goulian knife are suboptimal, and this procedure tends to damage the surrounding graft or skin.

Hypertrophic Scarring

Hypertrophic scarring is a common problem after burn injury and usually occurs six to eight weeks after wound epithelialization. This complication is primarily limited to deep dermal wounds that are allowed to close spontaneously, the interstices of widely expanded meshed grafts, and the perimeter of sheet grafts. Hypertrophic scar rarely forms beneath narrowly meshed split-thickness skin grafts applied in sheets.

The scar's red to purple color reflects enhanced microvascular regeneration and the thick-walled capillaries that produce a hypoxic environment. The scar becomes elevated, firm, warm, hypersensitive, and pruritic, but (in contrast to keloids) the lesion remains within the confines of the original scar. A period of 6 to 18 months is required for scar maturation, at which time the erythema subsides and the scar contraction diminishes.

Hypertrophic scarring is an excessive reparative response whose mechanism is as yet not understood, although several theories about its development exist. One such theory is based on the presence of excessive collagen within the scars; this theory suggests that the hypertrophic scarring results from an imbalance between collagen synthesis and degradation (14,15). Histologically, hypertrophic scars contain less highly cross-linked collagen and more soluble collagen than normal scar tissues. In contrast to the collagen fibers in normal healing wounds, which have a parallel orientation, the collagen fibers in hypertrophic scars form a characteristic curvilinear whorl-like pattern. These patterns may progress to a nodular form separated from the subcutaneous tissue by parallel bands of connective tissue.

Pressure garments can provide precise amounts of pressure and can be custom-fit to the individual patient or wound. Interim garments provide circumferential pressure to the wound and are made of soft materials so as to protect the new epithelium. Once the wound edema has resolved and the wound can withstand shearing forces without breaking down, custom-fitted pressure garments can be worn at all times. Silicone inserts can act as adjuncts to the pressure garments to provide effective pressure in contoured areas including the face, neck, axilla, sternum, palms, web spaces, and feet. The inserts require a catalyst and can be molded to contour the affected area, beginning with thin, pliable materials and progressing to more rigid inserts. The inserts are worn for only a few hours each day with progression, as tolerated, to 24-hour applications. The silicone inserts work to depress the height of the hypertrophic scar, to prevent shrinking of skin grafts, and to increase the elasticity of the scar. Patients who wear these inserts seem to have less pain. The inserts should be removed frequently to avoid skin maceration, and their use should be discontinued in cases of skin breakdown, contact dermatitis, or rash (16).

Although the ideal amount of pressure for this therapy has not been identified, as little as 10 mmHg may be effective; pressures greater than 40 mmHg may cause paresthesias and tissue destruction. The custom-made pressure garments apply approximately 24 to 28 mmHg of pressure, thus equaling the capillary pressure.

Once the scar is mature enough to tolerate shearing forces, massage therapy of the scars can aid in softening and remodeling. This technique can make the scars more pliable and elastic and can improve the motility of involved joints. Massage is believed to break fibrous bands and to improve the mobility of the skin over underlying tissues. Therapy initially consists of stationary pressure to mobilize the skin without friction. As the scar matures, friction can be applied in multiple directions with enough pressure to blanch the skin. Patients generally report relief from the itching associated with healing when massage is employed.

Graft Contraction

Contraction is part of the normal wound-healing process, but healing burns often leave residual pathologic contractures that produce disfigurement and functional deficits. Wounds continue to contract until the affected area achieves a comfortable position or until an opposing force balances the tendency toward contracture. The basis of physical therapy and rehabilitation techniques is to provide opposing forces to the contracting wound.

The first priority in dealing with wound contraction should be preventing deformities. This goal is achieved by active mobilization, pressure garments, and splinting. When pathologic contraction occurs, the main focus should turn to restoration of active function, followed by therapy directed at restoring passive function. Surgical treatment of pathologic contractures should generally be delayed until the wound has matured, usually after 18 to 24 months. When the contraction is causing a functional deficit, however, surgical correction of the deformity should be performed immediately. Once functionality has been maximized by conservative measures or surgical corrections, cosmetic procedures can be performed (17,18).

Burn contractures are best reconstructed with excision and primary approximation or Z-plasty. Split-thickness grafts are commonly used when these primary options are not feasible. Rotational flaps are also widely used in reconstructive surgery, and they are preferable to free grafts when the area to be covered lacks adequate vascular supply. Examples of such areas include bony surfaces, tendons, cartilage, and irradiated tissue. With the development of microsurgical techniques allowing vascular anastomosis of vessels less than 1 mm in diameter, the use of free grafts (full thickness) has also gained popularity. Free-tissue transfer techniques are rarely used in acute burn–wound management.

Pruritus

Many patients with large, healing skin wounds develop significant pruritus during the weeks and months after the injury. This morbidity is most common among children and affects the lower extremities more than the upper extremities. It rarely affects facial wounds. Pruritic intensity is greater immediately after healing and can be triggered and enhanced by heat, physical activity, and stress. The intensity of pruritus generally diminishes gradually, and the condition rarely persists for more than 18 months. Prolonged pruritus beyond this time frame usually involves a psychogenic component.

The precise mechanism of pruritus is not fully understood, but the condition is related to the release of histamine, bradykinin, and other endopeptides from the wound. Pruritus is treated with a combination of antihistamine medications, skin lotions, and analgesics to decrease the central nervous system's perception of itching. The drug most commonly prescribed for this condition is diphenhydramine hydrochloride, which has a mild sedative effect that helps reduce the patient's pruritus-related anxiety. However, newer agents have yielded improved responses. The combination of the H1 blocker cetirizine (Zyrtec) and the H2 blocker cimetidine (Zantac), administered orally, has demonstrated dramatic improvement in itching for six hours and moderate improvement for 12 hours (19). Reports have also demonstrated the antipruritic effects of topical doxepin (a tricyclic antidepressant when given orally) and hydrocortisone (20–22). Although most of the patients in these studies had atopic dermatitis, anecdotal reports indicate that these agents are also effective for patients with healing skin wounds.

Although empirical evidence of their effectiveness is lacking, other treatments for pruritus are commonly used on the basis of anecdotal accounts of their success. Cool compresses may interrupt the itching cycle; additionally, patients seem to find air-conditioned spaces more comfortable than warmer spaces. Topical agents, including aloe vera, which has anti-inflammatory and antimicrobial properties, skin moisturizers, cocoa butter, and mineral oil, have also been effective.

DONOR-SITE COMPLICATIONS

Donor sites are surgically created, superficial, partial-thickness wounds, and as such may suffer complications similar to those associated with large skin injuries. These wounds usually heal relatively quickly; healing originates from remaining epithelial cells, along with adnexal hair follicles, dermal sweat glands, and sebaceous glands. Consequently, the thicker the residual dermis at the donor site, the faster the healing and the better the quality of the regenerated epithelium. Thick split-thickness skin grafts and full-thickness grafts result in deeper donor-site wounds. These wounds derive granulation tissue from the wound edges only; therefore, they require more time to healing and they heal more inconsistently. These deep wounds are subject to the same distortion to which other relatively deep skin wounds are subject to because of contraction and hypertrophic scar formation. The healing interval for donor areas of thin and medium-thickness skin grafts is 10 to 20 days, whereas that for deeper donor-site wounds is 20 to 90 days. Full-thickness grafts should be closed primarily.

Aside from the healing complications, donor sites are also subject to infections. Donor-site infection prolongs the hospital stay and increases the interval between harvesting opportunities for patients with limited potential donor areas. The diagnosis of infection is clinical and is based on the classic signs of tenderness, erythema, warmth, and swelling. Preoperative antibiotics decrease the risk of donor-site infection in patients with small- or medium-sized burns but not in patients whose burns cover a large surface area. Donor-site infections are treated with topical antimicrobial agents or with systemic therapy if the patient has systemic symptoms such as fever or leukocytosis.

SPECIAL ISSUES WITH SCALP DONOR SITES

The scalp has many advantages as a donor site. It has a rich vascular supply, which reduces healing time until the scalp tissue is available for reharvesting. Scalp donor sites are usually less painful than other sites, and the scar is often hidden by hair growth. The scalp is frequently used in facial plastic and reconstructive procedures because of its excellent color match. The potential disadvantages of scalp skin as donor tissue include staphylococcal folliculitis, the possibility of hair transfer to recipient areas, and excessive bleeding (sometimes requiring transfusion) because of the extensive blood supply. Hemorrhage is a particular concern with scalp donor sites in children.

Concrete Scalp Deformity

One complication unique to scalp donor sites is a thickened, hardened healed wound known as concrete scalp deformity. The underlying pathophysiology is not clear, but it seems that epithelialization does not occur promptly; instead, granulation tissue containing hairs forms at the donor site. This mass desiccates into a thick scab with the hairs embedded in it. As described by Carter et al. (23) in their series of 16 patients, the development of concrete scalp deformity is related only to the depth of the harvested skin and the type of wound care given during the postoperative period. Its development is not associated with the total body surface area of the burn, or the age or sex of the patient. Infection also seems to play no role in causing concrete scalp deformity. This complication is generally limited to hair-bearing donor sites (24).

Treatment of concrete scalp deformity consists of shaving the hair and removing the granulation tissue, after which epithelialization is allowed to occur. Occlusive dressings are used to promote more rapid epithelialization.

Scalp Donor-Site Alopecia

Permanent donor-site alopecia occurs in approximately 32% of patients with scalp donor sites, although the incidence approaches 60% in those with concomitant scalp burns (25). Larger burn surface area also increases the risk of scalp donor-site alopecia, even in patients with no burned scalp. Other risk factors include repeated harvests and, especially, shorter time intervals between harvests.

de Viragh and Meuli (26) suggested that alopecia after scalp harvesting may be caused by harvesting the graft below the hair follicle bulge. They developed a formula for estimating the depth of the bulge. However, the variability of the donor skin that is harvested limits the clinical utility of this formula.

Despite the fact that this seemingly simple operation of the skin is frequently relegated to junior house staff, it is one that can be fraught with complications and morbidity. Great care should be taken to avoid the many known complications.

REFERENCES

1. Rheinwald JG, Green H. Serial cultivation of strains of human epidermal keratinocytes: the formation of keratinizing colonies from single cells. Cell 1975; 6(3): 331–343.
2. Rheinwald JG, Green H. Formation of a keratinizing epithelium in culture by a cloned cell line derived from a teratoma. Cell 1975; 6(3):317–330.
3. Monafo WW, Bessey PQ. Wound care. In: Herndon D, ed. Total Burn Care. Philadelphia: W.B. Saunders, 2002:109–119.
4. Valencia IC, Falabella AF, Eaglstein WH. Skin grafting. Dermatol Clin 2000; 18(3):521–532.
5. Gomez M, Logsetty S, Fish JS. Reduced blood loss during burn surgery. J Burn Care Rehabil 2001; 22(2): 111–117.

6. Griswold JA, Grube BJ, Engrav LH, Marvin JA, Heimbach DM. Determinants of donor site infections in small burn grafts. J Burn Care Rehabil 1989; 10(6):531–535.

7. Smith DJ Jr., Thompson PD, Bolton LL, Hutchinson JJ. Microbiology and healing of the occluded skin-graft donor site. Plast Reconstr Surg 1993; 91(6):1094–1097.

8. Alexander JW, MacMillan BG, Law EJ, Krummel R. Prophylactic antibiotics as an adjunct for skin grafting in clean reconstructive surgery following burn injury. J Trauma 1982; 22(8):687–690.

9. Mozingo DW, McManus AT, Kim SH, Pruitt BA Jr. Incidence of bacteremia after burn wound manipulation in the early postburn period. J Trauma 1997; 42(6):1006–1011.

10. Steer JA, Papini RP, Wilson AP, McGrouther DA, Nakhla LS, Parkhouse N. Randomized placebo-controlled trial of teicoplanin in the antibiotic prophylaxis of infection following manipulation of burn wounds. Br J Surg 1997; 84(6):848–853.

11. Fasano D, Palu P, Papadia F. Use of aztreonam in the perioperative prevention in burned patients. Acta Biomed Ateneo Parmense 1990; 61(1–2):99–104.

12. Matsumura H, Meyer NA, Mann R, Heimbach DM. Melting graft-wound syndrome. J Burn Care Rehabil 1998; 19(4):292–295.

13. Engrav LH, Gottleib JR, Walkinshaw MD, Heimbach DM, Grube B. The "sponge deformity" after tangential excision and grafting of burns. Plast Reconstr Surg 1989; 83(3):468–470.

14. Reno F, Grazianetti P, Cannas M. Effects of mechanical compression on hypertrophic scars: prostaglandin E2 release. Burns 2001; 27(3):215–218.

15. Davey RB, Sprod RT, Neild TO. Computerised colour: a technique for the assessment of burn scar hypertrophy. A preliminary report. Burns 1999; 25(3):207–213.

16. Van den Kerckhove E, Stappearts K, Boeckx W, et al. Silicones in the rehabilitation of burns: a review and overview. Burns 2001; 27(3):205–214.

17. Serghiou MA, Evans EB, Ott S. Comprehensive rehabilitation in the burned patient. In: Herndon DN, ed. Total Burn Care. Philadelphia: W.B. Saunders, 2002:563–592.

18. Sheridan RL, Tompkins RG. Skin substitutes in burns. Burns 1999; 25(2):97–103.

19. Baker RA, Zeller RA, Klein RL, et al. Burn wound itch control using H1 and H2 antagonists. J Burn Care Rehabil 2001; 22(4):263–268.

20. Greiding L, Moreno P. Doxepin incorporated into a dermatologic cream: an assessment of both doxepin antipruritic action and doxepin action as an inhibitor of papules, in allergen and histamine-caused pruritus. Allergol Immunopathol (Madr) 1999; 27(5):265–270.

21. Millikan LE. Treating pruritus. What's new in safe relief of symptoms? Postgrad Med 1996; 99(1):173–176, 179–184.

22. Zhai H, Frisch S, Pelosi A, Neibart S, Maibach HL. Antipruritic and thermal sensation effects of hydrocortisone creams in human skin. Skin Pharmacol Appl Skin Physiol 2000; 13(6):352–357.

23. Carter YM, Summer GJ, Engrav LH, Hansen FL, Costa BA, Matsumura H. Incidence of the concrete scalp deformity associated with deep scalp donor sites and management with the Unna cap. J Burn Care Rehabil 1999; 20(2):141–144.

24. Engrav LH, Grube BJ, Bubak PJ. Treatment of the concrete scalp donor site. Ann Plast Surg 1990; 24(2):162–164.

25. Brou J, Vu T, McCauley RL, et al. The scalp as a donor site: revisited. J Trauma 1990; 30(5):579–581.

26. de Viragh PA, Meuli M. Human scalp hair follicle development from birth to adulthood: statistical study with special regard to putative stem cells in the bulge and proliferating cells in the matrix. Arch Dermatol Res 1995; 287(3–4):279–284.

45

Complications of Reconstructive Surgery

D. Narayan, J. H. Shin, and J. A. Persing
Section of Plastic Surgery, Yale University School of Medicine, New Haven, Connecticut, U.S.A.

The term "reconstruction" implies a restoration of form and function. Because many postsurgical and traumatic conditions result in loss of tissue, restoration of form and function frequently requires replacement of the lost tissue. Two general categories of tissue are used in reconstruction: flaps and grafts. Grafts may be composed of any kind of tissue (skin, cartilage, fat, etc.), but all are devoid of an active, functioning blood supply. Flaps, in contrast, carry their own blood supply and therefore have the advantage of bringing tissue and blood supply to an area that is deficient in both.

Depending on the anatomical components they contain, flaps may be cutaneous, fasciocutaneous, muscular, or osteomyocutaneous. Cutaneous or fasciocutaneous flaps may be oriented to incorporate a blood vessel running along their length (the so-called axial-pattern flap) or may depend entirely on the richly anastomosing network of dermal circulation (the random-pattern flap). The absence of a defined blood vessel renders random-pattern flaps more prone to complications than axial-pattern flaps. To paraphrase Sir Harold Gilles, we might state that surgical procedures involving flaps face a constant struggle between blood supply and coverage; the loss of blood supply is responsible for many of the complications that ensue after such procedures.

Flaps may also be described as pedicled flaps, which retain their original blood supply, or free flaps, which are completely detached from their native source of circulation and are later anastomosed to a feeding vessel by means of microsurgical techniques. Of these two types of flaps, pedicled flaps in general are easier to create, allow shorter operative procedures, and, unlike free flaps, are not subject to a myriad of complications related to surgical technique. Free flaps, however, have greatly increased the number of reconstructive techniques available to plastic surgeons. When coupled with advances in technology and patient care, free-flap reconstructions are now considered the standard of care in many situations; therefore, we will discuss these flaps in more detail than the pedicled flaps.

Flaps may be seen as a panacea for infected wounds, which they are not. Debridement, removal of foreign bodies (when appropriate), and provision of an adequate blood supply are crucial for the success of procedures involving

flaps. Antibiotic therapy is a vital adjunct. Persistent infections despite flap coverage, therefore, should not be construed as a failure of the flap but may instead be associated with a failure to adhere to the crucial principles enumerated above.

The reconstructive surgeon's goal of completely restoring preinjury form and function, although laudable, is rarely, if ever, achieved in practice. Realistic expectations on the part of the patient, the referring colleague, and the surgical team are necessary.

CUTANEOUS FLAPS

Many types of cutaneous flaps exist, including advancement, rotation, and rhomboid. The principal advantage of these local flaps is the ability to cover "like with like," i.e., the ability to match the color, thickness, and texture of the remaining tissue by reconstructing the defect with neighboring skin. Cutaneous flaps may be subject to a variety of mishaps: poor design, inability to cover the defect, tension on the flap with subsequent ischemic necrosis, etc. (Figs. 1–4). These complications can be amplified by the use of flaps in cosmetically sensitive areas. The "pin cushion" or trap-door deformity results when flap tissue bunches up because of a circular scar line at its base; this deformity can be obviated by the use of angular flaps such as the rhomboid flap. Random-skin flaps are much more prone to complications when the patient is a smoker, presumably because of the ischemic complications induced by nicotine and carbon monoxide (1).

MATHES–NAHAI CLASSIFICATION

Because many of the complications of flap surgery are related to vascularity, any paradigm that correlates anatomy with surgical application is useful. The Mathes–Nahai classification is one such paradigm in general use; it describes the vascular anatomy of muscles in a manner that can be correlated with their potential clinical use. This classification scheme defines five primary types of flaps (Table 1).

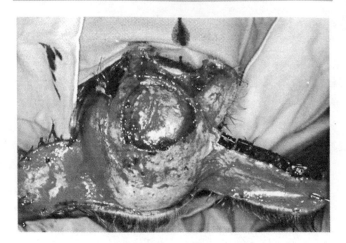

Figure 1 A 75-year-old woman was injured in a fall; the injury resulted in exposed hardware (placed for calvarial replacement after resection of a meningioma) on the vertex of the skull. Shown here is the defect (*center of the picture*) with scalp flaps raised circumferentially. *Source*: Courtesy of JG Thomson, Yale University.

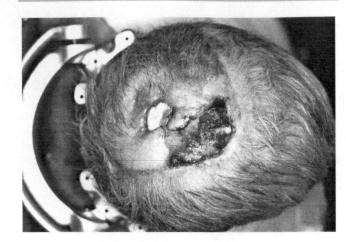

Figure 3 Ischemic necrosis of flaps with re-exposure of hardware. *Source*: Courtesy of JG Thomson, Yale University.

This classification scheme has practical applications. For example, a Type-4 muscle such as the sartorius has a limited arc of rotation (and, hence, limited transferability) because its blood supply is segmental. The blood vessel orientation of the medial head of the gastrocnemius (Type 1), in contrast, is much more axial and therefore allows a wider arc, as long as the main pedicle is not compromised. Two dominant blood vessels in the rectus abdominis muscle (the superior and inferior epigastric arteries), each of which can nourish the entire muscle and its overlying fasciocutaneous unit, allow either vessel to be divided for pedicled transfer. Dividing the inferior epigastric

artery allows the transverse rectus abdominis muscle (TRAM) flap to be inset into the chest wall with connection to the superior epigastric artery alone (see below).

PEDICLED FLAPS
Gracilis

The pedicled gracilis muscle, along with its overlying skin paddle, is often used for vaginal reconstructions. The muscle alone has been used to reconstruct the rectal sphincter. Abdominal, perineal, or groin wounds may also be covered with flaps composed of this muscle.

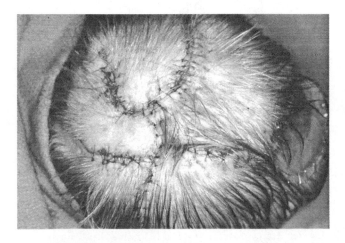

Figure 2 Immediate postoperative result with coverage of hardware. *Source*: Courtesy of JG Thomson, Yale University.

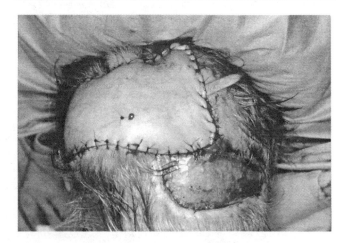

Figure 4 The wound was debrided, and a lateral arm flap was harvested (because the results of Allen's tests on both arms precluded the use of a radial forearm flap) to provide coverage. Here we see the lateral arm flap covering the defect. *Source*: Courtesy of JG Thomson, Yale University.

Table 1   Types and Examples of Muscle Flaps According to the Mathes–Nahai Classification Scheme

Type	Description	Example
1	Muscle with single dominant pedicle	Tensor fascia lata, gastrocnemius (each head)
2	Muscle with single dominant and minor pedicle(s)	Gracilis
3	Muscle with two dominant pedicles	Rectus abdominis
4	Muscle with segmental blood supply	Sartorius
5	Muscle with one main and multiple segmental branches	Latissimus dorsi

Table 2   Sources of Complications Affecting Free-Flap Reconstruction

1. Technical factors
   a. Surgical skill
   b. Position of the anastomosis
   c. Tension of the pedicle
   d. Redundant pedicle
2. Poor inflow (below stenotic lesions, use of vasoconstrictors)
3. Poor outflow (venous engorgement)
4. Inadequate immobilization
5. Poor pain control
6. Hypothermia
7. Constrictive dressings

Source: From Ref. 2

Lying between the adductor longus anteriorly and the semimembranosus posteriorly is the thin, flat gracilis, which is supplied predominantly by the ascending branch of the medial circumflex femoral artery, a branch of the profunda femoris. The distal end of the skin paddle, however, is not as a general rule reliable, and delay procedures have been used in an effort to avert avascular necrosis. The sartorius muscle (also thin and flat) is sometimes mistaken for the gracilis, especially in limbs with long-standing paralysis. Shearing off the skin paddle from the underlying muscle during overly aggressive attempts to tunnel the flap can also contribute to the loss of the accompanying skin paddle. Tunneling the muscle under unyielding skin or placing undue tension on the pedicle may also cause vascular compromise.

Gastrocnemius

The gastrocnemius is conveniently divided into two heads, each with its own blood supply. This muscle is particularly robust and is useful for covering defects around the knee joint and the upper-third of the leg. Unsightly contour donor defects can result if the muscle is used with a skin paddle. Therefore, the muscle is usually transferred without the overlying skin and is then covered by a split-thickness skin graft. Damage to the tibial and peroneal nerves can result during dissection of the popliteal fossa. Sural artery occlusion may compromise the vascularity of the flap; a preoperative angiogram can identify this arterial anatomy and may help prevent this mishap. Lower-extremity deep vein thrombosis is a relative contraindication to the use of this flap. So that plantar flexion can be preserved, the medial or lateral gastrocnemius muscle flap should not be used if the opposite head of the gastrocnemius and the soleus muscles are not functional.

FREE MICROVASCULAR FLAPS

Free flaps are more technically demanding than local or pedicled flaps. A free flap involves detaching a unit of tissue (which may contain skin, fascia, fat, muscle, bone, or various combinations of all of these tissues) with its blood supply, and anastomosing this unit to a new blood supply by using microvascular techniques. The main complications result from vascular compromise at either the arterial or the venous end (Table 2).

Technical factors are clearly the most important consideration, and many of these factors are interlinked. For instance, inadequate pain control may lead to excessive movement, which may lead to the mechanical shearing of the graft. Venous engorgement may produce thrombosis of the vessels in the graft, eventually causing ischemic damage. Constrictive dressings may compromise both venous outflow and arterial inflow, thus resulting in flap loss. Hypothermia may lead to vasospasm of the inflow vessel, as may the use of vasopressors.

A few commonly used free flaps and the complications associated with them are described below.

Radial Forearm Free Flap

The radial forearm free flap, usually constructed in its fasciocutaneous form, is applicable in diverse situations such as lower extremity coverage, resurfacing of the floor of the mouth, pharyngeal reconstruction, and penile reconstruction. A preoperative Allen's test to ascertain the patency of the radial and ulnar arteries is mandatory in all cases to prevent the devastating complications of an ischemic hand, brought about by removing the dominant (or only) vessel of the hand. The ulnar artery trap, which includes the anatomic anomaly of a superficial ulnar artery in addition to the radial artery, can lead to the same problem (3). Donor-site complications include exposed tendons and their subsequent rupture, cold intolerance, and damage to the radial sensory nerve, which causes painful paresthesias. Harvesting the radius muscle in the form of an osteomyocutaneous flap may result in fracture of the radius. This complication can be avoided by harvesting less than 40% of the cross-sectional area of the radius muscle.

The skin graft used to cover the donor site is usually of a poor color match and does not address the contour defect in the more heavy-set patient. The flap is usually taken from the nondominant hand so that functional deficits can be minimized.

Fibular Free Flap

Since its original description by Taylor et al. (4), the fibular free flap has been adapted by plastic surgeons to become the workhorse of mandibular reconstruction. The specific advantages of this flap for mandibular reconstruction include the long length of available bone, the flap's ability to undergo segmental osteotomies (hence improving its malleability), the ready incorporation of dental implants, and the easily tolerated donor-site defect. The flap has also been used in this form to replace long bone defects resulting from either trauma or tumor ablation.

Assessment of the vascularity of the leg preoperatively by either angiography or magnetic resonance angiography (MRA) will help avert the consequences of critical limb ischemia. Thorough knowledge of the regional anatomy is a prerequisite for harvesting this flap, which is among the most demanding of flap procedures. The vascularity of the skin paddle incorporated in an osteomyocutaneous fibular flap may be unreliable because it relies on few and diminutive septocutaneous perforators. Incorporating a cuff of muscle from the lateral and anterior compartment muscles helps preserve the periosteum and, consequently, the blood supply to the bone.

Damage to the peroneal artery during osteotomy can compromise the viability of the flap. During flap harvest, care must be taken to avoid the peroneal nerve where it curves around the neck of the fibula. Similarly, leaving approximately 8 cm of the bone at the lower end of the fibula helps maintain the stability of the ankle mortise.

Rectus Abdominis Free Flap

This long, strap-like muscle is particularly useful in providing coverage for large defects, and it can be harvested with its overlying skin paddle if necessary. The muscle is usually harvested with the deep inferior epigastric artery; this procedure provides the advantages of a long pedicle and a large-diameter vessel, thus considerably easing the task of anastomosis. A slipped tie from this pedicle, however, can result in substantial yet initially "silent" retroperitoneal blood loss. Prosthetic mesh may be used to prevent the complications of hernia resulting from the harvest of muscle.

A variant of the rectus abdominis flap is the free TRAM flap, which has been widely used for breast reconstruction. The complications associated with the pedicled TRAM flap, such as ventral hernia or interference with the ability to cough, can be minimized with the free-flap transfer of a more limited segmental harvest of the rectus muscle. The free TRAM flap generally has a better blood supply than the pedicled TRAM flap; this advantage results in a lower incidence of fat necrosis because it is not necessary to include the blood flow, thus limiting mesh of vessels connecting the deep superior and inferior epigastric arterial systems. The procedure, however, requires a steep learning curve, in part because of the difficulty in performing a microvascular anastomosis to the thoracodorsal vessels deep in the axilla. Total flap loss, although uncommon when the surgeon is experienced, is more likely than when the pedicled form of the flap is used.

Latissimus Dorsi Free Flap

The large mass (area) of the latissimus dorsi muscle makes this muscle ideal for covering very large defects. Like the rectus abdominis flap, the latissimus dorsi flap is hardy and can be easily harvested with a skin paddle. Skin necrosis is unusual. Seromas at the donor site are a common problem when latissimus dorsi flaps are used, but reports indicate that using sharp dissection instead of electrocautery can reduce the incidence of this complication by half. More muscle mass can be harvested by including the serratus anterior muscle in the dissection. This procedure, however, increases the likelihood of injury to the long thoracic nerve and a resultant "winged scapula."

Using this flap to treat patients who are wheelchair bound can lead to a loss of strength in stabilization and in extending the shoulder. This condition may negatively affect the patients' ability to transfer to and from the wheelchair, thus decreasing their quality of life.

Jejunal Free Flap

Currently, the jejunal free flap is most commonly used to reconstruct the upper digestive tract after ablative resection of cancerous growths. Jejunal flaps are much more susceptible to ischemia than the flaps described above and therefore demand greater technical proficiency of the surgeon performing the anastomosis. Complications associated with jejunal flaps include anastomotic strictures; problems at the donor site, such as abdominal wound infection, dehiscence, and bowel obstruction due to adhesions; and volvulus. Necrosis of the jejunal segment used for esophageal reconstruction could lead to fistulae, abscess, and mediastinitis.

COMPLICATIONS OF RECONSTRUCTIVE SURGERY: MAXILLOFACIAL SURGERY

Reconstructive surgery for patients who have suffered serious facial injuries has improved greatly over the past several decades. Early intervention and rehabilitation, as well as advancements in bony fixation, have reduced the long-term sequelae of such injuries. Despite these improvements, surgical procedures can still cause complications, which fall into two broad categories: soft-tissue complications and skeletal complications.

Traumatic soft-tissue injuries to the head and face may result in a wide variety of secondary complications. The extent of these complications depends on the exact nature of both the inciting traumatic event and the specific tissue injured. Lacerations and abrasions should be thoroughly cleansed and vigorously debrided of foreign bodies because of the risk of substantial scarring and tattooing. However, overzealous debridement or removal of tissue may result in significant loss of tissue that is not easily replaced, such as that of the eyelid. Every effort should be made to meticulously remove foreign bodies and devitalized tissue, but maximal preservation of vital structures is standard. Scarring is generally inevitable in most cases of significant lacerations, but early closure with fine suture materials and meticulous wound care can minimize the extent of scarring and the need for surgical revision.

Soft-tissue injuries may affect additional structures of the head and face, which are crucial to function. Because of its course and superficial location, the facial nerve is easily damaged by a number of mechanisms of trauma to the face. Early intervention and repair of such injuries are important to assure the long-term function of the facial muscles. Once significant scarring and muscle atrophy have occurred, return of function is less than optimal. Injuries to the orbital and ocular region may cause substantial long-term complications. Such injuries may include unrecognized injuries to the lacrimal system, corneal abrasions with residual scarring, and orbital malposition or entrapment of the globe or the extraocular muscle with subsequent enophthalmos and diplopia. If recognized early, most of these injuries can be successfully treated with a minimum number of residual long-term complications. However, late repair of such problems is generally less satisfactory because scar formation in such delicate tissues may compromise function. Additional complications may involve neuropraxia to the sensory nerves, especially the infraorbital and inferior alveolar nerve. Proper alignment of fractures in the maxilla and mandible is generally sufficient to help restore function, if the nerve has not been lacerated. With blunt injury, however, chronic pain or complete loss of sensation may yield substantial morbidity.

Fractures of the facial skeleton are relatively common. The pattern of injury is generally reproducible related to the type and nature of the trauma. The likelihood of complications after repair of facial fractures has been greatly reduced as a result of early intervention and the use of vastly improved techniques of exposure and fixation. Although it was previously believed that repair of facial skeletal injuries should be delayed to allow soft-tissue swelling to decrease, subsequent studies have demonstrated that early intervention within 24 to 48 hours is beneficial in allowing more precise alignment of the bony segments because the ingrowth of fibroblasts and the process of scar healing will not yet have commenced.

Additionally, early fixation will allow the patient to begin all aspects of rehabilitation and mastication, thereby accelerating healing. The use of rigid fixation has improved not only early fixation but also long-term results. Traditional complications associated with fracture fixation in the facial skeleton include malunion, nonunion, and infection.

Of particular concern in the repair of facial fractures is proper maintenance of occlusion. Malunion or nonunion of the maxilla or mandible may lead to malocclusion of the teeth, which can be devastating for the patient. Significant reconstruction may be required to correct this postoperative complication. All efforts should be expended preoperatively to ascertain proper occlusal contact. Injuries to the temporomandibular joint (TMJ) and the condyle, if inadequately addressed, may result in ankylosis of the TMJ. Proper evaluation of such injuries with early mobilization of the jaw may improve functional outcome. Maxillary sinusitis may occur after fracture repair. Care should be taken to remove bone fragments and blood from the fractured sinus. Frontal sinus fractures may result in dural injuries and obstruction of the frontal sinus drainage. In such cases, care should be taken to properly address the frontal sinus fracture, and cranialization of the sinus may be required in certain cases. Patency of the frontal sinus duct should be ascertained. Complications may include cerebrospinal fluid leakage or late formation of mucocele.

REFERENCES

1. Sanders WE. Principles of microvascular surgery. In: Green DP, Pederson WC, Campert R, eds. Green's Operative Hand Surgery. 4th ed. New York: Elsevier Science 1998.
2. Kilaru S, Frangos SG, Chen AH, et al. Nicotine: a review of its role in atherosclerosis. J Am Coll Surg 2001; 193: 538–546.
3. Fatah MF, Nancarrow JD, Murray DS. Raising the radial artery forearm flap: the superficial ulnar artery "trap". Br J Plast Surg 1985; 38:394–395.
4. Taylor GI, Miler G, Ham FJ. The free vascularized bone graft. A clinical extension of microvascular techniques. Plast Reconstr Surg 1975; 55:533–544.

FURTHER READINGS

Mathes SJ, Nahai F. Reconstructive Surgery: Principles, Anatomy and Technique. New York: Elsevier Science, 1999.
Strauch B, Vasconez L, Findlay-Hall E, eds. Grabb's Encyclopedia of Flaps. 2nd ed. New York: Lippincott Williams and Wilkins, 1998.

46

Complications in Gynecologic Surgery

Emery M. Salom and Manuel Penalver

Division of Gynecologic Oncology, Department of Obstetrics and Gynecology, Sylvester Comprehensive Cancer Center, University of Miami/Jackson Memorial Medical Center, Miami, Florida, U.S.A.

The complexity of the female anatomy poses a challenge for the pelvic surgeon during gynecologic procedures. During both abdominal and vaginal surgery, the intimate embryological and anatomical relationships between the various pelvic organs can be a source of complications. Congenital and acquired conditions can inevitably distort the anatomy and lead to unforeseen injuries. The pelvic surgeon needs to attain a comfortable level of knowledge regarding the female anatomy and become technically skilled at abdominal and vaginal surgery. It is important to develop the ability of preventing, recognizing, and managing injuries during gynecologic surgery.

Complications during gynecologic surgery can be caused by a number of different factors. Vaginal procedures afford a limited operative field, and this limitation leads to poor visibility and increased technical difficulty. Multiple operative procedures, including cesarean deliveries and other procedures designed to improve, retain, and terminate reproductive potential, can also affect the likelihood of intraoperative and postoperative complications. The pathophysiology of certain disease processes, such as pelvic inflammatory disease, endometriosis, pelvic relaxation, and gynecologic malignancy, distorts the anatomy and inevitably increases the technical complexity of the treatment.

Appropriate preoperative evaluation and preparation are paramount to preventing intraoperative and postoperative morbidities. Patients should be evaluated for preexisting medical conditions, electrolyte imbalances should be corrected, infections should be cultured and treated, cytologic studies of the cervix should be completed, and other routine examinations should be performed as indicated by the patient's age and risk factors. Any suspicious pelvic mass or malignancy should be assessed with ultrasonography, barium enema, sigmoidoscopy, or computed tomography so that the likelihood of multiorgan involvement can be predicted. Preoperative bowel preparation, antithromboembolic measures, and prophylactic antibiotics have been shown to minimize perioperative morbidity for specifically indicated procedures (Table 1).

This chapter will outline the more common genitourinary, gastrointestinal, and neural injuries encountered during gynecologic surgery and trauma. It will also discuss the basic preventative and management strategies for these injuries. All surgeons performing pelvic procedures should have a thorough understanding of pelvic anatomy and the operative knowledge needed for managing any unforeseen complications.

ABDOMINAL GYNECOLOGIC SURGERY
Abdominal Hysterectomy, Salpingectomy, Ovarian Cystectomy, and Oophorectomy
Incision

When gynecologic surgery is performed for benign conditions, the Pfannenstiel, Maylard, and Cherney transverse incisions are usually chosen rather than midline incisions. These transverse incisions provide adequate exposure, excellent cosmetic results, decreased postoperative pain, and a more expedient return to activities of daily living after abdominal hysterectomies and cesarean deliveries. The choice of a transverse incision rather than a midline incision must be made only after a diligent assessment of medical conditions, comorbid factors, preoperative diagnosis, and the potential for malignancy. An inadequate incision in this area can compromise the operative procedure.

When compared to the midline incision, the Pfannenstiel incision, which is the most popular transverse incision, has several disadvantages. The midline incision provides the most rapid entry into the peritoneal cavity, minimizes blood loss, and, most importantly, provides optimal exposure of the upper abdomen. The midline incision is advocated for patients with abdominal trauma, upper abdominal disease, or coagulopathies, and for those who refuse blood transfusions. However, the incidence of wound dehiscence is higher when in association with midline incisions (2.94%) than in association with the

Table 1 Preoperative Indications for Bowel Preparation

Suspected gynecologic malignancy
Suspected gastrointestinal malignancy
Laparoscopic procedure
Endometriosis
Pelvic inflammatory disease
Previous abdominal surgery

Pfannenstiel incision (0.37%) (1). Although observational studies have shown that midline incisions are associated with a higher risk of wound infections, wound dehiscence, and incisional hernias, only a few randomized studies have shown such trends, and none have demonstrated a statistically significant difference (2–4).

The Maylard incision, which involves a transverse transection of the rectus muscle and the peritoneum, is associated with more complications than is the Pfannenstiel incision. Transverse Maylard incisions have been performed safely for certain procedures that require access to the upper abdomen such as radical hysterectomy, para-aortic lymph node dissection, and exenteration.

Although many pelvic surgeons believe that the Maylard incision rivals the vertical incision with respect to surgical exposure, the incision is associated with an increased risk of wound hematomas and seromas as the result of ligation and transection of the inferior epigastric artery and transection of the rectus abdominus muscle. In addition, patients with extensive vascular insufficiency may require collateral circulation from the inferior epigastric artery to the lower extremities, and if this artery is ligated, these patients may experience claudication and ischemia. The Maylard incision may also cause damage to the femoral nerve when inappropriate retractors are used because the protective medial tension of the rectus abdominus muscle is lost.

Rapid entry into the abdominal cavity can cause injury to both the gastrointestinal tract and the genitourinary tract. A patient with a history of other abdominal surgical procedures is at an increased risk of iatrogenic injury to the bowel and bladder because of adhesions to the previous scar. Becker and Stucchi (5) found that 93% of patients who had previously undergone abdominal surgery had substantial abdominal adhesions at the time of reoperation, whereas only 10% of patients undergoing first-time laparotomy had such adhesions. The authors reported adhesions from abdominal scars to the omentum (81%) and the small bowel (50%), from the target organ to the omentum (27%) and the small bowel (9%), and between loops of small bowel (15%). For this reason, we emphasize the importance of entering the peritoneal cavity cephalad to the previous incision by tenting and incising the translucent peritoneum down to the dome of the bladder.

It is important to select an adequate incision at the inception of the procedure. When a Pfannenstiel

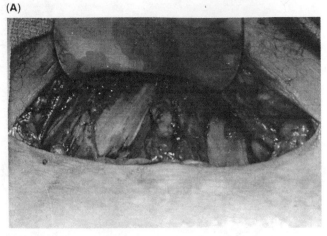

(A)

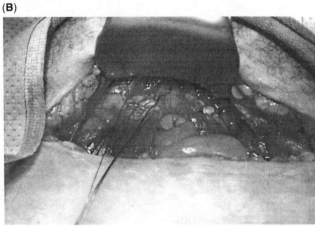

(B)

Figure 1 Cherney incision. **(A)** The tendon of the rectus muscle is easily accessible through a Pfannenstiel incision as it is attached to the superior pubic rami. **(B)** The right tendon has been transected; this procedure allows additional access to the pelvis because the rectus muscle on the right side retracts laterally. In the absence of the rectus muscle, the jejunum becomes visible. The left tendon has been reapproximated with #-0 interrupted figure-of-eight prolene sutures.

incision is performed but the procedure demands a larger operative field, the Pfannenstiel incision can be converted into a Cherney incision by transecting the tendinous insertion of the rectus muscle into the symphysis pubis (Fig. 1). Cherney advocated that transecting the tendon of the rectus would expand the operative field to two-thirds the size of the field created by a vertical infraumbilical incision (6).

Retraction, Packing, and Neurovascular Injury

Once an adequate incision has been made, the surgeon must ensure that the surrounding subcutaneous tissues have been freed before placing a self-retaining retractor. All adhesions of the omentum and bowel to the pelvis or to previous incisions should be cut so that crushing injuries to these areas can be avoided. The surgeon must palpate the underlying muscle to ensure that the retractor blades are held adjacent to the muscle and do not impinge on the psoas muscle, the bowel, or the vessels. If the retractor blades are inappropriately large, they will rest on the psoas muscle and the iliac vessels and may cause femoral, ilioinguinal, and iliohypogastric neuropathy.

The femoral nerve is the nerve most commonly injured during abdominal gynecologic surgery; the incidence of such a injury ranges from 7.7% to 11.6% (7,8). The symptoms include weakness during hip flexion and lower leg extension, numbness, and paresthesia of the medial and lateral thigh and medial leg. Most of these neuropathies are self-limiting and resolve within six weeks. These injuries occur most frequently in association with lengthy pelvic procedures, the use of self-retaining retractors and transverse incisions, and procedures performed on patients with a thin body habitus.

The sciatic nerve can be injured during abdominopelvic surgery when the patient is placed in an inappropriate lithotomy position or when pelvic bleeding occurs (9). The sciatic nerve can be compressed when a mattress suture is placed in the pelvic soft tissue to control severe pelvic hemorrhage. Damage results in weakness and paresthesias of the lower leg (10). Ilioinguinal and iliohypogastric neuropathies occur when the nerve is entrapped during suturing of the abdominal wound or during scar formation. The symptoms of nerve entrapment depend on the specific nerve affected. Injury to the ilioinguinal nerve causes loss of sensation to the inguinal area, the upper region of the labia majora, the area over the pubic symphysis, and the medial aspect of the thigh. Injury to the iliohypogastric nerve results in loss of sensation in the groin and the area of the symphysis pubis.

Urinary Tract Injury

One of the most serious complications associated with abdominal gynecologic procedures is injury to the urinary tract. The lower urinary tract is more prone to injuries than most other organs because of its intimate anatomical relationship to the reproductive tract. Injuries to the urinary tract most often affect the bladder; the ureter and the urethra are less frequently injured. Most injuries to the urinary tract are not life threatening, and 84% of such injuries are detected intraoperatively (11). If the injury remains undetected, the patient may experience urinoma, peritonitis, infection, ileus, fistulous tract, or loss of renal function on the ipsilateral side. Therefore, surgeons must understand the anatomic relationship of the urinary tract to the reproductive organs and must be familiar with techniques for avoiding, diagnosing, and treating these complications (Fig. 2).

Bladder

Injuries to the bladder occur five times more frequently than to the ureter. The incidence of bladder

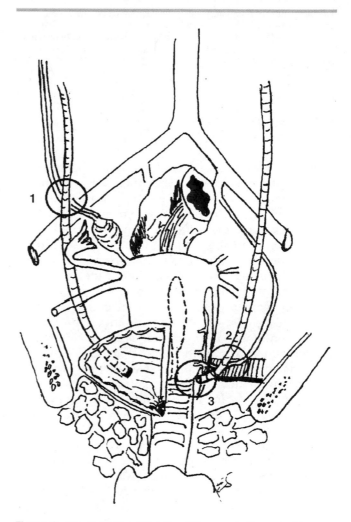

Figure 2 The anatomic relationship of the reproductive and urinary systems. The three most common sites of ureteral injury are (1) the section where the infundibulopelvic ligament meets the ureter near the pelvic sidewall; (2) the section where the ureter crosses under the uterine artery; and (3) the section where the ureter passes near the vaginal cuff as it enters the bladder.

injury ranges from 0.3% to 2.5%; recent studies report that bladder injury is associated with an average of 0.3% of simple abdominal hysterectomies and with 1.5% of radical abdominal hysterectomies (Tables 2 and 3) (12–15).

The bladder is a retroperitoneal organ that is adherent to the anterior vagina, the cervix, and the uterus via the vesicovaginal fascia. It meets the parietal peritoneum at the anterior abdominal wall. The

Table 2 Urinary Tract Injury During Simple Abdominal Hysterectomy

Author	Number of patients	Bladder injuries (%)	Ureteral injuries (%)
Harkki–Siren (14)	62,379	0.2	0.1
Dicker (16)	1851	0.3	0.2
Takamizawa (17)	923	0.5	0.5
Total (average)	229,153	(0.3)	(0.2)

Table 3 Urinary Tract Injury During Radical Abdominal Hysterectomy

Author	Number of patients	Bladder injuries (%)	Ureteral injuries (%)
Averette (18)	978	0.3	1.3
Christensen (19)	670	1.8	1.2
Rampone (20)	537	0.4	0.7
Mikuta (21)	242	3.7	1.7
Total (average)	2427	(1.5)	(1.2)

anatomic position of a bladder injury depends on whether the operation is performed via a vaginal or an abdominal approach. The area most frequently injured during abdominal hysterectomy is the dome of the bladder; this structure can be injured either upon entry into the parietal peritoneum or during the creation of the vesicovaginal space. The trigone can be damaged during dissection of the vesicovaginal space or during transection and ligation of the cardinal ligament and the vaginal cuff. Such complications can be avoided by draining the bladder with a continuous transurethral catheter, entering the peritoneum as cephalad as possible, and extending the incision toward the bladder while the peritoneum is transilluminated. The uterus and cervix should be kept under constant traction; the vesicovaginal flap should be sharply created and clearly separated from all pedicles.

If a complication is suspected, prompt recognition and repair of the bladder are necessary if more aggressive future therapy for fistula formation is to be avoided. Bladder injuries can be detected intraoperatively by using a transurethral catheter to fill the bladder in a retrograde manner with 500 mL of sterile water colored with methylene blue. As the bladder distends, small perforations, denuded areas, or portions of the bladder that have been crushed under a surgical clamp may become apparent. Needle injuries and crushing clamp injuries do not require repair. If an external sheath tear is visible through a denuded window of serosa, we recommend imbricating the serosa around the area with either a continuous or an interrupted layer of 3–0 delayed absorbable suture. When extravasation of urine results from a full-thickness tear or a laceration near the dome of the bladder, the repair should consist of a two-layer closure with interrupted stitches of 3–0 absorbable suture. For tears smaller than 4 cm, we have had excellent results with a continuous layered closure. Occasionally, an intentional cystotomy is required for evaluating the location and extent of the laceration. If the laceration is at the level of the trigone within 2 or 3 cm of the ureteral orifice, the tear is repaired with a two-layered interrupted stitch of 3–0 absorbable suture in the direction of the horizontal axis of the trigone (22). If the tear is closed vertically, the two ureteral orifices may be approximated and obstructed. Patency and integrity are confirmed by placing a 7- to 8-Fr catheter into each ureter; the catheters are removed after three or four weeks. Continuous bladder drainage with a suprapubic or transurethral catheter for 5 to 10 days is recommended. Repairs of cystotomies larger than 4 to 6 cm are drained with transabdominal suction catheters (Table 4).

Table 4 Corrective Surgeries for Urinary Tract Injuries

Organ	Type of injury	Corrective surgery	Stents	Suction drain
Bladder				
	Needle injury	Nothing unless bleeding or urine leakage	No	No
	Serosal tears	Imbrication of muscular layer	No	No
	Full thickness	Two-layered closure	Urethral	Optional
	Trigone area	Interrupted 1 or 2 layers	Both ureters and urethra	Yes
Ureter				
	Tears of external sheath	External sheath repair	Ureter	No
	Needle	Nothing unless bleeding or urine leakage	No	No
	Clamps, suture	Ureteral catheter only, if the tissue is intact	Ureter	No
	Transection without loss of ureteral segment			
	$\leq$5 cm from ureterovesical junction	Ureteroneocystostomy with or without bladder elongation	Ureter	Yes
	>5 cm from ureterovesical junction	Ureteroureterostomy		
	Transection with loss of ureteral segment	Ureteroneocystostomy with bladder elongation and/or mobilization of kidney	Ureter	Yes
		Ureteroneocystostomy with bladder flap with or without mobilization of kidney	Ureter	Yes
	Large segment and/or unhealthy organs	Ureteroileocystostomy	Ureter	Yes
		Transureteroureterostomy	Both ureters	Yes
		Urinary diversion	Both ureters	Yes
Urethra				
	External layer only	External layer only	Urethral	No
	Full thickness of the wall	Interrupted through the entire thickness of the wall	Urethral	No

Source: From Ref. 23.

Ureter

After the bladder, the genitourinary organ next most commonly injured during pelvic surgery is the ureter. The most recently reported incidence of ureteral injuries during abdominal hysterectomies is 0.2% (Table 2) (16,24). Ureteral injury is more common during radical hysterectomy; the reported average incidence is 1.2% (16,17,19,20,25,26). The highest risk of urinary injury is associated with procedures performed for ovarian remnant syndrome; injury occurs during as many as 25% of such cases (27). The three segments of the ureter that are most vulnerable to damage because of their relation to the reproductive tract are the segment of ureter adjacent to the infundibular pelvic ligament, the segment at the level of the uterine artery, and the segment adjacent to the attachment of the cardinal ligament and the vaginal cuff (Fig. 2). The ureter may be inadvertently clamped or transected when it is displaced by tumor, when it takes an anomalous course, or when it is involved with adhesions from pelvic inflammatory disease. The segment most commonly damaged is the segment located where the ureter crosses the uterine artery (28).

The pelvic surgeon must identify the normal ureteral anatomy at the initiation of the procedure. Before hysterectomies and oophorectomies proceed, the retroperitoneum is entered and dissected between the round ligament and the infundibulopelvic ligament until the course of the ureter has been identified on the medial aspect of the posterior leaf of the broad ligament. When a needle, suture, or clamp is placed on or near the ureter, it should be removed expeditiously and the patient should be given intravenous indigo carmine with 10 mL of furosemide so that the integrity of the ureter can be established. If the ureter is intact and the external sheath is well vascularized and not blanched, no further treatment will be required. If the external sheath is torn, a 4–0 or 5–0 interrupted delayed absorbable suture is placed with care to avoid the muscularis. A full-thickness tear or a break in the external sheath that is larger than 1 cm should be repaired as described above; an 8-Fr ureteral stent is guided into place through an intentional cystotomy. This stent may be removed 14 to 21 days postoperatively. A percutaneous suction catheter is positioned adjacent to the repair and is removed when the amount of drainage has decreased to less than 30 to 50 mL per day. The use of this catheter will assist with the diagnosis and therapy of a urinary leak.

The ureter can be transected when it is incorporated with the uterine artery or the vaginal cuff pedicle at the time of hysterectomy or upper vaginectomy. When the ureter is transected without segmental loss and within 5 cm of the bladder, ureteroneocystostomy can be performed (Fig. 3) (28–30). The remaining proximal ureteral stump is ligated with a permanent suture, and the distal portion of the ureter is mobilized so that tension on the anastomotic site can be prevented. An intentional cystostomy is created and

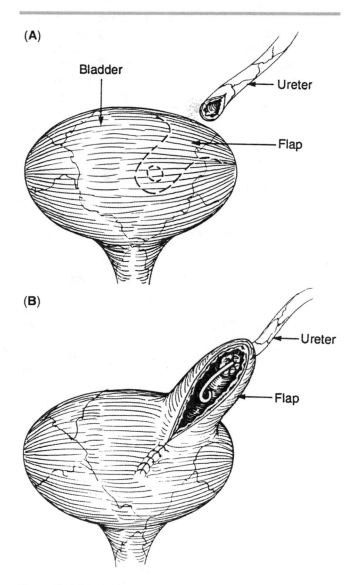

Figure 3 A bladder flap with ureteroneocystostomy. **(A)** The site of the bladder flap and the ureteroneocystostomy are identified. **(B)** The ureteroneocystostomy is shown with the ureteral catheter in place and the flap being closed with 3-0 or 4-0 absorbable suture. *Source*: From Ref. 31.

the distal end of the ureter is tunneled under the submucosa. The ureter is spatulated 0.5 to 1 cm from the end and is secured to the mucosa with 4–0 and 5–0 interrupted absorbable or delayed absorbable suture. On the serosal aspect of the bladder, two 4–0 interrupted delayed absorbable sutures are placed through the seromuscular surface of both the newly reimplanted ureter and the bladder so that the anastomotic tension can be decreased. If the anastomotic site between the ureter and the bladder is under undue tension, a bladder flap can be created, or a psoas hitch can be accomplished by suturing the seromuscular layer of the bladder to the psoas muscle (Fig. 3). A 7- or 8-Fr ureteral stent is passed into the bladder and is removed by cystoscopy after 14 to 21 days.

Alternatively, the stent can be passed through the urethra and removed externally. A suction drain is placed in the retroperitoneum, adjacent to the bladder and the ureter, so that any leaks can be detected. If the output from this retroperitoneal drain is high, the fluid should be tested for measurement of blood urea nitrogen and creatinine concentrations. The transurethral or suprapubic catheter can be removed after 7 to 10 days if no leak if present. After the stents have been removed, intravenous pyelography (IVP) is performed; this procedure ensures that there is no extravasation of contrast.

If a ureteral injury occurs at the level of the infundibulopelvic ligament, the ureter should be repaired end-to-end by ureteroureterostomy (Fig. 4).

The devitalized ends are excised and the end is spatulated for approximately 0.5 cm. A double J stent is passed from the renal pelvis to the bladder. A 4–0 to 5–0 delayed absorbable interrupted suture is placed circumferentially through the seromuscular surface, with care to avoid the mucosa. Finally, a suction drain is placed adjacent to the anastomosis. The stent is removed via cystoscopy, manually, or percutaneously after 14 to 21 days. Other techniques for repairing the ureter when there is segmental loss or when the injury is not adjacent to the ureterovesical junction are bladder flap augmentation, ureteroileocystostomy, and transureterostomy (Table 4).

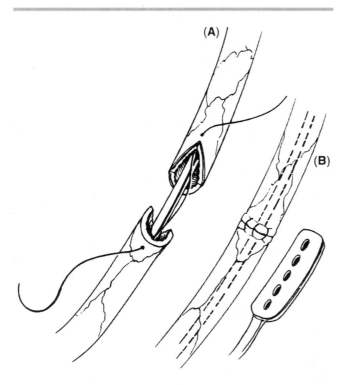

Figure 4 Ureteral end-to-end anastomosis (ureteroureterostomy). **(A)** A transected ureter with the spatulated ends. The anastomosis is performed with full-thickness interrupted stitches with a ureteral catheter in place. **(B)** Completed anastomosis and a suction drain close to the anastomotic site. *Source*: From Ref. 31.

Gastrointestinal Injury

The incidence of iatrogenic injuries to the gastrointestinal tract is low, but such injuries are possible because of the complexity of the surgical procedure and the disease process. The incidence of injury to the bowel during abdominal hysterectomy for a benign condition ranges from 0.3% to 0.5% (16,28–30). Most intestinal injuries occur upon entry into the peritoneal cavity when the bowel is adherent to the anterior abdominal wall, during lysis of adhesions, and during dissection of the rectovaginal space. We recommend preoperative bowel preparation for all patients who have undergone previous surgery or who have pelvic inflammatory disease, endometriosis, suspected malignancy, or gastrointestinal complaints. Such complications can be avoided by extending the skin incision above the previous incision and entering the peritoneum above that point. When dense abdominal adhesions are encountered, the agglutinated serosal interface must be identified. Once the surgeon has outlined the plane of agglutination, the adhesions can be easily separated by sharp and blunt dissection. We advocate sharp dissection when dense inflammatory adhesions have developed as a result of endometriosis, radiation therapy, or malignancy. In such cases, blunt dissection should be avoided because the approximated serosal surfaces lose their plane of demarcation.

Small-Bowel Injuries

The management of injuries to the gastrointestinal tract depends on the segment of bowel involved and the type and size of the tear. When a tear is superficial, involving only the serosa and muscularis, a 3–0 interrupted delayed absorbable or permanent suture can be used to close the defect. If the intestinal lumen is perforated, fecal contamination must be minimized by placing a moist laparotomy pack under the leak and occluding the intestinal lumen with proximal and distal linen–shod intestinal clamps.

A small full-thickness enterotomy can be repaired in a two-layer technique; the suture line must be maintained perpendicular to the axis of the lumen. The first layer is closed with a 3–0 interrupted absorbable or delayed absorbable suture, which runs the full thickness of the intestinal wall (32). A second 3–0 interrupted permanent imbricating suture is used to incorporate the seromuscular layers. Resection and primary anastomosis are indicated when the repair would constrict the intestinal lumen to less than 2 cm, when the vascular supply to a segment of bowel is sacrificed, or when there are multiple adjacent tears. We prefer to use an automatic stapling device to perform the resection and repair in a side-to-side functional end-to-end technique whenever feasible.

Large-Bowel Injuries

Although injury to the colon is less common than injury to the small bowel, colon injuries may be associated with more serious postoperative morbidity because of the increased bacterial colonization found in the large bowel. Dissecting adhesions between the rectum and the vagina, which have resulted from stage IV endometriosis, can be tedious and can result in damage to the rectosigmoid colon. Superficial tears can be repaired as previously outlined. Lacerations that result in full-thickness injuries can be repaired by the two-layer closure technique described above for the repair of small-bowel injuries. Simple injuries near the narrow sigmoid colon should be repaired with a single-thickness closure so that narrowing and postoperative obstruction can be prevented.

When lacerations affect more than 40% of the circumference of the large bowel, when there are multiple adjacent injuries, or when the vascular supply to the corresponding segment of bowel is compromised, we recommend resection and primary anastomosis. An automatic stapling device is used for performing a side-to-side functional end-to-end anastomosis; alternatively, a two-layer hand-sewn closure can be used. In the past, small lacerations to the colon were traditionally repaired with a protective colostomy so that wound dehiscence and peritonitis could be prevented. Several prospective and retrospective studies have found that primary repair without a protective colostomy is safe in the absence of fecal contamination (22,33–40). However, creating a protective colostomy is advisable whenever the anastomosis involves an irradiated segment of bowel or when ascites, an infectious process, or fecal contamination with spillage into more than one abdominal quadrant is present (34).

Abdominal Retropubic Procedures for Urinary Stress Incontinence: Burch and Marshal–Marchetti–Krantz Procedures

First described in the 1950s, the Marshal–Merchetti–Krantz (MMK) procedure and the Burch procedure are the retropubic vesicourethral suspension techniques most commonly used for treating genuine urinary stress incontinence. Both techniques entail dissection and identification of the retropubic space of Retzius, the Cooper ligament, the pubic symphysis, and the periurethral and paravaginal fascia. A supportive in situ sling is created by suturing the periurethral fascia and the perivaginal fascia under the urethra to either the Cooper ligament or the periosteum of the pubic symphysis. The surgeon must be familiar with the retropubic space so that injury to the engorged venous plexus, urethra, bladder, or ureter can be avoided.

The space of Retzius can be developed by using blunt or sharp dissection, but sharp dissection should be used only for patients who have undergone previous surgery and have dense adhesions. The bulb of a transurethral catheter is used to identify the vesicourethral junction. The index and middle finger of the surgeon's nondominant hand tent the lateral aspects of the vagina to allow placement of two

bilateral sutures 2 cm lateral to the midline at the level of the mid-urethra and the vesicourethral junction. The incidence of bladder and urethral injury associated with the MMK procedure reportedly ranges from 0.3% to 0.7% (41). Identification of the bladder margin can be facilitated by filling the bladder with 100 mL of indigo carmine. The incidence of ureteral obstruction ranges from 0.1% to 1.6% (41,42). For this reason, whenever obstruction or damage to the ureter is suspected, we recommend the use of cystoscopy to confirm the efflux of the dye from the ureteral opening. Transurethral or suprapubic catheters draining the bladder should be removed three to seven days postoperatively so that urinary retention can be minimized. Hemorrhage, which occasionally ensues from damage to the venous plexus during dissection of the retropubic space, can be controlled with constant pressure, electrocautery, figure eight sutures, or by simply tying down the sutures previously applied during the Burch or MMK procedure.

VAGINAL SURGERY
Patient Positioning and Nerve Injury

Improper alignment of a patient in the dorsal lithotomy position during vaginal surgery can result in nerve damage. The femoral, sciatic, and peroneal nerves can be injured by compression, although such injury occurs less frequently during vaginal surgery than during abdominal surgery. Excessive hip flexion, abduction, and external rotation damage the sciatic nerve during 0.4% of cases and the femoral nerve during 4.4% of cases (9,10). Both nerves can be damaged by stretch injuries when hip flexion and leg extension are extended; such extension compresses the femoral nerve under the inguinal ligament and traps the sciatic nerve within the greater sciatic notch. The peroneal nerve can be damaged if the knee is allowed to rest on the side of the stirrups because this positioning causes direct compression of the nerve against the tibia as the nerve courses into the lateral compartment. To avoid such complications, we use lithotomy boots that provide support and limit external rotation of the leg. These boots restrict external rotation, once the long axis of the lower leg has been properly aligned to the contralateral clavicular notch. The thigh should be flexed at an 80° angle to the pelvis, and the knee should be flexed at a 90° to 100° angle to the posterior thigh.

Dilation and Curettage

Dilation and curettage (D&C) is a simple and rapid procedure performed routinely across the United States each year for missed, inevitable, and therapeutic abortions and for irregular vaginal bleeding. The procedure is relatively simple but can result in many serious complications such as uterine perforation, hemorrhage, incompetent cervix, intrauterine synechiae, and cervical stenosis. Although D&C is perceived to be a simple procedure, the surgeon should always be vigilant so that the reported rate of 1 complication per 1000 cases and the reported mortality rate of 1 patient per 10,000 cases can be avoided (38).

The patient should undergo the preoperative preparation and receive antibiotics appropriate for limiting ascending infections that could result in salpingitis and decreased fertility. The size of the uterus should be gauged by a bimanual examination with the patient under anesthesia; the uterus should then be sounded so that the length of the endometrial cavity can be determined. A discrepancy between the depth of the uterus as measured by the uterine sound and the bimanual examination increases risk of uterine perforation during D&C. The anterior portion of the cervix is grasped with a single-toothed tenaculum, and gentle traction is placed so that the uterine cavity can be aligned in a straight configuration. Such alignment prevents the sound, the dilator, or the curette from perforating the posterior wall of an anteverted uterus or the anterior wall of a retroverted uterus (Fig. 5).

The reported incidence of uterine perforation during D&C ranges from 0.6% to 1.3%. The risk of perforation is as high as 2.6% for menopausal patients and as high as 5.1% for patients who experience postpartum bleeding (5.1%) (43). If perforation is suspected to have occurred, the surgeon can observe the patient for signs of perforation or consider diagnostic laparoscopy if there is active bleeding. In cases of anterior perforation, cystoscopy will confirm whether the bladder has been entered. Because the likelihood of perforation is highest when the uterus is gravid or infected, sounding the uterus in these cases is contraindicated. Aggressive dilation may also lead to cervical incompetence and cervical stenosis. Dilation should be no greater than the amount necessary for allowing entry of the smallest curette required for the procedure.

Hemorrhage is a rare complication of therapeutic curettage, but its likelihood is higher with a gravid uterus. If bleeding ensues, the surgeon must confirm that the product of conception has been completely evacuated from the cavity or verify that a perforation has occurred laterally at the level of the uterine arteries. If the injury occurs on the lateral wall of the uterine cavity, laparoscopy is necessary for confirming the perforation and controlling bleeding from the uterine artery. When bleeding is believed to have occurred as the result of an atonic uterus rather than a perforation, methergine (methyl ergonovine) should be administered by intramuscular injection. Alternatively, an intravenous infusion of 40 U oxytocin diluted in 1 L of normal saline can be administered. Recent pilot studies have shown that rectal administration of 600 to 1000 μg misoprostol is highly effective in decreasing blood loss by causing myometrial contractions.

The terms "Asherman syndrome" and "synechia" refer to intrauterine adhesions that can involve most of the endometrium and lead to amenorrhea and infertility. Aggressive curettage of a gravid or infected

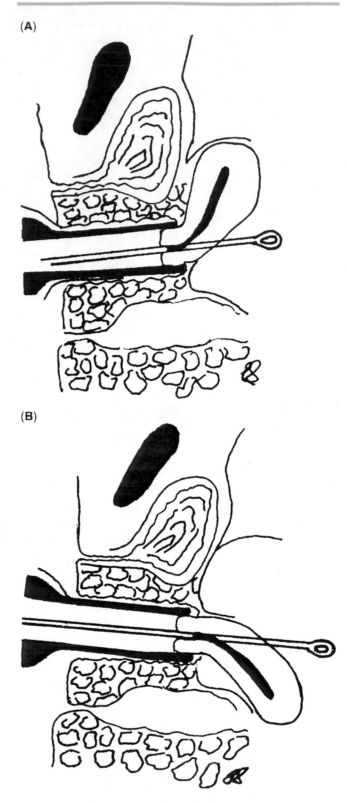

(A)

(B)

Figure 5 Perforation during dilation and curettage. A curette can perforate either the anterior or the posterior wall of the uterus and consequently injure the bladder, bowel, or rectum, depending on the orientation of the uterus. The uterus is perforated along the posterior wall when in the anteverted position **(A)** and along the anterior wall when in the retroverted position **(B)**.

endometrium has been associated with the development of this syndrome. If oligomenorrhea or amenorrhea develops after curettage, then synechiae should be confirmed hysteroscopically. Treatment consists of adhesionolysis, insertion of an intrauterine device, and estrogen therapy. Intrauterine pregnancies that occur following this procedure require careful monitoring due to the increased risk of uterine perforation.

Conization of the Cervix

Cervical dysplasia or carcinoma is diagnosed and treated by removing a cone-shaped biopsy from the uterine cervix with a loop electrocautery excisional procedure, a laser procedure, or a cold-knife conization. The complications associated with this procedure include hemorrhage, ascending infection, cervical stenosis, and cervical incompetence. Patients with high-grade dysplastic cells or carcinoma are predisposed to surgical hemorrhage as a result of angiogenesis and neovascularization. Obstetrical patients are also at a higher risk of intraoperative complications. For this reason, the surgeon must be aware of and able to perform several preventative and therapeutic options.

After the patient has been appropriately positioned and prepared, the cervix should be bathed with iodine solution for one minute. The iodine in the solution reacts with glycogen; because normal cells contain more glycogen than dysplastic cells, the normal cells become more darkly pigmented. This coloration clearly demarcates the lighter or hypopigmented dysplastic tissue from the darker normal tissue and allows the surgeon to excise the diseased tissue while avoiding the healthy tissue and the lateral extent of the cervix that contains the vascular supply. Before cold-knife conization is performed, the branches of the cervical artery can be ligated by placing #-0 absorbable or delayed absorbable figure-of-eight sutures into the cervix at 3 o'clock and 9 o'clock approximately 3 cm from the external os. Some gynecologists prefer to inject the cervix with vasopressin or saline circumferentially to provide a medical tourniquet. If bleeding is not controlled by electrocautery after the cone-shaped biopsy material has been excised, a piece of surgicel can be placed into the endocervix and held in place by approximating the lateral stitches that were previously placed. If the bleeding is more substantial, the anterior and posterior transected edges of the cervix can be sutured together with an interrupted #-0 absorbable or delayed absorbable suture.

During the early postoperative period, the patient may experience vaginal bleeding as a result of a loose suture and may require further treatment as outlined above. If the patient complains of a foul-smelling discharge, examination through a speculum may reveal a cervical infection that will require bacterial culture and antibiotic therapy. One long-term complication is cervical stenosis, which may lead to infertility or dysmenorrhea. If the cone margins involve the internal os of the cervix, the patient is at a higher risk of premature labor and cervical incompetence. In this scenario, placement of a cerclage may be required before the patient's next pregnancy.

Total Vaginal Hysterectomy

The preoperative assessment of the patient is essential for limiting the incidence of perioperative complications during vaginal hysterectomy. The technical difficulty of vaginal surgery is inherently greater than that of abdominal surgery because of the limited operative field. For this reason, the pubic arch, vaginal introitus, intertuberous diameter, and amount of uterine descensus and mobility must be evaluated preoperatively so that the surgeon can determine the accessibility of the planes of dissection and the vascular pedicles. Contraindications to the vaginal approach to hysterectomy are a history of active pelvic inflammatory disease, endometriosis, large immobile pelvic masses, suspected pelvic malignancy (not including endometrial cancer), chronic pelvic pain that requires abdominal visualization, and a contracted pelvis.

Vaginal hysterectomy is associated with all of the complications associated with abdominal hysterectomy such as infection, hemorrhage, and urinary and intestinal complications. However, Meltomaa et al. found that the incidence of bleeding complications requiring transfusions was twice as high during vaginal hysterectomy (2.9%) as during abdominal hysterectomy (1.1%) (28). The pelvic surgeon should not hesitate to convert a vaginal procedure to an abdominal approach when the source of bleeding cannot be identified vaginally. Published reports indicate that the incidence of urinary and intestinal complications is similar for vaginal and abdominal hysterectomy. However because abdominal hysterectomy is used to treat more complicated pathology, this similarity may be misleading, and vaginal hysterectomy may, in fact, be associated with a higher risk of complications.

The risk of intraoperative bleeding can be reduced by injecting diluted epinephrine (1:200,000) circumferentially around the cervix. The vasoconstriction caused by injecting 0.25% marcaine with epinephrine (1:200,000) will limit blood loss, increase visibility, and decrease postoperative pain. The hydrodissection produced by the injection may simplify localization and dissection of the surgical planes. Some surgeons believe that injecting marcaine with epinephrine into the pubovesical space facilitates the creation of the bladder flap and thereby decreases the risk of bladder injury.

Bladder injury occurs in association with vaginal hysterectomy when the bladder is dissected from the anterior portion of the cervix; the reported incidence ranges from 0% to 1.6% (14,16). We recommend sharp dissection for creating the surgical plane in the vesicouterine space by maintaining constant forceful downward traction on the uterus. Using finger dissection or blunt dissection with surgical gauze for separating the bladder may result in a shearing tear into the bladder lumen, especially when the patient has undergone previous surgery. Injury to the bladder during vaginal hysterectomy occurs in the area of the supratrigonal area of the bladder base. When such an injury is suspected because of the proximity of the trigone, spillage of indigo carmine and ureteral patency can be confirmed by cystoscopy. A simple incidental cystotomy should be repaired with a two-layer closure, and the bladder should be drained with a transurethral or suprapubic catheter for 7 to 10 days (Table 4).

Ureteral injury occurs less frequently than bladder injury during vaginal hysterectomy, and the incidence is 0.2% (14). During vaginal hysterectomy, downward traction on the uterus can bring the ureter into close proximity with the uterine artery. The surgical clamp must be applied at a right angle to the arterial insertion and flush to the uterus.

Ureteral compromise may also occur during uterosacral ligament suspension for support of the vaginal cuff when uterine prolapse is substantial. This complication occurs when the ureter is in close proximity to the uterosacral ligament as it nears the insertion to the bladder. Before sutures are placed, the uterosacral ligament must be identified and the ureter should be palpated 2 to 4 cm away. If ureteral compromise is suspected, cystoscopy should be performed to verify that indigo carmine is expressed through the ureterovesical orifice. A crushing clamp injury to the ureter can be simply released if the integrity of the lumen is not disrupted and no ischemic damage is noted. When the ureter is incorporated within a surgical pedicle and transected, a ureteroneocystostomy is used to reimplant the ureter, as described above.

An unrecognized ureteral obstruction that results from incorporation into a surgical pedicle during vaginal hysterectomy and uterosacral ligament suspension can lead to postoperative unilateral flank pain, a mild increase in the creatinine concentration, and eventual failure of the ipsilateral kidney. A nuclear medicine flow and function study or IVP can be used to diagnose ureteral obstruction. With complete obstruction, we prefer to insert percutaneous nephrostomy tubes and subsequently to perform ureterolysis. If a partial obstruction is detected, a transurethral nephroureteral stent can be inserted and then removed after four to six weeks with a follow-up IVP. If obstruction still persists at that time, we recommend ureterolysis or ureteral reimplantation (Table 4). Unrecognized tears or ischemic injuries to the ureter can lead to fistula formation 3 to 12 days after surgery (22).

Anterior Colporrhaphy

Anterior colporrhaphy is commonly used for reconstruction of the anterior wall of the vagina after prolapse of the bladder (cystocele), the urethra (urethrocele), or both into the vagina. Previously, anterior colporrhaphy was used to treat urinary stress incontinence, but it is currently used only in conjunction with other procedures because the success rate of this procedure alone is only 30% to 40%. Patients with large cystoceles, with advanced vaginal vault prolapse, and who have undergone previous surgery are at higher risk of injury and bleeding. Injecting epinephrine (1:200,000) or 0.25% marcaine with epinephrine (1:200,000) into the submucosa will facilitate the identification of dissection planes and thus decrease blood loss. Furthermore, sharp dissection and proper identification of the avascular vesicovaginal and pubocervical fascia will also decrease blood loss and prevent iatrogenic injuries to the bladder and urethra.

When a laceration to the seromuscular layer of the urethra is identified and the mucosa is intact, the laceration should be closed with an interrupted 3–0 or 4–0 absorbable or delayed absorbable suture with a protective imbricating second layer. A full-thickness laceration into the urethral lumen can be closed in two layers. The mucosa is closed with interrupted 3–0 to 4–0 absorbable suture through the mucosa and muscularis (22). The second layer closes the seromuscular tissue in an interrupted fashion and may include the surrounding periurethral tissue of the vesicovaginal fascia. Using transurethral bladder drainage for 7 to 10 days assists in the healing process (Table 4). Some early postoperative complications include infection and fistula formation. In a few cases, fibrosis can result in narrowing of the caliber of the urethral lumen; such narrowing in turn causes urinary retention, which may require prolonged transurethral drainage and urethral dilation. Injuries to the mid-urethra, if not repaired appropriately, can lead to urinary incontinence and fistula formation.

After anterior colporrhaphy, transurethral bladder drainage should be continued for three to four days postoperatively; such drainage avoids acute urinary retention, which is fairly common. Before the transurethral catheter is removed, a postvoid measurement of residual urine can be performed for assessing the risk of retention. Such a measurement is performed by filling the bladder with 300 to 400 mL of normal saline, removing the transurethral catheter, and encouraging the patient to void spontaneously. The voided amount is subtracted from the original amount instilled; if less than one-third of the original amount remains in the bladder, replacing the catheter is not necessary.

Posterior Colporrhaphy and Sacrospinous Colpopexy

The treatments of choice for the reconstruction of posterior vaginal compartment defects such as rectoceles and enteroceles are posterior colporrhaphy and sacrospinous colpopexy. These procedures should be performed during vaginal hysterectomy or vaginal vault prolapse repair. Patients who have undergone previous posterior repairs and patients with vaginal vault prolapse and enteroceles are at a greater risk of small bowel and rectal injury. Hoffman et al. (39) reported that the rate of rectal injury at the time of

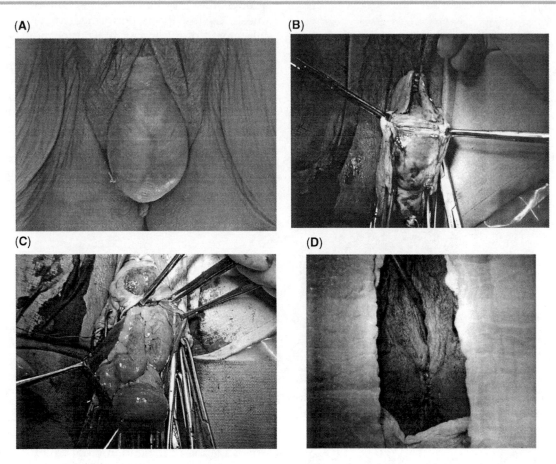

Figure 6 Vaginal vault prolapse, cystocele, rectocele, and enterocele. **(A)** Severe vaginal vault prolapse with a third-degree cystocele, rectocele, and enterocele. **(B)** The anterior vaginal mucosa is incised and the fascia is separated from the underlying peritoneum. **(C)** When the peritoneum is opened, herniation of the small bowel through the vagina is revealed. **(D)** The peritoneum is excised and closed. The defect is managed with a sacrospinous ligament fixation and an anterior and posterior colporrhaphy. Finally, the skin is closed with 3–0 absorbable suture.

posterior colpoperineorrhaphy is 0.07%. The incidence of rectal injury at the time of sacrospinous fixation has been reported to range from 0.4% to 4% (39,40). During vaginal hysterectomy, rectal injuries occur during entry into the posterior cul-de-sac, which may be obliterated by fibrosis resulting from endometriosis, inflammatory bowel disease, or diverticulitis.

Epinephrine or 0.25% marcaine with epinephrine (1:200,000) is injected as described earlier for anterior colporrhaphy, and the avascular plane between the vaginal mucosa and the rectovaginal fascia is developed. Rectal injuries occur during this portion of the procedure when fibrotic tissue from previous surgery or displacement of the normal anatomy because of severe vault prolapse distorts the surgical planes (Fig. 6). If the mucosa is intact, a single layer of interrupted 2–0 or 3–0 absorbable or delayed absorbable suture is used to imbricate the defect. When a full-thickness injury is found, a two-layer closure is performed. The overlying tissue is then plicated over the area so that the vaginal reconstruction can be completed without the added risk of breakdown and fistula formation. Unrecognized injuries lead to rectovaginal fistula formation.

Infrequent but significant hemorrhagic complications have been reported in association with sacrospinous colpopexy. At the University of Miami, we have found that when a Deschamps needle driver is used, vulvar hematoma occurs in 3% of cases and ischiorectal hematoma occurs in 0.1% of cases during the immediate postoperative period (Fig. 7) (40). If the patient remains hemodynamically normal, most of these complications can be treated conservatively by placing vaginal packing to tamponade the pararectal and ischiorectal spaces while serial hematocrit determinations are performed every 4 hours for 8 to 12 hours. If the vulvar hematoma continues to expand, or if the hematocrit continues to decrease because of bleeding into the retroperitoneum, surgical exploration is necessary. Control of bleeding in this area is difficult because the pudendal artery is encased in bone as it travels through the obturator foramen. One approach is incising the vulvar hematoma and placing tight vaginal packing. If bleeding continues, an exploratory laparotomy can be performed. The hypogastric arteries are ligated bilaterally and a large number of laparotomy packs are

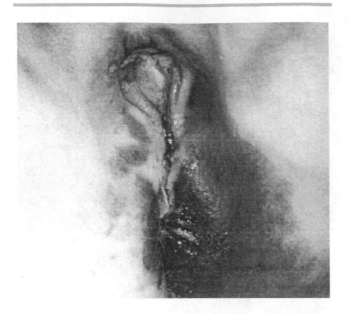

Figure 7 Ischiorectal hematoma.

placed into the pelvis; these packs are removed once the hemoglobin and hematocrit levels have been stabilized. Another therapeutic alternative for achieving hemostasis is catheterization and embolization of the pudendal artery.

Sling Procedures for Urinary Incontinence

The vaginal approaches to the treatment of urinary stress incontinence are the Pereyra, Stamey, Raz, and Gittes vaginal needle suspensions; the Kelly plication; and the tension-free vaginal taping (TVT) technique. Except for the TVT, which has a cure rate of 80%, these transvaginal urethral suspension techniques have fallen out of favor because of their poor five-year success rates. The TVT is performed by making bilateral incisions on the anterior wall of the vagina under the urethra and sharply dissecting the periurethral space to just under the pubic rami. Intraoperative bleeding and postoperative pain can be minimized by injecting marcaine with epinephrine into the periurethral and suprapubic areas. A sharp trocar is inserted into the periurethral space and passed just under the pubic rami, perforating the anterior fascia and exiting suprapubically. Although this procedure is relatively simple, it can result in a number of perioperative complications, including bladder perforation, urethral perforation, and hemorrhage.

Trocar insertion is the crucial portion of the operation and may lead to numerous complications. Precautions for avoiding urethral or bladder perforation include inserting a transurethral catheter with a stylet to deviate the urethra to the side opposite to that of trocar placement. The trocar is passed under the pubic rami and directed 2 to 3 cm lateral to the midline on the anterior abdominal wall; the trocar guides the positioning of the suburethral prolene mesh. Cystoscopy is performed for verifying proper placement of the trocar. If a perforation is noted, the trocar is simply removed and replaced. In our experience, no sequelae have been associated with conservative management of bladder perforations. After the procedure, the patient is observed for signs of hemorrhage, which can originate from the retropubic venous plexus or the external iliac artery as it enters the inguinal canal. If bleeding is substantial, exploratory laparotomy may be necessary. Another rare complication is urinary retention, which can be managed conservatively with transurethral bladder drainage. If the retention persists, surgical transection of the prolene mesh may be necessary.

HYSTEROSCOPY

Hysteroscopy as a Diagnostic and Therapeutic Method

Hysteroscopy has allowed advances in the treatment of intrauterine pathology and may be used to treat endometrial polyps, submucosal myomas, dysfunctional uterine bleeding with endometrial ablation, and synechiae with adhesiolysis. The conventional method of treatment, D&C, was a blind attempt at diagnosing and treating intrauterine abnormalities that would usually result in a hysterectomy. Direct visualization of the endometrial cavity has facilitated advances in diagnosis and therapeutic methods for endometrial abnormalities. Fertility is maintained because extirpation of the uterus is avoided. Although hysteroscopy is a relatively simple procedure, the surgeon should be well versed in correcting the intraoperative and postoperative complications that may be associated with it.

Complications During Insertion and Uterine Perforation

Laceration to the cervix can occur when traction is applied to the anterior portion of the cervix with a tenaculum while the dilator or the hysteroscope is inserted. Bleeding from such tears will usually stop when pressure is applied, but occasionally a fine 3–0 or 4–0 absorbable suture will be required. Bleeding can also be caused by abrasion to the endocervix; such bleeding can be stopped with electrocautery. The most troublesome complication is hemorrhage resulting from uterine perforation; the incidence of this complication is 0.1% during diagnostic procedures and 1% to 3% during operative hysteroscopy (43–45). Risk factors for such complications include distortion of the uterus, endometrial adhesions, uterine anomalies, hypoplastic uterus, and endometrial cancer. The hysteroscope should be inserted under direct vision with traction on the cervix; insertion should always follow the "dark spot" that represents the lumen. If a perforation occurs in the area of the fundus but no active bleeding ensues, treatment involves monitoring the patient's vital signs, watching for abdominal discomfort, and performing postoperative determinations of hematocrit. If the perforation occurs in the anterior or lateral portion of the uterus, or if active bleeding ensues, laparoscopy or cystoscopy is mandated.

Uterine Distention

The uterine cavity should be distended at a maximum pressure of 60 to 75 mmHg with Hyskon, dextrose solution, sorbitol, glycine, normal saline, or Ringer lactate solution (43). Higher pressures can cause rupture of the uterus and fallopian tubes or excessive absorption of the distention medium. Hyskon has a high viscosity but is no longer routinely used because it has been reported to cause coagulopathy and adult respiratory distress syndrome. Low-viscosity fluids are also associated with complications, depending on the specific properties of each solution. Nonisotonic solutions such as glycine, sorbitol, and dextrose in water may be associated with life-threatening hyponatremia if more than 1000 mL of fluid is absorbed. Isotonic and hypertonic solutions, such as normal saline and Ringer lactate, are associated with volume overload. Both conditions may be treated with diuretics and electrolyte replacement. Fluid balance must be monitored throughout the procedure, and the procedure will occasionally have to be aborted so that such complications can be avoided.

LAPAROSCOPY
Introduction

Laparoscopy has been a great advance in the treatment of gynecologic diseases because it reduces postoperative pain, morbidity, time off work, and overall cost. Procedures currently performed via this method include laparoscopically assisted vaginal hysterectomy, myomectomy, ovarian cystectomy, tubal ligation, pelvic reconstruction, urinary continence procedures, staging for pelvic malignancy, and lymphadenectomy. The complications associated with laparoscopy in terms of injury to blood vessels, bladder, ureter, and bowel are similar to those associated with open abdominal and vaginal surgery. However, certain injuries are unique to laparoscopy, and their incidence depends on the expertise of the surgeon. Management strategies are similar to those used during open procedures. The surgeon must always be cognizant of the increased technical difficulty involved in the laparoscopic management of iatrogenic injuries and should not hesitate to convert the procedure to laparotomy when the situation demands.

Vascular Injuries

Most injuries to major vessels occur during initial entry with a needle or trocar during the creation of pneumoperitoneum. The true incidence of vascular injuries is unknown, but the following steps can be taken to prevent such complications. After the skin incision has been made, the anterior abdominal wall can be elevated so that the distance between the fascia and the major vessels can be increased. The Veress needle or trocar should be inserted with the angle of entry directed toward the pelvis or the uterine fundus. If the intra-abdominal pressure produced by the Veress needle exceeds 15 mmHg and the patient's blood pressure decreases dramatically, or if blood returns from the needle, the surgeon should withdraw the needle and perform a midline incision to explore the abdomen.

The inferior epigastric vessels may be lacerated when the lateral lower quadrant ports are inserted, especially when patients are at high risk because of obesity or previous abdominal surgery. Traumatic entry can be avoided by identifying and transilluminating the inferior epigastric vessel with the superior port and placing the trocars at least 4 cm lateral to the midline. If a laceration ensues, the vessel can be cauterized with the contralateral port, the area can be tamponaded with a Foley catheter bulb, or the epigastric vessel can be ligated by placing a conventional suture or a J-needle suture either transabdominally or intra-abdominally (46).

Urinary Tract Injuries

The incidence of urinary tract injury during laparoscopy is reported to be 0.5% (47,48). Before the trocar or needle is placed, the bladder is decompressed by the insertion of a transurethral Foley catheter. Transillumination can be used in patients at high risk of adhesions to view and avoid these areas. In general, a Veress needle approach should not be used in these patients and a open technique is employed. However, should a Veress needle puncture occur, it can usually be treated simply by removing the needle. In contrast, the repair of a laceration or trocar injury must be accomplished by a traditional closure. Failure to diagnose an intraoperative bladder injury may result in oliguria, anuria, hematuria, suprapubic pain, and ileus during the patient's postoperative course. The diagnosis of bladder injury is suggested by infusing 300 mL of normal saline into the bladder and aspirating less fluid. A retrograde cystourethrogram will demonstrate the defect.

Ureteral injuries can occur during laparoscopically assisted vaginal hysterectomy, supracervical hysterectomy, or ovarian cyst resection for endometriosis. Complications involving the ureter are treated as described earlier for the abdominal approach. Ureteroureterostomy and ureteroneocystostomy have been performed laparoscopically, but these procedures are technically challenging and should be attempted only by surgeons who are comfortable with performing them.

Intestinal Injuries

The incidence of needle or trocar injury to the small or large bowel ranges from 0.1% to 0.6% (47,49,50).

Mechanical injuries to the gastrointestinal tract occur more frequently during adhesiolysis than during trocar or needle entry. The risk of such injuries is greatest for patients who have undergone previous surgery and those with a history of pelvic inflammatory disease, ruptured appendicitis, or pelvic malignancies. Such complications can be prevented by placing the initial port in the left upper quadrant or by beginning the procedure with the open technique.

If a Veress needle injury occurs, simply removing the needle is usually sufficient. Electrocautery can cause injuries that require treatment. Any blanched area should always be repaired and imbricated with a 3–0 absorbable or delayed absorbable suture. Superficial and full-thickness lacerations can be repaired laparoscopically, as described above (51). When laparoscopic injuries are undiagnosed, they can lead to postoperative fever, nausea, vomiting, abdominal pain, peritonitis, and sepsis. If such a complication is suspected, exploratory laparotomy is indicated.

RADICAL PELVIC SURGERY FOR GYNECOLOGIC MALIGNANCY
Radical Abdominal Hysterectomy, Cytoreductive Surgery for Ovarian Cancer, Pelvic and Para-Aortic Lymph Node Dissection, Pelvic Exenteration, and Urinary Diversion

The incidence of complications increases inherently when a gynecologic malignancy is treated because of the aggressive nature of the disease process and the radical procedures used to achieve a cure. Many patients with such malignancies are at high risk of complications because they have undergone multiple previous laparotomies or radiation therapy or because their pelvic anatomy has been distorted by the malignant process (52,53).

The gynecologic oncologist routinely performs a wide array of both curative and palliative surgeries for treating these destructive tumors. The traditional treatment for vulvar cancer has been radical vulvectomy. This approach is associated with a high incidence of wound breakdown and infection as a consequence of the en bloc butterfly resection of the entire vulva and inguinal area. Consequently, this procedure has been replaced with localized resection and separate-incision unilateral inguinal lymph node dissection; this newer surgical procedure produces comparable outcomes but is associated with a lower morbidity rate. Late complications of inguinal lymphadenectomy include chronic lymphedema and venous stasis.

Radical hysterectomy for the treatment of cervical cancer is associated with higher rates of pelvic hemorrhage, injuries to the ureters, and intestinal injuries than is simple hysterectomy (18,53). Late complications of radical hysterectomy include vaginal prolapse and bladder dysfunction caused by nerve injury during the radical dissection. Resection of retroperitoneal tumors and pelvic exenteration with resection of the bladder, rectosigmoid, vagina, and perineum may be associated with pelvic hemorrhage, infections, respiratory distress, and presacral bleeding.

Pelvic Hemorrhage

One of the most ominous and life-threatening complications encountered during surgery for gynecologic malignancies is intractable pelvic bleeding. Because of the generous amount of blood flow to the pelvic organs, the large vessels in the area, and the complex venous plexus in the retroperitoneal space, a simple vascular injury during resection of a tumor or endometriosis can cause copious bleeding. The extent and location of pelvic bleeding depend on the site of the tumor and the surgical procedure being performed. For example, presacral bleeding can occur during pelvic exenteration for recurrent cervical cancer or during the removal of a retroperitoneal tumor such as a schwannoma. During a cytoreductive or debulking procedure for ovarian cancer, the resection of a tumor that extends into the retroperitoneal space may precipitate a venous hemorrhage that quickly pools and obscures the visual field. Performing para-aortic and pelvic lymphadenectomy for treating cervical cancer can result in catastrophic bleeding from the vena cava or the obturator fossa—the most difficult areas in which to obtain hemostasis. Even pelvic surgery for benign conditions such as sacrocolpopexy can be associated with presacral hemorrhage. The surgeon must be aware of the potential complications and, even more importantly, must be prepared to execute the proper life-saving procedures.

In most cases, pelvic bleeding can be controlled by routine maneuvers such as applying firm pressure or hemoclips, cauterization, and suture ligation. When such maneuvers are not sufficient for controlling hemorrhage, the surgeon must be able to perform certain intraoperative alternatives that will allow hemodynamic stabilization. During such an event, the surgeon must always inform the anesthesiologist about the circumstances surrounding the blood loss, so that fluid resuscitation, blood transfusions, and the administration of blood products can be planned. In the following sections, we detail some of the techniques performed at our institution for treating catastrophic bleeding, including bilateral ligation of the hypogastric artery, mass suture, presacral thumbtack placement, pelvic packing, and arterial embolization.

Bilateral Ligation of the Hypogastric Artery

Bilateral ligation of the hypogastric artery minimizes the hemorrhaging and generalized oozing that occur after complicated radical hysterectomy, radical vulvectomy, ovarian cancer debulking, complicated gynecologic conditions, and even obstetrical operations. Ligation of the internal hypogastric artery controls hemorrhagic events by reducing the pelvic blood pressure by 24% and the blood flow by 50%;

this reduction gives the normal coagulation system an opportunity to work (54). Minimal sequelae have been reported after bilateral ligation of the internal hypogastric artery, and full-term deliveries have even been achieved. However, this procedure is associated with known hazards. Intraoperative complications have been reported to occur in as many as 15.7% of cases; these complications include ureteral injuries and injuries to the internal iliac vein (55). Postoperative complications include fistula formation, gluteal cramping, and ischemia as the result of inadequate perfusion.

The abdominal approach for the ligation of the hypogastric artery is accomplished by entering the retroperitoneal space through an incision in the posterior parietal peritoneum over the common iliac artery. After dissecting and reflecting the peritoneum, the surgeon identifies the hypogastric artery at its bifurcation by clearing away the surrounding connective areolar tissue. The ureter should always be identified and moved away from the iliac vessels. The tips of a long right-angle clamp are passed under the internal iliac artery (the hypogastric artery) on the lateral aspect of the vessel 2 cm distal to the bifurcation of the common iliac artery, so that ligation of the posterior branch of the internal iliac artery can be avoided (Fig. 8). After the long right-angle clamp is placed under the vessel to be ligated, it is tilted and pushed from lateral to medial so that the tips are visible on the medial side of the vessel. Next, a 0-silk suture is used to tie the vessel, and a second silk suture is placed 0.5 to 1 cm caudal to the first. The same procedure is performed on the contralateral side. The pulses of the external and femoral arteries should be palpated before the suture is secured so that the patency of the external iliac vessel can be verified and the surgeon can be confident that this vessel has not been ligated in error. If ligation of the internal iliac artery fails to control the bleeding, the ovarian artery can also be ligated before the surgeon commits to performing a hysterectomy (56).

Mass Suture

The extensive venous plexus that drains the pelvic floor can be damaged during lymph node dissection or resection of a retroperitoneal tumor. Because the source of bleeding is rarely a single vessel, it is usually futile to attempt to locate a single bleeding site and place a hemoclip or suture. Clamping and ligating the bleeding venous plexus is difficult and may require placement of a mass suture. Before proceeding, the surgeon must identify the adjacent pelvic anatomy, including the ureter, bladder, rectum, major vessels, and nerves, so that any injury to these structures can be avoided. At this point, a #-0 absorbable or delayed absorbable suture on a CT-1 needle is placed as a large figure-of-eight that incorporates the soft tissue around the bleeding site; this suture is tied firmly. If space is limited, a CT-2 needle can be chosen. Multiple mass sutures are often necessary for controlling the bleeding. If bleeding continues after the mass sutures have been placed, administering pressure with warm disposable lap sponges should be attempted for a few minutes. In addition, the surgeon can consider the use of thrombostatic agents. Finally, packing the pelvis can be the final attempt at stabilizing the patient so that coagulopathy can be corrected and further resuscitation can be performed.

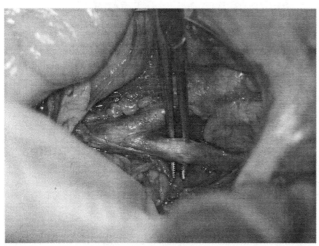

(A)

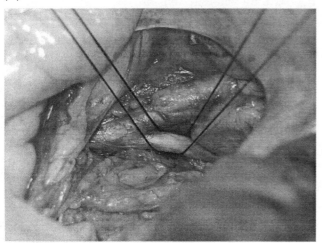

(B)

Figure 8 Bilateral hypogastric artery ligation. **(A)** A right-angle clamp is placed under the hypogastric artery 2 cm from the bifurcation of the common iliac artery. The surgeon standing on the contralateral side passes the instrument from lateral to medial to avoid injury to the hypogastric vein. **(B)** Two #-0 silk sutures are placed proximally and distally from the 2-cm mark and secured.

Thumbtack for Presacral Bleeding

Pelvic exenteration, abdominal sacral colpopexy, and resection of retroperitoneal malignancies can cause

CASE STUDY

A 39-year-old woman with an intrauterine pregnancy at 36 weeks gestation came to the hospital for an elective cesarean delivery. She was found to have multiple large uterine fibroids and a complete placenta previa, a condition in which the placenta overlies the birth canal and predisposes the patient to third-trimester bleeding. During her pregnancy, the patient had been admitted to the hospital twice for vaginal spotting and degenerating fibroids. Before the operative delivery was scheduled, fetal lung maturity was confirmed by amniocentesis.

A healthy baby girl was delivered by cesarean section. Immediately after delivery, the patient experienced a substantial uterine hemorrhage from the abnormally attached placental tissue. At this time, an emergency hysterectomy was begun; packed red blood cells and fresh frozen plasma were administered to correct clinically evident disseminated intravascular coagulopathy and a 3-L blood loss. The patient was transferred to the surgical intensive care unit, where her condition stabilized. The patient was discharged from the hospital on postoperative day 10.

Three weeks after discharge, the patient complained of urinary incontinence that was continuous but increased with the Valsalva maneuver. An examination through a speculum showed a clear watery discharge with no visible mucosal defects. The patient underwent specialized urodynamic studies as part of the work-up for urinary incontinence; the results were negative. When urinary incontinence continued, voiding cystourethrography was performed; the results were normal. IVP showed extravasation of contrast into the vagina but no clear source of the leak (Fig. 9). Computed tomography of the pelvis confirmed a persistent ureterovaginal fistula causing the symptoms of urinary incontinence (Fig. 10). A nephroureteral stent was placed for bypassing the fistula tract and allowing spontaneous healing. After 12 weeks of conservative management with no resolution, we performed ureteroneocystostomy. The patient remains free of symptoms.

laceration of the presacral vessels (57). Once these presacral vessels have been damaged, they retract and recoil into the bony surfaces of the sacrum; this retraction renders the conventional methods of controlling hemorrhage ineffective. Occasionally, applying pressure or temporarily packing the pelvis can achieve hemostasis, but once the packing is removed, bleeding may resume and blood can rapidly pool in the pelvis. Attempts at applying mass sutures onto the bony structures of the sacrum are usually futile and risk further vascular injury. When uncontrollable bleeding occurs in this area, a stainless steel thumbtack on the tips of a long Kelly or Kocher clamp can be applied to the source of the hemorrhage. Timmons et al. (58) used a 12-inch stainless steel rod with a recessed magnet at the end for securing and delivering the thumbtack.

Pelvic Packing

Another method of achieving hemostasis and stabilization for patients with extensive and intractable bleeding from raw surfaces, venous plexuses, and inaccessible areas is the prolonged use of abdominal and pelvic laparotomy packing. Various techniques are used for packing the pelvis, depending on the

experience of the surgeon. We place warm laparotomy packs, starting from the deepest portion of the pelvis, until enough tension has been obtained to maintain constant compression on the bleeding site.

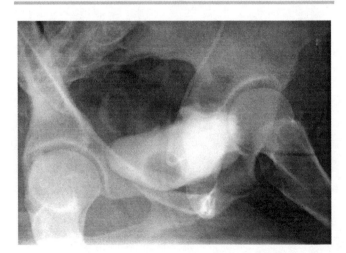

Figure 9 Intravenous pyelography demonstrates extravasation of the intravenous contrast material into the vagina.

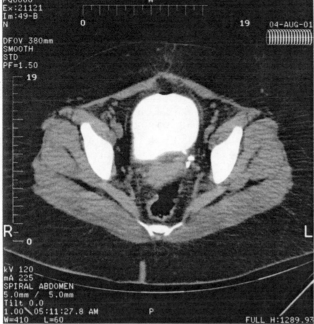

(A)

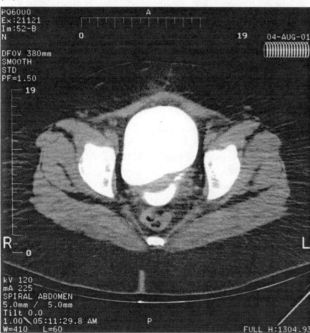

(B)

Figure 10 Computed tomography of the pelvis. **(A)** The contrast material within the fistula is seen tracking toward the vagina posterior to the ureter. **(B)** The fistula is seen entering and filling the vagina.

The number of laparotomy packs used depends on the size of the patient and the depth of the pelvis. Next, we close the fascia, but intra-abdominal pressures must be closely monitored for compartment syndrome. The skin incision is left open and packed so that intra-abdominal bleeding can be monitored and unnecessary wound closure can be avoided. Determining whether hemostasis has been achieved by placing a Jackson–Pratt drain in the area; however, this drain may not allow accurate monitoring of ongoing hemorrhage. The packing should be removed after 24 to 48 hours, provided the patient's hemodynamic condition is stable and the bleeding has stopped. To remove the packing, we reopen the abdomen to allow for proper visualization of the pelvic cavity and the bowel, thereby avoiding shearing tears and perforation.

SUMMARY

The complexity of the female pelvic anatomy, the small field of vision, and the distortion created by disease processes all contribute to the challenges faced by the pelvic surgeon. Innovations such as laparoscopy have advanced the quality of medical care provided in this field. However, careful preoperative preparation, surgical expertise, and familiarity with the prevention, recognition, and therapy of potential complications in this area are needed to achieve the best outcomes.

REFERENCES

1. Mowat J, Bonnar J. Abdominal wound dehiscence after cesarean delivery. Br Med J 1971; 2:256–257.
2. Ellis H, Coleridge-Smith PD, Joyce AD. Abdominal incisions—vertical or transverse? Postgrad Med J 1984; 60:407–410.
3. Stone HH, Hoefling SJ, Strom PR, Dunlop WE, Fabian TC. Abdominal incisions: transverse vs vertical placement and continuous vs interrupted closure. South Med J 1983; 76:1106–1108.
4. Guillon PJ, Hall TJ, Donaldson DR, Broughton AC, Brennan TG. Vertical abdominal incisions—a choice? Br J Surg 1980; 67:395–399.
5. Becker JM, Stucchi AF. Intra-abdominal adhesion prevention: are we getting any closer? Ann Surg 2004; 240:202–204.
6. Cherney LS. A modified transverse incision for low abdominal operations. Surg Gynecol Obstet 1941; 72:92–95.
7. Kvist-Poulsen H, Borel J. Iatrogenic femoral neuropathy subsequent to abdominal hysterectomy: incidence and prevention. Obstet Gynecol 1982; 60:516–520.
8. Goldman JA, Feldberg D, Dicker D, Samuel N, Dekel A. Femoral neuropathy subsequent to abdominal hysterectomy. A comparative study. Eur J Obstet Gynecol Reprod Biol 1985; 20:385–392.
9. Burkhart F, Daly JW. Sciatic and peroneal nerve injury: a complication of vaginal operations. Obstet Gynecol 1966; 28:99–102.
10. McQuarrie HG, Harris JW, Ellsworth HS, Stone RA, Anderson AE III. Sciatic neuropathy complicating vaginal hysterectomy. Am J Obset Gynecol 1972; 113:223–232.
11. Morey SS. ACOG issues report on management of operative injuries of the urinary tract. Am Fam Physician 1998; 57:870.

12. Benson RC, Hinman F Jr. Urinary tract injuries in obstetrics and gynecology. Am J Obstet Gynecol 1955; 70: 467–485.

13. Schmidt JD. Management of urinary tract injuries. In: Buchsbaum HJ, Schmidt JD, eds. Gynecologic and Obstetric Urology. 3rd ed. Philadelphia: WB Saunders, 1993:155–162.

14. Harkki-Siren P, Sjoberg J, Tiitinen A. Urinary tract injuries after hysterectomy. Obstet Gynecol 1998; 92: 113–118.

15. Johnson N, Barlow D, Lethaby A, Tavender E, Curr L, Garry R. Methods of hysterectomy: systematic review and meta-analysis of randomized controlled trials. BMJ 2005; 330:1478–1486.

16. Dicker RC, Greenspan JR, Strauss LT, et al. Complications of abdominal and vaginal hysterectomy among women of reproductive age in the United States. The Collaborative Review of Sterilization. Am J Obstet Gynecol 1982; 144:841–848.

17. Takamizawa S, Minakami H, Usui R, et al. Risk of complications and uterine malignancies in women undergoing hysterectomy for presumed benign leiomyomas. Gynecol Obstet Invest 1999; 48:193–196.

18. Averette HE, Nguyen HN, Donato DM, et al. Radical hysterectomy for invasive cervical cancer. A 25-year prospective experience with the Miami technique. Cancer 1993; 71:1422–1437.

19. Christensen A, Foglmann R. Cervical carcinoma stage I and II treated by primary radical hysterectomy and pelvic lymphadenectomy, 320 cases by the method of Meigs-Taussig and 350 by the method of Okabayaschi. Acta Obstet Gynecol Scand Suppl 1976; 58:1–44.

20. Rampone JF, Klem V, Kolstad P. Combined treatment of stage Ib carcinoma of the cervix. Obstet Gynecol 1973; 41:163–167.

21. Mikuta JJ, Giuntoli RL, Rubin EL, Mangan CE. The "problem" radical hysterectomy. Am J Obstet Gynecol 1977; 128:119–127.

22. Holley RL, Kilgore LC. Urologic complications. In: Orr JW Jr., Shingleton HM, eds. Complications in Gynecologic Surgery: Prevention, Recognition and Management. Philadelphia: Lippincott, 1994:131–166.

23. Angioli R, Penalver M. Urinary tract injuries. In: Hurt WG, ed. Urogynecologic Surgery. 2nd ed. Philadelphia: Lippincott-Raven, 2000:177–186.

24. Dowling RA, Corriere JN Jr., Sandler CM. Iatrogenic ureteral injury. J Urol 1986; 135:912–915.

25. Dorairajan G, Rani PR, Habeebullah S, Dorairajan LN. Urologic injuries during hysterectomies: a 6-year review. J Obstet Gynecol Res 2004; 30:430–435.

26. Kuno K, Menzin A, Kauder HH, Sison C, Gal D. Prophylactic ureteral catheterization in gynecologic surgery. Urology 1998; 52:1004–1008.

27. Lafferty HW, Angioli R, Rudolph J, Penalver MA. Ovarian remnant syndrome: experience at Jackson Memorial Hospital, University of Miami, 1985 through 1993. Am J Obstet Gynecol 1996; 174:641–645.

28. Meltomaa SS, Makinen JI, Taalikka MO, Helenius HY. One-year cohort of abdominal, vaginal, and laparoscopic hysterectomies: complications and subjective outcomes. J Am Coll Surg 1999; 189:389–396.

29. Mattlingly RF, Borkowf HI. Acute operative injury to the lower urinary tract. Clin Obstet Gynaecol 1978; 5: 123–149.

30. Fry DE, Milholen L, Harbrecht PJ. Iatrogenic ureteral injury. Options in management. Arch Surg 1983; 118: 454–457.

31. Angioli R, Penalver M. Ureteral injury at the time of radical pelvic surgery. Op Techniques Gynecol Surg 1998; 3:132–140.

32. Burke TW, Levenback C. Gastrointestinal tract. In: Orr JW Jr., Shingleton HM, eds. Complications in Gynecologic Surgery: Prevention, Recognition and Management. Philadelphia: Lippincott, 1994:103–130.

33. Sasaki LS, Allaben RD, Golwala R, Mittal VK. Primary repair of colon injuries: a prospective randomized study. J Trauma 1995; 39:895–901.

34. Gonzalez RP, Merlotti GJ, Holevar MR. Colostomy in penetrating colon injury: is it necessary? J Trauma 1996; 41:271–275.

35. Frame SB, Ridgeway CA, Rice JC, McSwain NE Jr., Kerstein MD. Penetrating injuries to the colon: analysis by anatomic region of injury. South Med J 1989; 82:1099–1102.

36. George SM Jr., Fabian TC, Mangiante EC. Colon trauma: further support for primary repair. Am J Surg 1988; 156:16–20.

37. Murray JJ, Schoetz DJ Jr., Coller JA, Roberts PL, Veidenheimer MC. Intraoperative colonic lavage and primary anastomosis in nonelective colon resection. Dis Colon Rectum 1991; 34:527–531.

38. Houston MC, Ratcliff DG, Hays JT, Gluck FW. Preoperative medical consultation and evaluation of surgical risk. South Med J 1987; 80:1386–1397.

39. Hoffman MS, Lynch C, Lockhart J, Knapp R. Injury of the rectum during vaginal surgery. Am J Obset Gynecol 1999; 181:274–277.

40. Salom EM, Penalver MA. Pelvic extenteration and reconstruction. Cancer J 2003; 9:415–424.

41. Mainprize TC, Drutz HP. The Marshall–Marchetti–Krantz procedure: a critical review. Obstet Gynecol Surv 1988; 43:724–729.

42. Maulik TG. Kinked ureter with unilateral obstructive uropathy complicating Burch colposuspension. J Urol 1983; 130:135.

43. Shirk GJ. Uterine perforation: endoscopic complications and treatment. In: Corfman RS, Diamond MP, DeCherney AH, eds. Complications of Laparoscopy and Hysteroscopy. Boston: Blackwell, 1997:221–225.

44. Lindelmann HJ, Mohr J. CO2-hysteroscopy: diagnosis and treatment. Am J Obstet Gynecol 1976; 124:129–133.

45. Hulka JF, Peterson HB, Phillips JM, Surrey MW. Operative hysteroscopy. American Association of Gynecologic Laparoscopists 1991 membership survey. J Reprod Med 1993; 38:572–573.

46. John DA. Perforation of the inferior epigastric vessels. In: Corfman RS, Diamond MP, DeCherney AH, eds. Complications of Laparoscopy and Hysteroscopy. Boston: Blackwell, 1997:30–35.

47. Loffer FD, Pent D. Indications, contraindications and complications of laparoscopy. Obstet Gynecol Surv 1975; 30:407–427.

48. Schanbacher PD, Rossi LJ Jr., Salem MR, Joseph NJ. Detection of urinary bladder perforation during laparoscopy by distention of the collection bag with carbon dioxide. Anesthesiology 1994; 80:680–681.

49. Krebs HB. Intestinal injury in gynecologic surgery: a ten-year experience. Am J Obstet Gynecol 1986; 155: 509–514.

50. Peterson HB, Hulka JF, Phillips JM. American Association of Gynecologic Laparoscopists' 1988 membership survey on operative laparoscopy. J Reprod Med 1990; 35:587–589.

51. Nezhat CR, Nezhat FR, Nezhat C, Luciano AA, Siegler AM, Metzger DA. Complications. In: Siegler A, Nezhat FR, Nezhat C, Siedman DS, Luciano AA, Nezhat CR, eds. Operative Gynecologic Laparoscopy: Principles and Techniques. 2nd ed. New York: McGraw-Hill, 2000:287–311.

52. Morley GW, Seski JC. Radical pelvic surgery versus radiation therapy for stage I carcinoma of the cervix (exclusive of microinvasion). Am J Obstet Gynecol 1976; 126:785–798.

53. Benedetti-Panici P, Scambia G, Baiocchi G, Maneschi F, Greggi S, Mancuso S. Radical hysterectomy: a randomized study comparing two techniques for resection of the cardinal ligament. Gynecol Oncol 1993; 50:226–231.

54. Burchell RC. Physiology of internal iliac artery ligation. J Obstet Gynaecol Br Commonw 1968; 75: 642–651.

55. Chattopadhyay SK, Deb Roy B, Edrees YB. Surgical control of obstetric hemorrhage: hypogastric artery ligation or hysterectomy? Int J Gynaecol Obstet 1990; 32:345–351.

56. Fehrman H. Surgical management of life-threatening obstetric and gynecologic hemorrhage. Acta Obstet Gynecol Scand 1988; 67:125–128.

57. Sutton GP, Addison WA, Livengood CH III, Hammond CB. Life-threatening hemorrhage complicating sacral colpopexy. Am J Obstet Gynecol 1981; 140: 836–837.

58. Timmons MC, Kohler MF, Addison WA. Thumbtack use for control of presacral bleeding, with description of an instrument for thumbtack application. Obstet Gynecol 1991; 78:313–315.

47

Complications of Bladder and Prostate Surgery

Adam J. Bell, Josh M. Randall, and Raymond J. Leveillee
*Division of Endourology and Laparoscopy, Department of Urology, University of Miami
Miller School of Medicine, Miami, Florida, U.S.A.*

Reports of surgical procedures involving the bladder date back to 200 B.C., when Ammonius wrote about perineal lithotomy for bladder stone removal. Since that time, a wide range of additional indications for bladder surgery have developed. Malignancy is the most common reason for surgical intervention involving the bladder. The most common urinary tract malignancy derived from the urothelial lining of the urinary system is bladder cancer in which transitional cell carcinoma accounts for approximately 90% of these tumors. In the United States, bladder cancer is the fourth leading cause of cancer death for men, after lung, prostate, and colon cancer. The remaining bladder tumors are accounted for by squamous cell carcinoma (3–7%), adenocarcinoma (2–3%), and metastatic lesions (1–2%) (1).

This chapter presents surgical treatment options for bladder cancer, as well as surgical intervention for other disease processes, such as neurogenic bladder, urinary incontinence, genitourinary anomalies, infections, intractable hematuria, ureteral and renal pathology, and trauma. To treat these conditions, surgeons may use a wide range of operative (and nonoperative) techniques, tools, and talents, but they must also be able to deal with a multitude of potential surgical complications. This chapter discusses the diagnosis, treatment, and prevention of complications associated with bladder surgery.

BLADDER CANCER
Transurethral Resection of Bladder Tumor

Endoscopic management of genitourinary pathology has become a cornerstone of urologic surgery (2). Cystoscopy allows for complete evaluation of the urethra, prostate, and bladder, and it is used as both a diagnostic and a therapeutic procedure. For example, cystourethroscopy is performed as part of the initial workup for hematuria; if a bladder tumor is discovered, it may be resected transurethrally. Approximately 55% to 60% of cases of transitional cell carcinoma (TCC) are diagnosed when they are still considered superficial disease, i.e., tumor confined to the mucosa (stage Ta or Cis) or the submucosa (stage T1) (1). Initial management requires performing transurethral resection of the bladder tumor (TURBT) so that a good amount of tissue can be obtained in order to make a diagnosis of cancer as well as stage the patient appropriately. This technique also adequately provides hemostasis and assesses the uninvolved urothelium and bladder tissue (2). The rate of recurrence of these superficial bladder tumors is approximately 75%, but only 10% to 15% will progress to muscle-invasive disease (1).

The technique of transurethral resection has been well described and essentially involves performing initial endoscopic inspection of the bladder and noting the area(s) of suspected pathology, resecting the bladder tumor, removing the specimen, and obtaining hemostasis (2). Although infrequent, complications may occur in association with transurethral resection; these complications can be characterized as major or minor and as early or late.

One potential early complication is postoperative bleeding. Although some degree of hematuria can be expected after transurethral resection, failure to achieve sufficient hemostasis after the procedure can result in postoperative gross hematuria, clot retention, and acute anemia. Initial treatment involves placing a three-way Foley catheter, irrigating the bladder by hand, removing the blood clot, initiating continuous bladder irrigation with close observation, and administering blood transfusions when indicated. A second surgical procedure may be required if bleeding does not subside. This complication can be prevented by meticulous electrosurgical hemostasis at the conclusion of the resection.

Free perforation through the bladder wall during resection of the bladder tumor is a worrisome and serious complication. The risk of perforation can be reduced by performing precise, controlled "swipes" of the tumor with the resectoscope loop, noting the depth of resection each time and limiting the bladder inflow (the bladder wall thins as it becomes progressively fuller). When perforation does occur, it may be either extraperitoneal or intraperitoneal. Most small extraperitoneal bladder perforations can be managed expectantly by placing a Foley catheter for 7 to 10 days so that complete healing can occur; a gravity cystogram is performed before the catheter is removed so that healing can be demonstrated (2). Substantial extravasation of perivesical fluid and suprapubic fullness may occur with large defects and can be treated by placing a drain through a small suprapubic incision. Small intraperitoneal bladder perforations can also be managed conservatively, but if the patient experiences any signs or symptoms of acute peritonitis, open surgical exploration and closure are indicated; this is because intraperitoneal bladder perforation indicates that the bowel is at risk of injury and delayed perforation as the result of thermal necrosis (2). The tumor may recur locally or distantly after bladder perforation, but the risk is relatively low. In one report, metastatic disease developed after intraperitoneal bladder perforation in only 1 of 16 patients with extravesical tumor recurrence (3).

Vesicoureteral reflux (VUR) or stenosis may occur after tumor resection over or near the ureteral orifice. This risk can be minimized by limited use of electrical coagulation in this area. As is the case with any transurethral manipulation, iatrogenic injury to the urethra and bladder neck can result in either acute or chronic urethral strictures. Proper lubrication and direct visual insertion of instruments is crucial. A situation unique to TURBT is the obturator reflex (Fig. 1). This reflex most commonly occurs during resection of a lateral wall tumor: electrical stimulation of the obturator nerve results in a sudden abduction of the leg. Bladder perforation and neurovascular injury have resulted from the obturator reflex. One strategy for prevention is neuromuscular paralysis with general anesthesia.

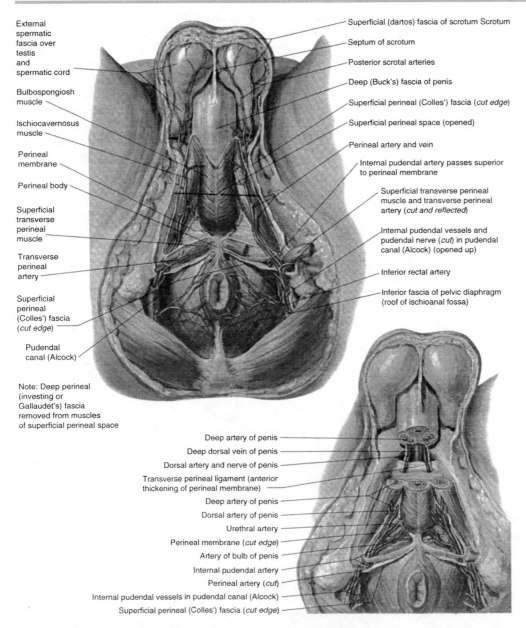

Figure 1 Pelvic anatomy. *Source:* From Netter, Frank H. *Atlas of Human Anatomy* plate 385.

Lasers have been used for some time as an alternative treatment for superficial bladder tumors, usually those less than 2 cm in diameter. The most frequently used lasers [neodymium + yttrium–aluminum–garnet (Nd:YAG) and holmium:YAG] offer several advantages: less bleeding, subjectively less pain, lower incidence of bladder spasms and dysuria, absence of obturator nerve stimulation, reduced need for Foley catheter, and substantially lower risk of bladder perforation (4). Specific laser training and safety issues must be addressed, and the lack of pathological tissue for review must be recognized. Because of the "forward scatter" effects of the Nd:YAG laser, the risk of bowel perforation exists, even when the bladder is apparently intact (5). If bowel perforation occurs, the signs and symptoms of peritonitis, such as free air under the diaphragm and pain, usually begin within the first 24 hours postoperatively. Ultimately, patients require laparotomy with resection of the damaged bowel segment. The risk of bowel injury can be reduced by avoiding excessive application of the laser energy in any given area and avoiding overdistention of the bladder, which thins the bladder wall. The risk of postoperative urinary tract infection (UTI) or urosepsis is reduced by ensuring negative preoperative urine cultures and perioperative antibiotic therapy. Rapid recognition of postoperative urosepsis before hospital discharge will allow treatment with appropriate empiric intravenous antibiotic therapy, intravenous fluid hydration, and definitive therapy based on culture and sensitivity results.

Radical Cystoprostatectomy

Invasive bladder cancer refers to tumor penetration through the lamina propria and into the muscularis propria (muscle layer of the bladder), with or without extension into the perivesical soft tissue (1). Most clinical urologists agree that bilateral pelvic lymph node dissection together with en bloc single-stage radical cystectomy and the creation of a continent or cutaneous urinary diversion is the treatment of choice for muscle-invasive bladder cancer (6). Exenterative pelvic surgery is rarely required. Alternative treatments exist for selected patients with locally advanced bladder cancer, such as various combinations of deep TURBT (7), partial cystectomy (8), radiation therapy (1), and chemotherapy (1). Although the survival rates associated with these alternative procedures may be lower than those associated with radical cystectomy, such treatments may be an alternative for high-risk patients or those who, for other reasons, are poor surgical candidates; these treatments may also be palliative (6,9,10). During the past few decades, improvements in anesthesia, antibacterial agents, and surgical techniques have dramatically decreased the morbidity and 30-day mortality rates associated with radical cystectomy. The morbidity rates have declined from approximately 35% to less than 10%, and the 30-day mortality rates have declined from

approximately 20% to less than 2% (11). Several reports have classified the surgical complications associated with radical cystectomy as acute or chronic and as minor or major (10–16).

Most muscle-invasive bladder cancers are diagnosed after endoscopic tumor resection. Imperative to the success of surgery for this type of cancer is the preoperative education of the patient about the type of urinary diversion that will be created. After a detailed review of all pathologic specimens and in-depth patient counseling, a metastatic evaluation is performed. This evaluation includes assessment of the upper urinary tract, urethral sampling, chest radiographs, renal and hepatic function examinations, and determination of cardiopulmonary risk status (12). Other important considerations are the patient's history of radiation exposure, other abdominal surgery, conditions such as inflammatory bowel disease and diverticulitis, hand–eye coordination, and manual dexterity. The stoma site is marked preoperatively in conjunction with an enterostomal nurse, and preoperative bowel preparation and antibiotic coverage are undertaken.

Briefly, the following general steps are involved in radical cystoprostatectomy: (i) laparotomy and exclusion of grossly metastatic intraperitoneal disease; (ii) bilateral pelvic–iliac lymphadenectomy; (iii) ligation and division of the anterolateral and dorsolateral vesical pedicles with subsequent ligation of Santorini's plexus; (iv) ureteral mobilization, tagging, and transection at the level of the iliac vessels; (v) incision of the peritoneum of the rectovesical pouch and blunt mobilization of the bladder posteriorly between Denonvillier's fascia and the rectum; (vi) ligation and transection of the dorsomedial pedicles; (vii) transection of Santorini's plexus and the urethra just distal to the prostate; and (viii) retrograde mobilization of the prostate with preservation of the neurovascular bundles, followed by excision of the gland (12). Routine removal of the appendix is associated with low morbidity rates and avoids future appendicitis but precludes the use of the appendix in any future reconstructive surgery that may be required (17).

A urethrectomy is indicated at the time of cystectomy if prostatic urethral biopsies indicate TCC or if gross carcinoma is detected at the prostatic urethral margin during excision; however, urethrectomy precludes construction of a neobladder (6,12,18,19,. A delayed urethrectomy may be performed after initial cystectomy and urinary diversion if urethral recurrence is discovered during routine follow-up. In addition, there is a 1% to 9% risk of upper-tract TCC after cystectomy; therefore, routine follow-up is encouraged (20). Either a cutaneous (e.g., ileal conduit) or a continent (e.g., neobladder) urinary diversion is performed. Additional maneuvers may include placing temporary stents across the ureteral anastomosis, inserting a closed suction drain, and performing appropriate urinary diversion drainage.

Urinary Diversion

The popularity of the various methods of urinary diversion has varied throughout the last century. An ideal reservoir should preserve upper urinary tract function by avoiding reflux and obstruction; allow high capacity with low pressure, thereby providing adequate compliance; and provide a continence mechanism that will allow achievable continence yet ease of emptying (Table 1) (21).

The oldest form of urinary diversion is the ureterosigmoidostomy; in this procedure, the ureters are anastomosed directly to the sigmoid colon (22). Before the antibiotic era, free reflux of urine contaminated with stool resulted in substantial morbidity and mortality rates related to repeated bouts of pyelonephritis and upper-tract deterioration (21). In response to this complication, antireflux procedures such as the Mainz II pouch were developed (23). Ureterosigmoidostomy is further complicated by a hyperchloremic metabolic acidosis, which is amplified by renal failure, and by an increased rate of colonic neoplasms (5–40%), especially among younger patients who require diversion for benign conditions and who have a long life expectancy (21). Although many of these young patients have already undergone rediversion, the risk of malignancy at the anastomotic site remains and lifelong surveillance is required (24–27).

Another form of urinary diversion is continent or incontinent cutaneous diversion. The ileal conduit popularized by Bricker anastomoses the ureters to an isolated segment of mid to distal ileum and then brings them through the abdominal wall as a stoma (28). An external appliance is required for collecting freely draining urine. A continent cutaneous diversion, in contrast, uses an isolated detubularized segment of bowel, usually ileum with or without cecum, to store adequate amounts of urine (typically 600–700 cc) at low pressures ($< 25\,cmH_2O$). This storage pouch (detubularized segment of bowel) prevents reflux; it is drained through a catheterizable continent stoma brought out to the skin. Many variations of this procedure use different segments of bowel to construct different stoma mechanisms, such as the Kock pouch (29), the Indiana pouch (30), the Mainz pouch (21,31), and the University of California Los Angeles (UCLA) right colonic pouch (21). Examples of such reservoirs are shown in Figure 2.

The overall rate of complications associated with "pouch" reservoirs is estimated at 10% to 35%; the rates of reoperation range from 10% to 20% (21,31–34). Corrective surgery may be indicated for urinary leakage through the efferent limb, difficulty in catheterizing the stoma, parastomal hernia, or afferent limb problems, such as stenosis or reflux leading to hydronephrosis and compromised renal function (34). The surgeon contemplating reoperation must have a thorough knowledge of the type of diversion and the segment of bowel used, so that damage to the diversion itself and inadvertent enterotomies can be avoided. Proper construction of the intussuscepted nipple valve and fixation of the distal efferent segment to the abdominal wall are crucial to preventing some of these complications (35). Removing a portion of the mesenteric fat before bringing the ileum through the stoma site may reduce the risk of parastomal hernia (32,34).

Other common complications are incontinence (most commonly nocturnal), stones in the pouch,

Table 1 Long-term complications in 198 of 675 patients treated with cystectomy and urinary diversion

Complication	No. (%)
Small bowel obstruction	50 (7.4)
Ureteroenteric stricture	47 (7.0)
Renal calculi	26 (3.9)
Acute pyelonephritis	21 (3.1)
Parastomal hernia	19 (2.8)
Stomal stenosis	19 (2.8)
Incisional hernia	15 (2.2)
Fistula	9 (1.8)
Colobic obstruction	8 (1.2)
Radiation proctitis	6 (0.9)
Hepatitis	3 (0.4)
Chronic renal failure	2 (0.3)
Pelvic abscess	2 (0.3)
Abdomincal wall abscess	2 (0.3)
Stomal prolapse	2 (0.3)
Other	6 (0.8)

Note: Total number of patients with one or more long-term complications 198 (29.3%).
Source: From Ref. 21.

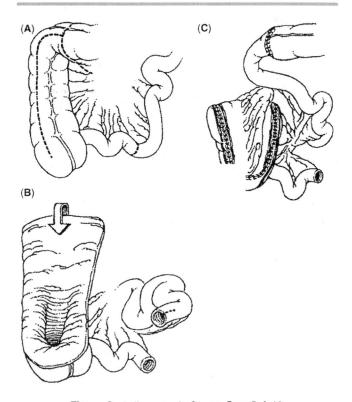

Figure 2 Indiana pouch. *Source*: From Ref. 10.

metabolic acidosis, and chronic bacteruria leading to "pouchitis." The risk of pouch stone formation can be reduced by eliminating staples from the exposed end of the nipple valves and replacing nonabsorbable sutures with absorbable sutures (34). Treatment of bladder stones is discussed below; however, options such as endoscopic lithotripsy (36), extracorporeal shock wave lithotripsy (37), percutaneous lithotripsy (38,39), and open stone removal (40) have been advocated for removing calculi from continent urinary diversions. Cases of malignancy within a pouch reservoir have also been documented (41,42).

Complications similar to those listed above are also possible after ileal conduit diversion (43). However, the complication rate associated with this procedure has steadily declined with improvements in preoperative nutritional assessment, surgical technique, antibiotic prophylaxis, absorbable suture material, and intensive care. Meticulous care during manipulation of the bowel and the ureter is necessary for preserving maximum blood supply. In addition, watertight ureterointestinal anastomoses, internal drainage with silicone stents, external drainage with Jackson Pratt or Penrose drains, and stoma drainage with red rubber catheters help to decrease the risk of early postoperative leakage.

Ureterointestinal leakage should be suspected when the patient is well hydrated, but stomal output decreases with a concurrent increase in drain output. The initial workup should include a measurement of the creatinine concentration in the drain fluid and either a loopogram or an intravenous pyelogram. Maintenance of the drains already in place is essential, but a certain percentage of patients may require additional urinary diversion, such as nephrostomy tubes or percutaneous drainage of a urinary collection. Definitive surgical management with open revision will often be necessary if conservative measures fail.

Early urinary leakage may lead to later ureterointestinal anastomotic stricture. Management techniques described for such a problem include endoscopic incision and stenting with open revision (44). Prolonged ileus, wound infection, sepsis, myocardial infarction, pulmonary embolism, and small-bowel obstruction are potential problems after any open abdominal procedure, and typical medical and surgical management is initiated. In cases of prolonged ileus or small-bowel obstruction, consultation with a general surgeon is often helpful. When concurrent bowel and urinary complications are encountered, such as a bowel leak and a urinary leak, treatment of the bowel condition should take precedence over treatment of the urinary condition because bowel complications are more likely to result in pelvic abscess, sepsis, and even death. Finally, adenocarcinoma has been reported to occur in the created ileal conduit diversion (45), but the rates are much lower than those associated with adenocarcinoma after ureterosigmoidostomy.

A final type of urinary diversion is an orthotopic bladder substitution or a neobladder. Usually, a

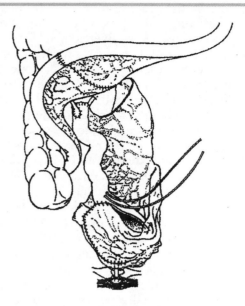

Figure 3 Studer neobladder. *Source:* From Ref. 32.

segment of distal ileum is isolated and detubularized for constructing a low-pressure, high-volume reservoir that is anastomosed to the native urethra. Continence is maintained via the external sphincter under voluntary control. Initially described by Camey et al. (46), orthotopic diversion may be performed by using any of the various techniques described by Elmajian et al. (47,48), Hautman et al. and Flohr et al. (49,50), Ghoneim et al. (51), Studer et al. (52), and others (53–55). Examples of orthotopic urinary diversion are shown in Figures 3 and 4. The Kock pouch has also been modified for emptying via the urethra.

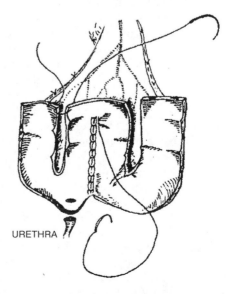

URETHRA

Figure 4 Ileal (Hautmann) neobladder. *Source:* From Ref. 32.

Some of the complications associated with orthotopic bladder substitution are similar to those associated with cutaneous diversion, such as urinary leakage, infection with urosepsis, pouch stones, ileus, obstruction, and incisional hernia. In one report, urinary continence was achieved by 85% of Kock neobladder substitutes; continence was defined as dryness or the use of no more than one pad during the day and night. This high rate of continence may be related to minimal anterior urethral dissection at the time of prostatic dissection (47). According to Schiff and Lytton (56), continence rates are mainly related to the pressure generated by the reservoir, the outflow resistance of the outlet, and the use of bowel detubularization to reduce uninhibited involuntary bowel contractions.

A secure, tension-free anastomosis between the urethra and the neobladder will reduce the likelihood of enterourethral fistula; however, if this complication does occur, it can usually be treated conservatively with drainage through a Foley catheter. Rupture of the neobladder must be included in the differential diagnosis of any patient who experiences acute abdomen and peritonitis during the postoperative period (57). Routine irrigation of the neobladder with saline is important because such irrigation will reduce the accumulation of intestinal mucus. The use of a neobladder is generally associated with a lower rate of reoperation during the late postoperative period.

Erectile dysfunction may occur after radical cystoprostatectomy, regardless of the type of diversion used (58). Preoperative assessment of erectile function is crucial for managing postoperative difficulties (59). The introduction of the nerve-sparing cystoprostatectomy by Walsh and Mostwin (60) has led to improved postoperative potency rates (60). Treatments for patients for whom erectile dysfunction persists include Viagra®, vacuum erection devices, injectable intracavernosal agents, transurethral agents, and, ultimately, penile prosthesis (61).

Metabolic complications of urinary diversion are always of concern to the urologist and are often an important cause of morbidity for the patient (62–64). Such consequences are mainly related to the type and length of bowel used, the type of diversion created, the patient's overall general health, and a history of abdominal surgery or irradiation (64). The pathophysiology of these metabolic derangements has been studied in depth and may be beyond the scope of this chapter, but a brief review of the therapeutic options and metabolic consequences associated with each bowel segment is provided below.

Parietal cells are stimulated to produce gastric acid (HCl) under the influences of the vagus nerve, histamine, and gastrin. Normally, the stomach exhibits a negative feedback loop through which increased production of acid decreases the antral production of gastrin. If this portion of the stomach is incorporated into the urinary reconstruction, a hypokalemic, hypochloremic metabolic alkalosis may occur and may lead to ulcerations in the pouch (62). This systemic alkalosis may be worsened by severe renal failure, which impairs the kidney's ability to secrete bicarbonate. Ulcerations may be part of the reason for the hematuria–dysuria syndrome (HDS) associated with gastrocystoplasty (see below). Treatment involves histamine receptor blockers, such as cimetidine or ranitidine, and proton pump inhibitors, such as omeprazole or lansoprazole (62).

Prolonged exposure of the jejunum to urine results in severe and possibly fatal electrolyte abnormalities; thus, the use of the jejunum for urinary diversion has generally been abandoned. A hyponatremic, hypochloremic, hyperkalemic metabolic acidosis results from the enhanced secretion of sodium and chloride and the increased absorption of potassium and hydrogen (62). Patients soon become dehydrated because water follows sodium down its equilibrium gradient, and this dehydration results in increased production of aldosterone. Increased reabsorption of sodium by the kidney results in urine low in sodium and high in potassium. When the jejunal mucosal surface is exposed to urine with these concentrations, the cycle is perpetuated as more sodium is lost and more potassium is absorbed. In the severe form of this condition, known as the jejunal conduit syndrome, patients may experience nausea, vomiting, anorexia, dehydration, lethargy, muscle weakness, and fever (63). Correction of the acidosis with administration of bicarbonate, infusion of saline, and drainage of the reservoir via a catheter are the initial treatment steps, and prolonged oral supplementation of sodium chloride is usually required (63).

The incorporation of ileum into urinary diversions is associated with much less severe metabolic abnormalities than is the incorporation of jejunum. A hypokalemic, hyperchloremic metabolic acidosis occurs; the extent of this acidosis may depend on the amount of ileum resected, the method of diversion used, and certain patient characteristics (64). A severe potential side effect of chronic acidosis is bone demineralization, which appears among children as rickets and among adults as osteomalacia. Osteoid replaces bone mineral because calcium and carbonate act as hydrogen ion buffers. Acidosis also impairs the activation of vitamin D and stimulates the activity of osteoclasts. These complications may be more evident among growing children and postmenopausal women than among other patients. The administration of sodium or potassium citrate is usually effective in correcting the acidosis, but supplemental chlorpromazine or nicotinic acid may be necessary for preventing chloride reabsorption because these two agents inhibit cyclic adenosine monophosphate, which impedes chloride reabsorption (62). Possible side effects of these medications include tardive dyskinesia (chlorpromazine) and exacerbation of liver dysfunction and peptic ulcer disease (nicotinic acid) (62). When large sections of the terminal ileum are resected, malabsorption of vitamin B12, bile acid, fatty acid, and fat-soluble vitamins may occur (64). Monthly injections of vitamin B12 are recommended once a deficiency has been detected. Excessive concentrations of bile salts and fatty acids may lead to soponification with calcium and resultant steatorrhea and selective oxalate reabsorption; in such cases, treatment begins with cholestyramine (62).

The use of large segments of colon in urinary diversion generally results in few major metabolic disturbances. Maintenance of the ileocecal valve is important for preventing the rapid transit of feces through the small bowel and colon and the reflux of large amounts of bacteria into the small intestine (64). Hypomagnesemia occasionally occurs because of malabsorption and renal tubular loss as the result of acidosis, and neuromuscular symptoms such as muscle fasciculation, tremor, tetany, and seizures may become evident (64). Treatment involves magnesium replacement. An increased ammonia load (because of increased absorption) in a patient with impaired hepatic function may result in hyperammonemia and hepatic coma (62). This rare syndrome is most commonly associated with ureterosigmoidostomy because urease-producing bacteria in the colon split urea to produce ammonia. Treatment involves draining the reservoir, administering lactulose, limiting protein intake, and administering antibiotics (62). Finally, adjustments in dosage may prevent the toxic effects of certain drugs, such as methotrexate, phenytoin, and theophylline, which are secreted unchanged in the urine and absorbed by the intestinal tract (62).

Partial Cystectomy

A final method of bladder tumor resection is partial cystectomy (8). Several indications for partial cystectomy are a solitary, primary, muscle-invasive tumor in an area of the bladder that will allow for adequate surgical margins (usually 2 cm); inability to achieve complete transurethral resection because of location or size of the tumor; tumor in a bladder diverticulum; or the inability to perform urinary diversion, either because the patient refuses it or because the patient is not a candidate for such a procedure (65). The ideal indications for partial cystectomy include tumor along the posterior wall or tumors in the dome of the bladder; the dome is a common site for urachal adenocarcinomas. In addition, certain metastatic lesions to the bladder, such as colon cancer, may be amendable to partial cystectomy (66). Several important contraindications to partial cystectomy are multiple tumors, carcinoma in situ or cellular atypia, trigonal or prostatic invasion, the inability to obtain adequate surgical margins, the inability to maintain functional bladder capacity, and the presence of extravesical tumor extension (65). If ureteral reimplantation is necessary after resection, strict adherence to surgical margin requirements is essential (66).

The general steps involved in partial cystectomy are transurethral resection or biopsy with pathological review; bimanual examination; peritoneal exploration to rule out tumor spread with subsequent closure of the peritoneum before the procedure continues; dissection of pelvic lymph nodes; mobilization of the bladder and excision of the tumor with wide, 2-cm margins; frozen-section analysis of full-thickness bladder wall and adjacent perivesical fat so that surgical margin status can be assessed; bladder closure in two layers with absorbable sutures, with placement of a closed-suction drain near the surgical site; and bladder drainage with a Foley catheter (65). Placing a suprapubic tube should be avoided because the development of a vesicocutaneous fistula may lead to tumor recurrence in this area; the recurrence rate for TCC after partial cystectomy ranges from 0% to 18% (65). Neoadjuvant and adjuvant chemotherapy or radiation after bladder-sparing surgery has been advocated for reducing the risk of wound recurrence (66). Most complications associated with partial cystectomy are considered minor and include wound hematoma or infection, urinary leak, transient hydronephrosis, and diminished bladder capacity. The overall complication rates range from 11% to 29% (65). Before the Foley catheter is removed, a cystogram should be performed so that the completeness of healing can be assessed. Indications for partial cystectomy other than malignancy include severe vesical endometriosis, refractory interstitial cystitis, and traumatic repair.

BLADDER AUGMENTATION

Another important procedure associated with potential urologic complications is bladder augmentation. Decades of work, mostly with pediatric patients, have provided various alternatives for increasing bladder capacity and compliance, improving bladder emptying, and strengthening outlet resistance. Initially described in the 1890s, bladder augmentation was performed to correct small, contracted bladders that resulted from tuberculosis cystitis (67). This condition remained the primary indication for bladder augmentation throughout the first half of the 20th century, until Lapides et al. (68) introduced clean intermittent catheterization and McGuire et al. (69) described the concept of bladder pressure and compliance. A wide range of subsequent indications for bladder augmentation soon developed, such as congenital anomalies (myelodysplasia, tethered spinal cord, posterior urethral valves, prune belly syndrome, bladder extrophy, and cloacal extrophy), spinal cord injury, multiple sclerosis, refractory interstitial and radiation cystitis, previous radical pelvic surgery, and traumatic injury (70).

Patients, especially children, may exhibit severe frequency, urgency, incontinence, upper and lower UTIs, VUR, various degrees of renal scarring or impaired renal growth, and, most importantly, a low-volume, poorly compliant, high-pressure bladder, as demonstrated by urodynamic evaluation (71). Usually, a conservative trial of behavioral training, intermittent self-catheterization, and anticholinergic medications is attempted, but when these measures fail to alleviate symptoms, surgical intervention is often required (71). Preoperative evaluation may include a voiding diary, urinalysis and urine culture, cytology (for adult patients), determination of serum blood count and chemistries for ruling out renal failure, liver function tests for ruling out hepatic insufficiency, video urodynamics, cystoscopy, and an evaluation of urinary tract anatomy and function. Examinations may include intravenous pyelogram, voiding cystourethrogram, and radionuclide scans (67).

The selection of tissue for the augmentation may depend on several factors. A severely dilated ureter, as seen in some cases of VUR or posterior urethral valves, may be used after ipsilateral nephrectomy for a poorly functioning or nonfunctioning kidney (72–74). Although such a ureter is rarely available, ureterocystoplasty results in no production of mucus and no electrolyte abnormalities because enteric segments are kept free of exposure to urine (72).

Using the stomach for gastrocystoplasty has been advocated for patients with renal dysfunction and acidosis because of the net secretion of hydrogen and chloride ions and the lack of absorption of ammonium (Fig. 5) (75–77). Some patients, however, are at risk of hypokalemic, hypochloremic metabolic alkalosis after gastrocystoplasty (74,78,79). The production of mucus and the occurrence of UTIs and stones are limited after gastrocystoplasty (76). As many as one-third of patients who undergo this type of augmentation experience repeated bouts of coffee-brown or red urine, suprapubic pain, cutaneous irritation, and burning with urination. This unique condition is referred to as the HDS (78–80). It is probably related to the lowered urinary pH that results from excessive secretion of HCl or from hypergastrinemia (76,79,80).

Most patients experience mild to moderate symptoms that are treatable with oral hydration and H-2 blockers or proton pump inhibitors. A small percentage of patients with intractable symptoms will require surgical revision for removing the gastric segment and replacing it with another intestinal segment (80).

As with continent urinary diversion, augmentation cystoplasty may use either small or large intestine. Described by Bramble (81), the "clam" enterocystoplasty, which uses a terminal ileal patch, provides relief of retractable bladder instability, increased compliance, and functional bladder capacity; it is associated with minimal early and late complications (81). Another option is ileocystoplasty, provided that no short-gut syndrome or other ileal pathology exists (67,70,82). Problems such as the production of mucus and electrolyte abnormalities (hypokalemia, hyperchloremia, and metabolic acidosis) are similar to those associated with ileal neobladders and ileal conduits. Treatment, especially for children, is important so that the development of osteomalacia and possible growth delay can be prevented (82). Daily bladder irrigation is essential during the early postoperative period because excessive production of mucus can obstruct urinary drainage, increase the risk of UTI, and act as a nidus for stone formation (83–85). Rates of stone formation as high as 52% have been reported after augmentation cystoplasty (84). The management of bladder stones is discussed below. Sigmoid colonic segments are also used for bladder augmentation because for some patients, especially children with myelodysplasia, leaving the ileocecal valve intact is imperative so that diarrhea can be prevented and fecal continence can be maintained (67).

An alternative technique, known as seromuscular colocystoplasty lined with urothelium, involves

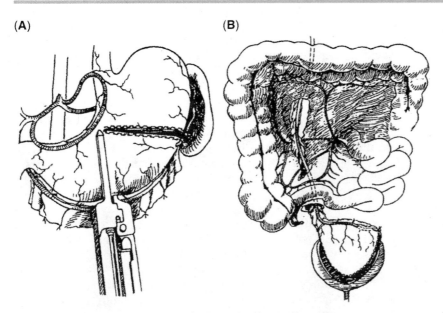

(A)   **(B)**

Figure 5 Gastrocystoplasty. *Source:* From Ref. 75.

removing the detrusor while sparing the urothelium; this is followed by an onlay of detubularized bowel void of its mucosa (74). The urodynamic results and continence rates associated with this procedure are similar to those associated with standard augmentation; however, this procedure avoids morbidity related to excessive production of mucus, metabolic derangement, and spontaneous perforation (86,87).

Regardless of the tissue segment used, most patients will require life-long intermittent self-catheterization because the bladder remains hypo-contractile. During follow-up, routine ultrasound measurement of postvoid residual urine will help gauge how well the bladder is emptying. When urethral catheterization is difficult, uncomfortable, or impossible, a catheterizable stoma is constructed, usually from the appendix, and is brought from the augmented bladder to the skin (88,89). The Mitrofanoff flap valve stoma (90) has provided durable results with respect to continence rates and stomal stenosis or stricture.

Perforation of the augmented bladder is always a feared complication; it occurs in as many as 3% to 6% of cases (67,71). Suspected causes of perforation are ischemia of the bowel segment wall as the result of overdistension with urine, trauma resulting from self-catheterization, chronic UTI, and a competent bladder outlet (91,92). Patients may exhibit acute abdomen or florid urosepsis or may simply complain of nausea with vague abdominal pain and distension; therefore, the physician must maintain a high degree of suspicion with regard to perforation. Although this complication usually occurs during the early post-operative period, an increasing number of cases of delayed perforation have been reported (92). If the situation permits, administering intravesical contrast and performing a cystogram will aid in the diagnosis of a leak or rupture. Intravenous hydration, the administration of broad-spectrum antibiotics, and urgent operative exploration and repair are generally the rule, although small leaks may be treated with urethral or suprapubic catheter drainage (92). Perforation sites may include the bowel segment, the anastomosis, and the native bladder. Preventing bladder overdistension by using strictly timed bladder emptying is encouraged.

Postoperative incontinence may be related to transposition of too short an intestinal segment and persistent low bladder capacity, a poorly constructed stoma, repeated bouts of UTI, or an incompetent bladder neck and external urethral sphincter (56). Therapeutic options for patients with poor outlet resistance are concomitant bladder neck sling or suspension, periurethral injection of a bulking agent, artificial urinary sphincter, bladder neck tubularization such as the Kropp procedure or Pippi Salle procedure, or bladder neck closure (93). After reviewing the available literature, Kryger et al. (93) suggested that placing an artificial urinary sphincter may be the procedure of choice for treating neurogenic sphincteric

incontinence with the goal of preserving spontaneous voiding (93). Some patients may be affected by nocturnal incontinence resulting from a full bladder (94). A strict sterile technique is crucial for preventing infection of an artificial urinary sphincter; such infection would require surgical removal.

Small-bowel obstruction related to intra-abdominal adhesions usually requires operative intervention. Although the true incidence of tumor occurrence is not known, several cases of malignancy within augmented bladders created with various intestinal segments have been reported (95–99). Life-long tumor surveillance with annual cystoscopy is recommended and should begin 10 years after surgery, especially for younger patients with long life expectancies (96).

BLADDER STONES

Reports of and references to bladder calculi are numerous throughout medical history. Stones have been found in Egyptian mummies, were mentioned in the Hippocratic oath, and were removed from the bladder by the earliest surgeons via perineal lithotomy around the first century, via suprapubic lithotomy in the 1500s, and via transurethral lithotomy in the 1800s (100). Various minimally invasive procedures are used today for removing bladder stones. Open surgery is reserved for the largest stones and is performed during concurrent open prostatectomy.

In the past, bladder stones resulted primarily from malnutrition, dietary inadequacies, and UTI (100). Throughout much of the developed world, the incidence of bladder stones related to these causes has decreased dramatically; however, the incidence of bladder stones remains high in certain areas of Southeast Asia, Northern Africa, and the Middle East, mainly among children (100). For adults, the development of bladder stones is mainly related to urinary stasis, as seen with outlet obstruction and neurogenic bladder (101). Leading causes of bladder stones among men are benign prostatic hypertrophy, urethral stricture disease, and bladder neck contracture after prostatectomy; among women, the primary causes of bladder stones are cystoceles and obstruction after incontinence surgery (100,101). The encrustation of foreign bodies may lead to stone formation, as has been reported with retained ureteral stents, long-term indwelling Foley catheters (especially for patients with spinal cord injury), suture material, and materials placed by the patient. Patients may have no symptoms or may experience suprapubic pain, dysuria, frequency, hesitancy, terminal gross hematuria, or sudden interruption of voiding by the obstructing stone. Examination may provide evidence of suprapubic fullness, enlarged prostate, cystocele, neurologic abnormalities, or elevated postvoid residual volumes (100). Workup includes urinalysis for detecting infection (with subsequent antibiotic therapy if the results are positive); kidney, ureter, and bladder radiography to detect calcifications; and possibly renal–bladder ultrasound, spiral noncontrast computed tomography (CT), or cystourethroscopy for confirmation (100). Initial medical therapy with urinary alkalinization may be attempted for stone dissolution, but operative intervention will probably be necessary. Before surgical treatment is planned, the physician must recognize the underlying cause of stone formation. For example, a middle-aged man with a bladder stone probably has some degree of prostatic obstruction that may or may not require transurethral resection of the prostate (TURP) or open prostatectomy.

Transurethral Cystolitholapaxy and Shockwave Lithotripsy

The initial approach for most patients is transurethral bladder stone destruction (100). In the operating room, a cystoscope can be placed and subsequent litholapaxy can be accomplished with a variety of lithotrites, such as mechanical lithotripsy, the Swiss Lithoclast®, electrohydrolic lithotripsy, ultrasound, and laser energy (102). The use of the holmium:YAG laser has been shown to be effective, technically feasible, and safe, even for bladder calculi larger than 4 cm in diameter (102,103).

Potential perioperative complications associated with transurethral procedures are urinary infection or urosepsis, bleeding, and bladder perforation (100). Prophylactic antibiotic coverage is essential because many of these stones are inherently infected. Excessive postoperative hematuria can be prevented by careful instrumentation and avoidance of torque on the prostate; when this condition occurs, it can be managed with continuous vigorous bladder irrigation by hand or via a three-way catheter. Bladder perforations can be managed according to the procedures discussed above for TURBT.

Late complications include urethral stricture after prolonged cystoscopic manipulation and recurrence of the bladder stone after inadequate treatment of the underlying cause (100). If concurrent TURP is to be performed, the lithotripsy portion should be performed first so that the potential complications of excessive blood loss and hypotonic fluid resorption associated with TURP can be avoided (100). Endoscopic treatment of bladder stones is reported to be safe and effective for children after augmentation cystoplasty (104).

An alternative, minimally invasive procedure for treating bladder stones is shockwave lithotripsy (SWL). Adequate stone clearance with minimal complications has been reported when calculi are less than 3 cm in diameter and patients are treated in the prone position (105). SWL has also been used to treat larger calculi (4–6 cm in diameter) with patients in the seated position (106). Bladder outlet obstruction resulting from prostatic enlargement or urethral stricture must be treated initially so that fragment impaction can be prevented after SWL.

Percutaneous and Open Stone Removal

An alternative to transurethral stone destruction, especially for children and patients with surgically reconstructed bladders, is percutaneous suprapubic cystolitholapaxy (107–111). A shorter instrument with a larger diameter is used for this procedure; this instrument allows rapid stone destruction and evacuation of stone fragments. Different means of percutaneous access have been described; the important step is avoidance of bowel injury, especially for patients who have previously undergone lower abdominal or pelvic surgery (107–111). The lithotrites used in this procedure are similar to those used in the transurethral approach; combinations of the two may also be used. When the bladder stone is accompanied by a large adenomatous prostate gland (more than 100 g) or a large bladder diverticulum, open suprapubic cystotomy with possible diverticulectomy may be the procedure of choice (100). Bladder calculi are removed with 100% accuracy before surgical removal of the enlarged prostatic lobe. Recuperation may be somewhat longer for open surgery. Prevention and treatment of potential postoperative complications such as sepsis and hemorrhage are similar to those for complications of transurethral cystolitholapaxy. Fistula formation is always a concern when the bladder is explored; its incidence can be reduced by meticulous two- or three-layer closure of the cystotomy site. Placing a drain may help detect any urinary leakage.

VESICOURETERAL REFLUX AND URETEROCELES

VUR and ureteroceles are two common urologic anomalies that occur most frequently among children. VUR is the retrograde flow of urine from the bladder through the ureter, the kidney, or both (112). VUR may be primary, due to a congenital lack of longitudinal muscle of the intravesical ureter, or it may be secondary, due to elevated bladder pressure with bladder outlet obstruction or voiding dysfunction (113). A ureterocele is a congenital dilatation of the distal segment of the ureter. Ureteroceles have been traditionally categorized as intravesical or ectopic in location, unilateral or bilateral, and associated with a single or a duplicated collecting system (114). Surgical intervention with its associated potential complications is often necessary for treating both disease processes.

Prenatal hydronephrosis often leads to VUR after birth. Alternatively, when newborns or young children exhibit symptoms of a UTI, renal–bladder ultrasonography and voiding cystourethrography will help confirm the presence of hydronephrosis and urinary reflux (113). Repeated bouts of infection may lead to renal scarring and subsequent loss of renal function. Thus, the primary objective of treating children with VUR is preventing these episodes of pyelonephritis and preserving renal function (112).

Initial antibiotic prophylaxis is the medical treatment of choice for most grades of VUR because the reflux often spontaneously resolves. Indications for surgical intervention include breakthrough UTIs, high-grade reflux associated with renal scarring, noncompliance with antibiotic prophylaxis, persistence of reflux in girls approaching puberty, and worsening in the grade of reflux over time (113).

The mainstay of surgical treatment is ureteral reimplantation, which can be performed as an open or a laparoscopic procedure and either intravesically or extravesically (113). Subureteral polytetrafluoroethylene injection has been described as an alternative endoscopic approach for correcting VUR, but the likelihood of durable results may be lower than that associated with primary reimplantation (115). The primary complication of ureteral reimplantation is subsequent urinary obstruction, mainly as a result of the technical intricacies of the procedure. However, when ureteral reimplantation is performed by experienced pediatric urologists, the associated rate of obstruction is relatively low (113). Postoperative stenting may aid in preventing early, transient ureteral obstruction by allowing edema and spasm to resolve. Late ureteral obstruction may be a result of tissue ischemia or ureteral angulation and compression during bladder filling. In such cases, surgical revision is often necessary (113).

Ureteroceles may be diagnosed by prenatal ultrasonography; alternatively, young infants may exhibit bladder outlet obstruction or urosepsis (114). In most cases, intravesical ureteroceles may be initially treated with endoscopic incision, but such treatment may not be possible for extravesical (ectopic) ureteroceles because controversy exists about the initial therapeutic intervention (114,116). Ectopic ureteroceles are often associated with an ipsilateral duplicated collecting system, and the upper pole moiety is often substantially dilated as a result of the distal obstruction. Initial transurethral puncture may temporarily stabilize renal function, but as many as 70% of patients will require secondary reconstructive surgery (117). Complete recovery of renal function is usually not possible even after the obstruction has been relieved; therefore, one initial surgical option is upper pole partial nephrectomy with or without ureterectomy (114,116). In addition to the upper pole obstruction, as many as 50% of patients will have VUR of the lower pole moiety or the contralateral kidney (116). An alternative surgical option, therefore, is a combination of upper tract surgery (e.g., heminephrectomy) with lower tract surgery (e.g., ureteral reimplantation) (114,116). Because not all patients with VUR will require reimplantation, patient selection is important and is based on the degree of reflux, the presence or absence of renal scarring, and the patient's age (118).

Potential complications of partial nephrectomy are acute vascular injury to the functioning lower pole; hemorrhage; the formation of urinary leak, urinoma, or both; and UTI. Careful dissection, knowledge of renal vascular anatomy, and placement of a drain postoperatively will aid in preventing such complications. Incomplete excision or inaccurate puncture of the ureterocele may cause the formation of an obstructing urethral flap, whereas excessive excision may damage the urinary sphincter, thereby causing incontinence (114).

URINARY INCONTINENCE

Urinary incontinence is frequently a reason for patients' visits to a urology clinic; this condition may be a result of dysfunctional bladder filling or emptying. A complete review of incontinence is beyond the scope of this chapter, and the forms of incontinence (stress, urge, overflow, and mixed) have been meticulously described in textbooks and in the medical literature. A careful history and physical examination will usually uncover the underlying cause. Medical therapy with agents such as tolterodine and oxybutynin is useful in treating the "overactive" bladder by relieving the symptoms of urgency and frequency. Various options for surgical treatment of urinary incontinence have been advocated.

The administration of periurethral bulking agents may be used as an initial attempt at treating incontinence related to intrinsic urinary sphincter deficiency if the patient is reluctant to undergo an open procedure. Alternatively, the administration of such agents may be attempted as an adjuvant treatment for persistent leakage after an open procedure (119). The agents are usually placed transurethrally under direct cystoscopic vision. Agents approved by the U.S. Food and Drug Administration include bovine collagen, autologous fat, and carbon beads (Durasphere®) (119). Bulking agents are an attractive alternative for patients because their placement is relatively simple, the associated morbidity rates are low, and patients often notice immediate results. Although bulking agents do not usually provide a permanent cure, repeated injections may leave many patients satisfied with the results (119). Temporary postoperative urinary retention is the most frequently encountered complication; it probably results from urethral edema along the injection site or from sphincter spasm. Treatment usually involves intermittent self-catheterization for a few days until the edema has resolved. Symptomatic UTIs may occur and are best prevented by ensuring that the results of preoperative urine cultures are negative for infection and by maintaining sterile technique through out the performance of the procedure.

Open surgical procedures for urinary incontinence include transvaginal bladder neck suspensions, retropubic urethropexy, pubovaginal sling, and artificial urinary sphincters (120). Retropubic urethropexy and its associated complications are discussed in chapter 48 of this textbook. An in-depth comparison of specific anti-incontinence procedures, with a review of expected results and reasons for selection, is not the focus of this chapter. Therefore, documented complications associated with the surgical treatment of urinary incontinence will be discussed as a whole.

Intraoperative complications may be recognized during the procedure or shortly thereafter. Injuries to the bladder or the urethra may occur during dissection or when a needle or trocar is passed to position the suspending material (121). Cystoscopy will often rule out such injuries. Some authors advocate immediate repair or repositioning the needle or trocar and continuing the procedure (121). Failure to recognize such an injury may result in vesicovaginal or urethrovaginal fistulas. When transvaginal fistulas occur, their repair may be early or delayed, with similar results (122,123). In addition, any retained material, such as permanent suture, may result in recurrent UTI or bladder stone formation. Inadvertent bowel injury may occur during trocar placement, suprapubic dissection, or placement of a suprapubic catheter, and the subsequent risk of infection is increased when artificial materials are used (120). Mild bleeding is frequently the result of transvaginal dissection, but serious hemorrhage and severe pelvic or vaginal hematomas are relatively uncommon (121). Infiltration of the anterior vaginal wall with normal saline will facilitate development of the proper plane for dissection. Direct pressure may be temporarily applied, but suture-ligature of the bleeding vessels under direct vision may be necessary if the procedure is to continue. Postoperative vaginal packing often controls venous oozing. Most patients are placed in the dorsal lithotomy position for anti-incontinence procedures; such positioning creates the risk of postoperative nerve damage (121). Careful patient positioning and padding of pressure points may reduce the risk of damage to the peroneal nerve; this damage manifests itself postoperatively by ipsilateral foot drop.

Acute and chronic postoperative complications are also well known. One of the most frequently experienced complications after any type of anti-incontinence procedure is postoperative urinary retention (121). This condition often results from transient inflammation and edema at the dissection site, the effects of general anesthesia, or the patient's perception of pain on urination immediately after the procedure (121). In addition, suture or sling material may have been fashioned or secured too tightly, and this problem results in compression of the urethra or the bladder neck (120). Placing a suprapubic catheter during the procedure helps prevent acute retention. Alternatively, patients may need to learn to perform intermittent self-catheterization. If outlet obstruction persists, urethrolysis may be indicated (124). Approximately 5% to 10% of patients experience persistent stress urinary incontinence, which may occur if the sling material is tied too loosely, is positioned improperly, is separated from its anchoring tissue, or undergoes breakage or degradation (120). Approximately 10% to 30% of

patients may experience de novo urgency symptoms as the result of a sudden change in bladder outlet resistance induced by the anti-incontinence procedure itself (120). Symptoms are usually transient and are best managed with usual anticholinergic therapy. Finally, some patients who undergo artificial urinary sphincter implantation may require revision for erosion, malfunction, or infection (125).

LAPAROSCOPY

Some physicians have advocated increased use of the laparoscopic approach to bladder surgery because laparoscopy is associated with less postoperative pain, shorter hospital stays, and improved cosmetic results (126). In fact, several of the previously described procedures have been performed laparoscopically, such as pelvic lymphadenectomy, simple and radical cystectomy, ileal conduit diversion, bladder augmentation, ureteral reimplantation, and bladder neck suspension (126–130). Complication rates decrease as operative experience increases; however, certain complications are unique to laparoscopy (128).

More than a decade ago, the laparoscopic procedure most commonly performed was pelvic lymph node dissection before radical prostatectomy. At that time, if the results of intraoperative frozen-section examination were positive for lymph node involvement, consideration was given to not performing prostatectomy. Changes in clinical management have limited the role of isolated laparoscopic pelvic lymph node dissection, but many of the reports of complications in the literature include this procedure for analysis and discussion. In one review of 372 patients who underwent laparoscopic pelvic lymph node dissection, vascular injuries were the most common complication, followed by visceral injury to the bowel, bladder, and ureter (129). The mechanism of injury was usually traumatic trocar insertion or sharp dissection. The epigastric vessels, distal aorta, and common iliac vessels are at greatest risk of injury, and these vessels can best be avoided by careful midline insertion of the Veress needle or the Hasson cannula (128,129,131). When a vascular injury is immediately recognized, control and repair may be attempted laparoscopically, but conversion to laparotomy should occur without hesitation if initial attempts are unsuccessful (132). Inspecting the abdomen with lower insufflation pressures, both before and at the end of the case, will help identify possible injuries. When the operation proceeds near small or large bowel, the use of bipolar coagulation or ultrasonic dissectors and limiting the use of monopolar coagulation may decrease the risk of injury or perforation to the bowel (128).

A complication that is unique to laparoscopy is carbon dioxide (CO_2) absorption. Elevated CO_2 absorption during laparoscopic pelvic procedures occurs when subcutaneous emphysema is present,

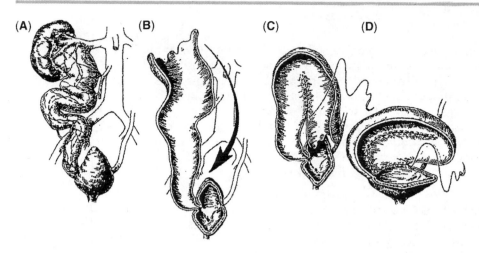

Figure 6 Control of bleeding from anterior wall vessel injured during port placement. *Source:* From Ref. 132.

when extraperitoneal insufflation is performed, and when the duration of insufflation is prolonged (133). Increased absorption may place patients with pulmonary compromise (chronic obstructive pulmonary disease, obesity, etc.) at an added risk of intraoperative or postoperative complications. Meticulous fascial closure of all port sites larger than 5 mm will help reduce the risk of postoperative incisional hernia (Fig. 6) (128). Finally because the likelihood of complications associated with laparoscopic surgery is higher when the procedure is performed by inexperienced surgeons, formal urologic residencies and fellowship training should include training in such skills (128,134).

BLADDER TRAUMA

An important topic of discussion regarding bladder complications is traumatic bladder injury. Again, a substantial volume of literature about urologic injury is available for review; therefore, this chapter will contain only a brief overview of mechanisms of injury, diagnosis, treatment, and potential complications.

Traumatic injuries to the bladder include contusions, extraperitoneal rupture, and intraperitoneal rupture. Such injuries account for approximately 22% of all urologic injuries (135). Blunt trauma (e.g., motor vehicle accidents, falls, and assault) to the pelvis and abdomen is the most common mechanism of bladder injury, accounting for 60% to 85% of injuries, whereas penetrating bladder trauma (e.g., gunshot wounds and stabbings) accounts for the remainder (136). Approximately 95% of patients with a ruptured bladder will exhibit gross hematuria, and 50% to 85% of the perforations will be extraperitoneal (137). Other important findings include suprapubic pain, anuria, blood at the urethral meatus, perineal swelling and hematoma, or the presence of a high riding prostate detected by digital rectal examination. Careful consideration must be given to an injury in the lower urinary tract when a severe pelvic fracture has been detected because 5% to 10% of patients with a fractured pelvis

will also have a ruptured bladder (137). If the patient's condition is hemodynamically stable, the key radiographic study is retrograde urethrography plus cystography or CT-guided cystography (135–141). When performed properly, static cystography involves instilling 300 to 500 cc of a water-soluble contrast solution under gravity, with slight overinjection at the end

(A)

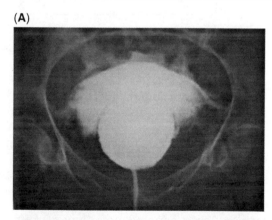

(B)

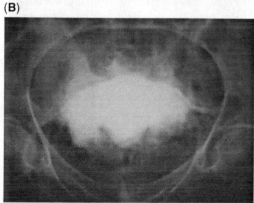

Figure 7 Intraoperative cystogram showing **(A)** filling and **(B)** drainage films.

CASE STUDY

An 82-year-old woman visited a urologist. She had a history of low-grade, low-stage papillary transitional cell carcinoma of the bladder with several recurrences over a 10-year period. The disease had not progressed during this time period. She had missed several scheduled appointments for routine follow-up. At the time of the current presentation, she was not experiencing gross hematuria or other lower urinary tract symptoms. Given her history, flexible cystoscopy was performed in the physician's office. Several large (4–5 cm) bladder tumors with a papillary appearance were detected on the right lateral wall and the dome of the bladder. The patient was scheduled for TURBTs.

In the operating room, the patient was given spinal anesthesia and was placed into the lithotomy position. The entire bladder was thoroughly inspected with the 12° and the 70° lens. The previously identified bladder tumors were readily visible. Transurethral resection was begun with the tumor located along the lateral wall of the bladder. An attempt was made to resect the tumor at its base and along the bladder wall. After resection, perivesical fat was readily identified, a finding suggestive of bladder perforation. Further tumor resection was discontinued, and intraoperative gravity cystography was performed. The contrast material surrounded the exterior of the bladder but did not enter the peritoneal cavity (Fig. 7). An extraperitoneal bladder perforation was diagnosed. Hemostasis was achieved, and a 20-Fr Foley catheter was placed for drainage. The patient remained in the hospital overnight for observation and was discharged home the following morning. Oral antibiotics were prescribed. Twelve days later, follow-up formal cystography showed no evidence of extravasation. The Foley catheter was removed, and the patient was free of symptoms. She was scheduled for subsequent TURBT.

of filling under pressure and appropriate anterior–posterior, oblique (if feasible), and postdrainage views (137). Extravasation confined to the pelvis appears as whisks, streaks, or sunbursts and indicates extraperitoneal bladder rupture, whereas extravasation that diffuses throughout the abdominal cavity and outlines bowel or settles in the paracolic gutters indicates intraperitoneal bladder rupture.

Most penetrating injuries require surgical exploration so that associated injuries to other organs and structures can be detected (140). When intraperitoneal bladder rupture is diagnosed after blunt injury, surgical exploration and repair are usually indicated because concomitant visceral injury is usually present (137,141). For extraperitoneal bladder rupture, nonoperative conservative management is recommended because minimal morbidity has been reported (137–142). Therapy consists of Foley catheter drainage and administration of broad-spectrum antibiotics for 7 to 10 days, at which time a follow-up cystogram is performed for documenting complete bladder healing before the catheter is removed. Persistent gross hematuria with obstructing clots, evidence of urosepsis, or persistent extraperitoneal extravasation should alert the clinician to the need for surgical exploration. Surgical principles of repair of traumatic bladder rupture include dissection through the peritoneum to the bladder dome, inspection of the entire bladder for injury, identification of the course of the ureters, avoidance of exploration of pelvic hematomas,

water-tight closure of the bladder in two or three layers with 2–0 or 3–0 absorbable sutures, placement of a suprapubic catheter through a separate cystotomy incision, and possible placement of a pelvic drain (136,137). Again, administering antibiotics will decrease the risk of pelvic abscess, especially if a pelvic hematoma or orthopedic hardware is present.

Potential complications that may result from the trauma itself or during the recovery period include persistent urinary extravasation, hemorrhage, pelvic infection, wound dehiscence, small capacity bladder, de novo urge incontinence, and erectile dysfunction (136,143). A large volume of output from the pelvic drain may indicate a persistent urinary leak, usually due to unrecognized lacerations or leakage along the suture line. This leakage usually resolves with continued catheter drainage but may occasionally place the fascia at risk of separation. During surgical exploration, avoiding pelvic hematomas will decrease the risk of serious bleeding. Antibiotic coverage is essential for preventing pelvic infection or UTI. Excessive debridement of the bladder injury can result in loss of functional bladder capacity and the development of bothersome lower urinary tract symptoms. Finally, neurovascular injury resulting from the trauma or from radical surgical exploration can lead to erectile dysfunction. If erectile dysfunction occurs, its evaluation should be delayed until all serious injuries have been addressed and stabilized (143).

CONCLUSIONS

A wide variety of indications exist for bladder surgery. Inherent to the techniques described above are potential associated complications. Thorough knowledge of patient selection, pathophysiology, anatomy, surgical technique, and potential complications will reduce the morbidity and mortality rates associated with bladder surgery.

REFERENCES

1. Walsh PC, Retik AB, Vaughan ED, Wein AJ. Urothelial tumor of the urinary tract. In: Walsh PC, Wein AJ, Retik AB, Vaughan ED, Vaughan ED Jr, eds. Campbell's Urology. 7th ed. Vol. 3. Philadelphia: Saunders, 1998: 2327–2410.
2. Holzbeierlein JM, Smith JA Jr. Surgical management of noninvasive bladder cancer (stages Ta/T1/CIS). Urol Clin North Am 2000; 27:15–24, vii–viii.
3. Mydlo JH, Weinstein R, Shah S, Solliday M, Macchia RJ. Long-term consequences from bladder perforation and/or violation in the presence of transitional cell carcinoma: results of a small series and a review of the literature. J Urol 1999; 161:1128–1132.
4. Smith JA Jr. Laser surgery for transitional-cell carcinoma. Technique, advantages, and limitations. Urol Clin North Am 1992; 19:473–483.
5. Smith JA Jr. Laser treatment of urologic cancers. Semin Surg Oncol 1989; 5:30–37.
6. Lerner SP, Skinner E, Skinner DG. Radical cystectomy in regionally advanced bladder cancer. Urol Clin North Am 1992; 19:713–723.
7. Herr HW. Transurethral resection in regionally advanced bladder cancer. Urol Clin North Am 1992; 19:695–700.
8. Hinman F Jr. Partial cystectomy. In: Hinman F, Donley S, Stempen PH, eds. Atlas of Urologic Surgery. 2nd ed. New York: Elsevier, 1998:501–520.
9. Droller MJ. Bladder cancer: state of the art care. CA Cancer J Clin 1998; 48(5):269–284.
10. Bales GT, Kim H, Steinberg GD. Surgical therapy for locally advanced bladder cancer. Semin Oncol 1996; 23:605–613.
11. Gschwend JE, Fair WR, Vieweg J. Radical cystectomy for invasive bladder cancer: contemporary results and remaining controversies. Eur Urol 2000; 38:121–130.
12. Turner WH, Studer UE. Cystectomy and urinary diversion. Semin Surg Oncol 1997; 13:350–358.
13. Frazier HA, Robertson JE, Paulson DF. Complications of radical cystectomy and urinary diversion: a retrospective review of 675 cases in 2 decades. J Urol 1992; 148:1401–1405.
14. Skinner DG, Crawford ED, Kaufman JJ. Complications of radical cystectomy for carcinoma of the bladder. J Urol 1980; 123:640–643.
15. Johnson DE, Lamy SM. Complications of a single stage radical cystectomy and ileal conduit diversion: review of 214 cases. J Urol 1977; 117:171–173.
16. Brannan W, Fuselier HA Jr, Ochsner M, Randrup ER. Critical evaluation of 1-stage cystectomy—reducing morbidity and mortality. J Urol 1981; 125:640–642.
17. Neulander EZ, Hawke CK, Soloway MS. Incidental appendectomy during radical cystectomy: an interdepartmental survey and review of the literature. Urology 2000; 56:241–244.
18. Hardeman SW, Soloway MS. Urethral recurrence following radical cystectomy. J Urol 1990; 144:666–669.
19. Freeman JA, Esrig D, Stein JP, Skinner DG. Management of the patient with bladder cancer. Urethral recurrence. Urol Clin North Am 1994; 21:645–651.
20. Braslis KG, Soloway MS. Management of ureteral and renal pelvic recurrence after cystectomy. Urol Clin North Am 1994; 21:653–659.
21. Walsh PC, Retik AB, Vaughan ED, Wein AJ. Use of intestinal segments and urinary diversion. In: Campbell's Urology. Vol. 3. 1998:3121.
22. Hendren WH. Historical perspective of the use of bowel in urology. Urol Clin North Am 1997; 24: 703–713.
23. Fisch M, Wammack R, Müller SC, Hohenfellner R. The Mainz pouch II (sigma rectum pouch). J Urol 1993; 149:258–263.
24. Spence HM, Hoffman WW, Fosmire GP. Tumour of the colon as a late complication of ureterosigmoidostomy for exstrophy of the bladder. Br J Urol 1979; 51: 466–470.
25. Husmann DA, Spence HM. Current status of tumor of the bowel following ureterosigmoidostomy: a review. J Urol 1990; 144:607–610.
26. Sohn M, Fuzesi L, Deutz F, Lagrange W, Kirkpatrick JC, Braun JC. Signet ring cell carcinoma in adenomatous polyp at site of ureterosigmoidostomy 16 years after conversion to ileal conduit. J Urol 1990; 143:805–807.
27. Gittes RF. Carcinogenesis in ureterosigmoidostomy. Urol Clin North Am 1986; 13:201–205.
28. Bricker EM. Bladder substitution after pelvic evisceration. Surg Clin North Am 1950; 30:1511–1521.
29. Kock NG, Nilson LO, Nilsson LJ, Norlen LJ, Philipson BM. Urinary diversion via a continent ileal reservoir: clinical results in 12 patients. J Urol 1982; 128:469–475.
30. Rowland RG, Mitchell ME, Bihrle R, Kahnoski RJ, Piser JE. Indiana continent urinary reservoir. J Urol 1987; 137:1136–1139.
31. Razor BR. Continent urinary reservoirs. Semin Oncol Nurs 1993; 9:272–285.
32. Benson MC, Olsson CA. Urinary diversion. Urol Clin North Am 1992; 19:779–795.
33. Killeen KP, Libertino JA. Management of bowel and urinary tract complications after urinary diversion. Urol Clin North Am 1988; 15:183–194.
34. Lieskovsky G, Skinner DG, Boyd SD. Complications of the Kock pouch. Urol Clin North Am 1988; 15: 195–205.
35. Stein JP, Freemen JA, Esrig D, et al. Complications of the afferent antireflux valve mechanism in the Kock ileal reservoir. J Urol 1996; 155:1579–1584.
36. Cohen TD, Streem SB. Minimally invasive endourologic management of calculi in continent urinary reservoirs. Urology 1994; 43:865–868.
37. Boyd SD, Everett RW, Schiff WM, Fugelso PD. Treatment of unusual Kock pouch urinary calculi with extracorporeal shock wave lithotripsy. J Urol 1988; 139:805–806.
38. Seaman EK, Benson MC, Shabsigh R. Percutaneous approach to treatment of Indiana pouch stones. J Urol 1994; 151:690–692.

39. Jarrett TW, Pound CR, Kavoussi LR. Stone entrapment during percutaneous removal of infection stones from a continent diversion. J Urol 1999; 162:775–776.

40. Sait K, Stuart G, Nation J, Ghatage P. Urolithiasis following formation of a continent urostomy: case report and review of the literature. Gynecol Oncol 2000; 77:330–333.

41. L'Esperance JO, Lakshmanan Y, Trainer AF, Jiang Z, Blute RD Jr., Ayvazian PA. Adenocarcinoma in an Indiana pouch after cystectomy for transitional cell carcinoma. J Urol 2001; 165:901–902.

42. Wang DS, Silverman ML, Bihrle W III. Stomal recurrence of bladder carcinoma after cystectomy. J Urol 1999; 162:157.

43. Schmidt JD, Hawtrey CE, Flocks RH, Culp DA. Complications, results and problems of ileal conduit diversions. J Urol 1973; 109:210–216.

44. Cornud F, Lefebvre JF, Chretien Y, Helenon O, Moreau JF. Percutaneous transrenal electro-incision of ureterointestinal anastomotic strictures: long-term results and comparison of fluoroscopic and endoscopic guidance. J Urol 1996; 155:1575–1578.

45. Sakano S, Yoshihiro S, Joko K, Kawano H, Naito K. Adenocarcinoma developing in an ileal conduit. J Urol 1995; 153:146–148.

46. Camey M, Botto H, Richard E. Complications of the Camey procedure. Urol Clin North Am 1988; 15:249–255.

47. Elmajian DA, Stein JP, Esrig D, et al. The Kock ileal neobladder: updated experience in 295 male patients. J Urol 1996; 156:920–925.

48. Elmajian DA, Stein JP, Skinner DG. Orthotopic urinary diversion: the Kock ileal neobladder. World J Urol 1996; 14:40–46.

49. Hautmann RE, Egghart G, Frohnberg D, Miller K. The ileal neobladder. J Urol 1988; 139:39–42.

50. Flohr P, Hefty R, Paiss T, Hautmann R. The ileal neobladder—updated experience with 306 patients. World J Urol 1996; 14:22–26.

51. Ghoneim MA, Kock NG, Lycke G, el-Din AB. An appliance-free, sphincter-controlled bladder substitute: the urethral Kock pouch. J Urol 1987; 138:1150–1154.

52. Studer UE, Danuser H, Hochreiter W, Springer JP, Turner WH, Zingg EJ. Summary of 10 years' experience with an ileal low-pressure bladder substitute combined with an afferent tubular isoperistaltic segment. World J Urol 1996; 14:29–39.

53. Reddy PK, Lange PH, Fraley EE. Total bladder replacement using detubularized sigmoid colon: technique and results. J Urol 1991; 145:51–55.

54. Benson MC, Seaman EK, Olsson CA. The ileal ureter neobladder is associated with a high success and a low complication rate. J Urol 1996; 155:1585–1588.

55. Cancrini A, De Carli P, Pompeo V, et al. Lower urinary tract reconstruction following cystectomy: experience and results in 96 patients using the orthotopic ileal neobladder substitution of Studer et al. Eur Urol 1996; 29:204–209.

56. Schiff SF, Lytton B. Incontinence after augmentation cystoplasty and internal diversion. Urol Clin North Am 1991; 18:383–392.

57. Haupt G, Pannek J, Knopf HJ, Schulze H, Senge T. Rupture of ileal neobladder due to urethral obstruction by mucous plug. J Urol 1990; 144:740–741.

58. Melman A. Iatrogenic causes of erectile dysfunction. Urol Clin North Am 1988; 15:33–39.

59. Lue TF. Impotence after radical pelvic surgery: physiology and management. Urol Int 1991; 46:259–265.

60. Walsh PC, Mostwin JL. Radical prostatectomy and cystoprostatectomy with preservation of potency. Results using a new nerve-sparing technique. Br J Urol 1984; 56:694–697.

61. Kirby R, Carson C, Goldstein I. Treatment. In: Kirby RS, Carson CC III, Goldstein I, eds. Erectile Dysfunction: A Clinical Guide. London: Taylor and Francis, 1999: 49–87.

62. McDougal WS. Metabolic complications of urinary intestinal diversion. J Urol 1992; 147:1199–1208.

63. Stampfer DS, McDougal WS, McGovern FJ. The use of bowel in urology. Metabolic and nutritional complications. Urol Clin North Am 1997; 24:715–722.

64. Mills RD, Studer UE. Metabolic consequences of continent urinary diversion. J Urol 1999; 161:1057–1066.

65. Sweeney P, Kursh ED, Resnick MI. Partial cystectomy. Urol Clin North Am 1992; 19:701–711.

66. Weinstein RP, Grob BM, Patcher EM, Soloway S, Fair WR. Partial cystectomy during radical surgery for nonurological malignancy. J Urol 2001; 166(1): 79–81.

67. Cranidis A, Nestoridis G. Bladder augmentation. Int Urogynecol J Pelvic Floor Dysfunct 2000; 11:33–40.

68. Lapides J, Diokno AC, Silber SJ, Lowe BS. Clean, intermittent self-catheterization in the treatment of urinary tract disease. J Urol 1972; 107:458–461.

69. McGuire EJ, Woodside JR, Borden TA, Weiss RM. Prognostic value of urodynamic testing in myelodysplastic patients. J Urol 1981; 126:205–209.

70. Goldwasser B, Webster GD. Augmentation and substitution enterocystoplasty. J Urol 1986; 135:215–224.

71. Duel BP, Gonzalez R, Barthold JS. Alternative techniques for augmentation cystoplasty. J Urol 1998; 159(3):998–1005.

72. Churchill BM, Aliabadi H, Landau EH, et al. Ureteral bladder augmentation. J Urol 1993; 150:716–720.

73. Bellinger MF. Ureterocystoplasty update. World J Urol 1998; 16:251–254.

74. Duel BP, Gonzalez R, Barthold JS. Alternative techniques for augmentation cystoplasty. J Urol 1998; 159: 998–1005.

75. Nguyen DH, Mitchell ME. Gastric bladder reconstruction. Urol Clin North Am 1991; 18:649–657.

76. Kurzrock EA, Baskin LS, Kogan BA. Gastrocystoplasty: is there a consensus? World J Urol 1998; 16:242–250.

77. Carr MC, Mitchell ME. Gastrocystoplasty. Sci World J 2004; 4(suppl 1):48–55.

78. Gosalbez R Jr., Woodard JR, Broecker BH, Warshaw B. Metabolic complications of the use of stomach for urinary reconstruction. J Urol 1993; 150:710–712.

79. Mingin GC, Stock JA, Hanna MK. Gastrocystoplasty: long-term complications in 22 patients. J Urol 1999; 162:1122–1125.

80. Nguyen DH, Bain MA, Salmonson KL, Ganesan GS, Burns MW, Mitchell ME. The syndrome of dysuria and hematuria in pediatric urinary reconstruction with stomach. J Urol 1993; 150:707–709.

81. Bramble FJ. The clam cystoplasty. Br J Urol 1990; 66: 337–341.

82. Shekarriz B, Upadhyay J, Demirbilek S, Barthold JS, Gonzalez R. Surgical complications of bladder augmentation: comparison between various enterocystoplasties in 133 patients. Urology 2000; 55:123–128.

83. Blyth B, Ewalt DH, Duckett JW, Snyder HM III. Lithogenic properties of enterocystoplasty. J Urol 1992; 148:575–579.

84. Palmer LS, Franco I, Kogan SJ, Reda E, Gill B, Levitt SB. Urolithiasis in children following augmentation cystoplasty. J Urol 1993; 150:726–729.

85. Nurse DE, McInerney PD, Thomas PJ, Mundy AR. Stones in enterocystoplasties. Br J Urol 1996; 77: 684–687.

86. Gonzalez R, Buson H, Reid C, Reinberg Y. Seromuscular colocystoplasty lined with urothelium: experience with 16 patients. Urology 1995; 45:124–129.

87. Jednak R, Schimke CM, Barroso U Jr, Barthold JS, Gonzalez R. Further experience with seromuscular colocystoplasty lined with urothelium. J Urol 2000; 164:2045–2049.

88. Cendron M, Gearhart JP. The Mitrofanoff principle. Technique and application in continent urinary diversion. Urol Clin North Am 1991; 18:615–621.

89. Kaefer M, Retik AB. The Mitrofanoff principle in continent urinary reconstruction. Urol Clin North Am 1997; 24:795–811.

90. Filipas D, Fisch M, Leissner J, Stein R, Hohenfellner R, Thuroff JW. Urinary diversion in childhood: indications for different techniques. BJU Int 1999; 84:897–904.

91. Bauer SB, Hendren WH, Kozakewich H, et al. Perforation of the augmented bladder. J Urol 1992; 148:699–703.

92. Couillard DR, Vapnek JM, Rentzepis MJ, Stone AR. Fatal perforation of augmentation cystoplasty in an adult. Urology 1993; 42:585–588.

93. Kryger JV, Gonzalez R, Barthold JS. Surgical management of urinary incontinence in children with neurogenic sphincteric incompetence. J Urol 2000; 163:256–263.

94. Herschorn S, Hewitt RJ. Patient perspective of long-term outcome of augmentation cystoplasty for neurogenic bladder. Urology 1998; 52:672–678.

95. Golomb J, Klutke CG, Lewin KJ, Goodwin WE, deKernion JB, Raz S. Bladder neoplasms associated with augmentation cystoplasty: report of 2 cases and literature review. J Urol 1989; 142:377–380.

96. Filmer RB, Spencer JR. Malignancies in bladder augmentations and intestinal conduits. J Urol 1990; 143:671–678.

97. Gregoire M, Kantoff P, DeWolf WC. Synchronous adenocarcinoma and transitional cell carcinoma of the bladder associated with augmentation: case report and review of the literature. J Urol 1993; 149:115–118.

98. Fernandez-Arjona M, Herrero L, Romero JC, Nieto S, Martin R, Pereira I. Synchronous signet ring cell carcinoma and squamous cell carcinoma arising in an augmented ileocystoplasty. Case report and review of the literature. Eur Urol 1996; 29:125–128.

99. Lane T, Shah J. Carcinoma following augmentation ileocystoplasty. Urol Int 2000; 64:31–32.

100. Lipke M, Schulsinger D, Sheynkin Y, Frischer Z, Waltzer W. Endoscopic treatment of bladder calculi in post-renal transplant patients: a 10-year experience. J Endourol 2004; 18(8):787–790.

101. Schwartz BF, Stoller ML. The vesicle calculus. Urol Clin North Am 2000; 27:333–346.

102. Teichman JM, Rogenes VJ, McIver BT, Harris JM. Holmium:yttrium-aluminum-garnet laser cystolithotripsy of large bladder calculi. Urology 1997; 50:44–48.

103. Grasso M. Experience with the holmium laser as an endoscopic lithotrite. Urology 1996; 48:199–206.

104. Palmer LS, Franco I, Reda EF, Kogan SJ, Levitt SB. Endoscopic management of bladder calculi following augmentation cystoplasty. Urology 1994; 44:902–904.

105. Bhatia V, Biyani CS. Vesical lithiasis: open surgery versus cystolithotripsy versus extracorporeal shock wave therapy. J Urol 1994; 151:660–662.

106. Husain I, el-Faqih SR, Shamsuddin AB, Atassi R. Primary extracorporeal shockwave lithotripsy in management of large bladder calculi. J Endourol 1994; 8:183–186.

107. Badlani GH, Douenias R, Smith AD. Percutaneous bladder procedures. Urol Clin North Am 1990; 17:67–73.

108. Ikari O, Netto NR Jr, D'Ancona CA, Palma PC. Percutaneous treatment of bladder stones. J Urol 1993; 149: 1499–1500.

109. Franzoni DF, Decter RM. Percutaneous vesicolithotomy: an alternative to open bladder surgery in patients with an impassable or surgically ablated urethra. J Urol 1999; 162:777–778.

110. Salah MA, Holman E, Toth C. Percutaneous suprapubic cystolithotripsy for pediatric bladder stones in a developing country. Eur Urol 2001; 39:466–470.

111. Elder JS. Percutaneous cystolithotomy with endotracheal tube tract dilation after urinary tract reconstruction. J Urol 1997; 157:2298–2300.

112. Elder JS, Peters CA, Arant BS Jr, et al. Pediatric Vesicoureteral Reflux Guidelines Panel summary report on the management of primary vesicoureteral reflux in children. J Urol 1997; 157:1846–1851.

113. Ellsworth PI, Cendron M, McCullough MF. Surgical management of vesicoureteral reflux. AORN J 2000; 71:498–505, 508–513, 517–520, 523–524.

114. Coplen DE, Duckett JW. The modern approach to ureteroceles. J Urol 1995; 153:166–171.

115. Engel JD, Palmer LS, Cheng EY, Kaplan WE. Surgical versus endoscopic correction of vesicoureteral reflux in children with neurogenic bladder dysfunction. J Urol 1997; 157:2291–2294.

116. Coplen DE, Barthold JS. Controversies in the management of ectopic ureteroceles. Urology 2000; 56:665–668.

117. Jayanthi VR, Koff SA. Long-term outcome of transurethral puncture of ectopic ureteroceles: initial success and late problems. J Urol 1999; 162:1077–1080.

118. Shekarriz B, Upadhyay J, Fleming P, Gonzalez R, Barthold JS. Long-term outcome based on the initial surgical approach to ureterocele. J Urol 1999; 162:1072–1076.

119. Chapple RW, Wein AJ, Brubaker L, et al. Stress incontinence injection therapy: what is best for our patients? Eur Urol 2005; 48(4):552–565.

120. Choe JM. Suprapubic sling adjustment: minimally invasive method of curing recurrent stress incontinence after sling surgery. J Urol 2002; 168(5):2059–2062.

121. Kelly MJ, Zimmern PE, Leach GE. Complications of bladder neck procedures. Urol Clin North Am 1991; 18:339–348.

122. Little NA, Juma S, Raz S. Vesicovaginal fistulae. Semin Urol 1989; 7:78–85.

123. Woo HH, Rosario DJ, Chapple CR. The treatment of vesicovaginal fistulae. Eur Urol 1996; 29:1–19.

124. Sweeney DD, Leng WW. Treatment of postoperative voiding dysfunction following incontinence surgery. Curr Urol Rep 2005; 6(5):365–370.

125. Stanton SL. Surgical treatment of sphincteric incontinence in women. World J Urol 1997; 15:275–279.

126. Parra RO, Boullier JA. Laparoscopic surgery for bladder carcinoma. Semin Surg Oncol 1996; 12:145–152.

127. Anderson KR, Clayman RV. Laparoscopic lower urinary tract reconstruction. World J Urol 2000; 18: 349–354.

128. Fahlenkamp D, Rassweiler J, Fornara P, Frede T, Loening SA. Complications of laparoscopic procedures in urology: experience with 2,407 procedures at 4 German centers. J Urol 1999; 162:765–771.

129. Kavoussi LR, Sosa E, Chandhoke P, et al. Complications of laparoscopic pelvic lymph node dissection. J Urol 1993; 149:322–325.

130. Mendoza D, Newman RC, Albala D, et al. Laparoscopic complications in markedly obese urologic patients (a multi-institutional review). Urology 1996; 48:562–567.

131. Nordestgaard AG, Bodily KC, Osborne RW Jr, Buttorff JD. Major vascular injuries during laparoscopic procedures. Am J Surg 1995; 169:543–545.

132. McGinnis DE, Strup SE, Gomella LG. Management of hemorrhage during laparoscopy. J Endourol 2000; 14: 915–920.

133. Wolf JS Jr, Clayman RV, Monk TG, McClennan BL, McDougall EM. Carbon dioxide absorption during laparoscopic pelvic operation. J Am Coll Surg 1995; 180:555–560.

134. See WA, Cooper CS, Fisher RJ. Predictors of laparoscopic complications after formal training in laparoscopic surgery. JAMA 1993; 270:2689–2692.

135. Godec CJ. Genitourinary trauma. Urol Radiol 1985; 7:185–191.

136. Gomez RG, Ceballos L, Coburn B, et al. Consensus statement on bladder injuries. BJU Int 2004; 94(1):27–32.

137. Bodner DR, Selzman AA, Spirnak JP. Evaluation and treatment of bladder rupture. Semin Urol 1995; 13: 62–65.

138. Spirnak JP. Pelvic fracture and injury to the lower urinary tract. Surg Clin North Am 1988; 68:1057–1069.

139. Coburn M. Damage control for urologic injuries. Surg Clin North Am 1997; 77:821–834.

140. Baniel J, Schein M. The management of penetrating trauma to the urinary tract. J Am Coll Surg 1994; 178:417–425.

141. Carroll PR, McAninch JW. Major bladder trauma: mechanisms of injury and a unified method of diagnosis and repair. J Urol 1984; 132:254–257.

142. Corriere JN Jr, Sandler CM. Management of the ruptured bladder: seven years of experience with 111 cases. J Trauma 1986; 26:830–833.

143. Matthews LA, Herbener TE, Seftel AD. Impotence associated with blunt pelvic and perineal trauma: penile revascularization as a treatment option. Semin Urol 1995; 13:66–72.

144. Golomb J, Klutke CG, Raz S. Complications of bladder substitution and continent urinary diversion. Urology 1989; 34:329–338.

48

Urethral, Scrotal, and Penile Surgery

Angelo E. Gousse and Robert R. Kester
Department of Urology, Miller School of Medicine at the University of Miami, Miami, Florida, U.S.A.

Patricia M. Byers
Division of Trauma, Burns, and Critical Care, The DeWitt Daughtry Family Department of Surgery, University of Miami, Miller School of Medicine, Miami, Florida, U.S.A.

The avoidance, recognition, and management of complications in the lower genitourinary tract require a thorough understanding of the anatomy of the pelvis and genitalia. The focus in the female is primarily the avoidance of fistulae and incontinence. In the male, due to the shared function and location of the urethra, the focus is to maintain continence, fertility, and erectile function.

URETHRA
Anatomy of the Urethra

The male urethra can be divided into four areas: the prostatic, membranous, bulbous, and penile or pendulous urethra (1). For the purposes of treatment, urethral injuries are classified as either posterior or anterior. Posterior injuries include prostatic and membranous injuries above or including the urogenital diaphragm, and anterior injuries affect the bulbous or penile urethra (Fig. 1).

The female urethra consists of a 4-cm tube of inner epithelium surrounded by an outer muscularis layer (2). The muscularis includes both smooth muscle in continuity with the trigonal musculature and striated muscle oriented circularly. The circular striated muscle fibers are most prominent in the middle-third of the urethra. As is true of the male urethra, the female urethra contains an inner mucosal layer composed of transitional cells at the bladder neck and squamous cells at the meatus. Additionally, the female urethra has posterior and anterior portions; the demarcation between the two portions is the urogenital diaphragm. The region above the urogenital diaphragm is the posterior portion, and the region below the diaphragm is the anterior portion.

Injuries to the Posterior Urethra
Presentation and Classification of Injuries

Posterior urethral injuries are the most serious injuries to the lower urinary tract. Such injuries are generally caused by a severe external force, such as a high-speed blunt injury or a penetrating injury (1). The injury tears the attachments of the prostate, the puboprostatic ligaments, from the pelvic floor and often

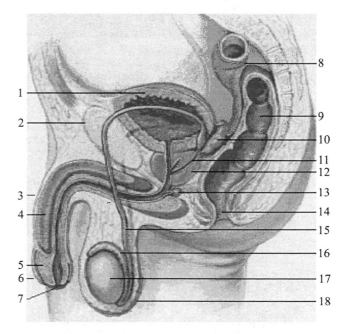

Figure 1 Male genitourinary system. 1, bladder; 2, pubic bone; 3, penis; 4, corpus cavernosa; 5, glans penis; 6, prepuce; 7, urethral opening; 8, sigmoid colon; 9, rectum; 10, seminal vesicle; 11, ejaculation duct; 12, prostate gland; 13, cowper gland; 14, anus; 15, vas deferens; 16, epididymis; 17, testicle; and 18, scrotum.

tears the urethra. Pelvic fractures cause more than 90% of traumatic urethral ruptures. Patients may experience an inability to urinate. Physical examination rarely demonstrates substantial genital swelling because neither Buck fascia nor Colles' fascia is violated. Most patients experience gross hematuria, but the absence of this symptom does not rule out serious injury. When the prostate has been completely disrupted, digital rectal examination will disclose a boggy fluid collection, composed of blood and urine, in the normal location of the prostate. In such cases, the prostate and bladder will ascend above their normal anatomic location.

When a patient is uninjured and is in stable condition, urologic diagnostic testing is directed by the type of suspected injury: external injuries are detected first, followed by urethral injury, bladder injury, and finally ureteral and renal injury (3). Retrograde urethrography (RUG) is indicated whenever urethral injury is suspected. Initial anteroposterior radiographs of the pelvis will demonstrate any associated pelvic fractures. Injection studies are performed after 20 to 25 mL of a water-soluble contrast agent has been injected into the male urethra while the patient is in a 25° to 30° oblique position. The injection is facilitated by holding the tip of the injection syringe in the penile meatus, inserting a small Foley catheter no deeper than the fossa navicularis with the balloon partially inflated with 1 to 2 mL of water, or using a specialized clamp such as the Brodney clamp.

When properly performed, RUG will clearly diagnose injuries to the male urethra. Such injuries are classified by types. Type I injuries, the mildest, involve elongation of the prostatic urethra without actual rupture. Type II injuries involve partial or complete rupture of the prostatomembranous urethra, with extravasation of contrast material confined below the urogenital diaphragm, as demonstrated by RUG. Type III injuries, the most common posterior urethral injuries, involve partial or complete rupture of the prostatomembranous urethra and disruption of the urogenital diaphragm. In such cases, RUG demonstrates extravasation of contrast material above the urogenital diaphragm, in the pelvis or the peritoneal cavity (4).

Posterior urethral obliterative stricture is a late complication associated with trauma, transurethral resection of the prostate, radical retropubic prostatectomy for prostate cancer, or radiation therapy for either prostate or bladder cancer. Clearly, such injuries occur much more frequently among men than among women. When they do occur, their diagnosis may be more difficult when only conventional radiographic contrast studies such as RUG, voiding cystourethrography (VCUG), and double-balloon catheter urethrography are used. Such studies do not clearly demonstrate the anatomy of the posterior urethra or the anatomic derangement of adjacent structures. Because the anatomic details of both the urethra and the periurethral tissues can be evaluated noninvasively with magnetic resonance (MR) imaging, this method can be used as an adjunctive tool for evaluation of urethral abnormalities (5). In cases of female urethral trauma, MR imaging is helpful in assessing the presence and the extent of anterior or posterior urethral injury and injury to adjacent structures.

Treatment

For Type I injuries, urethral Foley catheterization is recommended for three to five days so that acute urinary retention can be avoided. These injuries will resolve spontaneously.

The management of Type II or Type III posterior urethral injuries remains controversial and difficult. Initial goals should include designing a treatment plan that will minimize the long-term complications of urethral stricture, incontinence, and, for male patients, erectile dysfunction. For less severe injuries, when possible, urethral Foley catheterization is used for 10 to 14 days. VCUG is performed before the catheter is removed. For more serious injures, particularly those for which placing a Foley is impossible, the standard of care has become suprapubic catheter placement and delayed urethral reconstruction (6). However, primary repair may be advocated in certain situations, such as when there is concomitant vascular or rectal injury or when there is severe prostatic laceration or dislocation (7,8). In addition, some authors advocate passing a urethral catheter over a guidewire at the time of surgery by cystoscopic techniques. This procedure has been shown to reduce the incidence of delayed stricture formation that requires formal urethroplasty from 89% in cases managed by suprapubic catheter alone to 23% in cases managed with cystoscopically guided catheter placement (4).

For female patients, a recent study (9) advocates early drainage via cystostomy and deferred surgical reconstruction when immediate surgical repair is precluded by life-threatening clinical conditions or extensive traumatized tissue in the affected area (9). For children, initial treatment with open vesicostomy has been advocated (10).

Delayed repair of disruption of the male posterior urethra is carried out after a minimum of six to eight weeks of suprapubic drainage. The repair is made via a midline perineal approach and involves isolation and removal of the diseased segment and direct end-to-end suturing of the distal urethral segment to the membranous urethra. Patients are counseled about the possibility of postoperative incontinence and erectile dysfunction. Although delayed open repair by perineal urethroplasty is the standard of care, short strictures (less than 3 cm) can be managed by cystoscopic incision and postoperative urethral self-dilatation (11,12).

Injuries to the Anterior Male Urethra
Presentation and Diagnostic Imaging

Injuries to the anterior male urethra are more common than posterior urethral injuries. They commonly result from straddle injuries of the perineum, such as those caused by falling astride a fence rail or a bicycle crossbar (7). Unlike posterior urethral injuries, anterior urethral injuries are seldom caused by pelvic fractures. Less common causes of anterior urethral injury are associated penile fractures during sexual intercourse, gunshot and other penetrating wounds, iatrogenic causes, and self-mutilation.

Urethral disruption contained by Buck fascia causes a sleeve-like swelling of the penile shaft, with no swelling of the scrotum. More extensive penile extravasation can pass beyond Buck fascia and be limited by Colles' fascia; in such cases, the classic perineal butterfly hematoma configuration occurs (1). The mainstay of diagnosis is RUG.

Treatment

The management of blunt anterior urethral contusions without laceration involves observation and urethral Foley catheter drainage for three to five days. If any laceration is present, however, immediate surgical exploration and primary repair are indicated, whether the injury is blunt or penetrating in origin. For proximal injuries, a perineal approach is favored. For injuries distal to the proximal pendulous urethra, a circumcision incision is created and the penile shaft skin is degloved proximally.

A partial injury is surgically repaired over a urethral Foley catheter that is left in place for 7 to 10 days. For complete injuries, direct end-to-end anastomosis is preferred and the catheter is left in place for 10 to 14 days. Before the catheter is removed after either type of repair, urethrography is performed alongside the catheter, so that additional extravasation can be excluded.

Reconstructive Surgery of the Male Urethra
Anterior Urethral Strictures

Urethral stricture disease refers to the formation of scar tissue within the spongy erectile tissue of the anterior urethra (13). Such strictures may be caused by any disease process of this spongy tissue or of the urethral epithelium overlying it. Although these strictures are most commonly caused by straddle or iatrogenic injuries due to instrumentation, they may also be caused by infection or may be idiopathic.

The diagnosis of anterior urethral stricture begins with clinical suspicion when a male patient exhibits obstructive voiding symptoms, particularly if urinary infection is present. RUG and cystoscopy are indicated. With the patient under anesthesia, the stricture is gently dilatated and the urethra proximal to it is examined. This evaluation is important for appropriately staging the extent of the disease because missed proximal strictures can result in postoperative recurrent scarring proximal to the original stricture. In such cases, the proximal scar was present but was held open hydrostatically by the dilatation proximal to the original stricture.

Urethral strictures are treated surgically. Urethral dilatation is the oldest and simplest treatment for strictures. The use of metal urethral sounds or balloon dilators has been successful. Another option is internal urethrotomy, which involves transurethral incision of the stricture, most commonly with a cold endoscopic Collins knife.

The goal of therapy after any of these approaches is the maintenance of the enlarged urethral lumen after complete healing. This goal may be accomplished by leaving an indwelling urethral Foley catheter in place for three days and then requiring a program of self-catheterization for three to six months.

The most common surgical complication of operative treatment is recurrent stricture. The stricture recurs after 65% to 80% of internal urethrotomy procedures (14,15). Because of the high rate of stricture recurrence associated with urethrotomy, alternative energy sources have been sought, including various types of lasers such as the CO_2 laser, the potassium titanyl phosphate laser, the neodymium yttrium-aluminum-garnet laser, the argon laser, and the holmium: yttrium-aluminum-garnet laser. However, the results of laser therapy have been disappointing (13).

The most dependable technique for repairing anterior urethral strictures is excision and primary reanastomosis. This technique, which is suitable for shorter strictures of 1 to 2 cm, depends on adequate urethral mobilization and tension-free suturing. Durable success for more than one year has been reported in as many as 95% of cases (16).

For longer strictures, free grafts have been successful. Tissues that can be used for such grafts are full-thickness and partial-thickness skin, bladder epithelium, and buccal mucosa. Tubularized-free grafts should be avoided because they are associated with a high rate of stricture recurrence. Another treatment option for longer, more severe strictures is a two-staged repair. During the first stage, a urethral plate is constructed by using a meshed split-thickness skin graft. At a later date, another surgical procedure is performed for tubularizing the graft, thereby forming a neourethra (17). An alternative to skin grafts is the genital skin island flap based on the dartos fascia of the penis or on the tunica dartos of the scrotum (18). The success rate associated with onlay island flaps is higher than that associated with either tubularized-free grafts or island procedures.

Urinary Incontinence

Urinary incontinence is a well-recognized and serious health problem for 3% to 60% of patients after radical prostatectomy (19–21). The cause of the incontinence is the radical removal of the passive continence mechanism with its internal sphincter at the level of the bladder neck. This mechanism is removed as part of the surgical specimen, and there is an associated loss of cooptation of the membranous urethra. Historically, such incontinence has been treated with passive and active surgical procedures, culminating in the artificial urinary sphincter (AUS), first developed by Kaufman in 1972 as a silicone gel prosthesis (22,23).

The Artificial Urinary Sphincter

The AUS is an implantable prosthetic device that is placed surgically and can restore urinary control for patients with sphincteric incontinence. Via an open abdominal approach, the AUS is placed either circumferentially around the urethra at the level of the bulbar urethra or around the bladder neck. A control valve is placed in the scrotum and a reservoir is placed posterior to the rectus abdominis musculature (24).

The AUS currently in use is the American Medical Systems (AMS, Minnetonka, Minnesota, U.S.) AMS 800™, first introduced in 1982. Compared with its predecessor, the AMS 791™, it incorporates improved features. These features include a control valve and a reservoir as a single component, and a narrow-backed cuff design that decreases the incidence of tissue pressure atrophy and cuff erosion. The AMS 800 is well tolerated and offers men who are incontinent after prostatectomy a reasonable chance for obtaining long-term urinary control. Satisfactory continence is reported by 73% to 83% of men after device implantation (25,26). A recent telephone survey of patients found that the narrow-backed design was associated with a statistically significant decrease in the need for surgical revision due to cuff erosion (27).

Congenital and neurogenic conditions may also cause incontinence among men, women, and children. As long as the bladder volume is adequate, an AUS is indicated for any case of sphincteric incontinence. In cases that involve reduction in bladder volume, concomitant procedures may be required for augmenting bladder volume. For men, the cuff is placed at the bulbar urethra or the bladder neck; for children and women, the cuff is placed only around the bladder neck. For children, an open abdominal approach is recommended for placing the cuff around the vesical neck. For women, either an abdominal or a transvaginal approach can be used for placing the cuff around the vesical neck (24).

The cuff is left deactivated in the open position for six to eight weeks postoperatively. The cuff is then activated in the physician's office by the application of firm pressure that compresses the pump. The deactivation pin "pops" into the activated position; its positioning can be monitored by radiography because diluted contrast agent is used as the internal fluid. After activation, patients are taught how to cycle the device by compressing the pump, thereby opening the urethral cuff for voiding. After three to five minutes of micturation, the cuff will automatically refill, closing the urethra and restoring continence.

Complications of the Artificial Urinary Sphincter

The AUS may be associated with complications. Hematomas may occur and, when large, may require surgical drainage. In addition, the patient may experience early urinary retention during the immediate postoperative period. In such cases, it is necessary to confirm that the pump mechanism is in the open, deactivated position. If the incontinence is not due to a mechanical problem with the device, the patient may require gentle, intermittent urethral catheterization with a 10- or 12-Fr straight or Coude catheter. Delayed urinary retention due to recurrent bladder neck contracture is also possible.

Infections may occur days, months, or years after the insertion of an AUS despite the appropriate use of perioperative antibiotics. Early infections are commonly due to skin flora or airborne organisms, whereas late infections are more likely to be due to gram-negative bacteria of urinary tract origin. After an AUS has been placed, patients will require the administration of prophylactic antibiotics before undergoing any surgical, urological, or dental procedure, so that the risk of bacterial seeding can be decreased. Unfortunately, treating a prosthetic infection almost always requires removal of the device; reimplantation can be attempted three to six months later, although the likelihood of infection or cuff erosion is increased in such cases (24).

Cuff erosion may also occur either immediately or as a delayed complication; however, this condition most commonly occurs three to four months postoperatively. Symptoms of cuff erosion are pain and swelling of the perineum or scrotum, urinary infection, bloody discharge, and recurrent urinary incontinence. When cuff erosion is detected during the immediate postoperative period, the most likely cause is inadvertent and unrecognized iatrogenic injury at the time of surgery. The use of properly selected low-pressure and narrow-backed cuffs has lessened the incidence of the delayed form of this complication.

Persistent or recurrent incontinence may occur in association with an AUS. This complication is most often due to mechanical failure, tissue atrophy, unrecognized bladder urodynamic instability, cuff infection, or cuff erosion. The five-year reliability rate of the AMS 800 device is estimated at more than 90%. Mechanical failure due to fluid loss can be verified by radiography, although surgical exploration is necessary for locating the site of leakage. According to Barrett and Licht, the most common sites of leakage are the cuff, the tubing connectors, and the pump (24).

Tissue atrophy is another important cause of postoperative incontinence; this condition can be diagnosed by urodynamic studies and cystoscopy. Tissue atrophy may be treated by reoperation for increasing the pressure of the balloon reservoir pressure or for decreasing the size of the cuff, initially by 0.5 cm. Postoperative incontinence can also be caused by failure to recognize involuntary bladder contractions before an AUS is placed. Urodynamic studies are crucial for diagnosing this problem. Contractions may then be managed with pharmacologic therapy. However, if the problem is poor bladder compliance, surgery may be necessary for increasing bladder capacity.

Reconstructive Surgery of the Female Urethra
Pelvic Anatomy

The pelvic diaphragm is divided into the coccygeus muscles and the levator ani with its pubococcygeus, iliococcygeus, and ischiococcygeus muscles. These muscles form the primary inferior support for the urethra, vagina, and rectum, all of which pass through a hiatus formed by the pubococcygeus muscle. The lateral margins of these muscles are formed by the arcus tendineus, which extends from the posterior-inferior pubic ramus to the ischial spines. The endopelvic fascia covers the pelvic organs and is composed of an intrapelvic abdominal leaf and an extrapelvic vaginal leaf, which come together laterally and fuse into a common insertion along the arcus tendineus (28).

The levator fascia is central in the pelvic floor and consists of four specialized condensations: the pubourethral ligament, which anchors the urethra to the inferior pubic ramus; the urethropelvic ligaments, which attach the urethra and bladder neck to the arcus tendineus; the vesicopelvic fascia, which attaches the bladder base to the arcus tendineus and the pelvic sidewall; and the cardinal ligaments, the most posterior condensation of levator fascia, which are continuous with the vesicopelvic fascia and attach the uterine isthmus to the lateral pelvic wall. The cardinal ligaments are important because their laxity can lead to cystocele, uterine prolapse, or enterocele when the uterus has been surgically removed. Adequate surgical correction of any weakness of the cardinal ligament is required concomitant with grade IV cystocele repair so that recurrent pelvic floor prolapse can be prevented.

The three main support structures for the uterus are the cardinal ligaments, the sacrouterine ligaments, and the broad ligaments. The sacrouterine ligaments are located posteriorly and attach the cervix contiguous with the cardinal ligaments to either side of the sacrum. The broad ligaments are two superior peritoneal folds that contain the fallopian tubes, the round ligaments, the ovarian ligaments, and the ovarian vessels.

Stress Urinary Incontinence
Clinical Manifestations

Stress urinary incontinence among women is defined as the spontaneous loss of urine upon maneuvers such as coughing or straining that allow for the transmission of abdominal pressure within the bladder. The cause may be urethral hypermobility or intrinsic sphincter deficiency. Stress urinary incontinence should be corrected only when it adversely affects the patient's daily activities, personal hygiene, social interactions, financial status, or psychological well-being (29–32).

Corrective surgery for stress urinary incontinence among women is performed via either a vaginal or a retropubic approach and requires a comprehensive plan for pelvic reconstruction. Preoperative considerations are the type and severity of the stress incontinence, the degree of any associated cystocele, and the presence of other pelvic floor abnormalities, including enterocele, uterine hypermobility, or rectocele (28). Severe grades of cystocele can paradoxically cause urinary retention because of the hyperacute change in the vesicourethral angle.

Vaginal Repair of Stress Urinary Incontinence

When the vaginal approach is used for the surgical repair of stress urinary incontinence, the surgeon can also repair an associated enterocele or rectocele or can perform a vaginal hysterectomy, as indicated. In addition, complex pelvic prolapse can be corrected, either by sacrospinal fixation or by vaginal sacrocolporrhaphy (McCall culdoplasty procedure).

Currently, vaginal repair is an area of evolving clinical development; many types of repairs are possible, including anterior colporrhaphy, an anterior vaginal wall sling, a pubovaginal sling (PVS) incorporating autologous or cadaveric fascia, or porcine dermal grafts (Pelvicol®) (33–36). In addition, synthetic materials such as tension-free vaginal tape (TVT) and SPARC™ have been fashioned into grafts that are placed suburethrally via minimally invasive techniques (37,38). TVT is placed with vaginal needles, whereas SPARC is placed with retropubic needles. The advent of newer techniques has seen a decline in the frequency of bladder neck suspension procedures such as the Peyrera, Stamey, and Raz procedures (39,40). The overall cure rate of 67% and the improvement rate of 82% associated with these older procedures are inferior to those associated with the PVS procedure or the retropubic approaches. One study found that for PVS procedures the rate of cure is 83% and the rate of improvement is 87% after 48 months (41). Another found that for TVT the cure rate is 85% and the improvement rate is 96% at 56 months (42). Long-term data for SPARC are not yet available.

In addition to the low cure and improvement rates cited above, complications may also be associated with any procedure used to suspend the female urethra. Patients may develop pain, bleeding, infection, de novo urgency incontinence, prolongation of urinary retention, and secondary prolapse such as enterocele. A theoretical advantage of a synthetic material, such as TVT, is the ease with which it can be released if urinary retention is prolonged. In one study of TVT, the urinary retention rate was 3%; these cases resolved, with complete bladder emptying by 100% of the patients, after surgical release of the TVT (43).

Retropubic Repair of Stress Urinary Incontinence

Although its long-term results compare favorably with those of PVS techniques, open retropubic urethropexy is a much more invasive procedure. It can be performed either as a Marshall-Marchetti-Kranz procedure or as a Burch procedure (44,45). For open retropubic urethropexy, the rate of cure is 84% and the rate of improvement is 90% for more than two years (41).

As is true of PVS procedures, open retropubic urethropexy may be complicated by pain, bleeding, infection, de novo urgency incontinence, secondary prolapse such as enterocele, and prolongation of urinary retention. Patients who experience a recurrence of urinary incontinence should undergo urodynamic studies. If a postoperative intrinsic sphincter deficiency is found, an attempt at surgical repair is indicated (46).

Repair of Urethrovaginal Fistula

The spectrum of anatomic defects in the female urethra ranges from small urethrovaginal fistulas, which cause vaginal voiding, to the loss of the entire urethra and bladder neck, which causes total incontinence (47). The most common cause of urethrovaginal fistula is previous gynecologic or urologic surgery; anterior colporrhaphy and urethral diverticulectomy are the most common antecedent procedures (48,49).

Preoperative evaluation includes a thorough history and physical examination and an evaluation of the extent of urethral loss. Careful cystoscopy usually confirms the diagnosis. The extent of urethral loss will dictate the type of procedure needed for surgical repair. Distal fistulae beyond the external sphincter can be managed with simple excision. Extensive loss or very large fistulae will require complete urethral reconstruction. Anti-incontinence procedures are often performed simultaneously with extensive repairs.

The operation is begun by placing the patient in the lithotomy position. A 14-Fr urethral Foley catheter and a 24-Fr suprapubic Foley catheter are placed with a Lowsley tractor clamp. An inverted "U" incision is created, the fistula is circumscribed, and the scarred margins are used to provide a secure closure of the fistula tract. A vaginal advancement flap is used to prevent an overlapping suture line. When there is concern about the quality of the vaginal repair because of previous irradiation, a Martius labial fat pad may be used to bolster the repair (50).

Large defects of the female urethra present a challenging urological problem. An abdominal approach allows omental interposition and is preferred when ureteral implantation is required. The usefulness of the vaginal approach has been well described and has the advantage of allowing closure of all urethral fistulas without the attendant risks of major abdominal surgery (48–55). With urethral loss, the preferred approach is the use of vaginal flaps for transvaginal reconstruction of the urethra. Again, the patient is placed in the lithotomy position. An inverted "U" incision is created by making two parallel incisions on either side of the meatus and

extending them distally. Flaps are mobilized laterally and then medially; such mobilization allows tubularization of the neourethra around a 14-Fr catheter. The suture line is reinforced with a Martius graft, and the vagina and labia are closed. If a PVS was previously performed for incontinence, it must be secured before the vaginal mucosa is closed. Postoperatively, the Foley catheter is kept in place for 7 to 10 days. The catheter is then removed and VCUG is performed. If extravasation or retention is noted, a suprapubic catheter is placed for one to two weeks of drainage.

Complications of urethrovaginal fistula repair include elevated urinary residuals and urinary retention. Urinary retention is more common when a concomitant PVS procedure is performed. Prolonged drainage with a suprapubic catheter or long-term intermittent catheterization may be necessary. Another potential complication is urinary incontinence as a consequence of stress incontinence, detrusor instability, or urethral fistula recurrence. If stress urinary incontinence occurs, it should be treated in the standard fashion. Some patients may benefit from periurethral injection of collagen (56).

Repair of Urethral Diverticulum

The diagnosis of urethral diverticulum is often overlooked for women with lower urinary tract symptoms (57,58). The mean age of women with this condition is 45 years. The population incidence of urethral diverticulum among adult women ranges from 1.4% to 5% (59,60). Many cases are asymptomatic. The most widely held theory is that these lesions are acquired, and they probably develop from infected periurethral glands (58,61). Urethral diverticula may be complicated by infection, bladder outlet obstruction, paradoxical urinary incontinence, and malignancy, most commonly adenocarcinoma. Periurethral stones form in 1% to 10% of cases (62).

The common presentation is referred to as the three Ds: dysuria, dribbling, and dyspareunia. Frequency, urgency, and dysuria are the most common symptoms, occurring in approximately 50% of cases (47). Because these symptoms commonly result in visits to the urologist's office, urethral diverticulum should be considered whenever a patient's symptoms persist and do not respond therapy. In 63% of cases, the diagnosis can be made with a careful physical examination (63). In some cases, tenderness will be found without a palpable mass.

Preoperative evaluation should include cystoscopy performed with a 0° lens. VCUG is the most helpful imaging study and will be useful in diagnosing 95% of cases (47). Intravenous pyelography should be performed preoperatively for ruling out the diagnosis of ectopic ureterocele (64). Urodynamic testing is indicated for any woman with symptoms of stress urinary incontinence because these symptoms occur among 72% of patients with urethral diverticulum (58). If stress incontinence is present, it should be treated with a simultaneous anti-incontinence procedure at the time of diverticulectomy.

Multiple surgical procedures have been developed for treating urethral diverticulum. One method, transurethral saucerization, is generally reserved for distal diverticula (65). Transvaginal repair with excision of the diverticulum and the use of vaginal flaps is another recommended approach (66,67). With the patient in the dorsal lithotomy position, an 18-Fr suprapubic Foley catheter is placed with a Lowsley tractor clamp. A 12-Fr urethral Foley catheter is also placed. An inverted "U" incision is made in the anterior vaginal vault, with its apex distal to the urethral meatus. The flap is raised and the diverticulum is dissected circumferentially. The diverticulum sac is freed and excised by sharp dissection. At this point, the catheter is seen in the lumen of the urethra. The operculum of the diverticulum is closed in a longitudinal fashion over the urethral Foley catheter, and the periurethral tissues are closed transversely. At this point, if the quality of the repair is questionable, a Martius labial graft can be used between the periurethral and vaginal wall layers. The final vaginal wall layer is closed by reapproximating the inverted "U" incision.

Postoperatively, the Foley catheter is left for drainage for 10 to 14 days, after which time VCUG is performed. The suprapubic catheter is removed when the patient can void successfully. Postoperative complications include pain, bleeding, and infection. When bladder spasms occur, anticholinergic medications are indicated. In addition, stress incontinence may be unmasked postoperatively. Urethral strictures may occur if too much urethral wall is removed, particularly in the dissection of a large diverticulum. Recurrent diverticulum and urethrovaginal fistula formation are recognized late complications.

SCROTUM
History and Physical Examination

The adult scrotum is a loose sac containing testicles and spermatic cord structures (Fig. 1). Swelling can occur as the result of traumatic, infectious, or other inflammatory conditions. Pain can be local in the testes, the epididymides, or the scrotum itself, or it can be referred in origin. Referred pain can result from an incarcerated inguinal hernia or from colic caused by the passage of a renal calculus through the ureter. Evaluating and treating chronic orchalgia may be difficult (68). During scrotal examination, the physician should palpate the testicles, epididymides, and spermatic cords. This examination can also detect an inguinal hernia. If a scrotal mass is present, transillumination is helpful in determining whether the mass is solid or cystic. A solid mass is consistent with a diagnosis of tumor, whereas a cystic mass is consistent with a diagnosis of hydrocele or spermatocele (69).

Scrotal Conditions
Scrotal Injury

The scrotum is susceptible to trauma because of its external position (13). Degloving injuries of the scrotum occur when the skin is trapped and stripped from its underlying structures; such injuries are commonly associated with like injuries to the penis. With partial injuries, the remaining scrotal skin can be mobilized for quite a distance for use in coverage (1). Although some complete degloving injuries require burying the testicles in the thigh and later performing skin grafting, most of these injuries can be managed with immediate or delayed split-thickness skin grafting. For burn injuries, the ability to reconstruct the damage depends on how well the normal structures have been maintained. In cases in which the urethra is also burned and the phallus's integrity is severely compromised, a gracilis myocutaneous flap transfer with staged skin grafting or a complete phalloplasty may be required.

Infection

The scrotum contains sebaceous and apocrine sweat glands that are susceptible to infection. In addition, the moist intertriginous space between the scrotum and the medial thigh promotes tinea cruris infections. These infections are readily treated with local care and antimicrobial agents.

Necrotizing fasciitis or Fournier's gangrene is a serious infection of the male genitalia, usually the scrotum and perineum. First described in 1883, it was initially characterized as a fulminating genital gangrene of idiopathic origin among healthy young patients (70). Today it primarily affects older patients. In 95% of cases, a predisposing factor can be identified, such as diabetes mellitus, local trauma, periurethral extravasation of urine, paraphimosis, or perirectal or perianal infections. It is also a complication of surgical procedures such as circumcision or herniorrhaphy (71). Patients often have a history of recent perianal trauma, urological instrumentation, urethral stricture associated with a sexually transmitted disease, or urethrocutaneous fistula. The infection commonly starts as a cellulitis near the site of entry.

Fournier gangrene is a true urological emergency. Early in the course of the infection, pain, fever, and toxicity occur as deeper tissues become involved. Skin crepitus and necrosis rapidly ensue. Laboratory findings often point to a septic cause; the diagnosis is confirmed by radiography or ultrasonography, which will show subcutaneous air in the scrotum and adjacent areas of the abdominal wall and thighs (Fig. 2).

Successful treatment depends on prompt diagnosis. The presence of toxicity out of proportion to the clinical findings should raise clinical suspicion of the diagnosis of Fournier gangrene. Intravenous fluids and antibiotics are given in preparation for

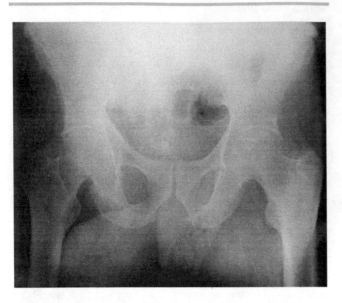

Figure 2 Radiograph showing subcutaneous emphysema in a patient with Fournier gangrene.

surgery. Wound cultures generally yield multiple organisms, and this finding indicates anaerobic–aerobic synergy (72). Immediate and extensive wide debridement is essential, and the incision should extend beyond the areas of involvement. Often, a suprapubic catheter is left in place. Postoperatively, aggressive fluid and antibiotic management is mandatory. A second procedure is almost always necessary within 24 to 48 hours of the first procedure. Some authors have reported that hyperbaric oxygen therapy is beneficial (73). Even with maximum medical and surgical intervention, the overall mortality rate is 20%, ranging from 7% to 75% (72,74,75). The fatality rates are higher among patients with diabetes or alcoholism and those for whom treatment has been delayed.

TESTICLE
Anatomy

The testicles are paired structures located in the scrotum. Each is invested in a vestige of the parietal and visceral peritoneum, which forms the tunica vaginalis testis. The testicle receives its blood supply from vessels within the spermatic cord structures, including the gubernaculum.

Traumatic Injury

Testicular rupture can be caused by either blunt or penetrating injury (76,77). Physical examination reveals swelling, tenderness, and signs of hematoma. Ultrasonography can be performed if the diagnosis is in doubt, but its sensitivity is only 64% and its specificity is only 75% (78). Immediate exploration is indicated; any extruded or necrotic tissue should be debrided and irrigated with copious amounts of warm

saline solution. Failure to close the tunica albuginea will result in the continued extrusion of seminiferous tubules. A small Penrose drain is placed beneath the tunica vaginalis for 24 to 36 hours, and antibiotics are administered for preventing postoperative infection.

Orchiectomy

The reasons for orchiectomy are surgical treatment of testicular tumor, torsion, abscess, or advanced prostate cancer. The therapeutic benefits of bilateral orchiectomy and androgen ablation for metastatic prostate cancer were first recognized by Huggins and associates at the University of Chicago (79). For the excision of testicular tumor, an inguinal incision is preferred; for cases of torsion, abscess, or prostate cancer, a scrotal incision is preferred. The primary complications after orchiectomy are bleeding and infection.

Hydrocele

A hydrocele is a fluid collection within the tunica vaginalis testis of the testicle. This condition is not uncommon among newborn boys, especially when the infant is premature; it is caused by a patent processus vaginalis of peritoneum. Generally, in such cases, the hydrocele will resolve spontaneously by the end of the first year of life (80). Hydrocele may also occur after inguinal hernia repair, varicocele repair, or vasectomy; it may also occur spontaneously later in life. Communicating hydroceles occur when there is a persistent communication between the peritoneum and the tunica vaginalis testis. Surgical repair is indicated in all of these cases. An inguinal incision with high ligation of the hydrocele tract is the preferred technique for repairing a communicating hydrocele. For hydrocele without communication, a scrotal approach with a plication or bottle technique is preferred.

   Complications associated with surgical repair of hydrocele are bleeding, infection, and recurrence. The most common complication is hematoma, which is minimized by meticulously suturing all of the raw edges of the hydrocele sac and draining the scrotum whenever necessary. Inadvertent injury of adjacent scrotal structures may also occur and may adversely affect male fertility (81).

Varicocele

The spermatic veins that drain the testis can dilate to form a varicocele. This process nearly always occurs on the left side, presumably because of incompetence of the spermatic vein as it drains into the left renal vein. This mass of veins has been described as a "bag of worms." Varicocele is graded along a scale from 0, which is a subclinical grade, through 4, in which the varicocele is very prominent on visual inspection. Normally, blood flows through either spermatic vein into a low-pressure venous system; thus, a varicocele will almost always decrease or disappear when the patient is placed in the supine position. In contrast, when the varicocele is caused by obstruction of venous drainage, as is the case with left renal cell cancer with renal vein extension, the vein will not drain and there will be no change when the patient is placed in the supine position. Varicocele can be associated with infertility and is the most common surgically correctable cause of male infertility (82).

Complications associated with varicocele repair are bleeding, infection, and recurrence. The most common complication is the formation of a secondary hydrocele because of lymphatic obstruction (83). The intraoperative use of magnification can reduce the risk of this complication (84). Another serious complication is injury or inadvertent ligation of the testicular artery, which may result in testicular atrophy and infertility.

EPIDIDYMIS AND VAS DEFERENS

Anatomy

The vas deferens is the main secretory duct of the testicle. Sperm cells from the testicle pass through a collection area called the epididymis and then travel via the vas deferens to the seminal vesicles, entering the ejaculatory duct in the prostatic urethra (Fig. 1).

Traumatic Injury

Direct trauma to the epididymis and the vas deferens can occur at the same time as injury to the testicle. Generally, in cases of epididymal injury, precise reanastamosis of the microtubular structures is not possible. Optimal surgical care consists of appropriate debridement, control of bleeding, and reapproximation of tissue edges. Neither vasoepididymostomy, which connects the vas deferens to the epididymis, nor vasovasostomy, which reconnects the vas deferens, is recommended in a contaminated field. Delayed repair is performed several months later with the goal of a precise, unobstructed, water-tight repair.

Vasectomy

Bilateral vasectomy is an office-based procedure for creating male sterility. Traditionally, two small incisions are made, and the right and left vas deferens are delivered through the ipsilateral incisions. A recent advance in the technique of vasectomy is the no-scalpel technique (85).

Bleeding and infection can occur after vasectomy. Hematoma is the most common complication; its average incidence is 2% (86). The surgeon's experience is the most important factor related to the postoperative occurrence of hematoma. Sperm granuloma is caused by an inflammatory response to sperm leaking from the cut end of the vas deferens or from sperm extravasating from the rete testes as the result of an increase in intratubular pressure. Long-term complications associated with vasectomy are chronic epididymal pain and testicular pain. Antisperm antibodies develop among 60% to 80% of patients, but no clinical disease has been documented as associated with these antibodies (87).

PENIS

Penile Anatomy

The penile shaft is composed of three erectile bodies: two corpora cavernosa and one corpora spongiosum, which contains the urethra (Fig. 1). Covering these structures are fascial layers, blood vessels, lymphatic vessels, nerves, and skin. One of the fascial layers consists of Buck fascia, which encloses the deep dorsal structures of the penis. The other important fascial layer is Colles' fascia, which makes up the anterior triangle and attaches to the perineum at the perineal body. The cavernosal artery supplies blood for erections and arises from the common penile artery, a branch of the internal pudendal artery. Venous drainage follows the arterial supply. The lymphatic vessels generally go deep to Buck fascia dorsally and drain into the deep inguinal lymph nodes. Somatic innervation is supplied by the pudendal nerves (motor and sensory). Autonomic innervation is supplied by the pelvic plexus, which consists of preganglionic afferent parasympathetic fibers from the sacral center (S2-S4) and preganglionic and visceral afferent fibers from the thoracolumbar center (T11–L2) (13). The skin includes the prepuce that forms a fold over the glans penis.

Penile Trauma

Injuries to the penis are classified as superficial, deep, or degloving. Superficial injuries include those to the skin and subcutaneous structures such as lacerations and thermal injuries. Deep injuries occur when structures deep to Buck fascia are injured and include deep lacerations, gunshot wounds, and spontaneous rupture of the corpora cavernosa that may occur during sexual intercourse. Degloving injuries occur when the skin of the penis is caught in machinery; degloving injuries to the penis often occur at the same time as degloving injuries to the scrotum (1).

Treatment generally includes operative debridement, copious irrigation with saline solution, and meticulous reapproximation of healthy tissues. Often, it is wise to place a suprapubic tube for ensuring proper bladder drainage. Deep injuries may result in erectile dysfunction. Degloving injuries will often require staged procedures. The penis can be buried into healthy subcutaneous tissue or covered with split-thickness skin grafts, either during the initial surgical procedure or subsequently.

Circumcision

Circumcision, the removal of the prepuce, is generally performed for social or religious reasons. Circumcision

---

CASE REPORT

A 62-year-old man with adult-onset diabetes mellitus underwent an uneventful repair of a left inguinal hernia. At his return visit one week after surgery, he complained of ongoing pain and requested renewal of his prescription for narcotics. The wound was neither draining nor erythematous. Three days later, he called the surgeon, again complaining of increased pain in the wound; after a telephone interview, he was told to continue the narcotic therapy. The next day he was found unresponsive at home and was taken to the emergency department by ambulance. He was unresponsive, cold, clammy, and anuric. On physical examination, the hernia incision was noted; palpation demonstrated diffuse crepitus in the left lower quadrant, perineum, left flank, and left thigh. Radiography demonstrated subcutaneous gas, a finding consistent with a diagnosis of Fournier gangrene (Fig. 2). Endotracheal intubation, ventilator support, and large-bore intravenous access were initiated, and the patient was resuscitated with intravenous fluids. Broad-spectrum intravenous antibiotics were administered. Although a bed in the intensive care unit was reserved for the patient, he was taken directly to the operating room for wide debridement. The patient lost the full-thickness skin covering of the entire perineum, left flank, and left thigh. The anesthesia team continued aggressive resuscitation with fluids and blood, with careful attention to the patient's central pressures. The penis and testicles were wrapped in Vaseline® gauze, and the patient was taken to the intensive care unit. On the following day, further operative debridement was performed. On the next day, the wounds were found to be clean, and the patient's condition stabilized. One week later, he underwent surgery for coverage of the genitalia. The right testicle was buried into the right thigh, and the left testicle and the penis were covered with a split-thickness skin graft. The rest of the wounds were eventually covered with skin grafts, and the patient was discharged to a rehabilitation unit.

---

is perhaps the most common surgical procedure performed in the United States (88). For neonates, a bell clamp (Gomco clamp) is used without any sutures, whereas for older children and adults, a double-sleeve technique including sutures is used. There is controversy about the indications for pediatric circumcision. Those who support routine circumcision point to a reduction in the risk of neonatal urinary tract infection and the prevention of penile cancer. However, an absolute contraindication to circumcision is the presence of congenital disorders such as hypospadias because the intact prepuce is crucial for penile reconstruction. For older men, the most common indication for circumcision is the presence of phimosis.

Complications occur in as many as 2% of cases; the frequency of their occurrence is negatively correlated with the experience of the surgeon (89). Bleeding and infection are common. A devastating complication is the removal of excessive skin and deep structures such as the urethra or corporal bodies. In these situations, reconstruction efforts should be undertaken without genital reassignment.

Penectomy

Penectomy is indicated for penile cancer. Partial penectomy is performed for distal cancers, whereas total penectomy is performed for proximal cancers.

Complications of penectomy are bleeding, infection, and urethral strictures at the neourethra.

Penile Prosthesis
Indications

Penile prosthesis surgery is indicated for patients who desire to regain erectile function. In such cases, lesser treatments such as oral ingestion or penile injection of vasoactive substances have usually already failed. Occasionally, these other treatments are contraindicated and penile prosthesis surgery is selected as the primary therapy. Either semirigid or inflatable devices may be chosen for implantation. Device selection is dictated by the preferences of the surgeon and the patient. Mechanically, the semirigid device is simpler in design and is therefore easier to place than the modern inflatable prosthesis, which is composed of three or four different pieces. In addition, the semirigid device is associated with fewer complications than the inflatable device (90).

Technical Considerations

The operative placement of a penile prosthesis begins with either a penoscrotal or an infrapubic incision. The corpora cavernosa are then dissected. The corporal bodies are dilated, and the cylinders of the prosthesis, either rigid or inflatable, are placed. As an inflatable device, a mechanical pump is placed in the scrotum. Finally, a hydraulic reservoir is placed either in a retropubic position (AMS) or with the pump as a single unit within the scrotum (Mentor, Santa Barbara, California, U.S.).

Complications

In general, complications associated with penile prosthesis surgery can be divided into four distinct categories: intraoperative technical problems, infections, postoperative problems, and mechanical failure (91). A common intraoperative problem is perforation of the corpora cavernosa during dilation; this problem typically occurs at the proximal crura. Management involves closing the perforation or fashioning a sleeve of artificial material (such as Gore-Tex®) into a "sock" that is placed at the proximal aspect of the prosthesis (92,93).

One of the most dreaded complications associated with penile prosthesis surgery is infection; it occurs in 0.6% to 8.9% of all cases (94). Infection is more common among patients with diabetes mellitus, spinal cord injuries, or recent urinary tract infections and among those undergoing an operation for placement of a replacement device. When a prosthetic infection occurs, the device is removed, either partially or, in the case of multicomponent devices, completely. The surgeon must then decide whether to replace the prosthesis while performing a salvage procedure or to remove the entire prosthesis and place drains within the corporal chambers (95).

Other postoperative surgical complications are problems with positioning, pain, and pressure necrosis that can result in erosion of the prosthesis. Mechanical complications have improved with each new generation of prosthetic devices. Presently, a 5% rate of mechanical failure is expected within 5 to 10 years after implantation (91). Revision surgery is more difficult than the original procedure because of scar tissue. If the patient has experienced leakage of hydraulic fluid, the connector sites should be explored first because these sites are frequently associated with pressure-induced failure. The second most common site of fluid leakage is the cylinders themselves, at the point at which the tubing attaches to the cylinder. However, if mechanical failure occurs more than five years after implantation, the entire device should be replaced.

SUMMARY

Complications of genitourinary surgery include fistulae, incontinence, infertility, and erectile dysfunction. Expertise in the anatomy and physiology of this organ system, coupled with the knowledge of the rapidly evolving technology, which is available, can decrease the long-term morbidity in patients with these complications.

REFERENCES

1. Saglowsky AI, Peters PC. Genitourinary trauma. In: Walsh PC, Retik AB, Vaughan ED, Wein AJ, eds. Campbell's Urology. 8th ed. Philadelphia: Saunders, 2002:3085–3120.
2. Staskin DR, Hadley HR, Leach GE, Schmidbauer CP, Zimmern P, Raz S. Anatomy for vaginal surgery. Semin Urol 1986; 4:2–6.
3. Dreitlein DA, Suner S, Basler J. Genitourinary trauma. Emerg Med Clin North Am 2001; 19:569–590.
4. Herschorn S, Thijssen A, Radomski SB. The value of immediate or early catheterization of the traumatized posterior urethra. J Urol 1992; 148:1428–1431.
5. Ryu J, Kim B. MR imaging of the male and female urethra. Radiographics 2001; 21:1169–1185.
6. Morehouse D, Belitsky P, Mackinnon K. Rupture of the posterior urethra. J Urol 1972; 107:255–258.
7. Corriere JN. Trauma to the lower urinary tract. In: Gillenwater JY, Grayhack JT, Howards SS, Mitchell ME, eds. Adult and Pediatric Urology. 4th ed. Lippincott Williams and Wilkins, 2001:400–513.
8. Devine CJ, Jordan GH, Schlossberg SM. Surgery of the penis and urethra. In: Walsh PC, Retik AB, Vaughan ED, Wein AJ, eds. Campbell's Urology. 8th ed. Philadelphia: Saunders, 2002:2957–3032.
9. Podesta ML, Jordan GH. Pelvic fracture urethral injuries in girls. J Urol 2001; 165:1660–1665.
10. Boone TB, Wilson WT, Husmann DA. Postpubertal genitourinary function following posterior urethral disruptions in children. J Urol 1992; 148:1232–1234.
11. Quint HJ, Stanisic TH. Above and below delayed endoscopic treatment of traumatic posterior urethral disruption. J Urol 1993; 149:484–487.
12. Spirnak JP, Smith EM, Elder JS. Posterior urethral obliteration treated by endoscopic reconstitution, internal urethrotomy and temporary self-dilation. J Urol 1993; 149:766–768.
13. Jordan GH, Schlossberg SM, Devine CJ. Surgery of the penis and urethra. In: Walsh PC, Retik AB, Vaughan ED, Wein AJ, eds. Campbell's Urology. 8th ed. Philadelphia: Saunders, 2002:3316–3394.
14. McAninch JW, Laing FC, Jeffrey RB Jr. Sonourethrography in the evaluation of urethral strictures: a preliminary report. J Urol 1988; 139:294–297.
15. Pansadoro V, Emiliozzi P. Internal urethrotomy in the management of anterior urethral strictures: long-term follow-up. J Urol 1996; 156:73–75.
16. Morey AF, McAninch JW, Duckett CP, Rogers RS. American Urological Association symptom index in the assessment of urethroplasty outcomes. J Urol 1998; 159:1192–1194.
17. Schreiter F, Noll F. Mesh graft urethroplasty using split thickness skin graft or foreskin. J Urol 1989; 142:1223–1226.
18. Quartey JK. One-stage penile/preputial cutaneous island flap urethroplasty for urethral stricture: a preliminary report. J Urol 1983; 129:284–287.
19. Fowler FJ Jr, Barry MJ, Lu-Yao G, Roman A, Wasson J, Wennberg JE. Patient-reported complications and follow-up treatment after radical prostatectomy. The National Medicare Experience: 1988–1990 (updated June 1993). Urology 1993; 42:622–629.
20. Litwiller SE, Djavan B, Klopukh BV, Richier JC, Roehrborn CG. Radical retropubic prostatectomy for localized carcinoma of the prostate in a large metropo-

litan hospital: changing trends over a 10-year period (1984–1994). Dallas Outcomes Research Group for Urological Disorders. Urology 1995; 45:813–822.

21. Steiner MS, Morton RA, Walsh PC. Impact of anatomical radical prostatectomy on urinary continence. J Urol 1991; 145:512–515.

22. Madjar S, Raz S, Gousse AE. Fixed and dynamic urethral compression for the treatment of post-prostatectomy urinary incontinence: is history repeating itself? J Urol 2001; 166:411–415.

23. Kaufman JJ. Urethral compression operations for the treatment of post-prostatectomy incontinence. J Urol 1973; 110:93–96.

24. Barrett DM, Licht MR. Implantation of the artificial genitourinary sphincter in men and women. In: Walsh PC, Retik AB, Vaughan ED, Wein AJ, eds. Campbell's Urology. 8th ed. Philadelphia: Saunders, 2002:1121–1134.

25. Fishman IJ, Shabsigh R, Scott FB. Experience with the artificial urinary sphincter Model AS800 in 148 patients. J Urol 1989; 141:307–310.

26. Montague DK, Angermeier KW, Paolone DR. Long-term continence and patient satisfaction after artificial sphincter implantation for urinary incontinence after prostatectomy. J Urol 2001; 166:547–549.

27. Gousse AE, Madjar S, Lambert MM, Fishman IJ. Artificial urinary sphincter for post-radical prostatectomy urinary incontinence: long-term subjective results. J Urol 2001; 166:1755–1758.

28. Dupont MC, Albo ME, Raz S. Diagnosis of stress urinary incontinence. An overview. Urol Clin North Am 1996; 2323:407–415.

29. Stothers L. Reliability, validity and gender differences in the quality of life index of the SEAPI-QMM incontinence classification system. Neurourol Urodyn 2004; 23:223–228.

30. Fonda D, Woodward M, D'Astoli M, Chin WF. Sustained improvement of subjective quality of life in older community-dwelling people after treatment of urinary incontinence. Age Ageing 1995; 24:283–286.

31. Ekelund P, Grimby A, Milsom I. Urinary incontinence. social and financial costs high. BMJ 1993; 306:1344.

32. Diokno AC. Epidemiology and psychosocial aspects of incontinence. Urol Clin North Am 1995; 22:481–485.

33. Beck RP, McCormick S. Treatment of urinary stress incontinence with anterior colporrhaphy. Obstet Gynecol 1982; 59:269–274.

34. Raz S, Stothers L, Young GP, et al. Vaginal wall sling for anatomical incontinence and intrinsic sphincter dysfunction: efficacy and outcome analysis. J Urol 1996; 156:166–170.

35. Dwyer NT, Kreder KJ. An update on slings. Curr Opin Urol 2005; 15:244–249.

36. Abdel-Fattah M, Barrington JW, Arunkalaivanan AS. Pelvicol pubovaginal sling versus tension-free vaginal tape for treatment of urodynamic stress incontinence: a prospective, randomized three-year follow-up study. Eur Urol 2004; 46:629–635.

37. Ulmsten U, Henriksson L, Johnson P, Varhos G. An ambulatory surgical procedure under local anesthesia for treatment of female urinary incontinence. Int Urogynecol J Pelvic Floor Dysfunct 1996; 7:81–86.

38. Tseng LH, Wang AC, Lin YH, Li SJ, Ko YJ. Randomized comparison of the suprapubic arc sling procedure versus tension-free vaginal taping for stress incontinent women. Int Urogynecol J Pelvic Floor Dysfunct 2005; 16(3):230–235.

39. O'Leary MP, Gee WF, Holtgrewe HL, et al. 1999 American Urologic Association Gallup Survey: changes in physician practice patterns, treatment of incontinence and bladder cancer, and impact of managed care. J Urol 2000; 164:1311–1316.

40. Kim HL, Gerber GS, Patel RV, Hollowell CM, Bales GT. Practice patterns in the treatment of female urinary incontinence: a postal and internet survey. Urology 2001; 57:45–48.

41. Leach GE, Dmochowski RR, Appell RA, et al. Female stress urinary incontinence. Clinical Guidelines Panel summary report on surgical management of female stress urinary incontinence. The American Urological Association. J Urol 1997; 158:875–880.

42. Nilsson CG, Kuuva N, Falconer C, Rezapour M, Ulmsten U. Long-term results of tension-free vaginal tape (TVT) procedure for surgical treatment of female stress urinary incontinence. Int Urogynecol J Pelvic Floor Dysfunct 2001; 12(suppl 2):S5–S8.

43. Klutke C, Siegel S, Carlin B, Paszkiewicz E, Kirkemo A, Klutke J. Urinary retention after tension-free vaginal tape procedure: incidence and treatment. Urology 2001; 58:697–701.

44. Stamey TA. Endoscopic suspension of the vesical neck for urinary incontinence. Surg Gynecol Obstet 1973; 136:547–554.

45. Raz S. Modified bladder neck suspension for female stress incontinence. Urology 1981; 17:82–85.

46. McGuire EJ. Urodynamic findings in patients after failure of stress incontinence operations. Prog Clin Biol Res 1981; 78:351–360.

47. Leach GE, Trockman BA. Surgery for vesicovaginal and urethrovaginal fistula and urethral diverticulum. In: Walsh PC, Retik AB, Vaughan ED, Wein AJ, eds. Campbell's Urology. 8th ed. Philadelphia: Saunders, 2002:1135–1153.

48. Patil U, Waterhouse K, Laungani G. Management of 18 difficult vesicovaginal and urethrovaginal fistulas with modified Ingelman-Sundberg and Martius operations. J Urol 1980; 123:653–656.

49. Blaivas JG. Vaginal flap urethral reconstruction: an alternative to the bladder flap neourethra. J Urol 1989; 141:542–545.

50. Leach GE. Urethrovaginal fistula repair with Martius labial fat pad graft. Urol Clin North Am 1991; 18:409–413.

51. Goodwin WE, Scardino PT. Vesicovaginal and ureterovaginal fistulas: a summary of 25 years of experience. J Urol 1980; 123:370–374.

52. Webster GD, Sihelnik SA, Stone AR. Urethrovaginal fistula: a review of the surgical management. J Urol 1984; 132:460–462.

53. Zimmern PE, Hadley HR, Leach GE, Raz S. Transvaginal closure of the bladder neck and placement of a suprapubic catheter for destroyed urethra after long-term indwelling catheterization. J Urol 1985; 134:554–557.

54. Blaivas JG. Treatment of female incontinence secondary to urethral damage or loss. Urol Clin North Am 1991; 18:355–363.

55. Elkins TE, Ghosh TS, Tagoe GA, Stocker R. Transvaginal mobilization and utilization of the anterior bladder wall to repair vesicovaginal fistulas involving the urethra. Obstet Gynecol 1992; 79:455–460.

56. Lockhart JL, Walker RD, Vorstman B, Politano VA. Periurethral polytetrafluoroethylene injection following urethral reconstruction in female patients with urinary incontinence. J Urol 1988; 140:51–52.

57. Boyd SD, Raz S. Ectopic ureter presenting in midline urethral diverticulum. Urology 1993; 41:571–574.

58. Ganabathi K, Leach GE, Zimmern PE, Dmochowski R. Experience with the management of urethral diverticulum in 63 women. J Urol 1994; 152:1445–1452.

59. Aldridge CW Jr, Beaton JH, Nanzig RP. A review of office urethroscopy and cystometry. Am J Obstet Gynecol 1978; 131:432–437.

60. Robertson JR. Genitourinary Problems in Women. Springfield, IL: Charles C. Thomas, 1978.

61. Peters W III, Vaughan ED Jr. Urethral diverticulum in the female. Etiologic factors and postoperative results. Obstet Gynecol 1976; 47:549–552.

62. Leach GE, Bavendam TG. Female urethral diverticula. Urology 1987; 30:407–415.

63. Davis HJ, TeLinde RW. Urethral diverticula: an assay of 121 cases. J Urol 1958; 80:34–39.

64. Blacklock AR, Shaw RE, Geddes JR. Late presentation of ectopic ureter. Br J Urol 1982; 54:106–110.

65. Lapides J. Transurethral treatment of urethral diverticula in women. J Urol 1979; 121:736–738.

66. Burrows LJ, Howden NL, Meyn L, Weber AM. Surgical procedures for urethral diverticula in women in the United States, 1979–1997. Int Urogynecol J Pelvic Floor Dysfunct 2005; 16:158–161.

67. Leach GE, Schmidbauer CP, Hadley HR, Staskin DR, Zimmern P, Raz S. Surgical treatment of female urethral diverticulum. Semin Urol 1986; 4:33–42.

68. Granitsiotis P, Kirk D. Chronic testicular pain: an overview. Eur Urol 2004; 45:430–436.

69. Junnila, Lassen P. Testicular masses. Am Fam Physician 1998; 57:685–692.

70. Fournier JA. Jean-Alfred Fournier 1832–1914. Gangrenefoudroyante de la verge (overwhelming gangrene) Sem Med 1883; 3:345. Dis Colon Rectum 1988; 31:984–988.

71. Yeniyol CO, Suelozgen T, Arslan M, Ayder AR. Fournier's gangrene: experience with 25 patients and use of Fournier's gangrene severity index score. Urology 2004; 64:218–222.

72. Quatan N, Kirby RS. Improving outcomes in Fournier's gangrene. BJU Int 2004; 93:691–692.

73. Paty R, Smith AD. Gangrene and Fournier's gangrene. Urol Clin North Am 1992; 19:149–162.

74. Baskin LS, Carroll PR, Cattolica EV, McAninch JW. Necrotising soft tissue infections of the perineum and genitalia. Bacteriology, treatment and risk assessment. Br J Urol 1990; 65:524–529.

75. Clayton MD, Fowler JE Jr, Sharifi R, Pearl RK. Causes, presentation and survival of fifty-seven patients with necrotizing fasciitis of the male genitalia. Surg Gynecol Obstet 1990; 170:49–55.

76. Aboseif S, Gomez R, McAninch JW. Genital self-mutilation. J Urol 1993; 150:1143–1146.

77. Altarac S. Management of 53 cases of testicular trauma. Eur Urol 1994; 25:119–123.

78. Corrales JG, Corbel L, Cipolla B, et al. Accuracy of ultrasound diagnosis after blunt testicular trauma. J Urol 1993; 150:1834–1836.

79. Huggins C, Hodges CV. Studies on prostatic cancer: I. The effects of castration, of estrogen and of androgen injection of serum phospholipases in metastatic carcinoma of the prostate 1941. J Urol 2002; 168:9–12.

80. Benjamin K. Scrotal and inguinal masses in the newborn period. Adv Neonatal Care 2002; 2:140–148.

81. Ross LS, Flom LS. Azoospermia: a complication of hydrocele repair in a fertile population. J Urol 1991; 146:852–853.

82. Aafjes JH, van der Vijver JC. Fertility in men with and without a varicocele. Fertil Steril 1985; 43:901–904.

83. Szabo R, Kessler R. Hydrocele following internal spermatic vein ligation: a retrospective study and review of the literature. J Urol 1984; 132:924–925.

84. Goldstein M, Gilbert BR, Dicker AP, Dwosh J, Gnecco C. Microsurgical inguinal varicocelectomy with delivery of the testis: an artery and lymphatic sparing technique. J Urol 1992; 148:1808–1811.

85. Li SQ, Goldstein M, Zhu J, Huber D. The no-scalpel vasectomy. J Urol 1991; 145:341–344.

86. Kendrick J, Gonzales B, Huber D, Grubb GS, Rubin GL. Complications of vasectomy in the United States. J Fam Pract 1987; 25:245–248.

87. Schuman LM, Coulson AH, Mandel JS, Massey FJ Jr, O'Fallon WM. Health Status of American Men – A study of postvasectomy sequelae. 1993; 46:697–958.

88. Thompson HC, King LR, Knox E, Korones SB. Report of the ad hoc task force on circumcision. Pediatrics 1975; 56:610–611.

89. Williams N, Kapila L. Complications of circumcision. Br J Surg 1993; 80:1231–1236.

90. Lewis RW. Long-term results of penile prosthetic implantation. Urol Clin North Am 1995; 22:847–856.

91. Lewis R. Surgery for erectile dysfunction. In: Walsh PC, Retik AB, Vaughan ED, Wein AJ, eds. Campbell's Urology. 7th ed. Philadelphia: Saunders, 1998:1215–1235.

92. Fishman IJ. Corporeal reconstruction procedures for complicated penile implants. Urol Clin North Am 1989; 16:73–90.

93. Mulcahy JJ. A technique of maintaining penile prosthesis position to prevent proximal migration. J Urol 1987; 137:294–296.

94. Carson CC. Diagnosis, treatment and prevention of penile prosthesis infection. Int J Impot Res 2003; 15(suppl 5):S139–S146.

95. Wilson SK, Delk JR II. Inflatable penile implant infection: predisposing factors and treatment suggestions. J Urol 1995; 153:659–661.

49

Complications of Genitourinary Trauma

Yekutiel Sandman

*Department of Urology, Jackson Memorial Medical Center, University of Miami Miller School of
Medicine, Miami, Florida, U.S.A.*

Peter P. Lopez

*Division of Trauma and Surgical Critical Care, DeWitt Daughtry Family Department of
Surgery, University of Miami Miller School of Medicine, Miami, Florida, U.S.A.*

Injury to the genitourinary (GU) system is a common, but rarely life-threatening, injury after major trauma. Urologic trauma is associated with other, more serious, injuries. Overall, about 10% of all traumas have GU involvement (1). When presented with a trauma patient, the clinician needs to be attentive to potential GU trauma by knowing the mechanism of injury, anatomy, and signs and symptoms of GU trauma. Following initial evaluation according to advanced trauma life support (ATLS) standards, the possibility of GU injury should be addressed if certain signs and symptoms are present (2). Among these signs are hematuria, hypotension, pelvic fracture, and flank hematoma. An increased blood urea nitrogen (BUN) to creatinine ratio is consistent with spillage of urine into the peritoneal cavity, though many types of traumatic GU injuries have a normal ratio (3).

When GU trauma is suspected (Fig. 1), the first decision is whether to proceed to the operating room (OR) or to obtain imaging studies. If the patient is stable, radiologic evaluation may begin; however, if the patient is unstable, the patient should be taken directly to the OR. If the patient does go to the OR, the next decision is whether to obtain intraoperative imaging of the GU tract. Intraoperative images are obtained by injecting 2 mL/kg of contrast and acquiring a film 10 minutes after injection (4). Intraoperative images allow assessment of the GU tract in an unstable patient without delaying critical surgery. This data rules out serious renal injury, thereby negating the need for renal exploration in most circumstances and documents the presence of a second functioning kidney (which may be of medicolegal importance). However, intraoperative films are not always necessary.

In a stable patient, imaging is indicated with (i) gross hematuria; (ii) microhematuria and signs of shock; (iii) penetrating trauma consistent with injury to the GU system; or (iv) signs of renal trauma such as flank ecchymosis, pulsatile flank mass, lower rib fractures, or facture of the transverse spinous processes (2,5). In the pediatric patient, microscopic hematuria with greater than

50 red blood cells (RBCs) per high-powered field (HPF) should lead to evaluation of the GU tract even without signs of shock (6). The lower threshold in children is due to less perinephric fat protecting the kidney, the fact that children maintain normal pressure for longer time even with severe fluid loss, and the relatively larger size of their kidneys, which increases the possibility of renal trauma.

Ultrasound, though a popular imaging technique for abdominal trauma (7), is less helpful in imaging the GU system (8). In the past two decades, computerized tomography (CT) has replaced intravenous pyelogram (IVP) for imaging the GU tract when trauma is suspected (9). Among the advantages of CT, is the ability to distinguish patients requiring operative intervention from those who would benefit from conservative management (10). In addition, CT provides a baseline for later comparison. Spiral CT scans have been criticized by many for not having an excretory phase nephrogram due to the rapidity of the imaging (11,12); obtaining delayed images assures the GU tract is adequately assessed (13,14).

Those patients that do not require imaging, i.e., those without hematuria or adults with microscopic hematuria and stable blood pressure, may safely be followed with a standard urinalysis, three weeks after the initial trauma, to assure that there is no persistent hematuria (15).

RENAL

Epidemiology and Diagnosis

The kidneys are injured in about 5% to 10% of all trauma (16). Presenting signs, symptoms and clues include flank or abdominal pain, flank ecchymosis, rib fractures, penetrating injuries (usually bullet or stab wounds) to the flank, abdomen or lower chest and, like most other GU trauma, hematuria. However, there is no correlation between the amount of hematuria and the severity of the injury to the kidney. Moreover, pedicle injury, which potentially results in renal loss, may not have any hematuria at all as the

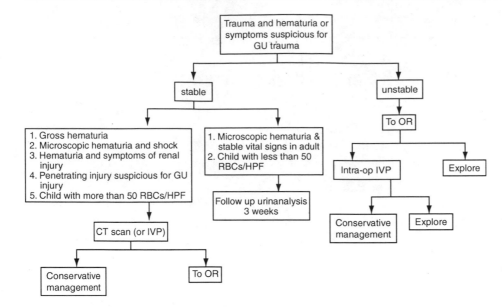

Figure 1 Flowchart. *Abbreviations*: GU, genitourinary; RBCs, red blood cells; HPF, high-powered field; IVP, intravenous pyelogram; OR, operating room; CT, computerized tomography.

injury is outside the collecting system. The most common mechanism of injury (10) to the kidney (about 90% of renal trauma) is blunt trauma. Blunt injury with rapid deceleration may cause injury to the renal vessels. Penetrating injuries account for only 10% of traumatic renal injuries, though urban trauma centers may see a 20% to 30% incidence of penetrating renal trauma.

In a stable patient with any of the indications discussed above, CT imaging of the GU tract is paramount because most renal injuries are managed nonoperatively (see below). CT scan allows radiographic grading of the injury assisting with formulation of a treatment plan.

Subtle differences exist between various authors on how to best perform a CT scan for GU trauma. According to Wah and Spencer (5), the scan should start from the dome of the diaphragm and continue to the iliac crests; patients receive contrast by mouth, as well as intravenous (IV) contrast. The scan begins at 65 seconds after the administration of 150 mL of 300 mg/mL nonionic IV contrast to obtain early phase films. Wah also obtains delayed films when renal injury is suspected, though others advocate regularly obtaining delayed films at three minutes to evaluate the renal system, regardless of suspicion of renal injury (17). To evaluate the collecting system, late films at 15 to 20 minutes are routinely done.

Management

The most accepted classification for renal trauma is the one developed by the American Association for the Surgery of Trauma (Fig. 2 and Table 1) (18,20). A review of 2483 patients with renal trauma at San Francisco General Hospital showed (19) that Grade I and II injuries (injuries of the kidney including hematoma and superficial lacerations) are managed

nonoperatively as are most (deeper) Grade III injuries (21). Grade IV injuries, (those with laceration to the kidney involving the collecting system or thrombosis of the main renal vessels), are managed operatively if there is hemodynamic instability. Other operative criteria include intractable renal bleeding (expanding renal hematoma, or a pulsatile renal hematoma), injury to the renal vessels, or the presence of a nonviable kidney segment associated with other injuries (22,23). Extravasation of urine alone has been an indication for operative intervention, although currently it is commonly handled nonoperatively (16,24). Grade V injuries, (avulsed renal pedicle or shattered kidney) should be managed operatively except in rare, select cases (when the criteria above are not met despite having a Grade V injury) (25). Nicol and Theunissen advocate exploring all penetrating renal trauma, if the patient is undergoing laparotomy for other injuries because it allows direct visualization and does not lead to higher rates of nephrectomy (26). Margenthaler et al. advocate nonoperative management of all renal trauma in children unless the patient is hemodynamically unstable (27).

Nonoperative management consists of bed rest until gross hematuria ceases. If hematuria recurs upon ambulation, the patient should be reconfined to bed. Once the patient can ambulate without hematuria, he or she can be safely discharged with follow-up (28).

Surgical options include primary repair, partial nephrectomy or, as a last resort, total nephrectomy. The approach to the kidney (29) is via the abdomen. After examining the abdominal contents and repairing any intra-abdominal injury, attention should be turned to the kidneys. The transverse colon is superiorly reflected. The small bowel is reflected off the field superiorly and to the right. At this point, the posterior peritoneum is incised (Fig. 3). Obtaining

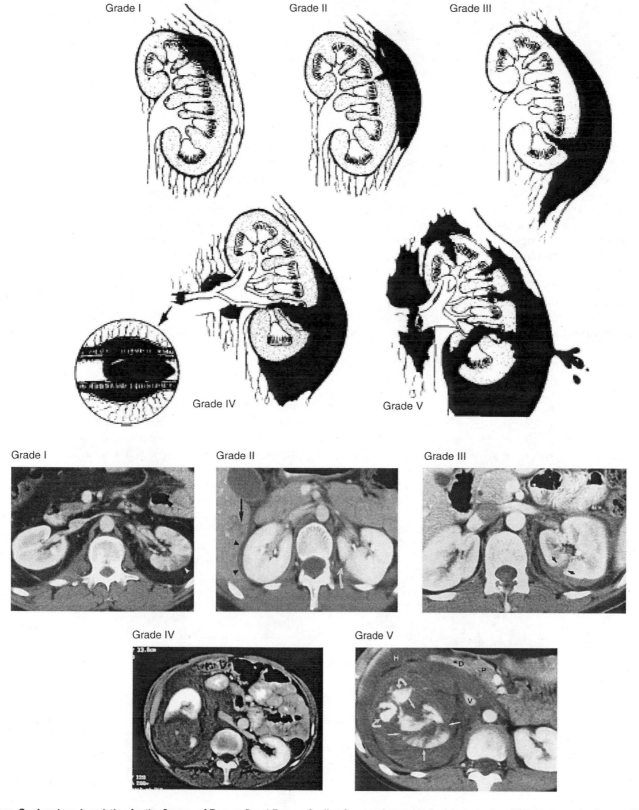

Figure 2 American Association for the Surgery of Trauma Renal Trauma Grading Score and computerized tomography of injuries by grade. *Source:* From Refs. 17–19.

Table 1   American Association for the Surgery of Trauma Classification of Renal Trauma

Grade	Type of injury	Management
I	Hematoma	Nonoperative
II	Laceration < 1 cm	Nonoperative
III	Laceration > 1 cm but not involving the collecting system	Nonoperative
IV	Laceration extending into the collecting system or main renal vessel thrombosis	At times nonoperative but usually operative
V	Multiple lacerations extending into the collecting system or devascularized kidney	Almost always operative

control of the aorta and vena cava at this point is the accepted next step (Fig. 4); however, the utility of this maneuver has recently come into question (30). To obtain control of the renal vessels, one should gently retract the left renal vein superiorly with a vessel loop. The left renal artery is identified and controlled with a nonocclusive vessel loop followed by identification and control of the right renal artery, which is found between the aorta and vena cava after retracting the left renal vein cranially and after incising between the aorta and vena cava. Finally, the right renal vein is identified and controlled. The vessels are not occluded unnecessarily since the warm ischemia time of the kidney is only 30 minutes. Next, the colon is reflected medially, Gerota's fascia incised, and the kidney and all its vessels should be explored.

Primary operative repair (Fig. 5) is an option if there is a Grade I, II, III, or IV injury to the kidney. It consists of individual control of parenchymal renal vessels with suture ligation (typically with 4-0 chromic sutures) and watertight closure of the collecting system with a running absorbable suture (such as 4-0 chromic). Partial nephrectomy follows the same principles and includes the sharp debridement of nonviable tissue. In both procedures, the surgeon should cover the kidney with intrinsic renal fascia or with the omentum in order to decrease extravasation and increase hemostasis (29). Total nephrectomy is indicated in select cases: an unstable patient with a normal second kidney, if the patient's instability is due to low body temperature and poor coagulation, a nonrepairable kidney, and warm ischemic time greater than six hours (31).

Complications

Complications of renal trauma, in addition to the morbidity and mortality attached to any traumatic injury, are either immediate or delayed (16). Immediate complications include extravasation, which can lead to urinoma, which, in turn, can lead to infection and abscess. Whitney and Peterson (32), in a series of 81 penetrating trauma victims who underwent operative intervention, found a urinary leak rate of 2% in minor injuries (injuries in which the surgical intervention proved needless) and 33% with major injuries (those where the operative intervention proved essential). Simple extravasation may be treated via internal stenting (33). In fact, in a series of 46 patients with Grade IV or V lesions that were treated nonoperatively, Matthews et al. found that 31 patients had extravasation. However, the leak resolved without any intervention in all but four patients. Those patients were treated with ureteral stenting. There were no complications

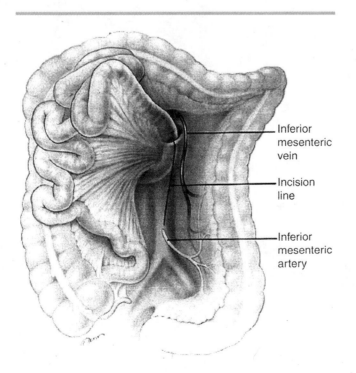

Figure 3   Exposure for renal trauma. *Source:* From Ref. 29.

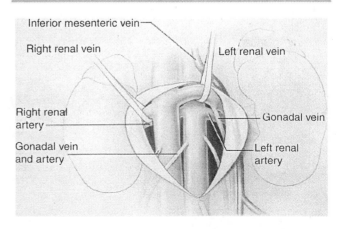

Figure 4   Method of renovascular control. *Source:* From Ref. 29.

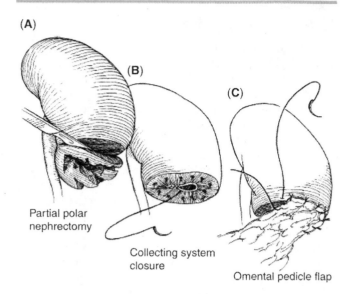

Figure 5 Primary renal repair: **(A)** Debridement of nonviable tissue. **(B)** Closure of collecting system (after tying off of parenchymal vessels). **(C)** Omental flap. *Source*: From Ref. 29.

Table 2 Complication Rate In Grade IV Injuries by Concurrent Intra-abdominal Injury and Management

Injury/management	Explored	Not explored
Intra-abdominal injury	3/13 (23%)	12/14 (85%)
No intra-abdominal Injury	6/38 (38%)	N/A

Abbreviation: N/A, not applicable.

with nonoperative management (no increased risk of hypertension or renal failure) and all 31 patients received prophylactic antibiotics (24).

The incidence of urinoma (Fig. 6) and infection can be stratified by grade of injury. The overall risk of surgery versus nonoperative complications falls in favor of nonintervention for Grades I to III (19). For Grade IV injuries, Husmann et al. (22) demonstrated that there is an 85% chance of complication including infected urinoma, hypertension, and hemorrhage if an abdominal injury coexists with a devitalized segment of kidney. In contrast, there was only a 23% risk of complication if the same type of patient was managed surgically. If there was no associated intra-abdominal injury, the likelihood of complication was 38%; however, the majority of these complications (five of six) were amenable to nonoperative management (Table 2).

Urinoma is diagnosed by CT scan obtained with delayed images, which allows the contrast to pass through the kidney and into the collecting system. Treatment for urinoma is based on the length of time since the operation and/or trauma and whether an abscess or fistula is present. If it has been a week or less and there is no active infection, operative drainage and repair is indicated. If the patient is actively infected or if the urinoma has been present for seven days or more, the patient should be managed nonoperatively as the inflammation will likely make for a difficult dissection and poorly healing tissue (28). Percutaneous drainage of the collection and placement of a nephroureteral stent is the treatment of choice in these instances (34–36). Infection should be treated with broad-spectrum antibiotics and other supportive treatment as needed. Definitive repair is undertaken when the patient is more stable.

Knudson et al. (37) found an overall 23% complication rate with renovascular injuries (all Grade IV or V

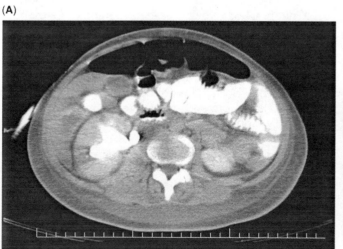
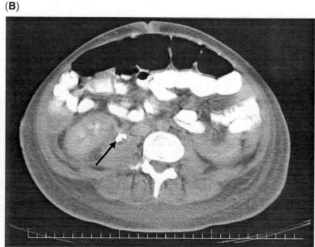

Figure 6 **(A)** Perinephric collection in a case of a ureteropelvic junction distraction injury on the right with **(B)** extension into the Psoas muscle (*solid black arrow*).

by definition). These complications included delayed nephrectomy, persistent hypertension, renal failure, and diminished renal function. Renovascular injuries have not shown to have statistically significant differences in repair versus nephrectomy except in Grade V arterial injuries. More patients develop complications in attempted repair of such an injury than do those that undergo nephrectomy (odds ratio of 15% increase in above complications). Knudson et al., therefore, recommend nephrectomy in Grade V renal artery injuries and repair in Grade IV renal artery injuries.

Hypertension has also been reported as a delayed complication of renal trauma (38). In a review of 158 patients with vascular and parenchymal renal trauma, Montgomery et al. found a 4.4% incidence of hypertension attributable to renal trauma. The onset of symptoms ranged from immediate (when still hospitalized for the trauma) to eight months after the initial event. The symptoms included headache, chest pain or tightness, and nosebleeds. There were several patients with no symptoms or vague complaints as well.

The need to obtain vascular control prior to exploration of the kidney for trauma has come into question recently. It has been thought that vascular control decreases the rate of nephrectomy while adding minimal time to the operation (39). However, recent studies have questioned the advantages of vascular control. For instance, Gonzalez et al. found no statistical difference in blood loss, rate of nephrectomy, or transfusions in a trial of patients randomized to either vascular control versus no early vascular control (30). The rate of nephrectomy was 31% and 30% in the vascular control and no-control groups, respectively. The no-control patients were transfused an average of 5.2 units of packed RBCs versus 5.5 units in the control group, while the blood loss was 0.9 and 1.1 L in the each of the above groups. A limitation of the above study was its small sample size. Our experience has been to gain vascular control if repair of the kidney is planned. However, if the patient is unstable and bleeding, we do not take the additional time required gaining vascular control; rather, we proceed directly to evaluation of the kidney.

Delayed bleeding has been noted following renal trauma as well (40). Carroll et al. reviewed 92 of the renal trauma cases that came into San Francisco General Hospital and found two cases that had delayed bleeding (41). Both of these cases were operatively reexplored. Neither required nephrectomy to control the bleeding. Teigen et al. described two cases of delayed hematuria in children where pseudoaneurysm developed in an area of the kidney that was devitalized (40). They advocate early angiography for evaluation of delayed hematuria and possible treatment via embolization of any pseudoaneurysm. Delayed bleeding occurs in adults as well and is usually managed by interventional radiologic techniques.

URETERAL
Epidemiology and Diagnosis

Traumatic ureteral injury is rare, usually occurring in coincidence with damage to other intra-abdominal structures (42). Iatrogenic injuries occur most commonly during ureteroscopic and gynecological procedures (43). Though ureteral injury is often accompanied by hematuria, typically microscopic, in one series, 15% of these injuries occurred without hematuria (44). Diagnosing ureteral trauma correctly depends on a high index of suspicion, which should be raised when the injury makes ureteral damage possible (a bullet's trajectory in proximity to the ureter) or when an intervention has occurred in proximity to the ureter. When such injury is missed, the patient will often present with a flank mass, or the signs and symptoms of an infected urinoma (e.g., rigors, tenderness, erythema, fevers, and hypotension). Regardless of the cause of ureteric injury, the principles of diagnosis and repair remain the same.

The most common mode of noniatrogenic injury to the ureter is gunshot wounds (GSW); however, only about 2.5% to 5% of GSW are accompanied by ureteral injury (45). Some GSW are not due to direct transection, but rather secondary to a "blast injury." This blast effect occurs when the force of the bullet is transmitted through the abdomen; the ureter is devascularized and becomes nonviable (28). Eventually, there is necrosis and breakdown of the ureter, which results in ureteral stricture or rupture. Another possible etiology of ureteral injury due to external trauma is ureteral-pelvic disruption secondary to violent hyperextension of the trunk, e.g., as during a motor vehicle crash. This type of injury occurs more frequently in children (46). Those patients who have suffered external trauma with ureteral damage, regardless of etiology, are often critically ill with multiple injuries (47).

Imaging of the ureters allows identification of injury (48). If CT scanning is used, it is paramount that a nephric excretory phase is obtained to make the diagnosis. It is in these instances that spiral CTs are criticized, due to their speed and the possibility that a ureteric injury may be missed due to the lack of an excretory phase. Therefore, when a CT scan is used for diagnosis of a possible GU injury, it is imperative that delayed films (at least five to eight minutes after the injection of contrast) are obtained (49). Extravasation of contrast (Fig. 7) if the ureter is disrupted or nonpassage of contrast if the ureter has ceased functioning without formal disruption (as in the first stages of a "blast" injury) would be seen. A ureteral contusion can be missed with intraoperative IVP (4). Therefore, Palmer et al. (42) as well as Medina et al. (50) maintain that diagnosis of ureteral injury should be made by direct observation when exploring the abdomen in the OR. They point out that methylene blue can be injected into the renal pelvis with subsequent observation for leaking to assist with the diagnosis. Care should be taken to use a large gauge

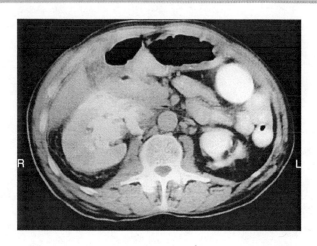

Figure 7 Extravasation of contrast after right ureteral injury. *Source:* From Ref. 48.

needle, such as a 25 gauge needle, to prevent iatrogenic damage to the collecting system.

Management

The first critical decision to make after diagnosing a ureteral injury is whether the patient is stable enough to undergo repair. As the consequences of GU damage are rarely life threatening, patients who are hemodynamically unstable will likely not benefit from an extended repair of a noncritical injury. In these instances, planned reoperation is the most reasonable course of action. If time permits, the ureter may be externalized by ureterostomy (Fig. 8) and corrected at a later point (52). If the patient is stable, immediate repair should be done.

The ureter is divided into three parts: proximal, mid and distal. All parts share the same basic

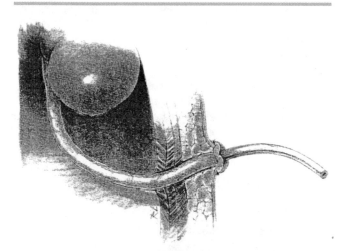

Figure 8 Pediatric feeding tube in proximal ureter brought out through the abdominal wall. *Source:* From Ref. 51.

principles of repair; the only difference is the type of anastomosis performed. The goal is to create a tension-free but watertight anastomosis (Fig. 9). Basic principles include mobilizing a large amount of ureter while giving a wide swath to the adventitia, dissecting the ureter back to its viable, bleeding edge, spatulating the ureter at the anastomosis, isolating the repair with omentum, especially if other organs are injured, and draining the area of repair (35,53). In addition, routine stenting is beneficial (31). These principles hold true whether the injury is due to penetrating or iatrogenic trauma.

In proximal injury, an end-to-end ureteroureterostomy, (reconnecting the ureter with primary closure), is usually performed if there is a simple injury with viable ureter, for example, caused by a stab wound (48). In cases of profound ureteral loss with preservation of only the most proximal ureter, options include extending the length of the ureter by interposition of ileum or decreasing the ureteral length needed by either mobilization of the kidney, autotransplantation, or via a transureteroureterostomy (connecting the injured ureter to the noninjured ureter on the contralateral side). Autotransplantation for severe proximal ureteral loss, advocated by Meng et al., has been met with success in six of seven attempts. Two of the six attempts had a direct ureterocystostomy (implanting the ureter into the bladder) and four had ureteropyeloplasties (fixing the ureter-renal pelvis area) (54). However, autotransplantation and ileal interposition have been criticized as too time-consuming to undertake in an acute trauma setting, and an expeditious transureteroureterostomy (Fig. 10) is advocated (53). In addition, Guerriero recommends a transureteroureterostomy to avoid fecal spillage in the case of contamination of the retroperitoneum (35).

Midureteral injuries are treated by ureteroureterostomy. Other options, if the mobilized segment does not allow for a tension-free anastomosis, include mobilization of the kidney or creation of either a Psoas bladder hitch or Boari flap (48), though the Boari flap has been criticized for decreasing the functional capacity of the bladder (55). These options are also possible with distal ureteral injuries, although a direct ureterocystostomy is preferable if there is sufficient ureteral length (52).

Due to the ability to span a large segment of nonfunctional ureter and the relative lack of complications, the Psoas hitch (Fig. 11) has gained widespread approval (55,57). It includes mobilization of the contralateral obliterated umbilical artery and the ipsilateral umbilical artery if needed, making a cystotomy to aid with pexing the bladder to the Psoas tendon, affixing the bladder to the Psoas with nonabsorbable sutures while avoiding the genitofemoral nerve and finally reanastomosing the ureter to the bladder. The ureter should be stented (56). A Boari flap (Fig. 12) consists of taking an ipsilateral bladder flap, after having filled the bladder to near capacity, and anastomosing the ureter to the flap. The flap/ureter area is

(A)   (B)

(C)   (D)   (E)

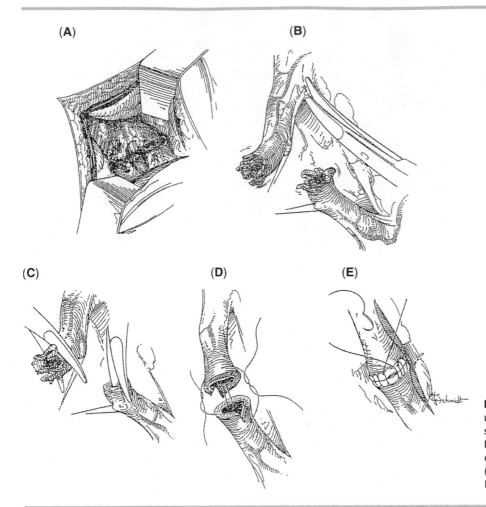

Figure 9 Ureteroureterostomy. **(A)** Exposure of ureteral injury. **(B)** Mobilization of ureter with wide swath given to adventitia to assure adequate blood supply. **(C)** Debridement to viable, bleeding edge. **(D)** Suturing of spatulated ureteral ends. **(E)** Final appearance of repaired ureter. *Source:* From Ref. 35.

then fixed to the Psoas muscle and the flap is tubularized and a stent is placed (56).

Complications

Complications of ureteral injury include stricture, which occurs if there is a devitalized segment. Stricture may eventually lead to permanent renal damage because of increased pressure. Treatment of a ureteral stricture depends on several factors including the length and the vascularity of the segment that is strictured. In a study by Richter et al., strictures that were short and vascularized were found to have a balloon dilatation success rate of 89% (58). The same study found that devascularized strictures had a 40% or less success rate while strictures with increased length, at the ureteral pelvic junction or at an ureteroenteric anastomosis, had a poor success rate regardless of vascularity.

If there is a leak from the anastomotic site or, more commonly, an unrecognized damaged ureter, a urinoma (Fig. 6) and all the consequences of a urinoma may occur; these include abscess formation, sepsis, and possible ureterocutaneous fistula (59). A urinoma requires drainage, as would an abscess. Access to drain them is often attained percutaneously.

Though rare, ureterovaginal fistulas or ureterocutaneous fistulas occur after unrecognized ureteral trauma as well (60). Stenting across the fistula is the treatment of choice for this type of complication (35,36). Selzman et al. found that stenting alone was adequate in patients who had the stent in place for a sufficient amount of time (seven of seven patients) (61). They found no difference in the results of two patients whose stent was placed in an anterograde fashion.

Ahn and Loughlin (57) reported that only 1 of 17 patients had any postoperative complications to their Psoas hitch method. This patient was 1 of 14 with a refluxing (nontunneled) ureteral-bladder anastomosis. This patient developed urosepsis that resolved with medical treatment and had no recurrences in the 16 months of follow-up and intact renal function as well.

BLADDER
Epidemiology and Diagnosis

Bladder rupture due to trauma is generally categorized as either intraperitoneal or extraperitoneal. The etiology and the management of each of these are unique, as are the ramifications of the particular

(A)

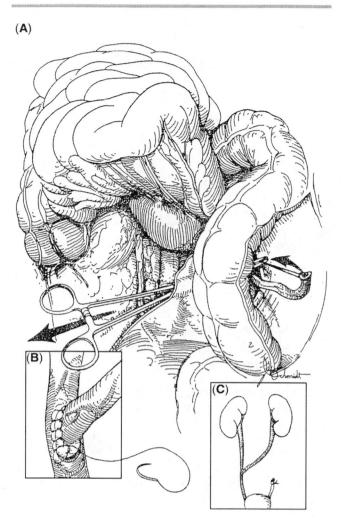

Figure 10 Transureteroureterostomy. **(A)** Injured ureter pulled (behind colon) to uninjured ureter. **(B)** Anastomosis. **(C)** Final appearance. *Source:* From Ref. 35.

injury. Close to 100% of blunt trauma bladder injuries are associated with pelvic fractures (62), though only one out of 10 pelvic fractures have an associated bladder injury (63). Fifteen percent of blunt trauma associated bladder injuries are intraperitoneal while 85% are extraperitoneal (64). The causes of bladder rupture into either of these areas is due to the fact that the peritoneal lining sits above the dome of the bladder and the force of the injury may be directed superiorly, yielding an intraperitoneal rupture, or elsewhere resulting in an extraperitoneal injury. Extraperitoneal bladder rupture is due to bursting of a full bladder, shearing from its areas of attachment or perforation of the bladder by bony spicules after pelvic fracture (65). Intraperitoneal bladder injury need not be associated with pelvic fracture; the blunt trauma force transmitted to a full bladder can be enough to result in intraperitoneal rupture (66).

The key to diagnosis of a bladder injury is hematuria. When associated with pelvic fracture, workup of the lower urinary tract (bladder and distal) is warranted (67). Injuries to associated areas, such as perineal hematoma or rectal bleeding, are also indicative of bladder injury (68). Morey et al. state the only absolute indication for cystography in the setting of blunt trauma is gross hematuria associated with pelvic fracture. They found 85% to 100% of patients with intra- or extraperitoneal bladder rupture had these two findings. They maintain that patients with gross hematuria without a pelvic fracture, microhematuria with a pelvic fracture, and isolated microhematuria only need to be imaged to rule out bladder rupture in the face of clinical indicators such as those mentioned above (69).

Diagnosis of bladder rupture is made by a *stress* retrograde cystourethrogram. The key element of this study is filling the bladder to the point where it is fully distended. This ensures the entire bladder is filled and there is no collapsed segment masking a tear that can

(A)   **(B)**

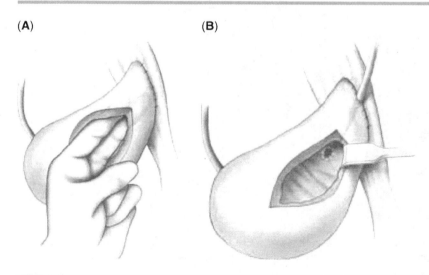

Figure 11 Psoas hitch: **(A)** Contralateral bladder freed, cystotomy made, and the bladder pexed. **(B)** Ureter anastomosed at area of psoas hitch (NB ureter yet to be stented). *Source:* From Ref. 56.

(A) (B) (C)

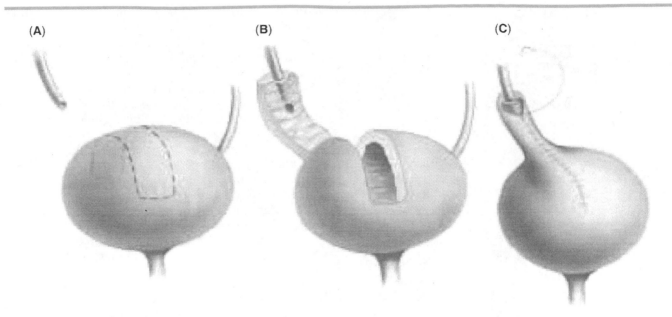

Figure 12 Boari flap: **(A)** Ipsilateral bladder flap identified, **(B)** raised and ureter reimplanted, and **(C)** bladder flap tabularized. *Source:* From Ref. 56.

yield a false negative test result. Deck et al. performed CT stress cystourethrogram in three steps (14). First, 100 mL of contrast was instilled into the bladder in a retrograde fashion and initial images obtained. Next, the bladder was filled to maximum capacity tolerated (with nonresponsive patients the bladder was filled to a water pressure of 40 cm and 350 mL of contrast) and repeat images were obtained. Last, postdrainage films were obtained. Plain films with anterior–posterior, oblique views, and postvoid films are acceptable (62). The advantage of CT is that it allows evaluation of the bladder concurrently, with the imaging commonly obtained after abdominal and GU trauma. On the other hand, plain films are significantly less expensive than CT scans.

On plain films, extraperitoneal rupture, a flame-like extravasation, would be seen, while intraperitoneal rupture distinguishes itself as superior extravasation from the dome of the bladder. On CT, extraperitoneal bladder rupture will outline the various extraperitoneal fascial planes (Figs. 13 and 14) while intraperitoneal rupture will outline abdominal contents such as bowel (Figs. 15 and 16) (71). Ultrasound imaging is often nondiagnostic as extraperitoneal rupture is not seen via sonography and intraperitoneal rupture is often missed (72). Diagnostic peritoneal lavage does not provide enough

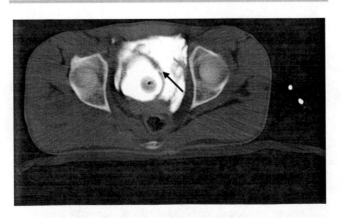

Figure 13 Extraperitoneal bladder rupture. Note wisp of contrast exiting left side of bladder (*arrow*) and feathery appearance of contrast.

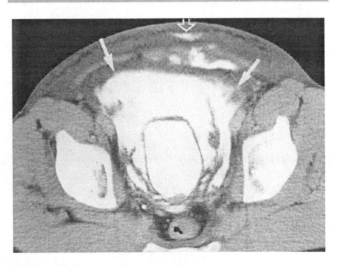

Figure 14 Contrast extravasating between the layers of the rectus and layers of the abdominal wall (*arrows*). *Source:* From Ref. 71.

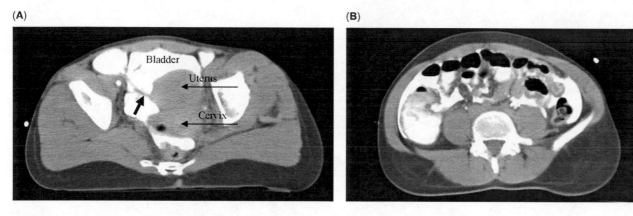

Figure 15 Intraperitoneal bladder rupture seen on CT scan with delayed imaging. Note the contrast exiting the dome of the bladder (*thick arrow* in **A**) and the multiple bowel loops outlined and contrast collections in pericolic gutters (**B**). *Abbreviation*: CT, computed tomography.

information to rule out bladder injury either as it does not sample the extraperitoneal area.

Management

Surgical intervention is generally not indicated in extraperitoneal rupture and urethral catheter drainage is the standard of care according to Corriere and Sandler, though they advocate surgical repair if the patient is going to the OR for other injuries (65,73). In one study (73), they present 39 patients with extraperitoneal bladder trauma due to blunt injury who were treated with either urethral catheter alone (30) or both a urethral and suprapubic catheter (SPC) (9). Extravasation was resolved in all the patients, 34 within 10 days, the other five ranging

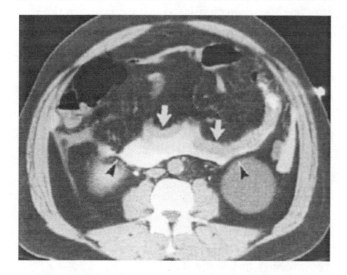

Figure 16 Contrast outlining small bowel loops (*arrows*) and the posterior peritoneal fascia (*arrowheads*). *Source*: From Ref. 71.

between 14 and 90 days. There were no complications and no prophylactic antibiotics were used. A follow-up cystogram was obtained after 10 to 14 days with nonoperative management and again after three weeks if there was persistent extravasation of contrast. When surgical closure was performed, the follow-up cystogram was done after one week. In both cases, the catheter was removed when there was no extravasation of contrast (74). Some authors believe all patients with bladder rupture should be started on empiric antibiotics despite the results in the study discussed above (1,75).

Intraperitoneal bladder ruptures are repaired with absorbable sutures in a two-layer, running fashion (Fig. 17). Operative repair is necessary due to the possibility of uroascites and the concomitant electrolyte disturbances that occur with intraperitoneal urine (73). Catheter drainage alone is believed to be insufficient because the urine will preferentially drain through the larger rent in the bladder. Standard approach to the bladder (70) is through a low vertical midline incision (Fig. 17). Taking care to avoid any possible pelvic hematoma, a midline cystotomy is created. Following inspection and identification of any lacerations, the outermost layer is repaired with an absorbable suture, followed by the same type of repair in the additional one or two layers (Fig. 18). If the ureteral orifices are in proximity to the wound, a stent should be placed. Placing both suprapubic and urethral catheters has been the standard practice; however, it is now believed that postoperative urethral catheterization alone may suffice with no increase in posttraumatic complications (77,78).

All penetrating trauma to the bladder should be explored, debrided, and repaired with absorbable sutures in a two-layer, running fashion. Treatment includes postoperative bladder decompression via suprapubic and urethral catheters or just urethral catheters, as described above (70).

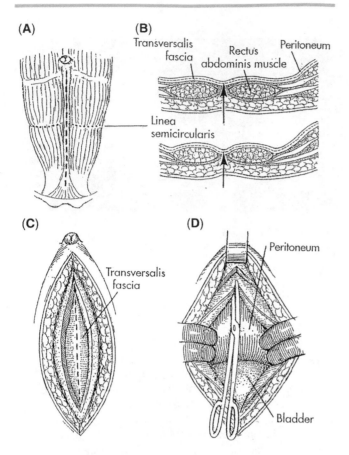

(A)

(B)
Transversalis fascia
Rectus abdominis muscle
Peritoneum
Linea semicircularis

(C)
Transversalis fascia

(D)
Peritoneum
Bladder

Figure 17 (**A** and **B**) The relationship of the rectus asdominis muscle to the linea alba and linea semicircularis. (**C** and **D**) The transversal is fascia is opened, and the peritoneum is reflected cranially. *Source*: From Ref. 76.

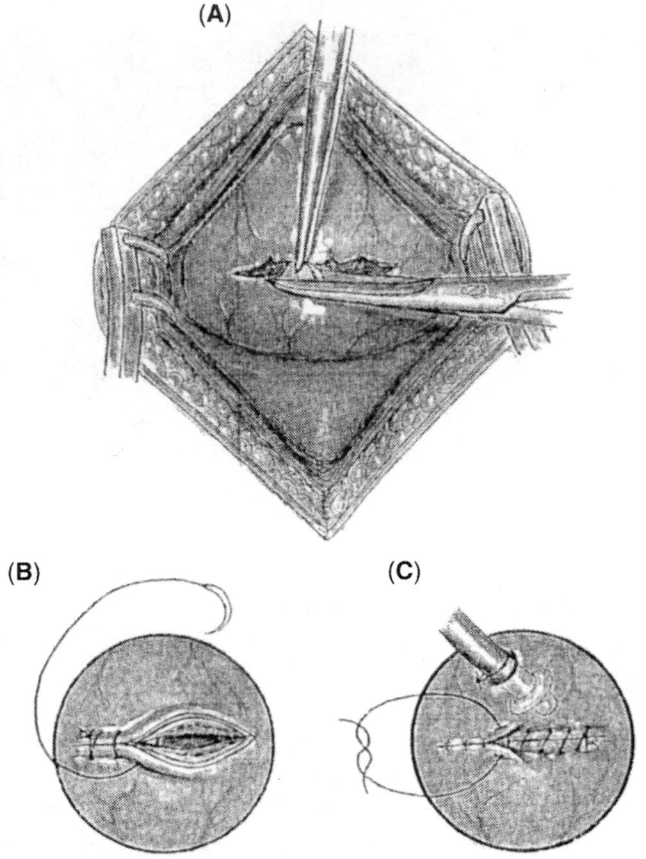

(A)

(B)

(C)

Figure 18 Repair of an intraperitoneal bladder rupture; (**A**) Debridement of devitalized tissue; (**B**) A simple, full-thickness running closure of the incision with a 3-0 absorbale stich; (**C**) A second, running Lambert suture is used to invert the anastomosis in a watertight fashion. *Source*: From Ref. 76.

Complications

A persistent leak occurs when there is incomplete closure of the bladder or misdiagnosis of an intraperitoneal rupture as extraperitoneal, or in the case of insufficient catheter drainage. With extraperitoneal bladder injuries, the morbidity associated with prolonged drainage is largely the inconvenience of prolonged catheterization and the possibility of bladder calculi (75). However, intraperitoneal bladder rupture may lead to uroascites and complications including peritonitis, increased breakdown of gastrointestinal anastomosis, respiratory difficulty, and sepsis (74). A pelvic hematoma may become infected, leading to septic complications. The chance of infection may be decreased by administration of broad-spectrum antibiotics if given prophylactically, though they are not always given after bladder repair or catheter treatment (75).

Fistula formation, either vesicocutaneous or vesicovaginal, is another possible complication. Kotkin and Koch (75) reported that 2 of their 36 patients with extraperitoneal rupture developed fistulas, though Corriere and Sandler (73) reported no fistulas in their 111 patients. With intraperitoneal rupture, the fistula may develop along the tract of the suprapubic tube. Peters advocates looking for causes of fistula formation (foreign body, infected tract) if the tract does not close with adequate bladder emptying (66). Definitive treatment for fistulas resistant to simple urinary diversion via urethral catheter is the excision of the tract and suturing the bladder in two layers (60). Newer options include fibrin sealant to close fistulous tracts after excision (79).

Incontinence, another possible complication of bladder injury, is usually not permanent after bladder laceration, unless the bladder neck is involved. Incontinence is usually transient, a result of irritation of the bladder mucosa, due to the catheter balloon, the catheter, or the laceration itself (60).

URETHRA
Epidemiology and Diagnosis

The urethra, from a trauma injury perspective, is divided into anterior, referring to the urethra distal to the pelvic diaphragm, and posterior, proximal to

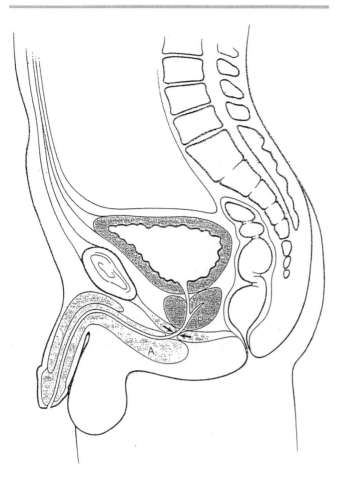

Figure 19 Proximal and distal urethra in male. *Source:* From Ref. 80.

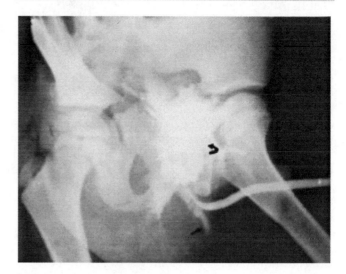

Figure 20 Complete rupture of the urethra with no contrast entering the bladder. *Source:* From Ref. 83.

the diaphragm. In the male, anterior includes the membranous and bulbous urethra, while the posterior includes the prostatic urethra (Fig. 19). Due to its short length in the female, the urethra is treated as a single entity. Urethral injuries are more common in males (64). Anterior urethral injuries are usually due to iatrogenic causes, for example, catheterization, straddle injuries, or penetrating injuries (81). Posterior urethral injuries most often occur with pelvic injuries; in fact, 80% to 90% have an associated pelvic fracture (64).

Presenting symptoms include blood at the penile meatus and an inability to void despite having the sensation of a "full" bladder. Anterior urethral injuries may also be associated with a butterfly (i.e., perineal) hematoma or a penile (sleeve) hematoma. Posterior urethral injury is associated with a "boggy" prostate caused by a hematoma occupying the prostatic fossa. In addition, a pelvic fracture associated with blood at the penile meatus should raise the suspicion of a posterior urethral fracture (82). Diagnosis of urethral injury is made by retrograde cystourethrogram. Complete interruption would demonstrate no contrast in the bladder and extravasation into the pelvis (Fig. 20), while incomplete disruption

would demonstrate extravasation with bladder filling (Fig. 21) (68).

Management

Urethral stretch injuries should be managed by Foley catheterization for three to four days (83). Incomplete rupture is treated with Foley catheterization. As long as there is a mucosal bridge, the urethra should regenerate and heal. After 10 to 14 days, the Foley catheter is removed and a voiding cystourethrogram to confirm

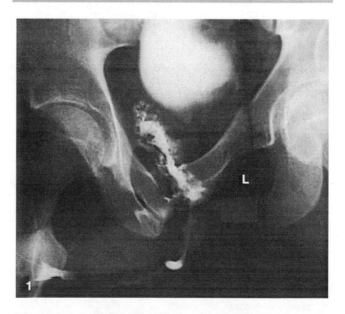

Figure 21 Retrograde cystourethrogram with extravasation of contrast as well as contrast in the bladder. *Source:* From Ref. 84.

healing should be obtained (85). Complete anterior disruption is treated by immediate repair, or delayed reconstruction with an SPC providing immediate urinary diversion. With most anterior urethral injuries, primary realignment is the method of choice, given the patient's clinical situation allows for repair and the tissue loss is not extensive enough to prevent a tension-free anastomosis (86). Straddle injuries to the anterior urethra and any other injury that obliterates the urethra are not amenable to primary repair because there is insufficient length to provide a tension-free anastomosis despite mobilization of the urethra. In these cases, the urine is drained via SPC and the urethra is reconnected at least six weeks after the trauma (81).

Management of posterior urethral injuries is more controversial. The goals of management are to correct the defect while minimizing complications, namely, incontinence, stricture, and impotence. The two most common strategies, primary realignment versus delayed reconstruction with urinary diversion via an SPC, minimize certain negative results while increasing others. In a study of 100 males with pelvic fractures and urethral disruption and a review of 771 patients discussed in the literature, Koraitim (87) found that formation of a stricture with the SPC method is almost guaranteed (97% stricture rate), though the rates of incontinence and impotence were the lowest of the various methods discussed (4% and 19%, respectively). The rate of stricture is markedly decreased with primary realignment (53%) and the rate of incontinence was similar to that of SPC (5%); however, patients were at a greater risk of impotence, with a rate of 36%. Primarily, reanastomosing the posterior urethra via direct vision and suturing was found to be unacceptable because this method had much higher rates of impotence (56%) and incontinence (21%) and a virtually identical rate of stricture (49%) when compared to primary realignment (Table 3).

Given this data, Koraitim (83) recommends SPC in situations where the patient is unstable, where the defect in the urethra is minimal or incomplete, or when the procedure is technically difficult either due to inexperience of the surgeon or due to anatomic issues. Primary realignment is appropriate in instances of widely separated urethral ends or associated rectal or bladder neck injury. Morey et al. echo these recommendations (85). Recently, performing endoscopic realignment after patient stabilization has been suggested (88,89). This follows the damage control philosophy: stabilization and immediate alleviation of any potential

life-threatening concerns, resuscitation, and then finally reoperation.

SPC is done via an open cystotomy, which allows for inspection of the bladder as well (85). Realignment has classically been via a "railroading" technique. This consists of placing one catheter in an antegrade manner through the cystotomy and a urethral via the urethral meatus, suturing the two together in the retropubic space, and bringing a second catheter into the bladder to bridge the defect (Fig. 22) (90). Another option is the sound technique, where one passes an antegrade Davis interlocking sound and has it meet a retrograde sound placed via the meatus. At that point, the antegrade sound is guided out the meatus and facilitates retrograde catheter placement.

More recently, endoscopic placement of a bridging catheter to achieve realignment has gained popularity (91,92). It is believed this method decreases disruption of any pelvic hematoma and less trauma to the nerves around the urethra, which, in turn, decreases the risk of infection or impotence. One endoscopic method, described by Kielb et al. (92), begins with performing a flexible cystoscopy to visualize the bladder and the "puckered opening" found after complete disruption of the posterior urethra. The bladder is entered with the cystoscope, a guidewire is passed into the bladder, and the scope is removed. Using the Seldinger technique, a Council

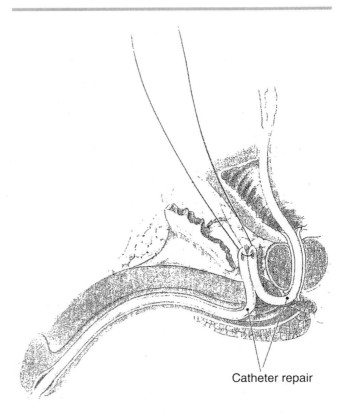

Catheter repair

Figure 22 Railroading of catheters to realign a distracted urethra. *Source:* From Ref. 51.

Table 3 Incidence of Complication and Type of Repair After Posterior Urethral Trauma

Complication/procedure	Stricture (%)	Incontinence (%)	Impotence (%)
Suprapubic catheter	97	4	19
Primary realignment	53	5	36
Primary suturing	49	21	56

tip catheter (or a Foley catheter with the tip cut off) is passed over a wire and left in place. If the operator is unable to find the bladder opening, a cystotomy is made and a second scope placed in an antegrade fashion, facilitating recognition of the bladder opening (92).

In women, Hemal et al. (93) found that primary repair had acceptable results requiring no reoperation in 17 of 17 patients, and with stricture amenable to nonsurgical resolution in 4 of 17 patients. SPC, on the other hand, was found to be a less desirable treatment modality as it has a high rate of urethrovaginal fistula (two of eight patients) as well as stricture requiring a second, delayed operation (eight of eight patients). They, therefore, advocate performing either realignment or a primary end-to-end reanastomosis. If these options are not feasible, due to the extensive urethral disruption or the patient's tenuous clinical state, the method of choice is SPC and eventual correction of the inevitable stricture and possible fistula that will follow.

Complications

As stated above, the complications of urethral injury include impotence, incontinence, and stricture, and the incidence of each is dependent on the immediate management modality taken (Table 2). The decisive factor leading to posttraumatic impotence seems to be the severity of the initial injury rather than management choice between SPC versus primary realignment. For instance, Asci et al. (94) found no statistically significant difference between initial treatment by SPC versus primary realignment for incontinence or impotence, though there was a difference for stricture (83.3% and 45.0%, respectively). In addition, Jenkins et al. (95) have shown that 10% of patients with small urethral displacement were impotent after suffering trauma, while 25% of those with a widely separated urethra were impotent, lending weight to the fact that initial injury is the determining factor for urethral injury complications.

Controversy remains whether the predominant etiology of posttraumatic impotence is due to neural or vascular injury (96–98). The significance of this difference is that the nature of the injury may dictate both initial and subsequent treatment; if neural factors determine later potency, primary realignment, which may damage the neurovascular bundle, would not be done; if there is extensive neural injury, there would be little gained from penile revascularization. Presently, treatment for impotence after urethral trauma tends to be conservative, including intracavernosal therapy and venoocclusive rings with vacuum devices. If evidence of vasculogenic impotence exists, the patient may benefit from penile revascularization (98).

If a stricture does develop, regardless of initial treatment, management depends on the length of the stricture. To determine the length of a stricture (99), retrograde urethrography along with antegrade cystourethrography may be performed (Fig. 23).

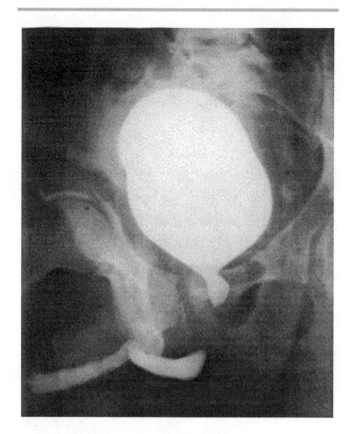

Figure 23 Cystogram and retrograde urethrogram showing large defect due to a stricture. *Source*: From Ref. 90.

Alternatively, sonourethrography can determine anterior stricture length, possibly more accurately than an urethrogram. For posterior strictures, magnetic resonance imaging in conjunction with retrograde urethrography and antegrade cystourethrography is helpful to determine stricture length and pelvic anatomy.

If the length is short, reconstructive options are either endoscopic or open. Open treatment consists of primary urethral reanastomosis, in the manner described above. Endoscopically, various options are available, including the "cut to the light" technique, with simultaneously placed antegrade and retrograde rigid cystoscopes, one with a urethrotome blade cutting to the second light source after assuring proper position fluoroscopically (100). Also available is the core technique consisting of passing a guidewire (or needle and then guidewire through the needle) through the stricture and then placing a urethral catheter in a retrograde fashion. The catheter is left in place for three to four weeks and then repeated endoscopy and urethrotomy is done when removing the catheter in order to stabilize the stricture walls (101). There is disagreement about the success of each method. Levine and Wessells (100) do not believe that endoscopic intervention improves upon the results of open urethroplasty. They point to the 100% repeat procedure requirement of the endoscopic group versus

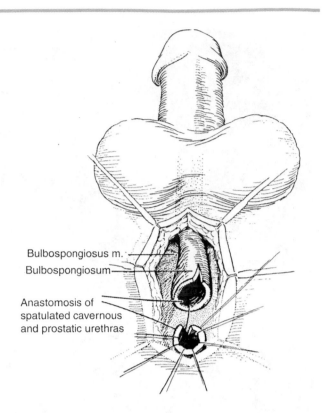

Bulbospongiosus m.

Bulbospongiosum

Anastomosis of
spatulated cavernous
and prostatic urethras

Figure 24 Cystogram and retrograde urethrogram showing a large defect due to a stricture. *Source*: From Ref. 102.

the 22% in the open group. On the other hand, Goel et al. (101) state the avoidance of an open procedure and its inherent morbidity, coupled with the long-term success rate of endoscopic procedures, regardless of minor reprocedures needed, justifies their use.

Open repair, generally undertaken three to six months after the initial injury, consists of several steps (90). First, an antegrade urethral sound is passed into the bladder and then into the urethra with the tip in the proximal stricture. After palpating the sound, the pelvic floor is opened and the sound is exposed. The prostatic urethra is spatulated posteriorly, exposing the verumontanum. If sufficient length is available to perform a tension-free, spatulated anastomosis, it is done at this time (Fig. 24). If not, to get more length, one can free up the distal urethra as far as the ligament of the penis circumferentially. If sufficient length still has not been achieved, the next option is to dissect between the corporal bodies and lay the urethra between the two. To obtain still more length, one may resect the pubis and lay the urethra in the space previously occupied by the bone. Between these three maneuvers (Fig. 25), an additional 7 cm or so can be obtained. Various grafts can be used to bridge the defect as well. The anastomosis should be spatulated and large enough to accommodate a 40-French catheter.

Incontinence is another potential complication after pelvic fracture and urethral injury. In men, continence is maintained by two mechanisms: the

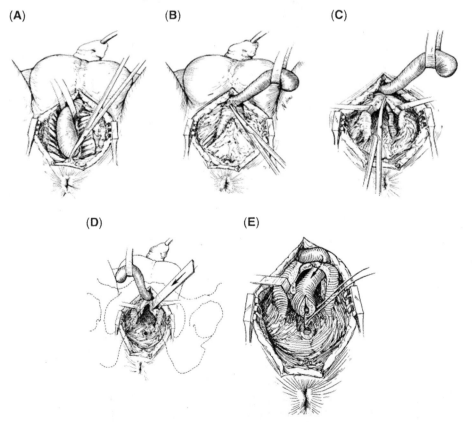

(A)   (B)   (C)

(D)   (E)

Figure 25 Diagram of various maneuvers to increase urethral length. *Source*: From Ref. 90.

internal sphincter, composed of the bladder neck, and the external sphincter, composed of intrinsic and extrinsic muscle. After urethral distraction defects, there is often compromise of the external urinary sphincter, either due to the initial insult or due to its subsequent repair (103,104). If compromise occurs, continence is maintained by the bladder neck only (Fig. 26). If the bladder neck is significantly compromised, continence will be affected adversely as well. Iselin and Webster (103) evaluated 15 men with pelvic fractures and four of five patients with incontinence had a bladder neck opening greater or equal to 1.5 cm prior to urethroplasty (the fifth had an opening 0.8 cm long). The six continent patients all had bladder neck lengths less than 1.5 cm. They concluded there was a higher rate of incontinence with greater bladder neck compromise. Treatment for incontinence due to trauma consists of repair of the bladder neck and freeing it from any surrounding fibrotic tissue that may be holding the bladder neck open. Artificial urinary sphincter placement is an option as well (90).

Pelvic hematoma is a likely occurrence after pelvic fracture (104). If contaminated through repeated attempts at catheterization, the hematoma may become infected. This in turn increases the likelihood of abscess or microabscess. Microabscess, in turn, cause fistula formation. Management of abscess is usually via percutaneous drainage. Fistulous tracts have to be excised entirely as described above (see section on "Complications" under "Bladder").

MALE REPRODUCTIVE ORGANS
Penis
Amputation (105)

Penile amputation may occur under various circumstances; however, most are self-inflicted. Self-amputation warrants a psychiatric evaluation. Regardless of etiology, the amputated penis has a warm ischemia time of about two to six hours. Management consists of determining whether the possibility of

reanastomosis exists. If so, a microvascular repair technique is used and the urine is diverted away from the anastomosis (usually via a suprapubic cystostomy catheter). If the penile remnant is unavailable or not amenable to reattachment, one should debride the penile stump to the bleeding edge with preservation of excess skin. The urethra should be spatulated and the excess skin brought down to cover the distal end of the penile stump (creating a "neo-corona").

Fracture (105)

Penile fracture occurs when an erect penis strikes a hard object, most commonly against a partner during vigorous intercourse, and bends at an acute angle resulting in a tear in Buck's fascia. The patient will experience a sudden "popping" sound and/or sensation accompanied by immediate detumescence of the penis. Treatment includes degloving the penis, evacuation of the hematoma, and primary repair of Buck's fascia. In addition, as a significant number of penile fractures are associated with urethral damage, evaluation of the urethra is necessary. This may include a urinalysis to evaluate for hematuria, radiologic evaluation, or direct inspection at the time of surgery.

Penetrating Injuries (105)

Penetrating injuries, regardless of etiology, should be managed by limited debridement of the devitalized area and primarily reanastomosing the urethra in a spatulated fashion. If the urethra cannot be reattached in a tension-free fashion, it should be marsupialized cutaneously at the distal limit of the proximal urethra. Further debridement should be undertaken as needed when the viable margins declare themselves. Prophylactic antibiotics should be used in all cases. Penetrating urethral trauma should be managed as stated above.

Scrotum and Testicle
Avulsion (105)

Scrotal avulsion can occur as a result of rotating machine accidents and/or after car or motorcycle accidents (as a form of "road rash"). Usually the external spermatic fascia is spared and only the dartos is affected. Initial management is conservative, waiting for the nonviable area to declare itself. At that point, usually 12 to 24 hours later, debridement is undertaken and assessment is made whether to primarily repair the scrotum or to perform a split thickness skin graft. While waiting for the demarcation, the exposed areas should be kept moist and cool with saline packs. There is no need to bury the penis or testicles in thigh pouches. The urethra should be evaluated for injury as well, in the method described above.

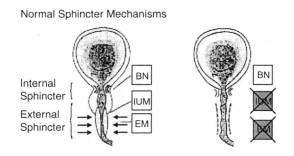

Figure 26 Normal and compromised sphincter in males. *Abbreviations*: BN, bladder neck; IUM, intrinsic urethral mechanism; EM, extrinsic muscles. *Source*: From Ref. 103.

Fracture (105)

Blunt or penetrating trauma may cause fracture of the testicles. On ultrasound examination, disruption of the tunica albuginea and tubules in a hematocele are seen. Operative management is indicated if the above-mentioned findings are confirmed or if lack of injury to the testicle is not assured. Treatment is surgical drainage of any peri- or intratesticular hematoma, debridement of any extruded or devitalized seminiferous tubules, and closure of the tunica albuginea with an absorbable suture. Conservative management has a significantly higher rate of orchiectomy and is, therefore, not an optimal choice. As a fresh hematocele is difficult to distinguish from a traumatic hydrocele, all traumatic hydroceles should be followed and observed to definitively differentiate it from hematocele.

REFERENCES

1. Skinner EC, Parisky YR, Skinner DG. Management of complex urologic injuries. Surg Clin N Am 1996; 76(4): 861–878.
2. Miller KS, McAninch JW. Radiographic assessment of renal trauma: our 15 year experience. J Urol 1995; 154(8):352–355.
3. Sullivan MJ, Lackner H, Banowsky LHW. Intraperitoneal extravasation of urine: BUN/serum creatinine disproportion. JAMA 1972; 221(5):491–492.
4. Morey AL, McAninch JW, Tiller BK, et al. Single shot intraoperative excretory urography for the immediate evaluation of renal trauma. J Urol 1999; 161:1088–1092.
5. Wah TM, Spencer JA. The role of CT in the management of adult urinary tract trauma. Clin Radiol 2001; 56(4):268–277.
6. Perez-Brayfield MR, Gatti JM, Smith EA, et al. Blunt traumatic hematuria in children. Is a simplified algorithm justified? J Urol 2002; 167(6):2543–2546; discussion 2546–2547.
7. Hoff WS, Holevar M, Nagy KK, et al. Practice Management Guidelines for the Evaluation of Blunt Abdominal Trauma. Eastern Association for the Surgery of Trauma, 2001.
8. Goldman SM, Sandler CM. Upper urinary tract trauma—current concepts. World J Urol 1998; 16: 62–68.
9. Sandler CM, et al. Diagnostic Approach to Renal Trauma. American College of Radiology ACR Appropriateness Criteria, 1998:727–731.
10. Carpio F, Morey AF. Radiographic staging of renal injuries. World J Urol 1999; 17(2):66–70.
11. Haas CA, Brown SL, Spirnak JP. Limitations of routine spiral computerized tomography in the evaluation of bladder trauma. J Urol 1999; 162(1):51–52.
12. Blankenship JC, Gavant ML, Cox CE, Chauhan RD, Gingrich JR. Importance of delayed imaging for blunt renal trauma. World J Surg 2001; 25(12):1561–1564.
13. Brown SL, Hoffman DM, Spirnak JP. Limitations of routine spiral computerized tomography in the evaluation of blunt renal trauma. J Urol 1998; 160(6 Pt 1): 1979–1981.
14. Deck AJ, Shaves S, Talner L, Porter JR. Computerized tomography cystography for the diagnosis of traumatic bladder rupture. J Urol 2000; 164(1):43–46.
15. Ahn JH, Morey AF, McAninch JW. Workup and management of traumatic hematuria. Emerg Med Clin N Am 1998; 16(1):145–164.
16. Brandes SB, McAninch JW. Renal trauma: a practical guide to evaluation and management. Digital Urol J 1996 (http://www.duj.com/Article/McAninch/McAninch.html).
17. Kawashima A, Sandler CM, Corl FM, et al. Imaging of renal trauma: a comprehensive review. Radiographics 2001; 21(3):557–574.
18. Santucci RA, McAninch JW, Safir M, Mario LA, Service S, Segal MR. Validation of the American Association for the Surgery of Trauma Organ Injury Severity Scale for the Kidney. J Trauma 2001; 50(2): 195–200.
19. Santucci RA, McAninch JW. Grade IV renal injuries: evaluation, treatment and outcome. World J Surg 2001; 25:1565–1572.
20. Moore E, Shackford S, Packter H, et al. Scaling: spleen, liver, and kidney. J Trauma 1989; 29:1664–1666.
21. Thall EH, Stone NN, Cheng DL, et al. Conservative management of penetrating and blunt type III renal injuries. Br J Urol 1996; 77(4):512–517.
22. Husmann DA, Gilling PJ, Perry MO, et al. Major renal lacerations with devitalized fragments following blunt abdominal trauma: a comparison between non-operative (expectant) versus surgical management. J Urol 1993; 150:1774–1777.
23. Moudouni SM, Patard JJ, Manunta A, Guiraud P, Guille F, Lobel B. A conservative approach to major blunt renal lacerations with urinary extravasation and devitalized renal segments. BJU Int 2001; 87(4): 290–294.
24. Matthews LA, Smith EM, Spirnak JP. Nonoperative treatment of major blunt renal lacerations with urinary extravasation. J Urol 1997; 157(6):2056–2058.
25. Altman AL, Haas C, Dinchman KH, Spirnak JP. Selective nonoperative management of blunt grade 5 renal injury. J Urol 2000; 164(1):27–30.
26. Nicol AJ, Theunissen D. Renal salvage in penetrating kidney injuries: a prospective analysis. J Trauma 2002; 53(2):351–353.
27. Margenthaler JA, Weber TR, Keller MS. Blunt renal trauma in children: experience with conservative management at a pediatric trauma center. J Trauma 2002; 52(5):928–932.
28. Wessells H, McAninch JW. Update on Upper Urinary Tract Trauma. AUA Update Series. Vol. XV. Lesson 14, 1996.
29. Meng MV, Brandes SB, McAninch JW. Renal trauma: indications and techniques for surgical exploration. World J Urol 1999; 17(2):71–77.
30. Gonzalez RP, Falimirski M, Holevar MR, Evankovich C. Surgical management of renal trauma: is vascular control necessary? J Trauma 1999; 47(6):1039–1042; discussion 1042–1044.
31. Kuo RL, Eachempati SR, Makhuli MJ, Reed RL II. Factors affecting management and outcome in blunt renal injury. World J Surg 2002; 26(4):416–419.
32. Whitney RF, Peterson NE. Penetrating renal injuries. Urology 1976; 7(1):7–11.

33. Moudouni SM, Hadj Slimen M, Manunta A, et al. Management of major blunt renal lacerations: is a non-operative approach indicated? Eur Urol 2001; 40(4): 409–414.

34. Toporoff B, Sclafani S, Scalea T, et al. Percutaneous antegrade ureteral stenting as an adjunct for treatment of complicated ureteral injuries. J Trauma 1992; 32(4): 534–538.

35. Guerriero WG. Ureteral injuries. Urol Clin N Am 1989; 16(2):237–248.

36. Al-Ali AF, Haddad LF. The late treatment of 63 over-looked or complicated ureteral missile injuries: the promise of nephrostomy and role of autotransplantation. J Urol 1996; 156(6):1918–1921.

37. Knudson MM, Harrison PB, Hoyt DB, et al. Outcome after major renovascular injuries: a Western Trauma Association Multicenter report. J Trauma 2000; 49(6): 1116–1122.

38. Montgomery RC, Richardson JD, Harty JI. Posttrau-matic renovascular hypertension after occult renal injury. J Trauma 1998; 45(1):106–110.

39. McAninch JW, Carroll PR. Renal trauma: kidney pre-servation through improved vascular control—a refined approach. J Trauma 1982; 22(4):285–290.

40. Teigen CL, Venbrux AC, Quinlan DM, Jeffs RD. Late massive hematuria as a complication of conservative management of blunt renal trauma in children. J Urol 1992; 147(5):1333–1336.

41. Carroll PR, Klosterman PW, McAninch JW. Surgical management of renal trauma: analysis of risk factors, technique and outcome. J Trauma 1998; 28(7):1071–1077.

42. Palmer LS, Rosenbaum RR, Gershbaum MD, Kreutzer ER. Penetrating ureteral trauma at an urban trauma center: 10-year experience. Urology 1999; 54(1):34–36.

43. Preston JM Iatrogenic ureteric injury: common medi-colegal pitfalls. BJU International 86(3):313–317.

44. Perez-Brayfield MR, Keane TE, Krishnan A, Lafontaine P, Feliciano DV, Clarke HS. Gunshot wounds to the ureter: a 40-year experience at Grady Memorial Hospital. J Urol 2001; 166(1):119–121.

45. Campbell EW Jr., Filderman PS, Jacobs SC. Ureteral injury due to blunt and penetrating trauma. Urology 1992; 40(3):216–220.

46. Ghali AM, El Malik EM, Ibrahim AI, Ismail G, Rashid M. Ureteric injuries: diagnosis, management, and outcome. J Trauma 1999; 46(1):150–158.

47. Azimuddin K, Milanesa D, Ivatury R, Porter J, Ehrenpreis M, Allman DB. Penetrating ureteric inju-ries. Injury 1998; 29(5):363–367.

48. Armenakas NA. Current methods of diagnosis and management of ureteral injuries. World J Urol 1999; 17(2):78–83.

49. Mulligan JM, Cagiannos I, Collins JP, Millward SF. Ureteropelvic junction disruption secondary to blunt trauma: excretory phase imaging (delayed films) should help prevent a missed diagnosis. J Urol 1998; 159(1):67–70.

50. Medina D, Lavery R, Ross SE, Livingston DH. Ureteral trauma: preoperative studies neither predict injury nor prevent missed injuries. JACS 1998; 186(6):641–644.

51. Thal, Weigelt, Carrico. Operative Trauma Manage-ment: An Atlas. 2nd ed. McGraw Hill, 2002.

52. Azimuddin K, Ivatury R, Porter J, Allman DB. Damage control in a trauma patient with ureteric injury. J Trauma 1997; 43(6):977–979.

53. Brandes SB, McAninch JW. Reconstructive surgery for trauma of the upper urinary tract. Urol Clin N Am 1999; 26(1):183–199.

54. Meng M, Friese CE, Stroller ML. Extended experience with laparoscopic nephrectomy and autotransplanta-tion for severe proximal ureter loss. J Urol 2003; 169(4):1363–1367.

55. Mathews R, Marshall FF. Versatility of the adult psoas hitch ureteral implantation. J Urol 1997; 158(6): 2078–2082.

56. Stief CG, Jonas U, Petry KU, et al. Ureteric reconstruc-tion. BJU Int 2003; 91(2):138–142.

57. Ahn M, Loughlin KR. Psoas hitch ureteral reimplanta-tion in adults—analysis of a modified technique and timing of repair. Urology 2001; 58:184–187.

58. Richter F, Irwin RJ, Watson RA, Lang EK. Endourolo-gic management of benign ureteral strictures with and without compromised vascular supply. Urology 2000; 55(5):652–657.

59. Cass AS. Ureteral contusion with gunshot wounds. J Trauma 1984; 24(1):59–60.

60. Brandes SB, McAninch JW. Complications of genitour-inary trauma. In: Taneja SS, Smith RB, Ehrlich RM, eds. Complications of Urologic Surgery: Prevention and Management : WB Saunders, 2001:205–225.

61. Selzman AA, Spirnak JP, Kursh ED. The changing management of ureterovaginal fistulas. J Urol 1995; 153(3):626–628.

62. Corriere JN Jr., Sandler CM. Bladder rupture from external trauma: diagnosis and management. World J Urol 1999; 17(2):84–89.

63. Sandler CM, Goldman SM, Kawashima A. Lower urinary tract trauma. World J Urol 1998; 16:69–75.

64. Dreitlein DA, Suner S, Basler J. Genitourinary trauma. Emerg Med Clin N Am 2001; 19(3):569–590.

65. Corriere JN Jr., Sandler CM. Mechanisms of injury, patterns of extravasation and management of extra-peritoneal bladder rupture due to blunt trauma. J Urol 1988; 139(1):43–44.

66. Peters PC. Intraperitoneal rupture of the bladder. Urol Clin N Am 1989; 16(2):279–282.

67. Iverson AJ, Morey AF. Radiographic evaluation of suspected bladder rupture following blunt trauma: critical review. World J Surg 2001; 25(12):1588–1591.

68. Brandes S, Borrelli J Jr.. Pelvic fracture and associated urologic injuries. World J Surg 2001; 25(12):1578–1587.

69. Morey AF, Iverson AJ, Swan A, et al. Bladder rupture after blunt trauma: guidelines for diagnostic imaging. J Trauma 2001; 51(4):683–686.

70. Carroll PR, McAninch JW. Major bladder trauma: mechanisms of injury and unified method of diagno-sis and repair. J Urol 1984; 132:254–257.

71. Vaccaro JP, Brody JM. CT cystography in the evalua-tion of major bladder trauma. Radiographics 2000; 20(5):1373–1381.

72. Bigongiari LR, et al. Trauma to the bladder and ure-thra. ACR Appropriateness Criteria. American College of Radiology, 1998:733–740.

73. Corriere JN Jr., Sandler CM. Management of the rup-tured bladder: seven years of experience with 111 cases. J Trauma 1986; 28(9):830–833.

74. Corriere JN Jr., Sandler CM. Management of extraperitoneal bladder rupture. Urol Clin N Am 1989; 16(2): 275–277.

75. Kotkin L, Koch MO. Morbidity associated with nonoperative management of extraperitoneal bladder injuries. J Trauma 1995; 38(6):895–898.

76. Libertino JA, ed. Reconstructive Urologic Surgery. 3rd ed. Mosby, 1998.

77. Volpe MA, Pachter EM, Scalea TM, et al. Is there a difference in outcome when treating traumatic intraperitoneal bladder rupture with or without a suprapubic tube? J Urol 1999; 161:1103–1105.

78. Parry NG, Rozycki GS, Feliciano DV, et al. Traumatic rupture of the urinary bladder: is the suprapubic tube necessary? J Trauma 2003; 54:431–436.

79. Evans LA, Ferguson KH, Foley JP, Rozanski TA, Morey AF. Fibrin sealant for the management of genitourinary injuries, fistulas and surgical complications. J Urol 2003; 169(4):1360–1362.

80. Gibbs MA, Schneider R. Genitourinary tract and renovascular trauma. In: Ferrera P, et al., eds. Trauma Management: An Emergency Medicine Approach. Vol 1. Mosby Year Book, 2000:317–329.

81. Hernandez J, Morey AF. Anterior urethral injury. World J Urol 1999; 17(2):96–100.

82. Dobrowolski ZF, Weglarz W, Jakubik P, Lipczynski W, Dobrowolska B. Treatment of posterior and anterior urethral trauma. BJU Int 2002; 89(7):752–754.

83. Koraitim MM. Pelvic fracture urethral injuries: the unresolved controversy. J Urol 1999; 161(5):1433–1441.

84. Mundy AR. Pelvic fracture injuries of the posterior urethra. World J Urol 1999; 17:90–95.

85. Morey AF, Hernandez J, McAninch JW. Reconstructive surgery for trauma of the lower urinary tract. Urol Clin N Am 1999; 26(1):49–60.

86. Hall SJ, Wagner JR, Edelstein RA, Carpinito GA. Management of gunshot injuries to the penis and anterior urethra. J Trauma 1995; 38(3):439–443.

87. Koraitim MM. Pelvic fracture urethral injuries: evaluation of various methods of management. J Urol 1996; 156(4):1288–1291.

88. Moudouni SM, Patard JJ, Manunta A, Guiraud P, Lobel B, Guille F. Early endoscopic realignment of post-traumatic posterior urethral disruption. Urology 2001; 57(4):628–632.

89. Jepson BR, Boullier JA, Moore RG, Parra RO. Traumatic posterior urethral injury and early primary endoscopic realignment: evaluation of long-term follow-up. Urology 1999; 53(6):1205–1210.

90. Webster GD, Guralnick ML. Reconstruction of posterior urethral disruption. Urol Clin N Am 2002; 29(2): 429–441, viii.

91. Gheiler EL, Frontera JR. Immediate primary realignment of prostatomembranous urethral disruptions using endourologic techniques. Urology 1997; 49(4):596–599.

92. Kielb SJ, Voeltz ZL, Wolf JS. Evaluation and management of traumatic posterior urethral disruption with flexible cystourethroscopy. J Trauma 2001; 50(1):36–40.

93. Hemal AK, Dorairajan LN, Gupta NP. Posttraumatic complete and partial loss of urethra with pelvic fracture in girls: an appraisal of management. J Urol 2000; 163(1):282–287.

94. Asci R, Sarikaya S, Buyukalpelli R, Saylik A, Yilmaz AF, Yildiz S. Voiding and sexual dysfunctions after pelvic fracture urethral injuries treated with either initial cystostomy and delayed urethroplasty or immediate primary urethral realignment. Scand J Urol Nephrol 1999; 33(4):228–233.

95. Jenkins BJ, Badenoch DF, Fowler CG, Slandy JP. Long-term results of treatment of urethral injuries in males caused by external trauma. Br J Urol 1992; 70(1):73–75.

96. Armenakas NA, McAninch JW, Lue TF, Dixon CM, Hricak H. Posttraumatic impotence: magnetic resonance imaging and duplex ultrasound in diagnosis and management. J Urol 1993; 149(5 Pt 2):1272–1275.

97. Machtens S, Gansslen A, Pohlemann T, Stief CG. Erectile dysfunction in relation to traumatic pelvic injuries or pelvic fractures. BJU Int 2001; 87(5):441–448.

98. Shenfeld OZ, Kiselgorf D, Gofrit ON, et al. The incidence and causes of erectile dysfunction after pelvic fractures associated with posterior urethral disruption. J Urol 2003; 169(6):2173–2176.

99. Gallentine ML, Morey AF. Imaging of the male urethra for stricture disease. Urol Clin N Am 2002; 29(2):361–372.

100. Levine J, Wessells H. Comparison of open and endoscopic treatment of posttraumatic posterior urethral strictures. World J Surg 2001; 25(12):1597–1601.

101. Goel MC, Kumar M, Kapoor R. Endoscopic management of traumatic posterior urethral stricture: early results and followup. J Urol 1997; 157(1):95–97.

102. Morey AF, McAninch JW. Reconstruction of posterior urethral disruption injuries: outcome analysis in 82 patients. J Urol 1997; 157(2):506–510.

103. Iselin CE, Webster GD. The significance of the open bladder neck associated with pelvic fracture urethral distraction defects. J Urol 1999; 162(2):347–351.

104. Turner-Warwick R. Prevention of complications resulting from pelvic fracture urethral injuries and from their surgical management. Urol Clin N Am 1989; 16(2):335–358.

105. Jordan GH. Lower Genitourinary Tract Trauma and Male External Genitalia Trauma Parts 2–3. Lessons 11 and 12. Vol. 19. AUA Update Series, 2000.

50

Surgical Complications of Kidney–Pancreas Transplantation

Gaetano Ciancio, Joshua Miller, and George W. Burke
Division of Transplantation, The DeWitt Daughtry Family Department of Surgery, University of Miami, Miller School of Medicine, Miami, Florida, U.S.A.

Patricia M. Byers
Division of Trauma, Burns, and Critical Care, The DeWitt Daughtry Family Department of Surgery, University of Miami, Miller School of Medicine, Miami, Florida, U.S.A.

Simultaneous pancreas–kidney (SPK) transplantation is becoming one of the standard treatment options for patients with type 1 diabetes and end-stage renal disease. More potent immunosuppression protocols, improvements in surgical techniques, and a better understanding of postoperative complications have made SPK transplantation a successful procedure of choice (1–3).

Currently, SPK transplantation is offered to patients with type 1 diabetes and end-stage renal disease if there are no absolute contraindications to the procedure. For safety reasons, at our center, we primarily drain the exocrine pancreas and duodenal segment into the bladder. This technique also allows us to measure urinary amylase activity so that we can monitor any changes in the function of the pancreas graft (4). The 10-year survival rates at our center—84% for patients and 76% for pancreas grafts—are among the best-reported long-term survival rates (4).

TRANSPLANTATION
Donor Operation

The standard donor operation generally includes procurement of the liver, both kidneys, and the whole pancreas with the duodenum. The nasogastric tube is advanced into the duodenum of the donor and is irrigated with 25 mL of 1% povidone-iodine solution, followed by 50 mL of cold saline solution. The duodenum is irrigated with an antibiotic solution that includes amphotericin B. The nasogastric tube is then pulled back into the stomach, the duodenal contents are gently milked out of the duodenal segments, and the proximal and distal segments are staple divided. Care is taken to ensure that there is no distention. A Y vascular graft, composed of the donor's common, external, and internal iliac arteries or the brachiocephalic trunk (Fig. 1), is stored in a separate container of University of Wisconsin (UW) solution on the back table (5). The composite pancreas graft is then taken to the back table for further dissection. However, staple lines are not opened. At this time, splenectomy is performed and the duodenal segment is shortened; only the second portion of the duodenum is kept. Both the proximal end and the distal end are divided with staples and oversewn with interrupted 4–0 silk or Prolene® sutures (Ethicon Suture Co., Sommerville, New Jersey, U.S.A.). Finally, the Y graft is fashioned, the internal iliac artery is anastomosed to the splenic artery of the pancreas, and the external iliac artery is anastomosed to the superior mesenteric artery of the pancreas with 6–0 Prolene sutures (Fig. 2). The portal vein is then dissected free from the pancreatic bed.

Recipient Operation

The recipient operation (Fig. 3) begins with a midline incision. The left kidney is revascularized by anastomosing the renal vein to the common or external iliac vein and the renal artery to the common or external iliac artery. A 4-cm opening is made in the dome of the bladder, where the ureteroneocystostomy anastomosis is performed with a short submucosal tunnel. Next, the pancreas–duodenal allograft is revascularized on the right side. The portal vein is anastomosed to the common iliac vein with a 5–0 Prolene suture, and the common iliac artery of the Y graft is anastomosed to the recipient's external or common iliac artery with a 6–0 Prolene suture. The duodenum is opened to allow drainage and prevent distention; a pancreatic duodenocystostomy (PDC) is then performed with a two-layer hand-sewn technique. Closure of the inner layer is performed with a running 4–0 Vicryl® suture (Ethicon Suture Co., Sommerville, New Jersey, U.S.A.). The outer layer is then closed with a running 4–0 Prolene suture. No external drains are used, and a Foley catheter is left in place for 7 to 10 days.

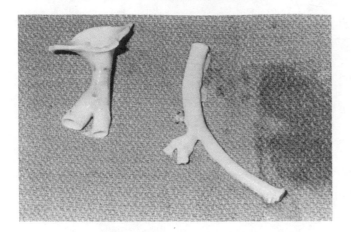

Figure 1 Brachiocephalic trunk with an aortic patch (*left*) or an iliac Y graft (*right*).

SURGICAL COMPLICATIONS AFTER PANCREAS TRANSPLANTATION

Surgical complications are more common after pancreas transplantation than after kidney transplantation. Nonimmunological complications of pancreas transplantation account for graft losses in 5% to 10% of cases. These complications usually occur within six months after the transplantation; their impact on loss of the pancreas graft is the same as that of acute rejection (6).

Thrombosis

Vascular thrombosis is a very early complication that typically occurs no later than 48 hours and usually within 24 hours after transplantation. Of all potential causes of technical failure, graft thrombosis is the most common; its incidence in association with SPK transplantation is 5.5% (7).

It may be difficult to determine precisely which risk factor is implicated in the pathogenesis of graft thrombosis because many causal factors have been described. Graft thrombosis may occur for many reasons, such as preterminal donor hypoperfusion, poor preservation, technical or mechanical issues, immunologic problems, sepsis, or hypercoagulable states. In addition, graft thrombosis has been attributed to the hemodynamic changes in blood flow from a high-flow to a low-flow state after ligation of the distal splenic vessels, the superior mesenteric vessels, and all nonpancreatic branches.

Graft salvage is unlikely after thrombosis and can occur only when parenchymal damage is minimal. For this reason, some surgeons have attempted to develop surgical techniques for preventing vascular thrombosis. Some have suggested creating a distal arteriovenous fistula (AVF) so that splenic artery flow is increased (8–11). Another alternative is transplanting the pancreas with the spleen so that physiological hemodynamic flow can be maintained (12). The disadvantage of this procedure is the risk of the potentially lethal complication of graft-versus-host disease (13). None of these techniques have consistently prevented early graft thrombosis (14), perhaps because graft perfusion probably remains unchanged despite attempts to increase flow through the larger vessels (15,16).

Partial Venous Thrombosis

We retrospectively reviewed our experience with the outcome and treatment options associated with partial venous thrombosis of pancreas allografts. From July 1994 to April 1997, 66 patients scheduled for SPK transplantation underwent antilymphocyte induction therapy with a monoclonal anti-CD3 preparation (OKT3) and oral or intravenous tacrolimus in the operating room. None of these patients experienced partial venous thrombosis. In contrast, from May 1997 to June 1999, 48 patients underwent induction therapy with intravenous tacrolimus alone or in conjunction with humanized monoclonal antibody to the interleukin (IL)-2 receptor (IL2-rmAb; Daclizumab®) (17). Of these 48 patients, 14 (29%) experienced partial venous thrombosis, which was detected during routine color Doppler ultrasonography. Twelve of these patients had thrombosis of the splenic vein, one had thrombosis of the superior mesenteric vein (Fig. 4), and one had partial thrombosis of the splenic and superior mesenteric veins. We administered tacrolimus intravenously so that we could ensure sufficient concentrations early in the posttransplantation period to avoid acute rejection (18–21).

Microvascular changes associated with pancreatic transplantation may also predispose patients to venous thrombosis. Prostacyclin (PGI_2) and thromboxane A_2 (TXA_2), prostanoid derivatives of eicosapolyenoic fatty

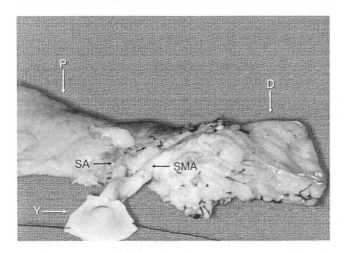

Figure 2 The composite pancreas and duodenal graft, demonstrating the Y graft. The portal vein has been dissected free of the pancreatic bed. *Key*: Y, brachiocephalic trunk anastomosed to the splenic artery and the superior mesenteric artery of the pancreaticoduodenal graft; P, pancreas; D, duodenum; SA, splenic artery; and SMA, superior mesenteric artery.

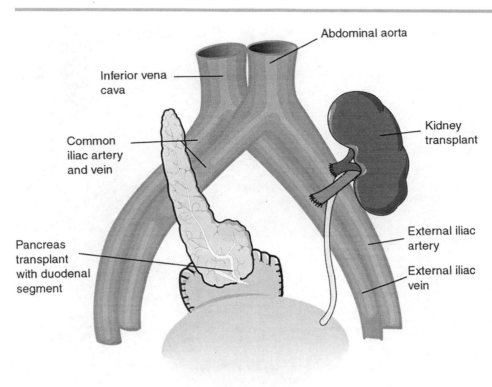

Figure 3 Surgical technique of simultaneous pancreas–kidney transplantation with bladder drainage through a midline intraperitoneal approach. The donor kidney is revascularized on the left side by anastomosing the renal vein to the external iliac vein and the renal artery to the external iliac artery. The dome of the bladder is shown with the ureteroneocystostomy and pancreaticoduodenocystostomy anastomoses. The pancreas–duodenal allograft is revascularized on the right side by anastomosing the portal vein to the common iliac vein and the common iliac artery of the Y graft to the recipient common iliac artery.

acids with opposing actions on vascular smooth muscle tone and platelet aggregation, provide a homeostatic mechanism for maintaining the integrity of the circulation (22–24). TXA_2 promotes platelet aggregation and causes vasospasm, whereas PGI_2 opposes these actions, inhibiting platelet aggregation and causing vasodilation. Experimental studies noted an increase in the production of TXA_2 by the pancreas and a decrease in the ratio of PGI_2 to TXA_2 after cold ischemia and reperfusion of the pancreas (25,26). Others have noted that the change in the ratio of these prostaglandins may result from the stasis of the blood flow in the splenic vessels (27). Tacrolimus may contribute to this problem by inducing vasospasm and causing microvascular injury (28). Alternatively, it may cause endothelial injury and thrombosis because of alterations in the ratio of TXA_2 to prostaglandin PGI_2 or because of the release of endothelin (29–31). The potential for increased adhesion of T cells that express IL-2 receptors bound by daclizumab, combined with the known low-flow state of the splenic vein, may provide the setting for venous thrombosis when the endothelial toxic effects of tacrolimus are added to the mix.

Studies have reported microvascular changes late in the course of oral tacrolimus-based immunosuppression therapy (32–35). Corry et al. (36) reported that 9 of their 123 patients experienced pancreas thrombosis while receiving intravenous tacrolimus, but the authors attributed the thrombosis to ischemia and reperfusion injury rather than to the use of intravenous tacrolimus. We have also described microangiopathy among recipients of kidney transplants or SPK transplants, who were treated with tacrolimus within two to four weeks after transplantation (31). In each case, the intravenous administration of tacrolimus was discontinued, and immunosuppression

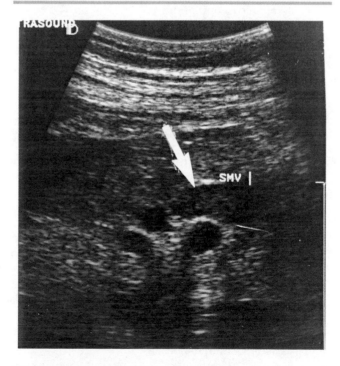

Figure 4 Partial thrombosis (*arrow*) of the superior mesenteric vein detected by routine color Doppler ultrasonography.

was maintained by oral tacrolimus, steroids, and mycophenolate mofetil.

Currently, there is limited information about the use of both tacrolimus and daclizumab for patients undergoing SPK transplantation. A multicenter retrospective analysis found only one case of pancreas thrombosis, which was probably not related to the use of tacrolimus and daclizumab as induction therapy (37). No clinical symptoms of thrombosis, such as graft tenderness, decreased or absent urinary amylase activity, sudden-onset hyperglycemia, hematuria, thrombocytopenia, leukocytosis, or intra-abdominal bleeding, were seen. None of the patients experienced any change in clinical parameters. Superior mesenteric or splenic vein thrombosis was detected incidentally during routine Doppler ultrasonography. Sonography, computed tomography (CT), magnetic resonance imaging, and nuclear medicine scanning have been used to diagnose pancreatic graft thrombosis (38–42). We have found color Doppler ultrasonography to be helpful and cost-effective in diagnosing and assessing venous thrombosis of the pancreatic allograft.

More recently, six patients with partial thrombosis of the splenic vein were treated with aspirin and followed up with serial Doppler ultrasonography. None of the partial thromboses progressed to complete splenic vein or pancreatic graft thrombosis. It is possible that partial splenic vein thrombosis is a self-limited process and does not require heparinization. The administration of aspirin may be sufficient (43).

Complete Venous Thrombosis

When partial thrombosis has progressed to complete venous thrombosis, attempts at salvaging the thrombosed pancreas graft have been disappointing (44). Immediate reoperation has been advised so that life-threatening sequelae can be avoided (44,45). Thrombectomy can be performed through a previous portal anastomosis or through a longitudinal or transverse venotomy in the portal vein (44,46,47). Another approach is resection of the thrombosed segment of the pancreas graft (48). Transplant pancreatectomy with immediate transplantation of a new donor pancreas has also been described in cases of graft thrombosis (47,49). This option requires the absence of infection and the availability of a suitable donor within 24 to 48 hours.

Recently, we reported our experience with three recipients of SPK transplants who experienced complete venous thrombosis of the pancreas (Fig. 5). All three underwent surgical thrombectomy followed by immediate systemic anticoagulation with heparin. The splenic vein was opened at the tail of the pancreas, and the superior mesenteric vein was opened at the level of the mesentery or the head of the pancreas. This procedure resulted in the successful salvage of the pancreas allografts (50). After resolution of the clot was demonstrated by Doppler ultrasonography, heparinization was converted to warfarin therapy for three months; after that, aspirin therapy was used. All of

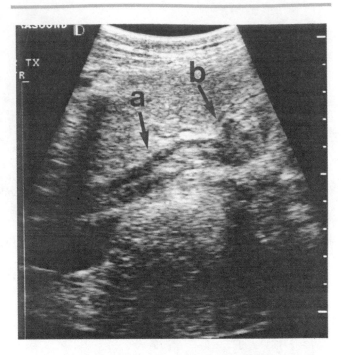

Figure 5   Doppler ultrasonogram showing complete venous thrombosis of the pancreas allograft, including the splenic vein (a) and the superior mesenteric vein (b).

these patients were monitored closely with Doppler ultrasonography and checks of serum and urinary amylase activity. One patient experienced recurrent thrombosis. The allograft was salvaged by percutaneous thrombectomy and urokinase infusion, followed by systemic anticoagulation.

Arterial Thrombosis

Arterial thrombosis is less common than venous thrombosis and is usually associated with anastomoses of atherosclerotic vessels. In our series, one patient experienced thrombosis of the superior mesenteric artery. Diagnosis was made by routine Doppler ultrasonography of the pancreas (Fig. 6). Surgical thrombectomy was performed successfully through the head of the pancreas allograft. We placed loops around the recipient iliac artery and the Y arterial graft, but did not have any need to occlude inflow; thus, we were able to avoid further ischemic injury to the pancreatic graft.

Another patient experienced late thrombosis of the Y graft, although the function of the pancreas allograft persisted. It is possible that pancreatic function was maintained by collateral flow or neovascularization between the donor graft and the recipient vessels. This patient required no treatment (51).

Prophylaxis of Graft Thrombosis

Thrombocytosis has been seen after pancreas transplantation without obvious pathophysiological explanations. Because multiple factors predispose the

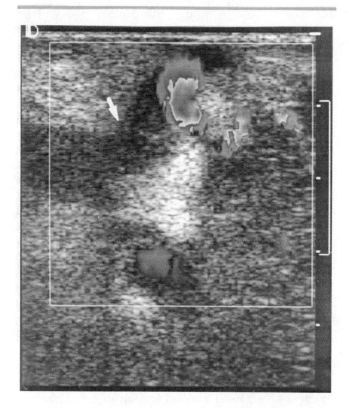

Figure 6 Doppler ultrasonogram of the pancreas allograft, showing thrombosis of the superior mesenteric artery (*arrow*).

vessels of the pancreas graft to thrombosis, platelet inhibitors should be administered during the first two postoperative months (52). Another option for preventing graft thrombosis is the use of prophylactic anticoagulant therapy.

Various transplant centers use different therapeutic protocols in an attempt to prevent thrombosis. For example, one group advocates the use of low-molecular-weight dextran, followed by intravenous heparin and antithrombin III supplementation in combination with long-term administration of acetylsalicylic acid (53,54). Another group uses dextran followed by low-dose aspirin, or a combination of aspirin and dipyridamole (55,56).

The routine use of systemic anticoagulation has been controversial. Systemic anticoagulation is accepted therapy when splenic vein thrombosis has been documented, when SPK grafts have come from live donors, and when only the pancreas has been transplanted (43,57,58). However, Sollinger has suggested that the use of systemic anticoagulation does not reduce the incidence of vascular graft thrombosis and may increase the likelihood of postoperative bleeding, which may in turn cause venous compression, thereby actually increasing the risk of graft thrombosis (59).

Arteriovenous Fistula

AVF has only recently been recognized as a complication of pancreas transplantation. AVF may cause pancreatic endocrine insufficiency, hematuria, or a bruit over the graft. The causes of this abnormality are congenital malformation, needle injury during procurement, injury during the back-table preparation, and injury during reperfusion hemostasis in the recipient. Doppler ultrasonography is indicated if endocrine function suddenly deteriorates or if the patient experiences hematuria and pain over the graft. The diagnosis is confirmed by abnormal flow in the pancreatic head (Fig. 7). In our series of patients, four have experienced AVF. Two were treated with surgical correction; the other two were treated with angiography and embolization. Pancreatic endocrine function has been preserved in all four patients (51,60).

Transplant Pancreatitis

Graft thrombosis may occur after the development of reperfusion-induced graft pancreatitis, which is caused when pancreatic blood flow is reduced to a critical level (61). Multiple factors may be related to graft pancreatitis, and Troppmann has described these in detail (62). Donor risk factors include hemodynamic instability, brain injury, and vasopressor administration; procurement injury may be due to excessive intraoperative manipulation. Perfusion injury may also occur when excessive flush volumes or perfusion pressures are used. Also, total cold and warm ischemia times may have an effect on preservation and the occurrence of reperfusion injury. Grewal et al. (63) demonstrated that postoperative treatment of the recipient with calcium-channel blockers, combined with the administration of steroids to the donor at the time of procurement, protects against the development of pancreatitis.

Animal models of pancreatitis demonstrate that the microcirculation is impaired as pancreatitis

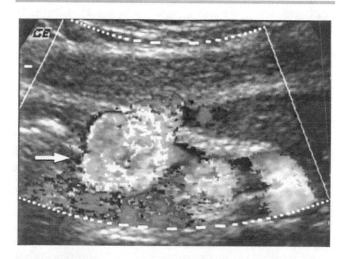

Figure 7 Doppler ultrasonogram of the pancreas allograft, showing increased pulsatile flow within the area of the body of the pancreas (*arrow*), a finding diagnostic of a arteriovenous fistula.

progresses, and this impairment leads to necrosis and thrombosis of the pancreas (64–66). Although these findings do not necessarily reflect allograft pancreatitis as associated with transplantation, they could explain some of the events that occur in association with pancreatic graft edema. With the introduction of UW (or Belzer) solution as a perfusate for pancreatic transplantation, pancreatic graft edema after reperfusion is less pronounced (67,68). The introduction of this solution was a pivotal contribution to the reduction of graft loss due to thrombosis during the early postoperative period (69).

Reduced preservation time may also help reduce the incidence and the severity of reperfusion injury and edema of the pancreas allograft; however, other large studies have not found that cold ischemia time affects graft survival (62,70). The incidence of allograft pancreatitis during the postoperative period has decreased because of improvements in procurement techniques that use the spleen and duodenum as handles that avoid pancreatic manipulation, the introduction of Belzer preservation solution, decompression of the portal system during in situ flushing, and intraperitoneal transplantation of the whole organ with exocrine drainage. However, allograft pancreatitis is still an important cause of morbidity.

When pancreatitis persists after transplantation, a thorough evaluation is necessary so that its cause can be determined (71,72). Reflux pancreatitis, high postvoid residual volumes, peripancreatic fluid collections, infectious pancreatitis, and leaks from the duodenal segment may cause hyperamylasemia. A Foley catheter should be placed so that postvoid residual volumes can be checked, and urodynamic studies should be performed so that high postvoid residual volumes and pressures can be detected (73). In addition, abdominal ultrasonography, CT of the abdomen, and cystography should be performed so that the cause of the pancreatitis can be determined. If the results of the work-up are nondiagnostic, a biopsy of the pancreas should be performed so that rejection can be ruled out as a cause of hyperamylasemia.

Complications Associated with Bladder-Drained Pancreas Transplantation

Bladder-drained pancreas transplantation is associated with multiple urologic (73,74) and metabolic complications. Published reports have shown that 14% to 50% of patients require enteric conversion; nearly 8% of our 200 consecutive patients who underwent SPK transplantation required enteric conversion.

Hematuria occurs very frequently and may be caused by the formation of a bladder stone on the staple or suture line. Approximately 30% of patients will require interventions such as Foley catheter placement, irrigation, and cystoscopy for evacuation of clots.

Urinary tract infections are common; they occur in as many as half of all cases and are probably induced by the irritating effect of the exocrine secretion on the bladder mucosa. Although the urinary pH is generally alkalotic and will maintain proenzymes in an inactive state, a urinary tract infection may reduce the pH enough to activate these digestive enzymes. In addition, enterokinase in the brush border of the duodenal mucosa may activate the proenzyme trypsinogen and thereby initiate the pancreatic enzyme–activation cascade. Other proteases, such as plasmin, thrombin, and fibrolysin, as well as bacterial enzymes, may also activate the conversion of trypsinogen to trypsin. The severe burning and dysuria caused by the resultant urethritis are attributed to urethral autodigestion by the activated pancreatic enzymes trypsinogen and chymotrypsinogen. If untreated, these symptoms may progress to urethral disruption or stricture. Treatment of urethral complications requires both enteric conversion and urological expertise (75). Fortunately, this complication has become less common during the last 15 years.

Metabolic acidosis is caused by the excretion from the bladder of large quantities of alkaline pancreatic secretions. Most patients require supplemental oral sodium bicarbonate once oral intake is tolerated; this treatment will minimize the degree of acidosis. With time, some of these patients may be able to decrease their need for oral sodium bicarbonate.

Fluid management can become problematic for these patients because of the potential for relatively large volume losses. Patients are at risk of episodes of dehydration, which can be worsened by poor intake as the result of gastric-motility problems commonly associated with diabetes. The symptoms from dehydration can be further increased when patients with diabetes have preexisting orthostatic hypotension because of autonomic neuropathy. Fluid balance can be improved in some patients by the postoperative administration of fludrocortisone acetate for three to six months. Of our 200 patients who underwent

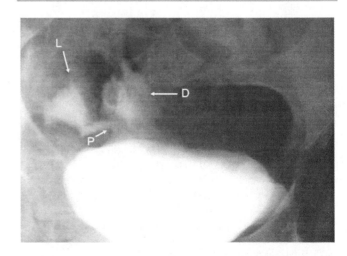

Figure 8 Cystogram showing a late leak from the duodenum of the pancreas allograft. *Key:* L, leak; D, duodenum; P, perforation.

CASE REPORT

A 42-year-old woman with type 1 diabetes mellitus and renal failure underwent SPK transplantation with drainage into the urinary bladder. Three weeks postoperatively, a decrease in urinary amylase activity was noted. Doppler ultrasonography demonstrated thrombosis of the superior mesenteric vein. The superior mesenteric vein was opened at the level of the head of the pancreas, and surgical thrombectomy was performed. The patient was treated with heparin after the procedure until a therapeutic level was achieved and then switch to Coumadin®. The patient was then kept on Coumadin for three months. The patient is now taking aspirin daily and the graft is functioning well.

SPK transplantation with bladder drainage, 30% to 40% were readmitted within the first year after transplantation for correction of acidosis and dehydration. Their serum creatinine concentrations usually returned to baseline after the administration of intravenous fluids with bicarbonate. Occasionally, patients will experience rejection exacerbated by episodes of dehydration with consequent increases in the serum concentrations of creatinine. These patients will require conversion to enteric drainage of the pancreatic secretions.

Urine leaks due to breakdown of the duodenal segment may occur years after transplantation, but this complication is usually encountered within the first two or three postoperative months. The causes of early urine leaks are technical in nature and usually require surgical correction with prolonged Foley catheter drainage. Late leaks (Fig. 8) can be caused by high pressure in the duodenum during urination. The onset of abdominal pain with elevated serum amylase activity, which can mimic reflux pancreatitis or acute rejection, is a typical presentation. Supporting imaging studies using cystography or CT may be necessary for confirming the diagnosis. Operative intervention may be required and includes reanastomosis to the bladder. Late leaks may develop as the result of rejection and can be treated successfully with Foley catheter drainage.

In our series of 200 patients, two patients experienced early postoperative leaks. One patient experienced a disruption of the PDC during cystoscopy for hematuria two weeks postoperatively. Another patient experienced a leak as the result of an episode of biopsy-proven acute rejection six weeks after transplantation. Both patients required operative treatment that included a revision of the PDC. Another of our patients experienced a late leak during an episode of rejection; this leak was successfully treated with Foley catheter drainage.

Despite these complications, bladder drainage of the pancreatic graft has many advantages. Early and late complications may cause morbidity; however, these complications are rarely lethal because enteroenterostomy can be avoided.

Another advantage of bladder drainage is the ability to monitor the patient for graft rejection.

The technique also allows cystoscopic access for biopsy of the duodenal or pancreatic graft and easy access to pancreatic fluid. An immediate decrease in urine amylase activity after pancreas transplantation signals early acute rejection. Six months after transplantation, a decrease in urinary amylase activity may signal late acute rejection. The decrease in urinary amylase activity may be the only clinical indication of a problem, with no change in the serum concentrations of creatinine or glucose or in the activity of serum amylase or lipase. A biopsy of the pancreas should be performed for confirming the diagnosis of rejection. Using this algorithm at our center, we have not yet lost a pancreas graft to rejection.

After the administration of rejection therapy with steroids, the need for repeat pancreatic biopsy can be determined by measuring urine amylase activity. If low urine amylase activity persists after rejection therapy, pancreatic biopsy is indicated. In contrast, if urine amylase activity is normal and the blood-glucose concentration remains high after therapy, the causative factor is steroid therapy rather than rejection, and pancreatic biopsy is not indicated.

Complications Associated with Enteric-Drained Pancreas Transplantation

When pancreas transplantation was first performed in the early 1970s, the results of enteric-drainage methods were poor. The small-bowel drainage procedure fell into disfavor because anastomotic leaks with abscess formation and sepsis caused high rates of morbidity and mortality. Recently, more centers are experiencing success with enteric drainage (Fig. 9) because of improvements in donor management, optimized surgical techniques during organ procurement, better preservation solutions, advances in the implantation procedure, and new immunosuppressive drugs (76–81). Enteric-drainage techniques vary in bowel arrangement, the level of anastomosis, the site of the recipient small bowel, and the choice of either a stapled or a hand-sewn anastomosis (79). The most serious complication of enteric-drained pancreas transplantation is a leak at the anastomotic site. This serious problem occurs one to six months

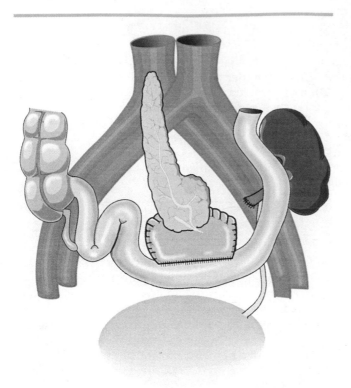

Figure 9 Surgical technique of simultaneous pancreas–kidney transplantation with enteric drainage through a midline intraperitoneal approach.

after transplantation and causes fever, abdominal discomfort, and leukocytosis. CT scans are helpful in diagnosing the problem. The mandatory treatment is surgical exploration and repair of the enteric leak.

Gastrointestinal bleeding may occur at the duodenoenteric suture line as a result of perioperative anticoagulation and inadequate hemostasis. Conservative management may not suffice, and reoperation is usually required (82,83).

Enteric drainage has advantages that balance the risk of serious complications associated with this procedure. First because metabolic acidosis and dehydration do not occur, bicarbonate supplementation is not needed. Second, this procedure is obviously not associated with urological complications such as urinary infections, hematuria, bladder stones, and urinary leaks. Third, fewer laboratory tests are required because there is no reason to monitor urinary activity. However, rejection episodes may progress undiagnosed before treatment is started, and this delay increases the possibility of allograft loss.

SUMMARY

The primary goal of therapy for type 1 diabetes mellitus is the optimal dosing of insulin and the restoration of normal metabolism. An ideal therapeutic choice for accomplishing this goal is the transplantation of endocrine pancreatic tissue, which can be achieved by transplanting an intact pancreas allograft. Many of the technical problems associated with this procedure have been solved, the incidence of associated thrombosis has diminished, and the management of exocrine secretions with bladder and enteric drainage now provides good results. Immunosuppression therapy aimed at preventing rejection has also improved with the advent of tacrolimus, mycophenolate mofetil, daclizumab, and thymoglobulin (21,84,85). These drugs, when used in combination, have been highly effective in decreasing the incidence of rejection among patients who undergo pancreas transplantation. In a recent study in which 30 patients who underwent SPK transplantation were treated with daclizumab and thymoglobulin as induction therapy in combination with tacrolimus and mycophenolate mofetil or rapamycin, no instances of rejection occurred.

REFERENCES

1. Burke G, Ciancio G, Alejandro R, et al. Cholesterol control: long-term benefit of pancreas-kidney transplantation with FK506 immunosuppression. Transplant Proc 1998; 30:513–514.
2. Burke GW, Ciancio G. The renal and pancreatic allograft recipient. In: Kirby RR, Taylor RW, Civetta JM, eds. Handbook of Critical Care. 3rd ed. Philadelphia: Lippincott, 1997:1311–1315.
3. Gruessner AC, Sutherland DE. Report for the International Pancreas Transplant registry-2000. Transplant Proc 2001; 33:1643–1646.
4. Burke GW, Ciancio G, Olson L, Roth D, Miller J. Ten-year survival after simultaneous pancreas/kidney transplantation with bladder drainage and tacrolimus-based immunosuppression. Transplant Proc 2001; 33:1681–1683.
5. Ciancio G, Olson L, Burke GW. The use of the brachiocephalic trunk for arterial reconstruction of the whole pancreas allograft for transplantation. J Am Coll Surg 1995; 181:79–80.
6. Ciancio G, Burke GW, Viciana AL, et al. Destructive allograft fungal arteritis following simultaneous pancreas-kidney transplantation. Transplantation 1996; 61: 1172–1175.
7. Gruessner RW, Burke GW, Stratta R, et al. A multicenter analysis of the first experience with FK506 for induction and rescue therapy after pancreas transplantation. Transplantation 1996; 61:261–273.
8. Calne RY, McMaster P, Rolles K, Duffy TJ. Technical observations in segmental pancreas allografting: observations on pancreatic blood flow. Transplant Proc 1980; 12:51–57.
9. Du Toit DF, Reece-Smith H, McShane R, Denton T, Morris PJ. A successful technique of segmental pancreatic autotransplantation in the dog. Transplantation 1981; 31:395–396.
10. Du Toit DF, Heydenrych JJ, Louw G, et al. Intraperitoneal transplantation of vascularized segmental pancreatic autografts without duct ligation in the primate. Surgery 1983; 94:471–477.
11. Duron JJ, Roux JM, Imbaud P, et al. The arteriovenous fistula in segmental pancreatic transplantation in dogs—a hemodynamic study. Transplantation 1987; 44:600–601.

12. Starzl TE, Iwatsuki S, Shaw BW Jr., et al. Pancreatico-duodenal transplantation in humans. Surg Gynecol Obstet 1984; 159:265–272.

13. Deierhoi MH, Sollinger HW, Bozdech MJ, Belzer FO. Lethal graft-versus-host disease in a recipient of a pancreas-spleen transplant. Transplantation 1986; 41:544–546.

14. Booster MH, Wijnen RM, van Hooff JP, et al. The role of the spleen in pancreas transplantation. Transplantation 1993; 56:1098–1102.

15. Gooszen HG, van Schilfgaarde R, Terpstra JL. Arterial blood supply of the left lobe of the canine pancreas. II. Electromagnetic flow measurements. Surgery 1983; 93:549–553.

16. Yun M, Inoue K, Kaji H, et al. The hemodynamic time course of the pancreas after segmental autotransplantation in dogs. Transplant Proc 1991; 23:1648–1650.

17. Ciancio G, Cespedes M, Olson L, Miller J, Burke GW. Partial venous thrombosis of the pancreatic allograft after simultaneous pancreas-kidney transplantation. Clin Transplant 2000; 14:464–471.

18. Ciancio G, Lo Monte A, Buscemi G, Miller J, Burke GW. Use of tacrolimus and mycophenolate mofetil as induction and maintenance in simultaneous pancreas-kidney transplantation. Transpl Int 2000; 13:S191–S194.

19. Ciancio G, Burke G, Viciana A, et al. Use of intravenous tacrolimus to reverse vascular rejection in kidney and simultaneous kidney-pancreas transplantation. Transplant Proc 1998; 30:1536–1537.

20. Ciancio G, Burke GW, Roth D, Miller J. Use of intravenous FK506 to treat acute rejection in simultaneous pancreas-kidney transplant recipients on maintenance oral FK506. Transplantation 1997; 63:785–788.

21. Burke GW, Ciancio G, Alejandro R, et al. Use of tacrolimus and mycophenolate mofetil for pancreas-kidney transplantation with or without OKT3 induction. Transplant Proc 1998; 30:1544–1545.

22. Moncada S, Gryglewski R, Bunting S, Vane JR. An enzyme isolated from arteries transforms prostaglandin endoperoxides to an unstable substance that inhibits platelet aggregation. Nature 1976; 263:663–665.

23. Hamberg M, Svensson J, Samuelsson B. Thromboxanes: a new group of biologically active compounds derived from prostaglandin endoperoxides. Proc Natl Acad Sci USA 1975; 72:2994–2998.

24. Moncada S, Vane JR. Arachidonic acid metabolites and interactions between platelets and blood-vessel walls. N Engl J Med 1979; 300:1142–1147.

25. Johnson BF, Thomas G, Wiley KN, et al. Thromboxane and prostacyclin synthesis in experimental pancreas transplantation. Changes in parenchymal and vascular prostanoids. Transplantation 1993; 56:1447–1453.

26. Kin S, Tamura K, Nagami H, Nakase A. Effect of preservation on blood flow and production of prostacyclin and thromboxane A_2 in canine segmental pancreatic autografts. Transplant Proc 1991; 23:1651–1653.

27. Kawai T, Teraoka S, Hayashi T, et al. The changes in prostaglandins after segmental pancreatic transplantation. Transplant Proc 1991; 23:1645–1647.

28. Lieberman KV, Lin WG, Reisman L. FK506 is a direct glomeruloconstrictor as determined by electrical resistance pulse sizing (ERPS). Transplant Proc 1991; 23:3119–3120.

29. Peters DH, Fitton A, Plosker GL, Faulds DT. A review of its pharmacology and therapeutic potential in hepatic and renal transplantation. Drugs 1993; 46:746–794.

30. Goodall T, Kind CN, Hammond TG. FK506-induced endothelin release by cultured rat mesangial cells. J Cardiovasc Pharmacol 1995; 26(suppl 3):S482–S485.

31. Burke GW, Ciancio G, Cirocco R, et al. Microangiopathy in kidney and simultaneous pancreas/kidney recipients treated with tacrolimus: evidence of endothelin and cytokine involvement. Transplantation 1999; 68:1336–1342.

32. Randhawa PS, Tsamandas AC, Magnone M, et al. Microvascular changes in renal allografts associated with FK506 (Tacrolimus) therapy. Am J Surg Pathol 1996; 20:306–312.

33. Antoine C, Thakur S, Daugas E, et al. Vascular microthrombosis in renal transplant recipients treated with tacrolimus. Transplant Proc 1998; 30:2813–2814.

34. Morphopathological findings of renal allografts under FK 506 therapy. Japanese FK 506 Study Group. Transplant Proc 1994; 26:1933–1936.

35. Randhawa PS, Shapiro R, Jordan ML, Starzl TE, Demetris AJ. The histopathological changes associated with allograft rejection and drug toxicity in renal transplant recipients maintained on FK506. Clinical significance and comparison with cyclosporine. Am J Surg Pathol 1993; 17:60–68.

36. Corry RJ, Egidi MF, Shapiro R, et al. Tacrolimus without antilymphocyte induction therapy prevents pancreas loss from rejection in 123 consecutive patients. Transplant Proc 1998; 30:521.

37. Bruce DS, Sollinger HW, Humar A, et al. Multicenter survey of daclizumab induction in simultaneous kidney-pancreas transplant recipients. Transplantation 2001; 72:1637–1643.

38. Yang HC, Neumyer MM, Thiele BL, Gifford RR. Evaluation of pancreatic allograft circulation using color Doppler ultrasonography. Transplant Proc 1990; 22:609–611.

39. Snider JF, Hunter DW, Kuni CC, Castaneda-Zuniga WR, Letourneau JG. Pancreatic transplantation: radiologic evaluation of vascular complications. Radiology 1991; 178:749–753.

40. Krebs TL, Daly B, Wong JJ, Chow CC, Bartlett ST. Vascular complications of pancreatic transplantation: MR evaluation. Radiology 1995; 196:793–798.

41. Sebastian A, Cuenca A, Li SF, et al. Pancreas transplant graft evaluation using MIBI scan—a useful tool. Transplant Proc 1998; 30:257–260.

42. Patel B, Markivee CR, Mahanta B, Vas W, George E, Garvin P. Pancreatic transplantation: scintigraphy, US, and CT. Radiology 1988; 167:685–687.

43. Kuo PC, Wong J, Schweitzer EJ, Johnson LB, Lim JW, Bartlett ST. Outcome after splenic vein thrombosis in the pancreas allograft. Transplantation 1997; 64:933–935.

44. Douzdjian V, Abecassis MM, Cooper JL, Argibay PF, Smith JL, Corry RJ. Pancreas transplant salvage after acute venous thrombosis. Transplantation 1993; 56:222–223.

45. Douzdjian V, Abecassis MM, Cooper JL, Smith JL, Corry RJ. Incidence, management and significance of surgical complications after pancreatic transplantation. Surg Gynecol Obstet 1993; 177:451–456.

46. Nghiem DD. Pancreatic allograft thrombosis: diagnostic and therapeutic importance of splenic venous flow velocity. Clin Transplant 1995; 9:390–395.

47. Gilabert R, Fernandez-Cruz L, Real MI, Ricart MJ, Astudillo E, Montana X. Treatment and outcomes of pancreatic venous graft thrombosis after kidney-pancreas transplantation. Br J Surg 2002; 89:355–360.

48. Fisher RA, Munda R, Madden R. Pancreas transplant functional salvage after segmental vascular thrombosis. Transplant Proc 1993; 25:2138–2140.

49. Ciancio G, Julian JF, Fernandez L, Miller J, Burke GW. Successful surgical salvage of pancreas allografts after complete venous thrombosis. Transplantation 2000; 70:126–131.

50. Boudreaux JP, Corry RJ, Dickerman R, Sutherland DE. Combined experience with immediate pancreas retransplantation. Transplant Proc 1991; 23:1628–1629.

51. Ciancio G, Lo Monte A, Julian JF, Romano M, Miller J, Burke GW. Vascular complications following bladder drained simultaneous pancreas-kidney transplantation; the University of Miami experience. Transpl Int 2000; 13(suppl 1):S187–S190.

52. Hunziker D. Thrombozytose nach Pankreastransplantation—eine retrospektive klinische Studie. Schweiz Rundsch Med Prax 1989; 78:191–196.

53. Hopt UT, Büsing M, Schareck W, et al. Prevention of early postoperative graft thrombosis in pancreatic transplantation. Transplant Proc 1993; 25:2607–2608.

54. Hopt UT, Büsing M, Schareck WD, Becker HD. The bladder drainage technique in pancreas transplantation—the Tübingen experience. Diabetologia 1991; 34:S24–S27.

55. Tibell A, Brattström, Kozlowski T, Tydén G, Groth CG. Management after clinical pancreatic transplantation with enteric exocrine drainage. Transplant Proc 1994; 26:1797–1798.

56. Bynon JS, Stratta RJ, Taylor RJ, Lowell JA, Cattral M. Vascular reconstruction in 105 consecutive pancreas transplants. Transplant Proc 1993; 25:3288–3289.

57. Gruessner RW, Kendall DM, Drangstveit MB, Gruessner AC, Sutherland DE. Simultaneous pancreas-kidney transplantation from live donors. Ann Surg 1997; 226:471–482.

58. Bartlett ST, Kuo PC, Johnson LB, Lim JW, Scheitzer EJ. Pancreas transplantation at the University of Maryland. In: Cecka JM, Teraski PI, eds. Clinical Transplants, 1996. Los Angeles: UCLA Tissue Typing Laboratory, 1997.

59. Sollinger HW. Pancreatic transplantation and vascular graft thrombosis. J Am Coll Surg 1996; 182:362–363.

60. Khan TF, Ciancio G, Burke GW III, Sfakianakis GN, Miller J. Pseudoaneurysm of the superior mesenteric artery with an arteriovenous fistula after simultaneous kidney-pancreas transplantation. Clin Transplant 1999; 13:277–279.

61. Schaapherder AF, van Oosterhout EC, Bode PJ, van der Woude FJ, Lemkes HH, Gooszen HG. Pancreatic graft survival after arterial thrombosis in simultaneous renal-pancreatic transplantation. Clin Transplant 1993; 7:37–42.

62. Troppmann C, Gruessner AC, Benedetti E, et al. Vascular graft thrombosis after pancreatic transplantation: univariate and multivariate operative and operative risk factor analysis. J Am Coll Surg 1996; 182:285–316.

63. Grewal HP, Garland L, Novak K, Gaber L, Tolley EA, Gaber AO. Risk factors for postimplantation pancreatitis and pancreatic thrombosis in pancreas transplant recipients. Transplantation 1993; 56:609–612.

64. Bassi D, Kollias N, Fernandez-del Castillo C, Foitzik T, Warshaw AL, Rattner DW. Impairment of pancreatic microcirculation correlates with the severity of acute experimental pancreatitis. J Am Coll Surg 1994; 179:257–263.

65. Fernandez-del Castillo C, Schmidt J, Warshaw AL, Rattner DW. Interstitial protease activation is the central event in progression to necrotizing pancreatitis. Surgery 1994; 116:497–504.

66. Klar E, Messmer K, Warshaw AL, Herfarth C. Pancreatic ischaemia in experimental acute pancreatitis: mechanism, significance and therapy. Br J Surg 1990; 77:1205–1210.

67. Belzer FO, Southard JH. Principles of solid-organ preservation by cold storage. Transplantation 1988; 45:673–676.

68. Wahlberg JA, Love R, Landegaard L, Southard JH, Belzer FO. 72-hour preservation of the canine pancreas. Transplantation 1987; 43:5–8.

69. D'Alessandro AM, Kalayoglu M, Sollinger HW, Pirsch JD, Southard JH, Belzer FO. Current status of organ preservation with University of Wisconsin solution. Arch Pathol Lab Med 1991; 115:306–310.

70. Morel P, Gillingham KJ, Moundry-Munns KC, Dunn DL, Najarian JS, Sutherland DE. Factors influencing pancreas transplant outcome: Cox proportional hazard regression analysis of a single institution's experience with 357 cases. Transplant Proc 1991; 23:1630–1633.

71. Ciancio G, Burke GW, Roth D, Luque CD, Coker D, Miller J. Reflux pancreatitis after simultaneous pancreas-kidney transplantation treated by α-1 blocker. Transplantation 1995; 60:760–761.

72. Ciancio G, Montalvo B, Roth D, Miller J, Burke GW. Allograft pancreatic duct dilatation following bladder drained simultaneous pancreas-kidney transplantation: clinical significance. JOP 2000; 1:4–12.

73. Ciancio G, Burke G, Lynne C, et al. Urodynamic findings following bladder-drained simultaneous pancreas-kidney transplantation. Transplant Proc 1997; 29:2912–2913.

74. Ciancio G, Burke GW, Nery J, et al. Urologic complications following simultaneous pancreas-kidney transplantation. Transplant Proc 1995; 27:3125–3126.

75. Ciancio G, Burke GW, Nery JR, Coker D, Miller J. Urethritis/dysuria after simultaneous pancreas-kidney transplantation. Clin Transplant 1996; 10:67–70.

76. Ciancio G, Burke G, Roth D, Miller J. Tacrolimus. Curr Opin Transplant 1997; 2:62–67.

77. Zucker K, Rosen A, Tsaroucha A, et al. Unexpected augmentation of mycophenolic acid pharmacokinetics in renal transplant patients receiving tacrolimus and mycophenolate mofetil in combination therapy, and analogous in vitro findings. Transpl Immunol 1997; 5:225–232.

78. Ciancio G, Burke GW, Miller J. Current treatment practices in immunosuppression. Expert Opin Pharcother 2000; 1:1307–1330.

79. Di Carlo V, Castoldi R, Cristallo M, et al. Techniques of pancreas transplantation through the world: an IPITA Center survey. Transplant Proc 1998; 30:231–241.

80. Ciancio G, Burke GW, Roth D, et al. Tacrolimus and Mycophenolate Mofetil as primary immunosuppression for renal allograft recipients. In: Racusen LC, Solez K, Burdick JF, eds. Kidney Transplant Rejection: Diagnosis and Treatment. New York: Marcel Dekker, 1998:519–529.

81. Stratta RJ, Gaber AO, Shokouh-Amiri MH, et al. A prospective comparison of systemic-bladder versus portal-enteric drainage in vascularized pancreas transplantation. Surgery 2000; 127:217–226.

82. Reddy KS, Stratta RJ, Shokouh-Amiri MH, Alloway R, Egidi MF, Gaber AO. Surgical complications after pancreas transplantation with portal-enteric drainage. J Am Coll Surg 1999; 189:305–313.

83. Ciancio G, Burke G, Roth D, Tzakis AG, Miller J. Update in transplantation 1997. In: Cecka JM, Terasaki PI, eds. Clinical Transplants, 1997. Los Angeles: UCLA Tissue Typing Laboratory, 1998:241–264.

84. Ciancio G, Miller J, Burke GW. The use of intravenous tacrolimus and mycophenolate mofetil as induction and maintenance immunosuppression in simultaneous pancreas-kidney recipients with previous transplants. Clin Transplantation 2001; 15:142–145.

85. Ciancio G, Miller A, Burke GW, et al. Dacliximab induction for primary kidney transplant recipients using tacrolimus, mycophenolate mofetil, and steroids as maintenance immunosuppression. Transplant Proc 2001; 33:1013–1014.

51

Complications of General Surgery During Pregnancy

Raymond P. Compton

Paris Surgical Specialists, Paris, Tennessee, U.S.A.

Although pregnancy is described as the most natural thing that can occur to a woman, it is unfortunately often complicated by events out of her control. Approximately 1 in 500 women will, during pregnancy, suffer some type of complication that must be addressed by a general surgeon (1). Such complications and their treatment are often affected by the altered physiology of pregnancy. The surgeon must now consider two lives instead of one. The well being of the mother and the treatment method that will least affect the fetus are of prime importance. The surgeon must always remember, however, that it is impossible to bring a fetus to term without a living mother.

The conditions affecting pregnant women that may require general surgery are, for the most part, the routine day-to-day conditions faced in the general surgery practice. These conditions include appendicitis, cholecystitis, bowel obstruction, pancreatitis, thyroid disorders, ulcer disease, breast cancer, melanoma, colon cancers, and anorectal disorders that are particular to the complications of delivery. For the most part, the best outcome can be expected when prudent treatment is administered in a fashion similar to that offered to women who are not pregnant.

GENERAL PRINCIPLES OF MANAGEMENT
Laparoscopy or Open Procedures

When general surgeons began performing laparoscopy, pregnancy was usually listed as an absolute contraindication for most procedures. Over the past 15 to 20 years, it has become clear that pregnant women can safely undergo laparoscopic procedures. Gouldman et al. (2) reported three spontaneous abortions, one occurring two months after surgery, and only one episode of preterm labor in association with 107 cholecystectomies performed on pregnant women. Their summary encompassed 30 published reports with 1 to 20 patients per study. Graham et al. (3) performed a review and reported similar outcomes. The preterm labor rate associated with open cholecystectomy may be as high as 40% (4). Barone et al. (5) reported eight episodes of premature labor associated with 26 open cholecystectomies and only one episode associated

with 20 laparoscopic procedures. In a more recent publication, Affleck et al. (6) reported a similar rate of preterm delivery in association with laparoscopic (10%) and open (12%) cholecystectomy. All of these reports stress that second-trimester procedures carry the lowest risk of preterm delivery or problems associated with processes such as symptomatic cholelithiasis. Often, surgery can be delayed until the second trimester. First-trimester laparoscopy has been established as quite safe, having been performed for many years to rule out ectopic pregnancies (7).

Unfortunately, the same results cannot be reported for appendicitis or other inflammatory conditions of the abdomen. Rates of preterm labor approach 20% in association with either open or laparoscopic appendectomy (8). The real risk of an open or a laparoscopic procedure during pregnancy seems to relate more to the disease process than to the actual technique involved. Certain inherent risks are, however, specific to laparoscopy, including the risk of uterine injury during placement of a trocar or a Veress needle, changes in end-tidal CO_2 measurements, and changes in maternal–fetal hemodynamics.

Hunter et al. (9) have described the effects of pneumoperitoneum on fetal dynamics in the model of a pregnant ewe. In this study, pneumoperitoneum induced by CO_2 caused increases in maternal CO_2 that led to fetal hypercapnia, tachycardia, and hypertension. End-tidal CO_2 was not found to correlate with measured arterial CO_2.

The Society of American Gastrointestinal and Endoscopic Surgeons (SAGES) has published a list of guidelines for laparoscopic surgery during pregnancy (10). These guidelines are listed in Table 1.

The three complications most frequently seen after nonobstetric operations during pregnancy are preterm labor, premature delivery, and spontaneous abortion or fetal demise. Clearly, the last of these complications is by far the worst. The incidence of these problems varies directly with the severity of the underlying disease process. This fact is well illustrated by the spectrum of appendicitis: rates of fetal complications extend from less than 1% in association with early appendicitis to well above 50% in association with frank rupture and peritonitis (11). The same increase

Table 1 SAGES Recommendations for Laparoscopic Surgery During Pregnancy

Pneumatic compression devices
Lead shield with selective fluoroscopy
Dependent positioning
Obstetric consultation
Intraoperative fetal and uterine monitoring
Serial arterial blood gas analyses with entitled CO_2 monitoring
Second-trimester deferment, if possible
Minimal pneumoperitoneum (8–12 mmHg)
Open (Hasson) technique

Abbreviation: SAGES, Society of American Gastrointestinal and Endoscopic Surgeons.

in fetal complications is seen when the outcomes of semielective procedures, such as laparoscopic cholecystectomy, are compared with those of emergent procedures such as bowel obstruction. In short, the worse the intra-abdominal inflammatory response, the higher the chance of a serious pregnancy-related complication. General surgeons must keep this underlying principle in mind when counseling patients and family members, both preoperatively and postoperatively. Laparoscopy is safe during pregnancy, but the inherent risks of the disease process remain ever present.

Prophylactic Tocolysis

The use of prophylactic tocolytic agents, such as progesterone, magnesium sulfate, and terbutaline, has decreased in the last 10 years. A study of 78 women at the University of North Carolina, Chapel Hill (11), found no measurable benefit in the use of prophylactic tocolytic agents. This study found that uterine contractions occurred twice as often when prophylactic perioperative tocolytic agents were used (84%) than when they were not (47%). These findings were unchanged when reviewed with respect to disease process. Likewise, Hill et al. (12) reported that their 17-year experience at the Mayo Clinic found no benefit in the use of prophylactic perioperative progesterone (12). Tocolytic agents should be used only at the discretion of the obstetrician, usually in response to actual contractions, and should not be used prophylactically.

Medications

When choosing medications for the pregnant patient, general surgeons must take into consideration not only the illness to be treated but also the effects on the fetus. Many antibiotics, including most penicillins, cephalosporins, and monobactam antibiotics, are not associated with teratogenic effects, nor are they associated with substantial risk to the developing fetus. Aminoglycosides, tetracycline, and chloramphenicol should be used with caution or not at all during pregnancy. Aminoglycosides are to be avoided because of the potential of ototoxic effects to the fetus. Tetracyclines rapidly cross the placenta and bind to the fetus's developing teeth and bones, causing discoloration of enamel, enamel hypoplasia, and bony

abnormalities. The administration of chloramphenicol to pregnant women is particularly worrisome; because the fetus can only poorly detoxify this antibiotic, high serum concentrations can result. These serum concentrations cause the gray baby syndrome, which often leads to fetal or neonatal demise. Other medications routinely used during the perioperative period may also carry risks to the fetus. Table 2 lists medications routinely used during the perioperative period, classified by risk stratification.

Imaging

Diagnostic imaging of pregnant patients can present some difficulty for the surgeon. Clearly, the imaging method of choice is ultrasound. Unfortunately, ultrasound cannot provide the general surgeon with all of the information that may be needed to make a diagnosis. Ultrasound is well accepted for diagnosing biliary and pancreatic pathology. It has also proved to be useful in diagnosing appendicitis. The safety of ultrasound for the pregnant patient and for the fetus is unquestioned.

Radiographic imaging must be chosen with somewhat more care. The National Counsel on Radiation Protection has set radiation exposure for the gestating fetus at an absolute limit of 0.5 rem, with a monthly exposure limit of no more than 0.05 rem. Most clinicians are more familiar with measuring X-ray dosage in rad. The term "rem" refers to the biologic affect of a radiation dose. It is the absorbed radiation dose (in rad) times a quality factor based on the biologic nature of the tissue exposure multiplied by a factor "n" that represents the type of radiation delivered. In terms of soft-tissue X-ray exposure, the rem and the rad are essentially equal (13,14). Table 3 lists common radiographs and the organ dose that can be expected for the uterus, fetus, or both (15,16).

This situation illustrates an important point of judgment. Although physicians are often reluctant to obtain radiologic studies during pregnancy, it must be remembered that the risk of radiation damage to the fetus is greatest during the first trimester when organogenesis occurs (17). Whenever shielding is possible, it should be used. But a radiographic study, even one that delivers more than the monthly limit of radiation, may be necessary for a decision about the absolute need for surgical exploration or intervention. A cholecystogram (with shielding) would yield a low dose of radiation, and, surprisingly, the helical computed tomography (CT) scan for appendicitis also yields a relatively low dose. The helical CT scan delivers an amount of radiation that is well above the recommended monthly exposure limit but lower than that recommended for the total gestation period.

The radiation dose to an embryo for a radiopharmaceutical, such as radiolabeled iodine or technetium, must be calculated on the basis of millicuries administered. These imaging technologies should be used only after consultation with a radiologist or a nuclear medicine physician.

Table 2 Medications Stratified by Class and the Published Risk of Fetal Complications

Drug class or drug[a]	Risk[b]
Penicillins	B
Cephalosporins	B
Quinolones	C
Aminoglycosides	D
Macrolides	
Azithromycin, erythromycin	B
Clarithromycin	C
Other antibiotics	
Aztreonam	B
Clindamycin	B
Metronidazole	B
Sulfamethoxazole/trimethoprim	C
Vancomycin	C
Doxycycline, tetracycline, minocycline	D
Antifungal agents	
Amphotericin B	B
Amphotericin B lipid complex	C
Fluconazole, itraconazole, ketoconazole	C
H2 blockers	B
Proton pump inhibitors	
Lansoprazole	B
Omeprazole	C
Anastrozole	D
Anesthetic agents	
Lidocaine	B
Atracurium, pancuronium	C
Cisatracurium, rocuronium	B
Desflurane, enflurane, sevoflurane	B
Ondansetron	B
Etomidate	C
Ephedrine	X
Anticoagulant or vascular agents	
Clopidogrel	B
Enoxaparin	B
Warfarin	X
Heparin	C
Other	
Levothyroxine	A
Glycopyrrolate	B
Albuterol	C
Pain medications	
Codeine, morphine, fentanyl	C
Acetaminophen	C
Ketorolac	B
Sedatives	
Propofol	B
Midazolam	D
Temazepam	X

[a]This is not meant to be an exhaustive list but rather to give an idea of classes that are available.
[b]Categories A through D: progressively increasing risk with progressively less knowledge about the drug–pregnancy interaction. Category X: unsafe for use by pregnant patients, should be completely avoided.

Table 3 Commonly Performed Radiographs and the Organ Dose that They Deliver to the Uterus, Fetus, or Both

Radiograph	mrad
Chest	0.06
Cervical spine[a]	0.01
Thoracic spine[a]	0.6
Cholecystogram	5
Lumbar spine	408
KUB	264
Pelvis	194
Helical-appendiceal CT	300
Computed tomographic pelvimetry	250

[a]The screening radiographs usually performed after trauma (cervical spine, chest, and pelvis radiographs with shielding) deliver less than the total exposure recommended for the gestational period (0.5 rem) but more than the recommended monthly exposure (0.05 rem).
Abbreviations: KUB, kidney, ureter, and bladder; CT, computed tomography.
Source: From Refs. 14–16.

physiologic changes during pregnancy may alter the usual presentation of these conditions and can affect the reliability of laboratory studies frequently used to help establish a diagnosis (18).

It has long been believed that the anatomic changes that affect the presentation of intra-abdominal problems usually occur because of displacement of the abdominal organs by the enlarging uterus. The enlarging uterus is definitely a factor in the ability to accurately diagnose intra-abdominal problems by physical examination. Baer et al. (19), in 1932, originally described the changes in the position of the normal appendix that were assumed to take place during pregnancy (19). Recently, Mourad et al. (20) reviewed 67,000 deliveries of which 67 were complicated by appendicitis. In this series, pain in the right lower quadrant was the most common presenting symptom despite gestational age (first trimester, 86%; second trimester, 83%; and third trimester, 78%). Nevertheless, the enlarging uterus must be kept in mind during physical examination of a pregnant woman. Physiologic changes that are usually present during pregnancy include an expanded intravascular volume, a relative anemia with a decreased heart rate, leukocytosis, and a mild increase in alkaline phosphatase and transaminase activity (18). Despite these changes, a high index of suspicion on the part of the surgeon and open communication between specialists will surely lead to the best outcome. In general, the health of the mother should be the first priority in the treatment of surgical diseases during pregnancy (18).

SPECIFIC DISORDERS IN PREGNANT WOMEN
Appendicitis

Appendicitis is the most common nonobstetrical surgical diagnosis during pregnancy. It occurs in approximately 1 in 1500 pregnancies (21). Although the incidence of appendicitis among pregnant women

Physiologic Changes

The accurate diagnosis of intra-abdominal problems is made more difficult by pregnancy because many of the signs and symptoms of these pathologic states mimic findings that are normal during pregnancy, especially during the first trimester. Anatomic and mirrors that among age-matched control subjects, perforated appendicitis is reported more frequently than would be expected (a rate of 43–55%) (22,23). This increased rate is believed to be primarily due to a relative delay in diagnosis. This delay is often attributed to the physiological changes that accompany pregnancy, such as relative leukocytosis, a high incidence of paroxysmal abdominal pain, and other changes occurring in the intra-abdominal anatomy (22). When diffuse peritonitis occurs with appendicitis, it is believed to be facilitated by the inability of the omentum to wall off the infection because of a relative obstruction by the gravid uterus (23). Clearly, the physical finding most frequently associated with appendicitis and pregnancy is pain in the right side of the abdomen. Some controversy exists between classic teaching and current reviews regarding the location of the physical findings in acute appendicitis in pregnancy. It has now been established that the finding of rebound tenderness and abdominal tenderness, whether localized to the right lower quadrant or higher, suggests the diagnosis of appendicitis.

The operative treatment may involve either laparoscopy or an open approach. During the third trimester, laparoscopy may be extremely difficult because of the enlarged uterus; the altered port placements may make laparoscopic exposure very difficult. Nonetheless, the number of reports of the use of laparoscopy for appendectomy during the last trimester is increasing (6). If any open procedure is contemplated, the incision is usually placed over the area of maximal tenderness. Maternal death is quite uncommon when appendectomy is performed during the first trimester, but increases in incidence with gestational age and is highly associated with delay in diagnosis and appendiceal perforation. Overall mortality rates should be less than 1% when appendicitis is found and treated in a timely fashion (24,25).

Postoperative complications associated with appendectomy during pregnancy include maternal morbidity and mortality, premature labor, and fetal loss. Factors most associated with an increased risk of these complications include the presence of symptoms for more than 24 hours, marked elevation of white blood cell count with significant left shift, and appendiceal perforation at the time of surgery (13). The likelihood of onset of premature labor is similar for both negative laparotomy and appendectomy for early acute appendicitis. When perforation has occurred, fetal loss may occur in as many as 20% of cases or more (13,20).

Cholelithiasis and Cholecystitis

Biliary tract disease is the second most common non-obstetrical surgical diagnosis during pregnancy. Neither a clear cause for the frequency of the disease nor a relationship between pregnancy and gall stone formation has been established. It appears that patients with gall stones who become pregnant are predisposed to symptomatic biliary disease (13). Pregnancy results in physiologic and hormonal changes that lead to an increase in bile stasis and decreased gall bladder contraction (18). Fortunately, the symptoms and physical findings of biliary tract disease are relatively similar for pregnant and nonpregnant women. As noted previously, changes in serum biochemistry that are inherent in pregnancy may make the diagnosis of biliary tract disease more difficult.

Ultrasound is the mainstay of imaging for biliary tract disease during pregnancy. Views of the pancreas are often limited because of overlying bowel gas and the relative decrease in the gastrointestinal tract motility that accompanies pregnancy. Although gall stone pancreatitis is not a frequent finding, it does occur and it carries a high rate of complications for both mother and fetus. If patients exhibit the signs and symptoms of cholecystitis, if an ultrasonogram shows stones, and if the biochemical findings are consistent with a diagnosis of pancreatitis, it is reasonable to treat pregnant women for biliary pancreatitis (13).

Typically, a patient with symptomatic biliary tract disease can be treated supportively until the second trimester of pregnancy. Barone et al. (5) retrospectively compared the outcomes of open and laparoscopic cholecystectomies performed on pregnant women over a five-year period. Complications were found among patients who underwent either procedure; these complications ranged from spontaneous hepatic rupture to premature contractions. The most frequently occurring complication was premature contraction; there was no statistically significant difference in the frequency of this complication between the open and laparoscopic groups (5). Similar findings have been published by Epstein (24). Barone's report (5) summarized and compared the results of reports of laparoscopic and open cholecystectomies during all trimesters of pregnancy that were published through March 1999. The rates of spontaneous abortion and premature labor associated with each procedure were similar, as would be expected. It should be stressed that when laparoscopy is performed for any reason during pregnancy, the open Hasson technique should be favored for access, and a low-pressure pneumoperitoneum (12 mmHg or less) should be used.

In short, the maternal mortality rates are low, and the rate of complications associated with emergent surgery for biliary tract disease is not substantially higher among pregnant women than among nonpregnant women (13). The overall management of biliary tract disease among pregnant women parallels the management of the disease among patients without symptoms. Indications for early operation include a lack of response to antibiotics, progression of the disease, and other complications of the disease process.

Endoscopic retrograde cholangiopancreatography (ERCP) is a valuable imaging tool even for pregnant women. ERCP is a useful adjunct to the treatment of cholecystitis and biliary tract disease, and the procedure can be undertaken without fluoroscopic exposure (26,27). There have even been reports describing the use of ultra-short fluoroscopy for imaging studies of pregnant patients (28). These techniques greatly increase the surgeon's ability to delay operative treatment until the second trimester.

The clinician must be alert to other conditions that may mimic cholecystitis, such as viral or alcoholic hepatitis and the HELLP (*h*emolysis, *e*levated *l*iver function, and *l*ow *p*latelet count) syndrome (29). A short review and case report by Watson et al. (29) has established the similarity of these conditions to cholecystitis (29). The findings associated with the HELLP syndrome may precede the features of preeclampsia.

Pancreatitis

Pancreatitis occurs in approximately 1 in 1500 pregnancies. It is more likely to occur during the third trimester and carries a rate of fetal loss of between 10% and 20% (30). The causes of acute pancreatitis during pregnancy are similar to its causes among the population as a whole, although alcohol is probably a less common cause among pregnant women than among the general population (30). The diagnosis of pancreatitis can usually be made by the biochemical measurement of amylase and lipase activity. The amylase-to-creatinine clearance ratio is also a useful marker among pregnant women (31). During pregnancy, pancreatitis should be managed supportively. Special attention should be paid to patients who experience pancreatitis in relation to hypertriglyceridemia. Pregnancy is known to relatively increase the incidence of hypertriglyceridemia as a cause of pancreatitis. This condition may make it very difficult to provide nutritional support for these patients. If total parenteral nutrition is needed, it may be necessary to delete intralipid from the regimen, using only carbohydrate and protein support for a short period of time until the triglyceride concentration falls to a more acceptable level (32).

Hepatic Rupture

If hepatitis is the most common liver disease during pregnancy, spontaneous hepatic rupture is the worst hepatic complication that can occur. It is often seen in association with a high-risk pregnancy and poor prenatal care. It is associated with eclampsia and preeclamptic syndromes (18,33). Hepatic rupture usually manifests itself during the third trimester of pregnancy. Hypertensive patients who complain of symptoms such as headache, third-trimester nausea and vomiting, and mild to moderate epigastric discomfort for several days to weeks are at risk. Mild jaundice and increased alkaline phosphatase concentrations may be seen. An ultrasound will often show a subcapsular hematoma or frank rupture.

The severity of these symptoms seems to be directly related to the severity of the hypertension (13).

Clearly, the management of spontaneous hepatic rupture is similar to that of a traumatic liver injury. This treatment often involves intra-abdominal packing and damage-control laparotomy. If the fetus is at a viable stage of development and has not succumbed to the events surrounding the hepatic rupture, then a Cesarean section at the time of damage-control laparotomy must be considered.

Intestinal Obstruction

Intestinal obstruction occurs infrequently, at a rate of 1 in 1500 to 1 in 60,000 pregnancies (18). The most common cause is adhesion. Interestingly, volvulus and intussusception cause intestinal obstruction much more frequently (5–25% of cases) among pregnant women than among nonpregnant patients (18). The surgical approach that provides the best exposure of an intestinal obstruction involves a midline laparotomy incision. Bowel strangulation is a common finding at the time of exploration (34). Studies have found a maternal mortality rate of 5% to 6% and a fetal mortality rate of 25% to 30% (34,35).

Breast Cancer

The incidence of breast cancer among pregnant women ranges from 1 in 3000 to 1 in 3500 (36). Many myths surround the treatment of breast cancer during pregnancy, including the value of negative mammographic results, the need for a therapeutic abortion or oophorectomy, and the relatively poorer prognosis associated with pregnancy at the time of diagnosis or subsequent to diagnosis. Negative results from mammography are not necessarily reassuring. A study performed at Memorial Sloan-Kettering Cancer Center found that 22% of women with pregnancy-associated breast cancers had mammographic results that did not demonstrate any radiologic signs of cancer (37). An older series found that six of eight pregnant patients with subsequent biopsy-proven cancer had negative mammographic results (38). Routine therapeutic abortion should not be recommended because no published series has demonstrated any additional benefit associated with this procedure (39). Women should undergo therapeutic abortion only if the issue is fetal damage due to proposed chemotherapy or radiation treatments. Women must make an informed decision about their pregnancies when possible. Oophorectomy cannot be uniformly recommended for the pregnant patient because this procedure is not associated with any survival benefit (40). It has long been held that breast cancer associated with pregnancy has a dismal prognosis and is often untreatable. Three frequently quoted early studies reported these findings. In 1929, Kilgore (41) found a five-year survival rate of only 17% for pregnancy-associated breast cancer. In 1937, Harrington (42) from the Mayo Clinic reported a five-year survival rate of only 5.7%; he was the first to begin to realize the marked difference in survival associated with nodal status (a five-year survival rate as high as 61% in patients without nodal involvement). In 1943, Haagensen and Stout (43) went so far as to suggest that the survival rate of pregnancy-associated breast cancer was so poor that mastectomy should not be considered. Unfortunately, these reviews were flawed by the late presentation of the disease and its comparison with the breast cancer population as a whole, among other factors. Finally, Petrek et al. (44) was able to demonstrate that the breast cancer survival rates were equivalent among pregnant women and premenopausal patients. In short, nodal status, not pregnancy, is the most significant predicator of 5- and 10-year survival rates (44). In addition, pregnancy after a diagnosis of breast cancer does not detrimentally affect long-term prognosis (45).

Most pregnancy-associated breast cancers are first detected as a painless mass. The physician may watch these masses to assess their clinical behavior, but only for a month or two. If the masses do not resolve spontaneously, biopsy is indicated; fine-needle aspiration, core biopsy, or open biopsy may be used. The treatment of choice for the pregnant woman with breast cancer is a modified radical mastectomy. Breast-conserving therapy with ionizing radiation is associated with a much higher risk to the fetus and cannot be considered safe. Most breast cancers that occur during pregnancy are hormone-receptor negative (46).

The treatment of pregnant women with breast cancer mirrors the treatment of breast cancer patients who are not pregnant. During the childbearing years, there is no statistically significant difference in survival, stage for stage, between women who are pregnant and those who are not (47). The current recommendation that breast cancer among pregnant women should be treated in the same way as breast cancer among nonpregnant women also holds for the treatment of melanoma and colon cancer among these populations. This treatment recommendation is well established but must incorporate a multidisciplinary approach (48–50).

Ulcer Disease

The true incidence of ulcers during pregnancy is unknown. The symptoms of this disease among pregnant women are similar to those among nonpregnant women. Surgical intervention is really reserved for the complications associated with the disease. Bleeding gastric or duodenal ulcers must be considered a surgical emergency. Given the increased intravascular volume of the pregnant patient and the relative increase in hematocrit, stress to the fetus may occur before hemodynamic changes are apparent in the mother.

For several reasons, ulcers are less common among pregnant women than among other populations (51).

First, the diagnosis of ulcer is often not definitive because pregnant women are fairly reluctant to undergo diagnostic studies to confirm the diagnosis. Next, there is an increase in plasma histaminase levels during pregnancy, but whether this increase is associated with a decreased incidence of ulcer disease is questionable (52). Finally, female sex hormones, namely progesterone, seem to increase gastric and duodenal mucosal protection against stomach acid by stimulating mucin production (51). However, it is important to stress that if a pregnant patient exhibits signs and symptoms of peptic ulcer disease, such as severe pain, vomiting, or bleeding, diagnostic (and possibly therapeutic) endoscopy should be undertaken.

The treatment of ulcer disease in a pregnant woman does present some problems. Pregnant women commonly take antacids because of gastroesophageal reflux, and these drugs seem to be safe. The use of sucralfate also seems to be relatively safe; this drug is listed as a category B drug for pregnant patients (Table 3). H2-receptor blockers are associated with variable risks, and proton pump inhibitors should be avoided during pregnancy (51). It is rare, though, that the pregnant patient will require surgery solely because of intractable symptoms. It is much more likely that surgery will be required because of perforation or hemorrhage. When perforation occurs, the risk to the unborn fetus is high. Some series report a fetal mortality rate of 21%, but this rate is much better than that associated with medical treatment of perforated ulcer, which approaches 65% (51). Likewise, the fetal mortality rate is much lower when pregnant women are treated surgically for bleeding peptic ulcers (14%) than when they are treated medically (44%) (51). Surgical options include exploration and endoscopic methods of control.

Anorectal Complications of Delivery

Five percent of women require third- or fourth-degree episiotomy during normal vaginal deliveries. These episiotomies are routinely repaired at the time of delivery, but 10% of these repairs will break down. The most common finding associated with such breakdown is complete disruption of the sphincter or the formation of a rectovaginal fistula. The treatment of sphincter disruption involves sphincteroplasty with reconstruction of the perineal body. The treatment of rectovaginal fistula usually involves an endorectal advancement flap of muscle tissue; success rates are good. When the patient is a good surgical risk, colostomy is frequently not needed. Most abscesses that occur will respond to local treatment, including incision and drainage. A fair number will drain spontaneously. Interestingly enough, as many as 30% of sphincter disruptions will heal with medical treatment along with satisfactory return of content rectal function (53).

Hyperparathyroidism

Hyperparathyroidism is a rare complication during pregnancy but can be catastrophic if not treated. The outcome of untreated maternal hyperparathyroidism is neonatal tetany in the infant because of the rapid placental transport of calcium. After birth, when maternal calcium is no longer available, the infant's parathyroid cannot mobilize calcium stores and hypocalcemic tetany results. Surgical resection should be undertaken, preferably during the second trimester, to cure hyperparathyroidism among pregnant women (54). Fewer than 150 cases of maternal hyperparathyroidism have been reported. The fetal complications include stillbirth and spontaneous abortion (54).

SUMMARY

The diagnosis and management of surgical complications in the pregnant patient challenge the general surgeon due to the altered physiology of pregnancy and the concern for the outcome of both the mother and the fetus. The concern for the fetus will sometimes necessitate a slightly altered approach in the selection of diagnostic modalities and pharmacologic agents. However, in general, the best outcome for the mother will ensure the best outcome for the fetus. A prudent therapeutic approach that would usually be selected for the woman who is not pregnant will result in the best outcome.

REFERENCES

1. Griffen WO Jr, Dilts PV Jr, Roddick JW Jr. Non-obstetric surgery during pregnancy. Curr Probl Surg 1969; Nov:1–56.
2. Gouldman JW, Sticca RP, Rippon MB, McAlhany JC Jr. Laparoscopic cholecystectomy in pregnancy. Am Surg 1998; 64:93–98.
3. Graham G, Baxi L, Tharakan T. Laparoscopic cholecystectomy during pregnancy: a case series and review of literature. Obstet Gynecol Surv 1998; 53:566–574.
4. McKellar DP, Anderson CT, Boynton CJ, Peoples JB. Cholecystectomy during pregnancy without fetal loss. Surg Gynecol Obstet 1992; 174:465–468.
5. Barone JE, Bears S, Chen S, Tsai J, Russell JC. Outcome study of cholecystectomy during pregnancy. Am J Surg 1999; 177:232–236.
6. Affleck DG, Handrahan DL, Egger MJ, Price RR. The laparoscopic management of appendicitis and cholelithiasis during pregnancy. Am J Surg 1999; 178:523–529.
7. Soper NJ, Hunter JG, Petrie RH. Laparoscopic cholecystectomy during pregnancy. Surg Endocs 1992; 6:115–117.
8. Al-Mulhim AA. Acute appendicitis in pregnancy. A review of 52 cases. Int Surg 1996; 81:295–297.
9. Hunter JG, Swanstrom L, Thornburg K. Carbon dioxide pneumoperitoneum induces fetal acidosis in a pregnant ewe model. Surg Endosc 1995; 9:272–279.
10. Board of Governors of the Society of American Gastrointestinal Endoscopic Surgeons (SAGES). Guidelines for laparoscopic surgery during pregnancy. Surg Endosc 1998; 12:189–190.
11. Kort B, Katz L, Watson WJ. The effect of nonobstetric operation during pregnancy. Surg Gynecol Obstet 1993; 177:371–376.
12. Hill LM, Johnson CE, Lee RA. Prophylactic use of hydroxyprogesterone caproate in abdominal surgery during pregnancy. A restrospective evaluation. Obstet Gynecol 1975; 46:287–290.
13. Fallon WF Jr, Newman JS, Fallon GL, Malangoni MA. The surgical management of intra-abdominal inflammatory conditions during pregnancy. Surg Clin North Am 1995; 75:15–31.
14. National Council on Radiation Protection and Measurements. Limitation of exposure to ionizing radiation: recommendations of the National Council on Radiation Protection and Measurements. Bethesda, MD: The Council. 1993; Report 116:9–21.
15. Dietrich MF, Miller KL, King SH. Determination of potential uterine (conceptus) doses from axial and helical CT scans. Health Phys 2005; 88:S10–S13.
16. Ames Castro M, Shipp TD, Castro EE, Ouzounian J, Rao P. The use of helical computed tomography in pregnancy for the diagnosis of acute appendicitis. Am J Obstet Gynecol 2001; 184:954–957.
17. Brent RL. The effect of embryonic and fetal exposure to x-rays, microwaves, and ultrasound: counseling the pregnant and nonpregnant patient about these risks. Semin Oncol 1989; 16:347–368.
18. Firstenberg MS, Malangoni MA. Gastrointestinal surgery during pregnancy. Gastroenterol Clin North Am 1998; 27:73–88.
19. Baer JL, Reis RA, Araens RA. Appendicitis in pregnancy with changes in position and axis of the normal appendix in pregnancy. JAMA 1932; 98:1359–1364.
20. Mourad J, Elliott JP, Erickson L, Lisboa L. Appendicitis in pregnancy: new information that contradicts long-held clinical beliefs. Am J Obstet Gynecol 2000; 182:1027–1029.
21. Babaknia A, Parsa H, Woodruff JD. Appendicitis during pregnancy. Obstet Gynecol 1977; 50:40–44.
22. Tracey M, Fletcher HS. Appendicitis in pregnancy. Am Surg 2000; 66:555–560.
23. Tamir IL, Bongard FS, Klein SR. Acute appendicitis in the pregnant patient. Am J Surg 1990; 160:571–576.
24. Epstein FB. Acute abdominal pain in pregnancy. Emerg Med Clin North Am 1994; 12:151–165.
25. Mahmoodian S. Appendicitis complicating pregnancy. South Med J 1992; 85:19–24.
26. Zagoni T, Tulassay Z. Endoscopic sphincterotomy without fluoroscopic control in pregnancy. Am J Gastroenterol 1995; 90:1028.
27. Berger Z. Endoscopic papillotomy without fluoroscopy in pregnancy. Endoscopy 1998; 30:313.
28. al Karawi M, Mohamed SA. Therapeutic endoscopic retrograde cholangiopancreatography with ultra-short fluoroscopy: report of two cases. Endoscopy 1997; 29:S31.
29. Watson CJ, Thompson HJ, Calne R. HELLP–It's not cholecystitis. Br J Surg 1990; 77:539–540.
30. Kline KB. Pancreatitis in pregnancy. In: Rustgi VK, Cooper JN, eds. Gastrointestinal and Hepatic Complications in Pregnancy. New York: John Wiley & Sons, 1986:138.

31. Ordorica SA, Frieden FJ, Marks F, Hoskins IA, Young BK. Pancreatic enzyme activity in pregnancy. J Reprod Med 1991; 36:359–362.

32. Scott LD. Gallstone disease and pancreatitis in pregnancy. Gastroenterol Clin North Am 1992; 21:803–815.

33. Cunningham FG, Clark SL, Gant NF, Leveno KJ, Hauth JC. Williams Obstetrics. 21st ed. New York: McGraw-Hill, 2001.

34. Perdue PW, Johnson HW Jr, Stafford PW. Intestinal obstruction complicating pregnancy. Am J Surg 1992; 164:384–388.

35. Watanabe S, Otsubo Y, Shinagawa T, Araki T. Small bowel obstruction in early pregnancy treated by jejunotomy and total parenteral nutrition. Obstet Gynecol 2000; 96:812–813.

36. Moore JL Jr, Martin JN Jr. Cancer and pregnancy. Obstet Gynecol Clin North Am 1992; 19:815–827.

37. Liberman L, Giess CS, Dershaw DD, Deutch BM, Petrek JA. Imaging of pregnancy-associated breast cancer. Radiology 1994; 191:245–248.

38. Max MH, Klamer TW. Pregnancy and breast cancer. South Med J 1983; 76:1088–1090.

39. Gemignani ML, Petrek JA, Borgen PI. Breast cancer and pregnancy. Surg Clin North Am 1999; 79:1157–1169.

40. Hoover HC Jr. Breast cancer during pregnancy and lactation. Surg Clin North Am 1990; 70:1151–1163.

41. Kilgore AR. Tumors and tumor-like lesions of the breast in association with pregnancy and lactation. Arch Surg 1929; 18:2079–2098.

42. Harrington SW. Carcinoma of the breast: results of surgical treatment when the carcinoma occurred in the course of pregnancy or lactation and when pregnancy occurred subsequent to operation (1910–1913). Ann Surg 1937; 106:690–700.

43. Haagensen CD, Stout AP. Carcinoma of the breast. Ann Surg 1943; 118:859–870.

44. Petrek JA, Dukoff R, Rogatko A. Prognosis of pregnancy-associated breast cancer. Cancer 1991; 67:869–872.

45. Donegan WL. Breast cancer and pregnancy. Obstet Gynecol 1977; 50:244–252.

46. Elledge RM, Ciocca DR, Langone G, McGuire WL. Estrogen receptor, progesterone receptor, and HER-2/neu protein in breast cancers from pregnant patients. Cancer 1993; 71:2499–2506.

47. DiFronzo LA, O'Connell TX. Breast cancer in pregnancy and lactation. Surg Clin North Am 1996; 76:267–278.

48. Walsh C, Fazio VW. Cancer of the colon, rectum, and anus during pregnancy. The surgeon's perspective. Gastroenterol Clin North Am 1998; 27:257–267.

49. Gallenberg MM, Loprinzi CL. Breast cancer and pregnancy. Semin Oncol 1989; 16:369–376.

50. Dillman RO, Vandermolen LA, Barth NM, Bransford KJ. Malignant melanoma and pregnancy: ten questions. West J Med 1996; 164:156–161.

51. Cappell MS, Garcia A. Gastric and duodenal ulcers during pregnancy. Gastroenterol Clin North Am 1998; 27:169–195.

52. Barnes LW. Serum histaminase during pregnancy. Obstet Gynecol 1957; 9:730–732.

53. Kort KC, Schiller HJ, Numann PJ. Hyperparathyroidism and pregnancy. Am J Surg 1999; 177:66–68.

54. Mestman JH. Parathyroid disorders of pregnancy. Semin Perinatol 1998; 22:485–496.

Index